Prescription for
NUTRITIONAL HEALING

THIRD EDITION

PHYLLIS A. BALCH, CNC

Every effort has been made to ensure that the information contained in this book is complete and accurate. However, neither the publisher nor the author is engaged in rendering professional advice or services to the individual reader. The ideas, procedures, and suggestions contained in this book are not intended as a substitute for consulting with your physician. All matters regarding health require medical supervision. Neither the author nor the publisher shall be liable for any loss, injury, or damage allegedly arising from any information or suggestion in this book.

Library of Congress Cataloging-in-Publication Data

Balch, Phyllis A., date.
   Prescription for nutritional healing / Phyllis A. Balch.
      p.   cm.
   Includes bibliographical references and index.
   ISBN 1-58333-077-1 (trade paperback)
       1-58333-083-6 (comb-bound)
       1-58333-228-6 (special markets edition)
   1. Nutrition—Popular works.   2. Diet therapy—Popular works.   3. Vitamin therapy—
Popular works.   4. Herbs—Therapeutic use—Popular works.   5. Food, Formulated—
Popular works.   6. Medicine, Herbal—Popular works.   7. Nutrition—Popular works.   8.
Vitamins—Therapeutic use—Popular works.   I. Title.
RA784.B248   2000   00-063936
615.8'54—dc21

Printed in the United States of America

10 9 8 7 6 5 4 3 2

In-house editor: Amy C. Tecklenburg
Typesetter: Gary A. Rosenberg
Cover designers: Martin Hochberg, William Gonzalez, and Rudy Shur

Contents

Preface, vii
How to Use This Book, viii

Part One   Understanding the Elements of Health

Introduction, 2
Nutrition, Diet, and Wellness, 3
Vitamins, 13
Minerals, 25
Water, 35

Amino Acids, 42
Antioxidants, 53
Enzymes, 59
Natural Food Supplements, 63
Herbs, 85

Part Two   The Disorders

Introduction, 116
Troubleshooting for Disorders, 117
Abscess, 120
Acid/Alkali Imbalance, 122
Acne, 125
Adrenal Disorders, 129
Age Spots, 131
Aging, 132
AIDS, 138
Alcoholism, 147
Allergies, 153
Aluminum Toxicity, 167
Alzheimer's Disease, 168
Anemia, 174
Anorexia Nervosa, 177
Anxiety Disorder, 179
Appendicitis, 183
Appetite, Poor, 184
Arsenic Poisoning, 185
Arteriosclerosis/Atherosclerosis, 186
Arthritis, 188
Asthma, 195
Athlete's Foot, 200
Attention Deficit Disorder (ADD)/
    Attention Deficit Hyperactivity
    Disorder (ADHD), 201
Autism, 205
Backache, 208
Bedsores, 212

Bed-Wetting, 214
Bee Sting, 215
Bladder Infection (Cystitis), 216
Boil, 219
Breast Cancer, 221
Breastfeeding-Related Problems, 229
    Engorgement, 229
    Mastitis (Breast Infection), 229
    Plugged Duct, 230
    Sore Nipples, 230
Bronchitis, 232
Bruising, 235
Bruxism, 237
Bulimia, 238
Burns, 241
Bursitis, 243
Cadmium Toxicity, 245
Cancer, 246
Candidiasis, 263
Canker Sores (Aphthous Ulcers), 266
Cardiovascular Disease, 267
Carpal Tunnel Syndrome, 275
Celiac Disease, 279
Chemical Allergies, 281
Chemical Poisoning, 283
Chickenpox, 283
Chlamydia, 285
Chronic Fatigue Syndrome, 286
Circulatory Problems, 290

Cirrhosis of the Liver, 292
Cold Sores (Fever Blisters), 295
Common Cold, 297
Constipation, 300
Copper Deficiency, 303
Copper Toxicity, 304
Corns and Calluses, 305
Crohn's Disease, 306
Croup, 310
Cystic Fibrosis, 311
Dandruff, 313
Depression, 314
Dermatitis, 319
Diabetes, 321
Diarrhea, 326
Diverticulitis, 328
Dog Bite, 330
Down Syndrome, 331
Drug Addiction (Substance Abuse), 334
Dry Skin, 337
Ear Infection, 340
Edema, 342
Emphysema, 343
Endometriosis, 346
Environmental Toxicity, 350
Epilepsy, 352
Eye Problems, 355
    Bags under the Eyes, 358
    Bitot's Spots, 358
    Blepharitis, 359
    Bloodshot Eyes, 359
    Blurred Vision, 359
    Cataracts, 360
    Colorblindness, 362
    Conjunctivitis (Pinkeye), 362
    Corneal Ulcer, 363
    Diabetic Retinopathy, 363
    Dimness or Loss of Vision, 363
    Dry Eyes, 364
    Eyestrain, 364
    Floaters, 365
    Glaucoma, 365
    Itchy or Tired Eyes, 366
    Macular Degeneration, 366
    Mucus in the Eyes, 367
    Photophobia, 367
    Retinitis Pigmentosa, 367
    Scotoma, 368
    Shingles (Herpes Zoster), 368
    Stye, 368
    Thinning Eyelashes, 369
    Ulcerated Eyelid, 369
    Xerophthalmia, 369
Fever, 369
Fibrocystic Breasts, 371

Fibroids, Uterine, 372
Fibromyalgia Syndrome, 374
Foodborne/Waterborne Disease, 378
Fracture, 384
Frigidity, 386
Fungal Infection, 387
Gallbladder Disorders, 389
Gangrene, 391
German Measles (Rubella), 392
Glaucoma, 394
Gout, 397
Growth Problems, 400
Hair Loss, 401
Halitosis (Bad Breath), 404
Hay Fever, 405
Headache, 408
Hearing Loss, 413
Heart Attack, 417
Heartburn/Gastroesophageal Reflux
    Disease (GERD), 422
Heel or Bone Spur, 424
Hemophilia, 425
Hemorrhoids, 426
Hepatitis, 429
Herpesvirus Infection, 433
High Blood Pressure (Hypertension), 436
High Cholesterol, 440
Hives, 443
Hyperthyroidism, 446
Hypoglycemia (Low Blood Sugar), 448
Hypothyroidism, 450
Hysterectomy-Related Problems, 453
Impotence, 455
Incontinence, 459
Indigestion (Dyspepsia), 460
Infertility, 463
Inflammation, 466
Influenza, 468
Insect Allergy, 470
Insect Bite, 471
Insomnia, 473
Irritable Bowel Syndrome, 476
Jaundice, 479
Kidney Disease (Renal Failure), 480
Kidney Stones, 483
Lactose Intolerance (Lactase
    Deficiency), 485
Lead Poisoning, 487
Leg Ulcers, 490
Legionnaires' Disease, 492
Lupus, 493
Lyme Disease, 496
Malabsorption Syndrome, 499
Manic-Depressive Disorder (Bipolar
    Mood Disorder), 502

Measles, 504
Memory Problems, 505
Ménière's Disease, 508
Meningitis, 510
Menopausal and Perimenopausal
    Problems, 511
Mercury Toxicity, 516
Migraine, 518
Mononucleosis, 521
Motion Sickness, 523
Multiple Sclerosis, 525
Mumps, 529
Muscle Cramps, 530
Nail Problems, 532
Narcolepsy, 535
Nickel Toxicity, 537
Nosebleed, 538
Obesity, 540
Oily Skin, 547
Osteoporosis, 549
Paget's Disease of Bone, 554
Pancreatitis, 556
Parkinson's Disease, 558
Peptic Ulcer, 561
Periodontal Disease, 564
Pneumonia, 567
Poison Ivy/Poison Oak/Poison
    Sumac, 570
Poisoning, 571
Polyps, 574
Pregnancy-Related Problems, 575
    Anemia, 576
    Asthma, 576
    Backache, 576
    Bladder Discomfort/Infection, 577
    Bleeding Gums, 577
    Constipation, 577
    Coughs and Colds, 577
    Depression, 577
    Diabetes, Gestational, 578
    Dizziness, 578
    Eclampsia and Preeclampsia, 578
    Ectopic Pregnancy, 579
    Edema (Swelling of the Hands
        and Feet), 579
    Gas (Flatulence), 579
    Groin Spasm, Stitch, or Pressure, 580
    Heartburn, 580
    Hemorrhoids, 580
    Insomnia, 580
    Leg Cramps, 581
    Miscarriage (Spontaneous Abortion), 581
    Morning Sickness, 581
    Nosebleeds and Nasal Congestion, 582

Sciatica, 582
Skin Problems, 582
Soreness in the Rib Area, 582
Stretch Marks, 583
Sweating, 583
Varicose Veins, 583
Premenstrual Syndrome, 587
Prolapse of the Uterus, 590
Prostate Cancer, 591
Prostatitis/Benign Prostatic Hyertrophy
    (BPH), 596
Psoriasis, 599
Radiation Exposure, 601
Raynaud's Disease/Raynaud's
    Phenomenon, 603
Reye's Syndrome, 604
Rheumatic Fever, 606
Rickets/Osteomalacia, 607
Rosacea, 608
Scabies, 610
Schizophrenia, 611
Sebaceous Cyst, 614
Seborrhea, 615
Senility (Dementia), 617
Sexually Transmitted Disease (STD), 619
Shingles (Herpes Zoster), 621
Sinusitis, 624
Skin Cancer, 627
Skin Rash, 632
Smoking Dependency, 635
Snakebite, 638
Sore Throat, 640
Spider Bite, 641
Sprains, Strains, and Other Injuries
    of the Muscles and Joints, 643
Stress, 646
Sunburn, 651
Thrombophlebitis, 653
TMJ Syndrome, 656
Tonsillitis, 658
Tooth Decay, 660
Tuberculosis, 662
Tumor, 664
Ulcerative Colitis, 666
Underweight/Weight Loss, 668
Vaginitis, 670
Varicose Veins, 672
Vertigo, 674
Vitiligo, 676
Warts, 677
Weakened Immune System, 679
Wilson's Disease, 684
Worms (Parasites), 686
Wrinkles, 688

Part Three   Remedies and Therapies

Introduction, 694
Aromatherapy and Essential Oils, 695
Ascorbic Acid Flush, 697
Ayurvedic Remedies, 698
Blood Purification, 698
Chelation Therapy, 699
    Oral Chelation Therapy, 700
    Intravenous Chelation Therapy, 701
Chinese Medicine, 701
Colon Cleansing, 702
Color Therapy (Chromotherapy), 703
Crystal and Gemstone Therapy, 704
DHEA Therapy, 704
Enemas, 705
    The Catnip Tea Enema, 705
    The Coffee or Wheatgrass Retention
        Enema, 706
    The Lemon Juice Cleansing
        Enema, 706
    The Pro-Flora Whey Enema, 707
Exercise, 707
Fasting, 708
Glandular Therapy, 710
Growth Hormone Therapy, 713
Hair Analysis, 713
Homeopathy, 714
Hydrotherapy, 715
Hyperbaric Oxygen Therapy, 716

Juicing, 717
Light Therapy, 719
Music and Sound Therapy, 719
Pain Control, 720
    Acupressure, 721
    Acupuncture, 721
    Biofeedback, 721
    Breathing Exercises, 721
    Chiropractic, 722
    Guided Imagery, 722
    Heat and Cold Therapy, 722
    Herbs, 723
    Hypnotherapy, 724
    Magnet Therapy, 724
    Massage, 724
    Medication, 725
    Meditation, 726
    Qi Gong, 726
    Relaxation Techniques, 726
    Tai Chi, 726
    TENS Unit Therapy, 727
Using a Poultice, 727
Sitz Bath, 728
Steam Inhalation, 728
Preparing for and Recovering
    from Surgery, 729
Therapeutic Liquids, 732
Yoga, 732

Appendix

Glossary, 737
Manufacturer and Distributor
    Information, 746

Health and Medical
    Organizations, 755
Suggested Reading, 764

Index, 767
Acknowledgments, 776
About the Authors, 776

Preface

"A wise man should consider that health is the greatest of human blessings."

—*Hippocrates*

Socrates once said, "There is only one good, knowledge, and one evil, ignorance." This statement should guide us in all of our actions, especially where our health is concerned. Too many of us do not have the slightest idea of how to maintain good health. When illness strikes, we rely on our doctors to cure us. What we fail to realize is that "the cure" comes from within. Nature has provided us with a wondrous immune system, and all we have to do is take proper care of this inner healing force.

Does this sound too simple? Basically, it is simple; our modern lifestyles have gotten us off the right track, with fast foods, alcohol abuse, drug dependencies, a polluted environment, and high-tech stress. Nature intended to fuel our inner healing force with the right natural substances to enable the body to function up to its fullest potential. Nature's resources—whole foods, vitamins, minerals, enzymes, amino acids, phytochemicals, and other natural bounties—are designed for use in our immune systems. However, because most of us have a profound lack of knowledge as to what our bodies need to function properly, we find ourselves out of balance and susceptible to all sorts of illnesses.

All individuals should take an active part in the maintenance of their health and in the treatment of their disorders with the guidance of a health care professional. The more we take it upon ourselves to learn about nutrition, the better prepared we will be to take that active role. Attitude is also an important factor in the processes of health maintenance and healing. We must have a positive state of mind in order to bring harmony to the body. The realization that body (lifestyle), spirit (desire), and mind (belief) must come together is the first step to better health.

This new edition has taken over twenty-five years of study, work, and research to put together. It is intended to provide you and your health care professional with a more natural approach to healing, which may be used in con-

junction with your current medical treatment. A number of the suggestions offered, such as intravenous therapy, can be administered only by or under the supervision of a licensed physician. Also, because our body chemistries differ, some of us may have allergic reactions to certain supplements. Before taking any nutritional supplement, check with your health care professional regarding its appropriateness. Should you experience an allergic reaction to any supplement, immediately discontinue use of the supplement. You should never attempt to treat yourself without professional advice.

No statement in this publication should be construed as a claim for cure, treatment, or prevention of any disease. It is also important to point out that you should not reject mainstream medical methods. Learn about your condition, and don't be afraid to ask questions. Feel free to get second and even third opinions from qualified health professionals. It is a sign of wisdom, not cowardice, to seek more knowledge through your active participation as a patient.

Every effort has been made to include the latest research available on nutritional healing. We also have added new sections on many health disorders at the suggestions of our readers. All the information in this book has been carefully researched, and the data have been reviewed and updated throughout the production process. Because this body of knowledge promises to continue growing and changing, we suggest that when questions arise, you refer to other current sources of information to verify textual material. We will strive to keep abreast of new scientific information, treatments, and supplements, and make this information available to you in future editions of this book.

Over 800 years ago, Moses Maimonides said, "The physician should not treat the ailment, but the patient who is suffering from it." This book was designed to meet the differing needs of individuals and to help each person create his or her own nutritional program.

How to Use This Book

This is a comprehensive in-home guide that will help you achieve and maintain the highest level of health and fitness through careful dietary planning and nutritional supplementation. Even if you are free from so-called disorders, you will benefit from this book because it gives advice on how to achieve optimum health, build up your immune system, and increase your energy level. Written by a certified nutritionist and a medical doctor, this book blends the latest scientific research with traditional treatments. It provides all the information you need to design your own personal nutritional program. In addition, the authors offer traditional and up-to-date home remedies, and suggest healthful modifications in diet and lifestyle.

It is important to stress that the suggestions offered in this book are not intended to replace appropriate medical investigation and treatment. The supplements and medications recommended for a particular disorder should be approved and monitored by your medical doctor or trained health care professional. If surgery or other conventional medical interventions are crucial and cannot be avoided, the nutritional supplements can shorten healing time.

The book is divided into three parts. Part One discusses the basic principles of nutrition and health, and lists and explains the various types of nutrients, food supplements, enzymes, antioxidants, and herbs found in health food shops and drugstores. Part Two is divided into sections on common disorders, from acne to cancer to yeast infection, arranged in alphabetical order. Each section discusses how to identify the symptoms and suggests ways to correct or treat the disorder through dietary guidelines and a supplementation program. Some contain helpful diagnostic self-tests to help you determine whether or not you have the condition in question. Part Three offers descriptions and explanations of traditional therapies and conventional treatments that can be used in conjunction with a nutritional program. Also discussed in Part Three are a number of alternative therapy approaches, such as acupressure and acupuncture, aromatherapy, Ayurvedic medicine, Chinese medicine, chiropractic, color therapy, fasting, glandular therapy, homeopathy, hydrotherapy, hyperbaric oxygen therapy, light therapy, magnet therapy, massage therapy, and music/sound therapy. In addition, there are insets throughout the book providing in-depth coverage of important topics. The ramifications of different drug therapies are discussed and the latest medical updates are provided.

Also included, in an appendix, are information on how to find some of the products recommended in this book; a recommended reading list; and a list of health organizations and the addresses and/or phone numbers at which they can be reached for information. A glossary is provided for easy reference.

Although a healthy diet is the backbone of any nutritional program, we believe that most if not all people should supplement their diets with the proper nutrients to achieve wellness. Nutritional deficiency diseases such as scurvy are rare, but these are only the tip of the iceberg when it comes to the problems a lack of adequate nutrition can cause. Nutritional deficiencies can cause a variety of symptoms, in addition to weakening the body's defenses against serious illness. Moreover, nutritional requirements may be increased by many things. People who are heavy alcohol drinkers, cigarette smokers, prescription or recreational drug users, and/or dieters are at a greater than normal risk for deficiencies, as are adolescents, elderly people, pregnant and nursing women, women who take oral contraceptives, people with certain genetic disorders, people who eat poor diets, and people with diabetes or other chronic illnesses. Unfortunately, a large percentage of the population fits into one or more of these categories.

The supplementation programs recommended in this book should be followed for three to twelve months, depending upon your individual needs and the recommendations of your health care provider. Start by taking nutrients classified "essential" and "very important" for the relevant disorder. Many times, the nutrients recommended for a particular disorder can be found in a single product. Before you start taking them on a regular basis, test the supplements one at a time to find out if you have a reaction to any of them. If you do not find relief within thirty days, add the supplements from the "helpful" list to your program. Each of us is unique; you may need all the nutrients listed, or you may be deficient in only a few. If you still do not notice an improvement after a month, consult your health care provider. You may suffer from malabsorption.

Always take supplements with a full glass of water. Nutritional supplements are concentrated and can overburden the liver if not enough liquid is consumed with the supplements. Water enhances absorption and is needed to aid in carrying the nutrients to the cells.

If you follow a nutritional supplementation program for longer than a year, change brands periodically so that you do not develop an intolerance or build up a resistance to one or more of the ingredients in one supplement. Remember, you can develop an intolerance to the ingredients in vitamins and other supplements just as you can to foods. Learn to listen to your body. Given time, you will notice changes in your body and be able to identify their cause. After the supplementation period for a certain disorder is completed, decrease supplement dosages gradually so that your body has a chance to adjust. Keep in mind, though, that virtually all of us need to supplement our diets with the basic nutrients for optimum wellness and illness prevention.

PART ONE

Understanding the Elements of Health

INTRODUCTION

The body is a complex organism that has the ability to heal itself—if only you listen to it and respond with proper nourishment and care. In spite of all the abuse our bodies endure—whether through exposure to environmental toxins, poor nutrition, cigarette smoking, alcohol consumption, or inactivity—they still usually serve us well for many years before signs of illness may start to appear. Even then, with a little help, they respond and continue to function.

The human body is the greatest machine on earth. Nerve signals travel through muscles at speeds as fast as 200 miles per hour. The brain puts out enough electric power to light a 20-watt light bulb. If your leg muscles moved as fast as your eye muscles, you could walk over fifty miles in one day. According to scientists, bone is among the strongest building materials known to humankind; it can withstand nearly as much stretching and bending stress as, and more compression stress than, steel-reinforced concrete can tolerate.

Think of your body as being composed of millions of tiny little engines. Some of these engines work in unison; some work independently. All are on call twenty-four hours a day. In order for the engines to work properly, they require specific fuels. If the type of fuel given is the wrong blend, the engine will not perform to its maximum capacity. If the fuel is of a poor grade, the engine may sputter, hesitate, and lose power. If the engine is given no fuel at all, it will stop.

The fuel we give our bodies' engines comes directly from the things we consume. The foods we eat contain nutrients. These nutrients come in the form of vitamins, minerals, enzymes, water, amino acids, carbohydrates, and lipids. It is these nutrients that sustain life by providing us with the basic materials our bodies need to carry on their daily functions.

Individual nutrients differ in form and function, and in the amount needed by the body; however, they are all vital to our health. The actions that involve nutrients take place on microscopic levels, and the specific processes differ greatly. Nutrients are involved in all body processes, from combating infection to repairing tissue to thinking. Although nutrients have different specific functions, their common function is to keep us going.

Research has shown that each part of the body contains high concentrations of certain nutrients. A deficiency of those nutrients will cause the body part to malfunction and eventually break down—and, like dominos, other body parts will follow. To keep this from happening, we need a proper diet and appropriate nutritional supplements. Brain function, memory, skin elasticity, eyesight, energy, the ratio of lean to fat tissue in the body, and overall health are all indications of how well the body is functioning. With the help of the proper nutrients, exercise, and a balanced diet, we can slow the aging process and greatly improve our chances for a healthier and pain-free—and possibly longer—life.

If we do not give ourselves the proper nutrients, we can impair the body's normal functions and cause ourselves great harm. Even if we show no signs of illness, we may not necessarily be healthy. It simply may be that we are not yet exhibiting any overt symptoms of illness. One problem most of us have is that we do not get the nutrients we need from our diets because most of the foods we consume are cooked and/or processed. Cooking at high temperatures and processing destroy vital nutrients the body needs to function properly. The organic raw foods that supply these elements are largely missing from today's diet.

The past decade has brought to light much new knowledge about nutrition and its effects on the body, and the role it plays in disease. Phytochemicals, also known as phytonutrients, are one example of the results of this research. These are compounds present in plants that make the plants biologically active. They are not nutrients in the classic sense, but they are what determines a plant's color, flavor, and ability to resist disease. Researchers have identified literally thousands of phytochemicals and also have developed the technology to extract these chemical compounds and concentrate them into pills, powders, and capsules. These are called nutraceuticals—the newest type of dietary supplement.

Your body's nutritional needs are as unique to you as your appearance is. The first essential step toward wellness, therefore, is to be sure you are getting the correct amounts of the proper nutrients. By understanding the principles of holistic nutrition and knowing what nutrients you need, you can improve the state of your health, ward off disease, and maintain a harmonious balance in the way nature intended. Part One should provide you with a clear understanding of the vitamins, minerals, amino acids, enzymes, phytochemicals, and other nutrients you need, as well as important information on natural food supplements, herbs, and products that enhance nutrient activity. Eating a healthful diet and supplementing your diet with appropriate nutrients will help to assure that your organs, cells, and tissues get the fuel they need to operate properly. The nutrients suggested in this book promote healing and wellness by allowing the body to heal and reinvigorate itself.

NUTRITION, DIET, AND WELLNESS

UNDERSTANDING THE BASICS OF NUTRITION

Good nutrition is the foundation of good health. Everyone needs the four basic nutrients—water, carbohydrates, proteins, and fats—as well as vitamins, minerals, and other micronutrients. To be able to choose the proper foods, and to better understand why those foods should be supported with supplements, you need to have a clear idea of the components of a healthy diet.

The Four Basic Nutrients

Water, carbohydrates, proteins, and fats are the basic building blocks of a good diet. By choosing the healthiest forms of each of these nutrients and eating them in the proper balance, you enable your body to function at its optimal level.

Water

The human body is two-thirds water. Water is an essential nutrient that is involved in every function of the body. It helps transport nutrients and waste products in and out of cells. It is necessary for all digestive, absorptive, circulatory, and excretory functions, as well as for the utilization of the water-soluble vitamins. It is also needed for the maintenance of proper body temperature. By drinking an adequate amount of water each day—at least eight 8-ounce glasses—you can ensure that your body has all it needs to maintain good health. (For details on choosing the best water, *see* WATER in Part One.)

Carbohydrates

Carbohydrates supply the body with the energy it needs to function. They are found almost exclusively in plant foods, such as fruits, vegetables, peas, and beans. Milk and milk products are the only foods derived from animals that contain a significant amount of carbohydrates.

Carbohydrates are divided into two groups—simple carbohydrates and complex carbohydrates. *Simple carbohydrates*, sometimes called simple sugars, include fructose (fruit sugar), sucrose (table sugar), and lactose (milk sugar), as well as several other sugars. Fruits are one of the richest natural sources of simple carbohydrates. *Complex carbohydrates* are also made up of sugars, but the sugar molecules are strung together to form longer, more complex chains. Complex carbohydrates include fiber and starches. Foods rich in complex carbohydrates include vegetables, whole grains, peas, and beans.

Carbohydrates are the main source of blood glucose, which is a major fuel for all of the body's cells and the only source of energy for the brain and red blood cells. Except for fiber, which cannot be digested, both simple and complex carbohydrates are converted into glucose. The glucose is then either used directly to provide energy for the body or stored in the liver for future use. If a person consumes more calories than his or her body is using, a portion of the carbohydrates consumed may be stored in the body as fat. Due to complex chemical reactions in the brain, eating carbohydrates has a mild tranquilizing effect, and can be beneficial for people who suffer from seasonal affective disorder and/or depression.

When choosing carbohydrate-rich foods for your diet, always select unrefined foods such as fruits, vegetables, peas, beans, and whole-grain products, as opposed to refined, processed foods such as soft drinks, desserts, candy, and sugar. Refined foods offer few, if any, of the vitamins and minerals that are important to your health. In addition, if eaten in excess, especially over a period of many years, the large amounts of simple carbohydrates found in refined foods can lead to a number of disorders, including diabetes and hypoglycemia (low blood sugar). Yet another problem is that foods high in refined simple sugars often are also high in fats, which should be limited in a healthy diet. This is why such foods—which include most cookies and cakes, as well as many snack foods—are usually loaded with calories.

A word is in order here regarding fiber, a very important form of carbohydrate. Referred to in the past as "roughage," dietary fiber is the part of a plant that is resistant to the body's digestive enzymes. As a result, only a relatively small amount of fiber is digested or metabolized in the stomach or intestines. Instead, most of it moves through the gastrointestinal tract and ends up in the stool.

Although most fiber is not digested, it delivers several important health benefits. First, fiber retains water, resulting in softer and bulkier stools that prevent constipation and hemorrhoids. A high-fiber diet also reduces the risk of colon cancer, perhaps by speeding the rate at which stool passes through the intestine and by keeping the digestive tract clean. In addition, fiber binds with certain substances that would normally result in the production of cholesterol, and eliminates these substances from the body. In this way, a high-fiber diet helps lower blood cholesterol levels, reducing the risk of heart disease.

It is recommended that about 60 percent of your total daily calories come from carbohydrates. If much of your diet consists of healthy complex carbohydrates, you should easily fulfill the recommended daily minimum of 25 grams of fiber.

Protein

Protein is essential for growth and development. It provides the body with energy, and is needed for the manufacture of hormones, antibodies, enzymes, and tissues. It also helps maintain the proper acid-alkali balance in the body.

When protein is consumed, the body breaks it down into amino acids, the building blocks of all proteins. Some of the amino acids are designated *nonessential*. This does not mean that they are unnecessary, but rather that they do not have to come from the diet because they can be synthesized by the body from other amino acids. Other amino acids are considered *essential*, meaning that the body cannot synthesize them, and therefore must obtain them from the diet.

Whenever the body *makes* a protein—when it builds muscle, for instance—it needs a variety of amino acids for the protein-making process. These amino acids may come from dietary protein or from the body's own pool of amino acids. If a shortage of amino acids becomes chronic, which can occur if the diet is deficient in essential amino acids, the building of protein in the body stops, and the body suffers. (For more information about amino acids, *see* AMINO ACIDS in Part One.)

Because of the importance of consuming proteins that provide all of the necessary amino acids, dietary proteins are considered to belong to two different groups, depending on the amino acids they provide. *Complete proteins*, which constitute the first group, contain ample amounts of all of the essential amino acids. These proteins are found in meat, fish, poultry, cheese, eggs, and milk. *Incomplete proteins*, which constitute the second group, contain only some of the essential amino acids. These proteins are found in a variety of foods, including grains, legumes, and leafy green vegetables.

Although it is important to consume the full range of amino acids, both essential and nonessential, it is not necessary to get them from meat, fish, poultry, and other complete-protein foods. In fact, because of their high fat content—as well as the use of antibiotics and other chemicals in the raising of poultry and cattle—most of those foods should be eaten in moderation only. Fortunately, the dietary strategy called *mutual supplementation* enables you to combine partial-protein foods to make *complementary protein*—proteins that supply adequate amounts of all the essential amino acids. For instance, although beans and brown rice are both quite rich in protein, each lacks one or more of the necessary amino acids. However, when you combine beans and brown rice with each other, or when you combine either one with any of a number of protein-rich foods, you form a complete protein that is a high-

quality substitute for meat. To make a complete protein, combine *beans* with any one of the following:

- Brown rice
- Corn
- Nuts
- Seeds
- Wheat

Or combine *brown rice* with any one of the following:

- Beans
- Nuts
- Seeds
- Wheat

Most Americans eat too much protein, largely as the result of a diet high in meat and dairy products. However, if you have reduced the amount of meat and dairy foods in your diet, you should make sure to get about 50 grams of protein a day. To make sure that you are getting a great enough variety of amino acids in your diet, add protein-rich foods to meals and snacks as often as possible. Eat bread with nut butters, for instance, or add nuts and seeds to salads and vegetable casseroles. Be aware that a combination of any grains, any nuts and seeds, any legumes (such as beans, peanuts, and peas), and a variety of mixed vegetables will make a complete protein. In addition, cornmeal fortified with the amino acid L-lysine makes a complete protein.

All soybean products, such as tofu and soymilk, are complete proteins. They contain the essential amino acids plus several other nutrients. Available in health food stores, tofu, soy oil, soy flour, soy-based meat substitutes, soy cheese, and many other soy products are healthful ways to complement the meatless diet.

Yogurt is the only animal-derived complete-protein source recommended for frequent use in the diet. Made from milk that is curdled by bacteria, yogurt contains *Lactobacillus acidophilus* and other "friendly" bacteria needed for the digestion of foods and the prevention of many disorders, including candidiasis. Yogurt also contains vitamins A and D, and many of the B-complex vitamins.

Do not buy the sweetened, flavored yogurts that are sold in supermarkets. These products contain added sugar and, often, preservatives. Instead, either purchase fresh unsweetened yogurt from a health food store or make the yogurt yourself, and sweeten it with fruit juices and other wholesome ingredients. Yogurt makers are relatively inexpensive and easy to use, and are available at most health food stores.

Fats

Although much attention has been focused on the need to reduce dietary fat, the body does need fat. During infancy and childhood, fat is necessary for normal brain development. Throughout life, it is essential to provide energy and support growth. Fat is, in fact, the most concentrated source of energy available to the body. However, after about two years of age, the body requires only small amounts of fat—much less than is provided by the average American diet. Excessive fat intake is a major causative factor in obesity, high blood pressure, coronary heart disease, and colon cancer, and has been linked to a number of other disorders as well. To understand how fat intake is related to these health problems, it is necessary to understand the different types of fats available and the ways in which these fats act within the body.

Fats are composed of building blocks called fatty acids. There are three major categories of fatty acids—saturated, polyunsaturated, and monounsaturated. These classifications are based on the number of hydrogen atoms in the chemical structure of a given molecule of fatty acid.

Saturated fatty acids are found primarily in animal products, including dairy items, such as whole milk, cream, and cheese, and fatty meats like beef, veal, lamb, pork, and ham. The fat marbling you can see in beef and pork is composed of saturated fat. Some vegetable products—including coconut oil, palm kernel oil, and vegetable shortening—are also high in saturates.

The liver uses saturated fats to manufacture cholesterol. Therefore, excessive dietary intake of saturated fats can significantly raise the blood cholesterol level, especially the level of low-density lipoproteins (LDLs), or "bad cholesterol." (For more information about cholesterol, *see* HIGH CHOLESTEROL in Part Two.) Guidelines issued by the National Cholesterol Education Program (NCEP), and widely supported by most experts, recommend that the daily intake of saturated fats be kept below 10 percent of total caloric intake. However, for people who have severe problems with high blood cholesterol, even that level may be too high.

Polyunsaturated fatty acids are found in greatest abundance in corn, soybean, safflower, and sunflower oils. Certain fish oils are also high in polyunsaturates. Unlike the saturated fats, polyunsaturates may actually lower your total blood cholesterol level. In doing so, however, large amounts of polyunsaturates also have a tendency to reduce your high-density lipoproteins (HDLs)—your "good cholesterol." For this reason—and because, like all fats, polyunsaturates are high in calories for their weight and volume—the NCEP guidelines state that an individual's intake of polyunsaturated fats should not exceed 10 percent of total caloric intake.

Monounsaturated fatty acids are found mostly in vegetable and nut oils such as olive, peanut, and canola. These fats appear to reduce blood levels of LDLs without affecting HDLs in any way. However, this positive impact upon LDL cholesterol is relatively modest. The NCEP guidelines recommend that intake of monounsaturated fats be kept between 10 and 15 percent of total caloric intake.

Although most foods—including some plant-derived foods—contain a combination of all three types of fatty acids, one of the types usually predominates. Thus, a fat or oil is considered "saturated" or "high in saturates" when it is composed primarily of saturated fatty acids. Such saturated fats are usually solid at room temperature. Similarly, a fat or oil composed mostly of polyunsaturated fatty acids is called "polyunsaturated," while a fat or oil composed mostly of monounsaturated fatty acids is called "monounsaturated."

One other element, *trans-fatty acids,* may play a role in blood cholesterol levels. Also called trans fats, these substances occur when polyunsaturated oils are altered through hydrogenation, a process used to harden liquid vegetable oils into solid foods like margarine and shortening. One recent study found that trans-monounsaturated fatty acids raise LDL cholesterol levels, behaving much like saturated fats. Simultaneously, the trans-fatty acids reduced HDL cholesterol readings. Much more research on this subject is necessary, as studies have not reached consistent and conclusive findings. For now, however, it is clear that if your goal is to lower cholesterol, polyunsaturated and monounsaturted fats are more desirable than saturated fats or products with trans-fatty acids. Just as important, your total calories from fat should not constitute more than 20 to 25 percent of daily calories.

The Micronutrients: Vitamins and Minerals

Like water, carbohydrates, protein, and fats, and the enzymes required to digest them, vitamins and minerals are essential to life. They are therefore considered nutrients, and are often referred to as *micronutrients* simply because they are needed in relatively small amounts compared with the four basic nutrients.

Because vitamins and minerals are so necessary for health, the U.S. Food and Drug Administration (FDA) has formulated recommended consumption levels for vitamins called recommended daily allowances (RDAs). But, as we will see in VITAMINS in Part One, these allowances do not account for the amount needed to maintain maximum health rather than borderline health, only the amount needed to prevent deficiency diseases. Therefore, the average adult who is not suffering from any specific disorder should obtain more than the RDAs of vitamins and minerals from food sources and/or from supplements. The table on page 6—which includes not just vitamin and mineral supplements, but other supplements as well—should be used as a guideline. Although the amounts listed are safe (they will not cause toxicity), they should be varied according to size and weight. People who are active and exercise; those who are under great stress, on restricted diets, or mentally or physically ill; women who take oral contraceptives; those on medication; those who are recovering from surgery; and smokers and those who consume alcoholic beverages all need higher than normal amounts of nutrients.

In addition to a proper diet, exercise and a positive attitude are two important elements that are needed to prevent sickness and disease. If your lifestyle includes each of these, you will feel good and have more energy—something we all deserve. Nature has the answers we need to maintain our health, but you need to know what nutrients you are taking to make sure all the pieces of the puzzle fit together.

Nutrients and Dosages for Maintaining Good Health

The nutrients listed below are recommended for good health. Daily dosages are suggested; however, before using any supplements, you should consult with your health care provider. The dosages given here are for adults and children weighing 100 pounds and over. Appropriate dosages for children vary according to age and weight. A child weighing between 70 and 100 pounds should be given three-fourths the adult dose; a child weighing under 70 pounds (and *over* the age of six years) should be given half the adult dose. A child under the age of six years should be given nutritional formulas designed specifically for young children. Follow the dosage directions on the product label.

Use only quality natural (not synthetic) supplements from a reputable source. Lower priced supplements can mean lower quality, with higher levels of fillers and other undesirable ingredients. Give your body the best—it deserves it. If you cannot locate one or more of the supplements recommended in this book, you can call or write to one of the sources listed in the Appendix.

Vitamins	Daily Dosages*
Vitamin A (retinol)	5,000–10,000 IU
A carotenoid complex containing beta-carotene	5,000–25,000 IU
Vitamin B$_1$ (thiamine)	50–100 mg
Vitamin B$_2$ (riboflavin)	15–50 mg
Vitamin B$_3$ (niacin)	15–50 mg
(niacinamide)	50–100 mg
Pantothenic acid (vitamin B$_5$)	50–100 mg
Vitamin B$_6$ (pyridoxine)	50–100 mg
Vitamin B$_{12}$	200–400 mcg
Biotin	400–800 mcg
Choline	50–200 mg
Folic acid	400–800 mcg
Inositol	50–200 mg
Para-aminobenzoic acid (PABA)	10–50 mg
Vitamin C with mineral ascorbates (Ester-C)	1,000–3,000 mg
Bioflavonoids (mixed)	200–500 mg
Hesperidin	50–100 mg
Rutin	25 mg
Vitamin D$_3$ (cholecalciferol)	400 IU
Vitamin E (d-alpha-tocopherol)	400–600 IU
Vitamin K (use natural sources such as alfalfa, green leafy vegetables)	100–500 mcg
Essential fatty acids (EFAs) (primrose oil, flaxseed oil, salmon oil, and fish oil are good sources)	As directed on label.

Minerals	Daily Dosages
Boron (picolinate or citrate)	3–6 mg
Calcium (citrate, ascorbate, or malate)	1,500–2,000 mg
Chromium (GTF, picolinate, or polynicotinate)	150–400 mcg
Copper	2–3 mg
Iodine (kelp is a good source)	100–225 mcg
Iron** (ferrous gluconate, fumarate, citrate, or amino acid chelate; avoid inorganic forms such as ferrous sulfate, which can oxidize vitamin E.)	18–30 mg
Magnesium	750–1,000 mg
Manganese	3–10 mg
Molybdenum (ascorbate, aspartate, or picolinate)	30–100 mcg
Potassium (citrate)	99–500 mg
Selenium	100–200 mcg
Vanadium (vanadyl sulfate)	200 mcg–1 mg
Zinc	30–50 mg

Amino Acids***	Daily Dosages
L-Carnitine	500 mg
Acetyl-L-Carnitine	100–500 mg
L-Cysteine	50–100 mg
Acetyl-L-Cysteine	100–500 mg
L-Lysine	50–100 mg
L-Methionine	50–100 mg
Taurine	100–500 mg
L-Tyrosine	500 mg

Optional Supplements****	Daily Dosages
Chondroitin sulfate	As directed on label.
Coenzyme Q$_{10}$	30–100 mg
Cryptoxanthin	110 mcg
Flavonoids (citrus fruits and berries)	As directed on label.
Garlic	As directed on label.
Ginkgo biloba (herb)	As directed on label.
Glucosamine sulfate	As directed on label.
Lecithin	200–500 mg
Lutein/lycopene	As directed on label.
Pectin	50–100 mg
Phosphatidyl choline	As directed on label.
Phosphatidyl serine	As directed on label.
Pycnogenol or grape seed extract (OPCs)	As directed on label.
Quercetin	70–140 mg
RNA-DNA	100 mg
Silicon	As directed on label.
Soy isoflavones (genistein)	As directed on label.
Superoxide dismutase (SOD)	As directed on label.
Zeaxanthin	90 mcg

*Be careful not to confuse milligrams (mg) with micrograms (mcg). A microgram is $^1/_{1,000}$ of a milligram.

**Iron should be taken only if a deficiency exists. Always take iron supplements separately, rather than in a multivitamin and mineral formula.

***See AMINO ACIDS for more information. Individual amino acids should not be taken on a regular basis unless used for treatment of a certain disorder.

****See NATURAL FOOD SUPPLEMENTS for more information.

Other supplements that you may wish to take for increased energy are:

- Bee pollen.
- Coenzyme A.
- Coenzyme 1 (nicotinamide adenine dinucleotide with high-energy hydrogen, or NADH; sold under the brand name Enada).
- Free-form amino acid complex.
- Kyo-Green from Wakunaga of America.
- N,N-Dimethylglycine (DMG).
- Octacosanol.
- Siberian ginseng.
- Spirulina.
- Wheat germ.

In addition, there are many good formulas on the market specifically formulated to help meet the nutritional needs of infants and children, among them Mycel Baby Vites from Ethical Nutrients, a highly absorbable liquid multivitamin formula.

Synergy and Deficiency

Data compiled by the U.S. Department of Agriculture indicate that at least 40 percent of the people in this country routinely consume a diet containing only 60 percent of the RDA of each of ten selected nutrients. This means that close to half of the population (and very likely more) suffer from a deficiency of at least one important nutrient. A poll of 37,000 Americans conducted by Food Technology found that half of them were deficient in vitamin B_6 (pyridoxine), 42 percent did not consume sufficient amounts of calcium, 39 percent had an insufficient iron intake, and 25 to 39 percent did not obtain enough vitamin C. Additional research has shown that a vitamin deficiency may not affect the whole body, but only specific cells. For example, those who smoke may suffer from a vitamin C deficiency, but only in the lung area.

Whenever you seek to correct a vitamin or mineral deficiency, you must recognize that nutrients work synergistically. This means that there is a cooperative action between certain vitamins and minerals, which work as catalysts, promoting the absorption and assimilation of other vitamins and minerals. Correcting a deficiency in one vitamin or mineral requires the addition of others, not simply replacement of the one in which you are deficient. This is why taking a single vitamin or mineral may be ineffective, or even dangerous, and why a balanced vitamin and mineral preparation should always be taken in addition to any single supplements. The following table indicates which vitamins and minerals are necessary to correct certain deficiencies.

Vitamin	Supplements Needed for Assimilation
Vitamin A	Choline, essential fatty acids, zinc, vitamins C, D, and E.
Vitamin B complex	Calcium, vitamins C and E.
Vitamin B_1 (thiamine)	Manganese, vitamin B complex, vitamins C and E.
Vitamin B_2 (riboflavin)	Vitamin B complex, vitamin C.
Vitamin B_3 (niacin)	Vitamin B complex, vitamin C.
Pantothenic acid (vitamin B_5)	Vitamin B complex, vitamins A, C, and E.
Vitamin B_6 (pyridoxine)	Potassium, vitamin B complex, vitamin C.
Biotin	Folic acid, vitamin B complex, pantothenic acid (vitamin B_5), vitamin B_{12}, vitamin C.
Choline	Vitamin B complex, vitamin B_{12}, folic acid, inositol.
Inositol	Vitamin B complex, vitamin C.
Para-aminobenzoic acid (PABA)	Vitamin B complex, folic acid, vitamin C.
Vitamin C	Bioflavonoids, calcium, magnesium.
Vitamin D	Calcium, choline, essential fatty acids, phosphorus, vitamins A and C.
Vitamin E	Essential fatty acids, manganese, selenium, vitamin A, vitamin B_1 (thiamine), inositol, vitamin C.
Essential fatty acids	Vitamins A, C, D, and E.

Mineral	Supplements Needed for Assimilation
Calcium	Boron, essential fatty acids, lysine, magnesium, manganese, phosphorus, vitamins A, C, D, and E.
Copper	Cobalt, folic acid, iron, zinc.
Iodine	Iron, manganese, phosphorus.
Magnesium	Calcium, phosphorus, potassium, vitamin B_6 (pyridoxine), vitamins C and D.
Manganese	Calcium, iron, vitamin B complex, vitamin E.
Phosphorus	Calcium, iron, manganese, sodium, vitamin B_6 (pyridoxine).
Silicon	Iron, phosphorus.
Sodium	Calcium, potassium, sulfur, vitamin D.
Sulfur	Potassium, vitamin B_1 (thiamine), pantothenic acid (vitamin B_5), biotin.
Zinc	Calcium, copper, phosphorus, vitamin B_6 (pyridoxine).

There are certain cautions that you should take into account when taking supplements. Antibiotics interfere with the natural balance of normal intestinal flora needed to produce vitamin K, which is necessary for normal blood clotting and maintaining the integrity of the bones. Too much coffee and/or caffeinated soft drinks can interfere with calcium metabolism. Aspirin can irritate the gastrointestinal tract, and may cause gastrointestinal bleeding. Aspirin can also interfere with the absorption of B vitamins and vitamin C. If you are taking aspirin daily for cardiovascular health, it is better to take baby aspirin—studies have shown that it is less irritating to the gastrointestinal tract, and it works just as well as ordinary aspirin.

GUIDELINES FOR SELECTING AND PREPARING FOODS

Clearly, a healthy diet must provide a proper balance of the four essential nutrients, as well as a rich supply of vitamins, minerals, and other micronutrients. However, it is not enough simply to purchase foods that are high in complex carbohydrates, fiber, and complementary proteins, and low in saturated fats. Food also must be free of harmful additives, and it must be prepared in a way that preserves its nutrients and avoids the production of harmful substances.

When nutritionists talk about diet, they are referring to live whole foods—unprocessed food with nothing added or taken away. Whole foods are more healthful because they contain no potentially harmful ingredients. In addition, plant foods are full of hundreds of phytochemicals that can help prevent disease and keep the body healthy. These are our front-line defenders against cancer and free radicals (see Phytochemicals, page 9). Foods known to supply important phytochemicals include soybeans and soy products, broccoli, citrus peels, flax, garlic, green tea, grapes, and tomatoes.

Avoid Foods that Contain Additives and Artificial Ingredients

Additives are placed in foods for a number of reasons: to lengthen shelf life; to make a food more appealing by enhancing color, texture, or taste; to facilitate food preparation; or to otherwise make the product more marketable. Certain additives, like sugar, are derived from natural sources. Other additives, like aspartame (NutraSweet), are made synthetically.

Although many additives are used in very small amounts, it has been estimated that the average American consumes about 5 pounds of additives per year. If you include sugar—the food-processing industry's most used additive—the number jumps to 135 pounds a year. Anyone whose diet is high in processed products clearly consumes a significant amount of additives and artificial ingredients.

At their best, additives and artificial ingredients simply add little or no nutritional value to a food product. At their worst, additives pose a threat to your health. The history of additive use includes a number of products that were once deemed safe but later were banned or allowed to be used only if accompanied by warnings. The artificial sweeteners cyclamate and saccharin are just two examples of such products. Other additives, like monosodium glutamate (MSG) and aspartame, are used without warnings, but have been known to cause problems ranging from headaches and diarrhea to confusion, memory loss, and seizures. (For more information on aspartame, see Is Aspartame a Safe Sugar Substitute? on page 10.)

The number of food additives now in use is staggering. To learn more about these substances, you can consult Michael Jacobson's Safe Food: Eating Wisely in a Risky World (Living Planet Press, 1991) or Unsafe at Any Meal by Earl Mindell (Warner Books, 1986).

Increase Your Consumption of Raw Produce

The most healthful fruits and vegetables are those that have been grown organically—without the use of insecticides, herbicides, artificial fertilizers, or growth-stimulating chemicals. Organic produce can be found in select health food stores, as well as in some supermarkets and greenmarkets and through food co-ops.

When choosing your produce, look for fruits and vegetables that are at the peak of ripeness. These contain more vitamins and enzymes than do foods that are underripe or overripe, or that have been stored for any length of time. Remember that the longer a food is kept in storage, the more nutrients it loses.

Once you get your organic produce home, running water and a vegetable brush are probably all that will be needed to get it ready for the table. If the produce is not organic, however, you will want to wash it more thoroughly to rid it of any chemical residues. Use a soft vegetable brush to scrub the foods, and then let them soak in water for ten minutes. You can also clean produce with nontoxic rinsing preparations, which are available in reputable health food stores. If the products are waxed, peel them, as wax cannot be washed away, but remove as thin a layer of peel as possible.

Most fruits and vegetables should be eaten in their entirety, as all of the parts, including the skin, contain valuable nutrients. When eating citrus fruits, remove the rinds, but eat the white part inside the skin for its vitamin C and bioflavonoid content.

Although most people usually cook their vegetables before eating, both fruits and vegetables should be eaten raw as much as possible. All enzymes and most vitamins are extremely sensitive to heat, and are usually destroyed in the cooking process.

If fresh produce is unavailable, use frozen foods instead. Do not use canned vegetables or boxed vegetable dishes, as they usually contain significant amounts of salt and other unhealthy additives. If raw produce does not agree with you, steam your vegetables lightly in a steamer, cooking pan, or wok just until slightly tender.

Phytochemicals

For many years, researchers have recognized that diets high in fruits, vegetables, grains, and legumes appear to reduce the risk of a number of diseases, including cancer, heart disease, diabetes, and high blood pressure when compared with diets high in meat. More recently, it was discovered that the disease-preventing effects of these foods are partly due to antioxidants—specific vitamins, minerals, and enzymes that help prevent cancer and other disorders by protecting cells against damage from oxidation. Now, researchers have discovered that fruits, vegetables, grains, and legumes contain yet another group of health-promoting nutrients. Called *phytochemicals,* these substances appear to be powerful ammunition in the war against cancer and other disorders.

Phytochemicals are the biologically active substances in plants that are responsible for giving them color, flavor, and natural disease resistance. To understand how phytochemicals protect the body against cancer, it is necessary to understand that cancer formation is a multistep process. Phytochemicals seem to fight cancer by blocking one or more of the steps that lead to cancer. For instance, cancer can begin when a carcinogenic molecule—from the food you eat or the air you breathe—invades a cell. But if sulforaphane, a phytochemical found in broccoli, also reaches the cell, it activates a group of enzymes that whisk the carcinogen out of the cell before it can cause any harm.

Other phytochemicals are known to prevent cancer in other ways. Flavonoids, found in citrus fruits and berries, keep cancer-causing hormones from latching on to cells in the first place. Genistein, found in soybeans, kills tumors by preventing the formation of the capillaries needed to nourish them. Indoles, found in cruciferous vegetables such as Brussels sprouts, cauliflower, and cabbage, increase immune activity and make it easier for the body to excrete toxins. Saponins, found in kidney beans, chickpeas, soybeans, and lentils, may prevent cancer cells from multiplying. P-coumaric acid and chlorogenic acid, found in tomatoes, interfere with certain chemical unions that can create carcinogens. The list of these protective substances goes on and on. Tomatoes alone are believed to contain an estimated 10,000 different phytochemicals.

Although no long-term human studies have shown that specific phytochemicals stop cancer, research on phytochemicals supports the more than 200 studies that link lowered cancer risk with a diet rich in grains, legumes, fruits, and vegetables. Moreover, animal and in vitro studies have demonstrated how some phytochemicals prevent carcinogens from promoting the growth of specific cancers. For instance, the phytochemical phenethyl isothiocyanate (PEITC), found in cabbage and turnips, has been shown to inhibit the growth of lung cancer in rats and mice. Among other things, PEITC protects the cells' DNA from a potent carcinogen found in tobacco smoke.

Researchers have been able to isolate some phytochemicals, and a number of companies are now selling concentrates that contain phytochemicals obtained from vegetables such as broccoli. These may be used as supplemental sources of some of these nutrients. However, such pills should *not* be seen as replacements for fresh whole foods. Because several *thousand* phytochemicals are currently known to exist, and because new ones are being discovered all the time, no supplement can possibly contain all of the cancer-fighters found in a shopping basket full of fruits and vegetables.

Fortunately, it is easy to get a healthy dose of phytochemicals at every meal. Almost every grain, legume, fruit, and vegetable tested has been found to contain these substances. Moreover, unlike many vitamins, these substances do not appear to be destroyed by cooking or other processing. Genistein, the substance found in soybeans, for instance, is also found in soybean products such as tofu and miso soup. Similarly, the phytochemical PEITC, found in cabbage, remains intact even when the cabbage is made into cole slaw or sauerkraut. Of course, by eating much of your produce raw or only lightly cooked, you will be able to enjoy the benefits not just of phytochemicals, but of all of the vitamins, minerals, and other nutrients that fresh whole foods have to offer.

Avoid Overcooking Your Foods

As just discussed, cooking foods for all but brief periods of time can destroy many valuable nutrients. More alarming is that when foods are cooked to the point of browning or charring, the organic compounds they contain undergo changes in structure, producing carcinogens.

Barbecued meats seem to pose the worst health threat in this regard. When burning fat drips onto an open flame, polycyclic aromatic hydrocarbons (PAHs)—dangerous carcinogens—are formed. When amino acids and other chemicals found in muscle are exposed to high temperatures, other carcinogens, called heterocyclic aromatic amines (HAAs), are created. In fact, many of the chemicals used to produce cancer in laboratory animals have been isolated from cooked proteins.

It is important to note, though, that cooked meats do not pose the only threat. Even browned or burned bread crusts contain a variety of carcinogenic substances.

The dangers posed by the practice of cooking foods at high temperatures or until browned or burned should not be dismissed. Although eating habits vary widely from person to person, it seems safe to assume that many people consume many grams of overcooked foods a day. By comparison, only half a gram of this same dangerous burned

Is Aspartame a Safe Sugar Substitute?

Due to America's obsession with dieting, the popularity of aspartame (NutraSweet) has soared. Because it is about 200 times sweeter than sugar, much smaller amounts of aspartame are needed to sweeten the taste of foods. This artificial sweetener pervades supermarket shelves. It is especially prevalent in diet foods, and can be found in the following products:

- Instant breakfasts.
- Breath mints.
- Cereals.
- Sugar-free chewing gum.
- Cocoa mixes.
- Coffee beverages.
- Frozen desserts.
- Gelatin desserts.
- Juice beverages.
- Laxatives.
- Milk drinks.
- Multivitamins.
- Nonprescription pharmaceuticals.
- Shake mixes.
- Soft drinks.
- Tabletop sweeteners.
- Tea beverages.
- Instant teas and coffees.
- Topping mixes.
- Wine coolers.
- Yogurt.

Aspartame consists of three components: the amino acids phenylalanine and aspartic acid, and methanol, which is also known as methyl alcohol or wood alcohol.

Although it has been claimed that the amino acids in aspartame are metabolized in the same way that their natural counterparts, found in foods, are metabolized, research suggests otherwise. Consumption of aspartame in sodas, for instance, appears to cause a flooding of the amino acids in the bloodstream—a prompt rise that does not occur after the ingestion of dietary protein. This rise, it is believed, may cause problems.

No one disputes that aspartame should be avoided by people with phenylketonuria (PKU). People with PKU lack the enzyme needed to convert phenylalanine into tyrosine, another amino acid. As a result, high concentrations of phenylalanine accumulate and can cause brain damage. It should be noted that a number of people who have disorders other than PKU—people with iron deficiencies and kidney disease, for instance—also may be prone to high levels of this amino acid. For such people, the consumption of aspartame may increase the risk of toxicity.

Methanol, the third ingredient in aspartame, is known to be poisonous even when consumed in relatively modest amounts. Disorders caused by toxic levels of methanol include blindness, brain swelling, and inflammation of the pancreas and heart muscle. Although the Food and Drug Administration (FDA) states that exposure to methanol through aspartame consumption is not of "sufficient quantity to be of toxicological concern," the cumulative effects of high doses of aspartame are unknown.

Regardless of any claims of the FDA, a significant number of people have reported suffering ill effects as a result of aspartame consumption. According to *Aspartame (NutraSweet): Is It Safe?* by H.J. Roberts (The Charles Press, 1990), reported reactions include headaches, mood swings, changes in vision, nausea and diarrhea, sleep disorders, memory loss and confusion, and even convulsions. Aspartame appears to be especially dangerous for children.

Needless to say, if you have experienced a reaction to aspartame, you should refrain from using foods that contain this additive. Better yet, avoid all additives, and enjoy a diet rich in fruits and fresh juices. These foods are naturally sweet, free of artificial coloring and preservatives, and full of the nutrients needed for good health.

material is inhaled by someone who smokes two packs of cigarettes a day. Clearly, by eating produce raw or only lightly cooked, and by greatly limiting your consumption of meat, you will be doing much to decrease your risk of cancer and, possibly, other disorders.

Use the Proper Cooking Utensils

Although raw foods have many advantages over cooked, nourishing soups and a variety of other dishes can be made healthfully. One of the ways to ensure wholesome cooked food is the careful selection of cookware.

When preparing foods, use only glass, stainless steel, or iron pots and pans. Do not use aluminum cookware or utensils. Foods cooked or stored in aluminum produce a substance that neutralizes the digestive juices, leading to acidosis and ulcers. Worse, the aluminum in the cookware can leach from the pot into the food. When the food is consumed, the aluminum is absorbed by the body, where it accumulates in the brain and nervous system tissues. Excessive amounts of these aluminum deposits have been implicated in Alzheimer's disease.

Other cookware to be avoided includes all pots and pans with nonstick coatings. Too often, the metals and other substances in the pots' finish flakes or leaches into the food. Ultimately, these chemicals end up in your body.

Basic Nutritional Guide

A diet high in nutrients is the key to good health. Use the following table as a guide when deciding which types of food to include in your diet and which ones to avoid in order to maintain good health.

Type of Food	Foods to Avoid	Acceptable Foods
Beans	Canned pork and beans, canned beans with salt or preservatives, frozen beans.	All beans (especially soy) cooked without animal fat or salt.
Beverages	Alcoholic drinks, coffee, cocoa, pasteurized and/or sweetened juices and fruit drinks, sodas, tea (except herbal tea).	Herbal teas, fresh vegetable and fruit juices, cereal grain beverages (often sold as coffee substitutes), mineral or distilled water.
Dairy products	All soft cheeses, all pasteurized or artificially colored cheese products, ice cream.	Raw goat cheese, nonfat cottage cheese, kefir, unsweetened yogurt, goat's milk, raw or skim milk, buttermilk.
Eggs	Fried or pickled.	Boiled or poached (limit of four weekly).
Fish	All fried fish, all shellfish, salted fish, anchovies, herring, fish canned in oil.	All freshwater white fish, salmon, broiled or baked fish, water-packed tuna.
Fruits	Canned, bottled, or frozen fruits with sweeteners added; oranges.	All fresh, frozen, stewed, or dried fruits without sweeteners (except oranges, which are acidic and highly allergenic), unsulfured fruits, home-canned fruits.
Grains	All white flour products, white rice, pasta, crackers, cold cereals, instant types of oatmeal and other hot cereals.	All whole grains and products containing whole grains: cereals, breads, muffins, whole-grain crackers, cream of wheat or rye cereal, buckwheat, millet, oats, brown rice, wild rice. (Limit yeast breads to three servings per week.)
Meats	Beef; all forms of pork; hot dogs; luncheon meats; smoked, pickled, and processed meats; corned beef; duck; goose; spare ribs; gravies; organ meats.	Skinless turkey and chicken, lamb. (Limit meat to three 3-oz servings per week.)
Nuts	All salted or roasted nuts; peanuts (if suffering from any disorder).	All fresh raw nuts (peanuts in moderation only).
Oils (fats)	All saturated fats, hydrogenated margarine, refined processed oils, shortenings, hardened oils.	All cold-pressed oils: corn, safflower, sesame, olive, flaxseed, soybean, sunflower, and canola oils; margarine made from these oils; eggless mayonnaise.
Seasonings	Black or white pepper, salt, hot red peppers, all types of vinegar except pure natural apple cider vinegar.	Garlic, onions, cayenne, Spike, all herbs, dried vegetables, apple cider vinegar, tamari, miso, seaweed, dulse.
Soups	Canned soups made with salt, preservatives, MSG, or fat stock; all creamed soups.	Homemade (salt- and fat-free) bean, lentil, pea, vegetable, barley, brown rice, onion.
Sprouts and seeds	All seeds cooked in oil or salt.	All slightly cooked sprouts (except alfalfa, which should be raw and washed thoroughly), wheatgrass, all raw seeds.
Sweets	White, brown, or raw cane sugar, corn syrups, chocolate, sugar candy, fructose (except that in fresh whole fruit), all syrups (except pure maple syrup), all sugar substitutes, jams and jellies made with sugar.	Barley malt or rice syrup, small amounts of raw honey, pure maple syrup, stevia, unsulfured blackstrap molasses.
Vegetables	All canned or frozen with salt or additives.	All raw, fresh, frozen (no additives), or home-canned without salt (undercook vegetables slightly).

Limit Your Use of Salt

Although some sodium is essential for survival, inadequate sodium intake is a rare problem. We need less than 500 milligrams of sodium a day to stay healthy. This is enough to accomplish all the vital functions that sodium performs in the body—helping maintain normal fluid levels, healthy muscle function, and proper acidity (pH) of the blood. Excessive sodium intake can cause fluid to be retained in the tissues, which can lead to hypertension (high blood pressure) and can aggravate many medical disorders, including congestive heart failure, certain forms of kidney disease, and premenstrual syndrome (PMS).

One of the best ways to limit the sodium in your diet is to limit your use of salt when cooking and dining. Just as important, stay away from processed foods, which often contain excessively high amounts of sodium.

VITAMINS

INTRODUCTION

Vitamins are essential to life. They contribute to good health by regulating the metabolism and assisting the biochemical processes that release energy from digested food. They are considered micronutrients because the body needs them in relatively small amounts compared with nutrients such as carbohydrates, proteins, fats, and water.

Enzymes are essential chemicals that are the foundation of human bodily functions. (*See* ENZYMES in Part One.) They are catalysts (activators) in the chemical reactions that are continually taking place within the body. As coenzymes, vitamins work with enzymes, thereby allowing all the activities that occur within the body to be carried out as they should. Whole, fresh raw foods are a good source of enzymes.

Of the major vitamins, some are water soluble and some are oil soluble. Water-soluble vitamins must be taken into the body daily, as they cannot be stored and are excreted within four hours to one day. These include vitamin C and the B-complex vitamins. Oil-soluble vitamins can be stored for longer periods of time in the body's fatty tissue and the liver. These include vitamins A, D, E, and K. Both types of vitamins are needed by the body for proper functioning.

RDA VERSUS RDI VERSUS ODI

Recommended Dietary Allowances (RDAs) were instituted over forty years ago by the National Academy of Sciences' U.S. Food and Nutrition Board as a standard for the daily amounts of vitamins needed by a healthy person. These RDAs were the basis for the U.S. Recommended Daily Allowances (U.S. RDAs) adopted by the Food and Drug Administration (FDA). The provisions of the Nutrition Labeling and Education Act and the Dietary Supplement Act of 1992 required a change in food product labeling to use a new reference term, Daily Value (DV), which began to appear on FDA-regulated product labels in 1994.

DVs are made up of two sets of references: Daily Reference Values (DRVs) and Reference Daily Intakes (RDIs). DRVs are a set of dietary references that apply to fat, saturated fat, cholesterol, carbohydrate, protein, fiber, sodium, and potassium. RDIs are a set of dietary references based on the Recommended Dietary Allowances for essential vitamins and minerals and, in selected groups, protein. The term *RDI* replaces *U.S. RDA*.

Unfortunately, the amounts of these nutrients defined by the Recommended Dietary Allowances give us only the bare minimum required to ward off vitamin deficiency diseases such as beriberi, rickets, scurvy, and night blindness. What they do not account for are the amounts needed to maintain maximum health, rather than borderline health.

Scientific studies have shown that taking dosages of vitamins above the RDIs helps our bodies work better. The RDIs therefore are not very useful for determining what our intake of different vitamins should be. We prefer to speak in terms of *optimum daily intakes* (ODIs)—the amounts of nutrients needed for vibrant good health. This entails consuming larger amounts of vitamins than the RDIs. The nutrient doses recommended on page 6 are ODIs. By providing our bodies with an optimum daily amount of necessary vitamins, we can enhance our health. The dosages outlined in this book will enable you to design a vitamin program that is custom-tailored for the individual.

BALANCE AND SYNERGY

Having the proper balance of vitamins and minerals is very important. Scientific research has proved that excesses of isolated vitamins or minerals can produce the same symptoms as deficiencies of vitamins or minerals. For example, high doses of isolated B vitamins have been shown to cause the depletion of other B vitamins. Similarly, if zinc is taken in excess, symptoms of zinc deficiency can result. Studies have shown that an intake of up to 100 milligrams of zinc daily enhances immune function, but an amount in excess of 100 milligrams daily may actually harm immune function.

Synergy is a phenomenon whereby two or more vitamins combine to create a stronger vitamin function than the sum of their individual effects would suggest. For example, in order for bioflavonoids to work properly (they prevent bruising and bleeding gums), they must be taken along with vitamin C. Recent studies show that bioflavonoids also may be a big factor in preventing cancer and many other diseases.

In addition, certain substances can block the absorption and effects of vitamins. For example, the absorption of vitamin C is greatly reduced by antibiotic drugs, so a person taking antibiotics requires a higher than normal intake of this vitamin.

SYNTHETIC VERSUS NATURAL

Ideally, all of us would get all of the nutrients we need for optimal health from fresh, healthful foods. In reality, however, this is often difficult, if not impossible. In our chemically polluted and stress-filled world, our nutritional requirements have been increasing, but the number of calories we require has been *decreasing,* as our general level of physical activity has declined. This means we are faced with needing somehow to get more nutrients from less food. At the same time, many of our foods are depleted of certain nutrients. Modern farming practices have resulted in soils that are lacking in selenium and other nutrients. Harvesting and shipping practices are dictated not by nutritional considerations but by marketing demands. Add to this extensive processing, improper storage, and other factors, and it is little wonder that many of the foods that reach our tables cannot meet our nutritional needs. Getting even the RDIs of vitamins from today's diet has become quite hard to do. This means that for optimum health, it is necessary to take nutrients in supplement form.

Vitamin supplements can be divided into two groups: synthetic and natural. Synthetic vitamins are vitamins produced in laboratories from isolated chemicals that mirror their counterparts found in nature. Natural vitamins are derived from food sources. Although there are no major chemical differences between a vitamin found in food and one created in a laboratory, synthetic supplements contain the isolated vitamins only, while natural supplements may contain other nutrients not yet discovered. This is because these vitamins are in their natural state. If you are deficient in a particular nutrient, the chemical source will work, but you will not get the benefits of the vitamin as found in whole foods. Supplements that are not labeled natural also may include coal tars, artificial coloring, preservatives, sugars, and starch, as well as other additives. You should beware of such harmful elements. However, you should also note that a bottle of "natural" vitamins may contain vitamins that have not been extracted from a natural food source. It is necessary to read labels carefully to make sure the products you buy contain nutrients from food sources, with none of the artificial additives mentioned above.

Studies have shown that protein-bonded vitamins, as found in natural whole food supplements, are absorbed, utilized, and retained in the tissues better than supplements that are not protein-bonded. Chemical-derived vitamins are not protein-bonded. Vitamins and minerals in food are bonded to proteins, lipids, carbohydrates, and bioflavonoids. Dr. Abram Hoffer, one of the "founding fathers" of orthomolecular medicine (a school of medicine that emphasizes the role of nutrition in health), explains:

> Components [of food] do not exist free in nature; nature does not lay down pure protein, pure fat, or pure carbohydrates. Their molecules are interlaced in very complex three-dimensional structures which even now have not been fully described. Intermingled are the essential nutrients such as vitamins and minerals, again not free, but combined in complex molecules.

Using a natural form of vitamins and minerals in nutritional supplements is the objective of the protein-bonding process. Taking supplements with meals helps to assure a supply of other nutrients needed for better assimilation as well.

WHAT'S ON THE SHELVES

Over-the-counter vitamin supplements come in various forms, combinations, and amounts. They are available in tablet, capsule, gel-capsule, powder, sublingual, lozenge, and liquid forms. They can also be administered by injection. In most cases, it is a matter of personal preference as to how you take them; however, due to slight variations in how rapidly the supplements are absorbed and assimilated into the body, we will sometimes recommend one form over another. These recommendations are given throughout the book.

Vitamin supplements are usually available as isolated vitamins or in combination with other nutrients. It is important to select your vitamins based upon what you really need. A program designed for health maintenance would be different from one designed to overcome a specific disorder. If you find one supplement that meets your needs, remember to take it daily. If it does not contain a large enough quantity of what you want, you may consider taking more than one. Just make sure that you are aware of the increased dosage of the other nutrients it may contain. If there is no single supplement that provides you with what you are looking for, consider taking a combination of different supplements. This book lists each supplement separately, so you will know what each does and the amount needed. But you may find a supplement that contains several needed nutrients in one tablet or capsule.

Because the potency of most vitamins may be decreased by sunlight, make sure that the container holding your vitamins is dark enough to shield its contents properly. Some people may be sensitive to plastic, and may need to purchase vitamins in glass containers. Vitamin supplements should be kept in a cool, dark place.

All vitamin supplements work best when taken in combination with food. Unless specified otherwise, oil-soluble vitamins should be taken before meals, and water-soluble ones should be taken after meals.

VITAMINS FROM A TO Z

Vitamin A and the Carotenoids

Vitamin A prevents night blindness and other eye problems, as well as some skin disorders, such as acne. It enhances immunity, may help to heal gastrointestinal ulcers, and is needed for the maintenance and repair of epithelial tissue, of which the skin and mucous membranes are composed. It is important in the formation of bones and teeth, aids in fat storage, and protects against colds, flu, and infections of the kidneys, bladder, lungs, and mucous membranes. Vitamin A acts as an antioxidant, helping to protect the cells against cancer and other diseases (*see* ANTIOXIDANTS in Part One) and is necessary for new cell growth. It guards against heart disease and stroke, and lowers cholesterol levels. This important vitamin also slows the aging process. Protein cannot be utilized by the body without vitamin A. Vitamin A is a well-known wrinkle eliminator. Applied topically in the form of tretinoin (the active ingredient in Retin-A and Renova), vitamin A reduces fine lines in the skin and helps fade age spots.

A deficiency of vitamin A can cause dry hair and/or skin, dryness of the conjunctiva and cornea, poor growth, and/or night blindness. Other possible results of vitamin A deficiency include abscesses in the ears; insomnia; fatigue; reproductive difficulties; sinusitis, pneumonia, and frequent colds and other respiratory infections; skin disorders, including acne; and weight loss.

The *carotenoids* are a class of compounds related to vitamin A. In some cases, they can act as precursors of vitamin A; some act as antioxidants or have other important functions. The best known subclass of the carotenoids are the carotenes, of which beta-carotene is the most widely known. Also included in this group are alpha- and gamma-carotene, and lycopene. When food or supplements containing beta-carotene are consumed, the beta-carotene is converted into vitamin A in the liver. According to recent reports, beta-carotene appears to aid in cancer prevention by scavenging, or neutralizing, free radicals. Other types of carotenoids that have been identified are the xanthophylls (including beta-cryptoxanthin, canthaxanthin, lutein, and zeaxanthin); the limonoids (including limonene); and the phytosterols (including perillyl alcohol). Science has not yet discovered all of the carotenoids, although one source documents 563 different carotenoids identified so far. Combinations of carotenoids have been shown to be more beneficial than individual carotenoids taken alone.

Taking large amounts of vitamin A, over 100,000 international units daily, over long periods can be toxic to the body, mainly the liver. Toxic levels of vitamin A are associated with abdominal pain, amenorrhea (cessation of menstruation), enlargement of the liver and/or spleen, gastrointestinal disturbances, hair loss, itching, joint pain, nausea and vomiting, water on the brain, elevated liver enzymes, and small cracks and scales on the lips and at the corners of the mouth. Excessive intake of vitamin A during pregnancy has been linked to birth defects, including cleft palate and heart defects. It is better to take beta-carotene during pregnancy. If you have a particular disorder that calls for taking high doses of vitamin A, use an emulsified form, which puts less stress on the liver.

No overdose can occur with beta-carotene, although if you take too much, your skin may turn slightly yellow-orange in color. Beta-carotene does not have the same effect as vitamin A in the body and is not harmful in larger amounts unless your liver cannot convert beta-carotene

into vitamin A. People with hypothyroidism often have this problem. It is important to take only *natural* beta-carotene or a natural carotenoid complex. Betatene is the trade name for a type of carotenoid complex extracted from sea algae. It is used as an ingredient in various products by different manufacturers.

Sources

Vitamin A can be found in animal livers, fish liver oils, and green and yellow fruits and vegetables. Foods that contain significant amounts include apricots, asparagus, beet greens, broccoli, cantaloupe, carrots, collards, dandelion greens, dulse, fish liver and fish liver oil, garlic, kale, mustard greens, papayas, peaches, pumpkin, red peppers, spinach, spirulina, sweet potatoes, Swiss chard, turnip greens, watercress, and yellow squash. It is also present in the following herbs: alfalfa, borage leaves, burdock root, cayenne (capsicum), chickweed, eyebright, fennel seed, hops, horsetail, kelp, lemongrass, mullein, nettle, oat straw, paprika, parsley, peppermint, plantain, raspberry leaf, red clover, rose hips, sage, uva ursi, violet leaves, watercress, and yellow dock. Animal sources of vitamin A are up to six times as strong as vegetable sources.

Comments

Antibiotics, laxatives, and some cholesterol-lowering drugs interfere with the absorption of vitamin A.

Cautions

If you have liver disease, do not take a daily dose of over 10,000 international units of vitamin A in pill form, or any amount of cod liver oil. If you are pregnant, do not take more than 10,000 international units of vitamin A daily because of reported problems in fetal development. Children should not take more than 18,000 international units of vitamin A on a daily basis for over one month. For most people, beta-carotene is the best source of vitamin A because it is converted by the liver into only the amount of vitamin A that the body actually needs. However, if you have diabetes or hypothyroidism, there is a good possibility your body cannot convert beta-carotene into vitamin A. Consuming large amounts of beta-carotene may therefore place unnecessary stress on your liver.

Vitamin B Complex

The B vitamins help to maintain the health of the nerves, skin, eyes, hair, liver, and mouth, as well as healthy muscle tone in the gastrointestinal tract and proper brain function. B-complex vitamins act as coenzymes, helping enzymes to react chemically with other substances, and are involved in energy production. They may be useful for alleviating depression or anxiety as well. Adequate intake of the B vitamins is very important for elderly people because these nutrients are not as well absorbed as we age. There have even been cases of people diagnosed with Alzheimer's disease whose problems were later found to be due to a deficiency of vitamin B_{12} plus the B complex. The B vitamins should always be taken together, but up to two to three times more of one B vitamin than another can be taken for a period of time if needed for a particular disorder. There are spray and sublingual forms that are absorbed more easily, which are good choices for older adults and those with absorption problems.

Because the B vitamins work together, a deficiency in one often indicates a deficiency in another. Although the B vitamins are a team, they will be discussed individually.

Vitamin B_1 (Thiamine)

Thiamine enhances circulation and assists in blood formation, carbohydrate metabolism, and the production of hydrochloric acid, which is important for proper digestion. Thiamine also optimizes cognitive activity and brain function. It has a positive effect on energy, growth, normal appetite, and learning capacity, and is needed for proper muscle tone of the intestines, stomach, and heart. Thiamine also acts as an antioxidant, protecting the body from the degenerative effects of aging, alcohol consumption, and smoking.

Beriberi, a nervous system disease that is rare in developed nations, is caused by a deficiency of thiamine. Other symptoms that can result from thiamine deficiency include constipation, edema, enlarged liver, fatigue, forgetfulness, gastrointestinal disturbances, heart changes, irritability, labored breathing, loss of appetite, muscle atrophy, nervousness, numbness of the hands and feet, pain and sensitivity, poor coordination, tingling sensations, weak and sore muscles, general weakness, and severe weight loss.

Sources

The richest food sources of thiamine include brown rice, egg yolks, fish, legumes, liver, peanuts, peas, pork, poultry, rice bran, wheat germ, and whole grains. Other sources are asparagus, brewer's yeast, broccoli, Brussels sprouts, dulse, kelp, most nuts, oatmeal, plums, dried prunes, raisins, spirulina, and watercress. Herbs that contain thiamine include alfalfa, bladderwrack, burdock root, catnip, cayenne, chamomile, chickweed, eyebright, fennel seed, fenugreek, hops, nettle, oat straw, parsley, peppermint, raspberry leaf, red clover, rose hips, sage, yarrow, and yellow dock.

Comments

Antibiotics, phenytoin (Dilantin, a drug used to prevent seizures), sulfa drugs, and oral contraceptives, and heavy alcohol or caffeine consumption may decrease thiamine levels in the body. A high-carbohydrate diet increases the need for thiamine. Alcoholics are among those most often deficient in thiamine.

Vitamin B_2 (Riboflavin)

Riboflavin is necessary for red blood cell formation, antibody production, cell respiration, and growth. It alleviates eye fatigue and is important in the prevention and treatment of cataracts. It aids in the metabolism of carbohydrates, fats, and proteins. Together with vitamin A, it maintains and improves the mucous membranes in the digestive tract. Riboflavin also facilitates the use of oxygen by the tissues of the skin, nails, and hair; eliminates dandruff; and helps the absorption of iron and vitamin B_6 (pyridoxine). Consumption of adequate amounts of riboflavin is important during pregnancy, because a lack of this vitamin can damage a developing fetus even if a woman shows no signs of deficiency. Riboflavin is needed for the metabolism of the amino acid tryptophan, which is converted into niacin in the body. Carpal tunnel syndrome may benefit from a treatment program that includes riboflavin and vitamin B_6.

Deficiency symptoms include cracks and sores at the corners of the mouth, eye disorders, inflammation of the mouth and tongue, and skin lesions, a group of symptoms collectively referred to as *ariboflavinosis*. Other possible deficiency symptoms include dermatitis, dizziness, hair loss, insomnia, light sensitivity, poor digestion, retarded growth, and slowed mental response.

Sources

High levels of vitamin B_2 are found in the following foods: cheese, egg yolks, fish, legumes, meat, milk, poultry, spinach, whole grains, and yogurt. Other sources include asparagus, avocados, broccoli, Brussels sprouts, currants, dandelion greens, dulse, kelp, leafy green vegetables, mushrooms, molasses, nuts, and watercress. Herbs that contain vitamin B_2 include alfalfa, bladderwrack, burdock root, catnip, cayenne, chamomile, chickweed, eyebright, fennel seed, fenugreek, ginseng, hops, horsetail, mullein, nettle, oat straw, parsley, peppermint, raspberry leaves, red clover, rose hips, sage, and yellow dock.

Comments

Factors that increase the need for riboflavin include the use of oral contraceptives and strenuous exercise. This B vitamin is easily destroyed by light, antibiotics, and alcohol. Taking too much riboflavin (over 50 milligrams daily) over a long period of time may lead to cataracts and retinal diseases.

Vitamin B_3 (Niacin, Nicotinic Acid, Niacinamide)

Vitamin B_3 is needed for proper circulation and healthy skin. It aids in the functioning of the nervous system; in the metabolism of carbohydrates, fats, and proteins; and in the production of hydrochloric acid for the digestive system. It is involved in the normal secretion of bile and stomach fluids, and in the synthesis of sex hormones. Niacin lowers cholesterol and improves circulation. It is helpful for schizophrenia and other mental illnesses, and is also a memory-enhancer.

Pellagra is a disease caused by niacin deficiency. Other symptoms of niacin deficiency include canker sores, dementia, depression, diarrhea, dizziness, fatigue, halitosis, headaches, indigestion, insomnia, limb pains, loss of appetite, low blood sugar, muscular weakness, skin eruptions, and inflammation.

Sources

Niacin and niacinamide are found in beef liver, brewer's yeast, broccoli, carrots, cheese, corn flour, dandelion greens, dates, eggs, fish, milk, peanuts, pork, potatoes, tomatoes, wheat germ, and whole wheat products. Herbs that contain niacin include alfalfa, burdock root, catnip, cayenne, chamomile, chickweed, eyebright, fennel seed, hops, licorice, mullein, nettle, oat straw, parsley, peppermint, raspberry leaf, red clover, rose hips, slippery elm, and yellow dock.

Comments

A flush, usually harmless, may occur after the ingestion of niacin supplements; a red rash appears on the skin and a tingling sensation may be experienced as well. Usually, these symptoms last only a few minutes. There are two forms of this vitamin: niacin (or nicotinic acid) and niacinamide. In the form of niacinamide, it does not cause flushing. However, niacinamide does not have all the same properties of niacin. Specifically, it is not effective for lowering blood cholesterol.

Cautions

People who are pregnant or who suffer from diabetes, glaucoma, gout, liver disease, or peptic ulcers should use niacin supplements with caution. Niacin may elevate blood sugar levels. Amounts over 500 milligrams daily may cause liver damage if taken for prolonged periods.

Vitamin B_5 (Pantothenic Acid)

Known as "the anti-stress vitamin," pantothenic acid plays a role in the production of the adrenal hormones and the formation of antibodies, aids in vitamin utilization, and helps to convert fats, carbohydrates, and proteins into energy. It is required by all cells in the body and is concentrated in the organs. It is also involved in the production of neurotransmitters. This vitamin is an essential element of coenzyme A, a vital body chemical involved in many nec-

essary metabolic functions. Pantothenic acid is also a stamina enhancer and prevents certain forms of anemia. It is needed for normal functioning of the gastrointestinal tract and may be helpful in treating depression and anxiety. A deficiency of pantothenic acid may cause fatigue, headache, nausea, and tingling in the hands. Pantothenic acid is also needed for proper functioning of the adrenal glands.

Sources

The following foods contain pantothenic acid: beef, brewer's yeast, eggs, fresh vegetables, kidney, legumes, liver, mushrooms, nuts, pork, royal jelly, saltwater fish, torula yeast, whole rye flour, and whole wheat.

Vitamin B_6 (Pyridoxine)

Pyridoxine is involved in more bodily functions than almost any other single nutrient. It affects both physical and mental health. It is beneficial if you suffer from water retention, and is necessary for the production of hydrochloric acid and the absorption of fats and protein. Pyridoxine also aids in maintaining sodium and potassium balance, and promotes red blood cell formation. It is required by the nervous system and is needed for normal brain function and for the synthesis of the nucleic acids RNA and DNA, which contain the genetic instructions for the reproduction of all cells and for normal cellular growth. It activates many enzymes and aids in the absorption of vitamin B_{12}, in immune system function, and in antibody production.

Vitamin B_6 plays a role in cancer immunity and aids in the prevention of arteriosclerosis. It inhibits the formation of a toxic chemical called homocysteine, which attacks the heart muscle and allows the deposition of cholesterol around the heart muscle. Pyridoxine acts as a mild diuretic, reducing the symptoms of premenstrual syndrome, and it may be useful in preventing oxalate kidney stones as well. It is helpful in the treatment of allergies, arthritis, and asthma.

A deficiency of vitamin B_6 can result in anemia, convulsions, headaches, nausea, flaky skin, a sore tongue, and vomiting. Other possible signs of deficiency include acne, anorexia, arthritis, conjunctivitis, cracks or sores on the mouth and lips, depression, dizziness, fatigue, hyperirritability, impaired wound healing, inflammation of the mouth and gums, learning difficulties, impaired memory or memory loss, hair loss, hearing problems, numbness, oily facial skin, stunted growth, and tingling sensations. Carpal tunnel syndrome has been linked to a deficiency of vitamin B_6 as well.

Sources

All foods contain some vitamin B_6; however, the following foods have the highest amounts: brewer's yeast, carrots, chicken, eggs, fish, meat, peas, spinach, sunflower seeds, walnuts, and wheat germ. Other sources include avocado, bananas, beans, blackstrap molasses, broccoli, brown rice and other whole grains, cabbage, cantaloupe, corn, dulse, plantains, potatoes, rice bran, soybeans, and tempeh. Herbs that contain vitamin B_6 include alfalfa, catnip, and oat straw.

Comments

Antidepressants, estrogen therapy, and oral contraceptives may increase the need for vitamin B_6. Diuretics and cortisone drugs block the absorption of this vitamin by the body. Prolonged use of high doses of vitamin B_6 (over 1,000 milligrams per day) can be toxic, and may result in nerve damage and loss of coordination.

Vitamin B_{12} (Cyanocobalamin)

Vitamin B_{12} is needed to prevent anemia. It aids folic acid in regulating the formation of red blood cells, and helps in the utilization of iron. This vitamin is also required for proper digestion, absorption of foods, the synthesis of protein, and the metabolism of carbohydrates and fats. It aids in cell formation and cellular longevity. In addition, vitamin B_{12} prevents nerve damage, maintains fertility, and promotes normal growth and development by maintaining the fatty sheaths that cover and protect nerve endings. Vitamin B_{12} is linked to the production of acetylcholine, a neurotransmitter that assists memory and learning. Vitamin B_{12} supplementation has been shown to enhance sleep patterns, allowing for more restful and refreshing sleep.

A vitamin B_{12} deficiency can be caused by malabsorption, which is most common in elderly people and in those with digestive disorders. Deficiency can cause abnormal gait, bone loss, chronic fatigue, constipation, depression, digestive disorders, dizziness, drowsiness, enlargement of the liver, eye disorders, hallucinations, headaches (including migraines), inflammation of the tongue, irritability, labored breathing, memory loss, moodiness, nervousness, neurological damage, palpitations, pernicious anemia, ringing in the ears, and spinal cord degeneration. Strict vegetarians must remember that they require vitamin B_{12} supplementation, as this vitamin is found almost exclusively in animal tissues. Although people adopting a strictly vegetarian diet may not see any signs of the deficiency for some time—the body can store up to five years' worth of vitamin B_{12}—signs will eventually develop.

Sources

The largest amounts of vitamin B_{12} are found in brewer's yeast, clams, eggs, herring, kidney, liver, mackerel, milk and dairy products, and seafood. Vitamin B_{12} is not found in many vegetables; it is available only from sea vegetables, such as dulse, kelp, kombu, and nori, and soybeans and soy products. It is also present in the herbs alfalfa, bladderwrack, and hops.

Comments

Anti-gout medications, anticoagulant drugs, and potassium supplements may block the absorption of vitamin B_{12} from the digestive tract. Taking vitamin B_{12} in sublingual tablets, which are dissolved under the tongue rather than swallowed, can be a good option for those who have difficulty absorbing this vitamin. *Intrinsic factor* is a protein produced in the gastrointestinal tract that is necessary for absorption of vitamin B_{12}. People who lack intrinsic factor must use a sublingual form for absorption.

Biotin

Biotin aids in cell growth; in fatty acid production; in the metabolism of carbohydrates, fats, and proteins; and in the utilization of the other B-complex vitamins. Sufficient quantities are needed for healthy hair and skin. One hundred milligrams of biotin daily may prevent hair loss in some men. Biotin also promotes healthy sweat glands, nerve tissue, and bone marrow. In addition, it helps to relieve muscle pain.

In infants, a condition called seborrheic dermatitis, or cradle cap, which is characterized by a dry, scaly scalp, may occur as a result of biotin deficiency. In adults, deficiency of this B vitamin is rare because it can be produced in the intestines from foods such as those mentioned below. However, if a deficiency does occur, it can cause anemia, depression, hair loss, high blood sugar, inflammation or pallor of the skin and mucous membranes, insomnia, loss of appetite, muscular pain, nausea, and soreness of the tongue.

Sources

Biotin is found in brewer's yeast, cooked egg yolks, meat, milk, poultry, saltwater fish, soybeans, and whole grains.

Comments

Raw egg whites contain a protein called avidin, which combines with biotin in the intestinal tract and depletes the body of this needed nutrient. Fats and oils that have been subjected to heat or exposed to the air for any length of time inhibit biotin absorption. Antibiotics, sulfa drugs, and saccharin also threaten the availability of biotin.

Choline

Choline is needed for the proper transmission of nerve impulses from the brain through the central nervous system, as well as for gallbladder regulation, liver function, and lecithin formation. It aids in hormone production and minimizes excess fat in the liver because it aids in fat and cholesterol metabolism. Without choline, brain function and memory are impaired. Choline is beneficial for disorders of the nervous system such as Parkinson's disease and tardive dyskinesia. A deficiency may result in fatty buildup in the liver, as well as in cardiac symptoms, gastric ulcers, high blood pressure, an inability to digest fats, kidney and liver impairment, and stunted growth. Research in the last decade indicates that choline plays an important role in cardiovascular health, as well as in reproduction and fetal development. One study showed a need for choline for both prevention and treatment of arteriosclerosis and the metabolism of homocysteine.

Sources

The following foods contain significant amounts of choline: egg yolks, lecithin (about 13 percent choline by weight), legumes, meat, milk, soybeans, and whole-grain cereals.

Folate

Also known as folacin, folic acid, or pteroylglutamic acid (PGA), folate is considered a brain food, and is needed for energy production and the formation of red blood cells. It also strengthens immunity by aiding in the proper formation and functioning of white blood cells. Because it functions as a coenzyme in DNA and RNA synthesis, it is important for healthy cell division and replication. It is involved in protein metabolism and has been used in the prevention and treatment of folic acid anemia. This nutrient may also help depression and anxiety, and may be effective in the treatment of uterine cervical dysplasia.

Folate may be the most important nutrient in regulating homocysteine levels. Homocysteine is an amino acid that is naturally formed in the body as the result of the breakdown of another amino acid, methionine. In recent years, high levels of homocysteine have been found to be associated with an increased risk of atherosclerosis (hardening of the arteries due to the accumulation of fatty plaques). Normally, homocysteine is converted to other, non-harmful amino acids in the body. In order for this conversion to take place as it should, the body needs an adequate supply of folate, as well as of vitamins B_6 and B_{12}. Homocysteine levels in red blood cells have been shown to have an inverse relationship to levels of these three important B vitamins—that is, the lower the levels of these vitamins, the higher the level of homocysteine.

Folate is very important in pregnancy. It helps to regulate embryonic and fetal nerve cell formation, which is vital for normal development. Studies have shown that a daily intake of 400 micrograms of folate in early pregnancy may prevent the vast majority of neural tube defects, such as spina bifida and anencephaly. It may also help to prevent premature birth. To be effective, this regimen must begin *before* conception and continue for at least the first three months of pregnancy; if a woman waits until she knows she is pregnant, it may be too late, because critical events in fetal development occur during the first six weeks of pregnancy—before many women know that they have conceived. This is why many experts recommend that every

woman of childbearing age take a folate supplement daily as a matter of course. Folate works best when combined with vitamin B_{12} and vitamin C.

A sore, red tongue is one sign of folate deficiency. Other possible signs include anemia, apathy, digestive disturbances, fatigue, graying hair, growth impairment, insomnia, labored breathing, memory problems, paranoia, weakness, and birth defects in one's offspring. Folate deficiency may be caused by inadequate consumption of fresh fruits and vegetables; consumption of only cooked or microwaved vegetables (cooking destroys folate); and malabsorption problems.

Sources

The following foods contain significant quantities of folate: asparagus, barley, beef, bran, brewer's yeast, brown rice, cheese, chicken, dates, green leafy vegetables, lamb, legumes, lentils, liver, milk, mushrooms, oranges, split peas, pork, root vegetables, salmon, tuna, wheat germ, whole grains, and whole wheat.

Comments

Oral contraceptives may increase the need for folate. Alcohol also can act as an enemy to folate absorption.

Cautions

Do not take high doses of folate for extended periods if you have a hormone-related cancer or seizure disorder.

Inositol

Inositol is vital for hair growth. This vitamin has a calming effect and helps to reduce cholesterol levels. It helps prevent hardening of the arteries and is important in the formation of lecithin and the metabolism of fat and cholesterol. It also helps remove fats from the liver. Deficiency can lead to arteriosclerosis, constipation, hair loss, high blood cholesterol, irritability, mood swings, and skin eruptions. Research has also shown that high doses of inositol may help in the treatment of depression, obsessive-compulsive disorder, and anxiety disorders, without the side effects of prescription medications.

Sources

Inositol is found in brewer's yeast, fruits, lecithin, legumes, meats, milk, unrefined molasses, raisins, vegetables, and whole grains.

Comments

The consumption of large amounts of caffeine may cause a shortage of inositol in the body.

Para-Aminobenzoic Acid (PABA)

PABA is one of the basic constituents of folate and also helps in the assimilation of pantothenic acid. PABA can be converted into folate by intestinal bacteria. This antioxidant helps protect against sunburn (through the absorption of ultraviolet-B [UVB] radiation) and, consequently, skin cancer; acts as a coenzyme in the breakdown and utilization of protein; and assists in the formation of red blood cells. PABA also aids in the maintenance of healthy intestinal flora. Supplementing the diet with PABA may restore gray hair to its original color if the graying was caused by stress or a nutritional deficiency. Other benefits of PABA include protection against secondhand smoke, ozone, and other air pollutants; reduced inflammation in arthritis; and enhanced flexibility.

A deficiency of PABA may lead to depression, fatigue, gastrointestinal disorders, graying of the hair, irritability, nervousness, and patchy areas of white skin.

Sources

Foods that contain PABA include kidney, liver, molasses, mushrooms, spinach, and whole grains.

Comments

Sulfa drugs may cause a deficiency of PABA.

Vitamin C (Ascorbic Acid)

Vitamin C is an antioxidant that is required for at least 300 metabolic functions in the body, including tissue growth and repair, adrenal gland function, and healthy gums. It also aids in the production of anti-stress hormones and interferon, an important immune-system protein, and is needed for the metabolism of folic acid, tyrosine, and phenylalanine. Studies have shown that taking vitamin C can reduce symptoms of asthma. It protects against the harmful effects of pollution, helps to prevent cancer, protects against infection, and enhances immunity. Vitamin C increases the absorption of iron. It can combine with toxic substances, such as certain heavy metals, and render them harmless so that they can be eliminated from the body. Even the venom of a black widow spider may be rendered harmless with the administration of very large doses of vitamin C. This vitamin also may reduce levels of low-density lipoproteins (LDL, the so-called "bad cholesterol"), while increasing levels of high-density lipoproteins (HDL, or "good cholesterol"), as well as lowering high blood pressure and helping to prevent atherosclerosis. Essential in the formation of collagen, vitamin C protects against abnormal blood clotting and bruising, may reduce the risk of cataracts, and promotes the healing of wounds and burns.

Vitamin C works synergistically with both vitamin E and beta-carotene—that is, when these vitamins work together, they have an effect even greater than the sum of their individual effects, and taking them together may counter potential adverse effects of taking these vitamins alone. Vitamin E scavenges for dangerous free radicals in cell membranes, while vitamin C attacks free radicals in biologic fluids. These vitamins reinforce and extend each other's antioxidant activity.

Because the body cannot manufacture vitamin C, it must be obtained through the diet or in the form of supplements. Unfortunately, most of the vitamin C consumed in the diet is lost in the urine. If larger amounts of vitamin C are required due to serious illness, such as cancer, it is more effective to take vitamin C intravenously, under the advisement and supervision of a physician, than it is to take high doses orally.

Scurvy is a disease caused by vitamin C deficiency. It is characterized by poor wound healing, soft and spongy bleeding gums, edema, extreme weakness, and "pinpoint" hemorrhages under the skin. Fortunately, this condition is rare in Western societies. More common are signs of lesser degrees of deficiency, including gums that bleed when brushed; increased susceptibility to infection, especially colds and bronchial infections; joint pains; lack of energy; poor digestion; prolonged wound healing time; a tendency to bruise easily; and tooth loss.

Sources

Vitamin C is found in berries, citrus fruits, and green vegetables. Good sources include asparagus, avocados, beet greens, black currants, broccoli, Brussels sprouts, cantaloupe, collards, dandelion greens, dulse, grapefruit, kale, lemons, mangos, mustard greens, onions, oranges, papayas, green peas, sweet peppers, persimmons, pineapple, radishes, rose hips, spinach, strawberries, Swiss chard, tomatoes, turnip greens, and watercress. Herbs that contain vitamin C include alfalfa, burdock root, cayenne, chickweed, eyebright, fennel seed, fenugreek, hops, horsetail, kelp, peppermint, mullein, nettle, oat straw, paprika, parsley, pine needle, plantain, raspberry leaf, red clover, rose hips, skullcap, violet leaves, yarrow, and yellow dock.

Comments

Alcohol, analgesics, antidepressants, anticoagulants, oral contraceptives, and steroids may reduce levels of vitamin C in the body. Smoking causes a serious depletion of vitamin C.

Diabetes medications such as chlorpropamide (Diabinese) and sulfa drugs may not be as effective if taken with vitamin C. Taking high doses of vitamin C may cause a false-negative reading in tests for blood in the stool.

For maximum effectiveness, supplemental vitamin C should be taken in divided doses, twice daily. Esterified vitamin C (Ester-C) is a remarkably effective form of vitamin C, especially for those suffering from chronic illnesses such as cancer and AIDS. It is created by having the vitamin C react with a necessary mineral, such as calcium, magnesium, potassium, sodium, or zinc. This results in a form of the vitamin that is nonacidic and that contains vitamin C metabolites identical to those produced by the body. Esterified vitamin C enters the bloodstream and tissues four times faster than standard forms of vitamin C because it moves into the blood cells more efficiently and also stays in the body tissues longer. The levels of vitamin C in white blood cells achieved by taking esterified vitamin C are four times higher than those achieved with standard vitamin C. Further, only one-third as much is lost through excretion in the urine. A variety of manufacturers produce supplements containing Ester-C, either by itself or in combination with other valuable nutrients, including the antioxidants Pycnogenol and proanthocyanidins, and the herbs echinacea and garlic.

Cautions

If aspirin and standard vitamin C (ascorbic acid) are taken together in large doses, stomach irritation can occur, possibly leading to ulcers. If you take aspirin regularly, use an esterified form of vitamin C, and take it separately from the aspirin.

If you are pregnant, do not take more than 5,000 milligrams of vitamin C daily. A developing infant may become dependent on this supplement and develop scurvy when deprived of the accustomed megadoses after birth.

Avoid using chewable vitamin C supplements, as these can damage tooth enamel.

Vitamin D

Vitamin D, a fat-soluble vitamin that has properties of both a vitamin and a hormone, is required for the absorption and utilization of calcium and phosphorus. It is necessary for growth, and is especially important for the normal growth and development of bones and teeth in children. It protects against muscle weakness and is involved in regulation of the heartbeat. It is also important in the prevention and treatment of breast and colon cancer, osteoarthritis, osteoporosis, and hypocalcemia, enhances immunity, and is necessary for thyroid function and normal blood clotting.

There are several forms of vitamin D, including vitamin D_2 (ergocaliciferol), which comes from food sources; vitamin D_3 (cholecalciferol), which is synthesized in the skin in response to exposure to the sun's ultraviolet rays; and a synthetic form identified as vitamin D_5. Of the three, vitamin D_3 is considered the natural form of vitamin D and is the most active.

The form of vitamin D that we get from food or supplements is not fully active. It requires conversion by the liver, and then by the kidneys, before it becomes fully active. This is why people with liver or kidney disorders are at a higher risk for osteoporosis. When the skin is exposed to the sun's ultraviolet rays, a cholesterol compound in the skin is transformed into a precursor of vitamin D. Exposing the face and arms to the sun for fifteen minutes three times a week is an effective way to ensure adequate amounts of vitamin D in the body. However, researchers have learned that people living in the upper third of the continental United States cannot produce adequate amounts of vitamin D from exposure to the limited available sunlight during the winter months.

Severe deficiency of vitamin D can cause rickets in children and osteomalacia, a similar disorder, in adults. Lesser degrees of deficiency may be characterized by loss of appetite, a burning sensation in the mouth and throat, diarrhea, insomnia, visual problems, and weight loss. In a study reported in *The New England Journal of Medicine,* there are indications that vitamin D deficiency is much more widespread than previously thought, especially in older adults. In a group of people of whom few had risk factors for vitamin D deficiency, 57 percent were found to have below-normal levels of vitamin D. Sixty-seven percent of those reporting a vitamin D intake below the RDI had deficiencies categorized as moderate to severe.

Sources

Fish liver oils, fatty saltwater fish, dairy products, and eggs all contain vitamin D. It is found in butter, cod liver oil, dandelion greens, egg yolks, halibut, liver, milk, oatmeal, salmon, sardines, sweet potatoes, tuna, and vegetable oils. Vitamin D is also formed by the body in response to the action of sunlight on the skin. Herbs that contain vitamin D include alfalfa, horsetail, nettle, and parsley.

Comments

Intestinal disorders and liver and gallbladder malfunctions interfere with the absorption of vitamin D. Some cholesterol-lowering drugs, antacids, mineral oil, and steroid hormones such as cortisone also interfere with absorption. Thiazide diuretics such as chlorothiazide (Diuril) and hydrochlorothiazide (Esidrix, HydroDIURIL, Oretic) disturb the body's calcium/vitamin D ratio. Taking excessive amounts of vitamin D (over 1,000 international units) daily may cause a decrease in bone mass.

Cautions

Do not take vitamin D without calcium. Toxicity may result from taking excessive amounts of supplemental vitamin D.

Vitamin E

Vitamin E is an antioxidant that is important in the prevention of cancer and cardiovascular disease. It improves circulation, is necessary for tissue repair, and is useful in treating premenstrual syndrome and fibrocystic disease of the breast. It promotes normal blood clotting and healing, reduces scarring from some wounds, reduces blood pressure, aids in preventing cataracts, improves athletic performance, and relaxes leg cramps. Vitamin E can enhance sperm production in some men. It also maintains healthy nerves and muscles while strengthening capillary walls. In addition, it promotes healthy skin and hair, and helps to prevent anemia and retrolental fibroplasia, an eye disorder that can affect premature infants. A 1998 study by the National Cancer Institute found that long-term use of vitamin E substantially reduced prostate cancer risk in smokers. Other studies suggest that this vitamin may slow the progression of Alzheimer's disease. Thus far, vitamin E has been shown to protect against approximately eighty diseases.

As an antioxidant, vitamin E prevents cell damage by inhibiting the oxidation of lipids (fats) and the formation of free radicals. It protects other fat-soluble vitamins from destruction by oxygen and aids in the utilization of vitamin A. It retards aging and may prevent age spots as well. Some studies have shown daily use of vitamin E to be more protective than aspirin for prevention of heart attacks, with no harmful side effects. The misuse of aspirin, in contrast, causes or contributes to an estimated 3,000 deaths in the United States each year.

Vitamin E deficiency may result in damage to red blood cells and destruction of nerves. Signs of deficiency can include infertility (in both men and women), menstrual problems, neuromuscular impairment, shortened red blood cell lifespan, spontaneous abortion (miscarriage), and uterine degeneration. Low levels of vitamin E in the body have been linked to both bowel cancer and breast cancer. Epidemiological links have been identified between the increase in the incidence of heart disease and the increasing lack of vitamin E in the American diet due to our reliance on overprocessed foods.

Vitamin E is actually a family of eight different but related molecules that fall into two major groups: the tocopherols and the tocotrienols. Within each group, there are alpha, beta, gamma, and delta forms. Of all eight of these molecules, it is the d-alpha-tocopherol form that is the most potent. Natural sources of vitamin E are better than synthetic vitamin E because natural vitamin E is more available for use by the body than the synthetic form. Synthetic vitamin E is only 67 percent as active as the natural form. Read labels closely. The natural form of vitamin E is listed as *d-alpha-tocopherol*; the synthetic form is listed as *dl-alpha-tocopherol* (watch out for the *l* after the *d*). The *dl* form costs only about half as much as the *d* form, but it has significantly less activity, or potency.

Sources

Vitamin E is found in the following food sources: cold-pressed vegetable oils, dark green leafy vegetables, legumes, nuts, seeds, and whole grains. Significant quanti-

ties of this vitamin are also found in brown rice, cornmeal, dulse, eggs, kelp, desiccated liver, milk, oatmeal, organ meats, soybeans, sweet potatoes, watercress, wheat, and wheat germ. Herbs that contain vitamin E include alfalfa, bladderwrack, dandelion, dong quai, flaxseed, nettle, oat straw, raspberry leaf, and rose hips.

Comments

The body needs zinc in order to maintain the proper level of vitamin E in the blood. Vitamin E that has oxidized a free radical can be revitalized by vitamin C and enabled to battle additional free radicals, according to Lester Packer, Ph.D., noted researcher and professor of molecular and cell biology at the University of California—Berkeley. Adding vitamin E to fats and oils prevents them from becoming rancid. The oxidation of fats is a key factor in the formation of plaque adhering to blood vessel walls.

If you take both vitamin E and iron supplements, take them at different times of the day. Inorganic forms of iron (such as ferrous sulfate) destroy vitamin E. Organic iron (ferrous gluconate or ferrous fumarate) leaves vitamin E intact.

Cautions

If you are taking an anticoagulant medication (blood thinner), do not take more than 1,200 international units of vitamin E daily. If you suffer from diabetes, rheumatic heart disease, or an overactive thyroid, do not take more than the recommended dose. If you have high blood pressure, start with a small amount, such as 200 international units daily, and increase slowly to the desired amount.

Vitamin K

Vitamin K is needed for the production of prothrombin, which is necessary for blood clotting. It is also essential for bone formation and repair; it is necessary for the synthesis of osteocalcin, the protein in bone tissue on which calcium crystallizes. Consequently, it may help prevent osteoporosis.

Vitamin K plays an important role in the intestines and aids in converting glucose into glycogen for storage in the liver, promoting healthy liver function. It may increase resistance to infection in children and help prevent cancers that target the inner linings of the organs. It aids in promoting longevity. A deficiency of this vitamin can cause abnormal and/or internal bleeding.

There are three forms of vitamin K: vitamin K_1 (phylloquinone or phytonactone), which comes from plants; vitamin K_2, a family of substances called menaquinones, which are made by intestinal bacteria; and vitamin K_3 (menadione), which is a synthetic substance.

Sources

Vitamin K is found in some foods, including asparagus,

blackstrap molasses, broccoli, Brussels sprouts, cabbage, cauliflower, dark green leafy vegetables, egg yolks, leaf lettuce, liver, oatmeal, oats, rye, safflower oil, soybeans, wheat, and yogurt. Herbs that can supply vitamin K include alfalfa, green tea, kelp, nettle, oat straw, and shepherd's purse. However, the majority of the body's supply of this vitamin is synthesized by the "friendly" bacteria normally present in the intestines.

Comments

Antibiotics increase the need for dietary or supplemental vitamin K. Because vitamin K is synthesized by bacteria in the intestines, taking antibiotics—which kill the bacteria—interferes with this process. Antibiotics also interfere with the absorption of vitamin K.

Cautions

Do not take large doses of synthetic vitamin K during the last few weeks of pregnancy. It can result in a toxic reaction in the newborn. If you are taking anticoagulant (blood thinning) drugs, consult with your health care provider before taking any supplemental vitamin K, as it can interfere with the action of these medications. Megadoses of this vitamin can accumulate in the body and cause flushing and sweating.

Bioflavonoids

Although bioflavonoids are not true vitamins in the strictest sense, they are sometimes referred to as vitamin P. Bioflavonoids are essential for the absorption of vitamin C, and the two should be taken together. There are many different bioflavonoids, including citrin, eriodictyol, flavones, hesperetin, hesperidin, quercetin, quercetrin, and rutin. The human body cannot produce bioflavonoids, so they must be supplied in the diet.

Bioflavonoids are used extensively in the treatment of athletic injuries because they relieve pain, bumps, and bruises. They also reduce pain located in the legs or across the back, and lessen symptoms associated with prolonged bleeding and low serum calcium. Bioflavonoids act synergistically with vitamin C to protect and preserve the structure of capillaries. In addition, bioflavonoids have an antibacterial effect and promote circulation, stimulate bile production, lower cholesterol levels, and treat and prevent cataracts. When taken with vitamin C, bioflavonoids also reduce the symptoms of oral herpes.

Quercetin, a bioflavonoid available in supplement form, may effectively treat and prevent asthma symptoms. Activated Quercetin from Source Naturals is a good source of quercetin. It also contains two other ingredients that increase its efficacy: bromelain, an enzyme from pineapple, and vitamin C, in the nonacidic form of magnesium ascorbate. Bromelain and quercetin are synergists, and should be taken in conjunction to enhance absorption.

Sources

Peppers, buckwheat, black currants, and the white material just beneath the peel of citrus fruits contain bioflavonoids. Sources of bioflavonoids include apricots, blackberries, cherries, grapefruit, grapes, lemons, oranges, plums, prunes, and rose hips. Herbs that contain bioflavonoids include chervil, elderberries, hawthorn berry, horsetail, rose hips, and shepherd's purse.

Comments

Extremely high doses may cause diarrhea.

Coenzyme Q$_{10}$

Coenzyme Q$_{10}$ is a vitamin-like substance found in all parts of the body whose actions resemble those of vitamin E. It may be an even more powerful antioxidant. It is also called ubiquinone. There are ten common substances designated coenzyme Qs, but coenzyme Q$_{10}$ is the only one found in human tissue. This substance plays a critical role in the production of energy in every cell of the body. It aids circulation, stimulates the immune system, increases tissue oxygenation, and has vital anti-aging effects. Deficiencies of coenzyme Q$_{10}$ have been linked to periodontal disease, diabetes, and muscular dystrophy.

Research has revealed that supplemental coenzyme Q$_{10}$ has the ability to counter histamine, and therefore is beneficial for people with allergies, asthma, or respiratory disease. It is used by many health care professionals to treat anomalies of mental function such as those associated with schizophrenia and Alzheimer's disease. It is also beneficial in fighting obesity, candidiasis, multiple sclerosis, and diabetes.

Coenzyme Q$_{10}$ appears to be a giant step forward in the treatment and prevention of cardiovascular disease. A six-year study conducted by scientists at the University of Texas found that people being treated for congestive heart failure who took coenzyme Q$_{10}$ in addition to conventional therapy had a 75-percent chance of survival after three years, compared with a 25-percent survival rate for those using conventional therapy alone. In a similar study by the University of Texas and the Center for Adult Diseases in Japan, coenzyme Q$_{10}$ was shown to be able to lower high blood pressure without medication or dietary changes.

In addition to its use in fighting cardiovascular disease, coenzyme Q$_{10}$ has been shown to be effective in reducing mortality in experimental animals afflicted with tumors and leukemia. Some doctors give their patients coenzyme Q$_{10}$ to reduce the side effects of cancer chemotherapy.

Coenzyme Q$_{10}$ is widely used in Japan. More than 12 million people in that country are reportedly taking it at the direction of their physicians for treatment of heart disease (it strengthens the heart muscle) and high blood pressure, and also to enhance the immune system. Research in

Japan has shown that coenzyme Q_{10} also protects the stomach lining and duodenum, and may help heal duodenal ulcers.

The amount of coenzyme Q_{10} present in the body declines with age, so it should be supplemented in the diet, especially by people who are over the age of fifty. A sublingual form containing 50 milligrams of this vital nutrient, available from FoodScience Laboratories, is an especially easy to assimilate supplement. Nature's Plus and Carlson Labs both make soft gel-capsules of coenzyme Q_{10} in dosage levels up to 100 milligrams. Oil-based forms are best.

Sources

Mackerel, salmon, and sardines contain the largest amounts of coenzyme Q_{10}. It is also found in beef, peanuts, and spinach.

Comments

Coenzyme Q_{10} is oil soluble and is best absorbed when taken with oily or fatty foods, such as fish. Be cautious when purchasing coenzyme Q_{10}. Not all products offer it in its purest form. Its natural color is dark bright yellow to orange, and it has very little taste in the powdered form. It should be kept away from heat and light. Pure coenzyme Q_{10} is perishable and deteriorates in temperatures above 115 °F. A liquid or oil form is preferable. Look for a product that includes a small amount of vitamin E, as this helps to preserve the coenzyme Q_{10}.

MINERALS

INTRODUCTION

Every living cell on this planet depends on minerals for proper function and structure. Minerals are needed for the proper composition of body fluids, the formation of blood and bone, the maintenance of healthy nerve function, and the regulation of muscle tone, including that of the muscles of the cardiovascular system. Like vitamins, minerals function as coenzymes, enabling the body to perform its functions, including energy production, growth, and healing. Because all enzyme activities involve minerals, minerals are essential for the proper utilization of vitamins and other nutrients.

The human body, as all of nature, must maintain its proper chemical balance. This balance depends on the levels of different minerals in the body and especially the ratios of certain mineral levels to one another. The level of each mineral in the body has an effect on every other, so if one is out of balance, all mineral levels are affected. If not corrected, this can start a chain reaction of imbalances that leads to illness.

Minerals are naturally occurring elements found in the earth. Rock formations are made up of mineral salts. Rock and stone are gradually broken down into tiny fragments by erosion, a process that can take literally millions of years. The resulting dust and sand accumulate, forming the basis of soil. The soil is teeming with microbes that utilize these tiny crystals of mineral salts, which are then passed from the soil to plants. The plants are eaten by herbivorous animals. We obtain these minerals by consuming plants or herbivorous animals.

Nutritionally, minerals belong to two groups: bulk minerals (also called macrominerals) and trace minerals (microminerals). Bulk minerals include calcium, magnesium, sodium, potassium, and phosphorus. These are needed in larger amounts than trace minerals. Although only minute quantities of trace minerals are needed, they are nevertheless important for good health. Trace minerals include boron, chromium, copper, germanium, iodine, iron, manganese, molybdenum, selenium, silicon, sulfur, vanadium, and zinc.

Because minerals are stored primarily in the body's bone and muscle tissue, it is possible to develop mineral toxicity if extremely large quantities are consumed. Such situations are rare, however, because toxic levels of minerals generally accumulate only if massive amounts are ingested for a prolonged period of time.

WHAT'S ON THE SHELVES

As with vitamins, it can be difficult, if not impossible, to obtain the amounts of minerals needed for optimum health through diet alone. Mineral supplements can help you to make sure you are getting all the minerals your body requires.

Minerals are often found in multivitamin formulas. Minerals can also be sold as single supplements. These are available in tablet, capsule, powder, and liquid forms. Some are available in chelated form, which means that the minerals are bonded to protein molecules that transport them to the bloodstream and enhance their absorption. When mineral supplements are taken with a meal, they are usually automatically chelated in the stomach during digestion. There is some controversy over which mineral supplements are best, but we prefer the chelated preparations. Our experience with the various chelated formulas available has shown that, in general, arginate forms of minerals make the most effective supplements.

Once a mineral is absorbed, it must be carried by the blood to the cells and then transported across the cell membranes in a form that can be utilized by the cells. After minerals enter the body, they compete with one another for absorption. For example, too much zinc can deplete the body of copper; excessive calcium intake can affect magnesium absorption. Consequently, supplemental minerals should always be taken in balanced amounts. Otherwise, they will not be effective and may even be harmful. The absorption of minerals can also be affected by the use of fiber supplements. Fiber decreases the body's absorption of minerals. Therefore, supplemental fiber and minerals should be taken at different times.

THE ABC'S OF MINERALS

Boron

Boron is needed in trace amounts for healthy bones and muscle growth because it assists in the production of natural steroid compounds within the body. It is also necessary for the metabolism of calcium, phosphorus, and magnesium. It enhances brain function, promotes alertness, and plays a role in how the body utilizes energy from fats and sugars. Most people are not deficient in boron. However, elderly people usually benefit from taking a supplement of 2 to 3 milligrams daily because they have greater problems with calcium absorption. Boron deficiency accentuates vitamin D deficiency.

Boron helps to prevent postmenopausal osteoporosis and build muscle. A study conducted by the U.S. Department of Agriculture indicated that within eight days of supplementing their daily diet with 3 milligrams of boron, a test group of postmenopausal women lost 40 percent less calcium, one-third less magnesium, and slightly less phosphorus through their urine than they had before beginning boron supplementation.

Sources

Boron is found in apples, carrots, grapes, dark green leafy vegetables, raw nuts, pears, and whole grains.

Cautions

Do not take more than 3 to 6 milligrams unless prescribed.

Calcium

Calcium is vital for the formation of strong bones and teeth and for the maintenance of healthy gums. It is also important in the maintenance of a regular heartbeat and in the transmission of nerve impulses. Calcium lowers cholesterol levels and helps prevent cardiovascular disease. It is needed for muscular growth and contraction, and for the prevention of muscle cramps. It may increase the rate of bone growth and bone mineral density in children. This important mineral is also essential in blood clotting and helps prevent cancer. It may lower blood pressure and prevent bone loss associated with osteoporosis as well. Calcium provides energy and participates in the protein structuring of RNA and DNA. It is also involved in the activation of several enzymes, including lipase, which breaks down fats for utilization by the body. In addition, calcium maintains proper cell membrane permeability, aids in neuromuscular activity, helps to keep the skin healthy, and protects against the development of preeclampsia during pregnancy, the number one cause of maternal death. If high blood pressure develops due to pregnancy, it can be reduced by calcium intake.

Calcium protects the bones and teeth from lead by inhibiting absorption of this toxic metal. If there is a calcium deficiency, lead can be absorbed by the body and deposited in the teeth and bones.

Calcium deficiency can lead to the following problems: aching joints, brittle nails, eczema, elevated blood cholesterol, heart palpitations, hypertension (high blood pressure), insomnia, muscle cramps, nervousness, numbness in the arms and/or legs, a pasty complexion, rheumatoid arthritis, rickets, and tooth decay. Deficiencies of calcium are also associated with cognitive impairment, convulsions, depression, delusions, and hyperactivity.

Sources

Calcium is found in dairy foods, salmon (with bones), sardines, seafood, and dark green leafy vegetables. Food sources include almonds, asparagus, blackstrap molasses, brewer's yeast, broccoli, buttermilk, cabbage, carob, cheese, collards, dandelion greens, dulse, figs, filberts, goat's milk, kale, kelp, milk, mustard greens, oats, prunes, sesame seeds, soybeans, tofu, turnip greens, watercress, whey, and yogurt. Herbs that contain calcium include alfalfa, burdock root, cayenne, chamomile, chickweed, chicory, dandelion, eyebright, fennel seed, fenugreek, flaxseed, hops, horsetail, kelp, lemongrass, mullein, nettle, oat straw, paprika, parsley, peppermint, plantain, raspberry leaves, red clover, rose hips, shepherd's purse, violet leaves, yarrow, and yellow dock.

Comments

The amino acid lysine is needed for calcium absorption. Food sources of lysine include cheese, eggs, fish, lima beans, milk, potatoes, red meat, soy products, and brewer's yeast. Lysine is also available in supplement form.

Female athletes and menopausal women need greater amounts of calcium than other women because their estrogen levels are lower. Estrogen protects the skeletal system by promoting the deposition of calcium in bone.

Heavy exercising hinders calcium uptake, but moderate exercise promotes it. Insufficient vitamin D intake, or the ingestion of excessive amounts of phosphorus and magnesium, also hinders the uptake of calcium.

If calcium is taken with iron, they bind together, preventing the optimal absorption of both minerals. It is therefore best to take calcium and iron at different times. Too much calcium can interfere with the absorption of zinc, and excess zinc can interfere with calcium absorption (especially if calcium intake is low). For most people, the best ratio between supplemental calcium and zinc is up to 2,500 milligrams of calcium with 50 milligrams of zinc daily. A hair analysis can determine the levels of these and other minerals in the body.

A diet that is high in protein, fat, and/or sugar affects calcium uptake. The average American diet of meats, refined grains, and soft drinks (which are high in phosphorus) leads to increased excretion of calcium. Consuming alcoholic beverages, coffee, junk foods, excess salt, and/or white flour also leads to the loss of calcium by the body. A diet based on foods such as vegetables, fruits, and whole grains, which contain significant amounts of calcium but lower amounts of phosphorus, is preferable.

Oxalic acid (found in almonds, beet greens, cashews, chard, cocoa, rhubarb, soybeans, and spinach) interferes with calcium absorption by binding with it in the intestines and producing insoluble salts that cannot be absorbed. The normal consumption of foods containing oxalic acid should not pose a problem, but overindulgence in these foods inhibits the absorption of calcium. Oxalic acid can also combine with calcium to form calcium-oxalate kidney stones. Studies have shown, however, that taking magnesium and potassium supplements can prevent the formation of this type of stone.

Calcium supplements are more effective when taken in smaller doses spread throughout the day and before bedtime. This mineral works less effectively when taken in a single megadose. Most experts agree that no more than 500 milligrams should be taken at one time, as this is the maximum amount the body can absorb in one dose. However, because calcium also promotes a sound sleep when taken at night, and because a high-fiber diet can interfere with calcium absorption, some recommend taking a single dose at bedtime.

Some vitamin companies use a compound called D_1-calcium-phosphate in their products. This form of calcium is insoluble and interferes with the absorption of the nutrients in a multinutrient supplement. Antacids such as Tums are not recommended as a source of calcium. While they do contain calcium, if taken in sufficient quantities to serve as a source of this mineral, they would also neutralize the stomach acid needed for calcium absorption. Additionally, a significant percentage (estimates range from 20 to 40 percent) of people over the age of sixty may have a condition called atrophic gastritis. This is a chronic inflammation of the stomach, and it reduces the ability to break down the calcium carbonate contained in Tums.

Calcium Absorption Formula from A. Vogel Homeopathic is a sublingual calcium supplement that is especially effective for growing children, older adults, pregnant women, and anyone who has difficulty swallowing pills.

Cautions

Calcium may interfere with the effects of verapamil (Calan, Isoptin, Verelan), a calcium channel blocker sometimes prescribed for heart problems and high blood pressure. Calcium can also interfere with the effectiveness of tetracycline, thyroid hormone, certain anticonvulsants, and steroids. Consult your health care provider before taking supplemental calcium if you must take any of these drugs.

Phenobarbital and diuretics may cause a deficiency of calcium. Although several major studies have shown that added calcium in the diet does not appear to increase the risk for either a first or repeat attack of kidney stones, persons with a history of kidney stones or kidney disease should not take calcium supplements except on the advice of a physician. The maximum safe dosage of supplemental calcium is now placed at 2,500 milligrams per day.

Chromium

Because it is involved in the metabolism of glucose, chromium (sometimes also called glucose tolerance factor or GTF) is needed for energy. It is also vital in the synthesis of cholesterol, fats, and proteins. This essential mineral maintains stable blood sugar levels through proper insulin utilization, and can be helpful both for people with diabetes and those with hypoglycemia. Studies have shown that low plasma chromium levels can be an indication of coronary artery disease. Additional chromium is needed during pregnancy because the developing fetus increases demand for this mineral. Chromium supplements can help an expectant mother maintain healthy blood sugar levels during pregnancy.

The average American diet is chromium deficient. Only one in ten Americans has an adequate amount of chromium in his or her diet. There are five main reasons for this: The form of chromium in many foods is not easily absorbed; not enough foods containing chromium are consumed; much of the chromium content is lost during processing; many people do not like the foods that are the best sources of chromium; and high quantities of sugar in the diet cause a loss of chromium from the body. Researchers estimate that two out of every three Americans are hypoglycemic, prehypoglycemic, or diabetic. The ability to maintain normal blood sugar levels is jeopardized by the lack of chromium in our soil and water supply and by a diet high in refined white sugar, flour, and junk foods.

A deficiency of chromium can lead to anxiety, fatigue, glucose intolerance (particularly in people with diabetes), inadequate metabolism of amino acids, and an increased risk of arteriosclerosis. Excessive intake (the level depends upon individual tolerance) can lead to chromium toxicity, which has been associated with dermatitis, gastrointestinal ulcers, and kidney and liver impairment.

Supplemental chromium is best absorbed by the body when it is taken in a form called *chromium picolinate* (chromium chelated with picolinate, a naturally occurring amino acid metabolite). Picolinate enables chromium to readily enter into the body's cells, where the mineral can then help insulin do its job much more effectively. Chromium picolinate has been used successfully to control blood cholesterol and blood glucose levels. It also promotes the loss of fat and an increase in lean muscle tissue. Studies show it may increase longevity and help to fight osteoporosis. Chromium polynicotinate (chromium bonded to niacin) is an effective form of this mineral as well.

Sources

Chromium is found in the following food sources: beer, brewer's yeast, brown rice, cheese, meat, and whole grains. It may also be found in dried beans, blackstrap molasses, calf liver, chicken, corn and corn oil, dairy products, dried liver, dulse, eggs, mushrooms, and potatoes. Herbs that contain chromium include catnip, horsetail, licorice, nettle, oat straw, red clover, sarsaparilla, wild yam, and yarrow.

Comments

Active, athletic individuals—people who engage in vigorous aerobic activities and consume higher amounts of carbohydrates than the general population—have higher chromium requirements than nonathletes. Chromium levels start to decrease as we age, starting in our early forties. Some smaller studies have confirmed that added chromium in the diet can reduce total body fat and increase the percentage of muscle.

Cautions

If you have insulin-dependent diabetes, you should not use chromium unless it is prescribed by your health care practioner. Chromium supplements can make insulin function more effectively and, in effect, reduce insulin requirements. People with diabetes therefore have to monitor their blood sugar levels very carefully when using chromium. Chromium requirements differ from person to person; consult your health care provider to determine the correct amount of this mineral for you.

Some people experience lightheadedness or a slight skin rash when taking chromium. If you feel lightheaded, stop taking the supplement and consult your health care provider. If you develop a rash, either try switching brands or discontinue use.

Copper

Among its many functions, copper aids in the formation of bone, hemoglobin, and red blood cells, and works in balance with zinc and vitamin C to form elastin, an important skin protein. It is involved in the healing process, energy production, hair and skin coloring, and taste sensitivity. This mineral is also needed for healthy nerves and joints.

One of the early signs of copper deficiency is osteoporosis. Copper is essential for the formation of collagen, one of the fundamental proteins making up bones, skin, and connective tissue. Other possible signs of copper deficiency include anemia, baldness, diarrhea, general weakness, impaired respiratory function, and skin sores. A lack of copper can also lead to increased blood fat levels. (*See* COPPER DEFICIENCY in Part Two.)

Excessive intake of copper can lead to toxicity, which has been associated with depression, irritability, nausea and vomiting, nervousness, and joint and muscle pain. Ingesting a quantity as small as 10 milligrams usually causes nausea. Sixty milligrams generally results in vomiting, and just 3.5 grams (3,500 milligrams) can be fatal. Children can be affected at much smaller dosage levels. (*See* COPPER TOXICITY in Part Two.)

Sources

Besides its use in cookware and plumbing, copper is also widely distributed in foods. Food sources include almonds, avocados, barley, beans, beets, blackstrap molasses, broccoli, garlic, lentils, liver, mushrooms, nuts, oats, oranges,

pecans, radishes, raisins, salmon, seafood, soybeans, and green leafy vegetables.

Comments

The level of copper in the body is related to the levels of zinc and vitamin C. Copper levels are reduced if large amounts of zinc or vitamin C are consumed. If copper intake is too high, levels of vitamin C and zinc drop.

The consumption of high amounts of fructose (fruit sugar) can make a copper deficiency significantly worse. In a study conducted by the U.S. Department of Agriculture, people who obtained 20 percent of their daily calories from fructose showed decreased levels of red blood cell superoxide dismutase (SOD), a copper-dependent enzyme critical to antioxidant protection within the red blood cells.

Cautions

Excessive copper in the body can promote destruction of eye tissue through oxidation. Persons with eye problems should be especially careful to balance their intake of copper with that of iron, zinc, and calcium.

Germanium

Germanium improves cellular oxygenation. This helps to fight pain, keep the immune system functioning properly, and rid the body of toxins and poisons. Researchers have shown that consuming foods containing organic germanium is an effective way to increase tissue oxygenation, because, like hemoglobin, germanium acts as a carrier of oxygen to the cells. A Japanese scientist, Kazuhiko Asai, found that an intake of 100 to 300 milligrams of germanium per day improved many illnesses, including rheumatoid arthritis, food allergies, elevated cholesterol, candidiasis, chronic viral infections, cancer, and AIDS.

Sources

Germanium is found in all organic material, of both plant and animal origin. The following foods contain the greatest concentrations of germanium: broccoli, celery, garlic, shiitake mushrooms, milk, onions, rhubarb, sauerkraut, tomato juice, and the herbs aloe vera, comfrey, ginseng, and suma.

Comments

Germanium is best obtained through the diet.

Cautions

Although it is rare, some individuals may develop kidney problems or have a toxic reaction to this mineral if they take it in excessive amounts.

Iodine

Needed only in trace amounts, iodine helps to metabolize excess fat and is important for physical and mental development. It is also needed for a healthy thyroid gland and for the prevention of goiter. Iodine deficiency in children may result in mental retardation. In addition, iodine deficiency has been linked to breast cancer and is associated with fatigue, neonatal hypothyroidism, and weight gain. Excessive iodine intake (sometimes as little as 750 micrograms daily) may inhibit the secretion of thyroid hormone and can produce a metallic taste and sores in the mouth, swollen salivary glands, diarrhea, and vomiting.

Sources

Foods that are high in iodine include dairy products (from cattle fed iodine-supplemented feed and salt licks), iodized salt, seafood, saltwater fish, and kelp. It may also be found in asparagus, dulse, garlic, lima beans, mushrooms, sea salt (which provides nature's own balance of minerals), sesame seeds, soybeans, spinach (but *see* Comments, below), summer squash, Swiss chard, and turnip greens.

Comments

Some foods block the uptake of iodine into the thyroid gland when eaten raw in large amounts. These include Brussels sprouts, cabbage, cauliflower, kale, peaches, pears, spinach, and turnips. If you have an underactive thyroid, you should limit your consumption of these foods.

Iron

Perhaps the most important of iron's functions in the body is the production of hemoglobin and myoglobin (the form of hemoglobin found in muscle tissue), and the oxygenation of red blood cells. Iron is the mineral found in the largest amounts in the blood. It is essential for many enzymes, including catalase, and is important for growth. Iron is also required for a healthy immune system and for energy production.

Iron deficiency is most often caused by insufficient intake. However, it may result from intestinal bleeding, a diet high in phosphorus, poor digestion, long-term illness, ulcers, prolonged use of antacids, excessive coffee or tea consumption, and other causes. Menstruating women may become iron deficient, especially if they have heavy or prolonged periods and/or short menstrual cycles. In some cases, a deficiency of vitamin B_6 (pyridoxine) or vitamin B_{12} can be the underlying cause of anemia. Strenuous exercise and heavy perspiration deplete iron from the body.

Iron deficiency symptoms include anemia, brittle hair, difficulty swallowing, digestive disturbances, dizziness, fatigue, fragile bones, hair loss, inflammation of the tissues of the mouth, nails that are spoon-shaped or that have ridges running lengthwise, nervousness, obesity, pallor, and slowed mental reactions.

Because iron is stored in the body, excessive iron intake can also cause problems. Too much iron in the tissues and organs leads to the production of free radicals and increases the need for vitamin E. High levels of iron have also been found in association with heart disease and cancer. The buildup of iron in the tissues has been associated with a rare disease known as hemochromatosis, a hereditary disorder of iron metabolism that is found mostly in men and that causes excessive absorption of iron from both foods and supplements, leading to bronze skin pigmentation, arthritis, cirrhosis of the liver, diabetes, and heart disorders.

Sources

Iron is found in eggs, fish, liver, meat, poultry, green leafy vegetables, whole grains, and enriched breads and cereals. Other food sources include almonds, avocados, beets, blackstrap molasses, brewer's yeast, dates, dulse, kelp, kidney and lima beans, lentils, millet, peaches, pears, dried prunes, pumpkins, raisins, rice and wheat bran, sesame seeds, soybeans, and watercress. Herbs that contain iron include alfalfa, burdock root, catnip, cayenne, chamomile, chickweed, chicory, dandelion, dong quai, eyebright, fennel seed, fenugreek, horsetail, kelp, lemongrass, licorice, milk thistle seed, mullein, nettle, oat straw, paprika, parsley, peppermint, plantain, raspberry leaf, rose hips, sarsaparilla, shepherd's purse, uva ursi, and yellow dock.

Comments

Unless you are diagnosed as anemic, you should not take iron supplements. If you take a multivitamin and mineral supplement, choose a product that does not contain iron. If you do need to take iron supplements, do not take them at the same time as vitamin E, and choose an organic form of iron such as ferrous gluconate or ferrous fumarate. Inorganic forms of iron, such as ferrous sulfate, can oxidize vitamin E.

There must be sufficient hydrochloric acid (HCl) present in the stomach in order for iron to be absorbed. Copper, manganese, molybdenum, vitamin A, and the B-complex vitamins are also needed for complete iron absorption. Taking vitamin C can increase iron absorption by as much as 30 percent.

Taking calcium with meals can inhibit the absorption of iron from dietary sources. If you are iron deficient, take calcium supplements at bedtime or at other times when you are not consuming foods containing iron. Excessive amounts of zinc and vitamin E can also interfere with iron absorption. The utilization of iron may be impaired by rheumatoid arthritis and cancer. These diseases can result in anemia despite adequate amounts of iron stored in the liver, spleen, and bone marrow. Iron deficiency is more prevalent in people with candidiasis or chronic herpes infections.

Cautions

Do not take iron supplements if you have an infection. Because bacteria require iron for growth, the body "hides" iron in the liver and other storage sites when an infection is present. Taking extra iron at such times encourages the proliferation of bacteria in the body.

Magnesium

Magnesium is a vital catalyst in enzyme activity, especially the activity of those enzymes involved in energy production. It also assists in calcium and potassium uptake. A deficiency of magnesium interferes with the transmission of nerve and muscle impulses, causing irritability and nervousness. Supplementing the diet with magnesium can help prevent depression, dizziness, muscle weakness and twitching, and premenstrual syndrome (PMS), and also aids in maintaining the body's proper pH balance and normal body temperature.

Magnesium is necessary to prevent the calcification of soft tissue. This essential mineral protects the arterial linings from stress caused by sudden blood pressure changes, and plays a role in the formation of bone and in carbohydrate and mineral metabolism. With vitamin B_6 (pyridoxine), magnesium helps to reduce and dissolve calcium phosphate kidney stones, and may prevent calcium-oxalate kidney stones. Research has shown that magnesium may help prevent cardiovascular disease, osteoporosis, and certain forms of cancer, and it may reduce cholesterol levels. It is effective in preventing premature labor and convulsions in pregnant women.

Studies have shown that taking magnesium supplements during pregnancy has a dramatic effect in reducing birth defects. A study reported by the *Journal of the American Medical Association* reported a 70-percent lower incidence of mental retardation in the children of mothers who had taken magnesium supplements during pregnancy. The incidence of cerebral palsy was 90 percent lower.

Possible manifestations of magnesium deficiency include confusion, insomnia, irritability, poor digestion, rapid heartbeat, seizures, and tantrums; often, a magnesium deficiency can be synonymous with diabetes. Magnesium deficiencies are at the root of many cardiovascular problems. Magnesium deficiency may be a major cause of fatal cardiac arrhythmia, hypertension, and sudden cardiac arrest, as well as asthma, chronic fatigue, chronic pain syndromes, depression, insomnia, irritable bowel syndrome, and pulmonary disorders. Research has also shown that magnesium deficiency may contribute to the formation of kidney stones. To test for magnesium deficiency, a procedure called an intracellular (mononuclear cell) magnesium screen should be performed. This is a more sensitive test than the

typical serum magnesium screen, and can detect a deficiency with more accuracy. Magnesium screening should be a routine test, as a low magnesium level makes nearly every disease worse. It is particularly important for individuals who have, or who are considered at risk for developing, cardiovascular disease.

Sources

Magnesium is found in most foods, especially dairy products, fish, meat, and seafood. Other rich food sources include apples, apricots, avocados, bananas, blackstrap molasses, brewer's yeast, brown rice, cantaloupe, dulse, figs, garlic, grapefruit, green leafy vegetables, kelp, lemons, lima beans, millet, nuts, peaches, black-eyed peas, salmon, sesame seeds, soybeans, tofu, torula yeast, watercress, wheat, and whole grains. Herbs that contain magnesium include alfalfa, bladderwrack, catnip, cayenne, chamomile, chickweed, dandelion, eyebright, fennel seed, fenugreek, hops, horsetail, lemongrass, licorice, mullein, nettle, oat straw, paprika, parsley, peppermint, raspberry leaf, red clover, sage, shepherd's purse, yarrow, and yellow dock.

Comments

The consumption of alcohol, the use of diuretics, diarrhea, the presence of fluoride, and high levels of zinc and vitamin D all increase the body's need for magnesium.

The consumption of large amounts of fats, cod liver oil, calcium, vitamin D, and protein decrease magnesium absorption. Fat-soluble vitamins also hinder the absorption of magnesium, as do foods high in oxalic acid, such as almonds, chard, cocoa, rhubarb, spinach, and tea.

Manganese

Minute quantities of manganese are needed for protein and fat metabolism, healthy nerves, a healthy immune system, and blood sugar regulation. Manganese is used in energy production and is required for normal bone growth and for reproduction. In addition, it is used in the formation of cartilage and synovial (lubricating) fluid of the joints. It is also necessary for the synthesis of bone.

Manganese is essential for people with iron-deficiency anemias and is needed for the utilization of vitamin B_1 (thiamine) and vitamin E. Manganese works well with the B-complex vitamins to give an overall feeling of well-being. It aids in the formation of mother's milk and is a key element in the production of enzymes needed to oxidize fats and to metabolize purines, including the antioxidant enzyme superoxide dismutase (SOD).

A deficiency of manganese (which is extremely rare) may lead to atherosclerosis, confusion, convulsions, eye problems, hearing problems, heart disorders, high cholesterol levels, hypertension, irritability, memory loss, muscle contractions, pancreatic damage, profuse perspiration, rapid pulse, tooth-grinding, tremors, and a tendency toward breast ailments.

Sources

The largest quantities of manganese are found in avocados, nuts and seeds, seaweed, and whole grains. This mineral may also be found in blueberries, egg yolks, legumes, dried peas, pineapples, and green leafy vegetables. Herbs that contain manganese include alfalfa, burdock root, catnip, chamomile, chickweed, dandelion, eyebright, fennel seed, fenugreek, ginseng, hops, horsetail, lemongrass, mullein, parsley, peppermint, raspberry, red clover, rose hips, wild yam, yarrow, and yellow dock.

Molybdenum

This essential mineral is required in extremely small amounts for nitrogen metabolism. It aids in the final stages of the conversion of purines to uric acid. It promotes normal cell function, aids in the activation of certain enzymes, and is a component of the metabolic enzyme xanthine oxidase. Molybdenum is found in the liver, bones, and kidneys. It supports bone growth and strengthening of the teeth. A low intake is associated with mouth and gum disorders and cancer. A molybdenum deficiency may cause impotence in older men. People whose diets are high in refined and processed foods are at risk for deficiency.

Sources

This trace mineral is found in beans, beef liver, cereal grains, dark green leafy vegetables, legumes, and peas.

Comments

Heat and moisture can change the action of supplemental molybdenum. A high intake of sulfur may decrease molybdenum levels. Excess amounts of molybdenum (over 15 milligrams daily) may interfere with copper metabolism.

Cautions

Do not take over 15 milligrams of molybdenum daily. Higher doses may lead to the development of gout.

Phosphorus

Phosphorus is needed for blood clotting, bone and tooth formation, cell growth, contraction of the heart muscle, normal heart rhythm, and kidney function. It also assists the body in the utilization of vitamins and the conversion of food to energy. A proper balance of magnesium, calcium, and phosphorus should be maintained at all times. If one of these minerals is present in either excessive or insufficient amounts, this will have adverse effects on the body.

Deficiencies of phosphorus are rare, but can lead to such symptoms as anxiety, bone pain, fatigue, irregular breathing, irritability, numbness, skin sensitivity, trembling, weakness, and weight changes.

Sources

Phosphorus deficiency is rare because this mineral is found in most foods, especially processed cooked foods and carbonated soft drinks. Significant amounts of phosphorus are contained in asparagus; bran; brewer's yeast; corn; dairy products; eggs; fish; dried fruit; garlic; legumes; nuts; sesame, sunflower, and pumpkin seeds; meats; poultry; salmon; and whole grains.

Comments

Excessive amounts of phosphorus interfere with calcium uptake. A diet high in processed cooked foods and junk food is a common culprit. Vitamin D increases the effectiveness of phosphorus.

Potassium

This mineral is important for a healthy nervous system and a regular heart rhythm. It helps prevent stroke, aids in proper muscle contraction, and works with sodium to control the body's water balance. Potassium is important for chemical reactions within the cells and aids in maintaining stable blood pressure and in transmitting electrochemical impulses. A 1997 review of earlier studies showed that low potassium intake may be a significant factor in the development of high blood pressure. Potassium also regulates the transfer of nutrients through cell membranes. This function of potassium has been shown to decrease with age, which may account for some of the circulatory damage, lethargy, and weakness experienced by older people. Together with magnesium, potassium can help prevent calcium-oxalate kidney stones.

Signs of potassium deficiency include abnormally dry skin, acne, chills, cognitive impairment, constipation, depression, diarrhea, diminished reflex function, edema, nervousness, insatiable thirst, fluctuations in heartbeat, glucose intolerance, growth impairment, high cholesterol levels, insomnia, low blood pressure, muscular fatigue and weakness, nausea and vomiting, periodic headaches, proteinuria (protein in the urine), respiratory distress, and salt retention.

Sources

Food sources of potassium include dairy foods, fish, fruit, legumes, meat, poultry, vegetables, and whole grains. High amounts are found in apricots, avocados, bananas, lima beans, blackstrap molasses, brewer's yeast, brown rice, dates, dulse, figs, dried fruit, garlic, nuts, potatoes, raisins, spinach, winter squash, torula yeast, wheat bran, yams, and yogurt. Herbs that contain potassium include catnip, hops, horsetail, nettle, plantain, red clover, sage, and skullcap.

Comments

Kidney disorders, diarrhea, and the use of diuretics or laxatives all disrupt potassium levels. Tobacco and caffeine reduce potassium absorption. Using large amounts of licorice over long periods can deplete the body's potassium supply.

Potassium is needed for hormone secretion. The secretion of stress hormones causes a decrease in the potassium-to-sodium ratio both inside and outside the cells. As a result, stress increases the body's potassium requirements.

Selenium

Selenium's principal function is to inhibit the oxidation of lipids (fats) as a component of the enzyme glutathione peroxidase. It is a vital antioxidant, especially when combined with vitamin E. It protects the immune system by preventing the formation of free radicals that can damage the body. (See ANTIOXIDANTS in Part One.) Selenium plays a vital role in regulating the effects of thyroid hormone on fat metabolism. It has also been found to function as a preventive against the formation of certain types of tumors. One study found that men who took 200 micrograms of selenium daily over a ten-year period had roughly half the risk of developing lung, prostate, and colorectal cancer as compared with men who did not.

Selenium and vitamin E act synergistically to aid in the production of antibodies and to help maintain a healthy heart and liver. This trace element is needed for pancreatic function and tissue elasticity. When combined with vitamin E and zinc, it may also provide relief from an enlarged prostate. Selenium supplementation has been found to protect the liver in people with alcoholic cirrhosis. Studies conducted at the University of Miami indicate that taking supplemental selenium may enhance the survival of people with AIDS by increasing both red and white blood cell counts. It has shown promise in the treatment of arthritis, cardiovascular disease, male infertility, cataracts, AIDS, and high blood pressure.

Selenium deficiency has been linked to cancer and heart disease. It has also been associated with exhaustion, growth impairment, high cholesterol levels, infections, liver impairment, pancreatic insufficiency, and sterility. Symptoms of excessively high selenium levels can include arthritis, brittle nails, garlicky breath odor, gastrointestinal disorders, hair loss, irritability, liver and kidney impairment, a metallic taste in the mouth, pallor, skin eruptions, tooth loss, and yellowish skin. Unless your health care provider prescribes it, do not take more than 400 micrograms daily.

Sources

Selenium can be found in meat and grains, depending on the selenium content of the soil where the food is raised. Because New Zealand soils are low in selenium, cattle and sheep raised there have suffered a breakdown of muscle tissue, including the heart muscle. However, human intake of selenium there is adequate because of imported Australian wheat. The soil of much American farm land is low in selenium, resulting in selenium-deficient produce.

Selenium can be found in Brazil nuts, brewer's yeast, broccoli, brown rice, chicken, dairy products, dulse, garlic, kelp, liver, molasses, onions, salmon, seafood, torula yeast, tuna, vegetables, wheat germ, and whole grains. Herbs that contain selenium include alfalfa, burdock root, catnip, cayenne, chamomile, chickweed, fennel seed, fenugreek, garlic, ginseng, hawthorn berry, hops, horsetail, lemongrass, milk thistle, nettle, oat straw, parsley, peppermint, raspberry leaf, rose hips, sarsaparilla, uva ursi, yarrow, and yellow dock.

Comments

Taking up to 200 micrograms of selenium per day is considered safe for most people. However, you should not take more than 40 micrograms of supplemental selenium daily if you are pregnant.

Silicon

Silicon is the second most abundant element on the planet (oxygen is the first). It is necessary for the formation of collagen for bones and connective tissue; for healthy nails, skin, and hair; and for calcium absorption in the early stages of bone formation. It is needed to maintain flexible arteries, and plays a major role in preventing cardiovascular disease. Silicon counteracts the effects of aluminum on the body and is important in the prevention of Alzheimer's disease and osteoporosis. It stimulates the immune system and inhibits the aging process in tissues. Silicon levels decrease with aging, so elderly people need larger amounts.

Sources

Foods that contain silicon include alfalfa, beets, brown rice, the herb horsetail, bell peppers, soybeans, leafy green vegetables, and whole grains.

Comments

Silicon is most commonly found in the form of silica, a compound of silicon and oxygen also known as silicon dioxide (SiO_2). Two good sources of silicon are Body Essential Silica Gel from Anton Huebner GmbH and BioSil from Jarrow Formulas.

Boron, calcium, magnesium, manganese, and potassium aid in the efficient utilization of silicon.

Sodium

Sodium is necessary for maintaining proper water balance and blood pH. It is also needed for stomach, nerve, and muscle function. Although sodium deficiency is rare—most people have adequate (if not excessive) levels of sodium in their bodies—it can occur. This condition is most likely to affect people who take diuretics for high blood pressure, especially if they simultaneously adhere to low-sodium diets. Some experts estimate that as many as 20 percent of elderly people who take diuretics may be deficient in sodium. In some cases of disorders such as fibromyalgia, studies have shown that moderate amounts of sodium may be needed as well (natural sea salt is recommended). Symptoms of sodium deficiency can include abdominal cramps, anorexia, confusion, dehydration, depression, dizziness, fatigue, flatulence, hallucinations, headache, heart palpitations, an impaired sense of taste, lethargy, low blood pressure, memory impairment, muscular weakness, nausea and vomiting, poor coordination, recurrent infections, seizures, and weight loss. Excessive sodium intake can result in edema, high blood pressure, potassium deficiency, and liver and kidney disease.

Sources

Virtually all foods contain some sodium.

Comments

A proper balance of potassium and sodium is necessary for good health. Since most people consume too much sodium, they typically need more potassium as well. An imbalance between sodium and potassium can lead to heart disease.

Sulfur

An acid-forming mineral that is part of the chemical structure of the amino acids methionine, cysteine, taurine, and glutathione, sulfur disinfects the blood, helps the body to resist bacteria, and protects the protoplasm of cells. It aids in necessary oxidation reactions in the body, stimulates bile secretion, and protects against toxic substances. Because of its ability to protect against the harmful effects of radiation and pollution, sulfur slows the aging process. It is found in all body tissues, and is needed for the synthesis of collagen, a principal protein that gives the skin its structural integrity.

Sources

Brussels sprouts, dried beans, cabbage, eggs, fish, garlic, kale, meats, onions, soybeans, turnips, and wheat germ contain sulfur, as do the herb horsetail and the amino acids cysteine, cystine, lysine, and methionine. Sulfur is also available in tablet and powder forms. Methylsufonyl-methane (MSM) is a good form of sulfur.

Comments

Moisture and heat may destroy or change the action of sulfur in the body. Sulfur is one of the key substances that makes garlic the "king of herbs."

Vanadium

Vanadium is needed for cellular metabolism and for the formation of bones and teeth. It plays a role in growth and reproduction, and inhibits cholesterol synthesis. Vanadium has been shown to have the ability to improve insulin utilization, resulting in improved glucose tolerance. A vanadium deficiency may be linked to cardiovascular and kidney disease, impaired reproductive ability, and increased infant mortality. Vanadium is not easily absorbed. Athletes may require more of this trace mineral than nonathletes.

Sources

Vanadium is found in dill, fish, olives, meat, radishes, snap beans, vegetable oils, and whole grains.

Comments

There may be an interaction between vanadium and chromium. If you take supplemental chromium and vanadium, take them at different times. Tobacco use decreases the uptake of vanadium.

Zinc

This essential mineral is important in prostate gland function and the growth of the reproductive organs. Zinc may help prevent acne and regulate the activity of oil glands. It is required for protein synthesis and collagen formation, and promotes a healthy immune system and the healing of wounds. Zinc also allows acuity of taste and smell. It protects the liver from chemical damage and is vital for bone formation. It is a constituent of insulin and many vital enzymes, including the antioxidant enzyme superoxide dismutase (SOD). It also helps to fight and prevent the formation of free radicals in other ways. A form of zinc called zinc monomethionine (zinc bound with the amino acid methionine), sold under the trademark OptiZinc, has been found to have antioxidant activity comparable to that of vitamin C, vitamin E, and beta-carotene. Zinc lozenges have been reported to be effective in relieving symptoms of the common cold and reducing the duration of colds.

Sufficient intake and absorption of zinc are needed to maintain the proper concentration of vitamin E in the blood. In addition, zinc increases the absorption of vitamin A. For optimum health, a proper 1-to-10 balance between copper and zinc levels should be maintained.

A deficiency of zinc may result in the loss of the senses of taste and smell. It can also cause fingernails to become thin, peel, and develop white spots. Other possible signs of zinc deficiency include acne, delayed sexual maturation, fatigue, growth impairment, hair loss, high cholesterol levels, impaired night vision, impotence, increased susceptibility to infection, infertility, memory impairment, a propensity to diabetes, prostate trouble, recurrent colds and flu, skin lesions, and slow wound healing.

Sources

Zinc is found in the following food sources: brewer's yeast, dulse, egg yolks, fish, kelp, lamb, legumes, lima beans, liver, meats, mushrooms, oysters, pecans, poultry, pumpkin seeds, sardines, seafood, soy lecithin, soybeans, sunflower seeds, torula yeast, and whole grains. Herbs that contain zinc include alfalfa, burdock root, cayenne, chamomile, chickweed, dandelion, eyebright, fennel seed, hops, milk thistle, mullein, nettle, parsley, rose hips, sage, sarsaparilla, skullcap, and wild yam.

Comments

Zinc levels may be lowered by diarrhea, kidney disease, cirrhosis of the liver, diabetes, or the consumption of fiber, which causes zinc to be excreted through the intestinal tract. A significant amount of zinc is lost through perspiration. The consumption of hard water also can upset zinc levels. Compounds called phytates that are found in grains and legumes bind with zinc so that it cannot be absorbed. If you take both zinc and iron supplements, take them at different times. If these two minerals are taken together, they interfere with each other's activity.

Cautions

Do not take a total of more than 100 milligrams of zinc daily. While daily doses under 100 milligrams enhance the immune response, doses of more than 100 milligrams can depress the immune system.

WATER

INTRODUCTION

Human beings can survive without food for thirty to forty days—about five weeks—but without water, life would end in three to five days. The average person's body is composed of approximately 70 percent water, although the water content varies considerably from person to person and even from one body part to another. The body's water supply is responsible for and involved in nearly every bodily process, including digestion, absorption, circulation, and excretion. Water is also the primary transporter of nutrients throughout the body and so is necessary for all building functions in the body. Water helps maintain normal body temperature and is essential for carrying waste material out of the body. Therefore, replacing the water that is continually being lost through sweating and elimination is very important.

A drop in the body's water content causes a decline in blood volume. The lowering of blood volume in turn triggers the hypothalamus, which is the brain's thirst center, to send out the demand for a drink. This causes a slight rise in the concentration of sodium in the blood. These changes quickly trigger a sensation of thirst. Unfortunately, people often consume only enough liquid to quench a dry or parched throat—not enough to cover all of their water loss. As a result, they can become dehydrated. As we age, the sense of thirst becomes dulled. At the same time, we have a lower percentage of reserve body water than we had when we were younger. This is why it is important to drink water even when you do not feel thirsty.

Quality water is beneficial for virtually all disorders known to humankind. Bowel and bladder problems, as well as headaches, can be reduced by drinking water. If not enough water is consumed, toxins can build up in the system, causing headaches. Water flushes these toxins out. Anxiety attacks, food intolerances, "acid stomach" and heartburn, muscle pains, colitis pain, hot flashes, and many other discomforts and disorders can be eased quickly by drinking a full glass of water. Chronic fatigue syndrome (CFS) is another disorder that necessitates consuming plenty of quality water daily to flush out toxins and other substances that contribute to muscle aches and extreme fatigue.

Without adequate water, we would poison ourselves with our own metabolic wastes. The kidneys remove waste products, such as uric acid, urea, and lactic acid, that must be dissolved in water. If there is not enough water available to remove these substances effectively, they may cause damage to the kidneys. Digestion and metabolism also rely on water for certain enzymatic and chemical reactions in the body. Water carries nutrients and oxygen to cells through the blood and is involved in the regulation of body temperature through perspiration. Water is especially important for people who have musculoskeletal problems such as arthritis, or who are athletic, as it lubricates the joints. Because lung tissue must be moist to facilitate oxygen intake and carbon dioxide excretion, water is essential for breathing. Approximately one pint of liquid is lost each day through exhaling. If you do not take in enough water to maintain fluid balance, every bodily function can be impaired. And the more active you are, the more water you must consume in order to keep your body's water level in balance.

Inadequate water consumption may contribute to excess body fat; poor muscle tone; digestive problems; poor functioning of many organs, including the brain; joint and muscle soreness; and, paradoxically, water retention. Consuming plenty of quality water can slow the aging process, and can prevent or improve arthritis, kidney stones, constipation, arteriosclerosis, obesity, glaucoma, cataracts, diabetes, hypoglycemia, and many other diseases. It is not expensive, and you should feel a difference quickly, but you must drink eight to ten full glasses of quality water daily.

Obtaining quality water would seem to be an easy matter. However, due to the numerous types of classifications water is given, the average consumer can easily be confused about what is available. This section offers a guide to understanding what the most commonly used classifications of water mean and how these different kinds of water may help or harm the body.

TAP WATER

Water that comes out of household taps or faucets is generally obtained either from surface water—water that has run off from ponds, creeks, streams, rivers, and lakes, and is collected in reservoirs—or from ground water—water that has filtered through the ground to the water table and is extracted by means of a well. Approximately half of the tap water in the United States comes from lakes, rivers, or other surface sources. Underground aquifers and municipal wells provide 35 percent of tap water, and the remaining 15 percent comes from private wells.

The Safety of Tap Water

Most people assume that when they turn on the kitchen tap, they are getting clean, safe, healthy drinking water. Unfortunately, this often is not the case. Regardless of the original source of tap water, it is vulnerable to a number of different types of impurities, and may be full of harmful chemicals and inorganic minerals that the body cannot use. Some undesirable substances found in water, including radon, fluoride, and arsenic, as well as iron, lead, copper, and other heavy metals, can occur naturally. Other contaminants, such as fertilizers, asbestos, cyanides, herbicides, pesticides, and industrial chemicals, may leach into ground water through the soil, or into any tap water from plumbing pipes. Many of these chemicals have been linked to cancer and other disorders. Water can also contain biological contaminants, including viruses, bacteria, and parasites. Still other substances, including chlorine, carbon, lime, phosphates, soda ash, and aluminum sulfate, are intentionally added to public water supplies to kill bacteria, adjust pH, and eliminate cloudiness, among other things.

A study conducted by the Natural Resources Defense Council found that 18,500 of the nation's water systems (serving some 45 million Americans) violated safe drinking water laws at some point during 1994 or 1995. The council's report blamed contaminated water for some 900,000 illnesses a year, including 100 deaths. Even if the levels of individual substances in water are well within "allowable" limits, the total of all contaminants present may still be harmful to your health. And private wells may not be regulated at all, except at the local level.

The greatest concerns about water quality today focus on chlorine, pesticides, and parasites. Chlorine has long been added to public water supplies to kill disease-causing bacteria. However, the levels of chlorine in drinking water today can be quite high, and some byproducts of chlorine are known carcinogens. As a result, the U.S. Environmental Protection Agency (EPA) is considering steps to reduce the level of chlorine in drinking water, but is facing opposition from industry groups.

Pesticides pose a risk in any area where the tap water is extracted from an underground source. These chemicals are suspected of causing, or at least contributing to, an increased incidence of cancer, especially breast cancer. Some scientists believe this may be because certain pesticides can mimic the action of the sex hormone estrogen in the body. Others point to the fact that toxins in the body tend to accumulate in fatty tissues, and the human breast is composed largely of fatty tissue. The pesticide problem is a particular concern in areas where agriculture is (or was) a major part of the economy. These chemicals are persistent. Residues from pesticides used decades ago may still be present in water coming out of the tap today, and may pose a risk to health.

Long considered a problem limited to poor, developing countries, the presence of bacteria and parasites in drinking water—especially a parasite called *cryptosporidium*—is becoming a serious problem in the United States today. In April 1993, as many as 370,000 people in and around Milwaukee, Wisconsin, were stricken by the parasite *Cryptosporidium parvum* from the city's water supply. Thousands suffered from severe diarrhea, and up to 100 deaths were attributed to the outbreak. These "unacceptable" levels of cryptosporidia, most likely from agricultural runoff, forced users of the public water system to boil their tap water before using it. The same organism has created controversy over the safety of the water in New York City; many people with weakened immune systems have charged that cryptosporidia in the city water have made them sick, even though local officials insist that the water is safe to drink. For people with HIV or AIDS, cryptosporidia can be lethal. The chlorine added to water to kill bacteria is not effective at killing these parasites. In addition to cryptosporidiosis, giardiasis, also caused by an intestinal parasite, can be contracted through drinking water and is an increasing problem. Like cryptosporidia, giardia resist the effects of chlorine (outbreaks have occurred in areas where the water is routinely chlorine-treated) and pose a more serious problem for people with diminished immune response. Indeed, because of increasing concern over the danger contaminated drinking water poses for people with compromised immune systems, the U.S. Centers for Disease Control and Prevention (CDC) and the EPA have issued suggestions that immunocompromised individuals boil tap water for at least one minute before use, use an appropriate filtration system, or buy quality bottled drinking water.

More than one-third of all community water systems have been cited for failure to meet the EPA's water safety standards or treatment technique, monitoring, or reporting requirements. Consumer activist Ralph Nader's Center for Study of Responsive Law issued a study in 1988 entitled *Troubled Waters On Tap: Organic Chemicals in Public Drinking Water Systems and the Failure or Regulation* that identified over 2,100 contaminants in tap water in the United States. And according to a study released in 1995, 54 million Americans drank tap water that was contaminated by feces, radiation, lead, or dangerous parasites at some time between 1993 and 1994.

If you receive your water from a municipal water source, that utility is now required to send an assessment of the water, including information about where it comes from, any contaminants that have been found in it, and any health risk associated with substances in the water. This should be sent to you in your water bill on an annual basis. Whatever the source of your water, it is important to know some warning signs of bad water. Watch for cloudiness or murkiness in water. Chlorination can cause some cloudiness, but it usually clears if the water is left to stand, whereas bacterial or sedimentary cloudiness will remain. Foaming may be caused by bacterial contamination, by floating particles of sediment, or by soaps or detergents. Bacteria can be destroyed by boiling water for at least five minutes, while sediment should settle out if you let the water stand for several hours. Strange smells or tastes in water that was previously fine could mean chemical contamination. However, many toxic hazards that work their way into water do not change its taste, smell, or appearance.

Hard Versus Soft Water

Hard water, found in various parts of the country, contains relatively high concentrations of the minerals calcium and magnesium. The presence of these minerals prevents soap from lathering and results in filmy sediment being deposited on hair, clothing, pipes, dishes, washtubs, and anything else that comes into regular contact with the water. It also affects the taste. Hard water can be annoying, and though some studies have shown that deaths from heart disease may be lower in areas where the drinking water is hard, we believe that the calcium found in hard water is not good for the heart, arteries, or bones. Hard water deposits its calcium and other minerals on the *outside* of these structures, while it is the calcium and magnesium found *within* these structures that are beneficial to the body.

Soft water can be naturally soft or it may be hard water that has been treated to remove the calcium and magnesium. Standard water-softening systems work by using pressure to pass the water through exchange media to exchange "hard" calcium and magnesium ions for "soft" sodium or potassium ions. Most use either sodium chloride

or potassium chloride for this purpose. The primary benefit of softening is in improved cleaning properties for the water and less mineral buildup inside household pipes and equipment. One potentially serious problem with artificially softened water is that it is more likely than hard water to dissolve the lining of pipes. This poses an especially significant threat if pipes are made of lead. Another threat comes from certain plastic and galvanized pipes, which contain cadmium, a toxic heavy metal. These types of pipes are rarely used in construction today, but they may be present in older buildings that have not undergone extensive renovation. But leaching from pipes can be a problem with today's copper pipes as well. Dangerous levels of copper, iron, zinc, and arsenic can leach into softened water from copper pipes. Another potential problem with artificially softened water is of concern to people with kidney failure. People with kidney failure must restrict their intake of potassium. Potassium-based water-softening systems can therefore pose a danger to such individuals.

Fluoridation

For many years now, controversy has raged over whether fluoride should be added to drinking water. As early as 1961, as recorded in the Congressional Record, fluoride was exposed as a lethal poison in our nation's water supply. Proponents say that fluoride occurs naturally and helps develop and maintain strong bones and teeth. Op-

MTBE and Drinking Water

Since 1979, methyl tertiary butyl ether (MTBE) has been added to gasoline to increase its oxygen content. It took the place of lead as an octane enhancer, and was supposed to reduce the problems of both smog and carbon monoxide in the atmosphere. The Clean Air Act of 1990 required the use of reformulated gasoline, or RFG, in certain parts of the country, with the goal of reducing air pollution in those areas. RFG accounts for some 30 percent of gasoline sold in the United States, and MTBE is now added to over 80 percent of RFG fuel.

According to a disturbing report aired on the CBS television program *60 Minutes* on January 16, 2000, this measure to improve air quality has, ironically, given Americans yet another reason to be concerned about the safety of their drinking water supply. MTBE has been seeping into all our water supplies, both surface and underground), at an alarming rate. It has been found in storm water in 592 samples collected in sixteen cities between 1991 and 1995. The primary sources of the MTBE that ends up in water systems are leaking gasoline tanks and reservoirs, drinking water lakes, and rivers where gasoline-powered recreational watercraft are permitted. Less than one-tenth of a gallon (roughly 12 ounces) of MTBE is capable of contaminating 13 million

gallons of drinking water. It is estimated that over 1 million gallons of fuel are deposited, unburned, into the water supply each year as a result of recreational boating.

Few long-term studies have been done on this chemical, but what little research there is indicates that MTBE is a likely human carcinogen and immune-system depressant. Certainly, tests on rats have provided evidence that MTBE is a cancer-causing agent. To date, drinking water supplies in the states of California, New York, Maine, Pennsylvania, Connecticut, and Rhode Island have been closed down due to contamination by MTBE (boiling drinking water does not help purge it of this agent). MTBE-contaminated tap water can cause problems even if you do not drink it. This chemical can also be absorbed through the skin when showering and can be inhaled as a vapor in the air. Possible effects of inhaling MTBE include headaches, burning of the nose and throat, dizziness, nausea, asthma, and respiratory problems. The possible effects on wildlife have not yet been documented.

Only recently has the Environmental Protection Agency (EPA) considered making it mandatory to test for MTBE in drinking water, but the likelihood is that it will not be until the year 2010 that the EPA will make a determination on the continued use of MTBE.

ponents to fluoridation contend that when fluoridated water is consumed regularly, toxic levels of fluorine, the poisonous substance from which fluoride is derived, build up in the body, causing irreparable harm to the immune system. The Delaney Congressional Investigation Committee, the government body charged with monitoring additives and other substances in the food supply, has stated that "fluoridation is mass medication without parallel in the history of medicine."

Meanwhile, no convincing scientific proof has ever been generated that fluoridated water makes for stronger bones and teeth. It is known, however, that chronic fluoride use results in numerous health problems, including osteoporosis and osteomalacia, and also damages teeth and leaves them mottled. The salts used to fluoridate our nation's water supply, sodium fluoride and fluorosalicic acid, are industrial byproducts that are never found in nature. They are also notoriously toxic compounds, so much so that they are used in rat poison and insecticides. The naturally occurring form of fluoride, calcium fluoride, is not toxic—but this form of fluoride is not used to fluoridate water.

Today, more than half the cities in the United States fluoridate their water supplies. In many states, it is required. Although many ailments and disorders—including Down syndrome, mottled teeth, and cancer—have been linked to fluoridated water, fluoridation has become the standard rather than the exception.

The fluoride added to tap water can be a problem. Individuals have different levels of tolerance for toxins such as fluoride. In addition, many water sources have levels of fluoride higher than one part per million, the level generally recognized as safe and originally set as the acceptable limit by the EPA. After the EPA learned that water in many towns had natural fluoride levels much higher than this, the permissible fluoride limit was raised—quadrupled, in fact—to four parts per million. And this is in addition to fluoride encountered from other sources. Fluoride is the thirteenth most widely distributed element on earth, so it can turn up just about anywhere—in vegetables and meats, for example. Since so many local water supplies are fluoridated, there is a good chance that virtually any packaged food product made with water, such as soft drinks and reconstituted juices, contains fluoride. Additional fluorides are widely used in toothpaste products, so it is easy to see how many Americans may be ingesting excessive amounts of this potentially toxic substance.

If your tap water contains fluoride, and you wish to remove it, you can use a reverse osmosis, distillation, or activated alumina filtration system to eliminate almost all of the fluoride from your water.

Water Analysis

Not all drinking water contains significant amounts of toxic substances. Some places rate higher in water safety than others. In addition, not all cities and towns process their water supplies the same way. Some do nothing at all to their water. Others add chemicals to the water to kill bacteria. Still others filter their water. It is up to the individual to find out how local drinking water is treated and to determine how safe the water coming out of the tap is.

The EPA has defined pure water as "bacteriologically safe" water, and it recommends—but does not require—that tap water have a pH between 6.5 and 8.5. This allows for a great deal of leeway in what passes as acceptable water. If you are concerned about the safety of the water coming out of your tap, you can contact your local water officials or local health department, which may test your tap water free of charge. In some cases, you may have to contact your state's water supply or health department. Typically, however, these agencies test the water only for bacteria levels, not for toxic substances. Therefore, you might want to contact a commercial laboratory or local state university laboratory to test your water for its chemical content. If you find that your tap water is unacceptable either because of its taste or because of its toxic chemical content, you may choose to use one of the alternative water supplies described in this section.

The Water Quality Association (see HEALTH AND MEDICAL ORGANIZATIONS in the Appendix) is prepared to answer questions about the various types of water and methods of water treatment. In addition, the EPA operates the toll-free Safe Drinking Water Hotline, which can help you to locate an office or laboratory in your area that does certified water testing. There are also a number of laboratories that will send a self-addressed container for you to fill and return by mail for testing. The cost starts at thirty-five to forty dollars per tap. Results are usually available in two to three weeks.

To help you understand the results of water testing, you should obtain information on the EPA's Recommended Maximum Contaminant Levels. This and other water-quality information is available from NSF International, Inc. (formerly the National Sanitation Foundation) and the Water Quality Association (again, see HEALTH AND MEDICAL ORGANIZATIONS in the Appendix for further information).

Improving Tap Water

Tap water can be improved in several ways. Heating tap water to a rolling boil and keeping it there for three to five minutes will kill bacteria and parasites. However, most people find boiling their drinking water too impractical and time-consuming. In addition, this procedure has the effect of concentrating whatever lead is present in the water, and the water must then be refrigerated if it is to be used for drinking. The taste of chlorinated tap water can be improved by keeping the water in an uncovered pitcher for several hours to allow the chlorine taste and odor to dissipate. Water can also be aerated in a blender to remove chlorine and other chemicals. Nevertheless, neither of these last two methods will improve the quality of the water—only the taste.

Filtration is a means by which contaminants in water are removed, rendering the water cleaner and better tasting. There are many different ways in which water can be filtered. Nature filters water as the water runs through streams and as it seeps down through the soil and rocks to the water table. As water passes through the earth or over the rocks in a stream, the bacteria in the water leech into the rocks and are replaced with minerals such as calcium and magnesium.

There are also man-made ways of filtering water. There are three basic types of filters available: absorbent types, which use materials such as carbon to pick up impurities; microfiltration systems, which run water through filters with tiny pores to catch and eliminate contaminants (the filter may be made of any of a number of different materials); and special media such as ion-exchange resins that are designed to remove heavy metals. Filters are often arranged in series, so that the filtering media that are most effective for specific types of contaminants can be used. The primary advantage of filters is relatively low cost and ease of use.

Water filtration systems vary in effectiveness. Two types that are considered good are reverse osmosis and ceramic filtration systems. In reverse osmosis filtering, the water is forced through a semipermeable membrane, while charged particles and larger molecules are repelled. It is the best system for treating water that is brackish (high in salt), high in nitrates, and loaded with inorganic heavy metals such as iron and lead. However, no filter can remove absolutely all contaminants. Each pore of even the finest filter is large enough for some viruses to permeate. To remove parasites such as cryptosporidia, the EPA and CDC recommend purchasing a filter that has an NSF rating for parasite reduction *and* that has an absolute pore size of one micron or smaller.

Other water treatment systems that remove various contaminants include distillers and ultraviolet treatment units. The latter are used to kill bacteria and viruses in water. Each treatment method has its advantages and disadvantages (*see* Home Water Treatment Methods, below), but using a combination of methods can result in the best overall quality drinking water. Even the quality and taste of distilled water can be improved by passing the water through a charcoal/carbon filter as a final step.

Before you purchase a water treatment unit, contact NSF International or the Water Quality Association. These nonprofit testing and certification organizations verify manufacturers' claims and certify that the materials used are

Home Water Treatment Methods

Treatment Type	Cost	How It Works	What It Does
Activated carbon	Faucet-mounted or pour-through unit: $20–$60 Countertop unit: $89–200 Under-sink unit: $75–$600 Whole-house system: $499–$1,250	Water is filtered through a carbon trap that absorbs the contaminants.	Reduces levels of chlorine, herbicides, lead, hydrogen sulfide, and volatile organic chemicals (VOCs). Also reduces color and turbidity.
Carbon filtration	Faucet-mounted unit: $25 Under-counter unit: $300 and up	Passes water through a charcoal or solid carbon block and captures contaminants. When carbon sites fill up, the filter cartridge is replaced.	Reduces levels of chlorine, organic chemicals, and pesticides. Also reduces bad taste and odors.
Distillation	Countertop unit: $99–$995 Free-standing unit: $599–$1,020 Whole-house system: $799–$4,500	Raises water temperature to boiling, leaving contaminants behind. Purified water vapor condenses to liquid.	Reduces levels of arsenic, cadmium, chromium, orin, lead, giardia cysts, nitrate, and sulfate. Also reduces turbidity.
Reverse osmosis	Countertop unit: $150–$250 Under-sink unit: $530–$1,500	Forces pressurized water through a contamination-rejecting membrane; sends improved water to holding tank.	Reduces levels of arsenic, cadmium, iron, chlorine, color, lead, giardia, giardia cysts, nitrate, radium, and sulfate. Also reduces color and turbidity.
Water softener	Whole-house system: $950–$3,500	Replaces calcium and magnesium with sodium to "soften" the water.	Reduces levels of calcium, iron, and radium.

nontoxic and structurally sound. They conduct periodic unannounced audits of the products they certify to ensure that the products still comply with standards.

One manufacturer of home distillation units that has certification for different models from both NSF International and the Water Quality Association is Waterwise, Inc. This company offers options combining both pre-distillation and post-distillation carbon filtration, and also manufactures a showerhead water filtration system that rids shower water of chlorine and various other contaminants. Pure Water, Inc. manufactures home and small business distillation systems that are in use throughout the world. Reverse osmosis system manufacturers whose products can claim certification by NSF International and the Water Quality Association include EcoWater Systems and Rainsoft. *See* HEALTH AND MEDICAL ORGANIZATIONS in the Appendix for more information about these companies.

BOTTLED WATER

Because of concerns over the safety and health effects of tap water, many people today are turning to bottled water. Bottled water is usually classified by its source (spring, spa, geyser, public water supply, etc.), by its mineral content (containing at least 250 parts per million of dissolved solids), and/or by the type of treatment it has undergone (deionized, steam-distilled, etc.). Because there is a lot of overlapping among these criteria, some water fits more than one classification. In addition, most states have no rules governing appropriate labeling, so some bottled water claims may be misleading or incorrect.

While the EPA is charged with the regulation of public water supplies, it is the U.S. Food and Drug Administration (FDA) that has responsibility for overseeing the quality and safety of bottled drinking water. The FDA defines the terms used to describe bottled drinking waters in specific requirements last revised in April 1997, making the choices for the consumer somewhat clearer than in the past. The FDA regulations for bottled water allow for the various terms that have been defined to be used with one another if bottled water meets more than one definition, so it is possible for some water labels to include a number of different terms.

All the terms that are legally necessary to describe bottled drinking water are discussed in the paragraphs that follow. Any term you find on a label that is *not* defined or included here is a marketing slogan added to entice the consumer to buy the product. It can mean anything that the manufacturer of the product says it means.

Artesian Water

Artesian water, or artesian well water, is water drawn from a well where the water is brought to the surface by natural pressure or flow.

Bottled Water

Bottled water, or bottled drinking water, is water that is intended for human consumption and that is sealed in bottles or other containers with no added ingredients except for optional antimicrobial agents. These must be identified on the label. If bottled water comes from a community water system or from a municipal source, this information must appear on the label. About 25 percent of bottled waters now sold come from the same water supplies that flow into some areas' household taps.

Deionized or Demineralized Water

When the electric charge of a molecule of water has been neutralized by the addition or removal of electrons, the resulting water is called *deionized* or *demineralized*. The deionization process removes nitrates and the minerals calcium and magnesium, in addition to the heavy metals cadmium, barium, lead, mercury, and some forms of radium.

Ground Water

This is water that comes from underground, in the water table, that is under pressure equal to or greater than atmospheric pressure, and that does not come into contact with surface water. Ground water must be pumped mechanically for bottling.

Mineral Water

Mineral water is water containing not less than 250 parts per million total dissolved solids (TDS), originating from a geologically and physically protected underground water source or spring that has been tapped at the spring opening or through a borehole. Mineral water is distinguished from other types of water by constant levels and relative proportions of minerals and trace elements at its source, allowing for seasonal variations. No minerals may be added to this water. If the TDS content of mineral water is below 500 parts per million, the water may be labeled *low mineral content*. If it is greater than 1,500 parts per million, the label *high mineral content* may be used.

Depending on where the source is, the minerals the water contains will vary. If you are suffering from a deficiency of certain minerals and are drinking mineral water for therapeutic reasons, you must be aware of which minerals are in the particular brand of water you drink. If you are drinking mineral water containing minerals that you do not lack, you could be doing yourself more harm than good.

Most mineral waters are carbonated. However, some sparkling waters, such as club soda, are called mineral waters because the manufacturer added bicarbonates, citrates, and sodium phosphates to filtered or distilled tap water.

Natural Spring Water

The term *natural spring water* on a bottled water label doesn't tell you where the water came from, only that the mineral content of the water has not been altered. It may or may not have been filtered or otherwise treated. While the number of gallons of "natural spring water" flowing through water coolers and from bottles has more than doubled in recent years, the meaning of these words on a label has been firmly defined only since the final changes in the FDA bottled drinking water regulations have been in place.

Spring water is water that comes from an underground formation from which water flows naturally to the surface of the earth. It must be collected at the spring or through a borehole tapping the underground formation that feeds the spring. To meet the definition of *spring*, there must be natural force bringing the water to the surface opening. The location of the spring must be identified on the label of any water labeled as spring water.

If you use a water cooler for bottled spring water, you should be sure to clean the cooler once a month to destroy bacteria. Run a 50-50 mixture of hydrogen peroxide and baking soda through the reservoir and spigots, then remove the residue by rinsing the cooler with four or more gallons of tap water.

Sparkling Water

This is bottled water that contains the same amount of carbon dioxide that it had at emergence from the water source. It can be a healthful alternative to soda and alcoholic beverages, but if it is loaded with fructose and other sweeteners, it may be no better than soda pop. Read labels before you buy. Soda water, seltzer water, and tonic water are *not* considered bottled waters. They are regulated separately, may contain sugar and calories, and are considered soft drinks.

Understanding where the carbonation in sparkling water comes from isn't always easy. A "naturally sparkling water" must get its carbonation from the same source as the water. If a water is "carbonated natural water," that means the carbonation came from a source other than the one that supplied the water. That doesn't mean the water is of poor quality. It can still be called "natural" because its mineral content is the same as when it came from the ground, even though it has been carbonated from a separate source. People suffering from intestinal disorders or ulcers should avoid drinking carbonated water because it may be irritating to the gastrointestinal tract.

Steam-Distilled Water

Distillation involves vaporizing water by boiling it. The steam rises, leaving behind most of the bacteria, viruses, chemicals, minerals, and pollutants from the water. The steam is then moved into a condensing chamber, where it is cooled and condensed to become distilled water.

Once consumed, steam-distilled water leaches inorganic minerals rejected by the cells and tissues out of the body.

We believe that only steam-distilled or reverse osmosis filtered water should be consumed. They should be used not only for drinking, but in cooking as well, because foods such as pasta, rice, and beans can absorb chemicals found in unpurified water.

Flavor can be added to distilled water by adding 1 to 2 tablespoons of raw apple cider vinegar (obtained from a health food store) per gallon of distilled water. Vinegar is an excellent solvent and aids in digestion. Lemon juice is another good flavoring agent, and has cleansing properties as well. For added minerals, you can add mineral drops to steam-distilled water. Concentrace from Trace Minerals Research is a good product for this purpose. Add 1¼ teaspoons of mineral drops to every 5 gallons of water.

AMINO ACIDS

INTRODUCTION

Amino acids are the chemical units or "building blocks," as they are popularly called, that make up proteins. They also are the end products of protein digestion, or *hydrolysis*. Amino acids contain about 16 percent nitrogen. Chemically, this is what distinguishes them from the other two basic nutrients, sugars and fatty acids, which do not contain nitrogen.

To understand how vital amino acids are, you must understand how essential proteins are to life. It is protein that provides the structure for all living things. Every living organism, from the largest animal to the tiniest microbe, is composed of protein. And in its various forms, protein participates in the vital chemical processes that sustain life.

Proteins are a necessary part of every living cell in the body. Next to water, protein makes up the greatest portion of our body weight. In the human body, protein substances make up the muscles, ligaments, tendons, organs, glands, nails, hair, and many vital body fluids, and are essential for the growth of bones. The enzymes and hormones that catalyze and regulate all bodily processes are proteins. Proteins help to regulate the body's water balance and maintain the proper internal pH. They assist in the exchange of nutrients between the intercellular fluids and the tissues, blood, and lymph. A deficiency of protein can upset the body's fluid balance, causing edema. Proteins form the structural basis of chromosomes, through which genetic information is passed from parents to offspring. The genetic "code" contained in each cell's DNA is actually information for how to make that cell's proteins.

Proteins are chains of amino acids linked together by what are called *peptide bonds*. Each individual type of protein is composed of a specific group of amino acids in a specific chemical arrangement. It is the particular amino acids present and the way in which they are linked together in sequence that gives the proteins that make up the various tissues their unique functions and characters. Each protein in the body is tailored for a specific need; proteins are not interchangeable.

The proteins that make up the human body are not obtained directly from the diet. Rather, dietary protein is broken down into its constituent amino acids, which the body then uses to build the specific proteins it needs. Thus, it is the amino acids rather than protein that are the essential nutrients.

In addition to those that combine to form the body's proteins, there are other amino acids that are important in metabolic functions. Some, such as citrulline, glutathione, ornithine, and taurine, can be similar to (or byproducts of) the protein-building amino acids. Some act as neurotransmitters or as precursors of neurotransmitters, the chemicals that carry information from one nerve cell to another. Certain amino acids are thus necessary for the brain to receive and send messages. Unlike many other substances, neurotransmitters are able to pass through the *blood-brain barrier*. This is a kind of defensive shield designed to protect the brain from toxins and foreign invaders that may be circulating in the bloodstream. The endothelial cells that make up the walls of the capillaries in the brain are much more tightly meshed together than are those of capillaries elsewhere in the body. This prevents many substances, especially water-based substances, from diffusing through the capillary walls into brain tissue. Because certain amino acids can pass through this barrier, they can be used by the brain to communicate with nerve cells elsewhere in the body.

Amino acids also enable vitamins and minerals to perform their jobs properly. Even if vitamins and minerals are absorbed and assimilated by the body, they cannot be effective unless the necessary amino acids are present. For example, low levels of the amino acid tyrosine may lead to iron deficiency. Deficiency and/or impaired metabolism of the amino acids methionine and taurine has been linked to allergies and autoimmune disorders. Many elderly people suffer from depression or neurological problems that may be associated with deficiencies of the amino acids tyrosine, tryptophan, phenylalanine, and histidine, and also of the *branched-chain amino acids*—valine, isoleucine, and leucine. These are amino acids that can be used to provide energy directly to muscle tissue. High doses of branched-chain amino acids have been used in hospitals to treat people suffering from trauma and infection. Some people are born with an inability to metabolize the branched-chain amino acids. This potentially life-threatening condition, branched-chain ketoaciduria (often referred to as *maple syrup urine disease* because keto acids released into the urine cause it to smell like maple syrup) can result in neurological damage and necessitates a special diet, including a synthetic infant formula that does not contain leucine, isoleucine, or valine.

There are approximately twenty-eight commonly known amino acids that are combined in various ways to create the hundreds of different types of proteins present in all living things. In the human body, the liver produces about 80 percent of the amino acids needed. The remaining

20 percent must be obtained from the diet. These are called the *essential amino acids.* The essential amino acids that must enter the body through diet are histidine, isoleucine, leucine, lysine, methionine, phenylalanine, threonine, tryptophan, and valine. The nonessential amino acids, which can be manufactured in the body from other amino acids obtained from dietary sources, include alanine, arginine, asparagine, aspartic acid, citrulline, cysteine, cystine, gamma-aminobutyric acid, glutamic acid, glutamine, glycine, ornithine, proline, serine, taurine, and tyrosine. The fact that they are termed "nonessential" does not mean that they are not necessary, only that they need not be obtained through the diet because the body can manufacture them as needed. And nonessential amino acids can become "essential" under certain conditions. For instance, the nonessential amino acids cysteine and tyrosine are made from the essential amino acids methionine and phenylalanine. If methionine and phenylalanine are not available in sufficient quantities, cysteine and tyrosine then become essential in the diet.

The processes of assembling amino acids to make proteins, and of breaking down proteins into individual amino acids for the body's use, are continuous ones. When we need more enzyme proteins, the body produces more enzyme proteins; when we need more cells, the body produces more proteins for cells. These different types of proteins are produced as the need arises. Should the body become depleted of its reserves of any of the essential amino acids, it would not be able to produce the proteins that require those amino acids. An inadequate supply of even one essential amino acid can hinder the synthesis, and reduce body levels, of necessary proteins. This can result in negative nitrogen balance, an unhealthy condition in which the body excretes more nitrogen than it assimilates. Further, *all* of the essential amino acids must be present simultaneously in the diet in order for the other amino acids to be utilized—otherwise, the body remains in negative nitrogen balance. A lack of vital proteins in the body can cause problems ranging from indigestion to depression to stunted growth.

How could such a situation occur? More easily than you might think. Many factors can contribute to deficiencies of essential amino acids, even if you eat a well-balanced diet that contains enough protein. Impaired absorption, infection, trauma, stress, drug use, age, and imbalances of other nutrients can all affect the availability of essential amino acids in the body. Insufficient intake of vitamins and minerals, especially vitamin C, can interfere with the absorption of amino acids in the lower part of the small intestines. Vitamin B_6 is needed also, for the transport of amino acids in the body.

If your diet is *not* properly balanced—that is, if it fails to supply adequate amounts of the essential amino acids—sooner or later, this will become apparent as some type of physical disorder. This does not mean, however, that eating a diet containing enormous amounts of protein is the answer. In fact, it is unhealthy. Excess protein puts undue stress on the kidneys and the liver, which are faced with processing the waste products of protein metabolism. Nearly half of the amino acids in dietary protein are transformed into glucose by the liver and utilized to provide needed energy to the cells. This process results in a waste product, ammonia. Ammonia is toxic to the body, so the body protects itself by having the liver turn the ammonia into a much less toxic compound, urea, which is then carried through the bloodstream, filtered out by the kidneys, and excreted.

As long as protein intake is not too great and the liver is working properly, ammonia is neutralized almost as soon as it is produced, so it does no harm. However, if there is too much ammonia for the liver to cope with—as a result of too much protein consumption, poor digestion, and/or a defect in liver function—toxic levels may accumulate. Strenuous exercise also tends to promote the accumulation of excess ammonia. This may put a person at risk for serious health problems, including encephalopathy (brain disease) or hepatic coma. Abnormally high levels of urea can also cause problems, including inflamed kidneys and back pain. Therefore, it is not the quantity but the quality of protein in the diet that is important (*see* DIET AND NUTRITION in Part One).

It is possible to take supplements containing amino acids, both essential and nonessential. For certain disorders, taking supplements of specific amino acids can be very beneficial. When you take a specific amino acid or amino acid combination, it supports the metabolic pathway involved in your particular illness. Vegetarians, especially vegans, would be wise to take a formula containing all of the essential amino acids to ensure that their protein requirements are met.

WHAT'S ON THE SHELVES

Supplemental amino acids are available in combination with various multivitamin formulas, as protein mixtures, in a wide variety of food supplements, and in a number of amino acid formulas. They can be purchased as capsules, tablets, liquids, and powders. Most amino acid supplements are derived from animal protein, yeast protein, or vegetable protein. Crystalline free-form amino acids are generally extracted from a variety of grain products. Brown rice bran is a prime source, although cold-pressed yeast and milk proteins are also used.

Free-form means the amino acid is in its purest form. Free-form amino acids need no digestion and are absorbed directly into the bloodstream. These white crystalline amino acids are stable at room temperature and decompose when heated to temperatures of 350°F to 660°F (180°C to 350°C). They are rapidly absorbed and do not come from potentially allergenic food sources. For best results, choose encapsulated powders or powder.

When choosing amino acid supplements, look for products that contain USP (U.S. Pharmacopeia) pharmaceutical-grade L-crystalline amino acids. Most of the amino acids (except for glycine) can appear in two forms, the chemical structure of one being the mirror image of the other. These are called the D- and L- forms—for example, D-cystine and L-cystine. The "D" stands for *dextro* (Latin for "right") and the "L" for *levo* (Latin for "left"); these terms denote the direction of the rotation of the spiral that is the chemical structure of the molecule. Proteins in animal and plant tissue are made from the L-forms of amino acids (with the exception of phenylalanine, which is also used in the form of DL-phenylalanine, a mixture of the D- and L- forms). Thus, with respect to supplements of amino acids, products containing the L- forms of amino acids are considered to be more compatible with human biochemistry.

Each amino acid has specific functions in the body. The many functions and possible symptoms of deficiency of twenty-eight amino acids and related compounds are described below. When taking amino acids individually for healing purposes, take them on an empty stomach to avoid making them compete for absorption with the amino acids present in foods. When taking individual amino acids, it is best to take them in the morning or between meals, with small amounts of vitamin B6 and vitamin C to enhance absorption. When taking an amino acid complex that includes all of the essential amino acids, it is best to take it one-half hour away from a meal, either before or after. If you are taking individual amino acids, it is wise also to take a full amino acid complex, including both essential and non-essential amino acids, at a different time. This is the best way to assure you have adequate amounts of all the necessary amino acids.

Be aware that individual amino acids should not be taken for long periods of time. A good rule to follow is to alternate the individual amino acids that fit your needs and back them up with an amino acid complex, taking the supplements for two months and then discontinuing them for two months. Moderation is the key. Some amino acids have potentially toxic effects when taken in high doses (over 6,000 milligrams per day) and may cause neurological damage. These include aspartic acid, glutamic acid, homocysteine, serine, and tryptophan. Cysteine can be toxic if taken in amounts over 1,000 milligrams per day. Do not give supplemental amino acids to a child, or take doses of any amino acid in excess of the amount recommended unless specifically directed to do so by your health care provider.

Some recommended amino acid products include the following:

• A/G-Pro from Miller Pharmacal Group, a complete amino acid and mineral supplement.

• Anabolic Amino Balance and Muscle Octane from Anabol Naturals. Anabolic Amino Balance is a complex of twenty-three free-form amino acids. Muscle Octane is a blend of free-form branched-chain amino acids (L-leucine, L-valine, and L-isoleucine). Anabol Naturals also produces free-form single amino acids.

• Amino Blend from Carlson Laboratories, a complex containing twenty amino acids, both essential and non-essential.

THE ABC'S OF AMINO ACIDS

Alanine

Alanine plays a major role in the transfer of nitrogen from peripheral tissue to the liver. It aids in the metabolism of glucose, a simple carbohydrate that the body uses for energy. It also guards against the buildup of toxic substances that are released in the muscle cells when muscle protein is broken down to quickly meet energy needs, such as happens with aerobic exercise. Epstein-Barr virus and chronic fatigue have been associated with excessive alanine levels and low levels of tyrosine and phenylalanine. One form of alanine, beta-alanine, is a constituent of pantothenic acid (vitamin B5) and coenzyme A, a vital catalyst in the body. Research has found that for people with insulin-dependent diabetes, taking an oral dose of L-alanine can be more effective than a conventional bedtime snack in preventing nighttime hypoglycemia.

Arginine

Arginine retards the growth of tumors and cancer by enhancing immune function. It increases the size and activity of the thymus gland, which manufactures T lymphocytes (T cells), crucial components of the immune system. Arginine may therefore benefit those suffering from AIDS and malignant diseases that suppress the immune system. It is also good for liver disorders such as cirrhosis of the liver and fatty liver; it aids in liver detoxification by neutralizing ammonia. It may reduce the effects of chronic alcohol toxicity. Seminal fluid contains arginine. Studies suggest that sexual maturity may be delayed by arginine deficiency; conversely, arginine is useful in treating sterility in men. It is found in high concentrations in the skin and connective tissues, making it helpful for healing and repair of damaged tissue.

Arginine is important for muscle metabolism. It helps to maintain a proper nitrogen balance by acting as a vehicle for transportation and storage, and aiding in the excretion of excess nitrogen. Studies have shown that it also reduces nitrogen losses in people who have undergone surgery, and improves the function of cells in lymphatic tissue. This amino acid aids in weight loss because it facilitates an increase in muscle mass and a reduction of body fat. It is also involved in a variety of enzymes and hormones. It aids in stimulating the pancreas to release insulin, is a component of the pituitary hormone vasopressin, and assists in the release of growth hormones. Because arginine is a component of collagen and aids in building new bone and tendon cells, it can be good for arthritis and connective tissue disorders. Scar tissue that forms during wound healing is made up of collagen, which is rich in arginine. A variety of functions, including insulin production, glucose tolerance, and liver lipid metabolism, are impaired if the body is deficient in arginine.

This amino acid can be produced in the body; however, in newborn infants, production may not occur quickly enough to keep up with requirements. It is therefore deemed essential early in life. Foods high in arginine include carob, chocolate, coconut, dairy products, gelatin, meat, oats, peanuts, soybeans, walnuts, white flour, wheat, and wheat germ.

People with viral infections such as herpes should *not* take supplemental arginine, and should avoid foods rich in arginine and low in the amino acid lysine (see below), as this appears to promote the growth of certain viruses. L-Arginine supplements should be avoided by pregnant and lactating women. Persons with schizophrenia should avoid amounts over 30 milligrams daily. Long-term use, especially of high doses, is not recommended. One study found that several weeks of large doses may result in thickening and coarsening of the skin.

Asparagine

Asparagine, created from another amino acid, aspartic acid, is needed to maintain balance in the central nervous system; it prevents you from being either overly nervous or overly calm. As it is converted back into aspartic acid, asparagine releases energy that brain and nervous system cells use for metabolism. It promotes the process by which one amino acid is transformed into another in the liver.

Aspartic Acid

Because aspartic acid increases stamina, it is good for fatigue and depression, and plays a vital role in metabolism. Chronic fatigue may result from low levels of aspartic acid, because this leads to lowered cellular energy. In proper balance, aspartic acid is beneficial for neural and brain disorders; it has been found in increased levels in persons with epilepsy and in decreased levels in people with some types of depression. It is good for athletes and helps to protect the liver by aiding in the removal of excess ammonia. Aspartic acid combines with other amino acids to form molecules that absorb toxins and remove them from the bloodstream. It helps to move certain minerals across the intestinal lining and into the blood and cells, aids cell function, and aids the function of RNA and DNA, which are the carriers of genetic information. It enhances the production of immunoglobulins and antibodies (immune system proteins). Plant protein, especially that found in sprouting seeds, contains an abundance of aspartic acid. The artificial sweetener aspartame is made from aspartic acid and phenylalanine, another amino acid.

Carnitine

Carnitine is not an amino acid in the strictest sense (it is actually a substance related to the B vitamins). However, because it has a chemical structure similar to that of amino acids, it is usually considered together with them.

Unlike true amino acids, carnitine is not used for protein synthesis or as a neurotransmitter. Its main function in the body is to help transport long-chain fatty acids, which are burned within the cells, mainly in the mitochondria, to provide energy. This is a major source of energy for the muscles. Carnitine thus increases the use of fat as an energy source. This prevents fatty buildup, especially in the heart, liver, and skeletal muscles. Carnitine may be useful in treating chronic fatigue syndrome (CFS), because a disturbance in the function of the mitochondria (the site of energy production within the cells) may be a factor in fatigue. Studies have shown decreased carnitine levels in many people with CFS.

Carnitine reduces the health risks posed by poor fat metabolism associated with diabetes; inhibits alcohol-induced fatty liver; and lessens the risk of heart disorders. Studies have shown that damage to the heart from cardiac surgery can be reduced by treatment with carnitine. According to *The American Journal of Cardiology,* one study showed that proprionyl-L-carnitine, a carnitine derivative, helps to ease the severe pain of intermittent claudication, a condition in which a blocked artery in the thigh decreases the supply of blood and oxygen to leg muscles, causing pain, especially with physical activity. Carnitine has the ability to lower blood triglyceride levels, aid in weight loss, improve the motility of sperm, and improve muscle strength in people with neuromuscular disorders. It may be useful in treating Alzheimer's disease. Conversely, carnitine deficiency may be a contributor to certain types of muscular dystrophy, and it has been shown that these disorders lead to losses of carnitine in the urine. People with such conditions need greater than normal amounts of carnitine. Carnitine also enhances the effectiveness of the antioxidant vitamins E and C. It works with antioxidants to help slow the aging process by promoting the synthesis of carnitine acetyl-transferease, an enzyme in the mitochondria of brain cells that is vital for the production of cellular energy there.

Carnitine can be manufactured by the body if sufficient amounts of iron, vitamin B_1 (thiamine), vitamin B_6 (pyridoxine), and the amino acids lysine and methionine are available. The synthesis of carnitine also depends on the presence of adequate levels of vitamin C. Inadequate intake of any of these nutrients can result in a carnitine deficiency. Carnitine can also be obtained from food, primarily meats and other foods of animal origin.

Many cases of carnitine deficiency have been identified as partly genetic in origin, resulting from an inherited defect in carnitine synthesis. Possible symptoms of deficiency include confusion, heart pain, muscle weakness, and obesity. Because of their generally greater muscle mass, men need more carnitine than women do. Vegetarians are more likely than nonvegetarians to be deficient in carnitine because it is not found in vegetable protein. Moreover, neither methionine nor lysine, two of the key constituents from which the body makes carnitine, are obtainable from vegetable sources in sufficient amounts. To ensure adequate production of carnitine, vegetarians should take supplements or should eat grains, such as cornmeal, that have been fortified with lysine.

Supplemental carnitine is available in different forms, including D-carnitine, L-carnitine, and DL-carnitine. DL-carnitine is not recommended, as it may cause toxicity. Acetyl-L-carnitine (ALC), a carnitine derivative produced naturally in the body, is involved in carbohydrate and protein metabolism and in the transport of fats into the mitochondria. It increases levels of carnitine in tissues and even surpasses the metabolic potency of carnitine. ALC has become one of the most studied compounds for its anti-aging effects, particularly with regard to degeneration of the brain and nervous system. Several major studies have shown that daily supplementation with ALC significantly slows the progression of Alzheimer's disease, resulting in less deterioration in memory, attention and language, and spatial abilities. It also can be used to treat other cognitive disorders, as well as depression.

ALC provides numerous other benefits to many of the body's systems. It helps to limit damage caused by oxygen starvation, enhance the immune system, protect against oxidative stress, stimulate the antioxidant activity of certain enzymes, protect membranes, slow cerebral aging, prevent nerve disease associated with diabetes and sciatica, modulate hormonal changes caused by physical stress, and increase the performance-enhancing benefits of branched-chain amino acids.

Total brain levels of ALC (and carnitine) decline with age. In most of the studies of ALC done with humans, subjects took 500 to 2,500 milligrams daily, in divided doses. No toxic or serious side effects have been reported.

Citrulline

The body makes citrulline from another amino acid, ornithine. Citrulline promotes energy, stimulates the immune system, is metabolized to form L-arginine, and detoxifies ammonia, which damages living cells. Citrulline is found primarily in the liver. It is helpful in treating fatigue.

Cysteine and Cystine

These two amino acids are closely related; each molecule of cystine consists of two molecules of cysteine joined together. Cysteine is very unstable and is easily converted to L-cystine; however, each form is capable of converting into the other as needed. Both are sulfur-containing amino acids that aid in the formation of skin and are important in detoxification.

Cysteine is present in alpha-keratin, the chief protein constituent of the fingernails, toenails, skin, and hair. Cysteine aids in the production of collagen and promotes the proper elasticity and texture of the skin. It is also found in a variety of other proteins in the body, including several of the digestive enzymes.

Cysteine helps to detoxify harmful toxins and protect the body from radiation damage. It is one of the best free radical destroyers, and works best when taken with selenium and vitamin E. Cysteine is also precursor to glutathione, a substance that detoxifies the liver by binding with potentially harmful substances there. It helps to protect the liver and brain from damage due to alcohol, drugs, and toxic compounds in cigarette smoke.

Since cysteine is more soluble than cystine, it is used more readily in the body and is usually best for treating most illnesses. This amino acid is formed from L-methionine in the body. Vitamin B_6, vitamin B_{12}, and folate are necessary for cysteine synthesis, which may not take place as it should in the presence of chronic disease. Therefore, people with chronic illnesses may need higher than normal doses of cysteine, as much as 1,000 milligrams three times daily for a month at a time.

Supplementation with L-cysteine is recommended in the treatment of rheumatoid arthritis, hardening of the arteries, and mutogenic disorders such as cancer. It promotes healing after surgery and severe burns, chelates heavy metals, and binds with soluble iron, aiding in iron absorption. This amino acid also promotes the burning of fat and the building of muscle. Because of its ability to break down mucus in the respiratory tract, L-cysteine is often beneficial in the treatment of bronchitis, emphysema, and tuberculosis. It promotes healing from respiratory disorders and plays an important role in the activity of white blood cells, which fight disease.

Cystine or the N-acetyl form of cysteine (N-acetylcysteine, or NAC) may be used in place of L-cysteine. NAC aids in preventing side effects from chemotherapy and radiation therapy. Because it increases glutathione levels in the lungs, kidneys, liver, and bone marrow, it has an anti-aging effect on the body—reducing the accumulation of age spots, for example. NAC has been shown to be more effective at boosting glutathione levels than supplements of cystine or even of glutathione itself.

People who have diabetes should be cautious about taking supplemental cysteine because it is capable of inactivating insulin. Persons with cystinuria, a rare genetic condition that leads to the formation of cystine kidney stones, should not take cysteine.

Gamma-Aminobutyric Acid

Gamma-aminobutyric acid (GABA) is an amino acid that acts as a neurotransmitter in the central nervous system. It is essential for brain metabolism, aiding in proper brain function. GABA is formed in the body from another amino acid, glutamic acid. Its function is to decrease neuron activity and inhibit nerve cells from overfiring. Together with niacinamide and inositol, it prevents anxiety- and stress-related messages from reaching the motor centers of the brain by occupying their receptor sites.

GABA can be taken to calm the body in much the same way as diazepam (Valium), chlordiazepoxide (Librium), and other tranquilizers, but without the fear of addiction. GABA has been used in the treatment of epilepsy and hypertension. It is good for depressed sex drive because of its ability as a relaxant. It is also useful for enlarged prostate, probably because it plays a role in the mechanism regulating the release of sex hormones. GABA is effective in treating attention deficit disorder and may reduce cravings for alcohol. It is also thought to promote growth hormone secretion.

Too much GABA, however, can cause increased anxiety, shortness of breath, numbness around the mouth, and tingling in the extremities. Further, abnormal levels of GABA unbalance the brain's message-delivery system and may cause seizures.

Glutamic Acid

Glutamic acid is an excitatory neurotransmitter that increases the firing of neurons in the central nervous system. It is a major excitatory neurotransmitter in the brain and spinal cord. It is converted into either glutamine or GABA.

This amino acid is important in the metabolism of sugars and fats, and aids in the transportation of potassium into the spinal fluid and across the blood-brain barrier. Although it does not pass the blood-brain barrier as readily as glutamine does, it is found at high levels in the blood and may infiltrate the brain in small amounts. The brain can use glutamic acid as fuel. Glutamic acid can detoxify ammonia by picking up nitrogen atoms, in the process creating another amino acid, glutamine. The conversion of glutamic acid into glutamine is the only means by which ammonia in the brain can be detoxified.

Glutamic acid helps to correct personality disorders and is useful in treating childhood behavioral disorders. It is used in the treatment of epilepsy, mental retardation, muscular dystrophy, ulcers, and hypoglycemic coma, a complication of insulin treatment for diabetes. It is a component of folate (folic acid), a B vitamin that helps the body break down amino acids. Because one of its salts is monosodium glutamate (MSG), glutamic acid should be avoided by anyone who is allergic to MSG.

Glutamine

Glutamine is the most abundant free amino acid found in the muscles of the body. Because it can readily pass the blood-brain barrier, it is known as brain fuel. In the brain, glutamine is converted into glutamic acid—which is essential for cerebral function—and vice versa. It also increases

the amount of GABA, which is needed to sustain proper brain function and mental activity. It assists in maintaining the proper acid/alkaline balance in the body, and is the basis of the building blocks for the synthesis of RNA and DNA. It promotes mental ability and the maintenance of a healthy digestive tract.

When an amino acid is broken down, nitrogen is released. The body needs nitrogen, but free nitrogen can form ammonia, which is especially toxic to brain tissues. The liver can convert nitrogen into urea, which is excreted in the urine, or nitrogen may attach itself to glutamic acid. This process forms glutamine. Glutamine is unique among the amino acids in that each molecule contains not one nitrogen atom but two. Thus, its creation helps to clear ammonia from the tissues, especially brain tissue, and it can transfer nitrogen from one place to another.

Glutamine is found in large amounts in the muscles and is readily available when needed for the synthesis of skeletal muscle proteins. Because this amino acid helps to build and maintain muscle, supplemental glutamine is useful for dieters and bodybuilders. More important, it helps to prevent the kind of muscle-wasting that can accompany prolonged bed rest or diseases such as cancer and AIDS. This is because stress and injury (including surgical trauma) cause the muscles to release glutamine into the bloodstream. In fact, during times of stress, as much as one third of the glutamine present in the muscles may be released. As a result, stress and/or illness can lead to the loss of skeletal muscle. If enough glutamine is available, however, this can be prevented.

Supplemental L-glutamine can be helpful in the treatment of arthritis, autoimmune diseases, fibrosis, intestinal disorders, peptic ulcers, connective tissue diseases such as polymyositis and scleroderma, and tissue damage due to radiation treatment for cancer. L-glutamine can enhance mental functioning and has been used to treat a range of problems, including developmental disabilities, epilepsy, fatigue, impotence, depression, schizophrenia, and senility. It preserves glutathione in the liver and protects that organ from the effects of acetaminophen overdose. It enhances antioxidant protection. L-glutamine decreases sugar cravings and the desire for alcohol, and is useful for recovering alcoholics.

Many plant and animal substances contain glutamine, but it is easily destroyed by cooking. If eaten raw, spinach and parsley are good sources. Supplemental glutamine must be kept absolutely dry or the powder will degrade into ammonia and pyroglutamic acid. Glutamine should *not* be taken by persons with cirrhosis of the liver, kidney problems, Reye's syndrome, or any type of disorder that can result in an accumulation of ammonia in the blood. For such individuals, taking supplemental glutamine may only cause further damage to the body. Be aware that although the names sound similar, glutamine, glutamic acid (also sometimes called glutamate), glutathione, gluten, and monosodium glutamate are all different substances.

Glutathione

Like carnitine, glutathione is not technically one of the amino acids. It is a compound classified as a tripeptide, and the body produces it from the amino acids cysteine, glutamic acid, and glycine. Because of its close relationship to these amino acids, however, it is usually considered together with them.

Glutathione is a powerful antioxidant that is produced in the liver. The largest stores of glutathione are found in the liver, where it detoxifies harmful compounds so that they can be excreted through the bile. Some glutathione is released from the liver directly into the bloodstream, where it helps to maintain the integrity of red blood cells and protect white blood cells. Glutathione is also found in the lungs and the intestinal tract. It is needed for carbohydrate metabolism and appears to exert anti-aging effects, aiding in the breakdown of oxidized fats that may contribute to atherosclerosis. It can mitigate some of the damage caused by tobacco smoke because it modifies the harmful effects of aldehydes, chemicals present in cigarette smoke that damage cells and molecules, and it may protect the liver from alcohol-induced damage.

A deficiency of glutathione first affects the nervous system, causing such symptoms as lack of coordination, mental disorders, tremors, and difficulty maintaining balance. These problems are believed to be due to the development of lesions in the brain. A study sponsored in part by the National Cancer Institute found that people with HIV disease who had low glutathione levels had a lower survival rate over a three-year period than those whose glutathione levels were normal. As we age, glutathione levels decline, although it is not known whether this is because we use it more rapidly or produce less of it to begin with. Unfortunately, if not corrected, the lack of glutathione in turn accelerates the aging process.

Supplemental glutathione is expensive, and the effectiveness of oral formulas is questionable. To raise glutathione levels, it is better to supply the body with the raw materials it uses to make this compound: cysteine, glutamic acid, and glycine. The N-acetyl form of cysteine, N-acetylcysteine (NAC), is considered particularly effective for this purpose.

Glycine

Glycine retards muscle degeneration by supplying additional creatine, a compound that is present in muscle tissue and is utilized in the construction of DNA and RNA. It improves glycogen storage, thus freeing up glucose for energy needs. Glycine is essential for the synthesis of nucleic acids, bile acids, and other nonessential amino acids in the body. It is used in many gastric antacid agents. Because high concentrations of glycine are found in the skin and connective tissues, it is useful for repairing damaged tissues and promoting healing.

Glycine is necessary for central nervous system function and a healthy prostate. It functions as an inhibitory neurotransmitter and as such can help prevent epileptic seizures. It has been used in the treatment of manic (bipolar) depression, and can also be effective for hyperactivity.

Having too much of this amino acid in the body can cause fatigue, but having the proper amount produces more energy. If necessary, glycine can be converted into the amino acid serine in the body.

Histidine

Histidine is an essential amino acid that is significant in the growth and repair of tissues. It is important for the maintenance of the myelin sheaths, which protect nerve cells, and is needed for the production of both red and white blood cells. Histidine also protects the body from radiation damage, helps lower blood pressure, aids in removing heavy metals from the system, and may help in the prevention of AIDS.

Histidine levels that are too high may lead to stress and even psychological disorders such as anxiety and schizophrenia; people with schizophrenia have been found to have high levels of histidine in their bodies. Inadequate levels of histidine may contribute to rheumatoid arthritis and may be associated with nerve deafness. Methionine has the ability to lower histidine levels.

Histamine, an important immune system chemical, is derived from histidine. Histamine aids in sexual arousal. Because the availability of histidine influences histamine production, taking supplemental histidine—together with vitamins B_3 (niacin) and B_6 (pyridoxine), which are required for the transformation from histidine to histamine—may help improve sexual functioning and pleasure. Because histamine also stimulates the secretion of gastric juices, histidine may be helpful for people with indigestion resulting from a lack of stomach acid.

Persons with manic (bipolar) depression should not take supplemental histidine unless a deficiency has been identified. Natural sources of histidine include rice, wheat, and rye.

Homocysteine

Homocysteine is an amino acid that is produced in the body in the course of methionine metabolism. This amino acid has been the focus of increasing attention in recent years, because high levels of homocysteine in the blood are associated with an increased risk of cardiovascular disease. Further, it is known that homocysteine has a toxic effect on cells lining the arteries, makes the blood more prone to clotting, and promotes the oxidation of low-density lipoproteins (LDL, the so-called "bad cholesterol"), which makes it more likely that cholesterol will be deposited as plaque in the blood vessels.

Like other amino acids, homocysteine does perform a necessary function in the body. It is then usually broken down quickly into the amino acid cysteine and other important compounds, including adenosine triphosphate (ATP, an important source of cellular energy) and S-adenosylmethionine (SAMe). However, a genetic defect or, more commonly, deficiencies of vitamins B_6 and B_{12} and folate (folic acid) can prevent homocysteine from converting rapidly enough. As a result, high levels of the amino acid accumulate in the body, damaging cell membranes and blood vessels, and increasing the risk of cardiovascular disease, particularly atherosclerosis. Vitamins B_6 and B_{12} and folate work together to facilitate the breakdown of homocysteine, and thus help protect against heart disease.

Isoleucine

Isoleucine, one of the essential amino acids, is needed for hemoglobin formation and also stabilizes and regulates blood sugar and energy levels. It is metabolized in muscle tissue. It is one of the three branched-chain amino acids. These amino acids are valuable for athletes because they enhance energy, increase endurance, and aid in the healing and repair of muscle tissue.

Isoleucine has been found to be deficient in people suffering from many different mental and physical disorders. A deficiency of isoleucine can lead to symptoms similar to those of hypoglycemia.

Food sources of isoleucine include almonds, cashews, chicken, chickpeas, eggs, fish, lentils, liver, meat, rye, most seeds, and soy protein. It is also available in supplemental form. Supplemental L-isoleucine should always be taken with a correct balance of the other two branched-chain amino acids, L-leucine and L-valine—approximately 2 milligrams each of leucine and valine for each milligram of isoleucine. Combination supplements that provide all three of the branched-chain amino acids are available and may be more convenient to use.

Leucine

Leucine is an essential amino acid and one of the branched-chain amino acids (the others are isoleucine and valine). These work together to protect muscle and act as fuel. They promote the healing of bones, skin, and muscle tissue, and are recommended for those recovering from surgery. Leucine also lowers elevated blood sugar levels and aids in increasing growth hormone production.

Natural sources of leucine include brown rice, beans, meat, nuts, soy flour, and whole wheat. Supplemental L-leucine must be taken in balance with L-isoleucine and L-valine (see Isoleucine in this section), and it should be taken in moderation, or symptoms of hypoglycemia may result. An excessively high intake of leucine may also contribute to pellagra, and may increase the amount of ammonia present in the body.

Lysine

Lysine is an essential amino acid that is a necessary building block for all protein. It is needed for proper growth and bone development in children; it helps calcium absorption and maintains a proper nitrogen balance in adults. This amino acid aids in the production of antibodies, hormones, and enzymes, and helps in collagen formation and tissue repair. Because it helps to build muscle protein, it is good for those recovering from surgery and sports injuries. It also lowers high serum triglyceride levels.

Another very useful ability of this amino acid is its capacity for fighting cold sores and herpesviruses. Taking supplemental L-lysine, together with vitamin C with bioflavonoids, can effectively fight and/or prevent herpes outbreaks, especially if foods containing the amino acid arginine are avoided (see HERPESVIRUS INFECTION in Part Two). Supplemental L-lysine also may decrease acute alcohol intoxication.

Lysine is an essential amino acid, and so cannot be manufactured in the body. It is therefore vital that adequate amounts be included in the diet. Deficiencies can result in anemia, bloodshot eyes, enzyme disorders, hair loss, an inability to concentrate, irritability, lack of energy, poor appetite, reproductive disorders, retarded growth, and weight loss. Food sources of lysine include cheese, eggs, fish, lima beans, milk, potatoes, red meat, soy products, and yeast.

Methionine

Methionine is an essential amino acid that assists in the breakdown of fats, thus helping to prevent a buildup of fat in the liver and arteries that might obstruct blood flow to the brain, heart, and kidneys. The synthesis of the amino acids cysteine and taurine may depend on the availability of methionine. This amino acid helps the digestive system; helps to detoxify harmful agents such as lead and other heavy metals; helps diminish muscle weakness, prevent brittle hair, and protect against radiation; and is beneficial for people with osteoporosis or chemical allergies. It is useful also in the treatment of rheumatic fever and toxemia of pregnancy.

Methionine is a powerful antioxidant. It is a good source of sulfur, which inactivates free radicals and helps to prevent skin and nail problems. It is also good for people with Gilbert's syndrome, an anomaly of liver function, and is required for the synthesis of nucleic acids, collagen, and proteins found in every cell of the body. It is beneficial for women who take oral contraceptives because it promotes the excretion of estrogen. It reduces the level of histamine in the body, which can be useful for people with schizophrenia, whose histamine levels are typically higher than normal.

As levels of toxic substances in the body increase, the need for methionine increases. The body can convert methionine into the amino acid cysteine, a precursor of glutathione. Methionine thus protects glutathione; it helps to prevent glutathione depletion if the body is overloaded with toxins. Since glutathione is a key neutralizer of toxins in the liver, this protects the liver from the damaging effects of toxic compounds.

An essential amino acid, methionine is not synthesized in the body and so must be obtained from food sources or from dietary supplements. Good food sources of methionine include beans, eggs, fish, garlic, lentils, meat, onions, soybeans, seeds, and yogurt. Because the body uses methionine to derive a brain food called choline, it is wise to supplement the diet with choline or lecithin (which is high in choline) to ensure that the supply of methionine is not depleted.

Ornithine

Ornithine helps to prompt the release of growth hormone, which promotes the metabolism of excess body fat. This effect is enhanced if ornithine is combined with arginine and carnitine. Ornithine is necessary for proper immune-system and liver function. This amino acid also detoxifies ammonia and aids in liver regeneration. High concentrations of ornithine are found in the skin and connective tissue, making it useful for promoting healing and repairing damaged tissues.

Ornithine is synthesized in the body from arginine, and in turn serves as the precursor of citrulline, proline, and glutamic acid. Supplemental L-ornithine should *not* be taken by children, pregnant women, nursing mothers, or anyone with a history of schizophrenia, unless they are specifically directed to do so by a physician.

Phenylalanine

Phenylalanine is an essential amino acid. Because it can cross the blood-brain barrier, it can have a direct effect on brain chemistry. Once in the body, phenylalanine can be converted into another amino acid, tyrosine, which in turn is used to synthesize two key neurotransmitters that promote alertness: dopamine and norepinephrine. Because of its relationship to the action of the central nervous system, this amino acid can elevate mood, decrease pain, aid in memory and learning, and suppress the appetite. It can be used to treat arthritis, depression, menstrual cramps, migraines, obesity, Parkinson's disease, and schizophrenia.

Phenylalanine is available in three different forms, designated L-, D-, and DL-. The L- form is the most common type and is the form in which phenylalanine is incorporated into the body's proteins. The D- type acts as a painkiller. The DL- form is a combination of the D- and the L-. Like the D-form, it is effective for controlling pain, especially the pain of arthritis; like the L- form, it functions as a building block for proteins, increases mental alertness, suppresses the appetite, and helps people with Parkinson's disease. It has been used to alleviate the symptoms of premenstrual syndrome (PMS) and various types of chronic pain.

Supplemental phenylalanine, as well as products containing aspartame (an artificial sweetener made from phenylalanine and another amino acid, aspartic acid) should *not* be taken by pregnant women or by people who suffer from anxiety attacks, diabetes, high blood pressure, phenylketonuria (PKU), or preexisting pigmented melanoma, a type of skin cancer.

Proline

Proline improves skin texture by aiding in the production of collagen and reducing the loss of collagen through the aging process. It also helps in the healing of cartilage and the strengthening of joints, tendons, and heart muscle. It works with vitamin C to promote healthy connective tissue. Proline is obtained primarily from meat sources, dairy products, and eggs.

Serine

Serine is needed for the proper metabolism of fats and fatty acids, the growth of muscle, and the maintenance of a healthy immune system. It is a component of brain proteins and the protective myelin sheaths that cover nerve fibers. It is important in RNA and DNA function, cell membrane formation, and creatine synthesis. It also aids in the production of immunoglobulins and antibodies. However, too-high serine levels in the body may have adverse effects on the immune system.

Serine can be made from glycine in the body, but this process requires the presence of sufficient amounts of vitamins B_3 and B_6 and folic acid. Food sources of serine include meat and soy foods, as well as many foods that often cause allergic reactions, such as dairy products, wheat gluten, and peanuts. It is included as a natural moisturizing agent in many cosmetics and skin care preparations.

Taurine

High concentrations of taurine are found in the heart muscle, white blood cells, skeletal muscle, and central nervous system. It is a building block of all the other amino acids as well as a key component of bile, which is needed for the digestion of fats, the absorption of fat-soluble vitamins, and the control of serum cholesterol levels. Taurine can be useful for people with atherosclerosis, edema, heart disorders, hypertension, or hypoglycemia. It is vital for the proper utilization of sodium, potassium, calcium, and magnesium, and it has been shown to play a particular role in sparing the loss of potassium from the heart muscle. This helps to prevent the development of potentially dangerous cardiac arrhythmias.

Taurine has a protective effect on the brain, particularly if the brain is dehydrated. It is used to treat anxiety, epilepsy, hyperactivity, poor brain function, and seizures. Taurine is found in concentrations up to four times greater in the brains of children than in those of adults. It may be that a deficiency of taurine in the developing brain is involved in seizures. Zinc deficiency also is commonly found in people with epilepsy, and this may play a part in the deficiency of taurine. Taurine is also associated with zinc in maintaining eye function; a deficiency of both may impair vision. Taurine supplementation may benefit children with Down syndrome and muscular dystrophy. This amino acid is also used in some clinics for breast cancer treatment.

Excessive losses of taurine through the urine can be caused by many metabolic disorders. Cardiac arrhythmias, disorders of platelet formation, intestinal problems, an overgrowth of candida, physical or emotional stress, a zinc deficiency, and excessive consumption of alcohol are all associated with high urinary losses of taurine. Excessive alcohol consumption also causes the body to lose its ability to utilize taurine properly. Taurine supplementation may reduce symptoms of alcohol withdrawal. Diabetes increases the body's requirements for taurine; conversely, supplementation with taurine and cystine may decrease the need for insulin.

Taurine is found in eggs, fish, meat, and milk, but not in vegetable proteins. It can be synthesized from cysteine in the liver and from methionine elsewhere in the body, as long as sufficient quantities of vitamin B_6 are present. For vegetarians, synthesis by the body is crucial. For individuals with genetic or metabolic disorders that prevent the synthesis of taurine, taurine supplementation is required.

Threonine

Threonine is an essential amino acid that helps to maintain the proper protein balance in the body. It is important for the formation of collagen, elastin, and tooth enamel, and aids liver and lipotropic function when combined with aspartic acid and methionine. A precursor of the amino acids glycine and serine, threonine is present in the heart, central nervous system, and skeletal muscle, and helps to prevent fatty buildup in the liver. It enhances the immune system by aiding in the production of antibodies, and may be helpful in treating some types of depression.

Because the threonine content of grains is low, vegetarians are more likely than others to have deficiencies.

Tryptophan

Tryptophan is an essential amino acid that is necessary for the production of vitamin B_3 (niacin). It is used by the brain to produce serotonin, a necessary neurotransmitter that transfers nerve impulses from one cell to another and is responsible for normal sleep. Consequently, tryptophan helps to combat depression and insomnia and to stabilize moods. It helps to control hyperactivity in children, alleviates stress, is good for the heart, aids in weight control by reducing appetite, and enhances the release of growth hormone. It is good for migraine headaches and may reduce some of the effects of nicotine. Sufficient amounts of vita-

mins B_6 (pyridoxine) and C, folate, and magnesium are necessary for the formation of tryptophan, which, in turn, is required for the formation of serotonin. A study reported in the *Archives of General Psychiatry* found that women with a history of bulimia nervosa, an eating disorder, experienced relapses after they took an amino acid mixture lacking tryptophan. Researchers believe that insufficient tryptophan altered brain serotonin levels and, consequently, the transmission of nerve impulses. A lack of tryptophan and magnesium may contribute to coronary artery spasms.

The best dietary sources of tryptophan include brown rice, cottage cheese, meat, peanuts, and soy protein. This amino acid is not available in supplement form in the United States. In November of 1989, the U.S. Centers for Disease Control (CDC) reported evidence linking L-tryptophan supplements to a blood disorder called eosinophilia-myalgia syndrome (EMS). Several hundred cases of this illness—which is characterized by an elevated white blood cell count and can also cause such symptoms as fatigue, muscular pain, respiratory ailments, edema, and rash—were reported. After the CDC established an association between the blood disorder and products containing L-tryptophan in New Mexico, the U.S. Food and Drug Administration (FDA) first warned consumers to stop taking L-tryptophan supplements, then recalled all products in which L-tryptophan was the sole or a major component. Subsequent research showed that it was contaminants in the supplements, *not* the tryptophan, that was probably responsible for the problem, but tryptophan supplements are still banned from the market in the United States. According to the FDA, at least thirty-eight deaths were attributable to the tryptophan supplements.

Tyrosine

Tyrosine is important to overall metabolism. It is a precursor of adrenaline and the neurotransmitters norepinephrine and dopamine, which regulate mood and stimulate metabolism and the nervous system. Tyrosine acts as a mood elevator; a lack of adequate amounts of tyrosine leads to a deficiency of norepinephrine in the brain, which in turn can result in depression. It also acts as a mild antioxidant, suppresses the appetite, and helps to reduce body fat. It aids in the production of melanin (the pigment responsible for skin and hair color) and in the functions of the adrenal, thyroid, and pituitary glands. It is also involved in the metabolism of the amino acid phenylalanine.

Tyrosine attaches to iodine atoms to form active thyroid hormones. Not surprisingly, therefore, low plasma levels of tyrosine have been associated with hypothyroidism. Symptoms of tyrosine deficiency can also include low blood pressure, low body temperature (such as cold hands and feet), and restless leg syndrome.

Supplemental L-tyrosine has been used for stress reduction, and research suggests it may be helpful against chronic fatigue and narcolepsy. It has been used to help individuals suffering from anxiety, depression, low sex drive, allergies, and headaches, as well as persons undergoing withdrawal from drugs. It may also help people with Parkinson's disease.

Natural sources of tyrosine include almonds, avocados, bananas, dairy products, lima beans, pumpkin seeds, and sesame seeds. Tyrosine can also be produced from phenylalanine in the body. Supplements of L-tyrosine should be taken at bedtime or with a high-carbohydrate meal so that it does not have to compete for absorption with other amino acids.

Persons taking monoamine oxidase (MAO) inhibitors, commonly prescribed for depression, must strictly limit their intake of foods containing tyrosine and should *not* take any supplements containing L-tyrosine, as it may lead to a sudden and dangerous rise in blood pressure. Anyone who takes prescription medication for depression should discuss necessary dietary restrictions with his or her physician.

Valine

Valine, an essential amino acid, has a stimulant effect. It is needed for muscle metabolism, tissue repair, and the maintenance of a proper nitrogen balance in the body. Valine is found in high concentrations in muscle tissue. It is one of the branched-chain amino acids, which means that it can be used as an energy source by muscle tissue. It may be helpful in treating liver and gallbladder disease, and it is good for correcting the type of severe amino acid deficiencies that can be caused by drug addiction. An excessively high level of valine may lead to such symptoms as a crawling sensation in the skin and even hallucinations.

Dietary sources of valine include dairy products, grains, meat, mushrooms, peanuts, and soy protein. Supplemental L-valine should always be taken in balance with the other branched-chain amino acids, L-isoleucine and L-leucine (*see* Isoleucine in this section).

ANTIOXIDANTS

INTRODUCTION

Antioxidants are natural compounds that help protect the body from harmful free radicals. These are atoms or groups of atoms that can cause damage to cells, impairing the immune system and leading to infections and various degenerative diseases such as heart disease and cancer. Antioxidants therefore play a beneficial role in the prevention of disease. Free radical damage is thought by scientists to be the basis for the aging process as well. (*See* Free Radicals on page 54.)

There are a number of known free radicals that occur in the body, the most common of which are oxygen-derived free radicals, such as superoxide radicals and hydroxyl radicals, hypochlorite radicals, hydrogen peroxide, various lipid peroxides, and nitric oxide. They may be formed by exposure to radiation, including exposure to the sun's rays; exposure to toxic chemicals such as those found in cigarette smoke, polluted air, and industrial and household chemicals; and various metabolic processes, such as the process of breaking down stored fat molecules for use as an energy source.

Free radicals are normally kept in check by the action of *free radical scavengers* that occur naturally in the body. These scavengers neutralize the free radicals. Certain enzymes serve this vital function. Four important enzymes that neutralize free radicals are superoxide dismutase (SOD), methionine reductase, catalase, and glutathione peroxidase. The body makes these as a matter of course. There are also a number of phytochemicals and nutrients that act as antioxidants, including vitamin A, beta-carotene and other carotenoids, flavonoids, vitamins C and E, and the mineral selenium. Another antioxidant is the hormone melatonin, which is a powerful free radical neutralizer. Certain herbs have antioxidant properties as well.

Although many antioxidants can be obtained from food sources such as sprouted grains and fresh fruits and vegetables, it is difficult to get enough of them from these sources to hold back the free radicals constantly being generated in our polluted environment. We can minimize free radical damage by taking supplements of key nutrients. A high intake of antioxidant nutrients appears to be especially protective against cancer.

Antioxidants work synergistically in giving protection against free radical damage, so it is better to take smaller doses of several different antioxidants than a large amount of only one. For example, while beta-carotene by itself is an excellent antioxidant, a mix of natural carotenoids provides more health benefits than beta-carotene alone. There are many good combination formulas available that make it easy to take multiple antioxidants every day.

THE ANTIOXIDANTS

Alpha-Lipoic Acid

Alpha-lipoic acid (ALA) is a powerful antioxidant—both on its own and as a "recycler" of vitamin E and vitamin C. It can restore the antioxidant properties of these vitamins after they have neutralized free radicals. ALA also stimulates the body's production of glutathione and aids in the absorption of coenzyme Q_{10}, both important antioxidants. Because ALA is soluble in both water and fat, it can move into all parts of cells to deactivate free radicals.

Supplemental ALA has been used for almost three decades in Europe to treat peripheral nerve degeneration and to help control blood sugar levels in people with diabetes. It also helps to detoxify the liver of metal pollutants, block cataract formation, protect nerve tissues against oxidative stress, and reduce blood cholesterol levels. According to Lester Packer, Ph.D., Professor of Molecular and Cell Biology at the University of California—Berkeley and a leading antioxidant researcher, ALA could play an important role in the prevention and treatment of chronic degenerative diseases such as diabetes and cardiovascular disease. ALA is known also as a metabolic antioxidant, because without it, cells cannot use sugar to produce energy. The body does not produce large amounts of ALA, and since it is found primarily in only a few foods, including spinach, broccoli, and organ meats, supplementation may be necessary.

Bilberry

The herb bilberry (*Vaccinium myrtillus*), a European relative of the American blueberry, contains natural antioxidants that keep capillary walls strong and flexible. They also help to maintain the flexibility of the walls of red blood cells and allow them to pass through the capillaries better. Bilberry contains anthocyanidins, phytochemicals that help to lower blood pressure, inhibit clot formation, and enhance blood supply to the nervous system. Studies indicate that anthocyanidins can provide up to fifty times the antioxidant protection of vitamin E and ten times the protection of vitamin C. In addition, this herb protects the eyes and may enhance

Free Radicals

A free radical is an atom or group of atoms that contains at least one unpaired electron. Electrons are negatively charged particles that usually occur in pairs, forming a chemically stable arrangement. If an electron is unpaired, another atom or molecule can easily bond with it, causing a chemical reaction. Because they join so readily with other compounds, free radicals can effect dramatic changes in the body, and they can cause a lot of oxidative damage. Each free radical may exist for only a tiny fraction of a second, but the damage it leaves behind can be irreversible, particularly damage to heart muscle cells, nerve cells, and certain immune system sensor cells.

Free radicals are normally present in the body in small numbers. Biochemical processes naturally lead to the formation of free radicals, and under normal circumstances the body can keep them in check. Indeed, not all free radicals are bad. Free radicals produced by the immune system destroy viruses and bacteria. Other free radicals are involved in producing vital hormones and activating enzymes that are needed for life. We need free radicals to produce energy and various substances that the body requires. If there is excessive free radical formation, however, damage to cells and tissues can occur. The formation of a large number of free radicals stimulates the formation of more free radicals, leading to even more damage.

Many different factors can lead to an excess of free radicals. Exposure to radiation, whether from the sun or from medical x-rays, activates the formation of free radicals, as does exposure to environmental pollutants such as tobacco smoke and automobile exhaust. Diet also can contribute to the formation of free radicals. When the body obtains nutrients through the diet, it utilizes oxygen and these nutrients to create energy. In this oxidation process, oxygen molecules containing unpaired electrons are released. These oxygen free radicals can cause damage to the body if produced in extremely large amounts. A diet that is high in fat can increase free radical activity because oxidation occurs more readily in fat molecules than it does in carbohydrate or protein molecules. Cooking fats at high temperatures, particularly frying foods in oil, can produce large numbers of free radicals.

The presence of a dangerous number of free radicals can alter the way in which the cells code genetic material. Changes in protein structure can occur as a result of errors in protein synthesis. The body's immune system may then see this altered protein as a foreign substance and try to destroy it. The formation of mutated proteins can eventually damage the immune system and lead to leukemia and other types of cancer, as well as to many other diseases.

In addition to damaging genetic material, free radicals can destroy the protective cell membranes. Calcium levels in the body may be upset as well. Over time, the body produces more free radicals than it does scavengers. The resulting imbalance is what causes us to age.

Substances known as antioxidants neutralize free radicals by binding to their free electrons. Antioxidants available in supplement form include the enzymes superoxide dismutase and glutathione peroxidase; vitamin A, beta-carotene, and vitamins C and E; the minerals selenium and zinc; and the hormone melatonin. By destroying free radicals, antioxidants help to detoxify and protect the body.

---

vision; supports and strengthens collagen structures; inhibits the growth of bacteria; acts as an anti-inflammatory; and has anti-aging and anticarcinogenic effects. Tests have shown that the compound glucoquinine, found in bilberry leaves, helps to lower blood sugar levels.

Burdock

The herb burdock (*Arctium lappa*) was tested by researchers at the Chia Nan College of Pharmacy and Science in Taiwan for its antioxidant properties. They found that burdock is a powerful antioxidant, capable of scavenging hydrogen peroxide and superoxide radicals. It also showed a marked scavenging effect against hydroxyl radicals. The study showed also that burdock and vitamin E quench more free radicals when used in combination. Burdock also protects against cancer by helping to control cell mutation.

Carotenoids

See under Vitamin A and the Carotenoids.

Coenzyme Q_{10}

Coenzyme Q_{10} is an antioxidant that is structurally similar to vitamin E. It plays a crucial role in the generation of cellular energy, is a significant immunologic stimulant, increases circulation, has anti-aging effects, and is beneficial for the cardiovascular system. Also known as *ubiquinone* (from *quinone*, a type of coenzyme, and *ubiquitous*, because it exists everywhere in the body), coenzyme Q_{10} is found in highest concentrations in the heart, followed by the liver, kidney, spleen, and pancreas. Within the mitochondria, the cells' energy-production centers, coenzyme Q_{10} helps to metabolize fats and carbohydrates. It also helps to maintain the flexibility of cell membranes.

In Japan, coenzyme Q_{10} has been approved for use in treating congestive heart failure. Various research reports suggest that coenzyme Q_{10} also may be beneficial in treating cancer, AIDS, muscular dystrophy, allergies, gastric ulcers, myopathy, periodontal disease, diabetes, and deafness.

Curcumin (Turmeric)

Found in the spice turmeric, the phytochemical curcumin has antioxidant properties that prevent the formation of and neutralize existing free radicals. It stops precancerous changes within DNA and interferes with enzymes necessary for cancer progression. Curcumin stops the oxidation of cholesterol, thus protecting against the formation of plaque in the arteries. In a study of chronic smokers, those who took curcumin excreted a substantially lower level of mutagens (substances that induce cells to mutate) in their urine, a reflection of how well the body is dealing with these cancer-causing substances. Curcumin also blocks toxic compounds from reaching or reacting with body tissues, and may prevent cataracts.

Curcumin should not be taken by anyone who has biliary tract obstruction or is taking anticoagulants, as curcumin stimulates bile secretion and acts as a blood-thinner.

Flavonoids

Flavonoids are especially potent antioxidants and metal chelators. They are chemical compounds that plants produce to protect themselves from parasites, bacteria, and cell injury. More than 4,000 chemically unique flavonoids are known; they occur in fruits, vegetables, spices, seeds, nuts, flowers, and bark. Wine (particularly red wine), apples, blueberries, bilberries, onions, soy products, and tea are some of the best food sources of flavonoids. Certain flavonoids in fruits and vegetables have much greater antioxidant activity than vitamins C and E or beta-carotene. In fact, flavonoids protect the antioxidant vitamins from oxidative damage.

Numerous medicinal herbs contain therapeutic amounts of flavonoids; they often are a major component of an herb's medicinal activity.

Garlic

This versatile healing herb also has antioxidant properties. The sulfhydryl (sulfur and hydrogen) compounds in garlic are potent chelators of toxic heavy metals, binding with them so that they can be excreted. These same compounds are effective protectants against oxidation and free radicals. Garlic aids in the detoxification of peroxides such as hydrogen peroxide and helps to prevent fats from being oxidized and deposited in tissues and arteries. Garlic also contains antioxidant nutrients such as vitamins A and C and selenium.

Studies on aged garlic extract (AGE) have shown that the aging process substantially boosts garlic's antioxidant potential. AGE protects against DNA damage, keeps blood vessels healthy, and guards against radiation and sunlight damage. According to researcher and nutritionist Robert I-San Lin, Ph.D., aged garlic extract can prevent liver damage caused by carbon tetrachloride, a common indoor pollutant and free radical generator. Overall, aged garlic supplements provide a greater concentration of garlic's beneficial compounds. If you're worried about "garlic breath" putting a strain on your social life, choose an odorless and tasteless form such as Kyolic aged garlic extract from Wakunaga of America. Aged garlic extract reduces blood cholesterol levels, thus lowering the risk of heart attack; provides protection from heart disease by preventing clots that can lead to heart attacks and strokes; and helps lower high blood pressure.

Ginkgo Biloba

Ginkgo biloba is an herb with powerful antioxidant effects in the brain, retina, and cardiovascular system. It is well known for its ability to enhance circulation, and a study reported in the *Journal of the American Medical Association* showed that it has a measurable effect on dementia in people with Alzheimer's disease and people recovering from strokes. Other studies indicate that it can improve both long- and short-term memory, and enhance concentration. Gingko biloba has also been used to treat hearing problems, impotence, and macular degeneration.

Anyone who takes prescription anticoagulant (blood-thinning) medication or who uses over-the-counter pain-killers regularly should consult a health care provider before using gingko biloba, as the combination may result in internal bleeding.

Glutathione

Glutathione is a protein that is produced in the liver from the amino acids cysteine, glutamic acid, and glycine. It is a powerful antioxidant that inhibits the formation of, and protects against cellular damage from, free radicals. It helps to defend the body against damage from cigarette smoking, exposure to radiation, cancer chemotherapy, and toxins such as alcohol. As a detoxifier of heavy metals and drugs, it aids in the treatment of blood and liver disorders.

Glutathione protects cells in several ways. It neutralizes oxygen molecules before they can harm cells. Together with selenium, it forms the enzyme glutathione peroxidase, which neutralizes hydrogen peroxide. It is also a component of another antioxidant enzyme, glutathione-S-transferase, which is a broad-spectrum liver-detoxifying enzyme.

Glutathione protects not only individual cells but also the tissues of the arteries, brain, heart, immune cells, kidneys, lenses of the eyes, liver, lungs, and skin against oxidant damage. It plays a role in preventing cancer, especially liver cancer, and may actually target carcinogens, make them water-soluble, and then help escort them from the body. It may also have an anti-aging effect. The rate at which we age is directly correlated with reduced concentrations of glutathione in cellular fluids; as we grow older, glutathione levels drop, resulting in a decreased ability to deactivate free radicals.

Glutathione can be taken in supplement form. The production of glutathione by the body can be boosted by taking supplemental dehydroepiandrosterone (DHEA), a hormone; N-acetylcysteine or L-cysteine; and L-methionine. Studies suggest that this may be a better way of raising glutathione levels than taking glutathione itself.

Grape Seed Extract

See under Oligomeric Proanthocyanidins in this section.

Green Tea

Green tea contains compounds known as polyphenols, including phytochemicals that have antioxidant, antibacterial, antiviral, and health-enhancing properties. Tests on epigallocatechin gallate (EGCG), a particular type of polyphenol in green tea, have shown that it is able to penetrate the body's cells and shield DNA from hydrogen peroxide, a potent free radical. Green tea protects against cancer, lowers cholesterol levels, and reduces the clotting tendency of the blood. It also shows promise as a weight-loss aid that can promote the burning of fat and help to regulate blood sugar and insulin levels.

Green tea is simply the dried leaves of the tea plant. Black tea undergoes natural fermentation, which converts tannins, astringent phytochemicals, into more complex compounds. This fermentation process destroys most of black tea's polyphenols, rendering it less effective as an antioxidant.

Melatonin

The hormone melatonin is an efficient free radical scavenger and singlet oxygen quencher. Singlet oxygen is an "excited" oxygen molecule whose excessive discharge of energy causes damage to other body molecules. While most antioxidants work only in certain parts of certain cells, melatonin can permeate any cell in any part of the body. More important, melatonin is one of the few antioxidants that can penetrate the mitochondria, the cells' "power plants," which produce energy. Melatonin does seem to protect the mitochondria from free radical damage. In laboratory experiments, melatonin supplementation has been found to extend the lifespan of mice. Other non-human laboratory studies have shown that supplemental melatonin can inhibit cancer growth, help modulate the immune system, and protect against degenerative diseases. Melatonin also stimulates the enzyme glutathione peroxidase, another antioxidant.

Methionine

A unique amino acid, methionine neutralizes hydroxyl radicals, one of the most dangerous types of free radicals. Most often a byproduct of reactions between heavy metals and

less toxic free radicals, hydroxyl radicals can be formed also during strenuous exercise or exposure to high levels of radiation, and can damage any type of body tissue.

N-Acetylcysteine (NAC)

The sulfur-containing amino acid cysteine is needed to produce the free radical fighter glutathione and to help maintain it at adequate levels in the cells. N-acetylcysteine (NAC) is a more stable form of cysteine that can be taken in supplement form.

NAC is used by the liver and the lymphocytes to detoxify chemicals and other poisons. It is a powerful detoxifier of alcohol, tobacco smoke, and environmental pollutants, all of which are immune suppressors. Taking supplemental NAC can boost the levels of protective enzymes in the body, thus slowing some of the cellular damage that is characteristic of aging. NAC supplementation may also decrease both the frequency and duration of infectious diseases. It has been used to treat AIDS and chronic bronchitis.

People with diabetes should not take supplemental NAC without first consulting a health care provider, as it can interfere with the effectiveness of insulin.

Nicotinamide Adenine Dinucleotide (NADH)

Also known as coenzyme 1, nicotinamide adenine dinucleotide with high-energy hydrogen, or NADH, is the "spark" that ignites energy production in the body's cells. NADH's high antioxidant capacity derives from its ability to reduce levels of substances. NADH plays a central role in DNA repair and maintenance, and in the cellular immune defense system. Studies report that NADH also can inhibit the auto-oxidation of the neurotransmitter dopamine, which causes the release of toxic chemicals that may damage sensitive parts of the brain.

Oligomeric Proanthocyanidins

Oligomeric proanthocyanidins (OPCs) are naturally occurring substances present in a variety of food and botanical sources. They are unique phytochemicals known as flavonoids that have powerful antioxidant capabilities. OPCs are highly water soluble, so the body is able to absorb them rapidly. Clinical tests suggest that OPCs may be as much as fifty times more potent than vitamin E and twenty times more potent than vitamin C in terms of bioavailable antioxidant activity. What's more, OPCs work with the antioxidant glutathione to recycle and restore oxidized vitamin C, thus increasing the vitamin's effectiveness. Because they are able to cross the blood-brain barrier, OPCs can protect the brain and spinal nerves against free radical damage. In addition to their antioxidant activity, OPCs protect the liver from damage caused by toxic doses of acetaminophen, a non-prescription pain reliever; they strengthen and repair connective tissue, including that of the cardiovascular system; and they support the immune system and slow aging. They also moderate allergic and inflammatory responses by reducing histamine production.

OPCs are found throughout plant life; however, the two main sources are pine bark extract (Pycnogenol), produced from the French maritime pine tree, and grape seed extract, made from the seeds of the wine grape (*Vitis vinifera*). Pycnogenol was the first source of OPCs discovered, and the process for extracting it was patented in the 1950s. Pycnogenol is a trademarked name for pine bark extract, not a generic term for OPCs from other sources.

Pycnogenol

See under Oligomeric Proanthocyanidins in this section.

Selenium

Selenium is an essential trace mineral that functions as an antioxidant in partnership with vitamin E to protect tissues and cell membranes. Among other things, it increases antioxidant enzyme levels in cells. Selenium is also an integral component of the antioxidant enzyme glutathione peroxidase (each molecule of this enzyme contains four atoms of selenium). Glutathione peroxidase targets harmful hydrogen peroxide in the body and converts it into water. It is a particularly important guardian of blood cells and of the heart, liver, and lungs.

Numerous plants contain selenium, including garlic, asparagus, and grains, but the levels depend on soil content, which varies from one geographic region to another.

Use caution when taking supplemental selenium. Amounts higher than 1,000 micrograms (1 milligram) daily may be toxic.

Silymarin

Extracted from the seeds of the herb milk thistle, silymarin has been used for centuries to treat liver disease. The active ingredients in milk thistle are several types of flavonoids (powerful antioxidants), known collectively as silymarin. Silymarin guards the liver from oxidative damage. It also protects the liver from toxins, drugs, and the effects of alcohol, and promotes the growth of new liver cells. In addition, silymarin increases levels of glutathione, a potent antioxidant enzyme produced in the liver.

Superoxide Dismutase

Superoxide dismutase (SOD) is an enzyme. SOD revitalizes cells and reduces the rate of cell destruction. It neutralizes the most common, and possibly the most dangerous, free radicals—superoxide radicals. Superoxide radicals instigate the breakdown of synovial fluid, the lubricant for the body's joints. This leads to friction and, ultimately, inflammation. SOD works synergistically with the enzyme catalase, which is abundant throughout the body. Catalase removes hydrogen peroxide byproducts created by SOD reactions.

SOD also aids in the body's utilization of zinc, copper, and manganese. Its levels tend to decline with age, while free radical production increases. Its potential as an anti-aging treatment is currently being explored.

Chemically speaking, there are two forms of this enzyme. The copper/zinc form (known as Cu/Zn SOD) exerts its antioxidant properties in the cytoplasm of cells. This is the watery fluid that surrounds all the other cellular components. Metabolic activity that takes place in the cytoplasm results in the production of free radicals; Cu/Zn neutralizes them. The manganese form (Mn SOD) is active in the mitochondria, structures within cells where energy is produced. The production of cellular energy also leads to the creation of free radicals.

SOD occurs naturally in barley grass, broccoli, Brussels sprouts, cabbage, wheatgrass, and most green plants. It is also available in supplement form. SOD supplements in pill form must be enteric coated—that is, coated with a protective substance that allows the pill to pass intact through the stomach acid into the small intestines to be absorbed. Cell Guard from Biotec Food Corporation and KAL SOD-3 from Nutraceutical International Corporation are good sources of SOD.

Vitamin A and the Carotenoids

A class of phytochemicals, carotenoids are fat-soluble pigments found in yellow, red, green, and orange vegetables and fruits. They are a potent family of antioxidants that include alpha-carotene, beta-carotene, lycopene, lutein, and zeaxanthin. Of the more than 500 carotenoids found in nature, about 50 can be converted into vitamin A in the body.

Carotenoids quench singlet oxygen, which is not, chemically speaking, a free radical, but is nevertheless highly reactive and can damage body molecules. Carotenoids also act as anticancer agents, decrease the risk of cataracts and age-related macular degeneration, and inhibit heart disease. Studies have shown that carotenoids found in tomato juice (lycopene), carrots (alpha- and beta-carotene) and spinach (lutein) may help to protect against cancer by reducing oxidative and other damage to DNA.

Together, the antioxidants alpha-lipoic acid, coenzyme Q_{10}, vitamin C, and vitamin E help conserve carotenoids in tissues.

The body converts beta-carotene into vitamin A as needed. Any leftover beta-carotene then acts as an antioxidant, breaking free radical chain reactions and preventing the oxidation of cholesterol. It reduces the oxidation of DNA and disables reactive oxygen species molecules generated by exposure to sunlight and air pollution, preventing damage to eyes, lungs, and skin.

A recent laboratory study found that taking high doses

of supplemental of beta-carotene alone (50,000 international units or more daily) may interfere with the normal control of cell division. It is best to take a carotenoid complex containing a variety of carotenoids.

Vitamin C

Vitamin C is a very powerful antioxidant that also recharges other antioxidants, such as vitamin E, to keep them potent. Its water solubility makes it an efficient free radical scavenger in body fluids. Some studies have shown that vitamin C is the first line of antioxidant defense in plasma against many different kinds of free radicals. The cells of the brain and spinal cord, which frequently incur free radical damage, can be protected by significant amounts of vitamin C. This vitamin also guards against atherosclerosis by preventing damage to artery walls. Vitamin C acts as a more potent free radical scavenger in the presence of the phytochemical hesperidin.

Vitamin E

Vitamin E is a powerful antioxidant that prevents the oxidation of lipids (fats). Fat oxidation has been implicated in the process that leads to atherosclerosis. Vitamin E is fat soluble and, since cell membranes are composed of lipids, it effectively prevents the cells' protective coatings from becoming rancid as a result of the assault of free radicals. Vitamin E also improves oxygen utilization, enhances immune response, plays a role in the prevention of cataracts caused by free radical damage, and may reduce the risk of coronary artery disease.

The natural form of vitamin E (d-alpha tocopherol) is superior to the synthetic version (dl-alpha tocopherol). New evidence suggests that zinc is needed to maintain normal blood concentrations of vitamin E. Selenium enhances vitamin E uptake. These two nutrients work together in the body.

Zinc

Zinc's main antioxidant function is in the prevention of fat oxidation. In addition, it is a constituent of the antioxidant enzyme superoxide dismutase (SOD). Zinc is also needed for proper maintenance of vitamin E levels in the blood and aids in the absorption of vitamin A.

Combination Antioxidant Supplements

No single antioxidant protects all body systems; rather, each one has protective properties for particular body parts or functions. Products that combine two or more of these vital nutrients are available. You can easily find formulas that give you a balance of multiple antioxidants. Some recommended antioxidant combination products include the following:

- ACES + Zinc and ACES + Selenium from Carlson Laboratories.
- Advanced Carotenoid Complex from Solgar.
- Body Language Super Antioxidant from OxyFresh USA.
- Cell Guard from Biotec Food Corporation.
- Glutathione Booster from Carlson Laboratories.
- Juice Plus from Kelco.
- Life Guard from Thompson Nutritional Products.
- Oxy-5000 Forte from American Biologics.
- Revenol from Neways, Inc.

Using a combination supplement is often more convenient than taking many different products separately.

ENZYMES

INTRODUCTION

The late Dr. Edward Howell, a physician and pioneer in enzyme research, called enzymes the "sparks of life." These energized protein molecules play a necessary role in virtually all of the biochemical activities that go on in the body. They are essential for digesting food, for stimulating the brain, for providing cellular energy, and for repairing all tissues, organs, and cells. Life as we know it could not exist without the action of enzymes, even in the presence of sufficient amounts of vitamins, minerals, water, and other nutrients.

In their primary role, enzymes are catalysts—substances that accelerate and precipitate the hundreds of thousands of biochemical reactions in the body that control life's processes. If it were not for the catalytic action of enzymes, most of these reactions would take place far too slowly to sustain life. Enzymes are not consumed in the reactions they facilitate.

Each enzyme has a specific function in the body that no other enzyme can fulfill. The chemical shape of each enzyme is specialized so that it can initiate a reaction only in a certain substance, or in a group of closely related substances, and not in others. The substance on which an enzyme acts is called the *substrate*. Because there must be a different enzyme for every substrate, the body must produce a great number of different enzymes.

THE FUNCTIONS OF ENZYMES

Enzymes assist in practically all bodily functions. Digestive enzymes break down food particles for storage in the liver or muscles. This stored energy is later converted by other enzymes for use by the body when necessary. Iron is concentrated in the blood by the action of enzymes; other enzymes in the blood help the blood to coagulate in order to stop bleeding. Uricolytic enzymes catalyze the conversion of uric acid into urea. Respiratory enzymes aid in eliminating carbon dioxide from the lungs. Enzymes assist the kidneys, liver, lungs, colon, and skin in removing wastes and toxins from the body. Enzymes also utilize the nutrients ingested by the body to construct new muscle tissue, nerve cells, bone, skin, and glandular tissue. One enzyme can take dietary phosphorus and convert it into bone. Enzymes prompt the oxidation of glucose, which creates energy for the cells. Enzymes also protect the blood from dangerous waste materials by converting these substances to forms that are easily eliminated by the body. Indeed, the functions of enzymes are so many and so diverse that it would be impossible to name them all.

Enzymes are often divided into two groups: digestive enzymes and metabolic enzymes. Digestive enzymes are secreted along the gastrointestinal tract and break down foods, enabling the nutrients to be absorbed into the bloodstream for use in various bodily functions. There are three main categories of digestive enzymes: amylase, protease, and lipase. Amylase, found in saliva and in the pancreatic and intestinal juices, breaks down carbohydrates. It begins to act as soon as you start chewing (this is why it is important to chew your food well). Different types of amylase break down specific types of sugars. For example, lactase breaks down lactose (milk sugar), maltase breaks down maltose (malt sugar), and sucrase breaks down sucrose (cane and beet sugar). Protease, found in the stomach juices and also in the pancreatic and intestinal juices, helps to digest protein. Lipase, found in the stomach and pancreatic juices, and also present in fats in foods, aids in fat digestion. Another component of the digestive process is hydrochloric acid. While not technically an enzyme itself, it interacts with digestive enzymes as they perform their functions.

Metabolic enzymes are enzymes that catalyze the various chemical reactions within the cells, such as energy production and detoxification. The activities of all of the body's organs, tissues, and cells are governed by metabolic enzymes. They are the workers that build the body from proteins, carbohydrates, and fats. Metabolic enzymes are found doing their specific work in the blood, organs, and tissues. Each body tissue has its own specific set of metabolic enzymes.

Two particularly important metabolic enzymes are superoxide dismutase (SOD) and its partner, catalase. SOD is an antioxidant that protects the cells by attacking a common free radical, superoxide. (*See* Superoxide Dismutase *under* ANTIOXIDANTS in Part One.) Catalase breaks down hydrogen peroxide, a metabolic waste product, and liberates oxygen for the body to use.

Of the tens of thousands of enzymes needed, the body uses more of its enzyme-producing potential to produce the two dozen enzymes that control the breakdown and utilization of proteins, fats, and carbohydrates than it uses to create the hundreds of metabolic enzymes necessary to maintain the rest of the tissues and organs in their functions.

FOOD ENZYMES

While the body manufactures a supply of enzymes, it can also obtain enzymes from food. Unfortunately, enzymes are extremely sensitive to heat. Even low to moderate heat (118°F or above) destroys most enzymes in food, so to obtain enzymes from the diet, one must eat raw foods. Eating raw foods or, alternatively, taking enzyme supplements, helps prevent depletion of the body's own enzymes and thus reduces the stress on the body.

Enzymes can be found in many different foods, from both plant and animal sources. Avocados, papayas, pineapples, bananas, and mangos are all high in enzymes. Sprouts are the richest source. Unripe papaya and pineapple are excellent sources of enzymes. The enzymes extracted from papaya and pineapple—papain and bromelain, respectively—are proteolytic enzymes, which break down proteins

Many fat-containing foods also supply lipase, which breaks down fats. In fact, fat in food exposed only to pancreatic lipase (the lipase produced by the body) in the intestines is not as well digested as fat that is first worked on in the stomach by food lipase. Pancreatic lipase digests fat in a highly alkaline environment (the intestines), whereas lipase found in food fats works in a more acidic environment (the stomach). The optimal extraction of nutrients from fats depends on the work of different fat-digesting enzymes in successive stages.

Hydrochloric acid (HCl) comes in several different forms, including lysine HCl and betaine HCl. Betaine HCl is derived from sugar beets. When new, HCl capsules and tablets are almost white in color, but sometimes they can turn a deep purple color when they age. Supplemental HCl is not sold in powder or liquid form because contact with the teeth can damage tooth enamel. HCl has a sulfur-like odor.

Superoxide dismutase occurs naturally in a variety of food sources, including alfalfa, barley grass, broccoli, Brussels sprouts, cabbage, wheatgrass, and most dark green plants.

As powerful as they are, enzymes cannot act alone. They require adequate amounts of other substances, known as coenzymes, to be fully active. Among the most important coenzymes are the B-complex vitamins, vitamin C, vitamin E, and zinc.

COMMERCIALLY AVAILABLE ENZYMES

The majority of commercially available enzymes are digestive enzymes extracted from various sources. (Scientists are unable to manufacture enzymes synthetically.) Most commercial enzyme products are made from animal enzymes, such as pancreatin and pepsin, which help in the digestion of food once it has reached the lower stomach and the intestinal tract. Some companies make their supplements from enzymes extracted from aspergillus, a type of fungus.

These enzymes begin their predigestive work in the upper stomach. All of these products are used primarily to aid the digestion of foods and absorption of nutrients, especially protein.

If proteins are not completely digested, undigested protein particles may make their way into the bloodstream through the intestinal wall with other nutrients. This phenomenon is known as *leaky gut syndrome,* and it can result in allergic reactions that may be more or less severe, depending upon the strength of the immune system. This is one reason why the proper digestion of proteins is so important.

Any enzyme that acts on protein and prepares it for absorption is called a proteolytic enzyme. Proteolytic enzymes available in supplement form include pepsin, trypsin, rennin, pancreatin, and chymotrypsin. In addition to aiding digestion, proteolytic enzymes have been shown to be beneficial as anti-inflammatory agents. Pancreatin, derived from secretions of animal pancreas, is a focus of cancer research, because people with cancer are often deficient in this enzyme. Pancreatin is used in the treatment of digestive problems, viral infections, and sports injuries, as well as pancreatic insufficiency, food allergies, cystic fibrosis, autoimmune disorders, and other chronic illnesses.

Also available in supplement form are the antioxidant enzymes superoxide dismutase (SOD) and catalase.

The following table lists some common enzymes and their substrates.

Enzyme	Substrate
Amylase	Carbohydrates
Bromelain	Proteins
Cellulase	Fiber
Chymopapain	Proteins
Diastase	Carbohydrates
Glucoamylase	Carbohydrates
Hemicellulase	Carbohydrates
Hyaluronidase	Proteins, adhesions, fibrin
Invertase	Carbohydrates
Lactase	Lactose (milk sugar)
Lipase	Fats
Maltase	Carbohydrates
Pancreatin	Proteins, fats, carbohydrates
Papain	Proteins, fats, carbohydrates
Pectinase	Carbohydrates
Pepsin	Proteins
Phytase	Carbohydrates
Plasmin	Proteins
Protease	Proteins
Rennin	Proteins
Trypsin	Proteins

Enzyme supplements may not be for everyone, however. During pregnancy, it is a rule to be careful with supplements in general. Nursing mothers also should be careful about supplements, to avoid affecting their milk. People who have hemophilia or who take anticoagulants (blood-thinners) should consult their health care providers before taking large amounts of enzymes. Anyone contemplating surgery where there is high risk of bleeding should ask his or her physician for advice before taking any supplement.

WHAT'S ON THE SHELVES

Enzymes are available over the counter in tablet, capsule, powder, and liquid forms. They may be sold in combination with each other or as separate items. Some enzyme products also contain garlic to aid digestion.

For maximum benefit, any digestive enzyme supplement you choose should contain all of the major enzyme groups—amylase, protease, and lipase. Digestive enzymes should be taken after meals, unless you are eating processed and/or cooked foods, in which case it is best to take them during the meal. You can make your own digestive enzymes by drying papaya seeds, placing them in a pepper grinder, and sprinkling them on your foods. These have a peppery taste.

If you take supplemental superoxide dismutase, make sure to choose a product that is enteric coated—that is, coated with a protective substance that allows the SOD to pass intact through the stomach acid to be absorbed in the small intestine. Do not crush or chew these pills. All forms of enzymes should be kept in a reasonably cool place to insure potency because they are susceptible to moisture.

Research has shown that as we grow older, the body's ability to produce enzymes decreases. At the same time, malabsorption of nutrients, tissue breakdown, and chronic health conditions increase. Taking supplemental enzymes can help to ensure that you continue to get the full nutritional value from your foods. We believe that enzyme supplementation is vital for elderly persons.

The following are a few recommended enzyme complex products:

• AbsorbAid from Nature's Sources is made from plant enzymes and includes lipase, amylase, and protease from bromelain, as well as cellulase and lactase. It has been shown to significantly improve the absorption of nutrients, especially essential fatty acids and zinc.

• Acid-Ease from Prevail Corporation is a digestive aid from natural plant sources that includes amylase, lipase, and cellulase, as well as the soothing herbs marshmallow root and slippery elm.

• All Complete Enzymes from TriMedica, Inc. is a blend of plant enzymes that provide a full range of essential enzymes, plus coenzymes for added effectiveness. It is designed to adapt to various body temperatures and pH levels without losing potency. Ingredients include amylase, lipase, bromelain, papain, protease, cellulase, acidophilus, bifidus, and trace minerals.

• Bio-Gestin from Biotec Foods (a division of AgriGenic Food Corporation) is freeze-dried mature green papaya containing papain and chymopapain. The naturally sweet taste of the papaya makes these especially good capsules to open and sprinkle over food before eating.

• Bio-Zyme from Metagenics contains proteolytic enzymes, including chymotrypsin, trypsin, and raw pancreas concentrate, enteric coated for absorption in the intestines so that they may benefit inflammatory conditions.

• Cardio Enzyme Formula from Prevail Corporation contains a combination of enzymes, herbs, and nutrients, including protease 1 and 2, amylase, cellulase, and lipase; extracts of hawthorn berry, dan-shen root, arjun bark, passionflower, ginkgo leaf, ginkgo rhizome, and garlic; and magnesium, vitamin B_6, vitamin B_{12}, folic acid, vitamin C, taurine, L-carnitine, and L-lysine, all in a special blend to support the heart.

• Cholesterol Enzyme Formula from Prevail Corporation is an enzyme and antioxidant formula designed to promote cardiovascular health. Ingredients include pantothenic acid, beta-glycan, guggul, gamma-oryzanol, garlic, cellulase, amylase, protease 1 and 2, and lipase 2.

• D.A. #34 Food Enzymes from Carlson Laboratories contains pancreatin and ox bile, with enough capability in each tablet to digest 34 grams of protein, 120 grams of carbohydrates, and 21 grams of fat. Ox bile is a beneficial supplement for people with gallbladder disorders.

• Daily Essential Enzymes from Source Naturals is a full-spectrum digestive enzyme supplement containing protease (acid stable), lipase, amylase, cellulase, and lactase. The powder in the capsules has very little taste of its own, and the contents may be added to food that is not hot (over 110°F) by sprinkling over food (this is a good option for vegetarians who want to avoid gelatin capsules). This supplement is designed to work in both the acidic environment of the stomach and the more alkaline environment of the intestines.

• Digest Support from Natrol is a multi-enzyme formula containing all three classes of digestive enzymes (proteolytic, amyolytic, and lipolytic), including protease 1 and 2, amylase, cellulase, lipase, maltase, and sucrase. It also contains A-galactosidase, an enzyme that acts on galactose, a breakdown product of lactose (milk sugar), and fights gas.

• Elastase from Cardiovascular Research contains elastase, a proteolytic enzyme found in pancreatic juices.

• Infla-Zyme Forte from American Biologics is a combination of enzymes and antioxidants for people requiring supplemental digestive enzymes to aid in the breakdown of proteins, fats, and carbohydrates. It may also be helpful for chronic or acute inflammation. Its ingredients include amylase, bromelain, catalase, chymotrypsin, L-cysteine, lipase, pancreatin, papain, rutin, superoxide dismutase, trypsin, and zinc. If taken as a digestive aid, the recommended dosage is 1 to 3 tablets following each meal; if you use it for other purposes, such as illness, inflammation, and/or injury, take 3 to 6 tablets one hour before each meal or between meals. Infla-Zyme Forte may be taken by persons on sodium-restricted diets.

• Inflazyme from Ecological Formulas is a blend of bromelain and vitamin C.

• Lipothiamine from Cardiovascular Research contains a specially prepared form of vitamin B_1 (thiamine) plus lipoate (thioctic acid), both enzyme cofactors involved in the production of cellular energy.

• Mega-Zyme from Enzymatic Therapy is an extra-strength pancreatic and digestive enzyme tablet. Each tablet contains protease, amylase, lipase, trypsin, papain, bromelain, and lysozyme.

• MegaZymes from MegaFood is a vegetarian enzyme and herbal formula made from plant-based enzymes, including amylase, cellulase, glucoamylase, invertase, lactase, lipase, and protease, blended with the tonic herbs caraway, gentian, and ginger, plus acidophilus to support healthy intestinal flora.

• Metazyme from Metagenics is a plant-derived enzyme supplement that contains protease, amylase, lipase, and cellulase.

• Multi-Zyme from FoodScience Laboratories of Vermont is an enteric-coated tablet containing pepsin, bromelain, ox bile, pancreas extract, papain, proteases, amylase, lipases, cellulase, and hydrochloric acid (HCl). HCl is another component of the digestive process that works with enzymes to break down foods.

• Serraflazyme from Cardiovascular Research contains serrapeptase (serratio peptidase), a proteolytic enzyme with anti-inflammatory properties.

• Vegetarian Enzyme Complex from Futurebiotics contains protease, amylase, celluase, lipase, papain, and bromelain.

• Wobenzym N from Marlyn Nutraceuticals contains a combination of enzymes designed to interact synergistically with each other. Its ingredients include bromelain, chymotrypsin, pancreatin, papain, rutin, and trypsin.

Other sources for quality enzyme supplements include the National Enzyme Company and Miller Pharmacal Group. Miller Pharmacal products, available through health care professionals only, include:

• Milcozyme, a two-part enzyme supplement with glutamic acid HCl, betaine HCl, papain, pepsin, and an enteric-coated side of the same tablet with pancreatin, lipase, amylase, and bromelain.

• Carbozyme, which contains betaine HCl, trypsin, chymotrypsin, bromelain, pancreatin, mannitol, thymus extract, lipase, amylase, and papain.

• Proteolytic Enzymes, made with enteric-coated trypsin and chymotrypsin.

• Karbozyme (not to be confused with the sound-alike product above), which contains pancreatin, sodium bicarbonate, and potassium bicarbonate.

• MM-Zyme, which contains pancreatic lipase, bromelain, amylase, raw pancreas extract, papain, trypsin, chymotrypsin, and selenium.

Finally, while not technically an enzyme product, Bioperine 10 from Nature's Plus also enhances the digestion and absorption of nutrients. It contains an extract of black pepper (*Piper nigrum*), and when taken with food or with vitamin, mineral, or herbal supplements, it helps food to digest and accelerates the distribution of nutrients throughout the body.

NATURAL FOOD SUPPLEMENTS

INTRODUCTION

Natural food supplements include a wide variety of products. Almost all health food stores carry them, and a number of drug stores and supermarkets stock them on their shelves as well. In general, natural food supplements are composed of, derived from, or byproducts of foods that provide health benefits. In some cases, health benefit claims made by manufacturers are based upon a supplement's use in traditional healing; in other cases, they are based on modern scientific research.

Food supplements can be high in certain nutrients, contain active ingredients that aid digestive or metabolic processes, or provide a combination of nutrients and active ingredients. It is important to point out that some unscrupulous manufacturers make false promises. It is therefore vital to be an informed consumer. It is also necessary to be aware that many conservative "watchdog" organizations point to these few unsubstantiated products and label the whole industry as unreliable. This occurs in spite of the fact that many natural food supplements have been known to work for years; these products are medically endorsed only when they are "discovered" by researchers deemed acceptable by these groups. Such recent discoveries include garlic, aloe vera, fiber, and fish oils—substances that have been used for centuries in many parts of the world.

WHAT'S ON THE SHELVES

Food supplements come in many shapes and forms—tablets, capsules, powders, liquids, jellies, creams, biscuits, wafers, granules, and more. Product packaging depends entirely on the nature of the food supplement's composition. The potency of these products varies. Because they are made up of perishable foods, food derivatives, or food byproducts, their potency may be affected by the length of time they sit on a shelf or by the temperature at which they are kept. If you don't understand how a product is to be used, ask questions or read the available literature on the particular supplement.

If you have never used a natural food supplement, you may be uncomfortable about buying and using one for the first time. This is normal. Keep in mind that once you become familiar with its use and benefits, you won't give the idea of using it a second thought.

In this section, we describe some of the types of food supplements that are recommended for use in dealing with the various disorders discussed in Part Two of this book.

Acidophilus

See Lactobacillus Acidophilus in this section.

Adenosine Triphosphate (ATP)

Adenosine triphosphate (ATP) is a compound that serves as the immediate source of energy for the body's cells, notably muscle cells. It increases energy and stamina, builds muscular density, increases muscular strength, buffers lactic-acid buildup (the reason for sore, achy muscles after physical activity), delays fatigue, and preserves muscle fibers. ATP is produced naturally in the body from adenine, a nitrogen-containing compound; ribose, a type of sugar; and phosphate units, each containing one phosphorus atom and four oxygen atoms. ATP from Integrated Health is a good source of supplemental ATP.

Alfalfa

One of the most mineral-rich foods known, alfalfa has roots that grow as much as 130 feet into the earth. Alfalfa is available in liquid extract form and is good to use while fasting because of its chlorophyll and nutrient content. It contains calcium, magnesium, phosphorus, potassium, plus virtually all known vitamins. The minerals are in a balanced form, which promotes absorption. These minerals are alkaline, but have a neutralizing effect on the intestinal tract.

If you need a mineral supplement, alfalfa is a good choice. It has helped many arthritis sufferers. Alfalfa, wheatgrass, barley, and spirulina, all of which contain chlorophyll, have been found to aid in the healing of intestinal ulcers, gastritis, liver disorders, eczema, hemorrhoids, asthma, high blood pressure, anemia, constipation, body and breath odor, bleeding gums, infections, burns, athlete's foot, and cancer.

Aloe Vera

This plant is known for its healing effect and is used in many cosmetic and hair care products. There are over 200 different species of aloe that grow in dry regions around the world.

Aloe vera is commonly known as a skin healer, moisturizer, and softener. It is dramatically effective on burns of all types, and is also good for cuts, insect stings, bruises, acne and blemishes, poison ivy, welts, skin ulcers, and eczema. Taken internally, 98- or 99-percent pure aloe vera is known to aid in the healing of stomach disorders, ulcers, constipation, hemorrhoids, rectal itching, colitis, and all colon problems. It can also be helpful against infections, varicose veins, skin cancer, and arthritis, and is used in the treatment of AIDS.

We have had excellent results using colon cleansers containing psyllium husks in combination with aloe vera juice. We have found this combination to be good for food allergy and colon disorder sufferers. Psyllium keeps the folds and pockets in the colon free of toxic material that gathers there. The aloe vera not only has a healing effect, but if constipation or diarrhea is present, it will return the stools to normal. It takes a few weeks to cleanse the colon, but regular, periodic use will keep the colon clean. As with any substance, it is possible to develop an intolerance to aloe vera juice and/or psyllium husks, so this treatment should not be used on an ongoing basis.

Barley Grass

Barley grass is high in calcium, iron, all the essential amino acids, chlorophyll, flavonoids, vitamin B_{12}, vitamin C, and many minerals, plus enzymes. This food heals stomach, duodenal, and colon disorders as well as pancreatitis, and is an effective anti-inflammatory.

Bee Byproducts

See Bee Pollen, Bee Propolis, Honey, and Royal Jelly, all in this section.

Bee Pollen

Bee pollen is a powderlike material that is produced by the anthers of flowering plants and gathered by bees. It is composed of 10 to 15 percent protein and also contains B-complex vitamins, vitamin C, essential fatty acids, enzymes, carotene, calcium, copper, iron, magnesium, potassium, manganese, sodium, plant sterols, and simple sugars.

Like other bee products, bee pollen has an antimicrobial effect. In addition, it is useful for combating fatigue, depression, cancer, and colon disorders. It is also helpful for people with allergies because it strengthens the immune system.

It is best to obtain bee pollen from a local source, as this increases its antiallergenic properties. Fresh bee pollen should not cling together or form clumps, and it should be sold in a tightly sealed container. Some people (an estimated 0.05 percent of the population) may be allergic to bee pollen. It is best to try taking a small amount at first and watch for a developing rash, wheezing, discomfort, or any other signs of a reaction. If such symptoms occur, discontinue taking bee pollen.

Bee Propolis

Bee propolis is a resinous substance collected from various plants by bees. Bees use propolis, together with beeswax, in the construction of hives. As a supplement, it is an excellent aid against bacterial infections. Bee propolis is believed to stimulate phagocytosis, the process by which some white blood cells destroy bacteria.

Propolis is beneficial as a salve for abrasions and bruises because of its antibacterial effect. Good results have been reported on the use of propolis against inflammation of the mucous membranes of the mouth and throat, dry cough and throat, halitosis, tonsillitis, ulcers, and acne, and for the stimulation of the immune system.

Be sure that any bee products you use smell and taste fresh. All bee products should be in tightly sealed containers. It is best to purchase these products from a manufacturer who specializes in bee products. If you are using bee products for allergies, it is best to obtain products that are produced within a ten-mile radius of your home. This way, you get a minute dose of pollen to desensitize you to the local pollen in the area.

Beta-1,3-Glucan

Beta-1,3-glucan is a polysaccharide (a complex type of carbohydrate molecule) with immune-stimulating properties. Specifically, it stimulates the activity of macrophages, immune cells that destroy cellular debris, microorganisms, and abnormal cells by surrounding and digesting them. Beta-1,3-D-glucan is a supplemental form of beta-1,3-glucan made from the cell walls of baker's yeast. Despite its origin, it does not contain any yeast proteins. It is useful for treating many bacterial, viral, and fungal diseases. It can also kill tumor cells and increase bone-marrow production. Because of its ability to protect the immune system, beta-1,3-D-glucan may protect against the effects of aging. Studies done as early as the 1970s, have found that it can reduce the size of cancerous tumors in rats. Further investigation has shown beta-1,3-D-glucan to be a potent agent for healing sores and ulcers in women who have undergone mastectomies.

Bifidobacterium Bifidum

Bifidobacterium bifidum aids in the synthesis of the B vitamins by creating healthy intestinal flora. *B. bifidum* is the predominant organism in the intestinal flora and establishes a healthy environment for the manufacture of the B-complex vitamins and vitamin K.

When you take antibiotics, the "friendly" bacteria in your digestive tract are destroyed along with the harmful bacteria. Supplementing your diet with *B. bifidum* helps you maintain healthy intestinal flora. Unhealthy flora can result in the liberation of abnormally high levels of ammonia as protein-containing foods are digested. This irritates the intestinal membranes. In addition, the ammonia is absorbed into the bloodstream and must be detoxified by the liver, or it will cause nausea, a decrease in appetite, vomiting, and other toxic reactions. By promoting the proper digestion of foods, the friendly bacteria also aid in preventing digestive disorders such as constipation and gas, as well as food allergies. If digestion is poor, the activity of intestinal bacteria on undigested food may lead to excessive production of the body chemical histamine, which triggers allergic symptoms.

Yeast infections of the vaginal tract respond very favorably to douching with *B. bifidum* preparations. These microorganisms destroy the pathogenic organisms. When used as an enema, *B. bifidum* also helps establish a healthy intestinal environment. It improves bowel function by aiding peristalsis, and results in the production of a softer, smoother stool. Harmful bacteria are kept in check, and toxic wastes that have accumulated in the intestines are destroyed and/or eliminated from the body.

B. bifidum has proved useful in the treatment of cirrhosis of the liver and chronic hepatitis; by improving digestion, it reduces the strain on the liver. Many people who do not respond to *L. acidophilus* react positively to *B. bifidum*. Many experts consider *B. bifidum* to be preferable to *L. acidophilus* for children and for adults with liver disorders.

Brewer's Yeast

See Yeast in this section.

Bifidus

See Bifidobacterium Bifidum in this section.

Bovine Cartilage

Cleaned, dried, and powdered bovine cartilage is a supplement that helps accelerate wound healing and reduce inflammation. Like shark cartilage, it has been shown to be helpful for psoriasis, all types of arthritis, and ulcerative colitis. VitaCarte from Phoenix BioLabs contains pure bovine cartilage from range-raised, hormone-free cattle. Another cartilage supplement, shark cartilage, is also available, and may be preferred by some individuals.

Cellulose

See under Fiber in this section.

Cerasomal-cis-9-cetylmyristoleate

This is a modified version of a medium-chain fatty acid, cetylmyristoleate, which is found in nuts, vegetables, and animal tissue. It appears to be a very promising development in arthritis research. Studies in laboratory rats have shown it to have anti-inflammatory effects, and early clinical studies in people suggest it may be beneficial for many with osteoarthritis, rheumatoid arthritis, and psoriatic arthritis, as well as psoriasis. It is believed to work by normalizing the functioning of the immune system and reducing the production of pro-inflammatory prostaglandins.

While this supplement is often referred to simply as CMO, that is actually a trademarked name for a cerasomal-cis-9-cetylmyristoleate product, not a generic term. A good source of this supplement is CM+ from Metabolic Response Modifiers.

Chlorella

Chlorella is a tiny, single-celled water-grown alga containing a nucleus and an enormous amount of readily available chlorophyll. It also contains protein (approximately 58 percent), carbohydrates, all of the B vitamins, vitamins C and E, amino acids, and rare trace minerals. In fact, it is virtually a complete food. It contains more vitamin B_{12} than liver does, plus a considerable amount of beta-carotene. It has a strong cell wall, however, which makes it difficult to gain access to its nutrients. Consequently, it requires factory processing to be effective.

Chlorella is one of the few edible species of water-grown algae. The chlorophyll in chlorella can help speed the cleansing of the bloodstream. Chlorella is very high in RNA and DNA, and has been found to protect against the effects of ultraviolet radiation. Studies show that chlorella is an excellent source of protein, especially for people who cannot or who choose not to eat meat.

Chlorophyll

See under Chlorella and "Green Drinks" in this section.

Chondroitin Sulfate

Chondroitin sulfate is an important element in the creation of cartilage, the tough yet flexible connective tissue found in the joints, where it acts as a cushion, and in other parts of the body, such as the tip of the nose and the outer ear. Chemically, chondroitins belong to a group of substances classified as *glycosaminoglycans* (also referred to as *mucopolysaccharides*), which are complex types of carbohydrate molecules. Glycosaminoglycans in turn attach to proteins such as collagen and elastin, forming even more complex substances designated *proteoglycans*, which are a vital component of cartilage tissue. Chondroitin sulfate attracts water to the proteoglycans and holds it there, which is important for maintaining healthy joint cartilage. It can also protect existing cartilage from premature degeneration by blocking certain enzymes that destroy cartilage and prevent nutrients from being transported to the cartilage for repair.

Taking supplemental chondroitin sulfate, usually derived from powdered shark cartilage or cow-trachea cartilage, has been shown to be helpful in the treatment of osteoarthritis. Many times it is used in conjunction with glucosamine for even more effective therapy. The supplements are usually taken together in pill form. Neither chondroitin sulfate nor glucosamine has shown any toxic effects, but there are potential side effects for certain people. The Arthritis Foundation recommends exercising caution in taking these supplements for treatment of osteoarthritis. You should let your physician know you are taking these supplements, and discuss any allergies or potential reactions. Use caution in taking chondroitin sulfate if you are taking anticoagulants (blood-thinners) or daily aspirin, as it is chemically similar to the blood-thinner heparin. Pregnant women should not take these supplements, as there has not been sufficient study regarding their safety and potential side effects during pregnancy.

Twinlab manufactures a number of good products containing chondroitin sulfate. Glucosamine Chondroitin Sulfate from Only Natural, Inc. is a good combination source of glucosamine and chondroitin sulfate.

Citrin

Citrin is a trademarked name for a standardized herbal extract from the fruit of the *Garcinia cambogia* plant, also known as Indian berry. It inhibits the synthesis of fatty acids in the liver, promotes the burning of body fat as fuel, and suppresses the appetite. Its primary usefulness is in treating obesity, although it may also aid in preventing or slowing atherosclerosis and heart disease. It does not affect the nervous system or cause any known side effects. Citrin is an ingredient in a number of different products sold by various manufacturers.

Coenzyme A

Coenzyme A, a substance manufactured by body cells from pantotheic acid (vitamin B_5), is at the center of the whole metabolic process. It performs a vital role in the process by which the cells generate energy from glucose. Indeed, it helps produce around 90 percent of the energy the body needs to fuction. Coenzyme A also begins the metabolism of fatty acids. A lack of sufficient coenzyme A can result in stiff, sore muscles and a decrease in energy. Taken as a supplement, coenzyme A increases energy, supports the manufacture of substances critical for the brain and adrenal glands, helps with the manufacture of connective tissue, and supports the immune system. Studies suggest that coenzyme A may be as, if not more, beneficial than coenzyme Q_{10}.

Coenzyme Q$_{10}$

Coenzyme Q_{10} is present in the mitochondria of all the cells in the body. It is vital because it carries into the cells the energy-laden protons and electrons that are used to produce adenosine triphosphate (ATP), the immediate source of cellular energy (*see* Adenosine Triphosphate [ATP] on page 63). This is a constant process because the body can store only a small quantity of ATP at any one time. It is believed that as many as 75 percent of people over fifty may

be deficient in coenzyme Q_{10}. A lack of sufficient coenzyme Q_{10} can lead to cardiovascular disease because without it, the heart does not have not enough energy to circulate the blood effectively.

Colloidal Silver

Colloidal silver is an inexpensive healing agent and disinfectant that has a myriad of applications. It is a clear golden liquid composed of 99.9-percent pure silver particles approximately 0.001 to 0.01 microns ($\frac{1}{1,000,000}$ to $\frac{1}{100,000}$ millimeter) in diameter that are suspended in pure water. Colloidal silver can be mixed with either tap or distilled water and applied topically, taken by mouth, or administered intravenously.

Topically, it can be used to fight fungal infections of the skin or nails and to promote the healing of burns, wounds, cuts, rashes, and sunburn. It can be used on toothaches and mouth sores, as eyedrops, and as a gargle to fight tooth decay and bad breath. It can also be used as sterilizer and can even be sprayed on air-conditioning filters and air ducts and vents to prevent germs from growing. Taken internally, colloidal silver can be used to fight infection. It has been shown to be effective against more that 650 disease-causing organisms, including *Escherichia coli* (*E. coli*) bacteria and the fungus *Candida albicans*.

Micronic Silver from Lifestar Millennium is a good source of colloidal silver. Cold Combat! from TriMedica, Inc. is a combination of sublingual forms of colloidal silver, colloidal copper, zinc, and the homeopathic remedies *Cinnabaris* and *Rhus toxicodendron*. It is good for fighting colds and flu.

Colostrum

Colostrum is a thin, yellowish fluid secreted by the mammary glands of mammalian mothers in the first days after giving birth, before the production of true milk begins. It contains high levels of protein and growth factors, as well as immune factors that help to protect the newborn against infection. Taken as a supplement, colostrum can boost the immune system and help the body to burn fat and build lean muscle. It may also accelerate the healing of injuries, increase vitality and stamina, and have an anti-aging effect. Supplemental colostrum usually contains bovine (cow) colostrum. Good sources include New Life Colostrum from Symbiotics (both original and high-Ig formulas) and Colostrum Specific from Jarrow Formulas.

Corn Germ

Corn germ is made by a process that isolates the embryo of the corn plant, which contains the most usable nutrients. Corn germ has a longer shelf life than wheat germ and is higher in some nutrients, especially zinc. Corn germ contains ten times the amount of zinc found in wheat germ.

You can use corn germ to bread chicken or fish. It is also good when added to cereals and used as a topping.

Creatine

Creatine (creatine monohydrate) is a compound produced by metabolic processes in the body. When muscles are in use, the compound adenosine triphosphate (ATP) is broken down into two other compounds—adenosine diphosphate (ADP) and inorganic phosphate. This process produces the body's cellular energy, which, among other things, powers the muscles. Each such burst of energy is very fleeting. However, with the addition of creatine, ADP can be transformed back to ATP, the source of cellular energy. Taken as a supplement, creatine can increase both endurance and strength, making possible extended workout time. Longer workouts in turn can result in increased lean muscle mass.

Creatine is particularly popular with athletes. The use of creatine for muscle-depleting illnesses and the natural wasting of muscles that comes with age is also being studied. Creatine should be used in combination with a balanced, nutritionally complete diet. You should not take it with fruit juices, as this combination results in the production of creatinine, which is difficult for the kidneys to process. Never exceed the recommended dose.

Dehydroepiandrosterone (DHEA)

Dehydroepiandrosterone (DHEA) is a hormone that is produced primarily by the adrenal glands and is found naturally in the human body. It is an important base from which other key substances, including the hormones testosterone, progesterone, and corticosterone, can be derived, either directly or indirectly. The amount of DHEA produced by the body declines with age, particularly after age forty. Research indicates that taking DHEA supplements may help to prevent cancer, arterial disease, multiple sclerosis, and Alzheimer's disease; may be beneficial in the treatment of lupus and osteoporosis; may enhance the activity of the immune system; and may help to improve memory.

However, caution should be exercised when taking this supplement. Some physicians believe that taking high doses of DHEA suppresses the body's natural ability to synthesize this hormone. Further, laboratory studies have shown that high doses can lead to liver damage. If you take supplemental DHEA, it is important also to take supplements of the antioxidant vitamins C and E and the antioxidant mineral selenium to prevent oxidative damage to the liver. Possible side effects of taking DHEA include excess growth of facial hair in women. This can often be avoided by starting with a dose of 10 milligrams daily. 7-Keto DHEA is a derivative of DHEA that is not converted into estrogen or testosterone, which is good for women concerned about breast cancer and for men concerned about prostate cancer. 7-Keto DHEA is a good alternative to DHEA and has the same benefits.

Desiccated Liver

Desiccated liver is concentrated dried liver that is put into powdered or tablet form. This form of liver contains vitamins A, D, and C; the B-complex vitamins; and the minerals calcium, copper, phosphorus, and iron. Desiccated liver is good for people with anemia, and aids in building healthy red blood cells. It is known to increase energy, aid in liver disorders, and help relieve stress in the body. Use only a product made from liver derived from beef that is raised organically.

Dimethylglycine (DMG)

Dimethylglycine (DMG) is a derivative of glycine, the simplest of the amino acids. It acts as a building block for many important substances, including the amino acid methionine, choline, a number of important hormones and neurotransmitters, and DNA.

Low levels of DMG are present in meats, seeds, and grains. It is a safe, nontoxic food substance that does not build up in the body. No deficiency symptoms are associated with a lack of DMG in the diet, but taking supplemental DMG can have a wide range of beneficial effects, including helping the body maintain high energy levels and boosting mental acuity. DMG has been found to enhance the immune system and to reduce elevated blood cholesterol and triglyceride levels. It improves oxygen utilization by the body, helps to normalize blood pressure and blood glucose levels, and improves the functioning of many important organs. It may also be useful for controlling epileptic seizures. Some people have used DMG as a substitute for pangamic acid, a supplement that is no longer available in the United States but that is widely used in Russia to treat heart disease, liver disease, alcohol and drug addiction, and other problems. DMG is thought to increase pangamic acid levels in the body. Aangamik DMG from FoodScience Laboratories is a good source of supplemental DMG.

Dimethylaminoethanol (DMAE)

Dimethylaminoethanol (DMAE) is similar to choline, a chemical involved in the processes of learning and memory. It has been known to be beneficial for people with autism, memory deficiency, and dementia. It is best not to take it on a daily basis, but to reserve it for days when you need to increase alertness and focus. DMAE can have a slight mood- and vision-enhancing effect in some people. Lifespan 2000 from Country Life is a good source of supplemental DMAE.

Dimethylsulfoxide (DMSO)

Dimethylsulfoxide (DMSO) is a byproduct of wood processing for papermaking. It is a somewhat oily liquid that looks like mineral oil and has a slightly garlicky odor. Because it is an excellent solvent, it is widely used as a degreaser, paint thinner, and antifreeze. However, it also has remarkable therapeutic properties, especially for the healing of injuries. Applying DMSO on sprained ankles, pulled muscles, dislocated joints, and even at the site of simple fractures can virtually eliminate the pain. It also promotes immune-system activity.

DMSO is absorbed through the skin and enters the bloodstream by osmosis through capillary walls. It is then distributed through the circulatory system and ultimately is excreted through the urine. It has been used successfully in the treatment of brain and spinal cord damage, arthritis, Down syndrome, sciatica and other back problems, keloids, acne, burns, musculoskeletal problems, sports injuries, cancer, sinusitis, headaches, skin ulcers, herpes, and cataracts.

Essential Fatty Acids (EFAs)

Fatty acids are the basic building blocks of which fats and oils are composed. Contrary to popular myth, the body does need fat. It must be the right kind, however.

The fatty acids that are necessary for health and that cannot be made by the body are called *essential fatty acids* (EFAs). They are occasionally also referred to as *vitamin F* or *polyunsaturates*. EFAs must be supplied through the diet.

Essential fatty acids have desirable effects on many disorders. They improve the skin and hair, reduce blood pressure, aid in the prevention of arthritis, lower cholesterol and triglyceride levels, and reduce the risk of blood clot formation. They are beneficial for candidiasis, cardiovascular disease, eczema, and psoriasis. Found in high concentrations in the brain, EFAs aid in the transmission of nerve impulses and are needed for the normal development and functioning of the brain. A deficiency of essential fatty acids can lead to an impaired ability to learn and recall information.

Every living cell in the body needs essential fatty acids. They are essential for rebuilding and producing new cells. Essential fatty acids are also used by the body for the production of prostaglandins, hormonelike substances that act as chemical messengers and regulators of various body processes.

There are two basic categories of essential fatty acids, designated *omega-3* and *omega-6*, based on their chemical structures. Omega-3 EFAs, including alpha-linolenic and eicosapentaenoic acid (EPA), are found in fresh deepwater fish, fish oil, and certain vegetable oils, among them canola oil, flaxseed oil, and walnut oil. Omega-6 EFAs, which include linoleic and gamma-linolenic acids, are found primarily in raw nuts, seeds, and legumes, and in unsaturated vegetable oils, such as borage oil, grape seed oil, primrose oil, sesame oil, and soybean oil. In order to supply essential fatty acids, these oils must be consumed in pure liquid or supplement form and must not be subjected to heat, either in processing or cooking. Heat destroys essential fatty acids. Worse, it results in the creation of dangerous free radicals (see ANTIOXIDANTS in Part One). If oils are hydro-

genated (processed to make the oil more solid, as is commonly done in the production of margarine), the linoleic acid is converted into trans-fatty acids, which are not beneficial to the body.

The daily requirement for essential fatty acids is satisfied by an amount equivalent to 10 to 20 percent of total caloric intake. The most essential of the essential fatty acids is linoleic acid.

A number of sources of essential fatty acids are recommended in this book, among them fish oils, flaxseeds and flaxseed oil, grape seed oil, and primrose oil.

Emu Oil

Emu oil is an excellent source of linoleic acid, linolenic acid, and oleic acid, which have anti-inflammatory properties. It can be used topically for the relief of rashes, hemorrhoids, poison ivy, insect bites, arthritis, joint aches, muscle strains, and it has been known to stop the pain of burns. It can also be used as a facial moisturizer to reduce wrinkles and lines. Emu Oil and Emu Plus from Emu Country, Inc. are good sources of Emu oil.

Fish Oil

Fish oil is a good source of omega-3 essential fatty acids. Salmon, mackerel, menhaden, herring, and sardines are good sources of fish oil because they have a higher fat content and provide more omega-3 factors than other fishes. For instance, 4 ounces of salmon contains up to 3,600 milligrams of omega-3 fatty acids, while 4 ounces of cod (a low-fat fish) contains only 300 milligrams.

Carlson Laboratories markets a good Norwegian salmon oil that we recommend. Cod liver oil from Norway is the most commonly used fish oil and is more mild tasting than other varieties. Author Dale Alexander claims it is excellent for arthritis. He has marketed an oil containing 13,800 international units of vitamin A and 1,380 international units of vitamin D per tablespoon. However, we do not recommend that you rely on cod liver oil as a source of the essential fatty acids. You would have to overdose on vitamins A and D to obtain the amount of fatty acids you need.

People with diabetes should not take fish oil supplements because of the high fat content, but they should consume fish for its essential fatty acids.

Flaxseeds and Flaxseed Oil

Flaxseeds are rich in omega-3 essential fatty acids, magnesium, potassium, and fiber. They are also a good source of the B vitamins, protein, and zinc. They are low in saturated fats and calories, and contain no cholesterol. The nutty taste of ground flaxseeds is pleasant, and they can be mixed with water or any fruit or vegetable juice. They can also be added to salads, soups, yogurt, cereals, baked goods, or fresh juices. You can grind these tiny seeds in a coffee grinder.

If you prefer not to eat the seeds, you can use flaxseed oil as an alternative. Like the seeds from which it is extracted, organic cold-pressed flaxseed oil is rich in essential fatty acids. Several studies have shown that it can reduce the pain, inflammation, and swelling of arthritis. It has been found to lower blood cholesterol and triglyceride levels, and to help reduce the hardening effects of cholesterol on cell membranes.

Grape Seed Oil

Of the many natural sources of essential fatty acids, grape seed oil is among the highest in linoleic acid and among the lowest in saturated fats. It contains no cholesterol and no sodium. It has a light, nutty taste that brings out the flavor in many foods. Unlike most other oils, it can be heated to temperatures as high as 485°F without producing dangerous and possibly carcinogenic free radicals. These features make it good for use in cooking. Buy only grape seed oil that is cold-pressed and contains no preservatives, such as Salute Santé Grapeseed Oil from Lifestar International.

Primrose Oil

Primrose oil (also known as evening primrose oil) contains 9 to 10 percent gamma-linolenic acid (GLA). This fatty acid is known to help prevent hardening of the arteries, heart disease, premenstrual syndrome, multiple sclerosis, and high blood pressure. It relieves pain and inflammation; enhances the release of sex hormones, including estrogen and testosterone; aids in lowering cholesterol levels; and is beneficial for cirrhosis of the liver.

Many women have found that primrose oil supplements relieve unpleasant menopausal symptoms such as hot flashes. Because it promotes the production of estrogen, women suffering from breast cancer that is diagnosed as estrogen-receptor positive (estrogen-related) should avoid or limit their intake of primrose oil. Black currant seed oil is a good substitute.

Combination EFA Supplements

A product called Ultimate Oil from Nature's Secret contains a blend of cold-pressed organic oils that offers a good balance of both omega-3 and omega-6 fatty acids. A purely vegetable-based product, Ultimate Oil contains extra-virgin flaxseed oil, black currant seed oil, pumpkin seed oil, lecithin, and safflower oil. We also recommend Kyolic-EPA from Wakunaga of America, a blend of aged garlic extract and fish oil derived from northern Pacific sardines, and Cardiovascular Research's Essential Fatty Acid Complex.

Evening Primrose Oil

See Primrose Oil *under* Essential Fatty Acids in this section.

Fiber

Found in many foods, fiber helps to lower blood cholesterol levels and stabilize blood sugar levels. It helps prevent colon cancer, constipation, hemorrhoids, obesity, and many other disorders. Fiber is also good for removing certain toxic metals from the body. Because the refining process has removed much of the natural fiber from our foods, the typical American diet is lacking in fiber.

There are seven basic classifications of fiber: bran, cellulose, gum, hemicellulose, lignin, mucilages, and pectin. Each form has its own function. It is best to rotate among several different supplemental fiber sources. Start with small amounts and gradually increase your intake until your stools are the proper consistency. Also, be aware that while today's average diet is lacking in fiber, consuming excessive amounts may decrease the absorption of zinc, iron, and calcium. Always take supplemental fiber separately from other medications or supplements. Otherwise, it can lessen their strength and effectiveness.

In addition to using a fiber supplement, you should make sure to get fiber through your diet. Make sure your diet contains these high-fiber foods: whole-grain cereals and flours, brown rice, agar agar, all kinds of bran, most fresh fruit, dried prunes, nuts, seeds (especially flaxseeds), beans, lentils, peas, and fresh raw vegetables. Eat several of these foods daily. When eating organic produce, leave the skin on apples and potatoes. Coat chicken in corn bran or oats for baking. Add extra bran to cereals and breads. Unsalted, unbuttered popcorn is also excellent for added fiber.

Bran, Gums, and Mucilages

Both gums and mucilages help to regulate blood glucose levels, aid in lowering cholesterol, and help in the removal of toxins. They are found in oatmeal, oat bran, sesame seeds, and dried beans.

One of the following should be part of your daily dietary plan:

- *Fennel seed.* Fennel is an herb that is helpful for digestive purposes. The seeds of this plant help to rid the intestinal tract of mucus and aid in relieving flatulence.

- *Glucomannan.* Derived from the tuber of the amorphophallis plant, it picks up and removes fat from the colon wall. This substance is good for diabetes and obesity because it helps to get rid of fat. It has been recognized for normalizing blood sugar and is good for people with hypoglycemia. Glucomannan expands to sixty times its own weight, thereby helping to curb the appetite. Taking 2 to 3 capsules with a large glass of water thirty minutes before meals is helpful for reducing allergic reactions and some symptoms associated with high and low blood sugar disorders. Always be sure to drink a large glass of water when taking glucomannan in capsule or pill form, as capsules can lodge in the throat and expand there, causing breathing problems. Glucomannan is tasteless and odorless, and can be added to foods to help normalize blood sugar.

• *Guar gum.* Extracted from the seeds of the guar plant, guar gum is good for the treatment of diabetes and for curbing the appetite. It also has the ability to reduce the levels of cholesterol, triglycerides, and low-density lipoproteins in the blood, and binds with toxic substances and carries them out of the body. Guar gum tablets must be chewed thoroughly or sucked gradually, not swallowed whole, and should be taken with lots of water, because guar gum has a tendency to ball up in the throat when mixed with saliva. It should not be used by individuals who have difficulty swallowing or who have had gastrointestinal surgery. Some persons with colon disorders may have trouble using guar gum.

• *Oat bran and rice bran.* Bran is the broken coat of the seed of cereal grain that has been separated from the flour or meal by sifting or bolting. It helps to lower cholesterol.

• *Psyllium seed.* Psyllium is a grain grown in India that is utilized for its fiber content. A good intestinal cleanser and stool softener, it is one of the most popular fibers used. It thickens very quickly when mixed with liquid, and must be consumed immediately. Some doctors recommend Metamucil, which contains psyllium hydrophilic mucilloid, as a laxative and fiber supplement. However, we prefer less processing and all-natural products.

Cellulose

Cellulose is an indigestible carbohydrate found in the outer layer of vegetables and fruits. It is good for hemorrhoids, varicose veins, colitis, and constipation, and for the removal of cancer-causing substances from the colon wall. It is found in apples, beets, Brazil nuts, broccoli, carrots, celery, green beans, lima beans, pears, peas, and whole grains.

Hemicellulose

Hemicellulose is an indigestible complex carbohydrate that absorbs water. It is good for promoting weight loss, relieving constipation, preventing colon cancer, and controlling carcinogens in the intestinal tract. Hemicellulose is found in apples, bananas, beans, beets, cabbage, corn, green leafy vegetables, pears, peppers, and whole grain cereals.

Lignin

This form of fiber is good for lowering cholesterol levels. It helps to prevent the formation of gallstones by binding with bile acids and removing cholesterol before stones can form. It is beneficial for persons with diabetes or colon cancer. Lignin is found in Brazil nuts, carrots, green beans, peaches, peas, potatoes, strawberries, tomatoes, and whole grains.

Pectin

Because it slows the absorption of food after meals, pectin is good for people with diabetes. It also removes unwanted metals and toxins, reduces the side effects of radiation therapy, helps lower cholesterol, and reduces the risk of heart disease and gallstones. Pectin is found in apples, bananas, beets, cabbage, carrots, citrus fruits, dried peas, and okra.

Combination Fiber Supplements

There are many products available that combine two or more different types of fiber, or that combine fiber with other ingredients. Three products of this kind that we recommend are:

• Aerobic Bulk Cleanse (ABC) from Aerobic Life Industries. This product is an excellent source of fiber. It contains blond psyllium seed husks and the herbs licorice and hibiscus. This therapeutic drink aids in healing and cleansing the colon. It is excellent for diarrhea and constipation. Add it to a combination of one-half aloe vera juice and one-half fruit juice. Be sure to take this mixture on an empty stomach, first thing in the morning. Stir it well and drink it down quickly, before it thickens. Related products, also from Aerobic Life Industries, include 10-Day Colon Cleanse and 45-Day Cleanse for Colon, Blood, and Lymph.

• Aerobic Colon Care from Aerobic Life Industries. This formula contains psyllium and oat bran, and provides approximately 3 grams of soluble fiber and 4 grams of insoluble fiber per serving.

• A.M/P.M. Ultimate Cleanse from Nature's Secret. This formula combines gums with cellulose, hemicellulose, pectin, and lignin, plus herbs that support and cleanse the blood and internal organs. It is a two-part system for stimulating and detoxifying the entire body.

Fish Oil

See under Essential Fatty Acids in this section.

5-Hydroxy L-Tryptophan (5-HTP)

5-HTP is a substance that is created naturally in the body from the amino acid tryptophan, and that in turn is used by the body to produce serotonin, an important neurotransmitter. Supplemental 5-HTP is derived from the seeds of the griffonia plant (*Griffonia simplicifolia*), which is native to western Africa. It can be used to aid in weight loss, insomnia, and depression. In a sense, 5-HTP can be seen as a substitute for supplemental L-tryptophan, which is no longer available in the United States (*see* AMINO ACIDS in Part One). 5-HTP should be used together with a high-carbohydrate food or liquid such as orange juice, and as part of a comprehensive nutritional program. It may not benefit everyone who takes it. If you regularly take large doses of 5-HTP (more than 300 milligrams daily), you should undergo blood testing for eosinophil (a type of white blood cell) levels every three months. HTP.Calm from Natural Balance is a good source of 5-HTP. You should avoid this supplement if you are taking antidepressants.

Flaxseeds and Flaxseed Oil

See under Essential Fatty Acids in this section.

Garlic

Garlic is one of the most valuable foods on this planet. It has been used since Biblical times and is mentioned in the literature of the ancient Hebrews, Greeks, Babylonians, Romans, and Egyptians. The builders of the pyramids supposedly ate garlic daily for endurance and strength.

Garlic lowers blood pressure through the actions of one of its components, methyl allyl trisulfide, which dilates blood vessels. It thins the blood by inhibiting platelet aggregation, which reduces the risk of blood clots and aids in preventing heart attacks. It also lowers serum cholesterol levels and aids in digestion. Garlic is useful for many diseases and illnesses, including cancer. It is a potent immune system stimulant and a natural antibiotic. It should be consumed daily. It can be eaten fresh, taken in supplement form, or used to prepare garlic oil.

Garlic contains an amino acid derivative, alliin. When garlic is consumed, the enzyme alliinase, which converts alliin to allicin, is released. Allicin has an antibiotic effect; it exerts an antibacterial effect estimated to be equivalent to 1 percent of that of penicillin. Because of its antibiotic properties, garlic was used to treat wounds and infections and to prevent gangrene during World War I.

Garlic is also effective against fungal infections, including athlete's foot, systemic candidiasis, and yeast vaginitis, and there is some evidence that it may also destroy certain viruses, such as those associated with fever blisters, genital herpes, a form of the common cold, smallpox, and a type of influenza.

Garlic oil is good for the heart and colon, and is effective in the treatment of arthritis, candidiasis, and circulation problems. To make garlic oil, add peeled whole garlic cloves to a quart of olive or canola oil. Experiment to find the number of cloves that gives the degree of flavor you like. Be sure to wash your hands thoroughly and rinse the garlic after peeling and before placing it in the oil. The peel may contain mold and bacteria that can contaminate the oil. Keep this oil refrigerated. This mixture will keep for up to a month before you need to replace it with fresh oil. Garlic oil can be used for sautéing, in salad dressings, and in a variety of other ways. If you find the odor too strong after you eat garlic, chew some sprigs of parsley or mint, or caraway or fennel seeds.

An alternative to fresh garlic is Kyolic from Wakunaga of America. Kyolic is an odorless, "sociable" garlic product, and is available in tablet, capsule, and oil extract forms.

Ginkgo Biloba

The ornamental tree *Ginkgo biloba* originated in China thousands of years ago, and now grows in temperate climates throughout the world. The extract of its fan-shaped leaves is one of the world's most popular herbal products. It has been reported in scientific journals to enhance blood circulation and to increase the supply of oxygen to the heart, brain, and all bodily parts. This makes it useful for improving memory and relieving muscle pains. It also acts as an antioxidant, has anti-aging effects, reduces blood pressure, inhibits blood clotting, and is helpful for tinnitus, vertigo, hearing loss, impotence, and Raynaud's disease. Ginkgo biloba is widely known as the "smart herb" of our time. It has even been shown to slow the early progression of Alzheimer's disease in some individuals.

Ginseng

Ginseng is used throughout the Far East as a general tonic to combat weakness and give extra energy. There are a number of different types of ginseng: *Eleutherococcus senticosus* (Siberian ginseng), *Panax quinquefolium* (American ginseng), *Panax ginseng* (Chinese or Korean ginseng), and *Panax japonicum* (Japanese ginseng). *Panax ginseng* is the most widely used species.

Early Native Americans were familiar with ginseng. They called it *gisens* and used it for stomach and bronchial disorders, asthma, and neck pain. Russian scientists claim that the ginseng root stimulates both physical and mental activity, improves endocrine gland function, and has a positive effect on the sex glands. Ginseng is beneficial for fatigue because it spares glycogen (the form of glucose stored in the liver and muscle cells) by increasing the use of fatty acids as an energy source. It is used to enhance athletic performance, to rejuvenate, to increase longevity, and to detoxify and normalize the entire system.

In lower doses, ginseng seems to raise blood pressure, while higher amounts appear to reduce blood pressure. Research suggests that high doses of ginseng may be helpful for inflammatory diseases such as rheumatoid arthritis, without the side effects of steroids, and may also protect against the harmful effects of radiation. Ginseng is beneficial for people with diabetes because it decreases the level of the hormone cortisol in the blood (cortisol interferes with the function of insulin). However, people with hypoglycemia should avoid using large amounts of ginseng.

The root is sold in many forms: as a whole root or root pieces, which are either untreated or blanched; as a powder or powdered extract; as a liquid extract or concentrate; in granules for instant tea; as a tincture; in an oil base; and in tablets and capsules. These products should not contain sugar or added color, and should be pure ginseng. Many supplement manufacturers add ginseng to combination products, but these often contain such low amounts that they may not be effective. Wakunaga of America distributes several high-quality Korean and Siberian ginseng products.

We advise following the Russian approach to using ginseng: Take it for fifteen to twenty days, followed by a rest period of two weeks. Avoid long-term usage of high doses.

Glucomannan

See under Fiber in this section.

Glucosamine

This is one of a number of substances classified as an *amino sugar.* Unlike other forms of sugar in the body, amino sugars are components of carbohydrates that are incorporated into the structure of body tissues, rather than being used as a source of energy. Glucosamine is thus involved in the formation of the nails, tendons, skin, eyes, bones, ligaments, and heart valves. It also plays a role in the mucous secretions of the digestive, respiratory, and urinary tracts.

Glucosamine is made in the body from the simple carbohydrate glucose and the amino acid glutamine. It is found in high concentrations in joint structures. It is also available as a supplement, in the form of glucosamine sulfate, which helps to combat both the causes and symptoms of osteoarthritis. Glucosamine has been proven in over 300 studies and 20 clinical trials to actually build joint cartilage. It can also slightly reduce the destruction of cartilage and depression caused by taking nonsteroidal anti-inflammatory drugs (NSAIDs), which are commonly prescribed for people with arthritis. Glucosamine may be taken in conjunction with chondroitin sulfate for an even greater effect on osteoarthritis (*see* Chondroitin Sulfate in this section).

In addition to having benefits for people with osteoarthritis, supplemental glucosamine can be helpful for asthma, bursitis, candidiasis, food allergies, osteoporosis, respiratory allergies, tendinitis, vaginitis, and various skin problems. GS-500 from Enzymatic Therapy is a good source of glucosamine. GlucosaMend from Source Naturals, Glucosamine Plus from FoodScience Laboratories, and Glucosamine Sulfate Complex from PhytoPharmica are other recommended products. A related compound is N-acetylglucosamine (NAG), available as N-A-G from Source Naturals.

Grape Seed Oil

See under Essential Fatty Acids in this section.

"Green Drinks"

"Green drinks" are natural food formulas made from plants that are good detoxifiers and blood cleansers, as well as sources of chlorophyll, minerals, enzymes, and other important nutrients. Generally, they are sold in powdered form to be mixed just before use. Many different companies market green drink formulas. The following are some recommended products:

- Barley Green from AIM International. This product contains a combination of barley juice and kelp.

- Earthsource Greens & More from Solgar. This formula combines four organically grown grasses (alfalfa, barley, kamut, and wheat), Hawaiian blue-green spirulina, and Chinese chlorella with three potent immune-stimulating mushrooms (maitake, reishi, and shiitake), plus powdered broccoli, carrots, and red beets, which supply phytonutrients. Its fruit flavor comes from fresh fruit powders.

- Green Magma from Green Foods Corporation. Green Magma is a pure, natural juice of young barley leaves that are organically grown in Japan and are pesticide-free. Brown rice is added to supply vitamins B_1 (thiamine) and B_3 (niacin), and linoleic acid. Green Magma contains thousands of enzymes, which play an important role in the metabolism of the body (*see* ENZYMES in Part One), plus a high concentration of superoxide dismutase (SOD). The powdered product may be added to juice or quality water.

- Kyo-Green from Wakunaga of America. This is a combination of barley, wheatgrass, kelp, and the green algae chlorella. The barley and wheatgrass are organically grown. It is a highly concentrated natural source of chlorophyll, amino acids, vitamins and minerals, carotene, and enzymes. Chlorella is a rich natural source of vitamin A, and kelp supplies iodine and other valuable minerals. (*See* Chlorella and Kelp in this section.)

- ProGreens from NutriCology. ProGreens includes organic alfalfa, barley, oat, and wheatgrass juice powders; natural fiber; wheat sprouts; blue-green algae; sea algae; fructooligosaccharides (FOS); lecithin; standardized bioflavonoid extracts; royal jelly and bee pollen; beet and spinach extracts; acerola juice powder; natural vitamin E; and the herbs astragalus, echinacea, licorice, Siberian ginseng, and suma.

Green Papaya

Green (unripe) papaya is an excellent source of vitamins, minerals, and enzymes. Ounce for ounce, it contains more vitamin A than carrots and more vitamin C than oranges, as well as abundant B vitamins and vitamin E. The complex of enzymes it contains helps to digest proteins, carbohydrates, and fats.

Green papaya can be eaten fresh or taken in supplement form. Papain is the most abundant, most active enzyme in both the fresh fruit and the powdered supplement form. Papain possesses very powerful digestive action. A good source of green papaya is Mature Green Papaya Powder from Papaya John's. Papaya John's makes a variety of papaya bars, including Papaya Ginger & NONI Turmeric

Milk Thistle & Flax, which is a papaya bar that is very beneficial for the internal organs (especially the liver), Papaya Almond, and Papaya Macadamia Nut. The same company also produces a Papaya Honey concentrate that can be used as a replacement for sugar, honey, or syrup, or as a jam.

Guar Gum

See under Fiber in this section.

Hemicellulose

See under Fiber in this section.

Honey

Bees produce honey by mixing nectar, which is a sweet substance secreted by flowers, with bee enzymes. Honey is a highly concentrated source of many essential nutrients, including large amounts of carbohydrates (sugars), some minerals, B-complex vitamins, and vitamins C, D, and E.

Honey is used to promote energy and healing. It is a natural antiseptic and makes a good salve for burns and wounds. Honey is also used for sweetening other foods and beverages. It varies somewhat in color and taste depending on the origin of the flower and nectar, but in general it is approximately twice as sweet as sugar, so not as much is needed for sweetening purposes.

People who have diabetes or hypoglycemia should be careful when consuming honey and its byproducts. These substances affect blood sugar levels in the same way that refined sugars do. Tupelo honey contains more fructose than other types of honey and it is absorbed at a slower rate, so some people with hypoglycemia can use this type sparingly without ill effects.

Buy only unfiltered, unheated, unprocessed honey, and *never* give honey to an infant under one year of age. In its natural form, honey can contain spores of the bacteria that cause botulism. This poses no problem for adults and older children, but in infants, the spores can colonize the digestive tract and produce the deadly botulin toxin there. Honey is safe for babies after age one.

Inosine

Inosine occurs naturally in the human body. It is involved in the rebuilding of adenosine triphosphate (ATP; see page 63), and stimulates the production of a compound designated 2,3-disphosphoglycerate (2,3-DPG), which is needed in the transportation of oxygen to muscle cells for the production of energy. Weight and endurance trainers have found supplemental inosine to be beneficial; it is believed to increase muscle development and blood circulation. It also enhances immune function.

If you have kidney problems or gout, you should not take inosine because it contains nitrogen and can increase the production of uric acid. For best results, use the dosage recommended by the manufacturer for your body size, and take it forty-five to sixty minutes prior to exercising.

Inositol Hexaphosphate (IP$_6$)

Inositol hexaphosphate (IP$_6$, also known as phytic acid) is a compound consisting of the B vitamin inositol plus six phosphate groups. Found naturally in many foods, including wheat, rice, and legumes, it is a powerful antioxidant that has many positive effects on the body. Laboratory studies suggest it may fight cancer, prevent and treat heart disease, prevent kidney stones and liver disease, and also reduce cholesterol levels and prevent the inappropriate formation of blood clots, a major cause of heart attacks. IP$_6$ inhibits the activity of free radicals in the body, which slows the type of abnormal cell division associated with cancer and tumor growth. It works best very early in the development of malignant tumors, before the malignancy can even be recognized by the immune system. The cells are then normalized and begin to grow in the usual manner again.

IP$_6$ contains a substance designated beta-1,3-D-glucan, which helps to maintain a strong immune system in people undergoing chemotherapy and radiation. IP$_6$ protects the heart by preventing the formation of blood clots in blood vessels and reducing the levels of cholesterol and triglycerides (fats) in the bloodstream. It protects the liver by preventing fatty deposits from accumulating there. Studies have shown that a diet high in IP$_6$ is associated with a lower incidence of cancer of the breast, colon, and prostate.

Significant amounts of IP$_6$ are found in foods such as beans, brown rice, whole-kernel corn, sesame seeds, wheat bran, cornbread, grape juice, raisins, and mulberries. It can also be taken in supplement form. Some studies have shown that IP$_6$ may interfere with the body's absorption of minerals, so supplements should not be taken within one hour of meals. IP$_6$ from Jarrow Formulas and Cell Forté with IP-6 from Enzymatic Therapy are recommended sources of IP$_6$.

Kelp

Kelp is a type of seaweed that can be eaten raw, but it is usually dried, granulated, or ground into powder. It is also available in a liquid form that can be added to drinking water. Granulated or powdered kelp can be used as a condiment and for flavoring, as a salt substitute. If you find the taste unappealing, you can purchase it in tablet form.

Kelp is a rich source of vitamins, especially the B vitamins, as well as of many valuable minerals and trace elements. It is reported to be very beneficial to brain tissue, the membranes surrounding the brain, the sensory nerves, and the spinal cord, as well as the nails and blood vessels. It has been used in the treatment of thyroid problems because of its iodine content, and is useful for other conditions as varied as hair loss, obesity, and ulcers. It protects against the effects of radiation and softens stools. Kelp is recommended as a daily dietary supplement, especially for people with mineral deficiencies.

Kombucha Tea

The kombucha, or Manchurian, "mushroom" has reputedly been used in Asian countries and in Russia for centuries. The "mushroom" itself is not eaten. Rather, a tea is made by fermenting the "mushroom" for about a week in a mixture of water, sugar, and green or black tea, with apple cider vinegar or a bit of previously made tea added. Kept in this mixture, the "mushroom" reproduces, and the "daughter mushrooms" can then be used to produce more tea.

Although commonly referred to as a mushroom, the kombucha is actually a combination of a number of different elements, including lichen, bacteria, and yeast. Kombucha tea contains a variety of different nutrients and other health-promoting substances. It is a natural energy booster and detoxifier that may also help slow or reverse the aging process and fight such serious diseases as AIDS, cancer, and multiple sclerosis.

Because of the way in which it has traditionally been propagated (one at a time, by individual users), kombucha may be difficult to find. Many people who have them received a daughter "mushroom" as a gift from a friend, although there are some herbal companies that sell both the "mushrooms" and the bottled tea commercially.

Lactobacillus Acidophilus

Lactobacillus acidophilus is a type of "friendly" bacteria that assists in the digestion of proteins, a process in which lactic acid, hydrogen peroxide, enzymes, B vitamins, and antibiotic substances that inhibit pathogenic organisms are produced. Acidophilus has antifungal properties, helps to reduce blood cholesterol levels, aids digestion, and enhances the absorption of nutrients.

The flora in the healthy colon should consist of at least 85 percent lactobacilli and 15 percent coliform bacteria. However, the typical colon bacteria count today is the reverse. This can result in gas, bloating, intestinal and systemic toxicity, constipation, and malabsorption of nutrients, and is conducive to an overgrowth of candida. Taking an acidophilus supplement helps to combat all of these problems by returning the intestinal flora to a healthier balance. In addition, acidophilus may help to detoxify harmful substances.

There are many good acidophilus supplements available. Acidophilus products come in tablet, capsule, and powdered forms. We recommend using the powdered form. Natren markets quality products that contain very high numbers of organisms. Nondairy formulas are best for people who are allergic to dairy products, and they work well against candida. Probiata from Wakunaga of America

is a milk-free product that remains stable at high temperatures. Other good nondairy acidophilus supplements include Primadophilus from Nature's Way, Neo-Flora from New Chapter, and Flora from DaVinci Labs. In general, we believe it is not advisable to buy a product containing a combination of different strains of lactobacilli, as one organism may be antagonistic to another. A single-strain product with a count of at least 1 billion organisms per gram is often better than a combination.

Acidophilus can die at high temperatures. Whatever product you choose, keep it in a cool, dry place—refrigerate but do not freeze it. Take acidophilus on an empty stomach in the morning and one hour before each meal. If you are taking antibiotics, do not take the antibiotics and acidophilus simultaneously.

Lactoferrin

Lactoferrin is a protein that occurs naturally in human bile, tears, mucus, saliva, and milk. Because it binds with free iron in the body, it plays an important role in regulating iron levels (and, in turn, growth) and aids in preventing and fighting infection by depriving disease-causing organisms of the iron they need to grow and multiply. It also plays a role in the functioning of lymphocytes, a type of white blood cell important for immunity. Taken in supplement form, it may boost immune function and help in combating both infectious and inflammatory conditions. It may also benefit intestinal health.

Lecithin

Lecithin is a type of lipid that is needed by every living cell in the human body. Cell membranes, which regulate the passage of nutrients into and out of the cells, are largely composed of lecithin. The protective sheaths surrounding the brain are composed of lecithin, and the muscles and nerve cells also contain this essential fatty substance. Lecithin consists mostly of the B vitamin choline, and also contains linoleic acid and inositol. Although lecithin is a lipid, it is partly soluble in water and thus acts as an emulsifying agent. This is why many processed foods contain lecithin.

This nutrient helps to prevent arteriosclerosis, protects against cardiovascular disease, improves brain function, and aids in the absorption of thiamine by the liver and vitamin A by the intestine. It is also known to promote energy and is needed to help repair damage to the liver caused by alcoholism. Lecithin enables fats, such as cholesterol and other lipids, to be dispersed in water and removed from the body. The vital organs and arteries are thus protected from fatty buildup.

Lecithin would be a wise addition to anyone's diet. It is especially valuable for older adults. Anyone who is taking niacin for high serum cholesterol and triglycerides should also include lecithin in his or her program. Two tablespoons of lecithin granules can be sprinkled on cereals and soups or added to juices or breads. Lecithin also comes in capsule form. Taking one 1,200-milligram capsule before each meal helps in the digestion of fats and the absorption of fat-soluble vitamins.

Most lecithin is derived from soybeans, but recently egg lecithin has become popular. This type of lecithin is extracted from the yolks of fresh eggs. Egg lecithin may hold promise for those suffering from AIDS, herpes, chronic fatigue syndrome, and immune disorders associated with aging. Studies have shown that it works better for people with these disorders than soy lecithin does. Other sources of lecithin include brewer's yeast, grains, legumes, fish, and wheat germ.

Lignin

See under Fiber in this section.

Maitake

Maitake (*Grifola frondosa*) is a mushroom that has a long history of use in traditional Chinese and Japanese herbology and cooking. It grows wild in Japan, as well as in some wooded areas in eastern North America. Because maitake is difficult to cultivate, however, only relatively recently have the mushrooms become widely available.

Maitake is considered an adaptogen, which means that it helps the body adapt to stress and normalizes bodily fuctions. Its healing properties are thought to be related to its high content of a polysaccharide called beta-1,6-glucan, which is considered very powerful. In laboratory studies, this substance has been shown to prevent carcinogenesis, inhibit the growth of cancerous tumors, kill HIV, and enhance the activity of key immune cells known as T-helper cells or CD4 cells. Maitake may also be useful for diabetes, chronic fatigue syndrome, chronic hepatitis, obesity, and high blood pressure.

Research suggests that maitake is better absorbed than other mushrooms, such as shiitake, and it is almost as effective when taken orally as it is when taken intravenously. Maitake can be eaten in food or taken as a supplement. Buy organically grown dried mushrooms (when using them in cooking, soak them in water or broth for half an hour first), or purchase maitake in capsule, extract, or tea form. Some of the capsule supplements contain a small amount of vitamin C, which enhances the effectiveness of the active ingredient in maitake by aiding in its absorption.

Melatonin

The hormone melatonin is naturally produced by the pineal gland, a cone-shaped structure in the brain. The body's pattern of melatonin production is similar to that of the other "anti-aging" hormones, human growth hormone (HGH) and dehydroepiandrosterone (DHEA). Throughout early life, melatonin is produced in abundance. Shortly before puberty, though, the production of melatonin begins to drop, and then continues to decline steadily as we age.

Research has demonstrated that melatonin may have several profound long-term effects on the body. As one of the most powerful antioxidants ever discovered—with a greater range of effectiveness than vitamin C, vitamin E, or beta-carotene—melatonin helps prevent harmful oxidation reactions from occurring. In this way, melatonin may prevent the changes that lead to hypertension and heart attack, and may reduce the risk of certain kinds of cancer. Indeed, research has indicated that many age-related problems are caused by declining levels of melatonin, which leave the body less able to prevent and repair oxidative damage. Melatonin also has been found to stimulate the immune system; have a major role in the production of estrogen, testosterone, and possibly other hormones, helping to prevent cancers involving the reproductive system; and slow the growth of existing malignancies. Recent studies suggest that if melatonin is taken in the mornings, tumor growth may be stimulated, but if it is taken in the evenings, tumor growth tends to be slowed. In addition, as melatonin is secreted cyclically, in response to the fall of darkness at the end of each day, the hormone helps our bodies keep in sync with the rhythms of day and night. Thus, melatonin helps regulate sleep.

Research on melatonin continues, and with it, knowledge is increasing about the functions of melatonin in the body and the effects of melatonin supplementation. Both human research studies and anecdotal evidence indicate that melatonin supplements can be an effective and side-effect-free sleep aid both for adults suffering from insomnia and for children with autism, epilepsy, Down syndrome, cerebral palsy, and other problems that can cause sleep disorders. Animal and other laboratory research indicates that melatonin supplementation may help prevent age-related disorders, and perhaps extend life. Melatonin can be taken to ease PMS symptoms; stimulate the immune system; prevent memory loss, arteriosclerosis, and stroke; and treat cancer and Alzheimer's disease.

Although no toxic levels of melatonin have been found, some researchers feel that certain people probably should not use this supplement until further information is available. Included in this category are pregnant and nursing women; people with severe allergies or autoimmune diseases; people with immune system cancers, such as lymphoma and leukemia; and healthy children, who already produce sufficient amounts of the hormone. Since high doses of melatonin have been found to act as a contraceptive, women who wish to become pregnant also might want to avoid taking this supplement.

Melatonin should be taken two hours or less before bedtime. This schedule is designed to release the added hormone at the same time that natural production peaks. A sustained-release form is best if you frequently awaken after several hours' sleep; a sublingual form is best if you are very ill or suffer from malabsorption. When you

Maintaining Your Melatonin Level Naturally

As darkness falls at the end of each day, melatonin production rises. In the morning, when daylight hits the retina, neural impulses cause production of the hormone to slow. Clearly, light and darkness are the primary factors that set the rhythms of melatonin production. However, they are not the only factors involved. In fact, it has been found that a variety of regular daily routines can strengthen the rhythm of melatonin production. Here are a few simple ways in which you can help your body maintain high levels of this important hormone:

• Eat regular meals. The rhythm of melatonin production is strengthened by regular daily routines. Keep your mealtimes as regular as possible to keep your body in sync with the rhythms of the day.

• Keep your diet light at night. When melatonin production begins after nightfall, the digestive process is slowed. Thus, any heavy foods eaten close to bedtime may lead to digestive problems, which can make it difficult to sleep. To get the sleep you need, eat small, light meals in the late evening.

• Avoid stimulants. Stimulants like coffee, tea, and caffeine-containing medications and soft drinks can interfere with melatonin production by interfering with your sleep. As much as possible, eliminate these stimulants from your diet and lifestyle.

• Avoid exercising late at night. Vigorous activity delays melatonin secretion. If you exercise in the morning, you will reinforce healthful sleeping habits that lead to regular melatonin production. For best results, do your morning exercise outdoors, in the morning light.

---

awaken after melatonin-assisted sleep, you should feel refreshed—not tired or groggy. If you do experience grogginess, you should reduce the dosage. (To learn how you can maintain or increase your melatonin levels through daily routines, *see* Maintaining Your Melatonin Level Naturally, above.) For information on other anti-aging hormones, *see* DHEA THERAPY and GROWTH HORMONE THERAPY in Part Three.

Methylsulfonylmethane (MSM)

Methylsulfonylmethane (MSM, also known as dimethylsulfone) is a naturally occurring organic sulfur compound found in plant and animal tissues that is essential for optimum health. It is a derivative of dimethysulfoxide (DMSO), which has remarkable therapeutic properties, especially for the healing of injuries. It can also help to detoxify the body on a cellular level. MSM helps to nourish the hair, skin, and nails; relieve pain and inflammation; reduce allergy problems; and promote gastrointestinal health. It has also been found to aid immune function, and there have been reports of benefits to patients with heartburn, arthritis, lung problems, migraines, and muscle pain.

MSM is present naturally in foods such as fresh fish, meat, plants, fruit, and milk. However, it can be eliminated by even moderate processing, including drying or heating. Since most North Americans today eat considerable amounts of processed food, MSM is normally either not present at all or present only in very small amounts in the typical diet. Most people therefore would probably benefit from supplementation.

Research suggests that we require a constant supply of MSM for optimum good health, as sulfur is one of the essential minerals. Commonly recommended dosage levels are about 2,000 milligrams (2 grams) per day taken in divided doses, with the morning and evening meals, but it is best to start out at 1,000 milligrams (1 gram) per day to avoid a too-rapid rate of detoxification. Benefits usually become evident in two to twenty-one days, and can be enhanced by vitamin C supplementation. MSM from Aerobic Life Industries and OptiMSM from Cardinal Nutrition are good sources of this nutrient. Natrol produces a good MSM supplement as well.

Mucilage

See under Fiber in this section.

Nicotinamide Adenine Dinucleotide (NADH)

NADH is a form of vitamin B_3 (niacin) that is essential for the production of various neurotransmitters and cellular energy. NADH, which is also known as coenzyme 1, also acts as an antioxidant (*see under* ANTIOXIDANTS in Part One).

As we age, natural levels of NADH decline, which can lead to reduced levels of both energy and significant brain chemicals. Taking supplemental NADH can result in improvements in the biochemistry of energy production, especially in the brain and nervous systems. NADH shows promise as a therapy for Parkinson's disease because it results in an increase in brain levels of the neurotransmitter dopamine, which is deficient in people with this disorder. People with Alzheimer's disease may be helped by this supplement as well. Some people suffering from chronic fatigue syndrome (CFS) have shown significant improvement with NADH therapy. ENADA (NADH) from Kal Dietary Supplements is a good source of NADH.

Oat Bran

See under Fiber in this section.

Octacosanol

Octacosanol is a naturally derived wheat germ oil concentrate. (Although it would be possible to extract octacosanol from whole wheat, 10 pounds of wheat would be needed to obtain just 1,000 micrograms of octacosanol.) Wheat germ has long been known for its many benefits. Today, extracts of wheat germ weighing only 2 milligrams offer remarkable benefits as well.

Octacosanol has been clinically proven to increase oxygen utilization during exercise and improve glycogen stores in muscle tissue. As a result, it increases physical endurance, improves reaction time, reduces high-altitude stress, and aids in tissue oxygenation. This substance can greatly benefit those who experience muscle pain after exercise or have a lowered endurance level. It is good for muscular dystrophies and other neuromuscular disorders as well. It also reduces blood cholesterol levels.

Olive Leaf Extract

Olive leaf extract is an herbal supplement that has been shown to be effective against virtually all the viruses and bacteria on which it has been tested. Laboratory studies suggest that olive leaf extract interferes with viral infection becoming established and/or spreading, either by rendering viruses incapable of infecting cells or by preventing them from reproducing. It has been shown to help protect against infection by such viruses as human immunodeficiency virus (HIV), herpesviruses, and influenza viruses. It is useful for such disorders as pneumonia, sore throat, sinusitis, and skin diseases such as chronic infections and rashes, as well as for fungal and bacterial infections. Olivir from DaVinci Laboratories is a good source of olive leaf extract that has been tested in clinical trials.

Pectin

See under Fiber in this section.

Perilla

Perilla (*Perilla frutescens*) is an Asian plant that is a member of the mint family. It has been prescribed by Asian herbalists for the relief of cough and lung ailments, and for certain types of food poisoning, as well as to prevent the flu and restore energy balance. It may aid in increasing learning ability and is also used as a culinary herb.

Perilla comes in several forms, including seed oil. This is an unsaturated oil that contains linolenic, linoleic, and oleic acids. Perilla oil is available in capsule form. Studies suggest that it may be an effective and safe source of essential omega-3 fatty acids.

Phosphatidyl Choline

Phosphatidyl choline (PC) is a component of lecithin (*see* Lecithin in this section). Taken as a supplement, it helps to break down fats and can be helpful in preventing atherosclerosis (hardening of the arteries due to fatty plaques in the blood vessels), heart disease, gallstones, and liver problems. It is has also shown substantial benefits for people with neurological disorders, memory loss, and depression. PC is known to be safe and effective; however, people with manic-depressive disorder should not take large amounts.

Phosphatidyl Serine

Phosphatidyl serine (PS) is a substance classified as a phospholipid (a phosphorus-containing lipid) that is needed by every cell in the body, and is especially abundant in nerve cells. PS is the most important of the phospholipids and is crucial for the maintenance of healthy cell membranes. Although the brain normally produces enough PS, production dwindles as we age, which can result in deficiency.

Supplemental PS, which is compounded from soybean oil, has been found to reduce symptoms of depression and Alzheimer's disease, and to enhance memory and learning abilities. Some people have experienced nausea as a result of taking PS; however, taking it with food can help to avoid this. No danger has been reported with long-term use of this supplement. Its safety for pregnant women has not been determined.

Pregnenolone

Pregnenolone is a steroid hormone that the body normally manufactures from cholesterol, and that in turn can be metabolized into a variety of other vital hormones, including DHEA, progesterone, testosterone, and estrogen. The body's own pregnenolone levels decline with age, and many scientists believe that pregnenolone supplements may treat symptoms commonly associated with aging. Other benefits of using pregnenolone may include improved brain function that manifests itself as enhanced mood, memory, and thinking. Pregnenolone has also been known to lower cholesterol levels and alleviate the symptoms of conditions as varied as Alzheimer's disease, lupus, multiple sclerosis, premenstrual syndrome (PMS), rheumatoid arthritis, scleroderma, seizures, psoriasis, prostate disorders, stress, trauma, injuries, sleep disorders, and chronic fatigue syndrome. It also increases the effectiveness of hormone replacement therapy and the immune system.

It is important to use caution in taking supplemental pregnenolone. It has not yet been studied as thoroughly as other hormones that are available over the counter; consequently, its full effects on the body are not yet conclusively known. Until more information is available, it may be best to use the lowest effective dosage and to seek the supervision of a knowledgeable health care provider. Reported side effects of pregnenolone include headache, insomnia, irritability, anxiety, mood swings, irregularities of heartbeat, acne, growth of facial hair, and loss of scalp hair.

Primrose Oil

See under Essential Fatty Acids in this section.

Probiotics

Probiotics are beneficial bacteria normally present in the digestive tract. They are vital for proper digestion and also perform a number of other useful functions, such as preventing the overgrowth of yeast and other pathogens, and synthesizing vitamin K. The probiotics most often used as supplements are acidophilus and bifidobacteria (*see Lactobacillus acidophilus* and/or *Bifidobacterium bifidum* in this section). Cultured, or fermented, foods also contain various types and amounts of beneficial bacteria. These foods include buttermilk, cheese, kefir, miso, sauerkraut, tempeh, umeboshi, and yogurt.

Progesterone Cream

Progesterone is a hormone that is produced primarly by the ovaries and also by the adrenal glands. It works in partnership with estrogen to regulate menstrual cycles and is important for the maintenance of pregnancy. In addition to its role in the female reproductive system, it has a number of other important effects: it stimulates the activity of bone-building cells called osteoblasts; exerts an antidepressant and calming effect in the brain; helps to regulate blood sugar levels; and plays a role in maintaining the myelin sheaths that protect nerve cells. It can be used by the body to produce other hormones, including DHEA, estrogen, testosterone, and cortisol, as needed. A deficiency of progesterone, on the other hand, can exacerbate symptoms of premenstrual syndrome (PMS) and menopausal discomforts, and may increase the risk of osteoporosis. Progesterone deficiency becomes increasingly common in women as they approach menopause, and can start as early as age thirty five. Symptoms can include night sweats, hot flashes, depression, and premenstrual discomfort.

Supplemental progesterone is available in cream form. The hormone is absorbed through the skin after the cream is applied, and it passes directly into the bloodstream for transport to sites where progesterone is needed. Natural Woman Essential Body Cream from Products of Nature and Endocreme 900 Extra Strength from Wuliton Labs are recommended products.

Propolis

See Bee Propolis in this section.

Psyllium Seed

See under Fiber in this section.

Red Yeast Rice

Red yeast rice is a food product created by fermenting rice with a strain of red yeast (*Monascus purpureus* Went yeast). It is also sometimes referred to as Monascus rice or, in Chinese, *Hung-chu* or *Hong-Qu*. It has long been used in China and Japan as a food and as a remedy for digestive ailments and poor circulation. More recently, red yeast rice extract, taken in supplement form, has been found both to reduce overall blood cholesterol levels and to improve the ratio of HDL ("good cholesterol") to LDL ("bad cholesterol"). A study conducted by the University of California—Los Angeles School of Medicine found that people who took red yeast rice and maintained a low-fat diet reduced their overall cholesterol levels by an average of 40 points over a period of twelve weeks. The extract contains a number of cholesterol-lowering compounds known as *statins*. One of these is lovastatin, a substance also sold as a prescription drug under the brand name Mevacor. Lovastatin acts to lower cholesterol by inhibiting the action of an enzyme designated HMG-CoA reductase, which in turn limits the rate at which the body produces cholesterol. Studies have shown statins to lower cholesterol levels and reduce the risk of heart attack. Unlike prescription products, red yeast rice extract has shown no serious adverse side effects in clinical trials.

Reishi

See Shiitake and Reishi in this section.

Rice Bran

See under Fiber in this section.

Royal Jelly

Royal jelly is a thick, milky substance that is secreted from the pharyngeal glands of a special group of young nurse bees between their sixth and twelfth days of life. When honey and pollen are combined and refined within the young nurse bee, royal jelly is naturally created. This substance contains all of the B-complex vitamins, including a high concentration of pantothenic acid (vitamin B_5) and vitamin B_6 (pyridoxine), and is the only natural source of pure acetylcholine. Royal jelly also contains minerals, enzymes, hormones, eighteen amino acids, antibacterial and antibiotic components, and vitamins A, C, D, and E. It is useful for bronchial asthma, liver disease, pancreatitis, insomnia, stomach ulcers, kidney disease, bone fractures, and skin disorders, and it strengthens the immune system.

This product must be combined with honey to preserve

its potency. Royal jelly spoils easily. Keep it refrigerated and make sure it is tightly sealed when purchased.

S-adenosylmethionine (SAMe)

S-adenosylmethionine (SAMe) is a derivative of the amino acid methionine that is formed in the body when methionine combines with adenosine triphosphate (ATP), the major source of cellular energy. Taken as a supplement, SAMe has a variety of positive effects: it is an effective antidepressant; it is beneficial for disorders of the joints and connective tissue, including arthritis and fibromyalgia; it promotes the health of the liver; and it may lower levels of homocysteine, a dangerous amino acid that is associated with cardiovascular disease. It may also help to slow the aging process. SAMe works closely with folic acid, choline, and vitamins B_6 and B_{12}. It is one of a class of substances called *methyl donors*. As the name implies, methyl donors are compounds that "donate" units called methyl groups, which contain hydrogen and carbon atoms, to other substances. This process is called *methylation,* and it is one way in which the body protects itself from damage on the cellular level. Among other things, methyl donors help to protect against such serious disorders as cancer, heart disease, neurological disorders, and many age-related problems, and facilitate the manufacture of DNA and brain neurotransmitters. Taking supplemental SAMe may also increase natural levels of glutathione, an antioxidant; phosphatidyl choline, which aids in the metabolism of fats; and the hormone melatonin. A small number of people have experienced minor nausea and gastrointestinal disturbances as a result of taking high doses, but otherwise no notable side effects have been reported. Although SAMe is considered very safe, anyone with manic-depressive disorder (bipolar mood disorder) should consult a physician before taking this supplement. SAMe should always be taken on an empty stomach.

Sea Cucumber

Sea cucumbers, also known as *bêche de mer* and *trepang,* are not actually cucumbers, but are marine animals related to starfishes and sea urchins. They have been used in China for thousands of years as a treatment for arthritis. Modern research has confirmed they are beneficial for musculoskeletal inflammatory diseases, especially rheumatoid arthritis, osteoarthritis, and ankylosing spondylitis, a rheumatic disease that affects the spine.

Researchers believe that sea cucumbers improve the balance of prostaglandins, which regulate the inflammatory process. They also contain substances known as chondroitins, which are often lacking in people with arthritis and connective tissue disorders (*see* Chondroitin Sulfate in this section). In addition, sea cucumbers provide vitamins A, B_1 (thiamine), B_2 (riboflavin), and B_3 (niacin), and C, as well as the minerals calcium, iron, magnesium, and zinc.

Sea Cucumber from Futurebiotics is a good source of this supplement.

Sea Mussel

The green-lipped mussel (*Perna canaliculus*) is a species of edible shellfish. They contain numerous amino acids, the building blocks of body proteins, in addition to enzymes and essential trace elements. The minerals they contain are present in a balance similar to that in blood plasma, and these minerals are naturally chelated by the amino acids, making for better assimilation into the body.

Sea mussel aids in the functioning of the cardiovascular system, the lymphatic system, the endocrine system, the eyes, connective tissues, and mucous membranes. They help to reduce inflammation and relieve the pain and stiffness of arthritis. They also promote the healing of wounds and burns.

Shark Cartilage

The tough, elastic material that makes up the skeleton of the shark is dried and pulverized (finely powdered) to make this food supplement. Shark cartilage contains a number of active components, the most important of which is a type of protein that acts as an angiogenesis inhibitor—that is, it acts to suppress the development of new blood vessels. This makes it valuable in fighting a number of disorders. Many cancerous tumors, for instance, are able to grow only because they induce the body to develop new networks of blood vessels to supply them with nutrients. Shark cartilage suppresses this process, so that tumors are deprived of their source of nourishment and, often, begin to shrink. There are also certain eye disorders, such as diabetic retinopathy and macular degeneration, that are characterized by the growth of new blood vessels within the eye; because they grow in inappropriate places, the presence of these blood vessels can lead to blindness. Such diseases also may respond well to shark cartilage. Other conditions for which shark cartilage is useful include arthritis, psoriasis, and regional enteritis (inflammation of the lining of the bowels). In addition to angiogenesis-inhibiting protein, shark cartilage contains calcium (approximately 16 percent) and phosphorus (approximately 8 percent), which are absorbed as nutrients, and mucopolysaccharides that act to stimulate the immune system.

Shark cartilage is available in powder and capsule forms. Exercise caution when buying shark cartilage, as the purity and correct processing of the product are vital to its effectiveness. Not all shark cartilage products contain only 100-percent pure shark cartilage, so read labels carefully. Pure shark cartilage is white in color. If you find the odor and/or taste of pure shark cartilage to be stronger than you can tolerate, look for a product called BeneFin, which has significantly less fishy taste and smell than most other products. BeneFin is a trademarked name for naturally processed shark cartilage manufactured by Lane Labs-USA and marketed by various companies under license. If you are taking large quantities of shark cartilage, it may be wise to increase your supplementation of certain minerals, especially magnesium and potassium, to maintain a proper mineral balance in the body. Shark cartilage should *not* be taken by pregnant women or children, or by persons who have recently undergone surgery or suffered a heart attack.

Shiitake and Reishi

Shiitake and reishi are Japanese mushrooms with a delicate texture, strong stems, and well-defined undersides. They are attractive and have impressive health-promoting properties.

Shiitake (*Lentinus edodes*) contain a polysaccharide, lentinan, that strengthens the immune system by increasing T cell function. Shiitake mushrooms contain eighteen amino acids, seven of which are essential amino acids. They are rich in B vitamins, especially vitamins B_1 (thiamine), B_2 (riboflavin), and B_3 (niacin). When sun-dried, they contain high amounts of vitamin D. Their effectiveness in treating cancer has been reported in a joint study by the Medical Department of Koibe University and Nippon Kinoko Institute in Japan. These mushrooms are considered delicacies and are entirely edible.

Reishi (*Ganoderma lucidum*) have been popular for at least 2,000 years in the Far East. They were rated number one on ancient Chinese lists of superior medicines, and were believed to give eternal youth and longevity.

Today, both shiitake and reishi mushrooms are used to treat a variety of disorders and to promote vitality. They are used to prevent high blood pressure and heart disease, to control and lower cholesterol, to build resistance to disease, and to treat fatigue and viral infections. They are also known to have anti-tumor properties valuable in treating cancer.

The mushrooms are available fresh or dried for use in foods (soak dried mushrooms in warm water or broth for thirty minutes before using), as well as in supplements in capsule, pill, and extract form.

Spirulina

Spirulina is a microalgae that thrives in hot, sunny climates and in alkaline waters around the world, and produces twenty times as much protein as soybeans growing on an equal-sized area of land. It contains concentrations of nutrients unlike any other single grain, herb, or plant. Among its valuable components are gamma-linolenic acid (GLA), linoleic and arachidonic acids, vitamin B_{12} (needed, especially by vegetarians, for healthy red blood cells), iron, a high level of protein (60 to 70 percent), essential amino acids, the nucleic acids RNA and DNA, chlorophyll, and phycocyanin, a blue pigment that is found only in blue-green algae and that has increased the survival rate of mice with liver cancer in laboratory experiments.

Spirulina is a naturally digestible food that aids in protecting the immune system, in cholesterol reduction, and in mineral absorption. Because it supplies nutrients needed to help cleanse and heal, while also curbing the appetite, it is beneficial for people who are fasting. A person with hypoglycemia may benefit from using this food supplement between meals because its high protein content helps stabilize blood sugar levels.

Torula Yeast

See Yeast in this section.

Wheat Germ

Wheat germ is the embryo of the wheat berry. It is a good source of vitamin E; most of the B vitamins; the minerals calcium, magnesium, and phosphorus; and several trace elements.

One problem with wheat germ is that it spoils easily. If you purchase wheat germ separately from the flour, make sure the product is fresh. It should be either vacuum packed or refrigerated, with a packing date or a label stating the date by which the product should be used. Toasted wheat germ has a longer shelf life, but the raw product is better because it is unprocessed. Wheat germ oil capsules are also available.

Wheatgrass

Wheatgrass is a rich nutritional food that was popularized by Dr. Ann Wigmore, an educator and founder of the Hippocrates Health Institute in Boston. Wheatgrass contains a great variety of vitamins, minerals, and trace elements. According to Dr. Wigmore, 1 pound of fresh wheatgrass is equal in nutritional value to nearly 25 pounds of the choicest vegetables.

Dr. Wigmore reported that wheatgrass therapy, along with "living foods," helped to eliminate cancerous growths and helped many other disorders, including mental health problems. The molecular structure of chlorophyll resembles that of hemoglobin, the oxygen-carrying protein of red blood cells, and this may be the reason for the effectiveness of wheatgrass. The key difference between the two is that the metallic atom in the middle of each molecule of human hemoglobin is iron, while the metallic atom at the center of a molecule of chlorophyll is magnesium. In experiments on anemic animals, blood counts returned to normal after four to five days of receiving chlorophyll.

Whey Protein

Whey is a normal byproduct of cheesemaking; it is the liquid that is left when the solids in milk come together and are pressed into solid form. Whey protein is produced by filtering and purifying whey, then removing the water to produce a powder that, while high in quality protein, is free of fat and lactose (milk sugar).

This supplement helps to build lean body mass by increasing the body's production of muscle protein. For this reason, it is popular among athletes and body-builders, and also helps to protect against muscle-wasting in people with such diseases as AIDS and cancer. In addition to its effect on muscles, it appears to inhibit the proliferation of cancer cells, protect against free radical damage, and enhance immune function. Some recommended whey protein supplements include Biochem Whey Pro 290 from Country Life, Molkosan Whey of Life from Bioforce A.G., ProFlora Whey from Healing Arts Association, and Whey to Go from Solgar.

Yeast

Yeast are single-celled organisms that can multiply at extremely rapid rates, doubling in number in two hours. Yeast is rich in many basic nutrients, such as the B vitamins (except for vitamin B_{12}), sixteen amino acids, and at least fourteen different minerals. The protein content of yeast is responsible for 52 percent of its weight. Yeast is also high in phosphorus.

There are various media on which yeast may be grown. Brewer's yeast, also known as nutritional yeast, is grown on hops, a bitter herb that is also used as an ingredient in beer. Torula yeast is grown on blackstrap molasses or wood pulp. A liquid yeast product from Switzerland called Bio-Strath, distributed by Bioforce of America, is derived from herbs, honey, and malt. It is a natural product that we highly recommend.

Live baker's yeast should be avoided. Live yeast cells actually deplete the body of B vitamins and other nutrients. In nutritional yeast, these live cells are destroyed, leaving the beneficial nutrients behind.

Yeast may be consumed in juice or water, and is a good energy booster between meals. It can also be added to the diet to aid in treating certain disorders. It helps in sugar metabolism and is good for eczema, heart disorders, gout, nervousness, and fatigue. By enhancing the immune system, yeast is useful for people undergoing radiation therapy or chemotherapy for cancer. Yeast also seems to increase mental and physical efficiency. Dr. William Crook, author of *The Yeast Connection* (Vintage Books, 1986), states that if a person with candida-related health problems is not specifically allergic to yeast, it is all right for him or her to take a food supplement containing yeast. However, we suggest avoiding yeast products if candidiasis is suspected. Because yeast contains significant amounts of phosphorus, people suffering from osteoporosis should avoid yeast products. (*See* OSTEOPOROSIS in Part Two.) Those who do take yeast should be sure to take extra calcium as well.

Specialty Supplements

In addition to the substances discussed above, there are many natural food supplements designed for specific circumstances. There are too many of these products for us to discuss all of them here, but several that we feel are to be highly recommended are the following:

• Allergy Relief formulas from bioAllers. These are eight homeopathic formulas designed to relieve allergies by combining homeopathic remedies with specific allergens to help strengthen resistance to those allergens. Formulas include Animal Hair/Dander; Grain/Dairy; Grass Pollen; Mold/Yeast/Dust; Pollen/Hayfever; Sinus & Allergy Nasal Spray; and Tree Pollen.

• Arthogesic from Enzymatic Therapy. This is a topical gel designed to provide temporary relief from minor muscle aches, joint pain associated with arthritis, backache, bruises, strains, and sprains. The active ingredient is capsaicin, a compound derived from cayenne pepper (capsicum).

• Artichoke from Nature's Plus Herbal Actives. This supplement contains artichoke extract standardized to a minimum of 2.5 to 5 percent caffeylquinic acids, and also contains sesquiterpene lactones and the highly active flavonoids scolymoside, inulin, and taraxasterol. It is designed to support the liver and circulatory system (*see* Artichoke under Herbs and Their Uses in HERBS in Part One).

• Betatene from NatureWorks. This is a dietary supplement of mixed carotenoids, including alpha- and beta-carotene, lutein, lycopene, zeaxanthin, and cryptoxanthin. It is intended to help maintain a healthy and strong immune system.

• Body Language Essential Green Foods from Oxyfresh USA. This is a combination that includes alfalfa, Atlantic kelp, kale, spinach, spirulina, bladderwrack, dulse, barley grass, chlorella, dunaliella, and wheatgrass, plus the enzymes maltase, amylase, protease, lipase, cellulase, and pectinase, to provide a green food concentrate rich in beta-carotene, chlorophyll, and trace minerals.

• Bone Maximizer from Metabolic Response Modifiers. This is a combination supplement that contains microcrystalline hydroxyapatite concentrate (MCHC). MCHC is a source of bone proteins and highly absorbable calcium. Other ingredients include glucosamine, pregnenolone, vitamin D, magnesium, methylsulfonylmethane (MSM, a source of bioavailable sulfur), and other nutrients vital for bone health.

• Bone Support with Ostivone from Twinlab. This is a combination supplement designed to help maintain healthy bones. Ingredients include ipriflavone, calcium, vitamin D, magnesium, boron, and purified soy phytoestrogen extracts.

• BotanImmune from Bodyonics. This is a hypoallergenic dietary supplement designed to boost the immune system. Ingredients include thymus fractions, olive leaf extract, raspberry-ellagic acid, soy isoflavones, beta-1,3-glucan, and indole-3-carbinol, a compound found in broccoli, cabbage, and other cruciferous vegetables that has shown promise as an immune-boosting and anticancer substance.

• Breast Health from NaturalMax. This supplement contains the soy isoflavone genistein, black currant blend, freeze-dried broccoli, indole-3-carbinol, the herbs gotu kola and saw palmetto, and lycopene.

• CamoCare cream from Abkit. This product contains chamomile and other active ingredients. It relieves pain associated with a variety of ailments involving the muscles and joints, such as backache, arthritis, and pain from inflamed joints.

• Cardiaforce from Bioforce AG. This hawthorn berry extract promotes healthy cardiovascular function, circulation, and heart-muscle strength. It is a liquid supplement that is meant to be added to water and taken three times a day, before meals. It has no known interactions with other medications, and should be taken over a period of several months, with periodic short interruptions.

• Chromium Picolinate from Superior Source. This is a sublingual form of chromium picolinate that is particularly good for children, older adults, and people with malabsorption problems. Chromium picolinate promotes the burning of fat by the body, increases lean muscle mass, and helps to speed up the metabolism (*see* MINERALS in Part One).

• Cold, flu and allergy season formulas from ZAND. This is a line of products designed to support health through the various allergy seasons of the year. Individual formulas include Insure Herbal, an echinacea and goldenseal formula; Decongest Herbal, a natural decongestant formula; HerbalMist throat spray; and Allergy Season, which contains bromelain, nettle extract, quercetin, and vitamin B_5 (pantothenic acid). These formulas can be used individually or on a rotating basis.

• Diamond Mind from Diamond-Herpanacine Associates. This product combines a number of herbal extracts and nutrients, including ginkgo biloba, goto kola, ginseng, garlic, phosphatidyl serine, and phosphatidyl choline, in a supplement intended to support and improve memory, concentration, and mental energy and alertness.

• Diamond Trim from Diamond-Herpanacine Associates. This is a supplement program intended to promote weight loss by helping control appetite, reduce food cravings, increase the burning of calories, and reduce the absorption of fats. It also contains minerals to replenish those often lost through dieting. Ingredients include fiber, digestive enzymes, the herbs St. John's wort and griffonia, the minerals calcium and potassium, and a trace mineral complex.

• Earth's Bounty NONI from Matrix Health Products. Noni (*Morinda citrifolia*) is a small tree that grows in Hawaii and other tropical regions. The fruit of this plant has a long history of use for a wide variety of problems, including joint problems, pain, inflammation, digestive problems, and cardiovascular disorders. Its active compounds include phytochemicals, designated anthraquinones, enzymes, and alkaloids.

• Echinaforce from Bioforce. This is a liquid echinacea supplement that promotes natural disease resistance during the winter season and helps to maintain a healthy immune system.

• EstroGentle from Bodyonics. This is an herbal supplement designed to help support women's health during and after menopause. Ingredients include phytoestrogen-containing botanicals such as black cohosh and soy isoflavones, as well as chaste tree berry (*Vitex agnus-castus*), dong quai, licorice root, red clover leaf extract, and wild yam root.

• Fibroplex from Metagenics. This supplement contains vitamins B_1 (thiamine) and B_6 (pyridoxine), magnesium, manganese, and malic acid. It is designed to provide nutritional support for the nerves and muscles.

• GastroSoothe from Enzymatic Therapy. GastroSoothe is a natural antacid that contains calcium carbonate, deglycyrrhizinated licorice extract (DGL), and the amino acid glycine for the relief of indigestion and heartburn.

• Herbal Mood Boost from Country Life. This supplement contains a complex of herbs and nutrients known for their positive effects on mood and anxiety, including St. John's wort, 5-hydroxytryptophan (5-HTP), Siberian ginseng, kava kava, and passionflower.

• Hyper-C Serum from Jason Natural Cosmetics. This is an oil-based moisturizing formula that contains vitamin C, an antioxidant, to protect the skin from free radical damage. It also reduces the appearance of existing fine lines and wrinkles, evens out skin tones, and makes the skin softer and smoother in texture.

• HyperiCalm from Enzymatic Therapy. This supplement contains St. John's wort extract standardized to provide 0.3 percent hypericin. It is designed to support mental and nervous system function (*see* St. John's Wort under Herbs and Their Uses in HERBS in Part One).

• Instant Enerjetz from Superior Source. This is a convenient, easy-to-take form of vitamin B_{12} that is placed on or under the tongue (not swallowed). Vitamin B_{12} is needed to prevent anemia and maintain a healthy nervous system, and it boosts energy and combats fatigue (*see* VITAMINS in Part One).

• Jerusalem artichoke tablets. Jerusalem artichoke whole tuber flour (JAF) tablets are a good source of fructooligosaccharides (FOS), which support the growth of healthy intestinal flora.

• Kava-30 from Enzymatic Therapy. This supplement provides kava kava extract standardized to contain 30 percent kavalactones. It is designed to soothe and support the central nervous system (see Kava Kava under Herbs and Their Uses in HERBS in Part One).

• Kolorex from Forest Herbs. Kolorex is an herbal antifungal product that contains extract of the native New Zealand shrub *Pseudowintera colorata* and anise seed oil. Taken in capsule form, it aids in balancing the bacteria in the gastrointestinal tract, preventing an overgrowth of candida. There is also a topical cream form that can be applied directly to surface fungal infections, including athlete's foot, jock itch, and nail infections. The manufacturer recommended that the two forms of this product be used in combination for best results.

• Kyolic Neuro Logic from Wakunaga of America. This supplement contains aged garlic extract, ginkgo biloba extract, lecithin, acetyl-L-carnitine, and phosphatidyl serine in a formula designed to improve memory and mental activity.

• Maxi-Calm from Prevail Corporation. Maxi-Calm is a dietary supplement containing kava kava, valerian, passion flower, skullcap, and wild lettuce, each of which has traditionally been used to support the nervous system.

• Micellized Multiple Vitamin and Minerals from Earth Science, Inc. This is a liquid multivitamin and mineral supplement that is easily absorbed and utilized by the body.

• Miracle 2000 from Century Systems, Inc. is a combination supplement that contains twenty-seven vitamins and minerals, eighteen herbs, eight amino acids, and numerous ionic trace minerals.

• Nature's Answer FOR KIDS. This is a line of herbal extracts designed for children. They are made using alcohol, like standard extracts, but the alcohol is then removed and replaced with glycerin, which is a preservative and a natural sweetener. Formulas include Bubble B-Gone, a combination colic remedy containing catnip, chamomile, fennel, and lemon balm; KID Catnip; KID Chamomile; E-KID-nacea, an echinacea extract; E-KID-nacea Plus, which contains echinacea and goldenseal; Ginger KID; KID B-Well Tonic, an immune-system tonic containing astragalus, burdock, and dandelion; NAT-Choo: a cold and flu remedy containing a blend of boneset, catnip, echinacea, eyebright, and peppermint; and Tummie Tonic, an indigestion remedy including angelica, chamomile, fennel, ginger, meadowsweet, and slippery elm.

• Osteo-Max from Metabolic Response Modifiers. This supplement contains ipriflavone, an isoflavone similar to those found in soybeans and soy products, and microcrystalline hydroxyapatite concentrate (MCHC; see under Bone

Maximizer, above). It is designed to support both bone metabolism and the maintenance of bone density.

• Phytodolor from Enzymatic Therapy. This liquid supplement contains extracts of common ash, aspen, and goldenrod; the key compounds include salicylic acid derivatives, phenolic acid, flavonoids, and triterpene saponins. Phytodolor is intended to support muscle and joint function without causing stomach irritation, as many other products used for the relief of arthritis and similar disorders do.

• PreNatal Care from Natrol. This is a combination supplement designed for pregnant women and nursing mothers. Ingredients include essential vitamins, minerals, and antioxidants, among them the B vitamin folic acid and the omega-3 essential fatty acid docosahexaenoic acid (DHA), that are necessary for a healthy pregnancy and healthy prenatal development.

• Quick Cleanse Program from ZAND. This is a program utilizing three separate supplements: Cleansing Fiber formula, a fiber supplement containing psyllium seed and husk, plus bentonite and kaolin; Cleansing Laxative formula, with cascara sagrada (an herbal stimulant laxative) and kaolin; and Thistle Cleanse formula, a milk thistle supplement. This combination of formulas is designed to cleanse the intestinal tract, eliminate toxins, and support liver function.

• Remifemin and Remifemin Plus from Enzymatic Therapy. Remifemin is a standardized extract of black cohosh that has been used in Europe for over forty years for the treatment of menopausal symptoms. Remifemin Plus also contains standardized St. John's wort extract, which has been found to combat depression and improve the sense of emotional well-being (see Black Cohosh and St. John's Wort under Herbs and Their Uses in HERBS in Part One). These supplements do not affect hormone levels.

• Smart Longevity from E'Ola Products. This liquid supplement is designed to bolster brain function. It contains nutrients to enhance brain function and antioxidants to protect against free radical damage. Ingredients include vitamin C, ginseng extract, schizandra extract, dimethylaminoethanol (DMAE), choline, and vitamin E.

• Soy-Licious from Country Life. This dietary supplement is a high-protein soy-based drink mix with added genistein and daidzein (soy isoflavones), essential vitamins and minerals, antioxidants, and adaptogenic herbs (adaptogens are herbs that help the body adapt to and cope with the effects of stress).

• Sub-Adrene from American Biologics. This is a highly concentrated whole adrenal-cortical extract of bovine origin. Designed for sublingual administration, it has a peppermint taste and supplies a balance of natural steroids.

• Super Green Tea Extract from Prolongevity. This supplement contains 95 percent green tea extract standardized to 35 percent epigallocatechin gallate. It is available in two forms, regular and decaffeinated. Studies have indicated that green tea can help to protect against stroke and heart attack, and may even inhibit the growth of cancer cells (*see* Green Tea under Herbs and Their Uses in HERBS in Part One).

• Ultra High Performance Dietary Supplement from Excel. This supplement contains a blend of energizing herbs and is designed to provide the body with a quick boost of energy without caffeine.

• Ultra Juice Green from Nature's Plus. This is a supplement based on marine algae and containing a total of twenty different green foods in tablet form. It contains a wide range of vitamins, minerals, and phytonutrients.

• VitaSerum from ABRA Therapeutic Skin Care. This is a skin-care product designed to protect against free radicals, stimulate cell renewal, and reduce the visible signs of aging. It contains vitamin C from acerola berries; herbal extracts of elder flower, green tea, grape seed, and horsetail; citrus and cranberry bioflavonoids; hyaluronic acid; zinc sulfate; and essential oils of lavender, rose geranium, and sweet lavender.

• Vita Synergy for Men from The Synergy Company. This is a combination nutritional supplement that contains a balanced blend of all major vitamins and minerals, trace elements, and a variety of herbal extracts used to support men's health.

• Wellness Formula from Source Naturals. This supplement is designed to support optimal health in cold weather. Its ingredients include vitamins A and C, beta-carotene, and bioflavonoids; the immune-boosting mineral zinc; bee propolis; and the herbs angelica, astragalus, boneset, cayenne, echinacea, garlic, goldenseal, hawthorn berry, horehound, mullein, pau d'arco, and Siberian ginseng.

HERBS

INTRODUCTION

The medicinal benefits of herbs have been known for centuries. Records of Native American, Roman, Egyptian, Persian, and Hebrew medical practices show that herbs were used extensively to cure practically every known illness. Many herbs contain powerful ingredients that, if used correctly, can help heal the body. The pharmaceutical industry was originally based upon the ability to isolate these ingredients and make them available in a purer form. Herbalists, however, contend that nature provides other ingredients in the same herbs to balance the more powerful ingredients. These other components, though they may be less potent, may help to act as buffers, synergists, or counterbalances working in harmony with the more powerful ingredients. Therefore, when you use herbs in their complete form, your body's healing process utilizes a balance of ingredients provided by nature.

In the United States, herbal remedies were used widely until the early 1900s, when what was to become the modern pharmaceutical industry began isolating individual active compounds and producing drugs based on them. American medicine became almost exclusively committed to a medical system some practitioners call *allopathy*, which seeks to treat illness by producing a condition in the body that does not allow the disease to live or thrive. Over the years, most Americans have become conditioned to rely on synthetic, commercial drugs for relief.

Today, however, scientists are taking a second look at herbal remedies. Particularly in the past fifteen years, a growing body of research (much of it done in Europe) has pointed to the therapeutic potential of numerous herbs. But a lot of work remains to be done; only about 15 percent of the estimated plant species on earth have been investigated for possible medicinal uses.

Today's renewed interest in herbs reflects increasing concern about the side effects of powerful synthetic drugs, as well as the desire of many people to take charge of their own health, rather than merely submitting themselves to a sometimes impersonal health care system. We are also rediscovering the healthful benefits of tasty herbs for cooking and aromatic herbs for enhancing and helping to balance mental, spiritual, and physical health.

Nature's pharmacy is an abundant one. Many herbs are rich in compounds that have a beneficial effect on certain tissues and organs, and, therefore, can be used as medicines to treat, cure, or prevent disease. Herbal remedies can help nourish your immune system, stimulate the regeneration of damaged liver tissue, build the strength of the adrenal glands, counter the adverse side affects of chemotherapy, balance the endocrine system, stimulate milk production, and improve night vision, among other things.

Generally, medicinal herbs fall into two basic categories: tonic and stimulating.

Tonics help cells, tissues, and organs to maintain tone, or balance, throughout the body. Some tonics activate and invigorate bodily processes or parts. Other tonics supply important nutrients that cells, tissues, and organs need to function properly. Tonics ordinarily are taken regularly for three to nine months at a time to gently strengthen and improve overall health and/or certain organ functions.

Stimulating herbs have much stronger actions and are used to treat particular ailments. They should be taken in smaller doses than tonic herbs, and for shorter periods of time.

PHYTOMEDICINALS: THE HEALING POWER OF HERBS

Ancient cultures had no idea why herbs worked—they simply knew that certain plants produced certain desired results. Only in the last 100 years or so have chemists and pharmacists been isolating and purifying the beneficial chemical compounds in plants to produce reliable pharmaceutical drugs. About 25 percent of the prescription medicines sold today are (or were originally) derived from plants. For example, morphine and codeine come from the opium poppy; aspirin originated from willow bark; digitalis, a heart muscle strengthener, is derived from the foxglove plant; and paclitaxel (Taxol), used in cancer chemotherapy, comes from the Pacific yew tree.

Phytomedicine, a recently coined term, refers to an herbal medicine that is a whole-plant preparation, rather than a single isolated chemical compound. (The prefix *phyto* comes from the Greek word *phyton*, meaning "plant.") The herbal preparation derived from a whole plant or plant part is considered the active entity, even though it may actually contain hundreds of individual active components. Phytomedicines are standardized, however—that is, they contain set percentages of specified active components—and their therapeutic values are backed by pharmacological and clinical studies and experience.

Phytomedicines are widely recognized in Europe, where they are categorized as plant-derived drugs. In Germany, for example, phytomedicines are considered "ethical drugs," and physicians prescribe them and pharmacists dispense them. In the United States, phytomedicines are sold as over-the-counter dietary supplements in health food stores and in some pharmacies. A few mainstream doctors, however, have begun prescribing herbal remedies along with standard drugs. Some health insurance companies cover the cost of herbal medicines when they are prescribed by health care professionals. And the Office of Alternative Medicine, part of the National Institutes of Health, is funding research on herbal remedies. According to an article published in *USA Today*, nearly 50 million Americans regularly use herbal supplements.

OTHER HERBAL HEALING SYSTEMS

The World Health Organization estimates that 80 percent of the earth's population today depends on plants to treat common ailments. Herbalism is an essential part of Ayurvedic (Indian), traditional Asian, Native American, and naturopathic medicines. Many homeopathic remedies are derived from plants as well.

Oriental herbs are a recent addition to the American herb scene, with the influx of several popular Chinese herbs. The Chinese are today's foremost herbalists, drawing on thousands of years of experience in compounding and processing roots and herbs. In the Asian tradition, herbs are used to bring the whole body into balance and harmony. They are taken daily as a preventive measure, rather than as a treatment once illness has occurred. In the Orient, medicinal herbs often find their way into foods as seasoning and ingredients. Indeed, according to the late Chinese writer and scholar Lin Yutang, the Chinese view medicine and food as the same thing, believing that what is good for the body is medicine and at the same time is also food. Some of the Chinese herbs most readily found in U.S. herb and natural food stores include astragalus, Chinese ginseng, ginkgo biloba, gotu kola, licorice root, dong quai, ginger, and schizandra.

Every Native American nation has its own herbal medicine tradition based on the plants growing in the geographic area where it lives. Common among all Native American cultures is the spirituality attached to the gathering and use of herbs, and many peoples use the same herbs both medicinally and ceremonially. For the Navajos, for example, herbalism is a complex and specialized religion, in which the Navajo healer serves as both doctor and priest. Before plants are collected, prayers and offerings are made to the earth and the plant spirit. Herbs used in healing ceremonies are not thrown away, but are reverently placed back into the earth. Much like the Asian approach, Native American herbalism aims to achieve balance within the total person. Medicinal and ceremonial herbs commonly used by Native American cultures include American ginseng, yarrow, black cohosh, boneset, echinacea, goldenseal, nettles, juniper, wild buckwheat, and dogwood.

As they have for centuries, indigenous rainforest tribes around the world rely on the forests for virtually all their medicines. They too have incorporated herbs into their religions and everyday lives. Researchers estimate that the world's rainforests contain literally thousands of potentially useful medicinal plants. Rainforests exist on every continent, though most research attention is currently directed at the rainforests of South America, particularly in the Amazon, and of the South Pacific Islands. Out of this rich storehouse of natural remedies, only a handful are now commonly found in health food stores, among them pau d'arco, boldo, cat's claw, kava, yerba maté, suma, yohimbe, guarana, and passionflower. More and more rainforest remedies are becoming available, however.

USING MEDICINAL HERBS

Commercial herbal preparations are available in several different forms, including bulk herbs, medicinal herb blends, teas, oils, tinctures, fluid extracts, and tablets or capsules. Following are some of the ways in which herbal remedies can be used.

Essential Oils

Essential oils are highly concentrated extracts—typically obtained either by steam distillation or cold pressing—from the flowers, leaves, roots, berries, stems, seeds, gums, needles, bark, or resins of numerous plants. They contain natural hormones, vitamins, antibiotics, and antiseptics. Known also as *volatile oils* because they evaporate easily in air, essential oils are soluble in vegetable oil, partially soluble in alcohol, and not soluble in water. Because they are so concentrated, they are likely to irritate mucus membranes and the stomach lining if taken internally. It is therefore best to use essential oils externally only, such as in poultices, inhalants, bath water, or on the skin (a few drops). The therapeutic properties of essential oils can help to remedy ailments ranging from insomnia to respiratory disorders to impotence to arthritis.

Extracts

An extract is a concentrate that results when crude herb is mixed with a suitable solvent, such as alcohol and/or water. Of the different herbal forms, extracts are generally the most effective because their active ingredients are more highly concentrated, and they can be standardized to a guaranteed potency. Extracts also have longer shelf lives than other herbal preparations. Fresh herbal extracts retain almost all of the original plant's benefits.

Alcohol-free extracts are available. When administered sublingually (drops are placed under the tongue), herbal extracts can be absorbed by the body quickly. This is an especially effective way for older adults and people with absorption problems to use herbs.

Plasters, Compresses, and Poultices

These are ways of applying herbal remedies directly to the skin. Plasters and compresses are cotton bandages soaked in infusions or decoctions and wrapped around the affected area or held on with pressure. Compresses are also warm. Poultices are made by moistening herbs, placing them on the skin, and holding them there with a bandage. Moistened and warmed herbal tea bags also help soothe and heal. Try using chamomile tea bags to relieve the itching and inflammation of insect bites and eczema.

Powders

Powders are dried herbs ground to a fine consistency. You can sprinkle them over food, stir them into a liquid such as juice or water for tonics, or add them to soup stocks. You also can take them in capsule or tablet form.

Salves, Ointments, and Creams

These preparations combine a medicinal herb with an oily base for external use. Creams are light and slightly oily, to blend with the skin's secretions and allow the active ingredients to penetrate the skin. The heavier and oilier salves and ointments apply protective remedies to the skin surface.

Syrups

Syrups are used to improve the taste of bitter herbal formulas and to administer soothing cough or throat medicines. Herbs often taken in syrup form include wild cherry, marshmallow root, and licorice.

Teas, Infusions, and Decoctions

People have been consuming herbal teas for as long as they have known how to heat water—since well before recorded history. Unlike green, black, and oolong teas, herbal teas can be made from virtually any plant, and from any part of the plant, including the roots, flowers, seeds, berries, or bark, although there are some herbs, such as echinacea, gingko leaf, saw palmetto, and milk thistle, that are not effective as healing when taken in tea form because their active components are not water soluble, and the concentration needed for medicinal potency is so high it can be obtained only from an extract, pill, or capsule.

Different herbal teas, which sometimes contain thousands of beneficial active compounds, have their own distinctive healing uses. According to Varro Tyler, Ph.D., distinguished professor emeritus of pharmacognosy (the study of natural drug properties) at Purdue University, herbal teas are very good for relieving mild to moderate ailments such as upset stomach, sore throat, coughs, stuffy nose, and insomnia.

Many herbal teas are available in tea bag form. They can also be prepared from the raw herb. To make an herbal tea, gently crumble leaves and flowers and break roots and barks into pieces (cutting the herbs causes the essential oils to dissipate) and place them in a ceramic or glass container. Cover the herb parts with boiling water (do not bring the herbs themselves to a boil), and allow them to steep. Most herbs should be steeped for four to six minutes, although some herbal teas, such as chamomile, need to be steeped for fifteen to twenty minutes in a covered container in order to deliver their full therapeutic effect. Other herbs, such as ginseng roots, can be boiled. Astragalus can be lightly simmered for several hours. In fact, in Asia, ginseng root, astragalus, dong quai, and other herbs are added to chicken broth to make a tonic soup that is both food and medicine.

Infusion is simply another term for tea. This is the easiest way to take herbal remedies. To make an infusion, you simply boil water and add leaves, stems, flowers, or powdered herbs—plant material whose active ingredients dissolve readily in hot water—then steep, strain, and drink the mixture as a tea.

A decoction is a tea made from thicker plant parts, such as bark, roots, seeds, or berries. These also contain lignin, a substance that is difficult to dissolve in water. Thus, decoctions require a more vigorous extraction method than infusions.

Tinctures

Plant components that are either insoluble or only partially soluble in water can be extracted with solvents such as alcohol or glycerol. The herb is soaked in the solvent for a period of time, then pressed to render the tincture. Tinctures can preserve extracted ingredients for twelve months or more.

Vinegars

Herbal vinegars can serve as both medicines and salad dressings. To make an herbal vinegar, add the herb or herbs of your choice to raw apple cider vinegar, balsamic vinegar, rice vinegar, or malt vinegar. Allow the herbs to steep for four days (agitate the container daily), strain, then press through a straining cloth and bottle in a dark glass container.

Wines

Steeping herbs in wine is a novel and pleasant way to use them medicinally. Wine does not keep as long as the stronger alcohols, so refrigeration is a good idea.

However they are used, most herbs act gently and subtly. They do not produce the kind of dramatic, immediate results we expect from prescription drugs. Basically, herbs are balancers that work with the body to help it heal and regulate itself. They work better together than they do singly because the effect of one herb is usually supported and reinforced when combined with others.

While most herbs aren't likely to be harmful, keep in mind that "natural" isn't a synonym for "safe." Like synthetic drugs, herbal preparations may be toxic, cause allergic reactions, or affect your response to other medications. Common sense, care, and forethought are needed when using herbs for either food or medicine. Here are some essential guidelines for herbal self-care:

• Use herbal self-care for minor ailments only, not for serious or life-threatening conditions.

• Use only recommended amounts for recommended periods of time.

• Use the correct herb. Buy your herbal remedies from a reputable company. If you collect or grow herbs on your own, be absolutely positive in your identification.

• Use the correct part of the plant. For instance, don't substitute roots for leaves. When buying fresh herbs, check to be sure which part of the herb is required for a remedy—the whole herb, flowers, fruit, leaves, stems, or roots.

• When using an herbal remedy for the first time, start with a small amount to test for possible allergic reactions.

• Don't take certain herbs if you are pregnant or planning to become pregnant.

• Don't take herbal remedies if you are nursing a baby.

• Don't give medicinal amounts of herbs to children without first consulting with your health care practitioner.

BUYING HERBAL REMEDIES

When choosing herbal remedies, it is important to select quality products from a reliable source. How do you know whether a manufacturer or supplier is reliable? Start by making a phone call to the manufacturer. Ask how long the company has been in business, what their quality control practices are, and how they determine the identity and potency of the herbs they sell. Membership in trade groups such as the American Herbal Products Association, while not a stamp of approval, does indicate the company's recognition of industry standards. We recommend purchasing herbs sold by reputable companies that have been in the herb business for at least ten years. A number of manufacturers and distributors specializing in herbal products, including herbal combinations for prevention or treatment of certain disorders, are listed under Manufacturer and Distributor Information in the Appendix.

If you wish to buy organically grown herbs, look for the "certified organic" label on the product. More than half of U.S. states have certification programs for organic farms and products. Federal standards that will be implemented through a nationwide certification system are now being formulated under the USDA's National Organic Program.

Finally, look for herbal products that are standardized to contain a specific percentage of active ingredient extracted from the specific herb part known to be effective.

HERBS AND THEIR USES

The following table describes some of the most commonly used medicinal herbs, including which parts of each herb are used, its chemical and nutrient content, and its various uses.

Herb (Scientific Name)	Parts Used	Phytochemical and Nutrient Content	Actions and Uses	Comments
Acerola (*Malpighia glabra*)	Fruit.	Phytochemicals: Beta-carotene. Nutrients: Calcium, iron, magnesium, phosphorus, potassium, vitamins A, B_1, B_2, B_3, B_5, B_6, and C.	Has antioxidant, antifungal, and astringent properties. Helps to support the liver and hydrate the skin. Useful for diarrhea and fever.	A rainforest herb similar to the cherry. One of the richest natural sources of vitamin C; found in numerous multivitamin supplements.
Alfalfa (*Medicago sativa*)	Flowers, leaves, petals, sprouted seeds.	Phytochemicals: Alpha-carotene, beta-carotene, beta-sitosterol, chlorophyll, coumarin, cryptoxanthin, daidzein, fumaric acid, genistein, limonene, lutein, saponin, stigmasterol, zeaxanthin. Nutrients: Calcium, copper, folate, iron, magnesium, manganese, phosphorus, potassium, silicon, zinc, vitamins A, B_1, B_2, B_3, B_5, B_6, C, D, E, and K.	Alkalizes and detoxifies the body. Acts as a diuretic, anti-inflammatory, and antifungal. Lowers cholesterol, balances blood sugar and hormones, and promotes pituitary gland function. Good for anemia, arthritis, ulcers, bleeding-related disorders, and disorders of the bones and joints, digestive system, and skin.	Must be used in fresh, raw form to provide all nutrients. Sprouts are especially effective (be sure to rinse them thoroughly before use to remove mold and bacteria).

Herb (Scientific Name)	Parts Used	Phytochemical and Nutrient Content	Actions and Uses	Comments
Aloe (Aloe vera)	Pulp from insides of succulent leaves.	Phytochemicals: Acemannan, beta-carotene, beta-sitosterol, campesterol, cinnamic acid, coumarin, lignins, p-coumaric acid, saponins. Nutrients: Amino acids, calcium, folate, iron, magnesium, phosphorus, potassium, zinc, vitamins A, B_1, B_2, B_3, C, and E.	Acts as an astringent, emollient, anti-fungal, antibacterial, and antiviral. Applied topically, heals burns and wounds; and stimulates cell regeneration. Ingested, helps to lower cholesterol, reduces inflammation resulting from radiation therapy, increases blood-vessel generation in lower extremities of people with poor circulation, soothes stomach irritation, aids healing, and acts as a laxative. Good for AIDS and for skin and digestive disorders.	Allergic reactions, though rare, may occur in susceptible persons. Before using, apply a small amount behind the ear or on the under-arm. If stinging or rash occurs, do not use. *Caution:* Should not be taken internally during pregnancy.
Anise (Pimpinella anisum)	Seeds, seed oil.	Phytochemicals: Alpha-pinene, apigenin, bergapten, caffeic acid, chlorogenic acid, eugenol, limonene, linalool, myristicin, rutin, scopoletin, squalene, stigmasterol, umbelliferone. Nutrients: Calcium, iron, magnesium, manganese, phosphorus, potassium, zinc, vitamins A, B_1, B_2, B_3, B_5, B_6, C, and E.	Aids digestion, clears mucus from air passages, combats infection, and promotes milk production in nursing mothers. Good for indigestion and for respiratory infections such as sinusitis. Also helpful for menopausal symptoms.	Used in many popular products as a fragrance and flavoring.
Annatto (Bixa orellana)	Leaves, roots, seeds.	Phytochemicals: Beta-carotene, bixin, cyanidin, ellagic acid, salicylic acid, saponin, tannins. Nutrients: Amino acids, calcium, iron, phosphorus, vitamins B_2, B_3, and C.	Has diuretic, antioxidant, antibacterial, anti-inflammatory, and expectorant properties. Helps to protect the liver and kidneys. May reduce blood sugar levels. Useful for indigestion, fever, coughs, burns, skin problems, and weight loss.	A rainforest herb used in skin care products as an emollient, and as an orange-yellow food coloring.
Ashwagandha (Withania somnifera)	Roots.	Phytochemicals: Alkaloids, beta-sitosterol, chlorogenic acid, scopoletin, withaferin. Nutrients: Amino acids, choline.	Rejuvenates and energizes the nervous system. Helps prevent stress-related disorders and stress-related depletion of vitamin C and cortisol. Increases physical endurance and improves sexual function. Has anti-inflammatory and anti-aging effects. In laboratory studies, has modulated and stimulated immune function.	An Ayurvedic herb also known as Indian ginseng and winter cherry. An important herb in Ayurvedic medicine.
Astragalus (Astragalus membranaceus)	Roots.	Phytochemicals: Betaine, beta-sitosterol, formononetin, isoliquiriti-genin. Nutrients: Calcium, choline, copper, essential fatty acids, iron, magnesium, manganese, potassium, zinc.	Acts as a tonic to protect the immune system. Aids adrenal gland function and digestion. Increases metabolism, produces spontaneous sweating, promotes healing, and provides energy to combat fatigue and prolonged stress. Increases stamina. Good for colds, flu, and immune-deficiency-related problems, including AIDS, cancer, and tumors. Effective for chronic lung weakness.	Also called huang qi. *Caution:* Should not be taken if fever is present.
Barberry (Berberis vulgaris)	Bark, berries, roots.	Phytochemicals: Berbamine, berberine, beta-carotene, caffeic acid, kaempferol, lutein, quercetin, sinapic acid, zeaxanthin. Nutrients: Calcium, iron, magnesium, manganese, phosphorus, potassium, selenium, silicon, zinc, vitamins B_1, B_2, B_3, and C.	Decreases heart rate, slows breathing, reduces bronchial constriction. Kills bacteria on the skin and stimulates intestinal movement.	*Caution:* Should not be used during pregnancy.

Herb (Scientific Name)	Parts Used	Phytochemical and Nutrient Content	Actions and Uses	Comments
Bayberry (*Myrica cerifera*)	Root bark.	Phytochemicals: Beta-carotene, gallic acid, myristic acid, phenol. Nutrients: Calcium, iron, magnesium, manganese, phosphorus, potassium, selenium, silicon, zinc, vitamins B_1, B_2, B_3, and C.	Acts as a decongestant and astringent. Aids circulation, reduces fever. Helps stop bleeding. Good for circulatory disorders, fever, hypothyroidism, and ulcers. Also good for the eyes and the immune system.	The wax of the berries is used to make fragrant candles. *Caution:* Should not be used at high dosages or for prolonged periods. May temporarily irritate sensitive stomachs.
Bilberry (*Vaccinium myrtillus*)	Entire plant.	Phytochemicals: Anthocyanosides, beta-carotene, caffeic acid, caryophyllene, catechin, chlorogenic acid, ferulic acid, gallic acid, hyperoside, lutein, quercetin, quercitrin, ursolic acid, vanillic acid. Nutrients: Calcium, inositol, magnesium, manganese, phosphorus, potassium, selenium, silicon, sulfur, zinc, vitamins B_1, B_2, B_3, and C.	Acts as an antioxidant, diuretic, and urinary tract antiseptic. Keeps blood vessels flexible, allowing increased blood flow. Helps control insulin levels and strengthen connective tissue. Supports and strengthens collagen structures, inhibits the growth of bacteria, and has anti-aging and anticarcinogenic effects. Useful for hypoglycemia, inflammation, stress, anxiety, night blindness, and cataracts. May help halt or prevent macular degeneration.	Also known as European blueberry. Related to the American blueberry. *Caution:* Interferes with iron absorption when taken internally. Should not be used by people with diabetes except under the supervision of a knowledgable health professional.
Birch (*Betula alba*)	Bark, leaves, sap.	Phytochemicals: Betulin, betulinic acid, hyperoside, luteolin and quercetin glycosides, methyl salicylate.	Acts as a diuretic, anti-inflammatory, and pain reliever. Good for joint pain and urinary tract infections. Applied topically, good for boils and sores.	Betulinic acid in birch bark has been found to kill cancer cells.
Black cohosh (*Cimicifuga racemosa*)	Rhizomes, roots.	Phytochemicals: Beta-carotene, cimicifugin, formononetin, gallic acid, phytosterols, salicylic acid, tannic acid, tannin. Nutrients: Calcium, chromium, iron, magnesium, manganese, phosphorus, potassium, selenium, silicon, zinc, vitamins B_1, B_2, B_3, and C.	Lowers blood pressure and cholesterol levels. Reduces mucus production. Helps cardiovascular and circulatory disorders. Induces labor and aids in childbirth (many herbalists recommend taking small amounts 2 weeks before expected delivery). Relieves menopausal symptoms, menstrual cramps with back pain, morning sickness, and pain. Helpful for poisonous snake bites. Good for arthritis.	Also known as black snakeroot. *Caution:* Should not be used during pregnancy (until just before birth) or in the presence of chronic disease.
Black walnut (*Juglans nigra*)	Husks, inner bark, leaves, nuts.	Phytochemicals: Beta-carotene, ellagic acid, juglone, myricetin, tannin. Nutrients: Calcium, iron, magnesium, manganese, phosphorus, potassium, selenium, silicon, zinc, vitamins B_1, B_2, B_3, and C.	Aids digestion and acts as a laxative. Helps heal mouth and throat sores. Cleanses the body of some types of parasites. Good for bruising, fungal infection, herpes, poison ivy, and warts. May help lower blood pressure and cholesterol levels.	When boiled, the hulls produce a dye that is used to color wool.
Blessed thistle (*Cnicus benedictus*)	Flowers, leaves, stems.	Phytochemicals: Beta-carotene, beta-sitosterol, cnicin, ferulic acid, kaempferol, luteolin, oleanolic acid, stigmasterol. Nutrients: Calcium, essential fatty acids, iron, magnesium, manganese, phosphorus, potassium, selenium, silicon, zinc, vitamins B_1, B_2, B_3, and C.	Stimulates the appetite and stomach secretions. Heals the liver. Lessens inflammation, improves circulation, cleanses the blood, and strengthens the heart. May act as brain food. Good for female disorders and increases milk flow in nursing mothers.	Also called St. Benedict thistle, holy thistle. *Caution:* Should be handled with care to avoid toxic skin effects.
Blue cohosh (*Caulophyllum thalictroides*)	Roots.	Phytochemicals: Anagyrine, beta-carotene, caulophylline, caulophyllo-saponin, caulosaponin, hederagenin, phytosterols, saponin. Nutrients: Calcium, iron, magnesium, manganese, phosphorus, potassium, selenium, zinc, vitamins B_1, B_2, B_3, and C.	Eases muscle spasms and stimulates uterine contractions for childbirth. Useful for memory problems, menstrual disorders, and nervous disorders.	*Caution:* Should not be used during the first two trimesters of pregnancy.

Herb (Scientific Name)	Parts Used	Phytochemical and Nutrient Content	Actions and Uses	Comments
Boldo (*Peumus boldus*)	Leaves.	Phytochemicals: Alpha-pinene, ascaridole, benzaldehyde, beta-pinene, boldin, boldine, camphor, coumarin, eugenol, farnesol, kaempferol, limonene, linalool, 1,8-cineole. Nutrients: Choline.	Acts as a diuretic, laxative, antibiotic, liver tonic, and anti-inflammatory. Aids in the excretion of uric acid and stimulates digestion.	Used by indigenous peoples of Chile and Peru for liver ailments and gallstones.
Boneset (*Eupatorium perfoliatum*)	Flower petals, leaves.	Phytochemicals: Astragalin, gallic acid, eufoliatin, eufoliatorin, eupatorin, euperfolin, euperfolitin, gallic acid, hyperoside, kaempferol, quercetin, rutin, tannic acid.	Acts as a decongestant, laxative, anti-inflammatory, and diuretic. Loosens phlegm, reduces fever, increases perspiration, calms the body. Useful for colds, flu, bronchitis, and fever-induced aches and pains.	Also called white snakeroot. *Caution:* Long-term use should be avoided, as it can result in toxicity.
Borage (*Borago officinalis*)	Leaves, seeds.	Phytochemicals: Beta-carotene, rosmarinic acid, silicic acid, tannin. Nutrients: Calcium, choline, essential fatty acids, iron, magnesium, phosphorus, potassium, zinc, vitamins B_1, B_2, B_3, and C.	Acts as an adrenal tonic and gland balancer. Contains valuable minerals and essential fatty acids needed for proper cardiovascular function and healthy skin and nails.	The flowers of the borage plant are edible.
Boswellia (*Boswellia serrata*)	Gum resin.	Phytochemicals: Borneol, boswellic acids, carvone, caryophyllene, farnesol, geraniol, limonene.	Acts as an anti-inflammatory, anti-arthritic, antifungal, and antibacterial. Used topically for pain relief. Lowers cholesterol, protects the liver. Useful for arthritis, gout, low back pain, myositis, and fibromyalgia. Helps repair blood vessels damaged by inflammation. Traditionally used as a remedy for obesity, diarrhea, dysentery, pulmonary diseases, ringworm, and boils.	An Ayurvedic herb also known as Indian frankincense. An important herb in Ayurvedic medicine.
Buchu (*Barosma betulina*)	Leaves.	Phytochemicals: Alpha-pinene, alpha-terpinene, barosma-camphor, diosphenol, hesperidin, limonene, menthone, pulegone, quercetin, quercetrin, rutin. Nutrients: Calcium, iron, magnesium, manganese, phosphorus, potassium, selenium, silicon, zinc, vitamins B_1, B_2, and B_3.	Lessens inflammation of the colon, gums, mucous membranes, prostate, sinuses, and vagina. Acts as a diuretic. Helps control bladder and kidney problems, diabetes, digestive disorders, fluid retention, and prostate disorders. A specific for bladder infections.	Do not boil buchu leaves.
Burdock (*Arctium lappa*)	Plant, roots, seeds.	Phytochemicals: Acetic acid, arctigenin, arctiin, beta-carotene, butyric acid, caffeic acid, chlorogenic acid, costic acid, inulin, isovaleric acid, lauric acid, lignin, myristic acid, propionic acid, sitosterol, stigmasterol. Nutrients: Amino acids, calcium, copper, chromium, iron, magnesium, manganese, phosphorus, potassium, selenium, silicon, zinc, vitamins B_1, B_2, B_3, and C.	Acts as an antioxidant. May help to protects against cancer by helping control cell mutation. Aids elimination of excess fluid, uric acid, and toxins. Has antibacterial and antifungal properties. Purifies the blood, restores liver and gallbladder function, and stimulates the digestive and immune systems. Helps skin disorders such as boils and carbuncles, and relieves gout and menopausal symptoms. Burdock root used as a hair rinse promotes scalp and hair health.	*Caution:* Interferes with iron absorption when taken internally.
Butcher's broom (*Ruscus aculeatus*)	Plant, roots, seeds.	Phytochemicals: Beta-carotene, chrysophanic acid, glycolic acid, neoruscogenin, rutin, saponin. Nutrients: Calcium, chromium, iron, magnesium, manganese, phosphorus, potassium, selenium, silicon, zinc, vitamins B_1, B_2, B_3, and C.	Reduces inflammation. Useful for carpal tunnel syndrome, circulatory disorders, edema, Ménière's disease, obesity, Raynaud's phenomenon, thrombophlebitis, varicose veins, and vertigo. Also good for the bladder and kidneys.	More effective if taken with vitamin C.

Herb (Scientific Name)	Parts Used	Phytochemical and Nutrient Content	Actions and Uses	Comments
Calendula (*Calendula officinalis*)	Flower petals.	Phytochemicals: Alpha-amyrin, beta-amyrin, beta-sitosterol, caffeic acid, campesterol, caryophyllene, chlorogenic acid, faradiol, galactose, gentisic acid, kaempferol, lutein, lycopene, malic acid, myristic acid, oleanolic acid, p-coumaric acid, phytofluene, quercetin, rutin, salicylic acid, saponin, stigmasterol, syringic acid, taraxasterol vanillic acid, zeta-carotene. Nutrients: Calcium, coenzyme Q_{10}, vitamins C and E.	Reduces inflammation and is soothing to the skin. Helps regulate the menstrual cycle and lower fever. Useful for skin disorders, such as rashes and sunburn, as well as for neuritis and toothache. Good for diaper rash and other skin problems in small children.	Also called pot marigold. Usually nonirritating when used externally.
Cascara sagrada (*Frangula purshiana*)	Bark.	Phytochemicals: Aloe-emodin, anthraquinones, barbaloin, beta carotene, casanthranol, chrysophanic acid, chrysophanol, frangulin, malic acid, myristic acid. Nutrients: Calcium, iron, linoleic acid, magnesium, manganese, phosphorus, potassium, selenium, silicon, zinc, vitamins B_1, B_2, B_3, and C.	Acts as a colon cleanser and laxative. Effective for colon disorders, constipation, and parasitic infestation.	Tastes very bitter taken as a tea.
Catnip (*Nepeta cataria*)	Leaves.	Phytochemicals: Alpha-humulene, beta-elemene, camphor, carvacrol, caryophyllene, citral, citronellal, geraniol, myrcene, nepetalactone, piperitone, pulegone, rosmarinic acid, thymol. Nutrients: Calcium, chromium, iron, magnesium, manganese, phosphorus, potassium, selenium, silicon, zinc.	Lowers fever (catnip tea enemas reduce fever quickly). Dispels gas and aids digestion and sleep; relieves stress; stimulates the appetite. Good for anxiety, colds and flu, inflammation, pain, and stress.	Can be given to children.
Cat's claw (*Uncaria tomentosa*)	Inner bark, roots.	Phytochemicals: Alloisopteropodine, allopteropodine, isomitraphylline, isopteropodine, mitraphylline, oleanolic acid, pteropodine, rhynchophylline, ursolic acid.	Acts as an antioxidant and anti-inflammatory. Stimulates the immune system. Cleanses the intestinal tract and enhances the action of white blood cells. Good for intestinal problems and viral infections. May help people with AIDS, arthritis, cancer, tumors, or ulcers.	Also called uña de gato. According to USDA research, cat's claw seeds contain an enzyme instrumental in converting saturated fats to unsaturated fats. *Caution:* Should not be used during pregnancy.
Cayenne (*Capsicum frutescens* or *C. annum*)	Berries.	Phytochemicals: Alpha-carotene, beta-carotene, beta-ionone, caffeic acid, campesterol, capsaicin, carvone, caryophyllene, chlorogenic acid, citric acid, cryptoxanthin, hesperidin, kaempferol, limonene, lutein, myristic acid, 1,8-cineole, p-coumaric acid, quercetin, scopoletin, stigmasterol, zeaxanthin. Nutrients: Amino acids, calcium, essential fatty acids, folate, iron, magnesium, phosphorus, potassium, zinc, vitamins B_1, B_2, B_3, B_5, B_6, C, and E.	Aids digestion, improves circulation, and stops bleeding from ulcers. Acts as a catalyst for other herbs. Good for the heart, kidneys, lungs, pancreas, spleen, and stomach. Useful for arthritis and rheumatism. Helps to ward off colds, sinus infections, and sore throats. Good for pain when applied topically. Used with lobelia for nerves.	Also called capsicum, hot pepper, red pepper. *Caution:* Avoid contact with the eyes.
Cedar (*Cedrus libani*)	Leaves, tops.	Phytochemicals: Borneol, quinic acid.	Acts as an antiviral, antifungal, expectorant, lymphatic cleanser, and urinary antiseptic. Stimulates the immune system. Increases venous blood flow. Can be used externally for warts.	

Herb (Scientific Name)	Parts Used	Phytochemical and Nutrient Content	Actions and Uses	Comments
Celery (*Apium graveolens*)	Plant, roots, seeds.	Phytochemicals: Alpha-pinene, apigenin, bergapten, beta-carotene, caffeic acid, carvone, chlorogenic acid, coumarin, eugenol, ferulic acid, isoquercitrin, limonene, linalool, luteolin, mannitol, myristic acid, myristicin, p-coumaric acid, rutin, scopoletin, shikimic acid, thymol. Nutrients: Amino acids, boron, calcium, choline, essential fatty acids, folate, inositol, iron, magnesium, manganese, phosphorus, potassium, selenium, sulfur, zinc, vitamins A, B_1, B_2, B_3, B_5, B_6, C, E, and K.	Reduces blood pressure, relieves muscle spasms, and improves appetite. Good for arthritis, gout, and kidney problems. Acts as an diuretic, antioxidant, and sedative.	*Caution:* The seeds should not be used during pregnancy, nor should large amounts of the herb.
Chamomile (*Matricaria recutita* or *M. chamomilla*)	Flowers, plant.	Phytochemicals: Alpha-bisabolol, apigenin, azulene, borneol, caffeic acid, chlorogenic acid, farnesol, gentisic acid, geraniol, hyperoside, kaempferol, luteolin, p-coumaric acid, perillyl alcohol, quercetin, rutin, salicylic acid, sinapic acid, tannin, umbelliferone. Nutrients: Choline, vitamins B_1, B_3, and C.	Reduces inflammation, stimulates the appetite, and aids digestion and sleep. Acts as a diuretic and nerve tonic. Helpful for colitis, diverticulosis, fever, headaches, and pain. Good for menstrual cramps. A traditional remedy for stress and anxiety, indigestion, and insomnia. Useful as a mouthwash for minor mouth and gum infections.	Also called German chamomile, wild chamomile. Roman chamomile (*Chamaemelum nobile*) is also available, but is less common. *Caution:* Should not be used daily for long periods of time, as this may lead to ragweed allergy. Should be used with caution by those who are allergic to ragweed. Should not be used with sedatives or alcohol.
Chanca piedra (*Phyllanthus niruri*)	Entire plant.	Phytochemicals: Limonene, lupeol, methyl salicylate, quercetin, quercitrin, rutin, saponins.	Fights inflammation and bacterial and viral infection. Acts as a diuretic. Useful for kidney stones, gallstones, colds, flu, digestion, asthma, bronchitis, diarrhea, pain relief, fever, sexually transmitted diseases, and muscle spasms.	A rainforest herb whose name means "stone crusher." Also known as seed-on-the-leaf.
Chaparral (*Larrea tridentata*)	Leaves.	Phytochemicals: Alpha-pinene, beta-carotene, borneol, camphene, camphor, gossypetin, limonene, nordihydroguaiaretic acid. Nutrients: Amino acids, calcium, magnesium, selenium, sulfur, zinc, vitamins B_1, B_2, B_3, and C.	Fights free radicals and chelates heavy metals. Has anti-HIV activity. Protects against harmful effects of radiation, sun exposure, and the formation of tumors and cancer cells. Relieves pain. Good for skin disorders.	*Caution:* Recommended for external use only. Taken internally, especially in large doses and/or for prolonged periods, can cause liver damage.
Chaste tree (*Vitex agnus-castus*)	Fruit, leaf.	Phytochemicals: Alpha-pinene, alpha-terpineol, chrysosplenol, flavonoids, limonene, linalool, myrcene, 1,8-cineole, pinene, progesterone, testosterone.	Has a calming and soothing effect. Relieves muscle cramps. Regulates and normalizes hormone levels and menstrual cycles. Increases and improves breast milk. Good for symptoms of PMS and menopause.	Also called chasteberry, vitex. *Caution:* Should not be used during pregnancy. Should not be given to children.
Chickweed (*Stellaria media*)	Leaves, stems.	Phytochemicals: Beta-carotene, genistein, rutin. Nutrients: Calcium, essential fatty acids, iron, magnesium, manganese, phosphorus, potassium, selenium, silicon, sulfur, zinc, vitamins B_1, B_2, B_3, C, and E.	Relieves nasal congestion. May lower blood lipids. Useful for bronchitis, circulatory problems, colds, coughs, skin diseases, and warts (applied topically). A good source of vitamin C and other nutrients.	Also called starweed.

Herb (Scientific Name)	Parts Used	Phytochemical and Nutrient Content	Actions and Uses	Comments
Chuchuhuasi (*Maytenus krukovit*)	Bark.	Anthocyanidins, catechin, maytensine, nocotinyl, sesquiterpenes, triterpenes, tannins.	Fights inflammation and stimulates the immune system. Supports the adrenal system and balances and regulates menstrual cycles. Good for arthritis, rheumatism, back pain, muscle spasms, fever, skin tumors, bronchitis, diarrhea.	A rainforest herb used traditionally to stimulate sexual desire.
Cinnamon (*Cinnamomum verum*)	Bark, plant.	Phytochemicals: Alpha-pinene, benzaldehyde, beta-carotene, beta-pinene, borneol, camphor, caryophyllene, cinnamaldehyde, coumarin, cuminaldehyde, eugenol, farnesol, geraniol, limonene, linalool, mannitol, mucilage, 1,8-cineole, phellandrene, tannin, terpinolene, vanillin. Nutrients: Calcium, chromium, copper, iodine, iron, manganese, phosphorus, potassium, zinc, vitamins A, B_1, B_2, B_3, and C.	Relieves diarrhea and nausea; counteracts congestion; aids peripheral circulation. Warms the body and enhances digestion, especially the metabolism of fats. Also fights fungal infection. Useful for diabetes, weight loss, yeast infection, and uterine hemorrhaging.	*Caution:* Should not be used in large amounts during pregnancy.
Clove (*Syzygium aromaticum*)	Flower buds, essential oil.	Phytochemicals: Beta-carotene, beta-pinene, beta-sitosterol, campesterol, carvone, caryophyllene, chavicol, cinnamaldehyde, ellagic acid, eugenol, gallic acid, kaempferol, linalool, methyleugenol, methylsalicylate, mucilage, oleanolic acid, stigmasterol, tannin, vanillin. Nutrients: Calcium, iron, magnesium, manganese, phosphorus, potassium, zinc, vitamins A, B_1, B_2, and C.	Has antiseptic and antiparasitic properties, and acts as a digestive aid. Essential oil is applied topically for relief of toothache and mouth pain.	*Caution:* Clove oil is very strong and can cause irritation if used in its pure form. Diluting the oil in olive oil or distilled water is recommended. Essential oil should not be taken internally except under the careful supervision of a health care professional.
Comfrey (*Symphytum officinale*)	Leaves, roots.	Phytochemicals: Allantoin, beta-carotene, caffeic acid, chlorogenic acid, rosmarinic acid, sitosterol, stigmasterol. Nutrients: Calcium, iron, magnesium, manganese, phosphorus, potassium, selenium, zinc, vitamins B_1, B_2, B_3, and C.	Speeds healing of wounds and many skin conditions. Beneficial for bedsores, bites and stings, bruises, inflamed bunions, burns, dermatitis, dry skin, bleeding hemorrhoids, leg ulcers, nosebleeds, psoriasis, scabies, skin rashes, and sunburn.	Also called knitbone. *Caution:* May cause liver damage if taken internally. Not recommended for internal use except under the careful supervision of a health care professional. External use is generally considered safe. Should not be used during pregnancy.
Corn silk (*Zea mays*)	Styles, stigmas ("tassels")	Phytochemicals: Benzaldehyde, beta-carotene, betaine, beta-sitosterol, caffeic acid, campesterol, carvacrol, caryophyllene, dioxycinnamic acid, geraniol, glycolic acid, limonene, 1,8-cineole, saponin, thymol, vitexin. Nutrients: Calcium, chromium, iron, magnesium, manganese, phosphorus, potassium, vitamins B_1, B_3, and C.	Acts as a diuretic. Aids the bladder, kidney, and small intestine. Lessens the incidence of bed-wetting when taken several hours before bedtime. Good for carpal tunnel syndrome, edema, obesity, premenstrual syndrome, and prostate disorders. Used in combination with other "kidney herbs," opens the urinary tract and removes mucus from the urine.	
Cramp bark (*Viburnum opulus*)	Bark, root.	Phytochemicals: Esculetin, scopoletin, valerianic acid. Nutrients: Calcium, iron, magnesium, manganese, phosphorus, potassium, selenium, zinc.	Relieves muscle spasms and pain. Good for menstrual cramps. Useful for lower back and leg spasms.	Also called guelder rose. Closely related to black haw, which has the same medicinal properties. *Caution:* Should be avoided during pregnancy.

Herb (Scientific Name)	Parts Used	Phytochemical and Nutrient Content	Actions and Uses	Comments
Cranberry (*Vaccinium macrocarpon*)	Fruit.	Phytochemicals: Alpha-terpineol, anthocyanosides, benzaldehyde, benzoic acid, beta-carotene, chlorogenic acid, ellagic acid, eugenol, ferulic acid, lutein, malic acid, quercetin. Nutrients: Calcium, folate, iron, magnesium, manganese, phosphorus, potassium, selenium, sulfur, zinc, vitamins A, B_1, B_2, B_3, B_5, C, and E.	Acidifies the urine and prevents bacteria from adhering to bladder cells. Good for the kidneys, bladder, and skin. Has anticancer properties. Helpful for infections of the urinary tract.	A good source of vitamin C. Cranberry juice cocktail products that contain sugar should be *avoided.*
Damiana (*Turnera diffusa*)	Leaves.	Phytochemicals: Alpha-pinene, beta-carotene, beta-pinene, beta-sitosterol, 1,8-cineole, tannins, thymol. Nutrients: Calcium, iron, magnesium, manganese, phosphorus, potassium, selenium, zinc, vitamins B_1, B_2, B_3, and C.	Stimulates muscular contractions of the intestinal tract and delivery of oxygen to the genital area. Used as an energy tonic and aphrodisiac, and to remedy sexual and hormonal problems. A "sexuality tonic" for women.	*Caution:* Interferes with iron absorption when taken internally.
Dandelion (*Taraxacum officinale*)	Flowers, leaves, roots, tops.	Phytochemicals: Beta-carotene, beta-sitosterol, caffeic acid, cryptoxanthin, lutein, mannitol, p-coumaric acid, saponin, stigmasterol. Nutrients: Calcium, iron, magnesium, manganese, phosphorus, potassium, selenium, zinc, vitamins B_1, B_2, B_3, and C.	Acts as a diuretic. Cleanses the blood and liver, and increases bile production. Reduces serum cholesterol and uric acid levels. Improves functioning of the kidneys, pancreas, spleen, and stomach. Relieves menopausal symptoms. Useful for abscesses, anemia, boils, breast tumors, cirrhosis of the liver, constipation, fluid retention, hepatitis, jaundice, and rheumatism. Believed to help prevent age spots and breast cancer.	Leaves can be boiled and eaten like spinach (young leaves can be used in salads). *Caution:* Should not be combined with prescription diuretics. Not recommended for people with gallstones or biliary tract obstruction.
Devil's claw (*Harpagophytum procumbens*)	Rhizome.	Phytochemicals: Chlorogenic acid, cinnamic acid, harpagide, harpagoside, kaempferol, luteolin, oleanolic acid. Nutrients: Calcium, iron, magnesium, manganese, phosphorus, potassium, selenium, zinc.	Relieves pain and reduces inflammation. Acts as a diuretic, sedative, and digestive stimulant. Good for back pain; arthritis; rheumatism; diabetes; allergies; liver; gallbladder and kidney disorders; arteriosclerosis; lumbago; gout; and menopausal symptoms.	Also called grapple plant, wood spider. *Caution:* Should not be used during pregnancy.
Dong quai (*Angelica sinensis*)	Roots.	Phytochemicals: Alpha-pinene, bergapten, beta-carotene, beta-sitosterol, carvacrol, falcarinol, ferulic acid, ligustilide, myristic acid, p-cymene, scopoletin, umbelliferone, vanillic acid. Nutrients: Calcium, folate, iron, magnesium, manganese, phosphorus, potassium, selenium, zinc, vitamins B_1, B_2, B_5, and C.	Acts as a mild sedative, laxative, diuretic, antispasmodic, and pain-reliever. Improves the blood. Strengthens the reproductive system. Assists the body in using hormones. Used to treat female problems such as hot flashes and other menopausal symptoms, premenstrual syndrome, and vaginal dryness.	Also known as Chinese angelica. *Caution:* Should not be used during pregnancy. Should not be used by people who have diabetes or are light-sensitive.
Echinacea (*Echinacea species*)	Leaves, roots.	Phytochemicals: Alpha-pinene, apigenin, arabinogalactan, beta-carotene, beta-sitosterol, betaine, borneol, caffeic acid, caryophyllene, chlorogenic acid, cichoric acid, cynarin, echinacoside, ferulic acid, kaempferol, luteolin, quercetin, rutin, stigmasterol, vanillin, verbascoside. Nutrients: Calcium, iron, magnesium, manganese, phosphorus, potassium, selenium, zinc, vitamins B_1, B_2, B_3, and C.	Fights inflammation and bacterial and viral infection. Stimulates certain white blood cells. Good for the immune system and the lymphatic system. Useful for allergies, colic, colds, flu, and other infectious illnesses. Also helpful for snakebite.	For internal use, a freeze-dried form or alcohol-free extract is recommended. *Caution:* Should be used with caution by people who are allergic to ragweed or to plants in the sunflower family. Should not be taken for prolonged periods by people with autoimmune disorders, as it stimulates the immune system.

Herb (Scientific Name)	Parts Used	Phytochemical and Nutrient Content	Actions and Uses	Comments
Elder (*Sambucus nigra*)	Flowers, fruit, inner bark, leaves, roots.	Phytochemicals: Alpha-amyrin, astragalin, beta-carotene, beta-sitosterol, betulin, caffeic acid, campesterol, chlorogenic acid, cycloartenol, ferulic acid, isoquercitrin, kaempferol, lupeol, malic acid, myristic acid, oleanolic acid, p-coumaric acid, pectin, quercetin, rutin, shikimic acid, stigmasterol, ursolic acid. Nutrients: Calcium, essential fatty acids, vitamins A, B_1, B_2, B_3, and C.	Combats free radicals and inflammation. Relieves coughs and congestion. Builds the blood, cleanses the system, eases constipation. Enhances immune system function. Increases perspiration, lowers fever, soothes the respiratory tract, and stimulates circulation. Effective against flu viruses. The flowers are used to soothe skin irritations.	Also called black elder, European elder. *Caution:* Should not be used during pregnancy. The stems of this plant should be *avoided.* They contain cyanide, and can be very toxic.
Ephedra (*Ephedra sinica*)	Stems.	Phytochemicals: Beta-carotene, d-norpseudoephedrine, ellagic acid, ephedrine, gallic acid. Nutrients: Calcium, iron, magnesium, manganese, phosphorus, potassium, selenium, zinc, vitamins B_1, B_2, B_3, and C.	Relieves congestion, aids in the elimination of fluids, relieves bronchial spasms, and stimulates the central nervous system. May decrease appetite and elevate mood. Useful for allergies, asthma, colds, and other respiratory complaints, as well as for depression and obesity.	Also known as ma huang. *Caution:* Should not be used by persons who have anxiety disorders (panic attacks), glaucoma, thyroid disease, diabetes, heart disease, or high blood pressure, or who are taking monoamine oxidase (MAO) inhibitor drugs.
Eucalyptus (*Eucalyptus globulus*)	Bark, essential oil, leaves.	Phytochemicals: Alpha-pinene, beta-pinene, caffeic acid, carvone, chlorogenic acid, ellagic acid, ferulic acid, gallic acid, gentisic acid, hyperoside, 1,8-cineole, p-cymene, protocatechuic acid, quercetin, quercitrin, rutin.	Acts as a decongestant and mild antiseptic. Reduces swelling by helping to increase blood flow. Relaxes tired and sore muscles. Good for colds, coughs, and other respiratory disorders. Inhaling vapor from a few drops of the oil helps to break up mucus.	Recommended for external use only. Should not be used on broken skin or open cuts or wounds.
Eyebright (*Euphrasia officinalis*)	Entire plant, except the root.	Phytochemicals: Beta-carotene, caffeic acid, ferulic acid, tannins. Nutrients: Calcium, chromium, iron, magnesium, manganese, phosphorus, potassium, selenium, zinc, vitamins B_1, B_2, B_3, and C.	Prevents secretion of fluids and relieves discomfort from eyestrain or minor irritation. Used as an eyewash. Good for allergies, itchy and/or watery eyes, and runny nose. Combats hay fever.	
False unicorn root (*Chamaelirium luteum*)	Roots.	Phytochemicals: Chamaelirin, helonin, saponins.	Balances sex hormones. Helps treat infertility, menstrual irregularities and pain, premenstrual syndrome, and prostrate disorders. May help prevent miscarriage.	Also called helonias.
Fennel (*Foeniculum vulgare*)	Fruit, roots, stems.	Phytochemicals: Alpha-pinene, benzoic acid, bergapten, beta-carotene, beta-phollandrene, beta-sitosterol, caffeic acid, camphor, cinnamic acid, cynarin, ferulic acid, fumaric acid, isopimpinellin, isoquercitrin, kaempferol, limonene, linalool, myristicin, 1,8-cineole, p-coumaric acid, pectin, protocatechuic acid, psoralen, quercetin, rutin, scopoletin, sinapic acid, stigmasterol, umbelliferone, vanillic acid, vanillin, xanthotoxin. Nutrients: Amino acids, calcium, choline, essential fatty acids, iron, magnesium, manganese, phosphorus, potassium, selenium, vitamins B_1, B_2, B_3, C, and E.	Used as an appetite suppressant and as an eyewash. Promotes the functioning of the kidneys, liver, and spleen, and also clears the lungs. Relieves abdominal pain, colon disorders, gas, and gastrointestinal tract spasms. Useful for acid stomach. Good after chemotherapy and/or radiation treatments for cancer.	The powdered plant can be used as a flea repellent.

Herb (Scientific Name)	Parts Used	Phytochemical and Nutrient Content	Actions and Uses	Comments
Fenugreek (*Trigonella foenum-graecum*)	Seeds.	Phytochemicals: Beta-carotene, beta-sitosterol, coumarin, diosgenin, kaempferol, luteolin, p-coumaric acid, quercetin, rutin, saponin, trigonelline, vitexin. Nutrients: Amino acids, calcium, essential fatty acids, folate, iron, magnesium, manganese, phosphorus, potassium, selenium, zinc, vitamins B_1, B_2, B_3, and C.	Acts as a laxative, lubricates the intestines, and reduces fever. Helps lower cholesterol and blood sugar levels. Helps asthma and sinus problems by reducing mucus. Promotes lactation in nursing mothers. Good for the eyes and for inflammation and lung disorders.	Oil of fenugreek has a maple-like flavor.
Feverfew (*Chrysanthemum parthenium*)	Bark, dried flowers, leaves.	Phytochemicals: Beta-carotene, parthenolide, santamarin. Nutrients: Calcium, iron, magnesium, manganese, phosphorus, potassium, selenium, zinc, vitamins B_1, B_2, B_3, and C.	Combats inflammation and muscle spasms. Increases fluidity of lung and bronchial tube mucus, promotes menses, stimulates the appetite, and stimulates uterine contractions. Relieves nausea and vomiting. Good for arthritis, colitis, fever, headaches, migraine headaches, menstrual problems, muscle tension, and pain.	Chewing the leaves is a folk remedy, but this may cause mouth sores. Also called featherfew, featherfoil. *Caution:* Should not be used during pregnancy. People who take prescription blood-thinning medications or who regularly take over-the-counter painkillers should consult a health care provider before using feverfew, as the combination can result in internal bleeding.
Flax (*Linum usitatissimum*)	Seeds, seed oil.	Phytochemicals: Apigenin, beta-carotene, beta-sitosterol, campesterol, chlorogenic acid, cycloartenol, lecithin, luteolin, myristic acid, squalene, stigmasterol, vitexin. Nutrients: Amino acids, calcium, essential fatty acids, iron, magnesium, manganese, phosphorus, potassium, sulfur, vanadium, zinc, vitamins B_1, B_2, B_3, B_5, and E.	Promotes strong bones, nails, and teeth, as well as healthy skin. Useful for colon problems, female disorders, and inflammation.	The seeds are an excellent addition to a diet that is low in fiber.
Garlic (*Allium sativa*)	Bulb.	Phytochemicals: Allicin, beta-carotene, beta-sitosterol, caffeic acid, chlorogenic acid, diallyl-disulfide, ferulic acid, geraniol, kaempferol, linalool, oleanolic acid, p-coumaric acid, phloroglucinol, phytic acid, quercetin, rutin, s-allyl cysteine, saponin, sinapic acid, stigmasterol. Nutrients: Calcium, folate, iron, magnesium, manganese, phosphorus, potassium, selenium, zinc, vitamins B_1, B_2, B_3, and C.	Detoxifies the body and protects against infection by enhancing immune function. Lowers blood pressure and improves circulation. Lowers blood lipid levels. Helps stabilize blood sugar levels. Aids in the treatment of arteriosclerosis, arthritis, asthma, cancer, circulatory problems, colds and flu, digestive problems, heart disorders, insomnia, liver disease, sinusitis, ulcers, and yeast infections. May prevent ulcers by inhibiting growth of *Helicobacter pylori*, the ulcer-causing bacterium. Good for virtually any disease or infection.	Garlic contains many sulfur compounds, which give it its healing properties. Odorless garlic supplements are available. Aged garlic extract (such as Kyolic) is good. *Caution:* Not recommended for people who take anticoagulants, as garlic has blood-thinning actions.
Gentian (*Gentiana lutea*)	Leaves, roots.	Phytochemicals: Caffeic acid, carvacrol, gentiopicrin, limonene, linalool, mangiferin, sinapic acid, swertiamarin. Nutrients: Calcium, iron, magnesium, manganese, phosphorus, potassium, selenium, zinc, vitamins B_1, B_2, B_3, and C.	Aids digestion, stimulates appetite, and boosts circulation. Kills plasmodia (organisms that cause malaria) and worms. Good for circulatory problems and pancreatitis.	

Herb (Scientific Name)	Parts Used	Phytochemical and Nutrient Content	Actions and Uses	Comments
Ginger (*Zingiber officinale*)	Rhizomes, roots.	Phytochemicals: alpha-pinene, beta-carotene, beta-ionone, beta-sitosterol, caffeic acid, camphor, capsaicin, caryophyllene, chlorogenic acid, citral, curcumin, farnesol, ferulic acid, geraniol, gingerols, lecithin, 1,8-cineole, zingerone. Nutrients: Amino acids, calcium, essential fatty acids, iron, magnesium, manganese, phosphorus, potassium, selenium, zinc, vitamins B_1, B_2, B_3, B_6, and C. Ground ginger also contains vitamin A.	Fights inflammation, cleanses the colon, reduces spasms and cramps, and stimulates circulation. A strong antioxidant and effective antimicrobial agent for sores and wounds. Protects the liver and stomach. Useful for bowel disorders, circulatory problems, arthritis, fever, headache, hot flashes, indigestion, morning sickness, motion sickness, muscle pain, nausea, and vomiting.	Can cause stomach distress if taken in large quantities. *Caution:* Not recommended for people who take anticoagulants or have gallstones. Not recommended for extended use during pregnancy.
Ginkgo (*Gingko biloba*)	Leaves, seed.	Phytochemicals: Amentoflavone, apigenin, beta-carotene, bilobalide, ginkgetin, isorhamnetin, kaempferol, luteolin, myristic acid, p-coumaric acid, procyanidin, quercetin, shikimic acid, stigmasterol, tannin, thymol. Nutrients: Amino acids, calcium, iron, magnesium, manganese, phosphorus, potassium, zinc, vitamins A, B_1, B_2, B_3, B_5, and C.	Improves brain functioning by increasing cerebral and peripheral circulation and tissue oxygenation. Has antioxidant properties. May slow the progression of Alzheimer's disease, and may relieve leg cramps by improving circulation. Beneficial for asthma, dementia, depression, eczema, headaches, heart and kidney disorders, memory loss, and tinnitis (ringing in the ears). Shows promise as a treatment for vascular-related impotence.	Can take at least 2 weeks to see results. *Caution:* People who take prescription blood-thinning medications or who regularly take over-the-counter painkillers should consult a health care provider before using ginkgo, as the combination can result in internal bleeding.
Ginseng (*Panax quinquefolius* [American ginseng], *P. ginseng* [Chinese or Korean ginseng])	Roots.	Phytochemicals: Beta-sitosterol, campesterols, caryophyllene, cinnamic acid, escin (*P. quinquefolius*), ferulic acid, fumaric acid, ginsenosides, kaempferol, oleanolic acid, panaxic acid, panaxin, saponin, stigmasterol, vanillic acid. Nutrients: Calcium, choline, fiber, folate, iron, magnesium, manganese, phosphorus, potassium, silicon, zinc, vitamins B_1, B_2, B_3, B_5, and C.	Strengthens the adrenal and reproductive glands. Enhances immune function, promotes lung functioning, and stimulates the appetite. Useful for bronchitis, circulatory problems, diabetes, infertility, lack of energy, and stress; to ease withdrawal from cocaine; and to protect against the effects of radiation exposure. Used by athletes for overall body strengthening. May help improve drug- or alcohol-induced liver dysfunction in older adults.	Siberian ginseng (*Eleutherococcus senticosus*) belongs to a different botanical family than American and Korean ginseng, but its properties are similar, and all are commonly referred to simply as ginseng. *Caution:* Should not be used by people with hypoglycemia, high blood pressure, heart disorders, asthma, or insomnia. Should not be used by pregnant women or nursing mothers.
Goldenseal (*Hydrastis canadensis*)	Rhizomes, roots.	Phytochemicals: Berberine, beta-carotene, canadine, chlorogenic acid. Nutrients: Calcium, iron, magnesium, manganese, phosphorus, potassium, selenium, zinc, vitamins B_1, B_2, B_3, and C.	Fights infection and inflammation. Cleanses the body. Increases the effectiveness of insulin and strengthens the immune system, colon, liver, pancreas, spleen, and lymphatic and respiratory systems. Improves digestion, regulates menses, decreases uterine bleeding, and stimulates the central nervous system. Good for allergies, ulcers, and disorders affecting the bladder, prostate, stomach, or vagina. Used at the first sign of possible symptoms, can stop a cold, flu, or sore throat from developing.	Alternating with echinacea or other herbs is recommended. Alcohol-free extract is the best form. *Caution:* Should not be used by pregnant women or nursing mothers. Should not be used for prolonged periods.

Herb (Scientific Name)	Parts Used	Phytochemical and Nutrient Content	Actions and Uses	Comments
Gotu kola (*Centella asiatica*)	Nuts, roots, seeds.	Phytochemicals: Beta-carotene, beta-sitosterol, campesterol, camphor, kaempferol, saponin, stigmasterol. Nutrients: Calcium, iron, magnesium, manganese, phosphorus, potassium, selenium, zinc, vitamins B_1, B_2, B_3, and C.	Helps eliminate excess fluids, decreases fatigue and depression, increases sex drive, shrinks tissues, and stimulates the central nervous system. May neutralize blood acids and lower body temperature. Promotes wound healing, and is good for varicose veins and for heart and liver function. Useful for cardiovascular and circulatory disorders, fatigue, connective tissue disorders, kidney stones, poor appetite, and sleep disorders.	May cause dermatitis if applied topically.
Gravel root (*Eupatorium purpureum*)	Flowers, root.	Phytochemicals: Euparin, eupatorin, resin.	Acts as a diuretic and urinary tract tonic. Combats prostate disorders, kidney stones, and problems related to fluid retention.	Also called joe-pye weed, queen-of-the-meadow.
Green tea (*Camellia sinensis*)	Leaves.	Phytochemicals: Apigenin, astragalin, benzaldehyde, beta-carotene, beta-ionone, beta-sitosterol, caffeic acid, caffeine, carvacrol, catechins, chlorogenic acid, cinnamic acid, cryptoxanthin, epicatechin, epigallocatechin, eugenol, farnesol, gallic acid, geraniol, hyperoside, indole, isoquercitrin, kaempferol, lutein, lycopene, myrcene, myricetin, myristic acid, naringenin, polyphenols, procyanidins, quercetin, quercitrin, rutin, salicylic acid, tannic acid, thymol, vitexin, zeaxanthin. Nutrients: Amino acids, calcium, iron, magnesium, manganese, phosphorus, potassium, zinc, vitamins B_1, B_2, B_3, B_5, and C.	Acts as an antioxidant and helps to protect against cancer. Lowers cholesterol levels, reduces the clotting tendency of the blood, stimulates the immune system, fights tooth decay, helps regulate blood sugar and insulin levels, combats mental fatigue, and may delay the onset of atherosclerosis. Good for asthma. Shows promise as a weight-loss aid. May help prevent enlarged prostate.	To get green tea's antioxidant benefits, drink it without milk (milk may bind with the beneficial compounds, making them unavailable to the body). *Caution:* Contains a small amount of caffeine. Should not be used in large quantities by pregnant women or nursing mothers. Persons with anxiety disorder or irregular heartbeat should limit their intake to no more than 2 cups daily.
Guarana (*Paullinia cupana*)	Seeds.	Phytochemicals: Adenine, caffeine, D-catechin, saponin, tannins, theobromine, theophylline.	Acts as a general tonic, stimulant, and intestinal cleanser. Increases mental alertness. Improves stamina and endurance. Reduces fatigue. Useful for headaches, urinary tract irritation, diarrhea.	Also called Brazilian cocoa, uabano. *Caution:* Due to guarana's caffeine content, taking more than 600 mg a day is not recommended. Not recommended for people with high blood pressure or heart conditions.
Hawthorn (*Crataegus laevigata*)	Flowers, fruit, leaves.	Phytochemicals: Acetylcholine, adenine, adenosine, anthocyanidins, beta-carotene, beta-sitosterol, caffeic acid, catechin, chlorogenic acid, epicatechin, esculin, hyperoside, pectin, quercitrin, rutin, ursolic acid, vitexin. Nutrients: Amino acids, calcium, choline, chromium, essential fatty acids, iron, magnesium, manganese, phosphorus, potassium, selenium, silicon, zinc, vitamins B_1, B_2, B_3, and C.	Dilates the coronary blood vessels, lowers blood pressure and cholesterol levels, and restores heart muscle. Decreases fat deposit levels. Increases intracellular vitamin C levels. Useful for anemia, cardiovascular and circulatory disorders, high cholesterol, and lowered immunity.	

Herb (Scientific Name)	Parts Used	Phytochemical and Nutrient Content	Actions and Uses	Comments
Hops (*Humulus lupulus*)	Flowers, fruit, leaves.	Phytochemicals: Alpha-pinene, alpha-terpineol, beta-carotene, beta-eudesmol, beta-sitosterol, caffeic acid, campesterol, catechin, chlorogenic acid, citral, eugenol, ferulic acid, limonene, p-cymene, piperidine, procyanidins, quercetin, tannins. Nutrients: Amino acids, calcium, chromium, magnesium, potassium, selenium, silicon, zinc, vitamins B_1, B_3, and C.	Relieves anxiety. Stimulates the appetite. Useful for cardiovascular disorders, hyperactivity, insomnia, nervousness, pain, restlessness, sexually transmitted diseases, shock, stress, toothaches, and ulcers.	Placed inside a pillowcase, aids sleep. *Caution:* Should not be used by people who take antidepressants.
Horehound (*Marrubium vulgare*)	Flowers, leaves.	Phytochemicals: Alpha-pinene, apigenin, beta-sitosterol, caffeic acid, gallic acid, limonene, luteolin, pectin, tannic acid, tannins, ursolic acid. Nutrients: B-complex vitamins, iron, potassium, vitamins A, C, and E.	Decreases thickness and increases fluidity of mucus in the bronchial tubes and lungs. Boosts the immune system. Useful for indigestion, loss of appetite, bloating, and hay fever, sinusitis, and other respiratory disorders.	*Caution:* Large doses may cause irregular heart rhythms.
Horse chestnut (*Aesculus hippocastanum*)	Bark, leaves, oil, seeds.	Phytochemicals: Allantoin, citric acid, epicatechin, escin, esculetin, esculin, fraxetin, fraxin, isoquercitrin, kaempferol, leucocyanidin, myricetin, quercetin, quercitrin, rutin, saponin, scopoletin, tannin.	Protects against vascular damage, makes capillary walls less porous, shields against UV radiation damage. Good for varicose veins, reducing excess tissue fluids, and easing night-time muscle spasms in the legs. Used topically, reduces pain and swelling, and prevents bruising.	
Horsetail (*Equisetum arvense*)	Stems.	Phytochemicals: Beta-carotene, beta-sitosterol, caffeic acid, campesterol, equisetonin, ferulic acid, gallic acid, isoquercitrin, isoquercitroside, kaempferol, luteolin, naringenin, p-coumaric acid, tannic acid, vanillic acid. Nutrients: Calcium, iron, magnesium, manganese, phosphorus, potassium, selenium, silicon, zinc, vitamins B_1, B_2, B_3, and C.	Acts as a diuretic, lessens inflammation, and reduces muscle cramps and spasms. Aids calcium absorption, which promotes healthy skin and strengthens bone, hair, nails, and teeth. Bolsters healing of broken bones and connective tissue. Strengthens the heart and lungs. Useful for the treatment of arthritis, bone diseases such as osteoporosis and rickets, bronchitis, cardiovascular disease, edema, gallbladder disorders, gout, muscle cramps, and prostate disorders. Used in poultice form to depress bleeding and accelerate healing of burns and wounds.	Also called bottle brush, shavegrass. If this herb is used for a prolonged period, supplemental vitamin B_1 (thiamin) should be taken, as horsetail interferes with the absorption of this vitamin.
Hydrangea (*Hydrangea arborescens*)	Rhizomes, roots.	Phytochemicals: Kaempferol, quercetin, rutin, saponin. Nutrients: Calcium, iron, magnesium, manganese, phosphorus, potassium, selenium, zinc.	Stimulates the kidneys and acts as a diuretic. Good for bladder infection, kidney disease, obesity, and prostate disorders. Combined with gravel root, good for kidney stones.	*Caution:* The leaves of this plant should *not* be consumed. They contain cyanide and can be toxic.
Hyssop (*Hyssopus officinalis*)	Flowers, leaves, shoots.	Phytochemicals: Alpha-pinene, benzaldehyde, beta-ionone, beta-sitosterol, borneol, caffeic acid, camphor, carvacrol, eugenol, ferulic acid, geraniol, hesperidin, limonene, linalool, marrubiin, oleanolic acid, 1,8-cineole, rosmarinic acid, thymol, ursolic acid. Nutrients: Choline.	Promotes expulsion of mucus from the respiratory tract, relieves congestion, regulates blood pressure, and dispels gas. Used externally, helpful for wound healing. Good for circulatory problems, epilepsy, fever, gout, and weight problems. Poultices made from fresh green hyssop help heal cuts.	*Caution:* Should not be used during pregnancy.

Herb (Scientific Name)	Parts Used	Phytochemical and Nutrient Content	Actions and Uses	Comments
Irish moss (Chondrus crispus)	Entire plant.	Phytochemicals: Beta-carotene. Nutrients: Calcium, iron, magnesium, manganese, phosphorus, potassium, selenium, zinc, vitamins B_1, B_2, B_3, and C.	Acts as an expectorant and aids in the formation of stools. Good for bronchitis and many intestinal disorders. Also used in skin lotions and in hair rinses for dry hair.	
Jaborandi (Pilocarpus jaborandi)	Leaves.	Phytochemicals: Alpha-pinene, limonene, myrcene, pilocarpine.	Fights inflammation and acts as a diuretic. Helps stimulate milk production and flow in nursing mothers. Beneficial for fever, colds and flu, bronchitis, colon disorders, and edema. Topically, useful for baldness and for promoting circulation in the capillaries.	A rainforest herb whose active compound, pilocarpine, has been used for over 120 years to relieve intraocular pressure in glaucoma.
Jatoba (Hymenaea courbaril)	Bark, leaves, fruit.	Phytochemicals: Beta-sitosterol, caryophyllene, delta-cadinene, epicatechin.	Fights inflammation, free radicals, and bacterial and fungal infection. Increases energy. Beneficial for asthma, bronchitis, bursitis, bladder infection, candida and other fungal infections, arthritis, and prostatitis.	A rainforest herb with a wide range of traditional uses.
Juniper (Juniperus communis)	Fruit.	Phytochemicals: Alpha-pinene, beta-carotene, beta-pinene, betulin, borneol, camphor, caryophyllene, catechin, farnesol, epicatechin, glycolic acid, limonene, linalool, menthol, rutin, tannins, umbelliferone. Nutrients: Calcium, chromium, iron, magnesium, manganese, phosphorus, potassium, selenium, zinc, vitamins B_1, B_2, B_3, and C.	Acts as a diuretic, anti-inflammatory, and decongestant. Helps regulate blood sugar levels. Helpful in treatment of asthma, bladder infection, fluid retention, gout, obesity, and prostate disorders.	Caution: May interfere with absorption of iron and other minerals when taken internally. Should not be used during pregnancy. Should not be used by persons with kidney disease.
Kava kava (Piper methysticum)	Roots.	Phytochemicals: Cinnamic acid, kavalactones (including kawain, dihydrokawain, methysticin, dihydromethysticin, yangonin).	Induces physical and mental relaxation. Acts as a diuretic, genitourinary antiseptic, and gastrointestinal tonic. Relieves muscle spasms and eases pain. Helpful for anxiety and anxiety disorders, insomnia, stress-related disorders, menopausal symptoms, and urinary tract infections.	Also called kava. Caution: Can cause drowsiness. If this occurs, discontinue use or reduce the dosage. Should not be combined with alcohol. Not recommended for persons under the age of 18, pregnant women, nursing mothers, or individuals who suffer from depression or take certain prescription drugs, especially antianxiety drugs.
Kudzu (Pueraria lobata)	Leaves, roots, shoots.	Phytochemicals: Daidzein, daidzin, genistein, p-coumaric acid, puerarin, quercetin. Nutrients: Calcium, iron, magnesium, phosphorus, potassium, vitamin B_2.	Suppresses alcohol cravings. Lowers blood pressure and relieves headache, stiff neck, vertigo, and tinnitus. Useful for treating alcoholism, colds, flu, and gastrointestinal problems.	In China and Japan, kudzu has been used as a food starch and medicine for centuries. The Chinese use kudzu extract to treat angina pectoris.
Lady's mantle (Achillea millefolium)	Entire plant, except the root.	Phytochemicals: Achilleine, alpha-pinene, apigenin, azulene, beta-carotene, betaine, beta-pinene, beta-sitosterol, betonicine, borneol, caffeic acid, camphor, caryophyllene,	Has anti-inflammatory, diuretic, and antiviral effects. Helps to heal mucous membranes, improve blood clotting, and increase perspiration. Helps to regulate menstruation, reduce	Also called soldier's herb, yarrow. Caution: Interferes with absorption of iron and

Herb (Scientific Name)	Parts Used	Phytochemical and Nutrient Content	Actions and Uses	Comments
Lady's mantle (continued)		chamazulene, coumarins, eugenol, guaiazulene, isorhamnetin, limonene, luteolin, mannitol, menthol, myrcene, myristic acid, 1,8-cineole, p-cymene, quercetin, quercitrin, rutin, salicylic acid, stigmasterol, tannin, thujone. Nutrients: Amino acids, calcium, fatty acids, folate, iron, magnesium, manganese, phosphorus, potassium, selenium, zinc, vitamins B_1, B_2, B_3, and C.	excessive bleeding, and ease cramps. Useful for muscle spasms, fever, gastrointestinal disorders, inflammatory disorders, and viral infections. Applied topically, stops bleeding and promotes healing. Good as a douche for vaginal irritation.	other minerals. Should not be used by individuals who are unusually sun sensitive. Should not be used during pregnancy.
Lavender (*Lavandula angustifolia*)	Flowers.	Phytochemicals: Alpha-pinene, beta-pinene, beta-santalene, borneol, camphor, caryophyllene, coumarin, geraniol, limonene, linalool, luteolin, 1,8-cineole, rosmarinic acid, tannin, umbelliferone, ursolic acid.	Relieves stress and depression. Beneficial for the skin. Good for burns, headaches, psoriasis, and other skin problems.	Essential oil of lavender is very popular in aromatherapy. *Caution:* Should not be used during pregnancy. Lavender oil should not be taken internally.
Lemongrass (*Cymbopogon citratus*)	Leaves, stems.	Phytochemicals: Alpha-pinene, beta-sitosterol, caryophyllene, citral, farnesol, geraniol, limonene, luteolin, myrcene, 1,8-cineole, quercetin, rutin, saponin, triacontanol. Nutrients: Calcium, iron, magnesium, manganese, phosphorus, potassium, selenium, zinc.	Acts as an astringent, tonic, and digestive aid. Good for the skin and nails. Useful for fever, flu, headaches, and intestinal irritations.	Used in perfumes and other products as a fragrance.
Licorice (*Glycyrrhiza glabra*)	Roots.	Phytochemicals: Apigenin, benzaldehyde, beta-carotene, beta-sitosterol, betaine, camphor, carvacrol, estriol, eugenol, ferulic acid, formononetin, geraniol, glabrene, glabridin, glabrol, glycyrrhetinic acid, glycyrrhizin, isoliquiritigenin, isoliquiritin, isoquercitrin, lignin, mannitol, phenol, quercetin, salicylic acid, sinapic acid, stigmasterol, thymol, umbelliferone, vitexin. Nutrients: Calcium, choline, iron, magnesium, manganese, phosphorus, potassium, selenium, silicon, zinc, vitamins B_1, B_2, B_3, and C.	Fights inflammation and viral, bacterial, and parasitic infection. Stimulates the production of interferon and may help inhibit replication of HIV. Cleanses the colon. Reduces muscle spasms, increases fluidity of mucus in the lungs and bronchial tubes, and promotes adrenal gland function. Has estrogen- and progesterone-like effects; may change the pitch of the voice. Helps to inhibit the formation of plaque and prevent bacteria from sticking to tooth enamel. Beneficial for allergies, asthma, chronic fatigue, depression, emphysema, enlarged prostate, fever, herpesvirus infection, hypoglycemia, glandular functions, inflammatory bowel disorders, premenstrual syndrome, menopausal symptoms, and upper respiratory infections. May prevent hepatitis C from causing liver cancer and cirrhosis and protect against atherosclerosis. Deglycyrrhizinated licorice may stimulate natural defense mechanisms that prevent the occurrence of ulcers by increasing the number of mucus-secreting cells in the digestive tract. This improves the quality of mucus, lengthens intestinal cell life, and enhances microcirculation in the gastrointestinal lining.	Licorice derivatives have been recommended as a standard support for ulcer sufferers in Europe. Licorice-flavored candy does not work for medicinal purposes because it is mostly made with anise, not licorice. *Caution:* Should not be used during pregnancy, nor by persons with diabetes, glaucoma, heart disease, high blood pressure, severe menstrual problems, or a history of stroke. Should not be used on a daily basis for more than seven days in a row, as this can result in high blood pressure in persons with previously normal blood pressure. Extended use can cause high blood pressure, water retention, and low potassium levels.

Herb (Scientific Name)	Parts Used	Phytochemical and Nutrient Content	Actions and Uses	Comments
Maca (*Lepidium meyenii*)	Roots.	Phytochemicals: Beta-sitosterol, saponin, stigmasterol, tannins. Nutrients: Amino acids, calcium, iron, magnesium, phosphorus, vitamins B_1, B_2, B_{12}, C, and E, zinc.	Increases energy and supports the immune system. Good for anemia, chronic fatigue syndrome, impotence, menopausal symptoms, and menstrual problems.	A rainforest herb that is a member of the potato family. An important food in the diet of native Peruvians, it is rich in amino acids and high in protein.
Macela (*Achyrocline satureoides*)	Aerial parts.	Phytochemicals: Alpha-pinene, caffeic acid, caryophyllene, chlorogenic acid, coumarin, delta-cadinene, galangin, luteolin, 1,8-cineole, quercetagetin, quercetin, scoparone.	Acts as an anti-inflammatory, antiseptic, antiviral, and antiparasitic. Stimulates and supports the immune system. Good for gastrointestinal and respiratory disorders. Useful in treating cancer, Crohn's disease, colds and flu, diabetes, menstrual problems and menopausal symptoms, and muscle aches and spasms.	A rainforest herb that has been found to have potential anti-HIV properties.
Marshmallow (*Althaea officinalis*)	Flowers, leaves, roots.	Phytochemicals: Beta-carotene, betaine, caffeic acid, chlorogenic acid, ferulic acid, kaempferol, mucilage, paraffin, p-coumaric acid, pectin, phytosterols, quercetin, salicylic acid, scopoletin, sorbitol, tannins, vanillic acid. Nutrients: Amino acids, calcium, iron, magnesium, manganese, phosphorus, potassium, selenium, zinc, vitamins B_1, B_2, B_3, and C.	Aids the body in expelling excess fluid and mucus. Soothes and heals skin, mucous membranes, and other tissues, externally and internally. Good for bladder infection, digestive upsets, fluid retention, headache, intestinal disorders, kidney problems, sinusitis, and sore throat.	Often used as a filler in the compounding of pills.
Meadowsweet (*Filipendula ulmaria*)	Leaves, flower tops.	Phytochemicals: Anthocyanidin, avicularin, coumarin, hyperoside, methyl salicylate, quercetin, rutin, salicin, salicylic acid, vanillin.	Tightens tissues and promotes elimination of excess fluid. Reduces inflammation and strengthens and tones the system. Good for colds, flu, nausea, digestive disorders, muscle cramps and aches, and diarrhea.	The word *aspirin* is derived from an old name for this plant, *spirea*. *Caution:* Because this plant contains compounds related to aspirin, it should not be used by pregnant women, and it should not be given to children with fever due to cold, flu, measles chicken-pox, or any other viral infection, as this increases the risk of Reye's syndrome, a dangerous complication that can alter or damage the liver, brain, and heart.
Milk thistle (*Silybum marianum*)	Fruit, leaves, seeds.	Phytochemicals: Apigenin, beta-carotene, fumaric acid, kaempferol, naringenin, quercetin, silandrin, silybin, silychristin, silydianin, silymarin, silymonin, taxifolin. Nutrients: Calcium, fatty acids, iron, magnesium, manganese, phosphorus, potassium, selenium, zinc.	Protects the liver from toxins and pollutants by preventing free radical damage and stimulates the production of new liver cells. Also protects the kidneys. Good for gallbladder and adrenal disorders, inflammatory bowel disorders, psoriasis, weakened immune system, and all liver disorders. Has shown anticancer effects against prostate cancer and breast cancer.	Also called Mary thistle, wild artichoke. Because milk thistle has poor water solubility, it is not effective as a tea. A concentrated capsule or extract form is best.

Herb (Scientific Name)	Parts Used	Phytochemical and Nutrient Content	Actions and Uses	Comments
Motherwort (*Leonurus cardiaca*)	Leaves, flowers, stems.	Phytochemicals: Alpha-pinene, benzaldehyde, caryophyllene, catechin, hyperoside, isoquercitrin, limonene, linalool, marrubiin, oleanolic acid, quercetin, quercitrin, rutin, saponin, stachydrine, tannin, ursolic acid. Nutrients: Vitamin C.	Traditionally used to relieve childbirth pain and as a tranquilizer. Helpful for menstrual disorders, menopausal symptoms, vaginitis, thyroid and rheumatic problems. Has a tonic effect on the heart. Useful for headache, insomnia, and vertigo.	*Caution:* Should not be used during pregnancy (until the onset of labor), as it can stimulate uterine contractions. Not recommended for persons with clotting disorders, high blood pressure, or heart disease.
Muira puama (*Ptychopetalum olacoides*)	Bark, roots.	Phytochemicals: Beta-sitosterol, campesterol, coumarin, lupeol.	Helps relieve pain, acts as a mild laxative and detoxifier, and supports the heart. Has a general tonic effect and balances sex hormones. Beneficial in treating nervous system disorders, impotence, depression, stress, rheumatism, hair loss, asthma, and menopausal and menstrual problems.	An alcohol-based extract is believed to be the best form of this rainforest herb, as the active constituents are neither water soluble nor broken down in the digestive process.
Mullein (*Verbascum thapsus*)	Leaves.	Phytochemicals: Beta-carotene, beta-sitosterol, coumarin, hesperidin, saponins. Nutrients: Calcium, iron, magnesium, manganese, phosphorus, potassium, selenium, zinc, vitamins B$_1$, B$_2$, B$_3$, and C.	Acts as a laxative, painkiller, and sleep aid. Taken internally, aids in getting rid of warts. Clears congestion. Useful for asthma, bronchitis, difficulty breathing, earache, hay fever, and swollen glands. Used in kidney formulas to soothe inflammation.	
Mustard (*Brassica nigra*)	Seeds.	Phytochemicals: Allyl isothiocyanate, caffeic acid, chlorogenic acid, ferulic acid, p-coumaric acid, protocatechuic acid, sinapic acid, vanillic acid.	Improves digestion and aids in the metabolism of fat. Applied externally, helpful for chest congestion, inflammation, injuries, and joint pain.	*Caution:* Can be irritating when applied directly to the skin. Not recommended for use on children under the age of six.
Myrrh (*Commiphora myrrha*)	Resin from stems.	Phytochemicals: Acetic acid, beta-sitosterol, campesterol, cinnamaldehyde, cuminaldehyde, dipentene, eugenol, limonene, m-cresol.	Acts as an antiseptic, disinfectant, expectorant, and deodorizer. Stimulates the immune system and gastric secretions. Tones and stimulates mucous tissue. Helps to fight harmful bacteria in the mouth. Good for bad breath, periodontal disease, skin disorders, asthma, bronchitis, colds, flu, sinusitis, sore throat, herpes simplex, and ulcers. Topically, useful for abscesses, boils, sores, and wounds.	Used in many perfumes and in incense for its aromatic properties. Guggul, the standardized extract of the Indian mukul myrrh tree, lowers both cholesterol and triglyceride levels.
Nettle (*Urtica dioica*)	Flowers, leaves, roots.	Phytochemicals: Acetic acid, beta-carotene, betaine, caffeic acid, ferulic acid, lecithin, lycopene, p-coumaric acid, scopoletin. Nutrients: Calcium, copper, fatty acids, folate, iron, magnesium, manganese, phosphorus, potassium, selenium, sulfur, zinc, vitamins B$_1$, B$_2$, B$_3$, B$_5$, C, and E.	Acts as a diuretic, expectorant, pain reliever, and tonic. Good for benign prostatic hyperplasia, anemia, arthritis, rheumatism, hay fever, and other allergic disorders, kidney problems, and malabsorption syndrome. Improves goiter, inflammatory conditions, and mucous conditions of the lungs. Used in hair care products, helps stimulate hair follicles and regulate scalp oil buildup.	Also called stinging nettle.

Herb (Scientific Name)	Parts Used	Phytochemical and Nutrient Content	Actions and Uses	Comments
Oat straw (*Avena sativa*)	Whole plant.	Phytochemicals: Benzaldehyde, beta-carotene, beta-ionone, beta-sitosterol, betaine, caffeic acid, campesterol, caryophyllene, chlorophyll, ferulic acid, lignin, limonene, p-coumaric acid, quercetin, scopoletin, sinapic acid, stigmasterol, vanillic acid, vanillin. Nutrients: Calcium, folate, iron, magnesium, manganese, phosphorus, potassium, selenium, zinc, vitamins A, B_1, B_2, B_3, B_5, B_6, and E.	Acts as an antidepressant and restorative nerve tonic. Increases perspiration. Helps to ease insomnia. Good for bed-wetting, depression, stress, and skin disorders.	
Olive leaf (*Olea europaea*)	Extract from leaves.	Phytochemicals: Apigenin, beta-sitosterol glucoside, cinchonidine, esculetin, kaempferol, luteolin, mannitol, maslinic acid, oleanic acid, oleuropein, quercetin, rutin, tannins. Nutrients: Calcium.	Fights all types of bacteria, viruses, fungi, and parasites. Helps stave off colds and flu. May have antioxidant properties. Has shown potential for lowering high blood pressure. Good for virtually any infectious disease, as well as for chronic fatigue syndrome, diarrheal diseases, inflammatory arthritis, and psoriasis.	
Oregon grape (*Mahonia aquifolia*)	Roots.	Berberine, tannins.	Purifies the blood and cleanses the liver. Acts as a laxative. Good for many skin conditions, from acne to psoriasis.	Has actions similar to those of goldenseal and barberry.
Papaya (*Carica papaya*)	Fruit, leaves.	Phytochemicals: Benzaldehyde, beta-carotene, caryophyllene, linalool, lycopene, malic acid, methyl salicylate, myristic acid, papain, phytofluene, zeaxanthin. Nutrients: Calcium, iron, magnesium, manganese, phosphorus, potassium, zinc, vitamins B_1, B_2, B_3, B_5, and C.	Stimulates the appetite and aids digestion. Good for heartburn, indigestion, and inflammatory bowel disorders.	The leaves can be used to tenderize meat.
Parsley (*Petroselinum crispum*)	Fruit, leaves, roots, stems.	Phytochemicals: Alpha-pinene, apigenin, apiole, benzaldehyde, bergapten, beta-carotene, caffeic acid, chlorogenic acid, geraniol, glycolic acid, kaempferol, limonene, linalool, lutein, myristic acid, myristicin, naringenin, p-coumaric acid, psoralen, quercetin, rosmarinic acid, rutin, xanthotoxin. Nutrients: Calcium, folate, iron, magnesium, manganese, phosphorus, potassium, selenium, zinc, vitamins A, B_1, B_2, B_3, B_5, C, and E.	Contains a substance that prevents the multiplication of tumor cells. Expels worms, relieves gas, stimulates normal activity of the digestive system, and freshens breath. Helps bladder, kidney, liver, lung, stomach, and thyroid function. Good for bed-wetting, fluid retention, gas, halitosis, high blood pressure, indigestion, kidney disease, obesity, and prostate disorders.	Contains more vitamin C than oranges by weight.
Passionflower (*Passiflora incarnata*)	Flowers, leaves, shoots, stems.	Phytochemicals: Apigenin, flavonoids, harmaline, kaempferol, luteolin, maltol, quercetin, rutin, scopoletin, stigmasterol, umbelliferone, vitexin. Nutrients: Amino acids, calcium.	Has a gentle sedative effect and helps lower blood pressure. Helpful for anxiety, hyperactivity, insomnia, neuritis, and stress-related disorders.	Also called maypop. *Caution:* Should not be used during pregnancy, as it may stimulate the uterus.
Pau d'arco (*Tabebuia heptaphylla*)	Inner bark.	Phytochemicals: Beta-carotene, beta-sitosterol, lapachol.	Fights bacterial and viral infection. Cleanses the blood. Good for candidiasis, smoker's cough, warts, and all types of infection. Helpful for AIDS, allergies, cancer, cardiovascular problems, inflammatory bowel disease, rheumatism, tumors, and ulcers.	Also called lapacho, taheebo.

Herb (Scientific Name)	Parts Used	Phytochemical and Nutrient Content	Actions and Uses	Comments
Peppermint (*Mentha piperita*)	Flowering tops, oil, leaves.	Phytochemicals: Acetic acid, alpha-carotene, alpha-pinene, azulene, beta-carotene, beta-ionone, betaine, caffeic acid, carvacrol, carvone, chlorogenic acid, coumarin, eugenol, hesperetin, limonene, linalool, luteolin, menthol, 1,8-cineole, p-coumaric acid, pectin, rosmarinic acid, rutin, tannin, thymol, vanillin. Nutrients: Calcium, choline, iron, magnesium, manganese, phosphorus, potassium, selenium, zinc, vitamins B_1, B_2, B_3, and E.	Increases stomach acidity, aiding digestion. Slightly anesthetizes mucous membranes and the gastrointestinal tract. Useful for chills, colic, diarrhea, headache, heart trouble, indigestion, irritable bowel syndrome, nausea, poor appetite, rheumatism, and spasms.	*Caution:* May interfere with iron absorption. Should not be used by nursing mothers. Do not ingest pure menthol or pure peppermint leaves.
Plantain (*Plantago major*)	Leaves.	Phytochemicals: Adenine, allantoin, aucubin, apigenin, benzoic acid, caffeic acid, chlorogenic acid, cinnamic acid, ferulic acid, fiber, luteolin, oleanolic acid, p-coumaric acid, salicylic acid, tannin, ursolic acid, vanillic acid. Nutrients: Potassium, vitamin A.	Acts as a diuretic and is soothing to the lungs and urinary tract. May slow the growth of tuberculosis bacteria. Has a healing, antibiotic, and styptic effect when used topically for sores and wounds. Useful for indigestion and heartburn. Applied in a poultice, good for bee stings and any kind of bite.	Young leaves are tasty and can be eaten in salads. *Caution:* Do not mistake plantain for foxglove (*Digitalis lanata*), which has a similar appearance.
Pleurisy root (*Asclepias tuberosa*)	Rhizome.	Phytochemicals: Alpha-amyrin, asclepiadin, beta-amyrin, isorhamnetin, kaempferol, lupeol, quercetin, rutin, viburnitol.	Reduces inflammation of the pleural membranes of the lungs, enhances secretion of healthy lung fluids, and stimulates the lymphatic system. Has antispasmodic properties. Induces sweating and aids expectoration. Beneficial for pleurisy, pneumonia, bronchitis, flu, and coughs.	Also called butterfly weed.
Primrose (*Oenothera biennis*)	Seed oil.	Phytochemicals: Beta-sitosterol, caffeic acid, campesterol, ellagic acid, gallic acid, kaempferol, lignin, p-coumaric acid, phytosterols, quercetin, tannin. Nutrients: Amino acids, calcium, essential fatty acids, iron, magnesium, manganese, phosphorus, potassium, vitamin E, zinc.	Promotes cardiovascular health. Aids in weight loss and reduces high blood pressure. Acts as a natural estrogen promoter. Helpful in treating alcoholism, arthritis, hot flashes, menstrual problems such as cramps and heavy bleeding, multiple sclerosis, and skin disorders.	Also called evening primrose. *Caution:* Primrose *root* should not be used during pregnancy.
Pumpkin (*Cucurbita pepo*)	Flesh, seed.	Phytochemicals: Astragalin, beta-carotene, beta-sitosterol, caffeic acid, chlorogenin, cryptoxanthin, diosgenin, ferulic acid, gitogenin, kaempferol, lutein, mannitol, myristic acid, phytosterols, quercetin, ruscogenin, salicylic acid, zeaxanthin. Nutrients: Amino acids, calcium, essential fatty acids, iron, magnesium, manganese, phosphorus, potassium, selenium, zinc, vitamins A, C, and E.	Useful for prostate disorders and irritable bladder.	
Puncture vine (*Tribulus terrestris*)	Flowers, fruit, leaves, stems.	Phytochemicals: Astragalin, beta-sitosterol, campesterol, chlorogenin, diosgenin, gitogenin, kaempferol, quercetin, ruscogenin, rutin, stigmasterol. Nutrients: Amino acids, calcium, essential fatty acids, iron, phosphorus, potassium, vitamin C.	Improves sex drive. Eases menopausal symptoms. Stimulates production of and balances male and female hormones. Enhances the immune system. Helps build muscles and increase stamina and endurance. Has antifungal, antibacterial, and anti-inflammatory actions. Useful as a general tonic and revitalizer for the liver, kidneys, and urinary tract.	Also called caltrop.

Herb (Scientific Name)	Parts Used	Phytochemical and Nutrient Content	Actions and Uses	Comments
Pygeum (Pygeum africanum)	Bark.	Phytochemicals: Beta-sitosterol, oleanic acid, ursolic acid.	Reduces inflammation and decongestion. Lowers levels of inflammatory compounds in the prostate. Effective in reducing prostate enlargement.	Used clinically in Europe to treat benign prostatic hyperplasia.
Red clover (Trifolium pratense)	Flowers.	Phytochemicals: Beta-carotene, beta-sitosterol, biochanin, caffeic acid, campesterol, chlorogenic acid, coumarin, coumestrol, daidzein, eugenol, formononetin, genistein, isorhamnetin, methyl salicylate, myricetin, p-coumaric acid, salicylic acid. Nutrients: Calcium, iron, magnesium, manganese, phosphorus, potassium, selenium, zinc, vitamins B_3, C, and E.	Fights infection, suppresses appetite, and purifies the blood. Has expectorant, antispasmodic, and relaxing effects. Good for bacterial infections, HIV and AIDS, coughs, bronchitis, inflamed lungs, inflammatory bowel disorders, kidney problems, liver disease, skin disorders, and weakened immune system.	
Red raspberry (Rubus idaeus)	Bark, leaves, roots.	Phytochemicals: Alpha-carotene, benzaldehyde, beta-carotene, beta-ionone, caffeic acid, ellagic acid, farnesol, ferulic acid, gallic acid, geraniol, lutein, tannin. Nutrients: Calcium, iron, magnesium, manganese, phosphorus, potassium, selenium, silicon, zinc, vitamins B_1, B_2, B_3, C, and E.	Reduces menstrual bleeding, relaxes uterine and intestinal spasms, and strengthens uterine walls. Promotes healthy nails, bones, teeth, and skin. Good for diarrhea and for female disorders such as morning sickness, hot flashes, and menstrual cramps. Also heals canker sores. Combined with peppermint, good for morning sickness.	
Rhubarb (Rheum rhabarbarum)	Roots, stalks.	Phytochemicals: Acetic acid, beta-carotene, caffeic acid, chrysophanol, emodin, epicatechin, ferulic acid, fumaric acid, gallic acid, isoquercitrin, lutein, p-coumaric acid, protocatechuic acid, rutin, sinapic acid, vanillic acid. Nutrients: Calcium, iron, magnesium, manganese, phosphorus, potassium, selenium, sulfur, zinc, vitamins B_1, B_2, B_3, B_5, C, and E.	Fights infection and eliminates worms. Enhances gallbladder function and promotes healing of duodenal ulcers. Good for constipation, malabsorption, and disorders of the colon, spleen, and liver.	Caution: Should not be used during pregnancy.
Rose (Rosa canina)	Fruit (hips).	Phytochemicals: Beta-carotene, betulin, catechin, epicatechin, flavonoids, isoquercitrin, lycopene, malic acid, pectin, tannin, vanillin, zeaxanthin. Nutrients: Calcium, iron, magnesium, manganese, phosphorus, potassium, selenium, zinc, vitamins B_1, B_2, B_3, C, and E.	Good for bladder problems and all infections. A good source of vitamin C when used fresh. Rose hip tea is good for diarrhea.	Many vitamin and other supplements are derived from rose hips.
Rosemary (Rosmarinus officinalis)	Leaves.	Phytochemicals: Alpha-pinene, apigenin, beta-carotene, beta-sitosterol, betulinic acid, borneol, caffeic acid, camphor, carnosol, carvacrol, carvone, caryophyllene, chlorogenic acid, diosmin, genkwanin, geraniol, hesperidin, limonene, linalool, luteolin, oleanolic acid, 1,8-cineole, phytosterols, rosmanol, rosmarinic acid, salicylates, squalene, tannin, thymol, ursolic acid. Nutrients: Calcium, iron, magnesium, manganese, phosphorus, potassium, zinc, vitamins B_1, B_3, and C.	Fights free radicals, inflammation, bacteria, and fungi. Relaxes the stomach, stimulates circulation and digestion, and acts as an astringent and decongestant. Improves circulation to the brain. Also helps detoxify the liver, and has anticancer and antitumor properties. Good for headaches, high and low blood pressure, circulatory problems, and menstrual cramps. Can be used as an antiseptic gargle.	Makes a good food preservative. Caution: Should not be used during pregnancy.

Herb (Scientific Name)	Parts Used	Phytochemical and Nutrient Content	Actions and Uses	Comments
Sage (Salvia officinalis)	Leaves.	Phytochemicals: Alpha-amyrin, alpha-pinene, alpha-terpineol, apigenin, beta-carotene, beta-sitosterol, betulin, borneol, caffeic acid, campesterol, camphene, camphor, carnosolic acid, caryophyllene, catechin, chlorogenic acid, citral, farnesol, ferulic acid, gallic acid, genkwanin, geraniol, hispidulin, limonene, linalool, luteolin, maslinic acid, oleanolic acid, 1,8-cineole, p-coumaric acid, pinene, rosmarinic acid, saponin, stigmasterol, tannins, terpineol, thymol, ursolic acid, vanillic acid. Nutrients: Boron, calcium, iron, magnesium, manganese, phosphorus, potassium, selenium, zinc, vitamins B_1, B_2, B_3, B_5, and C.	Stimulates the central nervous system and digestive tract, and has estrogenic effects on the body. Reduces sweating and salivation. Good for hot flashes and other symptoms of estrogen deficiency, whether in menopause or following hysterectomy. Beneficial for disorders affecting the mouth and throat, such as tonsillitis. In tea form, can be used as a hair rinse to promote shine (especially for dark hair) and hair growth. Also used to dry up milk when women wish to stop nursing.	*Caution:* Interferes with the absorption of iron and other minerals when taken internally, and decreases milk supply in nursing mothers. Should not be taken by individuals with seizure disorders. Should not be taken during pregnancy.
St. John's Wort (Hypericum perforatum)	Flowers, leaves, stems, oil.	Phytochemicals: Carotenoids, caryophyllene, chlorophyll, flavonoids, hyperoside, isoquercitrin, limonene, lutein, mannitol, myristic acid, phenol, phloroglucinol, phytosterols, quercetin, quercitrin, rutin, saponin, tannins. Nutrients: Vitamin C.	Good for depression and nerve pain. Helps control stress. In laboratory studies, protects bone marrow and intestinal mucosa from x-ray damage. Applied topically, the oil aids wound healing.	*Caution:* Large amounts can cause heightened sun sensitivity, especially in light-sensitive people. Should not be used by people who take prescription anti-depressants or any medication that interacts with MAO inhibitors. Should be used with caution during pregnancy.
Sangre de grado (Croton lechleri)	Bark, resin.	Alpha-pinene, betaine, beta-pinene, borneol, camphene, dipentene, eugenol, gamma-terpinene, lignin, linalool, myrcene, p-cymene, tannins, taspine, vanillin.	Fights free radicals, inflammation, and bacterial, viral, and fungal infection. Helps heal wounds and stop bleeding. Good for respiratory and skin disorders, mouth and skin ulcers, sore throat, colds and flu, candida, psoriasis, herpes, and vaginitis.	A rainforest herb whose name means "dragon's blood."
Sarsaparilla (Smilax species)	Roots, rhizomes.	Phytochemicals: Beta-sitosterol, saponin, stigmasterol. Nutrients: Iron, magnesium, manganese, phosphorus, potassium, selenium, zinc.	Promotes excretion of fluids, increases energy, protects against harm from radiation exposure, and regulates hormones. Useful for frigidity, hives, impotence, infertility, nervous system disorders, premenstrual syndrome, psoriasis, rheumatoid arthritis, and disorders caused by blood impurities.	Also called Chinese root, small spikenard.
Saw palmetto (Serenoa repens)	Berries, seeds.	Phytochemicals: Beta-carotene, beta-sitosterol, ferulic acid, mannitol, myristic acid, tannins, vanillic acid, vanillin.	Acts as a diuretic, urinary antiseptic, and appetite stimulant. Inhibits production of dihydrotestosterone, a form of testosterone that contributes to enlargement of the prostate. May also enhance sexual functioning and sexual desire.	Used clinically in Europe to treat benign prostate hyperplasia (BPH). Can be combined with nettle root for BPH also.

Herb (Scientific Name)	Parts Used	Phytochemical and Nutrient Content	Actions and Uses	Comments
Skullcap (*Scutellaria laterfolia*)	Leaves, shoots.	Phytochemicals: Beta-carotene, lignin, tannins. Nutrients: Calcium, iron, magnesium, manganese, phosphorus, potassium, selenium, zinc, vitamins B_1, B_2, B_3, and C.	Aids sleep, improves circulation, and strengthens the heart muscle. Relieves muscle cramps, pain, spasms, and stress. Good for anxiety, fatigue, cardiovascular disease, headache, hyperactivity, nervous disorders, and rheumatism. Useful in treating barbiturate addiction and drug withdrawal.	*Caution:* Should not be given to children under 6.
Slippery elm (*Ulmus rubra*)	Inner bark.	Phytochemicals: Beta-carotene, campesterol, mucilage, starch, tannin. Nutrients: Calcium, iron, magnesium, manganese, phosphorus, potassium, selenium, zinc, vitamins B_1, B_2, B_3, and C.	Soothes inflamed mucous membranes of the bowels, stomach, and urinary tract. Good for diarrhea and ulcers and for treatment of colds, flu, and sore throat. Beneficial for Crohn's disease, ulcerative colitis, diverticulosis, diverticulitis, and gastritis.	Also called moose elm, red elm.
Squawvine (*Mitchella repens*)	Leaves, stems.	Phytochemicals: Alkaloids, glycosides, mucilage, saponins, tannins.	Relieves pelvic congestion and soothes the nervous system. Good for menstrual cramps and preparation for childbirth.	Also called partridgeberry.
Stone root (*Collinsonia canadensis*)	Whole plant, fresh root.	Phytochemicals: Alpha-pinene, caffeic acid, caryophyllene, limonene. Nutrients: Magnesium.	Acts as a diuretic, sedative, antispasmodic, astringent, and tonic. Good for the urinary tract. Breaks up mucus. Helpful for bronchitis, headache, cramps, indigestion, and hemorrhoids.	
Suma (*Pfaffia paniculata*)	Bark, berries, leaves, roots.	Phytochemicals: Beta-sitosterol, saponin, stigmasterol. Nutrients: Iron, magnesium, zinc, vitamins A, B_1, B_2, B_5, E, and K.	Fights inflammation, boosts the immune system, and combats anemia, fatigue, and stress. Good for AIDS, arthritis, cancer, liver disease, menopausal symptoms, high blood pressure, Epstein-Barr virus and weakened immune system.	Also known as Brazilian ginseng.
Tea tree (*Melaleuca alternifolia*)	Essential oil.	Phytochemicals: Alpha-pinene, alpha-terpineol, aromadendrene, beta-pinene, camphor, caryophyllene, limonene, linalool, 1,8-cineole, p-cymene, terpinenes, terpinolene.	Used topically, disinfects wounds and heals virtually all skin conditions, including acne, athlete's foot, boils, cuts and scrapes, earache, fungal infections, hair and scalp problems, herpes outbreaks, insect and spider bites, scabies, and warts. Added to water, can be used as a douche for vaginitis and a gargle for colds, sore throats, and mouth sores (do not swallow it, however).	*Caution:* Should not be taken internally; can be toxic. If irritation occurs, discontinue use or dilute with distilled water, vegetable oil, primrose oil, or vitamin E oil. If irritation persists after dilution, discontinue use.
Thyme (*Thymus vulgaris*)	Berries, flowers, leaves.	Phytochemicals: Alpha-pinene, apigenin, beta-carotene, borneol, caffeic acid, camphor, caprylic acid, carvacrol, carvone, chlorogenic acid, cinnamic acid, citral, eugenol, ferulic acid, gallic acid, geraniol, kaempferol, lauric acid, limonene, linalool, luteolin, myristic acid, naringenin, oleanolic acid, p-coumaric acid, p-cymene, phytosterols, rosmarinic acid, salicylates, tannin, thymol, ursolic acid, vanillic acid. Nutrients: Amino acids, calcium, essential fatty acids, iron, magnesium, manganese, phosphorus, potassium, selenium, zinc, vitamins B_1, B_2, B_3, and C.	Eliminates gas and reduces fever, headache, and mucus. Has strong antiseptic properties. Lowers cholesterol levels. Good for asthma, bronchitis, croup and other respiratory problems, and for fever, headache, and liver disease. Eliminates scalp itching and flaking caused by candidiasis.	

Herb (Scientific Name)	Parts Used	Phytochemical and Nutrient Content	Actions and Uses	Comments
Turmeric (*Curcuma longa*)	Rhizomes.	Phytochemicals: Alpha-pinene, alpha-terpineol, azulene, beta-carotene, borneol, caffeic acid, caryophyllene, cinnamic acid, curcumin, eugenol, guaiacol, limonene, linalool, 1,8-cineole, p-coumaric acid, p-cymene, turmerone, vanillic acid. Nutrients: Calcium, iron, manganese, phosphorus, potassium, zinc, vitamins B_1, B_2, B_3, and C.	Fights free radicals, protects the liver against toxins, inhibits platelet aggregation, aids circulation, lowers cholesterol levels, and improves blood-vessel health. Has antibiotic, anticancer, and anti-inflammatory properties. Good for all arthritic conditions.	Used as a seasoning and the main ingredient in curry powder. Has inhibited the spread of HIV in laboratory tests. *Caution:* Extended use can result in stomach distress. Not recommended for persons with biliary tract obstruction, as curcumin stimulates bile secretion.
Uva ursi (*Arctostaphylos uva-ursi*)	Leaves.	Phytochemicals: Arbutin, beta-carotene, beta-sitosterol, ellagic acid, gallic acid, hyperin, isoquercitrin, myricetin, oleanolic acid, quercetin, quercitrin, ursolic acid. Nutrients: Calcium, iron, magnesium, manganese, phosphorus, potassium, selenium, zinc, vitamins B_1, B_2, B_3, and C.	Promotes excretion of fluids, fights bacteria, and strengthens heart muscle. Good for disorders of the spleen, liver, pancreas, and small intestine. Useful for bladder and kidney infections, diabetes, and prostate disorders.	Also called bearberry. *Caution:* Not recommended for women who are pregnant or nursing, nor for children under 12.
Valerian (*Valeriana officinalis*)	Rhizomes, roots.	Phytochemicals: Azulene, beta-carotene, beta-ionone, beta-sitosterol, borneol, bornyl acetate, caffeic acid, caryophyllene, chlorogenic acid, isovaleric acid, kaempferol, limonene, p-coumaric acid, quercetin, valepotriates, valerenic acid, valerenone, valeric acid. Nutrients: Calcium, choline, essential fatty acids, iron, magnesium, manganese, phosphorus, potassium, selenium, zinc, vitamins B_1, B_2, B_3, and C.	Acts as a sedative, improves circulation, and reduces mucus from colds. Good for anxiety, fatigue, high blood pressure, insomnia, irritable bowel syndrome, menstrual and muscle cramps, nervousness, pain, spasms, stress, and ulcers.	A water-soluble extract form is best. *Caution:* Should not be combined with alcohol.
Vervain (*Verbena officinalis*)	Flowers, leaves, shoots, stems.	Phytochemicals: Adenosine, aucubin, beta-carotene, caffeic acid, citral, tannin, ursolic acid, verbenalin, verbenin.	Strengthens the nervous system. Promotes liver and gallbladder health. Reduces tension and stress. Induces sweating. Promotes menstruation and increases mother's milk. Useful for mild depression, insomnia, headache, toothache, wounds, colds, fever.	*Caution:* Should not be used during pregnancy, as it stimulates uterine contractions.
White oak (*Quercus alba*)	Bark.	Phytochemicals: Beta-carotene, beta-sitosterol, catechin, gallic acid, pectin, quercetin, quercitrin, tannin. Nutrients: Calcium, iron, magnesium, manganese, phosphorus, potassium, selenium, zinc, vitamins B_1, B_2, B_3, and C.	Acts as an antiseptic. Good for skin wounds, bee stings, burns, diarrhea, fevers and cold, bronchitis, nosebleed, poison ivy, and varicose veins. Also good for the teeth. Can be used in enemas and douches.	
White willow (*Salix alba*)	Bark.	Phytochemicals: Apigenin, beta-carotene, catechin, isoquercitrin, lignin, p-coumaric acid, quercetin, rutin, salicin, salicylic acid, tannin. Nutrients: Calcium, iron, magnesium, manganese, phosphorus, potassium, selenium, zinc, vitamins B_1, B_2, B_3, and C.	Relieves pain. Good for allergies, headache, backache, nerve pain, joint pain, inflammation, menstrual cramps, toothache, and injuries.	Contains compounds from which aspirin was derived. *Caution:* Not recommended for use during pregnancy. May interfere with absorption of iron and other minerals when taken internally. Should not be used by people who are allergic to aspirin.

Herb (Scientific Name)	Parts Used	Phytochemical and Nutrient Content	Actions and Uses	Comments
Wild cherry (Prunus serotina)	Inner bark, root bark.	Phytochemicals: Benzaldehyde, caffeic acid, kaempferol, p-coumaric acid, quercetin, scopoletin, tannin, ursolic acid. Nutrients: Calcium, iron, magnesium, phosphorus, potassium, zinc.	Acts as an expectorant and mild sedative. Good for coughs, colds, bronchitis, asthma, digestive disorders, and diarrhea.	Also called choke cherry, wild black cherry, Virginia prune. _Caution:_ Wild cherry bark should not be used during pregnancy. Also, the leaves, bark, and fruit pits contain hydrocyanic acid, which can be poisonous. A commercially prepared syrup or tincture is best.
Wild oregano (Origanum vulgare)	Leaves, shoots, stems.	Phytochemicals: Alpha-pinene, apigenin, beta-carotene, borneol, caffeic acid, camphor, capric acid, carvacrol, caryophyllene, catechol, chlorogenic acid, cinnamic acid, eriodictyol, eugenol, geraniol, kaempferol, limonene, linalool, luteolin, myristic acid, naringenin, naringin, oleanolic acid, 1,8-cineole, p-coumaric acid, phytosterols, quercetin, rosmarinic acid, rutin, tannins, thymol, ursolic acid, vanillic acid, vitexin. Nutrients: Calcium, essential fatty acids, iron, magnesium, manganese, phosphorus, potassium, zinc, vitamins A, B_1, B_3, and C.	Fights free radicals, inflammation, and bacterial, viral, and fungal infection. Boosts the immune system. Useful for acne, allergies, animal bites, arthritis, asthma, athlete's foot, bee stings, bronchitis, chronic infections, cold, cough, diarrhea, digestive problems, earache, eczema, fatigue, gum disease, headache, menstrual irregularities, muscle pain, parasitic infections, psoriasis, sinusitis, skin infections, urinary tract disorders, and wounds.	Oregano sold in supermarkets is usually a combination of several oregano species, and does not have the medicinal benefits of _Origanum vulgare._
Wild yam (Dioscorea villosa)	Rhizomes, roots.	Phytochemicals: Beta-carotene, diosgenin. Nutrients: Calcium, chromium, iron, magnesium, manganese, phosphorus, potassium, selenium, zinc, vitamins B_1, B_2, B_3, and C.	Relaxes muscle spasms, reduces inflammation, and promotes perspiration. Contains compounds similar to the hormone progesterone. Good for colic, gallbladder disorders, hypoglycemia, irritable bowel syndrome, kidney stones, neuralgia, rheumatism, and female disorders, including premenstrual syndrome and menopause-related symptoms.	Many yam-based products are extracted from plants treated with fertilizers and pesticides, which may end up in the final products. The selection, cleansing, and processing of the raw materials is very important. _Caution:_ Should not be used during pregnancy.
Wintergreen (Gaultheria procumbens)	Leaves, roots, stems.	Phytochemicals: Caffeic acid, ferulic acid, gallic acid, p-coumaric acid, methyl salicylate, tannin, vanillic acid.	Relieves pain and reduces inflammation. Stimulates circulation. Good for arthritis, headache, toothache, muscle pain, and rheumatic complaints.	Oil distilled from the leaves is used in perfumes and as a flavoring. Contains a compound composed of 90 percent methyl salicylate, a substance similar to aspirin.
Witch hazel (Hamamelis virginiana)	Bark, leaves, twigs.	Phytochemials: Beta-ionone, gallic acid, isoquercitrin, kaempferol, leucodelphinidin, myrcetin, phenol, quercetin, quercetrin, saponins, tannins.	Applied topically, has astringent and healing properties, and relieves itching. Good for hemorrhoids, mouth and skin inflammation, and phlebitis. Very useful in skin care.	
Wood betony (Stachys officinalis)	Leaves.	Phytochemicals: Betaine, caffeic acid, chlorogenic acid, rosmarinic acid, stachydrine, tannin. Nutrients: Choline, magnesium, manganese, phosphorus.	Stimulates the heart and relaxes muscles. Improves digestion and appreciation of food. Good for cardiovascular disorders, hyperactivity, nerve pain, headaches, and anxiety attacks.	Also called betony. _Caution:_ Should not be used during pregnancy.

Herb (Scientific Name)	Parts Used	Phytochemical and Nutrient Content	Actions and Uses	Comments
Wormwood (Artemisia absinthium)	Leaves, tops.	Phytochemicals: Beta-carotene, chamazulene, chlorogenic acid, isoquercitrin, p-coumaric acid, rutin, salicylic acid, tannins, vanillic acid. Nutrients: Vitamin C.	Acts as a mild sedative, eliminates worms, increases stomach acidity, and lowers fever. Useful for loss of appetite and liver, gallbladder, gastric, and vascular disorders, including migraine. Applied topically, good for healing wounds, skin ulcers and blemishes, and insect bites.	Often used with black walnut for removal of parasites. *Caution:* Should not be used during pregnancy, as it can cause spontaneous abortion. Can be habit-forming with long-term use.
Yellow dock (Rumex crispus)	Roots.	Phytochemicals: Beta-carotene, hyperoside, quercetin, quercitrin, rutin, tannin. Nutrients: Calcium, iron, magnesium, manganese, phosphorus, potassium, selenium, zinc, vitamins B₁, B₂, B₃, and C.	Acts as a blood purifier and cleanser, and as a general tonic. Improves colon and liver function. Good for inflammation of the nasal passages and respiratory tract, anemia, liver disease, and skin disorders such as eczema, hives, psoriasis, and rashes. Combined with sarsaparilla, makes a tea for chronic skin disorders.	Also called curled dock. *Caution:* Yellow dock leaves should not be consumed in soups or salads. They are high in oxalates and may cause oxalic acid poisoning.
Yerba maté (Ilex paraguariensis)	Leaves.	Phytochemicals: Caffeine, chlorogenic acid, chlorophyll, rutin, tannin, theobromine, theophylline, ursolic acid, vanillin. Nutrients: Choline, inositol, nicotinic acid, pyridoxine, trace minerals, vitamins B₃, B₅, B₆, C, and E.	Fights free radicals, cleanses the blood, and suppresses appetite. Fights aging, stimulates the mind, stimulates the production of cortisone, and tones the nervous system. Enhances the healing powers of other herbs. Useful for allergies, constipation, and inflammatory bowel disorders.	Also called maté, Paraguay tea, South American holly. *Caution:* Should not be used by people who suffer from insomnia.
Yohimbe (Pausinystalia yohimbe)	Bark.	Phytochemicals: Ajmaline, corynantheine, corynanthine, tannin, yohimbine.	Increases libido and blood flow to erectile tissue. May increase testosterone levels.	Yohimbine, a key component of this herb, is sold as a prescription medication. *Caution:* May induce anxiety, panic attacks, and hallucinations in some individuals. May also cause elevated blood pressure and heart rate, headache, dizziness, and skin flushing. Should not be used by women or by anyone with high blood pressure; heart, kidney, or liver disease; or a psychological disorder. Should not be combined with foods rich in tyramine, such as cheese, red wine, and liver, as this may increase blood pressure to dangerous levels.
Yucca (Yucca baccata)	Roots.	Phytochemicals: Beta-carotene, sarsapogenin, tannin. Nutrients: Calcium, iron, magnesium, manganese, phosphorus, potassium, selenium, zinc, vitamins B₁, B₂, B₃, and C.	Purifies the blood. Beneficial in treating arthritis, osteoporosis, and inflammatory disorders.	Routinely prescribed for arthritis in some clinics. Can be cut up, added to water (1 cup of yucca in 2 cups of water), and used as a soap or shampoo substitute. Can be added to shampoo also.

MEDICINAL HERBS BY ACTIONS AND TARGETS IN THE BODY

Different medicinal herbs have different types of effects and tend to exert their activities on different body systems and organs. The following table classifies some of the best known herbs according to their actions and areas of prime activity.

Action(s)	Herbs
Antibacterial/antiviral	Aloe, anise, annatto, astragalus, black walnut, boneset, boswellia, burdock, catnip, cat's claw, cayenne, cedar, chanca piedra, chaparral, chickweed, echinacea, elder, ephedra, eucalyptus, garlic, goldenseal, jaborandi, jatoba, kudzu, lady's mantle, lemongrass, licorice, macela, meadowsweet, myrrh, olive leaf, pleurisy root, puncture vine, pau d'arco, red clover, rose, rosemary, sangre de grado, slippery elm, suma, tea tree, turmeric, uva ursi, valerian, white oak, wild oregano.
Anticancer/antitumor	Astragalus, birch, burdock, cat's claw, chaparral, chuchuhuasi, cranberry, dandelion, fennel, garlic, green tea, licorice, macela, milk thistle, parsley, pau d'arco, rosemary, suma, turmeric.
Antifungal	Acerola, alfalfa, aloe, black walnut, boswellia, burdock, cedar, cinnamon, jatoba, puncture vine, rosemary, sangre de grado, tea tree, wild oregano.
Anti-inflammatory	Alfalfa, aloe, annatto, ashwagandha, bilberry, birch, blessed thistle, boldo, boneset, boswellia, buchu, butcher's broom, calendula, catnip, cat's claw, chamomile, chanca piedra, chuchuhuasi, devil's claw, echinacea, elder, fenugreek, feverfew, flax, ginger, goldenseal, jaborandi, jatoba, juniper, lady's mantle, licorice, macela, meadowsweet, mullein, mustard, pleurisy root, puncture vine, pygeum, rosemary, sangre de grado, suma, turmeric, white willow, wild oregano, wild yam, wintergreen, witch hazel, yellow dock.
Antioxidant	Acerola, annatto, bilberry, burdock, cat's claw, celery, chaparral, elder, ginger, gingko, green tea, jatoba, milk thistle, olive leaf, rosemary, sangre de grado, turmeric, wild oregano, yerba maté.
Cleanser/detoxifer	Alfalfa, black walnut, blessed thistle, cascara sagrada, cat's claw, cedar, dandelion, elder, garlic, ginger, goldenseal, guarana, licorice, muira puama, oregon grape, pau d'arco, rosemary, yellow dock, yerba maté.

Body System/Organ	Herbs
Bones/joints	Alfalfa, black cohosh, boswellia, cat's claw, cayenne, celery, chuchuhuasi, dandelion, devil's claw, feverfew, flax, garlic, ginger, horsetail, jatoba, muira puama, nettle, olive leaf, pau d'arco, peppermint, primrose, red raspberry, St. John's wort, sarsaparilla, skullcap, suma, wild oregano, wild yam, wintergreen, yucca.
Brain/nervous system	Ashwagandha, astragalus, bayberry, bilberry, blessed thistle, blue cohosh, catnip, celery, chamomile, chaste tree, devil's claw, dong quai, ephedra, eyebright, fennel, fenugreek, feverfew, ginger, ginseng, goldenseal, gotu kola, guarana, hops, jaborandi, kava kava, kudzu, lavender, lemongrass, licorice, marshmallow, motherwort, muira puama, oat straw, passion flower, peppermint, plantain, rosemary, sage, St. John's wort, sarsaparilla, skullcap, squawvine, stone root, suma, thyme, valerian, vervain, white willow, wild cherry, wild oregano, wintergreen, wood betony, wormwood, yerba maté.
Circulatory/ cardiovascular system	Aloe, barberry, bayberry, bilberry, black cohosh, black walnut, blessed thistle, borage, boswellia, butcher's broom, cayenne, celery, chickweed, cinnamon, devil's claw, elder, garlic, gentian, ginger, gingko, ginseng, gotu kola, green tea, hawthorn, hops, horse chestnut, horsetail, hyssop, jaborandi, kudzu, licorice, motherwort, muira puama, olive leaf, parsley, passion flower, pau d'arco, peppermint, primrose, rosemary, skullcap, suma, uva ursi, valerian, white oak, wintergreen, wood betony.
Gastrointestinal/ digestive system	Acerola, alfalfa, aloe, anise, annatto, bilberry, black walnut, blessed thistle, boldo, boswellia, buchu, burdock, cascara sagrada, catnip, cayenne, chamomile, chanca piedra, chuchuhuasi, cinnamon, clove, dandelion, devil's claw, fennel, fenugreek, flax, garlic, gentian, ginger, ginseng, goldenseal, gotu kola, green tea, guarana, horsetail, horehound, jaborandi, juniper, kava kava, kudzu, lady's mantle, lemongrass, licorice, macela, marshmallow, meadowsweet, muira puama, mustard, olive leaf, oregon grape, papaya, parsley, pau d'arco, peppermint, plantain, puncture vine, red clover, red raspberry, rosemary, sage, slippery elm, stone root, suma, thyme, turmeric, uva ursi, valerian, vervain, white oak, wild cherry, wild oregano, wood betony, wormwood, yellow dock, yerba maté.
Hair/nails/teeth	Borage, burdock, clove, hops, horsetail, irish moss, lemongrass, muira puama, nettle, red raspberry, sage, tea tree, vervain, white willow, wintergreen.
Immune system	Ashwagandha, astragalus, bayberry, burdock, cat's claw, cedar, chuchuhuasi, devil's claw, echinacea, ephedra, eyebright, elder, garlic, ginseng, goldenseal, green tea, horehound, licorice, maca, macela, milk thistle, myrrh, pau d'arco, puncture vine, red clover, suma, white willow, wild oregano, yerba maté.

Body System/Organ	Herbs
Muscles	Blue cohosh, celery, chanca piedra, chuchuhuasi, eucalyptus, feverfew, ginger, hawthorn, horse chestnut, horsetail, kava kava, lady's mantle, licorice, macela, meadowsweet, puncture vine, skullcap, uva ursi, valerian, wild oregano, wild yam, wintergreen, wood betony.
Reproductive system	Menopause: Chaste tree, dandelion, devil's claw, kava kava, licorice, motherwort, puncture vine, sage, suma, wild yam.
	Menstruation: Black cohosh, blue cohosh, calendula, chamomile, chaste tree, chuchuhuasi, corn silk, crampbark, dong quai, false unicorn root, feverfew, licorice, maca, macela, motherwort, muira puama, primrose, red raspberry, rosemary, sarsaparilla, squawvine, valerian, white willow, wild oregano, wild yam.
	Prostate: buchu, goldenseal, gravel root, horsetail, hydrangea, juniper, licorice, milk thistle, parsley, pumpkin, pygeum, saw palmetto, uva ursi.
	Sexual function/hormones: alfalfa, ashwagandha, chaste tree, chuchuhuasi, damiana, dong quai, false unicorn root, gotu kola, muira puama, puncture vine, sarsaparilla, saw palmetto, yohimbe.
Respiratory tract	Anise, astragalus, boneset, boswellia, catnip, cayenne, chanca piedra, chuchuhuasi, chickweed, elder, ephedra, eucalyptus, fennel, fenugreek, feverfew, garlic, gingko, ginseng, goldenseal, green tea, horehound, horsetail, irish moss, jaborandi, jatoba, juniper, licorice, macela, muira puama, mullein, mustard, myrrh, nettle, parsley, plantain, pleurisy root, red clover, stone root, thyme, white oak, wild cherry, wild oregano, yellow dock.
Skin	Acerola, alfalfa, aloe, annatto, barberry, borage, boswellia, calendula, chaparral, chickweed, chuchuhuasi, comfrey, cranberry, elder, flax, green tea, horsetail, irish moss, lavender, lemongrass, marshmallow, milk thistle, myrrh, oat straw, olive leaf, oregon grape, primrose, red clover, red raspberry, sangre de grado, sarsaparilla, tea tree, white oak, wild oregano, witch hazel, wormwood, yellow dock.
Urinary tract	Annatto, bilberry, birch, buchu, butcher's broom, cayenne, cedar, celery, chanca piedra, corn silk, cranberry, dandelion, devil's claw, fennel, gingko, goldenseal, gotu kola, gravel root, guarana, hydrangea, jatoba, juniper, kava kava, marshmallow, milk thistle, mullein, nettle, parsley, plantain, puncture vine, pumpkin, rose, red clover, saw palmetto, slippery elm, stone root, uva ursi, wild oregano, wild yam.

PART TWO

THE DISORDERS

INTRODUCTION

Part One explored the nutritional and dietary needs of the body. In order to be well, the parts of the body must be fueled properly so that breakdown does not occur. With the growing number of stressors in the environment today, the body must obtain the proper nourishment in order to maintain a healthy immune system. If the immune system weakens, the body becomes susceptible to a number of harmful conditions.

Part Two offers an A-to-Z listing of disorders that can occur if the body is overcome by stress and suffering from insufficient nutritional intake due to poor eating habits. The descriptions of the conditions may help you identify whether you have a particular illness. If your symptoms match those given for a certain illness, confirm your suspicions by visiting your physician.

Your health care provider may recommend that certain diagnostic tests be performed to help in making a diagnosis. Some tests, such as amniocentesis or surgical biopsy, are invasive; others, such as urinalysis, are not. Many diagnostic tests—especially newer ones such as magnetic resonance imaging (MRI) and computerized tomography (CAT) scans—can be quite expensive. Always be sure you understand exactly what a test involves before agreeing to it—how it is done, what it will show, why it is necessary in your case, what the potential risks are, how much it will cost, and anything else you need to know to feel confident in making a choice. You should also inform your health care provider about all medications (including natural medicines) and supplements you take regularly; any known allergies to foods, medications, anesthetics, x-ray materials, and/or other substances; pregnancy, if applicable; and any other special concerns you may have.

Once a diagnosis has been confirmed, refer to the appropriate dietary guidelines, recommendations, and supplementation program in this book to help speed your recovery. Always be sure to learn as much as possible about the use of any supplement you take. (See Part One for more detailed supplement information.) Most of the suggestions in Part Two can be utilized either alone or in conjunction with other therapies. However, if you have any questions about the appropriateness of any suggested nutrients or other therapy, speak to your physician.

Finally, a word about brand names. From time to time, we recommend specific products by specific manufacturers. These recommendations may appear on their own or in parentheses following the generic term for the substance in question. This should not be taken to mean that these are the only such products available, or that they are the only ones that will work. There are many good supplements and other nutritional products available from many different manufacturers, and new products are being introduced to the market all the time. However, we occasionally choose to make specific recommendations for particular products because we have found them to be effective and of good quality.

Troubleshooting for Disorders

Some symptoms are indicative of a variety of illnesses. The following table lists some of the more common disorders that are associated with particular symptoms. It is not meant to serve as a substitute for professional diagnosis. Although you may experience one or more of the symptoms below, you may or may not have any of the illnesses cited.

Your body is simply sending a message that something may be wrong. Listening to your body can help stop a problem before it becomes serious. Moreover, the illnesses listed below are given in alphabetical order. Their inclusion here does not reflect your chances of having any of them. If you have any of these symptoms, consult with your health care provider.

Symptom	Possible Cause
Abdominal pain, cramping	Across the abdomen: bladder or kidney disorder; pelvic inflammatory disease; premenstrual syndrome; uterine prolapse. Around the navel: appendicitis; constipation; gas. Lower left side: colitis; Crohn's disease; diarrhea; diverticulitis; lactose intolerance; ovarian cyst; regional enteritis; uterine fibroids or polyps. Lower right side: acute appendicitis; colitis; Crohn's disease; uterine fibroids or polyps. Upper left side: food allergies; heartburn; hiatal hernia; irritable bowel syndrome; peptic ulcer. Upper right side of rib cage: liver or gallbladder problems. Any location: endometriosis; food poisoning; internal injury; indigestion; miscarriage; stress.
Anal bleeding, itching, pain, swelling	Abscess; allergies; anal fissure; bruising; cancer; candidiasis; Crohn's disease; cysts; diverticulitis; food poisoning; genital warts; hemorrhoids; infection; muscle spasms; pinworms; polyps; sexually transmitted diseases; tumor; ulcers; ulcerative colitis.
Back pain	Aortic aneurysm; arthritis; awkward sleeping/sitting position; cancer; disk disease; endometriosis; gallbladder disorders; heart attack; improper lifting; injury; kidney disease; lack of exercise; menstrual cramps; muscle spasms; obesity; osteoporosis; Paget's disease of bone; pelvic inflammatory disease; peptic ulcer; pneumonia; poor posture; pregnancy; scoliosis; spinal tumor; sprain; strained muscle and/or ligament; urinary tract infection; uterine fibroids.
Bad breath	Abscessed tooth; bulimia; constipation; diabetes; dry mouth; gum disease; indigestion; infection (especially sinus and lung infection); liver disease; lung disease; mouth ulcers; mouth-breathing; periodontal disease; poor oral hygiene; kidney failure; liver malfunction; disorders of the metabolism; sinusitis; tooth decay.
Bleeding, menstrual, heavy or irregular	Blood-clotting disorders; cancer; endometriosis; endocrine disorders; hormonal imbalance; menopause; miscarriage; obesity; overzealous dieting or exercise; urinary tract infection; use of improper oral contraceptives; thyroid disorder; uterine polyps or fibroids; vaginal infection; weight loss or gain.
Blinking, frequent	Anxiety; dry eyes; foreign body in the eye; injury; mimic spasm or tic (may occur in Tourette's syndrome); Parkinson's disease; stroke; use of contact lenses.
Bloating	Allergies; appendicitis; bowel or kidney obstruction; adrenal disorders; diverticulitis; edema; gallbladder disorders; heart failure; irritable bowel syndrome; kidney disease; lactose intolerance; menstruation; overeating; peptic ulcer; tumor.
Blood in sputum, vomit, urine, stools, or from vagina or penis	Blood clots and swelling of lung tissue; cancer; hemorrhoids; infection; peptic ulcer; polyps; prostatitis; prostate cancer; ruptured blood vessel; sexually transmitted disease; tumor.
Body aches	Arthritis; infection; influenza; lupus; Lyme disease; overexertion.
Body odor	Constipation; diabetes; excess toxins; gastrointestinal abnormalities; indigestion; infection; liver dysfunction; poor hygiene.
Breast lumps	Boils; cancer; cysts; fibrocystic disease; injury; infected milk duct; infected sweat gland or lymph node; premenstrual syndrome.
Breast tenderness	Blood clots in veins of breast; breastfeeding-related problems; cancer; estrogen therapy: excessive consumption of fat, salt, and/or caffeine; fibrocystic breast disease; hormonal imbalance; menopause; pregnancy; premenstrual syndrome; stress.
Breath, shortness of	Asthma; cardiovascular disease (especially in women); chronic bronchitis; cystic fibrosis; emphysema; obesity; panic attacks; pneumonia.

SYMPTOM	POSSIBLE CAUSE
Bruising, easy	AIDS; anemia; cancer; Cushing's syndrome; drug reaction; hemophilia; liver or kidney disorder; vitamin C or vitamin K deficiency; weakened immune system.
Chest pain	Angina; anxiety; bruised or broken rib; carditis (inflammation of the muscles of the heart); coronary artery disease; gas; heart attack; heartburn; hiatal hernia; hyperventilation; pleurisy; pneumonia; strained muscle; stress.
Chills	Acute infection; anemia; exposure to cold; fever; hypothermia; shock.
Cold sweats	AIDS; cancer; diabetes; food poisoning; influenza; menopause; mononucleosis; severe heart or circulatory disease; shock; tuberculosis.
Cough, persistent	Allergies; asthma; cancer; chronic bronchitis; emphysema; pneumonia; postnasal drip; tuberculosis.
Delirium	Alcohol abuse; appendicitis; diabetes; drug reaction; epilepsy; high fever; drug overdose; manic episode; stroke.
Disorientation	Alcohol abuse; Alzheimer's disease; anemia; acute anxiety (panic attack); drug reaction or overdose; hypoglycemia; poor circulation; schizophrenia; seizure; stroke; transient ischemic attack (TIA, temporary interference with blood flow to the brain).
Dizziness, lightheadedness	Acute anxiety (panic attack); allergies; anemia; brain tumor; inhaling chemical products; diabetes; drug reaction; heart disease; high blood pressure; hypoglycemia; infection; low blood pressure; Ménière's disease; motion sickness; stress; stroke or impending stroke; vertigo.
Double vision	Cataracts; concussion; excessive alcohol consumption; eye disorders; hyperthyroidism.
Drooling	Drug withdrawal; ill-fitting dentures; Parkinson's disease; pregnancy-related problems; salivary gland disorders; seizure; stroke.
Drowsiness	Acute kidney failure; allergies; caffeine withdrawal; drug reaction or overdose; encephalitis; narcolepsy; skull fracture; sleep disorders.
Dry mouth	Aging; breathing through the mouth; diabetes; dehydration; drug reactions; Sjögren's syndrome.
Ear discharge	Clogged eustachian tube; earwax buildup; immune system dysfunction; infection; middle-ear infection; ruptured eardrum; severe head injury; tumor.
Eye, bulging	Aneurysm; blood clot or hemorrhage; glaucoma; hyperthyroidism; infection.
Eyelid, drooping	Botulism; diabetes; head or eyelid injury; hypothyroidism; muscle weakness; stroke.
Fever, persistent	AIDS; autoimmune diseases; cancer (especially leukemia, kidney cancer, lymphoma); chronic bronchitis; chronic infection; diabetes; hepatitis; influenza; mononucleosis; rheumatic disorders.
Flushing	Alcohol consumption; anxiety; dehydration; diabetes; heart disease; high blood pressure; hyperthyroidism; menopause; pregnancy; rosacea; use of high doses of niacin or of cholesterol-lowering medications.
Gas, frequent burping	Allergies; candidiasis; digestive problems; gallbladder disorders; intestinal obstruction; intestinal parasites; irritable bowel syndrome; lactose intolerance; stomach acid deficiency; swallowing air.
Hands and/or feet, cold	Circulatory problems; exposure to cold; Raynaud's phenomenon; stress.
Headaches, persistent	Allergies; asthma; brain tumor; cluster headaches; drug reaction; eyestrain; glaucoma; high blood pressure; migrane; sinusitis; stress; vitamin deficiency.
Heartbeat, irregular or rapid	Anemia; anxiety; arteriosclerosis; asthma; caffeine, alcohol, or tobacco consumption; calcium, magnesium, and/or potassium deficiency; cancer; cardiovascular disease; drug reaction; fever; heart attack; high blood pressure; hormonal imbalance; low blood pressure; obesity; overeating; overzealous exercising.
Hot sweats, then chills	Acute infection; excessive alcohol or sugar consumption; fever; hypoglycemia; thyroid disorders; tuberculosis (mainly night sweats).
Incontinence	Advanced neurologic disease; Alzheimer's disease; atrophic vaginitis; bladder infection; diabetes; excessive liquid consumption; loss of muscle tone; multiple sclerosis; prostatitis; psychological problems; restricted mobility; spinal cord trauma; stroke; urinary tract infection.
Intercourse, painful	Endometriosis; inflammation or infection of the vulva; muscle spasms; unaccustomed position during sex; urinary tract infection; vaginal dryness.
Irritability, mood swings	Alcohol or drug abuse; Alzheimer's disease; anxiety; brain tumor; depression; diabetes; drug reactions; excessive sugar intake; food allergies; hormonal imbalance; hyperthyroidism; hypoglycemia; hypothyroidism; menopause; nutritional deficiencies; premenstrual syndrome; schizophrenia; stress; stroke; virtually any chronic or disabling illness.

SYMPTOM	POSSIBLE CAUSE
Joint pain, swelling	Arthritis; bone cancer; bone fracture; bone spur; bursitis; carpal tunnel syndrome; chronic overuse; cirrhosis of the liver; diabetes; edema; gout; hemophilia; hepatitis; hormonal imbalance; infection; injury; kidney disease; Lyme disease; lupus; neuritis; Paget's disease of bone; rheumatic fever; sprain; strained muscle and/or ligament; tendinitis.
Leg pain	Arteriosclerosis; bone fracture; cancer; fibromyalgia; injury; improper footwear; Lyme disease; obesity; osteomalacia; overuse; Paget's disease of bone; rickets; sciatica; tendinitis; thrombophlebitis; tumor or infection in intervertebral disk or spinal canal.
Lymph nodes, swollen	AIDS; any acute or chronic infection; cancer; lymphoma; metal toxicity.
Mouth sores	Allergies; cancer; canker sores; chickenpox; consumption of overly acidic foods or liquids; denture wearing; herpes; local trauma; measles; oral herpes; oral thrush; use of tobacco or aspirin.
Muscle control, loss of	Alcohol and/or drug abuse; extreme exhaustion; fibromyalgia; head injury; multiple sclerosis; muscular dystrophy; narcolepsy; overuse; Parkinson's disease; seizure; stroke.
Muscle cramps	Arthritis; calcium, magnesium, and/or potassium deficiency; dehydration; diabetes; hypothyroidism; injury; overuse; poor circulation.
Muscle pain, weakness	Anemia; arthritis; chronic fatigue syndrome; dehydration; diabetes; drug reaction; fever; fibromyalgia; infection; injury; lupus; multiple sclerosis; overuse.
Nausea	AIDS; alcohol consumption; allergies; anxiety; cancer; celiac disease; cirrhosis of the liver; copper toxicity; dehydration; drug withdrawal; endometriosis; extreme fatigue; food poisoning; gallbladder disorders; heart attack; hepatitis; hormonal imbalance; indigestion; influenza; kidney disease; kidney stones; Ménière's disease; migraine; morning sickness (pregnancy); motion sickness; pancreatitis; poisoning; sinusitis; stress; ulcerative colitis.
Neck pain, stiffness	Allergies; awkward sleeping position; disk disease; fibromyalgia; injury; meningitis; strained muscle and/or ligament; stress.
Night sweats	AIDS; anxiety; autoimmune disorders; bowel disease; cancer; cardiovascular disease; fever; hepatitis; menopause; sleep apnea; stress; tuberculosis; weakened immune system.
Numbness	Carpal tunnel syndrome; diabetes; hyperventilation; multiple sclerosis; pinched nerve; poor circulation; rheumatoid arthritis; stroke; transient ischemic attack.
Pulse, weak	Blood loss; dehydration; drug reaction; heart attack; low blood pressure; malnutrition; shock; trauma; vomiting.
Seizure	Alcoholism; Alzheimer's disease; drug abuse; drug reaction; encephalitis; epilepsy; head injury; high fever; meningitis; stroke; tumor.
Swallowing, difficult	Bulimia; cancer; dehydration; dry mouth; hiatal hernia; stress; tumor.
Sweating, excessive	Alcohol consumption; anxiety; cardiovascular disease; consumption of hot and/or spicy foods; cystic fibrosis; fever; food allergies; hormonal imbalance; hyperthyroidism; infection; kidney disease; liver disease; lymphoma; malaria; menopause; overexertion; pneumonia; stress.
Swelling of ankles, feet, legs, hands, abdomen	Arthritis; bursitis; cardiovascular disease; chronic overuse; cirrhosis of the liver; diabetes; drug reaction; edema; food allergies; gout; improper footwear; joint infection; kidney disease; lupus; lymphatic disorders; poor circulation; pregnancy; premenstrual syndrome; sprain; strained muscle and/or ligament; varicose veins.
Thirst, excessive	Dehydration; diabetes; diarrhea; drug reaction; fever; menopause-related problems; any viral or bacterial infection.
Tremors	Alcoholism; anxiety; caffeine consumption; drug reaction; hyperthyroidism; multiple sclerosis; muscle fatigue; Parkinson's disease; stroke; stress; tumor; withdrawal from drugs or alcohol.
Urination, frequent	Alcohol or caffeine consumption; bladder infection; cancer; Cushing's syndrome; diabetes; drug reaction; excessive liquid intake; kidney or bladder stones; pregnancy; prostatitis.
Vaginal discharge, itching	Allergies; cancer; chlamydia; genital herpes; pelvic inflammatory disease; polyps; sexually transmitted diseases; urinary tract infection; vaginitis; yeast infection.
Weight gain	Aging; congestive heart failure; depression; diabetes; drug reaction; edema; hormonal imbalance; hypothyroidism; kidney disease; lack of exercise; overeating; poor diet.
Weight loss	Aging; AIDS; Alzheimer's disease; anorexia nervosa; cancer; chronic infection; depression; diabetes; hepatitis; hyperthyroidism; malabsorption syndrome; mononucleosis; Parkinson's disease; stress; tuberculosis.
Wheezing	Allergies; asthma; bronchitis; cardiovascular disease; chronic bronchitis; croup; emphysema; lung cancer; pneumonia; tobacco; upper respiratory infection.

Abscess

When pus accumulates in a tissue, organ, or confined space in the body due to infection, an abscess forms. Abscesses may be located externally or internally, and may result from an injury or a lowered resistance to infection. An abscess can form in the brain, lungs, teeth, gums, underarms, abdominal wall, gastrointestinal tract, ears, tonsils, sinuses, bones, breasts, kidneys, prostate gland, rectum, scrotum, or almost any other body part. Infections are the most common human disorders and can be produced by bacteria, viruses, parasites, and fungi. A *boil* is an external (skin) abscess (*see* BOIL in Part Two).

The affected area may become swollen, inflamed, hot, red, and tender. The individual may also experience fatigue, loss of appetite, weight loss, and alternating bouts of fever and chills. In severe cases, bacteremia (blood infection) and/or rupture of the abscess can occur. The material inside an abscess consists of living and dead white blood cells, dead tissue, bacteria, and/or toxins—all of which need to be discarded from the body.

An abscess that appears suddenly (in a matter of a few hours or overnight) is said to be *acute*. If an abscess has been present for a period of days or weeks, it is termed chronic. Chronic abscesses are more resistant to treatment because the damage is more severe and/or widespread. Acute abscesses are less extensive and generally respond to treatment within a matter of days.

An abscess, if treated, should begin to heal in a few days. Usually there is complete healing in a week or two. An abscess that does not show any signs of healing within this time can be an indication of problems within the immune system. Complications, although rare, can include bleeding or recurrence of the abscess.

Acute dental abscesses can be characterized by inflamed, red, and tender gums. The affected tooth may be sensitive or loose, and a dull pain is often present. A periodontal abscess can cause an overall sick feeling accompanied by fever and swollen lymph glands. However, chronic dental abscesses often produce no symptoms and are harder to treat than acute abscesses, as they have been present longer and have had the chance to do more extensive damage.

Basically, an abscess is a sign that the body is trying to rid itself of impurities. The impurities may be half-starved cells, deficient in nutrients such as sulfur, or toxins that accumulate because of a failure of the normal eliminative processes. Such a situation often stems from poor diet and exposure to environmental pollutants, chemicals, and other harmful substances. Eating junk food not only clutters the system with foods lacking in nutrients, but prevents the cellular wastes from being eliminated efficiently by causing such problems as constipation and sluggish liver, spleen, and kidney function.

NUTRIENTS

SUPPLEMENT	SUGGESTED DOSAGE	COMMENTS
Very Important		
Zinc	80 mg daily, in divided doses. Do not exceed a total of 100 mg daily from all supplements.	Powerful immune system stimulant. Necessary for T lymphocyte function, which is needed to fight infection. Needed for all skin disorders.
Important		
Coenzyme A from Coenzyme-A Technologies	As directed on label.	Supports the immune system's detoxification of many dangerous substances.
Colloidal silver	Take orally or apply topically as directed on label.	Acts as a natural antibiotic and disinfectant. Destroys bacteria, viruses, fungi, and parasites.
Garlic (Kyolic)	2 capsules 3 times daily, with meals.	Acts as a natural antibiotic and stimulates the immune system and contains sulfur, needed for skin tissue repair.
Methylsulfonyl-methane (MSM)	As directed on label.	Naturally occurring organic sulfur compound.
Superoxide dismutase (SOD) or	As directed on label.	A potent antioxidant. Use a sublingual form for best absorption.
Cell Guard from Biotec Foods	As directed on label.	An antioxidant complex that contains SOD.
Vitamin A plus natural carotenoid complex (Betatene)	50,000 IU daily for 5 days, then 25,000 IU daily for 5 days, then reduce to 15,000 IU daily. If you are pregnant, do not exceed 10,000 IU daily. As directed on label.	Strengthens cell walls to protect against invasion by bacteria and promote tissue repair. Essential to the immune system. Use an emulsion form for easier assimilation and greater safety at high doses. Powerful antioxidants that promote healing.
Vitamin B complex	50 mg of each major B vitamin daily (amounts of individual vitamins in a complex will vary). Take with meals.	For repair and replacement of lost nutrients; aids in healing.
Vitamin C with bioflavonoids	5,000–20,000 mg daily, in divided doses. *See* ASCORBIC ACID FLUSH in Part Three.	Essential in immune function and tissue repair.
Vitamin E	400–600 IU daily. You can also open a capsule and apply it directly to the affected area.	Important in circulation and tissue oxygenation. Enhances the immune system and promotes healing. Use d-alpha-tocopherol form.
Helpful		
Bromelain	500 mg 3 times a day.	Reduces inflammation and swelling; speeds healing.
Multivitamin and mineral complex	As directed on label.	All nutrients are needed for healing.
Proteolytic enzymes or Inflazyme Forte from American Biologics or Intenzyme Forte from Biotics Research	As directed on label. Take between meals. As directed on label. As directed on label.	To aid in cleanup of the abscess. Powerful free radical scavengers.

HERBS

❏ The following herbs are beneficial for healing abscesses and cleansing the blood: burdock root, cayenne (capsicum), dandelion root, red clover, and yellow dock root.

❏ Chamomile tea is good for treating dental abscesses. Drink a cup three or four times daily. If your face is swollen from the infection, chamomile can be prepared as a poultice and applied to the outside of the cheek once or twice a day for five to ten minutes until the infection is gone.

❏ Consuming distilled water with fresh lemon juice, plus 3 cups of echinacea, goldenseal, and astragalus or suma tea every day is helpful. Goldenseal can also be made into a poultice and applied directly to the abscess. (*See* USING A POULTICE in Part Three.) Or apply alcohol-free goldenseal extract to sterile gauze and place the gauze over the abscess.

Caution: Do not use astragalus in the presence of a fever. Do not take echinacea if you have an autoimmune disorder. Do not take goldenseal on a daily basis for more than one week at a time, and do not use it during pregnancy. If you have a history of cardiovascular disease, diabetes, or glaucoma, use it only under a doctor's supervision.

❏ Echinacea tea or extract in warm water can be used as a mouthwash for dental abscesses. Be sure to prepare it warm and rinse your mouth with it every two hours.

Caution: Do not take echinacea if you have an autoimmune disorder.

❏ A poultice that combines lobelia and slippery elm bark is soothing and fights infection. (*See* USING A POULTICE in Part Three.)

❏ Milk thistle, taken in capsule form, is good for the liver and aids in cleansing the bloodstream.

❏ Tea tree oil, applied externally, is a potent natural antiseptic that kills infectious organisms without harming healthy cells. Mix 1 part tea tree oil with 4 parts water and apply the mixture with a cotton ball three times a day. This will destroy the bacteria, hasten healing, and prevent the infection from spreading.

RECOMMENDATIONS

❏ Eat fresh pineapple daily. Pineapple contains bromelain, an enzyme that fights inflammation and aids healing.

❏ Include garlic and onions in your diet. They are high in sulfur and can help to both cure and prevent abscesses.

❏ Add kelp to the diet for beneficial minerals.

❏ Perform a liquid fast using fresh juices for twenty-four to seventy-two hours. (*See* FASTING in Part Three.)

❏ For an external abscess, apply honey to the affected area. Honey destroys bacteria and viruses, apparently by drawing all the moisture out of them.

❏ To cleanse the affected area, apply chlorophyll liquid mixed with water several times a day.

❏ If you must take antibiotics, supplement your diet with the B vitamins and products containing "friendly" bacteria, such as acidophilus and yogurt.

❏ If pain, redness, swelling, bleeding, or discharge increases, call your doctor.

CONSIDERATIONS

❏ For very mild external abscesses, the application of heat from a warm-water soak, along with improved nutrition, can usually provide sufficient treatment. Most abscesses, however, require treatment with antibiotics or herbs. Taking acidophilus and B vitamins and increasing your intake of liquids can often aid in the healing process. In some cases, the abscess may have to be lanced (pierced), drained, deep-cleaned, and treated with antibiotics.

❏ To heal an abscess, you may have to get plenty of bed rest, drink plenty of fluids, and use warm-water packs, ice packs, hot baths, a heating pad, or a heat lamp to alleviate the pain.

❏ To aid healing, the blood must be cleansed and vitamin deficiencies that accompany skin eruptions must be corrected.

❏ Abscesses do not usually interfere with normal bathing or showering, but you should remove bandages first so the wound may be gently washed with surgical, antibacterial, or other mild, unscented soap. Afterward, apply a new bandage.

❏ If an abscess breaks open and drains without assistance, your doctor may still need to make sure the entire area is sufficiently clean to prevent recurrence. This minor surgery involves making an incision across and through the abscess so it can be opened enough to ensure that all pockets of pus are opened and thoroughly drained. Sterile gauze may be provided to absorb any additional fluids that may appear. This also allows healing to begin from the base up.

❏ If an abscess spreads to the blood, it may jeopardize the health of the rest of the system, and immediate treatment by a health care professional is necessary.

❏ Deep abscesses must be watched to ensure that they are not affecting or obstructing the function of deeper tissues and organs.

❏ Some abscesses may be prevented by good hygiene and careful cleansing of the skin to prevent a wound or injury from becoming infected.

❏ Appropriate treatment for a dental abscess depends on the type of abscess. Most often, the pus is drained from the infected area, antibiotics are prescribed, and deep-cleaning is necessary. In other cases, a tooth may have to be extracted or root-canal surgery performed. (*See* PERIODONTAL DISEASE in Part Two.)

❏ Good dental hygiene can help prevent dental abscesses. This includes regular brushing and flossing, as well as regular dental checkups.

Acid/Alkali Imbalance

Acidity and alkalinity are measured according to the pH (potential of hydrogen) scale. Water, with a pH of 7.0, is considered neutral—neither acid nor alkaline. Any substance with a pH below 7.0 is acid, while anything with a pH above 7.0 is alkaline.

The ideal pH range for the human body is between 6.0 and 6.8 (the human body is naturally mildly acidic). For the body, values below pH 6.3 are considered on the acidic side. Values above pH 6.8 are on the alkaline side.

ACID AND ALKALINE SELF-TEST

This test will determine whether your body fluids are either too acidic or too alkaline. Purchase litmus paper, and apply saliva and/or urine to the paper. The paper will change color to indicate if your system is overly acidic or alkaline. Red litmus paper turns blue in an alkaline medium and blue litmus paper turns red in an acid medium. Always perform the test either before eating or at least one hour after eating. If your test indicates that your body is too acidic, consult the recommendations under Acidosis, below. If your body is too alkaline, see Alkalosis on page 123.

ACIDOSIS

Acidosis is a condition in which body chemistry becomes imbalanced and overly acidic. Symptoms associated with acidosis include frequent sighing, insomnia, water retention, recessed eyes, arthritis, migraine headaches, abnormally low blood pressure, acid or strong perspiration, dry hard stools, foul-smelling stools accompanied by a burning sensation in the anus, alternating constipation and diarrhea, difficulty swallowing, halitosis, a burning sensation in the mouth and/or under the tongue, sensitivity of the teeth to vinegar and acidic fruits, and bumps on the tongue or the roof of the mouth.

There are two classifications of acidosis: respiratory and metabolic. *Respiratory acidosis* is caused by an interruption of the acid control of the body, resulting in an overabundance of acidic fluids or the depletion of alkali (base). Simply, it occurs if the lungs are unable to remove carbon dioxide. Respiratory acidosis can be a result of asthma, bronchitis, or obstruction of the airway. It can be either mild or severe.

Metabolic acidosis occurs when chemical changes in the body disturb the body's acid-base balance, creating an excessive amount of acid in the body fluids. Diabetes mellitus, kidney failure, the use of unusually large amounts of aspirin, and metabolic diseases are some of the conditions that can deplete the body's alkaline base. Other contributing factors can include liver and adrenal disorders, stomach ulcers, improper diet, malnutrition, obesity, ketosis, anger, stress, fear, anorexia, toxemia, fever, and the consumption of excessive amounts of niacin and vitamin C.

NUTRIENTS

SUPPLEMENT	SUGGESTED DOSAGE	COMMENTS
Very Important		
Tri-Salts from Ecological Formulas	As directed on label.	For acid-alkaline balance.
Helpful		
Buffer pH+ by Växa International, Inc.	As directed on label.	Helps to reduce the acidity in the body to normal.
Coenzyme A from Coenzyme-A Technologies	As directed on label.	Supports the immune system's detoxification of many dangerous substances.
Kelp	1,000–1,500 mg daily.	Reduces acid in the body. Aids in maintaining a proper balance of minerals.
Multi-Zyme from FoodScience of Vermont	As directed on label.	Contains HCl. Beneficial if you have too little stomach acid.
Oxy-Caps or Oxy-Max from Earth's Bounty	As directed on label. As directed on label.	Increases stamina and vitality. Nourishes the body's cells with added oxygen while reducing high acid content in the body. Has unique antiviral, antibacterial, and antifungal properties that help normalize friendly bacteria and keep the acid/alkali balance in check.
Phosphorus	As directed on label.	A mineral that helps in the conversion of food to energy.
Potassium	99 mg daily.	Increases metabolism. Aids in balancing the pH in the blood.
S-Adenosyl-methionine (SAMe)	As directed on label.	Helps reduce stress. Promotes a sense of well-being. *Caution:* Do not use if you have manic-depressive disorder or take prescription antidepressants.
Vitamin A	50,000 IU daily for 1 month, then reduce to 25,000 IU daily. If you are pregnant, do not exceed 10,000 IU daily.	Helps to protect mucous membranes.
Vitamin B complex	100 mg of each major B vitamin twice daily (amounts of individual vitamins in a complex will vary).	Needed for proper digestion.

Herbs

☐ Use elder bark, hops, and willow for acidosis.

☐ Externally, apply ginger compresses to the kidney area.

Recommendations

☐ Eat a diet of 50 percent raw foods. Raw foods not only maintain the correct acid/alkaline balance within the body, but they are also richer in nutrients that are easily assimilated into the body. Recommended foods include apples, avocados, bananas, bilberries, blackberries, grapefruit, grapes, lemons, pears, pineapples, strawberries, and all vegetables. Fresh fruits, especially citrus fruits and vegetables reduce acidosis. Start with small amounts of citrus fruits and gradually add larger amounts.

❏ Chew your food slowly, and do not overindulge. Make sure food is mixed well with saliva to form a liquid consistency before swallowing. Do not drink fluids during meals.

❏ Prepare cooked foods with care. Maintain clean working surfaces and wash vegetables and fruit. Keep meat and vegetables separate—you can contaminate vegetables with bacteria from raw meat. Do not overcook vegetables, as this makes them lose not only their flavor, but also their nutritional value. Eat processed foods in moderation only. They are low in nutrients and overexert the digestive system. Both cooked and processed foods tend to make the body more acid. Also avoid eating late at night, as this makes the body work more on digestion and less on restoration.

❏ Drink potato broth every day. (*See* THERAPEUTIC LIQUIDS in Part Three for the recipe.)

❏ Avoid animal protein (especially beef and pork), as they lead to acidity.

❏ Avoid beans, cereals, crackers, eggs, flour products, grains, oily foods, macaroni, and sugar. Plums, prunes, and cranberries do not oxidize and therefore remain acid to the body. Avoid these until the situation improves.

❏ Since excess vitamin C may lead to acidosis, reduce your intake of vitamin C for a few weeks. When taking vitamin C, use a non-acid-forming (buffered) variety.

❏ Heartburn and indigestion can be the result of food digesting poorly. If you suffer from heartburn, taking small swallows of a teaspoon or two of natural cider vinegar in a glass of water may be of some help. It may cause a burning sensation when you swallow it, but then, in approximately twenty minutes, you should feel relief. If the cider vinegar method works, this may indicate that you lack suffficient acid in your stomach and the cider vinegar compensated for this insufficiency. In this case, consider taking digestive enzyme supplements containing hydrochloric acid (HCl). Stomach acid is important for breaking down food, and also prevents germs from irritating the intestines.

❏ Practice deep breathing.

❏ Check your urine pH daily using pH paper. See the inset on page 124 for a list of acid-forming foods to avoid until your pH is corrected

Considerations

❏ Phosphorus and sulfur act as buffers to maintain pH. Sulfur can be taken in supplement form.

❏ Umeboshi plums contain many alkaline minerals that aid in treating acidosis. You can eat one plum every four hours (four plums per day) for three days, then reduce your intake to one per day.

ALKALOSIS

Alkalosis is the inverse of acidosis—it is a condition in which the body is too alkaline. Alkalosis is less common than acidosis and produces overexcitability of the nervous system. The peripheral nerves are affected first. The symptoms may be manifested as a highly nervous condition, including hyperventilation and even seizures. Other symptoms can include sore muscles, creaking joints, bursitis, drowsiness, protruding eyes, hypertension, hypothermia, seizures, edema, allergies, night cramps, asthma, chronic indigestion, night coughs, vomiting, too-rapid blood clotting and thick blood, menstrual problems, hard dry stools, prostatitis, and thickening of the skin, with burning, itching sensations. Alkalosis may cause calcium to build up in the body, as in bone or heel spurs.

Alkalosis is often the result of excessive intake of alkaline drugs such as sodium bicarbonate for the treatment of gastritis or peptic ulcers. It can also result from excessive vomiting, high cholesterol, endocrine imbalance, poor diet, diarrhea, and osteoarthritis.

NUTRIENTS

SUPPLEMENT	SUGGESTED DOSAGE	COMMENTS
Helpful		
Alfalfa		*See under* Herbs, below.
Betaine hydro-chloride (HCl)	As directed on label.	A digestive enzyme that releases acid in the digestive tract.
Coenzyme A from Coenzyme-A Technologies	As directed on label.	Supports the immune system's detoxification of many dangerous substances.
L-Cysteine	500 mg twice daily, on an empty stomach. Take with water or juice. Do not take with milk. Take with 50 mg vitamin B$_6$ and 100 mg vitamin C for better absorption.	Needed to produce glutathione, a major detoxifying chemical. Also aids in making the tissues more acid. *See* AMINO ACIDS in Part One.
Methylsulfonyl-methane (MSM)	As directed on label.	An acid-forming mineral that helps to correct pH balance.
Raw kidney glandular	500 mg daily.	Stimulates kidney function.
S-Adenosyl-methionine (SAMe)	As directed on label.	Good for the nervous system and chronic fatigue. *Caution:* Do not use if you have manic-depressive disorder or take prescription antidepressants.
Selenium	200 mcg daily. If you are pregnant, do not exceed 40 mcg daily.	Protects against free radicals produced in alkalosis.
Vitamin B complex	100 mg of each major B vitamin daily (amounts of individual vitamins in a complex will vary).	Essential for stable and normal pH.
plus extra vitamin B$_6$ (pyridoxine)	50 mg 3 times daily.	Needed for hydrochloric acid (HCl) production. Also relieves fluid retention.

Vitamin C with rose hips and citrus bioflavonoids	3,000–6,000 mg daily, in divided doses.	A potent antioxidant and free radical scavenger.
Vitamin D3	400 IU daily.	Necessary for the absorption and utilization of calcium and phosphorus by the intestinal tract.
Vitamin E	As directed on label.	A powerful antioxidant. Use d-alpha-tocopherol form.

Herbs

❑ Alfalfa is beneficial for the digestive tract. It is a good source of vitamin K and other nutrients. Use supplements plus natural sources, such as alfalfa sprouts.

Recommendations

❑ Adopt a diet that consists of 80 percent grains and includes beans, breads, brown rice, crackers, lentils, macaroni, nuts, soy sauce, and whole-grain cereals. The other 20 percent of the diet should include fresh fruits, vegetables, fish, chicken, eggs, and natural cheese.

❑ Do not use antacids or mineral supplements, except those mentioned above, for two weeks.

❑ Avoid sodium.

❑ Cut back on megadoses of vitamins and minerals for two weeks.

❑ Check your urine pH daily using litmus paper. See the self-testing section for a list of alkaline-forming foods to avoid until your pH is corrected.

Acid- and Alkaline-Forming Foods

A basic rule of thumb to follow to achieve and maintain pH balance is to eat 80 percent alkaline-forming foods and drinks and 20 percent acid-forming foods and drinks each day. If a pH test indicates that your body is too acidic, you should eat more alkaline-forming foods and omit acid-forming foods from your diet until another pH test shows you have returned to normal. Conversely, if your body is too alkaline, eat more acid-forming foods and omit alkaline-forming foods. Use the list below as a guide to which foods are acid-forming and which are alkaline-forming. Low-level acid-forming and low-level alkaline-forming foods are almost neutral.

Litmus paper may also be called nitrazine paper. It can be purchased at most local pharmacies. If your local pharmacy does not carry it or urine test strips for pH, check with a medical supply company (listed under *Medical Equipment, Supplies and Repair* in the yellow pages) or a hospital pharmacy. Or contact Trimedica or Växa International, Inc., listed under Manufacturer and Distributor Information in the Appendix. Trimedica also produces an Acid/Alkaline Placemat that charts the acidity and alkalinity of different foods.

Acid-Forming Foods
Alcohol
Asparagus
Beans
Brussels sprouts
Buckwheat
Catsup
Chickpeas
Cocoa
Coffee
Cornstarch
Cranberries
Eggs
Fish
Flour, flour-based products
Legumes
Lentils
Meat
Milk
Mustard
Noodles
Oatmeal
Olives
Organ meats

Pasta
Pepper
Plums
Poultry
Prunes
Sauerkraut
Shellfish
Soft drinks
Sugar, all foods with sugar added
Tea
Vinegar

Aspirin, tobacco, and most drugs are also acid forming.

Low-Level Acid-Forming Foods
Butter
Canned or glazed fruit
Cheeses
Dried coconut
Dried or sulfured fruit (most)

Grains (most)
Ice cream
Ice milk
Lamb's quarters
Nuts and seeds (most)
Parsley

Alkaline-Forming Foods
Avocados
Corn
Dates
Fresh coconut
Fresh fruits (most)
Fresh vegetables (most, especially kudzu, onions, potatoes, rutabagas)
Honey
Horseradish
Maple syrup
Molasses
Mushrooms
Onions
Raisins
Soy products

Sprouts
Umeboshi plums
Watercress

All vegetables, especially raw vegetables, balance the acidity and alkali levels in the blood. Although it might seem that citrus fruits would have an acidifying effect on the body, the citric acid they contain actually has an alkalinizing effect in the system.

Low-Level Alkaline-Forming Foods
Almonds
Blackstrap molasses
Brazil nuts
Chestnuts
Lima beans
Millet
Soured dairy products

Considerations

❑ Your breathing can affect the acid-alkali balance of your body. Prolonged hyperventilation may cause temporary alkalosis, resulting in anxiety and a feeling that one cannot get enough air, despite the fact that breathing itself is not actually restricted in any way. If this happens, breathe into a *paper* bag and rebreathe the air from the bag. This often helps to correct the chemical imbalance.

Acidosis

See under ACID/ALKALI IMBALANCE.

Acne

Acne is an inflammatory skin disorder characterized by pimples, blackheads, and whiteheads. To some degree, it affects about 80 percent of all Americans between the ages of twelve and forty-four. According to the American Academy of Dermatology, acne has become the most commonly treated skin abnormality. Perhaps modern lifestyles contribute to this change in statistics. For those that suffer from acne, it is not merely a cosmetic problem. The consequences include emotional stress that can have a strong impact on one's self-esteem.

Acne often arises at puberty, when the body dramatically increases its production of androgens (male sex hormones). These hormones stimulate the production of keratin (a type of protein) and sebum (an oily skin lubricant). If sebum is secreted faster than it can move through the pores, a blemish arises. The excess oil makes the pores sticky, allowing bacteria to become trapped inside. Blackheads form when sebum combines with skin pigments and plugs the pores. If scales below the surface of the skin become filled with sebum, whiteheads appear. In severe cases, whiteheads build up, spread under the skin, and rupture, which eventually spreads the inflammation. Although proper skin care is important in the treatment of acne, acne is not caused by uncleanliness, but is more likely to be a result of overactive oil glands.

Although more than 20 million teenagers suffer from this disorder, acne is not just affecting kids anymore—it is also affecting increasing numbers of adults. While teenage acne most commonly occurs on the face and/or upper body, adult acne is usually limited to the chin and jaw line, and involves fewer, but possibly more painful, blemishes. Many women suffer premenstrual acne flare-ups prompted by the release of progesterone after ovulation. Oral contraceptives high in progesterone can cause breakouts, too. The presence of candidiasis can also cause hormonal changes that encourage the liver to produce the wrong substances for healthy sebum. (*See* CANDIDIASIS in Part Two.)

Factors that can contribute to acne include heredity, oily skin, hormonal imbalance, monthly menstrual cycles, and candidiasis. Other possible contributing factors are allergies, stress, and the use of certain types of drugs, such as steroids, lithium, oral contraceptives, and some anti-epileptic drugs. Nutritional deficiencies and/or a diet high in saturated fats, hydrogenated fats, and animal products can also be involved. Exposure to industrial pollutants such as machine oils, coal tar derivatives, and chlorinated hydrocarbons are some environmental factors that can have an adverse effect on the condition. A body pH that is too acidic or too alkaline also fosters the nesting and breeding of acne-causing bacteria. (*See* ACID/ALKALI IMBALANCE in Part Two.)

The skin is the largest organ of the body. One of its functions is to eliminate a portion of the body's toxic waste products through sweating. If the body contains more toxins than the kidneys and liver can effectively discharge, the skin takes over. In fact, some doctors call the skin the "third kidney." As toxins escape through the skin, the skin's healthy integrity is disrupted. This is a key factor behind many skin disorders, including acne.

The skin also "breathes." If the pores become clogged, the microbes that are involved in causing acne flourish because they are protected against the bacteriostatic action of sunshine. Dirt, dust, oils, and grime from pollution clog the pores, but this can be eliminated by cleansing the skin properly, and with the proper products.

Unless otherwise specified, the dosages recommended here are for adults. For a child between the ages of twelve and seventeen, reduce the dose to three-quarters the recommended amount. For a child between six and twelve, use one-half the recommended dose.

NUTRIENTS

SUPPLEMENT	SUGGESTED DOSAGE	COMMENTS
Very Important		
Acidophilus (Probiata from Wakunaga)	As directed on label.	Replenishes essential bacterial to reduce outbreaks.
Chromium picolinate	As directed on label.	Aids in reducing infections of the skin.
Colloidal silver	As directed on label. Take orally and apply to the affected area with cotton.	Acts as a natural antibiotic.
Essential fatty acids (flaxseed oil and primrose oil are good sources)	As directed on label.	To supply essential gamma-linolenic acid. Needed to keep the skin smooth and soft, repair tissues, and dissolve fatty deposits that block pores. Also aids in healing.
Potassium	99 mg daily.	Deficiency has been associated with acne.

Vitamin A	25,000 IU daily until healed. Then reduce to 5,000 IU daily. If you are pregnant, do not exceed 10,000 IU daily.	To strengthen the protective epithelial (skin) tissue. Use emulsion form for easier assimilation.
with natural carotenoid complex (Betatene)	As directed on label.	Antioxidant and precursor of vitamin A.
Vitamin B complex	100 mg of each major B vitamin 3 times daily (amounts of individual vitamins in a complex will vary).	Important for healthy skin tone. The anti-stress vitamin. Deficiencies of B_6 (pyridoxine) have been associated with acne.
plus extra vitamin B_3 (niacinamide)	100 mg 3 times daily. Do not exceed this amount.	Improves blood flow to the surface of the skin. *Caution:* Do not substitute niacin for niacinamide. Do not take additional niacinamide if you have a liver disorder, gout, or high blood pressure.
Vitamin C with bioflavonoids	1,000–1,600 mg 3 times daily.	Promotes immune function and reduces inflammation. Needed for collagen repair of the skin tissue. Use a buffered type.
Vitamin D_3	400 IU daily.	Promotes healing and tissue repair.
Vitamin E	400 IU daily.	An antioxidant that enhances healing and tissue repair. Use d-alpha-tocopherol form.
Zinc	30–80 mg daily. Do not exceed a total of 100 mg daily from all supplements.	Aids in healing of tissue and helps to prevent scarring. A necessary element in the oil-producing glands of the skin.

Important

Garlic (Kyolic)	2 capsules 3 times daily, with meals.	Destroys bacteria and enhances immune function.

Helpful

Chlorophyll	As directed on label.	Aids in cleansing the blood, preventing infections. Also supplies needed nutrients.
Clear Skin Image from Coenzyme-A Technologies	As directed on label.	A nutrient formula that supports healthy skin by correcting imbalances to address deficiencies in fatty acid metabolism and balance production of adrenal and sex hormone production.
EFA Derma-Skin from Health From The Sun	As directed on label.	Helps to support healthy skin and dermatological function. Good for skin texture, moisture, and suppleness.
Herpanacine from Diamond-Herpanacine Associates	As directed on label.	Contains antioxidants, amino acids, and herbs that promote overall skin health.
Multienzyme complex with hydrochloric acid (HCl)	As directed on label. Take with meals.	To aid digestion. *Caution:* Do not use HCl if you have a history of ulcers.
L-Cysteine	500 mg daily, on an empty stomach. Take with water or juice. Do not take milk. Take with 50 mg vitamin B_6 and 100 mg vitamin C for better absorption.	Contains sulfur, needed for healthy skin. See AMINO ACIDS in Part One.
or		

Methylsulfonyl-methane (MSM) (MSM Capsules from Aerobic Life Industries)	As directed on label.	Makes cell walls permeable, allowing water and nutrients to freely flow into cells, and wastes and toxins to properly flow out.
Lecithin granules or capsules	1 tbsp 3 times daily, before meals. 1,200 mg 3 times daily, before meals.	Needed for better absorption of the essential fatty acids.
O_2 Spray from Earth's Bounty	As directed on label.	A skin cleanser with antibacterial and antifungal properties that aids in healing blemishes.
Oxy-Caps from Earth's Bounty	As directed on label.	Provides essential oxygen that allows cells to function at their optimum.
Proteolytic enzymes	As directed on label. Take with meals and between meals.	Free radical scavengers. Aid in breaking down undigested food particles in the colon.
Selenium	200 mcg daily. If you are pregnant, do not exceed 40 mcg daily.	Encourages tissue elasticity and is a powerful antioxidant.
Tretinoin (Retin-A)	As prescribed by physician.	Acts as a gradual chemical peel; speeds up sloughing off of top layers of skin, leaving new, smoother skin. Available by prescription only. Takes around 6 months to show results.

HERBS

❏ Burdock root, dandelion leaves, milk thistle, and red clover are good for acne. Burdock root and red clover are powerful blood cleansers. Milk thistle aids the liver in cleansing the blood. A good place to begin an acne program is herbal cleansing of the blood. Both burdock and dandelion can help cleanse the liver. A liver that is not performing at its best can worsen acne because it cannot break down and clear excess hormones from the body as it should. Burdock and dandelion also contain inulin, which can improve the quality of skin by removing bacteria.

❏ A poultice using chaparral, dandelion, and yellow dock root can be applied directly to the areas of skin with acne. (See USING A POULTICE in Part Three.)

Note: Chaparral is recommended for external use only.

❏ Chaste tree berry (*Vitex agnus-castus*) extract can aid in preventing premenstrual breakouts. Take it each morning as directed on the product label.

❏ Lavender, red clover, and strawberry leaves can be used as a steam sauna for the face. Lavender kills germs and stimulates new cell growth. Using a glass or enameled pot, simmer a total of 2 to 4 tablespoons of dried or fresh herbs in 2 quarts of water. When the pot is steaming, place it on top of a thick potholder on a table, and sit with your face at a comfortable distance over the steam for fifteen minutes. You can use a towel to trap the steam if you wish. After fifteen minutes, splash your face with cold water. Allow your skin to air dry or pat it dry with a towel. If desired, you may follow this treatment with the use of a clay mask: Blend together well 1 teaspoon of green clay powder (available in health food stores) and 1 teaspoon raw honey, and apply the mixture to your face, avoiding the eye area. Leave it on for fifteen minutes, then rinse with lukewarm water. Lavender essential oil is a good antibiotic and antiseptic that can be applied directly to individual blemishes.

Caution: If acne is extensive or badly inflamed, do not use steam treatments, as this may worsen the condition.

❑ Lavender essential oil is a good antibiotic and antiseptic that can be applied directly to individual blemishes.

❑ Tea tree oil is a natural antibiotic and antiseptic. Dab full-strength tea tree oil (sparingly) on blemishes three times a day, or add 1 dropperful of tea tree oil to $1/4$ cup warm water and pat it on the affected area with a clean cotton ball (be sure to use 100-percent cotton). Tea tree oil soap also works well. Discontinue it if a rash appears.

❑ Other beneficial herbs include alfalfa, cayenne (capsicum), echinacea, and yellow dock root.

Caution: Do not take echinacea if you have an autoimmune disorder.

RECOMMENDATIONS

❑ Eat a high-fiber diet. This is important for keeping the colon clean and ridding the body of toxins.

❑ Increase your intake of raw foods. The more natural raw foods consumed, the faster the skin will clear and heal. Especially include raw foods that contain oxalic acid, including almonds, beets, cashews, and Swiss chard. Exceptions are spinach and rhubarb; these contain oxalic acid, but should be consumed in small amounts only.

❑ Eat a lot of fruits. This is always good for the skin because of the nutritional value and water content of fruit. You can also use certain fruits as a tonic on the surface of the skin. Grapes, strawberries, and pineapple are rich in alpha-hydroxy acids (AHAs). These acids help to exfoliate the skin by removing the dead skin cells that can clog the oil glands.

❑ Eat more foods rich in zinc, including shellfish, soybeans, whole grains, sunflower seeds, and a small amount of raw nuts daily. Zinc is an antibacterial agent and a necessary element in the oil-producing glands of the skin. A diet low in zinc may promote flare-ups.

❑ Be sure your diet contains vitamins A, C, E, and essential fatty acids. Supplements of these vitamins can prove to be beneficial for acne sufferers. Although vitamin A is important in fighting acne, you must be sure not to take too much. Vitamin E can help regulate vitamin A levels and can also aid in scar prevention.

❑ Drink at least eight glasses of quality water per day.

❑ Avoid alcohol, butter, caffeine, cheese, chocolate, cocoa, cream, eggs, fat, fish, fried foods, hot and spicy foods, hydrogenated oils and shortenings, margarine, meat, poultry, wheat, soft drinks, and foods containing brominated vegetable oils.

❑ Try eliminating dairy products from your diet for one month. Acne may develop due to an allergic reaction to dairy products, and the fat content of the dairy products can worsen the condition. Modern dairy and other animal products often contain hormones and steroids that can upset the body's natural hormonal balance.

❑ If you are not allergic to dairy products, eat plenty of soured products, such as low-fat yogurt, to maintain healthy intestinal flora.

❑ Avoid all forms of sugar. Sugar impairs immune function. In addition, biopsies of individuals with acne have shown their tissues' glucose tolerance to be seriously flawed. One researcher calls this condition "skin diabetes." Sugar also promotes the growth of candida, which may be a contributing factor to acne (*see* CANDIDIASIS in Part Two).

❑ Eliminate all processed foods from the diet, and do not use iodized salt. Enzymes induce the nutrients in food to be used to construct muscle tissue, nerve cells, bone, skin, and glandule tissue. Because processed foods contain so few enzymes, they can result in damage to the skin and its collagen. Processed foods also contain high levels of iodine, which is known to worsen acne. For the same reason, avoid fish, kelp, and onions.

❑ Follow a fasting program. *See* FASTING in Part Three.

❑ Use cleansing enemas to removing toxic buildup in the system and promote faster healing. *See* ENEMAS in Part Three.

❑ Keep the affected area as free of oil as possible. Shampoo your hair frequently. Use an all-natural soap with sulfur that is designed for acne (available at health food stores). Wash your skin thoroughly but gently no more than twice daily; never rub hard. Overwashing, vigorous scrubbing, and repeated touching of the skin can make acne worse by overstimulating the sebaceous glands, causing them to produce excessive amounts of sebum.

❑ Avoid wearing makeup. If you feel you must use cosmetics, use only natural, water-based products. Do not use any oil-based formulas, and avoid any products containing harsh chemicals, dyes, or oils. Wash and dip makeup applicator brushes and sponges in alcohol after each use to avoid contamination.

❑ Use a mixture of organic apple cider vinegar and quality water to balance the skin's pH. Mix 1 part apple cider with 10 parts quality water, and apply the mixture on the affected area.

❑ Friction makes pimples more likely to rupture, so avoid wearing tight clothing like turtlenecks. Carefully adjust straps on sports equipment such as bicycle or football helmets. Even using the telephone can exacerbate inflammation if you hold the receiver against your cheek for long periods. Keep your hair away from your face to prevent excess oil and bacteria from being deposited on the skin.

❑ If you must shave an area of skin affected by acne, use a standard blade. Using an electric razor may lead to scarring. Always shave in the direction of hair growth.

❑ As much as possible, avoid stress. Stress can promote hormonal changes and cause flare-ups. Many dermatologists also recommend fifteen minutes of sunshine each day, regular exercise, and sufficient sleep for people with acne.

❑ Avoid the use of oral or topical steroids, which can aggravate acne.

❑ Do not squeeze the spots. To do so is to risk increasing the inflammation by causing breaks in the skin in which harmful bacteria can lodge. Do not touch the affected area unless your hands have been thoroughly cleaned.

CONSIDERATIONS

❑ Acne is a message that something may be wrong with your body chemistry, diet, and/or skin care routine. Proper diet, nutritional supplements, and finding the right skin care products may be all that is needed to correct the problem.

❑ For severe acne, the drug isotretinoin (Accutane) is the only reliable treatment. It disrupts plug formation, shrinks the sebaceous glands, and reduces the amount of sebum within the glands. Isotretinoin cures or greatly reduces acne in about 90 percent of the people who use it, but it can cause side effects like dry skin, nosebleeds, headaches, and joint and muscle pain. The most dangerous side effect of isotretinoin is that it can cause serious birth defects, such as fetal brain deformities, if taken during pregnancy. It can even cause birth defects if a woman becomes pregnant up to two months after it is discontinued. If a woman with acne is in her childbearing years, isotretinoin is not recommended unless she is using effective birth control. There have also been isolated cases of depression and other mental disorders among people using this drug, and a study published in the *Archives of Dermatology* found that it may cause a loss of bone density, raising questions regarding its effect on the risk of developing osteoporosis later in life.

❑ The weapon of choice against moderate cases of acne is topical tretinoin (Retin-A). It helps to keep the pores from becoming clogged by increasing the rate at which dead surface skin cells are shed. Like isotretinoin, tretinoin should not be used during pregnancy. Use it with caution, because it renders the skin extremely vulnerable to sun damage. In addition, the safety of long-term use of tretinoin has not been established. Some "sibling" forms of tretinoin are being studied in the hope that they may not be as drying to the skin.

❑ Research is being conducted on the development and use of androgen-blocking drugs to stop the oil glands from being turned on by hormonal functions.

❑ An antibiotic cream or an oral antibiotic, such as tetracycline, erythromycin, or clindamycin, is sometimes prescribed for acne. If these drugs are not effective, minocycline may be prescribed. Be aware that this drug can have such side effects as shortness of breath and joint pain. Antibiotics have been known to cause yeast infections (candidiasis) in some people, leading to worsened acne. If you must take antibiotics, it is wise to take some form of acidophilus because antibiotics kill "friendly" bacteria along with "unfriendly" bacteria.

❑ Benzoyl peroxide is the active ingredient in many over-the-counter acne products. It can be helpful, particularly in mild cases, but it is extremely drying and can cause allergic reactions. It should not be applied around the eyes or mouth.

❑ A study conducted by the Department of Dermatology of the Royal Prince Alfred Hospital in New South Wales, Australia, found that a 5-percent solution of tea tree oil was as effective as a 5-percent solution of benzoyl peroxide for most cases of acne, without the irritating side effects.

❑ Blackheads should be removed only with a specially designed instrument, a procedure best done by a professional. Picking, squeezing, or scratching the blemishes may cause scarring, according to dermatologists.

❑ Niacinamide is a major nutrient in the repair of any skin condition because it aids circulation. This increases the supply of fresh, healthy blood to the surface of the skin, which supplies the skin with blood and nutrients.

❑ Dimethylsulfoxide (DMSO), a byproduct of wood processing, can be applied to acne lesions to reduce inflammation and promote healing. If used regularly, it may also help minimize scarring from severe cystic acne.

Note: Only DMSO from a health food store should be used for therapeutic purposes. Commercial-grade DMSO such as that found in hardware stores is not suitable. The use of DMSO may result in a garlicky body odor. This is temporary and is not a cause for concern.

❑ An acne treatment program called Derma-Klear from Enzymatic Therapy may be helpful.

❑ In rare cases, acne may be a sign of a potentially serious hormonal disorder caused by tumors in the adrenal glands or ovaries. Other symptoms of such problems include irregular menstrual periods and excess facial hair. If such symptoms develop, consult your health care provider.

❑ *See also* OILY SKIN and ROSACEA, both in Part Two.

Acquired Immunodeficiency Syndrome

See AIDS.

Addison's Disease

See under ADRENAL DISORDERS.

Adrenal Disorders

The adrenal glands are a pair of triangular-shaped organs that rest on top of the kidneys. Each gland normally weighs about 5 grams (slightly less than $1/5$ ounce) and is composed of two parts. The cortex, or outer section, is responsible for the production of the hormones cortisone, cortisol, aldosterone, androstenedione, and dehydroepiandrosterone (DHEA). The medulla, or central section, secretes another hormone, adrenaline (also called epinephrine), and norepinephrine, which functions as both a hormone and a neurotransmitter.

Adrenaline, cortisol, DHEA, and norepinephrine are the body's four major stress hormones. The highest levels of these hormones are released in the morning and the lowest at night. Cortisol is also involved in the metabolism of carbohydrates and the regulation of blood sugar. Aldosterone helps to maintain electrolyte (salt) and water balance in the body. Androstenedione and DHEA are androgens, hormones that are similar to—and that can be converted into—testosterone. Adrenaline speeds up the rate of metabolism and produces other physiologic changes designed to help the body cope with danger. It is produced when the body is under stress. Under circumstances of extreme stress, large amounts of cortisol are released, which can lead to a host of health problems.

Reduced adrenal function may be indicated by the following: weakness, lethargy, dizziness, headaches, memory problems, food cravings, allergies, and blood sugar disorders. If the adrenal cortex is seriously underactive, a rare condition called *Addison's disease* may develop. Symptoms include fatigue, loss of appetite, dizziness or fainting, low blood pressure, nausea, diarrhea, depression, craving for salty foods, moodiness, a decrease in the amount of body hair, and an inability to cope with stress. The individual may also constantly complain about feeling cold. Discoloration and darkening of the skin is common in people with Addison's disease; discoloration of knees, elbows, scars, skin folds, and creases in the palms are more noticeable when these body parts are exposed to the sun. The mouth, the vagina, and freckles may appear darker. This disease is also characterized by the development of bands of pigment running the length of the nails and by darkening of the hair.

The most common type of this disorder is autoimmune Addison's disease. This comes about when the immune system mistakenly attacks the tissue of the adrenal glands, destroying them. It may be associated with other autoimmune diseases that affect other endocrine glands. The most common of these is hypothyroidism (an underactive thyroid). Addison's disease that coexists with hypothyroidism is known as *Schmidt's syndrome.* Less commonly, Addison's disease occurs together with insulin-dependent diabetes mellitus, another autoimmune disease, or insufficiencies of the parathyroid glands and/or gonads, or with pernicious anemia. Addison's disease is a chronic condition that requires lifelong treatment. Fortunately, people with Addison's disease can have a normal life expectancy if they stay on the proper medication as prescribed by an endocrinologist (a specialist in hormonal diseases).

Cushing's syndrome is a rare disorder caused by excessive production of cortisol or by excessive use of cortisol or similar glucocorticoid (steroid) hormones. Persons with Cushing's syndrome take on a characteristic appearance: They generally are heavy in the abdomen and buttocks but have very thin limbs, and they have rounded "moon" faces. Muscular weakness and wasting of muscles are also characteristic of this syndrome. Round, red marks mimicking acne may appear on the face, and the eyelids may appear swollen. An increased growth of body hair is common, and women may grow mustaches and beards. People with Cushing's syndrome generally are more susceptible to illness and have trouble healing properly. Thinning of the skin from Cushing's syndrome often leads to stretch marks and bruising. Other symptoms include fatigue, mood swings, depression, increased thirst and urination, and, in women, absence of menstrual periods. If untreated, Cushing's syndrome may cause extreme muscle weakness, poor skin healing, weakening of the bones that results in osteoporosis, and increased susceptibility to serious infections such as pneumonia and tuberculosis.

The functioning ability of the adrenal glands is most often impaired as a result of the extensive use of cortisone therapy for nonendocrine diseases, such as arthritis and asthma. The long-term use of cortisone drugs causes the adrenal gland to shrink in size, and can result in a "Cushinoid" appearance. Adrenocortical failure can also be caused by pituitary disease and tuberculosis. Poor nutritional habits, smoking, and alcohol and drug abuse can contribute to adrenal failure.

Unless otherwise specified, the dosages recommended in this section are for adults. For a child between the ages of twelve and seventeen, reduce the dose to three-quarters the recommended amount. For a child between six and twelve, use one-half the recommended dose, and for a child under the age of six, use one-quarter the recommended amount.

ADRENAL GLAND FUNCTION SELF-TEST

Normally, systolic blood pressure (the first number in the measurement of blood pressure—*120/80*) is approximately 10 points higher when you are standing than when you are lying down. If the adrenal glands are not functioning properly, however, this may not be the case.

Take and compare two blood pressure readings—one while lying down and one while standing. First, lie down and rest for five minutes. Then take your blood pressure. Stand up and immediately take your blood pressure again. If your blood pressure reading is lower after you stand up, suspect reduced adrenal gland function. The degree to which the blood pressure drops upon standing is often proportionate to the degree of hypoadrenalism.

NUTRIENTS

SUPPLEMENT	SUGGESTED DOSAGE	COMMENTS
Essential		
Vitamin B complex	100 mg of each major B vitamin twice daily (amounts of individual vitamins in a complex will vary).	All B vitamins are necessary for adrenal function.
plus extra pantothenic acid (vitamin B$_5$)	100 mg 3 times daily.	The adrenal glands do not function adequately without pantothenic acid.
Vitamin C with bioflavonoids	4,000–10,000 mg daily, in divided doses.	Vital for proper functioning of the adrenal glands.
Very Important		
Coenzyme A from Coenzyme-A Technologies	As directed on label.	Needed for proper functioning of the adrenal glands. Reduces stress.
L-Tyrosine	500 mg daily, on an empty stomach. Take with water or juice. Do not take with milk. Take with 50 mg vitamin B$_6$ and 100 mg vitamin C for better absorption.	Aids adrenal gland function and relieves excess stress put on the glands. *See* AMINO ACIDS in Part One. *Caution:* Do not take tyrosine if you are taking an MAO inhibitor drug.
Important		
Raw adrenal glandular and raw adrenal cortex glandular	As directed on label. As directed on label.	Protein derived from this adrenal gland substance helps to rebuild and repair the adrenal glands. *See* GLANDULAR THERAPY in Part Three.
Helpful		
Chlorophyll	As directed on label.	Cleanses the bloodstream.
Coenzyme Q$_{10}$	60 mg daily.	Carries oxygen to all glands.
Multivitamin and mineral complex with calcium and magnesium plus natural beta-carotene and copper and potassium and zinc	1,500 mg daily. 750 mg daily. 15,000 IU daily. 3 mg daily. 200 mg daily. 50 mg daily. Do not exceed a total of 100 mg daily from all supplements.	All nutrients are needed to support proper adrenal function. Use a high-potency formula. If you have diabetes, use a formula without beta-carotene. Needed to balance with sodium. Potassium is depleted with this disorder. Boosts immune function.
Raw liver extract	As directed on label.	Supplies natural B vitamins, iron, and enzymes.
Raw spleen glandular and raw pituitary glandulars	As directed on label.	Boosts immune function and aids healing process. (*See* GLANDULAR THERAPY in Part Three.)
S-adenosylmethio-nine (SAMe) (SAMe Rx-Mood from Nature's Plus or SAMe from Enzyme Process International)	As directed on label.	Helps reduce stress and depression. Gives a sense of well-being. *Caution:* Do not use if you have manic-depressive disorder or take prescription antidepressants.

HERBS

❏　The herb astragalus improves adrenal gland function and aids in stress reduction.
　Caution: Do not use this herb in the presence of a fever.

❏　China Gold from Aerobic Life Industries is a liquid herbal combination formula that helps to stimulate adrenal function and combat fatigue. It contains ten different varieties of ginseng plus twenty-six other valuable herbs.

❏　Using echinacea can increase white blood cell production and protect tissues from bacterial invasion.
　Caution: Do not take echinacea if you have an autoimmune disorder.

❏　Milk thistle extract aids liver function, which in turn helps adrenal function.

❏　Calming herbs such as kava kava, St. John's Wort, and valerian are good stress reducers.

❏　Siberian ginseng is an herb that helps the adrenal gland prepare the body for stressful situations.
　Caution: Do not use this herb if you have hypoglycemia, high blood pressure, or a heart disorder.

RECOMMENDATIONS

❏　Consume plenty of fresh fruits and vegetables—particularly green leafy ones. Brewer's yeast, brown rice, legumes, nuts, olive and safflower oils, seeds, wheat germ, and whole grains are healthy additions to the diet as well.

❏　Eat deep-water ocean fish, salmon, or tuna at least three times a week.

❏　Include in the diet garlic, onions, shiitake mushrooms, and pearl barley. These foods contain germanium, a powerful stimulant of the immune system.

❏　Avoid alcohol, caffeine, and tobacco as these substances are highly toxic to the adrenal and other glands.

❏　Stay away from fats, fried foods, ham, pork, highly processed foods, red meats, sodas, sugar, and white flour. These foods put unnecessary stress on the adrenal glands.

❏　Get regular, moderate exercise. This stimulates the adrenal glands and also helps relieve stress.

❏　As much as possible, avoid stress. Continuous and prolonged stress from a troubled marriage, job-related problems, illness, or feelings of low self-esteem or loneliness can be detrimental to the adrenal glands. Take positive action to relieve stressful situations. (*See* STRESS in Part Two.)

CONSIDERATIONS

❏　A person with Addison's disease must take medication

as prescribed and pay careful attention to diet. Nutritional supplements are recommended.

❑ Treatment of steroid excess involves management of high blood sugar with diet and medication, replacement of potassium, treatment of high blood pressure, early treatment of any infections, adequate calcium intake, and appropriate adjustments in steroid dosages at times of acute illness, surgery, or injury.

❑ Adrenocorticotropic hormone (ACTH), a hormone released by the pituitary gland when under stress, sets a sequence of biochemical events in motion resulting in the activation of substances that raise blood pressure. The presence of this hormone leads to sodium retention and potassium excretion. As a result of this mechanism, stress not only puts strain on the adrenal glands, but may also cause the body to retain water, which can lead to hypertension.

❑ Distress—that is, unresolved stress—is the most important factor in "adrenal burnout," with all its manifestations, including immune deficiency and degenerative diseases.

Age Spots

Age spots are flat brown spots that can appear anywhere on the body as it ages. They are also called liver spots. Most age spots appear on the face, neck, and hands. These brown spots in themselves are harmless, but they can be a sign of more serious underlying problems. They are the result of a buildup of wastes known as *lipofuscin accumulation*, a byproduct of free radical damage in skin cells (*see* Free Radicals *under* ANTIOXIDANTS in Part One). These spots are actually signs that the cells are full of the type of accumulated wastes that slowly destroy the body's cells, including brain and liver cells. In other words, they are a surface sign of free radical intoxication of the body that may affect many internal structures as well, including the heart muscle and the retina.

Factors leading to the formation of age spots include poor diet, lack of exercise, smoking, poor liver function, the ingestion of oxidized oils over a period of time, and, above all, *excessive sun exposure*. Exposure to the sun causes the development of free radicals that may damage the skin. Most people who have significant numbers of age spots live in sunny climates or have had excessive sun exposure. The formation of lipofuscin is associated with a deficiency of a number of important nutrients, including vitamin E, selenium, glutathione, chromium, and dimethylaminoethanol (DMAE). Consuming alcohol increases lipofuscin formation. One study found that animals fed alcohol over a period of eighteen months had twice the amount of lipofuscin on their brain cells as control animals in the control group.

NUTRIENTS

SUPPLEMENT	SUGGESTED DOSAGE	COMMENTS
Very Important		
ACES + Zn from Carlson Labs	As directed on label.	A combination of powerful antioxidants. Helps to protect against free radical damage.
Ageless Beauty from Biotec Foods	As directed on label.	A free radical destroyer.
Kyolic Super Formula 105 from Wakunaga	As directed on label.	Supplies an array of antioxidants that are potent cell protectors.
Vitamin B complex	100 mg of each major B vitamin 3 times daily. (amounts of individual vitamins in a complex will vary).	Needed by older adults for proper assimilation of all nutrients.
plus extra pantothenic acid (vitamin B$_5$)	50 mg 3 times daily.	Supports adrenal gland function.
Vitamin C with bioflavonoids	3,000–6,000 mg daily, in divided doses.	A powerful antioxidant and free radical scavenger necessary for tissue repair.
Important		
Kyo-Dophilus or Probiata from Wakunaga	As directed on label.	Aids in liver regeneration and digestion.
Vitamin E	600 IU daily.	A powerful antioxidant. Fights cellular aging by protecting cell membranes. Improves circulation and prolongs the life of red blood cells. Use d-alpha-tocopherol form.
Helpful		
Calcium and	1,500–2,000 mg daily.	Elderly people need these nutrients. Asporotate or chelate forms are best.
magnesium and	750–1,000 mg daily.	
vitamin D$_3$	400 IU daily.	
Coenzyme A from Coenzyme-A Technologies	As directed on label.	Supports the immune system's detoxification of many dangerous substances.
Grape seed extract	As directed on label.	A powerful antioxidant that helps prevent age spots.
Herpanacine from Diamond-Herpanacine Associates	As directed on label.	To provide antioxidants, amino acids, and herbs that promote overall skin health.
L-Carnitine	As directed on label. Take between meals.	Aids in breaking up fat in the bloodstream so it can be removed from the body.
Lecithin granules or capsules	1 tbsp 3 times daily, with meals. 1200 mg 3 times daily, with meals.	Needed for proper brain function and healthy cell membranes. Works well as an antioxidant when taken with vitamin E.
Superoxide dismutase (SOD) plus	As directed on label.	Powerful antioxidants. Good for reducing brown age spots.
selenium	As directed on label.	A powerful antioxidant.
Tretinoin (Retin-A)	As directed by physician.	Acts as a gradual chemical peel; speeds up sloughing off of top layers of skin. Also removes fine wrinkles. Available by prescription only. Takes around 6 months to show results.

HERBS

❑ Burdock, milk thistle, and red clover aid in cleansing the bloodstream.

❑ Ginkgo biloba improves circulation and is a potent antioxidant.

❑ Emu oil has shown good results on brown spots.

❑ Other herbs beneficial for age spots include ginseng, green tea, and licorice.

Caution: Ginseng and licorice can elevate blood pressure. Do not use them if you have high blood pressure.

RECOMMENDATIONS

❑ Eat a diet high in vegetable protein and that consists of 50 percent raw fruits and vegetables, plus fresh grains, cereals, seeds, and nuts. Be aware that seeds and nuts become rancid quickly when subjected to heat and/or exposed to the air. Purchase only raw nuts and seeds that have been vacuum sealed.

❑ Omit all animal protein from the diet for one month.

❑ Avoid caffeine, fried foods, saturated fats, red meat, processed foods, sugar, and tobacco.

❑ Follow a fasting program to cleanse the liver and rid the body of toxins. A properly functioning liver and a clean colon are important. Use black radish extract or dandelion root and beet juice along with three days of fasting a month with distilled water and fresh lemon, fruit, and vegetable juices. (*See* FASTING in Part Three.) Use cleansing enemas while fasting. (*See* ENEMAS in Part Three.)

❑ Limit sun exposure.

❑ Do not use cleansing creams, especially hydrogenated, hardened creams. Cleanse your skin with pure olive oil and a warm wet washcloth, then rinse with lemon juice and water.

❑ This has worked for some people: At night, saturate a cotton ball with pure lemon juice and put it over the spots (but do not apply it near the eyes). There may be some tingling, but only for a few minutes. If there is no sign of irritation, apply morning and night.

CONSIDERATIONS

❑ The prescription drug tretinoin (retinoic acid or Retin A) is being used for age spots with good results.

❑ Brown or yellow spots can usually be eliminated by freezing them off. During a painless in-office procedure, the doctor brushes liquid nitrogen on the spots with a cotton swab. In two seconds the cells freeze, and within five days, cells flake away, and permanent results occur. Alternatively, a doctor can burn the spots off with acid applied directly to the spots, or remove them using laser light. With this process, there is no lightening of the skin after removal is completed.

❑ *See* AGING in Part Two

Aging

Growing older is not an illness, but the passing years do make the body more vulnerable to disease. Our genes dictate that the body's cells stop dividing after they have divided between twenty and thirty times. New cells must be made to replace those that stop dividing, a process that slows with age. When there are no longer enough new cells to replace the ones that have died or suffered damage, the result is aging. Studies show that cells that stop dividing change form and release damaging proteins that harm bodily tissues, further contributing to the aging process. Many researchers still maintain that it is our chosen lifestyles that accelerate aging, rather than genetics or other factors.

The free radical theory of aging has been the subject of a great deal of research in recent years and has been gaining increasing acceptance. Free radicals are atoms or groups of atoms that are extremely unstable and highly reactive. If they are present in excessive amounts, they begin attacking the body on the cellular level. Free radicals attack the cells' protective membranes and genetic material (the nucleic acids DNA and RNA), causing cellular damage and malfunction. To make matters worse, the immune system may then attack the damaged cells as if they were foreign invaders.

Because they are so chemically reactive, free radicals exist for only one-millionth of a second each. This has made it difficult for researchers to study them directly. But there are millions of them, and even with their short life span, they do considerable damage to our cells. Denham Harman, M.D., Ph.D., of the University of Nebraska, is considered the founder of the free radical theory of aging. He postulated that many of the degenerative disorders we associate with aging, including cancer and hardening of the arteries, are not inevitable results of the passage of time, but rather are the result of the breakdown of nucleic acids, proteins, and cell structures caused by the presence of free radicals. He asserted that the phenomenon we refer to as aging is in fact nothing more than the ever-increasing accumulation of changes caused, or contributed to, by the presence of oxygen-based free radicals. Thus, though oxygen gives us life, it can also be our greatest enemy. (*See* ANTIOXIDANTS in Part One.)

A significant number of problems faced by people over the age of sixty may also be attributable to nutritional deficiencies. Many elderly people have malabsorption problems, in which the nutrients in food are not properly absorbed from the gastrointestinal tract. In addition, as we age, our bodies do not assimilate nutrients as well as they once did. At the same time, as the body ages, its systems slow down and become less efficient, so the correct nutrients are more important than ever for the support, repair, and regeneration of the cells.

There are many disorders associated with an inability to absorb nutrients successfully. One study of older people living in an urban area found that 90 percent of those examined had an inadequate intake of vitamins B_1 (thiamine) and B_6 (pyridoxine), and 30 to 40 percent demonstrated deficiencies of vitamin A, vitamin B_3 (niacin), vitamin B_{12}, vitamin C, calcium, and iron. Only 10 percent of the subjects consumed adequate amounts of protein. Many Americans in nursing homes and other confined environments are deprived of sunlight, making them deficient in Vitamin D. A diet that lacks essential nutrients over a long period of time leads to a greater risk of degenerative disease.

Vitamin B_{12} deficiency is a particular problem. A lack of vitamin B_{12} can lead to the development of neurologic symptoms ranging from tingling sensations, inability to coordinate muscular movements, weakened limbs, and lack of balance, to memory loss, mood changes, disorientation, and psychiatric disorders. Symptoms of vitamin B_{12} deficiency can easily be misinterpreted as signs of senility. Many older people become deficient in vitamin B_{12} because they do not produce adequate amounts of stomach acid for proper digestion. This creates a perfect environment for the overgrowth of certain bacteria that steal whatever vitamin B_{12} is extracted from protein in the digestive tract. Other people do not produce enough of a substance called *intrinsic factor*, without which vitamin B_{12} cannot travel from the stomach to the rest of the body, even if nothing else is standing in its way.

One can have vitality and a zest for living at any age. You should not assume that pain and illness are inevitable parts of aging. You can feel better at sixty than you did at thirty by making healthy changes in your diet and lifestyle. Adding the right supplements should give you the added power needed to boost immunity and prevent or cure most disorders—not to mention making you able to work or play longer than people much younger than you are. Looking youthful for your age is an added bonus. But remember: It takes years for these problems to develop, so it usually takes some time to resolve them as well. There are no silver bullets or magic potions, only the simple fact that if you give your body the correct fuel, it will perform for you and ward off illness.

Most of the supplements listed below can be found in complexes containing many nutrients. Be sure to check the amounts of different nutrients in your multinutrient supplements, and either exclude individual nutrients or adjust the dosages, as appropriate. For best absorption of nutrients, use as many sublingual, liquid, and powdered supplements as possible. It makes sense for older adults to use nutrients in drink form, but there are many good supplements in powder and liquid forms as well.

NUTRIENTS

SUPPLEMENT	SUGGESTED DOSAGE	COMMENTS
Essential		
Alpha-lipoic acid	As directed on label.	A powerful antioxidant. Aids proper blood sugar balance (diabetes) and liver function.
Coenzyme A from Coenzyme-A Technologies	As directed on label.	Supports the immune system's detoxification of many dangerous substances.
Coenzyme Q_{10}	100 mg daily.	Aids circulation, improves cellular oxygenation, and protects the heart.
Dimethylglycine (DMG) (Aangamik DMG from Food Science of Vermont)	As directed on label.	Improves cellular oxygenation. Use a sublingual form.
Glutathione	500 mg daily, on an empty stomach.	A potent free radical scavenger and mental booster that acts as a mood elevator. Also destroys ammonia, which interferes with brain function.
Inositol hexaphosphate (IP_6) from Enzymatic Therapy or Jarrow Formulas	As directed on label.	A powerful antioxidant that has many benefits (*see under* NATURAL FOOD SUPPLEMENTS in Part One).
L-Arginine and L-carnitine and L-lysine and L-methionine and L-ornithine and L-tyrosine plus N-acetylcysteine	500 mg each twice daily, on an empty stomach. Take with water or juice. Do not take with milk. Take with 50 mg vitamin B_6 and 100 mg vitamin C for better absorption. It is best to take a complex containing all the amino acids as well (but separately). 500 mg twice daily, on an empty stomach.	*See* AMINO ACIDS in Part One for the benefits of amino acids. Do not take single amino acids for longer than 2 months at a time. To avoid creating imbalances, alternate taking them for a month and then stopping for a month. Protects the heart and liver; decreases blood triglycerides; enhances the effectiveness of antioxidants; improves muscle strength and brain function. Attaches to heavy metals such as lead and mercury and removes them from the body. Also enhances brain function. Used by the body to produce glutathione, a powerful antioxidant and detoxifier.
Liquid Kyolic with B_1 and B_{12} from Wakunaga	As directed on label.	An excellent cell protector. *See under* ANTIOXIDANTS and NATURAL FOOD SUPPLEMENTS in Part One for its many benefits.
Multivitamin and mineral complex with vitamin A and natural beta-carotene and all the carotenoids and potassium and selenium and zinc	15,000 IU daily. 25,000 IU daily. 99–200 mg daily. 300 mcg daily. 50 mg daily. Do not exceed a total of 100 mg daily from all supplements.	All nutrients are needed. Use a high-potency formula with chelated trace minerals. Important antioxidants. Protect the lungs. Needed for growth and repair of body tissues. Promote smooth skin. Plays a role in cellular integrity and water balance. Prevents premature aging, boosts immunity, protects against cancer and heart disease. Needed for wound healing and healthy skin. Enhances immune function.

Omega-3 essential fatty acids (flaxseed oil, primrose oil, salmon oil, and Ultra Omega-3 Fish Oil from Health From The Sun are good sources)	As directed on label 3 times daily, with meals.	Plays an important role in cell formation. Essential for proper brain function. Protects the heart and helps keep plaque from adhering to the arteries.
Pycnogenol or grape seed extract	50 mg twice daily. As directed on label.	Possibly the most powerful free radical scavengers. They can pass the blood-brain barrier to protect brain cells.
Superoxide dismutase (SOD) or Cell Guard from Biotec Foods	As directed on label. As directed on label.	A potent antioxidant that destroys free radicals, which damage body cells and cause premature aging. Consider injections (under a doctor's supervision). An antioxidant complex containing SOD.
Taurine Plus from American Biologics	As directed on label.	A building block for all amino acids that improves white blood cell function. Use the sublingual form.
Vitamin B complex plus extra pantothenic acid (vitamin B) and choline and inositol and para-aminobenzoic acid (PABA)	50–100 mg of each major B vitamin 3 times daily, with meals (amounts of individual vitamins in a complex will vary). If you use sublingual forms, you need less. Follow label directions. 50 mg 3 times daily. 50 mg 3 times daily. 50 mg 3 times daily. 50 mg 3 times daily.	The B vitamins fight depression; aid in transforming proteins, fats, and carbohydrates into energy. Necessary for the formation of certain proteins and for the functioning of the nervous system. Essential for healthy red blood cells and the absorption of nutrients, including iron. Injections (under a doctor's supervision) are best. If injections are not available, use sublingual forms.
Vitamin B3 (niacinamide)	50–100 mg 3 times daily.	Important in proper functioning of the nervous system. A vasodilator that protects the heart and body cells. Caution: Do not substitute niacin for niacinamide. Niacin can be toxic in such high doses.
Vitamin C with bioflavonoids	4,000–10,000 mg daily, in divided doses.	A powerful antioxidant and immune system enhancer that reduces allergies, protects the brain and spinal cord, keeps white blood cells healthy, fights fatigue, and increases energy.
Vitamin E	Start with 200 IU daily and slowly increase to 800 IU daily. If you take blood-thinning medication, consult your physician before increasing the dose.	A potent antioxidant that fights cellular aging by protecting cell membranes. Also improves circulation and prolongs the life of red blood cells. Use d-alpha-tocopherol form.

Very Important

Boron	3–6 mg daily. Do not exceed this amount.	Aids calcium absorption and brain function.
Calcium and magnesium and	1,500–2,000 mg daily. 750 mg daily.	Necessary to prevent bone loss and for normal heart function. Use calcium chelate or calcium asporotate form. Needed to balance with calcium and for correct muscle and heart function.

vitamin D3 or Bone Defense from KAL	600–1,000 mg daily. As directed on label.	Enhances calcium absorption and bone formation. Contains calcium, magnesium, phosphorus, and other valuable bone-reinforcing nutrients.
Chromium picolinate	400–1,000 mcg daily.	Improves insulin efficiency, which maintains the health of the glands that control aging.
5-Hydroxy L-tryptophan (5-HTP) (Natural Balance is a good source)	As directed on label.	An important neurotransmitter.
Free-form essential amino acid complex (Amino Balance from Anabol Naturals)	As directed on label 3 times daily. Take with 50 mg vitamin B6 and 100 mg vitamin C for better absorption.	To supply needed protein. Elderly people often have difficulty assimilating dietary protein, and so are likely to have amino acid deficiencies.
Lecithin granules or capsules	1 tbsp 3 times daily, with meals. 1,200 mg 3 times daily, with meals.	Improves brain function and memory. Protects nervous system cells. A fat emulsifier.
Phosphatidyl serine	1,000 mg 3 times daily.	Improves brain function.
RNA and DNA	As directed on label.	Good for healthy cell reproduction. Use a sublingual form. Caution: Do not take this supplement if you have gout.

Helpful

Acidophilus (Probiata from Wakunaga)	As directed on label.	To improve liver function and aid in digestion by replacing bowel flora. Probiata is a nondairy formula requiring no refrigeration.
Dehydroepiandros-terone (DHEA) (7-Keto from Enzymatic Therapy)	As directed on label. Women should not take more than 15 mg daily except under medical supervision.	Studies show it slows the aging process. (See under NATURAL FOOD SUPPLEMENTS in Part One.)
Dimethylglycine (DMG)	As directed on label.	Boosts mental energy, enhances the immune system. (See under NATURAL FOOD SUPPLEMENTS in Part One.)
Glucosamine sulfate or N-Acetylglucosamine (N-A-G from Source Naturals) plus chondroitin	As directed on label. As directed on label. As directed on label.	Important for the formation of bones, skin, nails, connective tissues, and heart valves; also plays a role in the mucous secretions of the digestive, respiratory, and urinary tracts.
Lutein	As directed on label.	Protects the retinas from macular degeneration, the leading cause of blindness in older adults.
Melatonin or ChronoSet from Allergy Research Group	1.5–5 mg daily, taken 2 hours or less before bedtime. As directed on label.	Delays the aging process and improves sleep. Good for many disorders associated with aging. Contains melatonin.
Multienzyme complex with pancreatin and ox bile (D.A. #34 from Carlson Labs)	As directed on label, after meals.	To aid digestion. Most elderly people lack sufficient digestive enzymes. Caution: If you have a history of ulcers, do not use a formula containing HCl.

Raw thymus glandular	500 mg daily.	Enhances the immune system.
S-adenosylmethio-nine (SAMe)	As directed on label.	Aids in reducing stress and depression, giving a sense of well-being. *Caution:* Do not use if you have manic-depressive disorder or take prescription antidepressants.
Silica (BioSil from Jarrow Formulas or Body Essential silica from NatureWorks)	As directed on label.	Protects connective tissues and cells; keeps skin, bones, hair, nails, and other tissues youthful.
Zinc	50 mg daily. Do not exceed a total of 100 mg daily from all supplements.	Increases antibodies and protects the eyes against macular degeneration and vision loss. Very important for the prostate.
plus copper	3 mg daily.	Needed to balance with zinc.

HERBS

❑ Astragalus and echinacea help to boost the immune system.

Caution: Do not take echinacea if you have an autoimmune disorder.

❑ Bilberry and ginseng are good for giving extra energy, improving brain function, increasing circulation, and promoting better blood flow to supply oxygen to the cells. Bilberry also protects the eyes.

Caution: Do not use ginseng if you have high blood pressure.

❑ Burdock root and red clover cleanse the bloodstream. They can be used separately or in combination.

❑ Dandelion and milk thistle promote good liver function and bile flow.

❑ Garlic helps immune function and protects the heart.

❑ Ginkgo biloba has powerful antioxidant properties and increases the supply of oxygen to the brain cells, enhancing brain function.

❑ Green tea aids in cancer prevention and is a powerful antioxidant.

❑ Noni (*Morinda citrifolia*) is a plant that grows in Hawaii. Its fruit has many health benefits and has been used for thousands of years to ease pain and inflammation, relieve joint problems, promote cellular regeneration, boost the immune system, and improve digestion. Earth's Bounty NONI by Matrix Health Products is a good source of this herb.

❑ Horsetail, taken in tea or extract form, is an excellent source of silica, a form of the trace mineral silicon. Silicon is important for maintaining the strength of bones and connective tissue, and possibly the walls of blood vessels.

❑ Kava kava, St. John's wort, and valerian root are valuable as sleep aids and tranquilizers; St. John's wort is also a natural antidepressant.

❑ Licorice root is an effective anti-inflammatory and anti-allergenic agent that supports the organ systems.

Caution: Do not use this herb on a daily basis for more than seven days in a row. Avoid it completely if you have high blood pressure.

❑ Nettle is full of vital minerals and is good for hypoglycemia, allergies, arthritis, depression, prostate and urinary tract disorders, and a host of other problems.

❑ Saw palmetto aids in preventing cancer and, for men, in improving benign (noncancerous) prostate enlargement. It inhibits the production of dihydrotestosterone, a hormone that contributes to enlargement of the prostate.

❑ Wild yam contains natural steroids that have a rejuvenating effect. Steroids are what help exercise to melt off more weight and build muscle. This hormone is found in the human body as dehydroepiandrosterone (DHEA). Take larger amounts—2,400 mg daily, dropping to 1,600 mg daily—for two weeks, then stop for two weeks.

RECOMMENDATIONS

❑ Eat a balanced diet that includes raw vegetables, fruits, grains, seeds, nuts, and quality protein such as fish and soy foods. Consume less animal protein. Include in your diet broccoli, cabbage, cauliflower, fish, fruits, whole grains, nuts, oats, seeds, and soybeans. Avoid processed foods.

❑ Consume four or five small meals daily.

❑ A low-calorie diet is best for maintaining good health as you age. Eat only when you are hungry, and consume foods that are fresh and cooked in a fashion that maintains their nutritional content. A diet too high in carbohydrates may increase glucose levels (*See* DIABETES in Part Two).

❑ Decrease your overall food consumption, but increase your intake of raw foods.

❑ Consume steam-distilled water. Drink even when you don't feel thirsty—your body needs plenty of water. Dehydration has been identified as one of the most frequent causes of hospitalization among people over the age of sixty-five, according to a recent study published in the *American Journal of Public Health*. Common symptoms of dehydration include fatigue; headache; dry nasal passages; dry, cracked lips; and overall discomfort.

❑ Include in your diet garlic, onions, shiitake mushrooms, and pearl barley. These foods are good sources of germanium, potassium, and many other nutrients that lessen free radical damage and act as catalysts in the supply of oxygen to oxygen-poor tissue.

❑ An occasional glass of red wine is good for the heart, but limit your alcohol consumption otherwise.

❑ Cut back on salt.

❑ Avoid saturated fats.

❑ Avoid caffeine, red meat, white flour, white sugar, chemical food additives, drugs, pesticides, and tap water.

❑ Get regular exercise. Exercise is most important in

slowing the aging process because it increases the amount of oxygen available to body tissues, a key determinant of energy and stamina. Brisk walking and stretching exercises are good. Swimming is even better because it provides a low-impact exercise and exerts no pressure on the joints. For those with arthritic conditions, swimming is the ideal way to exercise. Exercise can ward off conditions such as arthritis, cardiovascular disease, diabetes, and osteoporosis, and because it releases endorphins into the body, exercise can also help overcome depression. Our brains need exercise as much as our bodies do. Bodily exercise increases the supply of oxygen to the brain. Studies have found that no matter how old you are—whether you are in your sixties, seventies, eighties, or even in your nineties—you can rebuild muscle. Science has found that brain cells do not die as we age if we keep our minds active. Hobbies, reading, and acquiring new skills exercise the brain and help prevent memory loss.

❏ Improve your blood's oxygenation and circulation with deep breathing exercises. Try holding your breath for thirty seconds every half hour. Inhale and hold for thirty seconds, then place your tongue on the roof of your mouth where your teeth meet your gums and release the air slowly. Repeat this exercise every day.

❏ Keep the colon clean. This is crucial for warding off degenerative diseases and slowing the aging process. Eat a high-fiber diet and use a cleansing enema once weekly. (See ENEMAS in Part Three.) Get extra fiber by eating plenty of fresh vegetables, whole grains, bran, and oats. Consider retention enemas, a potent way to assure that your body will assimilate and use needed nutrients.

❏ Learn how to relax. Keep active and be enthusiastic about life. By keeping up your appearance, exercising every day, and being involved in hobbies and other activities, you can keep your mind active. This is most important.

❏ Allow yourself sufficient sleep. Proper rest is important.

❏ Do not use harsh soaps on your skin. Use olive, avocado, or almond oil to cleanse the skin. Pat the oil on, then wash it off with warm water and a soft cloth. Use a facial loofah occasionally with the oil and warm water to remove dead skin. Use liquid creams and lotions (not solid creams) that contain nutrients and natural ingredients to keep your skin from becoming too dry. Do not use cold creams, cleansing creams, or solid moisturizing creams. These are hardened saturated fats that become rancid rapidly and then create free radicals, which can cause premature wrinkles. Free radicals can cause the brownish spots on the skin known as age spots. (See AGE SPOTS in Part Two.) Exposing the skin to the sun also promotes free radicals. To halt wrinkles, stay out of the sun and use all natural lotions or oils that contain nutrients and antioxidants.

❏ Don't smoke or overexpose yourself to harmful chemicals such as environmental pollutants.

CONSIDERATIONS

❏ Growing older is inevitable; however, we can try to slow the aging process and prolong our lives by taking measures to promote continuous cell division. If science could keep the cells from dying and doing bodily harm, the aging process could conceivably be suspended.

❏ Many older adults complain of sleep difficulties. One common cause is the consumption of sugar after dinner. Complex carbohydrates have a relaxing effect. A good nighttime snack is popcorn, or nut butter and crackers. Protein, on the other hand, promotes alertness, so it should be consumed earlier in the day.

❏ A burning sensation, mainly on the bottom of the feet, is not unusual among elderly people. A deficiency of the B vitamins, especially vitamin B_{12}, is often the cause. Since many older people have problems with absorption of the B vitamins, it is best to take supplements of these nutrients in a way that bypasses the digestive tract. Injections are best. Sublingual administration is also effective.

❏ The *American Journal of Clinical Nutrition* reported that up to 30 percent of people over the age of sixty-five are unable to absorb vitamin B_{12} and folic acid properly because they do not produce enough hydrochloric acid and/or they suffer from an overgrowth of bacteria in the intestinal tract. If injections are unavailable, use sublingual forms for best absorption.

❏ In laboratory experiments, the drug selegiline (Eldepryl [also known as Deprenyl]) has been shown to increase the life expectancy of adult rats by an astounding 210 percent. Researchers suggest that tiny doses of selegiline may rescue brain cells from death in the event of trauma or disease. Depending on the outcome of future research, selegiline may have a wide range of uses beyond the treatment of Parkinson's disease, the only condition for which it is now officially approved. There are other drugs currently under research as potential anti-aging treatments as well. These include substances known as N-tertiary-butyl-alpha-phenylnitrone (PBN), which appears to improve memory and block free radical damage; centrophenoxine, which blocks the accumulation of waste products and toxic substances in the cells; growth hormone-releasing hormone (GRH) and insulin, two hormones that stimulate the production of human growth hormone (See GROWTH HORMONE THERAPY in Part Three); isoprinosine, an immune booster and nerve growth factor that shows some promise against Alzheimer's disease; and thymosins, hormones from the thymus gland that boost immune function and play a role in the endocrine system.

❏ There are a number of substances available that have properties that make them "natural life extenders" such as the following:

• Coenzyme Q_{10} protects the heart, increases tissue oxygenation, and is vital for many bodily functions. The liver and heart muscle have the highest level of coenzyme Q_{10} of any tissue. Since the liver is the main detoxifying organ of the body, optimal liver function is vital for minimizing damage to all the body's tissues.

• Colostrum is referred to by its supporters as the ultimate anti-aging and immune supplement. It can help reduce the levels of hormones that promote aging and damage the immune system. Bovine colostrum is available in supplement form. Ask someone knowledgeable about the purity of individual brands.

• Dehydroepiandrosterone (DHEA) is an adrenal hormone that enhances immune function. It has been found to help prevent and treat many of the disorders associated with aging. 7-Keto DHEA is a form of DHEA that is not converted into estrogen or testosterone in the body. (*See* DHEA THERAPY in Part Three.)

Selected Prevention and Screening Recommendations for Adults

One of the keys to staying healthy as we age is to practice preventive health care. In addition to adhering to a healthy diet and lifestyle, with appropriate nutritional supplementation, doctors recommend undergoing certain routine screening procedures. The following is a summary of recommendations for some of the most important medical tests. If you are at risk of any particular illness due to heredity or personal history, you should probably undergo testing more frequently to ensure that all is well. Ask your physician what he or she recommends in your particular case.

Test	Why It's Done	Who Should Be Tested	How Often
Blood cholesterol	To look for signs of cardiovascular disease.	Men and women 40 and over.	Once every 5 years. If your tests show a high LDL (bad cholesterol) level, you may need more frequent testing. Ask your physician.
Blood pressure	To check heart function.	Men and women over 40.	Every visit to the physician, or at least once a year.
Breast self-exam and	To detect breast cancer.	Women 30 and over.	Once a month.
physician breast exam and		Women 30 and over.	Once a year.
mammogram		Women 40 and over (men too can get breast cancer, but it is so rare that routine screening is not done).	
Complete physical examination; may include	To assess overall health.	Men and women 20 and over.	From age 20 to 30, once every 5 years.
complete blood count (CBC) and/or	To check for anemia and leukemia.		From age 30 to 60, once every 2 years. Over age 60, once annually.
blood chemistry (Chem 7 [SMA7] or Chem 20 [SMA20])	To check for liver dysfunction, thyroid problems, kidney function, and diabetes.		
Pap smear/pelvic examination	To test for cervical cancer and other reproductive problems.	Women 18 and over, or younger if they become sexually active at an earlier age.	Once a year. After 3 consecutive negative tests, frequency may be decreased at physician's discretion.
PSA test and rectal examination	To look for signs of prostate cancer.	Men 40 and over.	Once a year.
Sigmoidoscopy	To detect colorectal cancer.	Men and women 40 and over.	Once every 3 to 5 years after initial exam.
Stool guaiac test	To test for blood in the stool.	Men and women over 40.	Once a year.

In addition, doctors recommend that all adults receive a tetanus vaccine booster every ten years.

- Dimethylaminoethanol (DMAE) is beneficial for memory and mental ability, acting to increase alertness and focus. It may also enhance mood and vision.

- Dimethylglycine (DMG) is a derivative of the amino acid glycine. It boosts immune function and improves tissue oxygenation.

- Glutathione is an amino acid compound that is a valuable antioxidant and detoxifier. Cellular glutathione levels tend to drop by 30 to 35 percent with age; increasing glutathione, particularly in the liver, lungs, kidneys, and bone marrow, may have an anti-aging effect. Glutathione can be taken in supplement form. Glutathione levels can also be increased by taking supplements of N-acetylcysteine, which is converted into glutathione in the body. (*See* AMINO ACIDS in Part One.)

- Human growth hormone (HGH or GH), also known as somatotropin, is the hormone that regulates growth. Administered to older adults, it rebuilds muscle mass and reduces the amount of fat tissue, reversing changes that occur with aging. It is available only under the supervision of a physician. (*See* GROWTH HORMONE THERAPY in Part Three.)

- Lipoic acid is critical in glycolysis and in the Kreb's cycle, two complex biochemical processes essential for the generation of cellular energy. The liver relies on these processes to meet its large energy demands. Lipoic acid is used extensively in Germany to enhance liver function and treat diabetes.

- Melatonin is a natural hormone that acts as an antioxidant. Early in life, the body produces an abundant supply, but as we age, production steadily declines. In one laboratory experiment, mice given melatonin lived almost one-third beyond normal life expectancy. Melatonin may also help prevent cancer, counteract insomnia, and boost immunity.

- Morel, reishi, shiitake, and maitake are mushrooms that were touted by the ancient Chinese as superior medicines that give eternal youth and longevity. They prevent high blood pressure and heart disease, lower cholesterol, prevent fatigue and viral infections, and much more. They are found in supplement form as well as fresh.

- Pantothenic acid (vitamin B_5) keeps hair healthy, with little graying, and prevents premature hair loss. It is also very important for normal adrenal and immune function.

- Para-aminobenzoic acid (PABA) is one of the B vitamins. It keeps skin healthy and delays wrinkles. In addition, the combination of PABA and dimethylaminoethanol (DMAE) has been found to enhance brain function, immunity, and cellular regeneration.

- Pregnenolone is a naturally occurring hormone that may improve brain function, enhancing mood, memory, and thinking ability. (*See under* NATURAL FOOD SUPPLEMENTS in Part One.)

- Pycnogenol is a powerful bioflavonoid and antioxidant.

- Superoxide dismutase (SOD) is an enzyme that is a powerful free radical scavenger that protects the cells.

As people age falls are all too common. Older adults are more likely to have weak muscles, poor vision, weaker legs, decreased sensation, or other medical conditions that make them more likely to fall easily, and with more troublesome consequences. They are also more likely than younger people to take prescription medications, some of which can slow reflexes, decrease perception, and/or impair mobility—in so doing, increasing the danger of injury through an accidental fall. Physical injury is only one potential consequence of a fall for older adults, especially those who are frail to begin with. Recovery is often prolonged even after relatively minor falls, and this can lead to complications such as bedsores, greater muscle weakness, and increased susceptibility to infection. Keeping physically active is important for maintaining strength and coordination, and is one of the best defenses against such accidental injuries. It is also important to discuss with your physician or pharmacist the possible side effects of any medications you are taking.

❑ Aging is not an illness, but it does increase one's chances of developing certain health problems. Constipation, depression, diarrhea, dizziness, heart palpitations, heartburn and indigestion, and weight gain are some of the more common complaints that accompany aging. Detailed information on the causes of and treatments for many problems that commonly affect older people may be found in the relevant sections of this book. *See* AGE SPOTS; ALZHEIMER'S DISEASE; APPETITE, POOR; ARTERIOSCLEROSIS/ATHEROSCLEROSIS; ARTHRITIS; BEDSORES; CANCER; CARDIOVASCULAR DISEASE; CIRCULATORY PROBLEMS; CONSTIPATION; DEPRESSION; DIABETES; EYE PROBLEMS; GLAUCOMA; HAIR LOSS; HEARING LOSS; HEART ATTACK; HIGH BLOOD PRESSURE; HIGH CHOLESTEROL; INDIGESTION; INSOMNIA; MEMORY PROBLEMS; MUSCLE CRAMPS; OBESITY; OSTEOPOROSIS; PROSTATITIS/ENLARGED PROSTATE; SENILITY; WEAKENED IMMUNE SYSTEM; and/or WRINKLES, all in Part Two.

❑ If you follow the suggestions in this section and do not feel a positive change in your energy level, *see* COLITIS; DIVERTICULITIS; and/or MALABSORPTION SYNDROME in Part Two.

AIDS (Acquired Immunodeficiency Syndrome)

AIDS is an immune system disorder in which the body's ability to defend itself is greatly diminished. When *human immunodeficiency virus* (HIV, the virus that causes AIDS) invades key white blood (immune) cells called T lymphocytes and multiplies, it causes a breakdown in the body's immune system, eventually leading to overwhelming infection and/or cancer—and, ultimately, to death. Most deaths among people with AIDS are not caused by AIDS itself, but by one of the many infections or cancers to which the syndrome makes the body vulnerable. Essentially, AIDS is experienced as a series of various illnesses made possible by the initial HIV infection. It is a monumental modern medical plague.

The origin of HIV is unknown. The earliest documented case of AIDS appeared in 1981; however, researchers acknowledge that there may have been unidentified cases in the 1970s. Some investigators have wondered if HIV might be a genetically engineered virus gone awry. Whatever its origin, HIV is a type of virus known as a retrovirus that is spread primarily through sexual or blood-to-blood contact, such as occurs with the sharing of needles by intravenous drug users. It can also be spread by blood transfusion (now rare) or the use of blood products such as clotting factors, if the blood used for these purposes is infected. Hemophiliacs, who require a specific coagulation factor from blood concentrates, have historically been especially vulnerable to HIV. In the United States, as well as in many other parts of the world, blood is routinely screened for the presence of HIV antibodies, the warning sign of HIV infection. It is possible HIV-infected blood may occasionally pass through the careful screening processes. HIV antibodies may not appear in the blood for as much as three to six months after a person is infected, so their presence in blood taken from a person who contracted the virus recently may not be detectable. Blood products are now subjected to heat to destroy the virus, although some AIDS advocates raise concerns that this process may not be 100-percent effective. Still, according to the American Association of Blood Banks, only 1 in 676,000 recipients currently become infected by HIV through blood transfusions.

It is possible for dentists and medical workers who come into close contact with the bodily fluids of infected persons to become infected under certain conditions. This is why paramedics, emergency medical technicians, dentists and dental hygienists, hospital and clinic employees, emergency room personnel, and law enforcement officers wear rubber gloves to prevent contact with blood products or saliva. The practice of wearing gloves also protects patients.

Babies of mothers with HIV can contract the virus during pregnancy or birth, or through breastfeeding, although this is not inevitable. In fact, statistics indicate that most such babies do not contract the virus themselves. A Surgeon General's report on HIV and AIDS estimated about 25 percent of these babies do become infected, either before or during birth. Scientists do not know what factors influence whether or not a child will become infected but are working diligently to find the answers. It is known that the use of drug therapy during pregnancy plus bottle-feeding after birth may dramatically decrease the likelihood of mother-to-baby transmission.

Many people who are infected with HIV are not even aware that they have it. While some people experience a

Risk Factors for AIDS

Since the beginning of the epidemic in the 1980s, a number of health conditions and lifestyle factors have been identified that increase an individual's risk of contracting HIV and developing AIDS. The more factors present, the greater the risk. They include the following:

- Overuse of certain drugs, especially antibiotics and steroids.
- High-risk sexual activity.
- Substance abuse, including the use of alcohol, cigarettes, cocaine, amyl nitrate, marijuana, and other recreational drugs, especially intravenous drug use.
- Preexisting herpes infection, hepatitis, and/or mononucleosis.
- Preexisting sexually transmitted disease, especially syphilis.
- A diet high in processed foods, refined sugars, and fat.
- Infection with yeast (Candida albicans) and/or parasites.

mild flulike illness within two to four weeks of exposure to the virus, it generally takes at least two to five years before any symptoms of HIV infection appear. The length of time between an initial HIV infection and a positive diagnosis of AIDS has been estimated to be between two and ten years or more. The virus does not lie dormant during this time, however. Instead, it immediately attacks the immune system. The virus quickly begins producing a billion copies of itself each day, which in turn forces the human immune system to produce the same number of antibodies as an attempted defense against the introducers. Year after year, the body struggles to beat the virus until finally, its overworked immune system simply wears out and AIDS results.

In many cases, the first symptoms of HIV and AIDS are nonspecific and variable. One of the most common is a tongue coated with white bumps. This is oral thrush, or candidiasis. Candidiasis indicates a compromised immune system. Intestinal parasites are another common problem. Other possible symptoms include:

- Prolonged, unexplained fatigue.
- Swollen glands (lymph nodes).
- Unexplained fever lasting more than ten days.
- Excessive sweating (especially at night).
- Mouth lesions, including thrush and painful, swollen gums.
- Sore throat.
- Cough.
- Shortness of breath.
- Changes in bowel habits, including constipation.

- Frequent diarrhea.
- Symptoms of a specific opportunistic infection.
- Tumor (Kaposi's sarcoma).
- Skin rashes or lesions of various types.
- Unintentional weight loss.
- General discomfort or uneasiness (malaise).
- Headache.

Additional symptoms that may be associated with HIV and/or AIDS include speech impairment, memory loss, joint swelling, joint pain, bone pain or tenderness, a lump or lumps in the groin, blurred vision, genital sores, muscle atrophy, decreasing intellectual function, joint stiffness, unusual or strange behavior, anxiety, stress, tension, pruritus (generalized itching), sensitivity to light, decreased vision or blindness, blind spots in the field of vision, and chest pain.

No one should assume he or she is infected with HIV just because he or she has one or more of the above symptoms. These symptoms can be related to many illnesses, so being tested for HIV is the only way to be sure. This can be done by a doctor or with a home HIV testing kit. Simple to perform, this test requires a very small blood sample, obtained by pricking a fingertip. The sample is mailed to a laboratory, which analyzes it and offers a diagnosis by telephone in a matter of days. Each test is identified by a code number (no personal information is attached to any sample), so the test and the results are completely confidential. To date, the FDA has approved only one home test kit, the Home Access Express HIV-1 Test System from Home Access Health Corporation (*see* Manufacturer and Distributor Information in the Appendix). Beware of fraudulent or unproven home HIV test kits. Doctors say if a kit claims to provide "instant" test results through a visual indicator such as a colored dot on a piece of paper after saliva has been applied, the outcome may be unreliable. If you believe you have used a questionable test kit, contact your doctor for another test or use the approved test kit.

Testing HIV-positive does *not* mean that one has AIDS. Rather, it means that one has been exposed to HIV, as demonstrated by the presence in the blood of antibodies to the virus. However, a confirmed positive HIV test result is often the earliest indication that the person may eventually develop AIDS. The medical criteria for a diagnosis of full-blown AIDS are quite specific, requiring the presence of one or more opportunistic infections or cancers known to be associated with HIV infection. According to the U.S. Centers for Disease Control and Prevention (CDC), these include:

- *Pneumoncystis carinii* pneumonia.
- Candidal esophagitis, esophagitis from herpes simplex or cytomegalo virus.
- Cryptosporidiosis of the intestine for more than four weeks.
- Primary lymphoma of the central nervous system.

- Kaposi's sarcoma.
- Herpes simplex ulcers, extensive in location, lasting for more than one month.
- Toxoplasmosis of the brain.

While this list is not all-inclusive, these are the more common AIDS-defining illnesses. *Pneumocystis carinii* pneumonia alone accounts for over 50 percent of initial AIDS-defining conditions.

Some authorities believe that, although strongly linked to HIV, AIDS must be considered a disease caused by many factors. It may be that HIV is necessary but not sufficient to cause the onset of AIDS; that is, the virus needs help in bringing about immune deficiency. For example, epidemiologists have observed that those infected with both HIV and another retrovirus, such as the less frequently seen but similarly transmitted human T cell lymphoma virus (HTLV), develop the disease far more quickly than those infected with HIV alone. Conversely, some people with signs of full-blown generalized immune deficiency, consistent with a diagnosis of AIDS, actually test *negative* for HIV antibodies.

To date, only 50 to 60 percent of individuals exposed to HIV, as documented by an antibody test, have actually developed AIDS. But some people carry the virus for many years and never develop *any* symptoms of immune deficiency. We believe a person who becomes infected with HIV is more likely to go on to develop AIDS if his or her immune system is severely suppressed by other factors at the time of exposure and later. The risk of developing AIDS is proportional to the degree of immune suppression and the amount and duration of exposure to HIV. If the immune system is functioning well, it may be possible to avoid developing AIDS, even if one is a member of a high-risk group. Studies have repeatedly shown that immune-compromised persons are at greatest risk of contracting AIDS.

HIV is highly adaptable and capable of changing its form. According to scientists at Oxford University in England, this may be the key to its survival. They say that through subtle mutations, or changes in its genetic structure, HIV evades and ultimately defuses the body's mechanisms for the elimination of infected cells. As a result, it continues to survive despite the immune system's aggressive attacks.

Meanwhile, studies conducted at the Pasteur Institute indicate that the virus may be more hardy and virulent than we have ever been told. Health authorities have long maintained that the AIDS virus cannot survive without a host, but the Pasteur Institute researchers demonstrated that HIV can survive outside the body, and that it can live for up to eleven days in untreated sewage. Apparently, HIV is not as fragile as has been thought. While there are varying points of view, we believe it is possible that the virus may live for many days outside the body, even in a dried, inactive state, and then become infectious again.

At this time, there is no cure for AIDS. In the United States alone, approximately 2 million people are infected with HIV. According to the U.S. Centers for Disease Control and Prevention, approximately 62 percent of Americans diagnosed with AIDS since 1981 have died. AIDS is now a leading cause of premature death among Americans. In this country, it tends to disproportionately affect members of minority communities, especially African-Americans and Hispanics, and men who have sex with other men. In 1999, AIDS was the leading cause of death among African-American males and the third leading cause of death among African-American females. Those who abuse drugs and those who engage in sexual intercourse (anal, oral, or vaginal) with persons whose sexual or drug history places them at risk of HIV, with persons whose sex or drug history is unknown, or who have had multiple partners, are likewise considered to be at risk for the disease. In all population groups, young males are more likely than others to have contracted HIV. AIDS education seems to have had some impact on the spread of the virus in the United States, but in recent years the number of new cases among young people has been rising again, even though they grew up in an atmosphere of widespread concern and awareness about AIDS. The highest percentage of AIDS infections in the United States occurs among the most sexually active age group, people between the ages of twenty-four and forty-four. Sadly, of the over 600,000 U.S. AIDS cases reported to date, approximately 8,400 were children under the age of thirteen. Among adolescents ages thirteen to nineteen, the number of cases is smaller—around 3,400. The statistic to note, unfortunately, is that, as of 1999, nearly 25,000 Americans aged twenty to twenty-four had been diagnosed with AIDS.

Worldwide, over 33 million people are carrying the HIV virus, and more than 15 million have died of complications of AIDS. In Africa and Southeast Asia, roughly 16,000 new infections occur each day. Alarmingly, *Time* magazine has reported that an estimated 20 million people living outside industrialized countries are infected with HIV, and most of these cases are due to a different strain of the virus than cases commonly studied in the United States and Europe.

Anyone with HIV or AIDS can make a major contribution to his or her survival and quality of life by getting into an early treatment program, especially a program in which immune enhancement is encouraged. People with HIV or AIDS need higher than normal amounts of all nutrients because malabsorption is a common problem. Those at risk of becoming infected with HIV or of developing AIDS can also be helped through the following program. For all nutritional supplements, we strongly recommend the use of sublingual and injectable forms, as well as rectal suppositories, if available, for improved absorption.

Many of the nutrients listed below can be found in combination formulas. A high-potency multivitamin and mineral supplement should be included as well. Be sure to check the amounts of different nutrients in the complex against those in the table below. Use sublingual, liquid, and powdered supplements for best absorption. (*See* MALABSORPTION SYNDROME in Part Two.)

Unless otherwise specified, the dosages recommended in this section are for adults. For a child between the ages of twelve and seventeen, reduce the dose to three-quarters the recommended amount. For a child between six and twelve, use one-half the recommended dose, and for a child under the age of six, use one-quarter the recommended amount.

NUTRIENTS

SUPPLEMENT	SUGGESTED DOSAGE	COMMENTS
Very Important		
Acetyl-L-carnitine	As directed on label.	An energy carrier, metabolic facilitator, and cell membrane protector. Also protects the heart.
AE Mulsion Forte from American Biologics	As directed on label. Reduce the dosage if you have liver disease.	To supply vitamins A and E, which destroy free radicals and enhance immune function. Avoid capsule forms of these vitamins.
Alpha-lipoic acid	As directed on label.	Appears to help slow the progression of HIV virus.
Bioperine 10 from Nature's Plus	As directed on label.	Aids in uptake of nutrients with meals and supplements.
Body Language Super Antioxidant from OxyFresh	As directed on label.	Protects the body from free radical damage, environmental stresses, and pollutants.
Bone Support from Synergy Plus	As directed on label.	Contains minerals needed for better absorption of calcium.
Bovine colostrum (New Life Colostrum from Symbiotics)	As directed on label.	Enhances immune function and controls AIDS-related diarrhea. New Life Colostrum is available in liquid form.
Coenzyme Q$_{10}$	100–200 mg daily.	Increases circulation and energy, and protects the heart. A powerful antioxidant and significant immune stimulant.
Colloidal silver	As directed on label.	A broad-spectrum antiseptic that subdues inflammation and promotes healing of skin lesions. Can also be used orally.
Dimethylglycine (DMG) (Aangamik DMG from FoodScience of Vermont)	As directed on label.	Good for breathing difficulties. Enhances oxygen transport, increases interferon production, and has antiviral and anticancer properties. Use a sublingual form.
Egg lecithin	20 g daily, in divided doses. Take on an empty stomach.	For cellular protection.
Free-form amino acid complex

plus extra | As directed on label. Take on an empty stomach with water or juice. Do not take with milk. Take with 50 mg vitamin B$_6$ and 100 mg vitamin C for better absorption. | Supplies protein for repair and rebuilding of body tissues. Use a formula containing all of the essential amino acids. |

Women and AIDS

The majority of people with HIV and/or AIDS in the United States are men, but the incidence of AIDS in women is rising nearly six times as fast as that in men. The AIDS epidemic disproportionately affects women who are members of racial and ethnic minorities. According to the U.S. Centers for Disease Control, 1 in 98 black women and 1 in 222 Hispanic women between the ages of twenty-seven and thirty-nine are infected, compared with only 1 in 1,667 white women. Being a member of a particular racial or ethnic group does not mean a woman is any more susceptible to AIDS, however. Instead, it reflects the fact that members of minority groups are more likely to live in places with a high incidence of HIV infection. In the early years of the epidemic, most women with AIDS contracted the disease through intravenous drug use, but sexual contact has now surpassed intravenous drug use as the leading means of AIDS transmission among women.

Most women remain undiagnosed as HIV-positive until after the onset of AIDS or until they give birth to a child with HIV who becomes ill. This delay in diagnosis can have grave consequences for survival, and has contributed to the continuing myth that women's expected survival time is shorter than that for men. Experts say that if women were diagnosed at the same point in the disease as men are, their average length of survival would be essentially the same. However, women *are* more easily infected by HIV than men are. Research conducted on couples with one HIV-infected partner continues to show the virus is more easily transmitted from males to females rather than the other way around. In addition, women have less control over "safer sex" practices, and it is more difficult for them to protect themselves.

Compounding the problems women with HIV face is the fact that the majority of them come from economically disadvantaged backgrounds, and their access to quality health care is often limited. In contrast, the gay men with HIV who were the primary ones affected in the early days of the epidemic were generally more affluent and lived in areas with better medical resources. This factor alone has helped to distort the figures kept by various advocacy groups and medical researchers. Moreover, until relatively recently, the list of opportunistic infections considered in diagnosing AIDS did not include diseases that are unique to women, such as chronic vaginal candidiasis (yeast infection). Thus, even a woman who was HIV-positive and had one or more opportunistic infections might not have qualified for an official diagnosis of AIDS.

Because recurrent vaginal candidiasis is the most common early indicator of HIV infection in women, the FDA mandated in 1992 that manufacturers of certain over-the-counter medications include a new warning label on their products. The warning states that frequent vaginal yeast infections, especially when persistent or recurrent, can be the result of a serious medical condition, such as HIV infection. The label advises women with these symptoms to consult their physicians.

Other infections and illnesses in women that should raise concern about possible HIV infection are pelvic inflammatory disease, cervical dysplasia (precancerous changes in the cervix), yeast infections of the mouth and throat, and any sexually transmitted disease, such as genital ulcers and warts, and herpesvirus infection.

L-arginine and L-ornithine plus L-cysteine and L-histidine and L-methionine	As directed on label, on an empty stomach. As directed on label, on an empty stomach. As directed on label, on an empty stomach. As directed on label, on an empty stomach. As directed on label, on an empty stomach.	Enhances the immune system and retards the growth of tumors. Necessary for the immune system. Protects against cancer. Destroys free radicals. Aids in healing. May help in the prevention of AIDS. An antioxidant and free radical scavenger.
Garlic (Kyolic from Wakunaga)	2 capsules 3 times daily, with meals. Or place 1 dropperful of Kyolic liquid in a 6- to 8-ounce glass of distilled water, add 5 drops of ConcenTrace mineral drops from Trace Mineral Research, and gradually sip the mixture. Do this 2 or 3 times daily.	A powerful immunostimulant that also aids in digestion, endurance, and strength. It is a natural antibiotic and is good for candida infections.
Glutathione	As directed on label, on an empty stomach.	Inhibits the formation of free radicals. Aids in red blood cell integrity and protects immune cells.
Hydrochloric acid (HCl)	As directed on label.	Replenishes stomach acid to aid digestion. *Caution:* Do not take this supplement if you have a history of ulcers.
Inflazyme Forte from American Biologics or Wobenzym N from Marlyn Nutraceuticals	4 tablets 3 times daily, with meals and between meals. 3–6 tablets 2 or 3 times daily, between meals and with meals.	Destroys free radicals and aids in proper breakdown and absorption of foods. Also good for inflammation.
Inositol hexaphos-phate (Cell Forté from Enzymatic Therapy or Cellular Forte with IP-6 from PhytoPharmica)	As directed on label. Take on an empty stomach.	Enhances natural killer cell (anticancer) activity.
Kyo-Dophilus or Probiata from Wakunaga	As directed on label.	To supply essential friendly bacteria for the intestinal tract and liver function. Fights candida infection, often associated with HIV. Probiata is a nondairy formula requiring no refrigeration.
Kyo-Green from Wakunaga	As directed on label.	Supplies nutrients and chlorophyll needed for repair. Important in immune response.

L-Lysine	As directed on label. Take on an empty stomach.	Aids in preventing mouth sores and herpes outbreaks. *Caution:* Do not take lysine for more than 6 months at a time.
Lycopene	As directed on label.	A strong cancer preventer.
Malic acid and magnesium	As directed on label.	Involved in energy production in many cells of the body, including muscle cells. Needed for sugar metabolism. Reduces pain.
Multimineral complex with copper and zinc	3 mg daily. 80 mg daily. Do not exceed a total of 100 mg daily from all supplements.	All nutrients are needed due to malabsorption. Use a high-potency, hypoallergenic powdered form. Use a formula without iron if fever is present.
Natural carotenoid complex (Betatene)	As directed on label.	Powerful antioxidant, free radical scavenger, potential cancer fighter, and immune enhancer. Also protects against heart disease.
Pycnogenol and/or grape seed extract or OPC-85 from Primary Source	As directed on label. As directed on label. As directed on label.	A unique bioflavonoid. A potent antioxidant and immune enhancer. One of the most potent antioxidants known. Protects the cells. A combination of grape seed and pine bark extracts.
Quercetin plus bromelain or Activated Quercetin from Source Naturals	As directed on label. As directed on label. Take on an empty stomach. As directed on label.	Aids in preventing allergic reactions and increases immunity. Increases absorption of quercetin and aids in reducing inflammation. Contains quercetin plus bromelain and vitamin C.
Raw thymus glandular plus multiglandular complex with raw spleen glandular	As directed on label. As directed on label.	Enhances T-cell production. (*See* GLANDULAR THERAPY in Part Three.) Glandulars from lamb source are best.
S-adenosylmethio-nine (SAMe)	As directed on label.	Good for depression and chronic fatigue. *Caution:* Do not use if you have manic-depressive disorder or take prescription antidepressants.
Selenium	400 mcg daily. If you are pregnant, do not exceed 40 mcg daily.	Free radical scavenger and powerful immune enhancer.
Shark cartilage (BeneFin)	As directed on label. Take on an empty stomach.	Inhibits tumor growth. Be sure to use 100-percent pure dried shark cartilage.
Superoxide dismutase (SOD)	As directed on label.	Free radical scavenger needed for cell protection.
Taurine Plus from American Biologics	As directed on label.	An important antioxidant and immune regulator necessary for white blood cell activation and neurological function. Use liquid sublingual form.

Vitamin B complex injections plus extra vitamin B6 (pyridoxine) and vitamin B12	As prescribed by physician. As prescribed by physician. As prescribed by physician.	Anti-stress vitamins, especially important for normal brain function. Injections (under a doctor's supervision) are most effective. If injections are not available, use sublingual forms such as Superior Source supplements from Continental Vitamin Company.
Vitamin C with bioflavonoids	10,000–20,000 mg daily, in divided doses. *See* ASCORBIC ACID FLUSH in Part Three.	Strengthens the immune system. Use buffered powdered ascorbic acid or Ester-C with minerals.
Vitamin D3	400 IU daily.	Necessary for proper immune function.
Vitamin E	600 IU daily. If you are taking blood-thinning medication, consult your physician before taking this supplement.	A powerful antioxidant that protects the joints from damage by free radicals. Use d-alpha-tocopherol form.

Helpful		
Acid-Ease from Prevail	As directed on label. Take with meals. Take between meals also if excess acid is a problem.	Contains pure plant enzymes that function in the breakdown and assimilation of foods.
Aerobic 07 from Aerobic Life Industries or Dioxychlor from American Biologics	9 drops in water 3 times daily. As directed on label 3 times daily.	For tissue oxygenation. Kills harmful bacteria and viruses.
Chromium picolinate	At least 600 mcg daily.	Helps to build and maintain muscle mass. Stabilizes blood sugar.
Maitake extract or reishi extract or shiitake extract	As directed on label. As directed on label. As directed on label.	Mushroom extracts that enhance the activity of T-helper cells in people with AIDS. Has been shown to kill HIV in the laboratory.
Nicotinamide adenine dinucleotide (NADH) (ENADA NADH from Kal or Menuco)	5 mg each morning on an empty stomach.	A naturally occurring coenzyme found in all living cells. Necessary for cellular development and energy production.
Shark liver oil	As directed on label.	Aids in the rebuilding and functioning of all cells, and has anticancer properties.
Ultimate Oil from Nature's Secret or Salmon oil with vitamin E from Carlson Labs	As directed on label. As directed on label.	Supplies essential fatty acids, a most important element of the diet.

HERBS

☐ Aloe vera contains carrisyn, which appears to inhibit the growth and spread of HIV. Take 2 cups twice daily. Use a pure, food-grade product. If diarrhea occurs, reduce the dosage.

☐ Astragalus boosts the immune system.
Caution: Do not use this herb if you have a fever.

❑ Black radish, dandelion root, and silymarin (milk this-tle extract) protect and aid in repairing the liver, and also cleanse the bloodstream. The liver is *the* organ of detoxifi-cation and must function optimally. Use these extracts as directed on the product labels.

❑ Burdock root, goldenseal, mullein, red clover, and suma are good for cleansing the blood and lymphatic systems, for viral and bacterial infections, and for boosting the immune system. Cayenne (capsicum) may also be helpful.

Caution: Do not take goldenseal on a daily basis for more than one week at a time, and do not use it during preg-nancy. If you have a history of cardiovascular disease, dia-betes, or glaucoma, use goldenseal only under a doctor's supervision.

❑ Cat's claw enhances immune function, and has been shown to be helpful for people with AIDS and AIDS-related cancers. Cat's Claw Defense Complex from Source Natu-rals is a combination of cat's claw and other herbs, plus an-tioxidants such as beta-carotene, N-acetylcysteine, vitamin C, and zinc.

Caution: Do not use cat's claw during pregnancy.

❑ The seeds and peels of the Chinese cucumber inhibit cancer. The root is currently being used in AIDS research.

❑ ClearLungs from RidgeCrest Herbals is a Chinese herbal formula that is good for all lung disorders.

❑ Ginkgo biloba extract is good for the brain cells and cir-culation.

❑ For mouth sores, place alcohol-free goldenseal extract on a piece of sterile gauze and apply the gauze between the lips and gums or to mouth sores before going to bed. Leave it on overnight. Sores and inflammation should heal in a few days with this treatment.

❑ Licorice and wild yam root are good for endocrine gland function.

Caution: Do not use licorice on a daily basis for more than seven days in a row. Avoid it completely if you have high blood pressure.

❑ Magnolia vine berries increase oxygen absorption and boost the immune system. They coordinate the activities of the internal organs and help control the balance of the body's physiological processes.

❑ Pau d'arco is a natural antibiotic and potentiates im-mune function. It is also a powerful antioxidant and is good for destroying candida in the colon.

❑ St. John's wort contains two substances, hypericin and pseudohypericin, that inhibit retroviral infections and could be useful in the treatment of AIDS.

❑ Siberian ginseng helps bronchial disorders and boosts energy.

Caution: Do not use this herb if you have hypoglycemia, high blood pressure, or a heart disorder.

❑ Echinacea is an immune stimulant, and should be *avoided.* In fact, it stimulates replication of T cells, which in turn enhances replication of the virus, according to Dr. Tieraona Low Dog, founder of the New Herb Center in Al-buquerque, New Mexico.

Caution: Do not take echinacea if you have an autoim-mune disorder.

RECOMMENDATIONS

❑ If you test positive for HIV, arrange for repeat testing as soon as you can to rule out the possibility of a false-positive result. If the initial result is confirmed, *immediately* begin taking measures to boost your immune system. *This is the single most important factor in disease prevention, and it is the best defense for the person with HIV.* Correct diet, appropriate supplements, exercise, stress reduction, a proper environ-ment, and a healthy mental outlook all play significant roles in keeping the immune system working adequately.

❑ Pay special attention to meeting your nutritional needs and requirements, and keep in mind that a higher than nor-mal intake of nutrients will probably be necessary.

❑ Increase your intake of fresh fruits and vegetables. Eat a diet consisting of 75 percent raw foods, organically grown if possible (avoid foods that have been treated with pesti-cides and other sprays), plus lentils, beans, seeds, nuts, and whole grains, including brown rice and millet, and also non-acid-forming fruit such as bananas, all berries, peaches, ap-ples, and melons. Raw foods are particularly important because cooking depletes foods of their vital enzymes.

❑ Eat plenty of cruciferous vegetables, such as broccoli, Brussels sprouts, cabbage, and cauliflower. Also consume yellow and deep-orange vegetables such as carrots, pump-kin, squash, and yams.

❑ Consume plenty of fresh live juices. Juicing is ex-tremely beneficial for supplying nutrients. (*See* JUICING in Part Three.) "Green drinks" made from leafy greens such as kale, spinach, and beet greens, and carrot and beet root juice, should be consumed on a daily basis, with garlic and onion added. Kyo-Green from Wakunaga is an excellent "green drink" product that contains chlorophyll, protein, vitamins, minerals, and enzymes. Take this drink three times a day.

❑ Cooking tomatoes rather than eating them raw has been shown to more than double the effectiveness of the ly-copene tomatoes contain. Lycopene, a phytochemical found in tomatoes, has been found to reduce the risk of prostate and lung cancer. The incidence of digestive can-cers, such as those of the mouth, esophagus, stomach, colon, intestines, and rectum, may also be lowered with correct dosages of lycopene. A study reported in the De-cember 1995 issue of the *Journal of the National Cancer Insti-tute* found a 45-percent lower risk of prostate cancer in men who regularly consumed ten or more servings of tomatoes or tomato-based foods per week than in those who did not.

❑ Drink steam-distilled water only (not tap water), and lots of it—eight or more 8-ounce glasses daily—to flush out toxins from the body. All cells and organ systems need water. Drink plenty of water even if you are not thirsty. The organs, and especially the brain, become dehydrated long before thirst develops.

❏ Eat unripened papaya (including a few of the seeds), fresh pineapple, and *Aspergillus oryzae* (a type of fungus) frequently. These foods are good sources of proteolytic enzymes, which are crucial for proper digestion of foods and assimilation of nutrients. Without enzymes, the body cannot be supplied with the energy it needs for its activities. Enzymes can also be taken in supplement form. These help in digestion in the lower stomach and intestinal tract.

❏ Eat onions and garlic, or take garlic in supplement form (*see under* Nutrients, above).

❏ Add shiitake, reishi, and maitake mushrooms to the diet, or take them in supplement form (*See under* Nutrients, above).

❏ Limit your intake of soybeans and soy products, which contain enzyme inhibitors. Do not completely eliminate them from your diet, however, as they are valuable sources of protein.

❏ Eliminate from your diet colas, foods with additives and colorings, junk foods, peanuts, processed refined foods, saturated fats, salt, sugar and sugar products, white flour, *all* animal protein, and anything containing caffeine.

❏ Take supplemental fiber daily. Alternate between psyllium husks and freshly ground flaxseeds. Take psyllium with a glass of water and drink it quickly before it thickens.

Note: Always take supplemental fiber separately from other supplements and medications.

❏ Exercise caution in your choice of foods so as to avoid exposure to foodborne illness. Food poisoning can be very dangerous for people with HIV or AIDS infection. (*See* FOODBORNE/WATERBORNE DISEASE in Part Two.)

❏ Do not smoke, and stay away from those who do.

❏ Avoid alcohol, noxious chemicals, and anything else that can damage the liver.

❏ Try using bee propolis and royal jelly to fight bacterial infections invading the lungs, mouth, throat, and mucous membranes.

❏ Obtain as much fresh air and rest as possible, and moderate amounts of sunshine.

❏ Use coffee or fresh wheatgrass retention enemas to eliminate toxins and supply nutrients. (*See* ENEMAS in Part Three.)

❏ Determine what food sensitivities or allergies may be present. The best way to do this is to have yourself tested by a health care professional. It is important to eliminate allergenic foods from the diet because they wreak havoc in the body, causing damage to the immune system (*see* ALLERGIES in Part Two).

❏ Always use a condom (latex, not sheepskin) and spermicide (spermicide kills HIV) for any sexual contact. If you use a lubricant with a latex condom, use only a water-based lubricant such as K-Y jelly. Do not use petroleum jelly (Vaseline), vegetable shortening (Crisco), hand lotion, or baby oil, as these substances can break down latex in a matter of minutes. Be aware, however, that even the proper use of a condom is not a guarantee against the transmission of HIV.

❏ Seek out the care of a qualified health care provider—if possible, one who has a great deal of experience, in treating people with HIV. Research shows the length of survival of a person with AIDS is closely linked to how much his or her physician knows about treating the condition. The median length of survival after diagnosis is twenty-six months for those whose doctors have the most experience with AIDS, compared with fourteen months for those whose doctors have the least experience with AIDS.

❏ Educate yourself. HIV and AIDS are complicated conditions, and treatment options are constantly changing and expanding. In order to stay well, it is vital to be as informed as possible.

CONSIDERATIONS

❏ Ever since the AIDS epidemic began, researchers have been looking for a "magic bullet"—a single miracle drug to combat the virus, or a vaccine to seek out and destroy the virus in the bloodstream and lymphatic system. Research into this field is promising, however, and existing therapies almost guarantee that people with AIDS will live much longer and more productive lives than was once the case.

❏ For persons infected with HIV, the most logical approach to staying well is to eliminate all known causes of immune suppression and to implement the use of therapies that inhibit viral activity and stimulate immune function.

❏ Research has shown that dehydroepiandrosterone (DHEA), a hormone, may enhance the functioning of the immune system. (*See* DHEA THERAPY in Part Three.)

❏ Human growth hormone (HGH) therapy has been shown to help prevent and/or reverse wasting syndrome. This treatment must be given under a doctor's supervision. (*See* GROWTH HORMONE THERAPY in Part Three.)

❏ Hyperbaric oxygen therapy is sometimes used, together with medications and other treatments, to help overcome opportunistic infections associated with AIDS. (*See* HYPERBARIC OXYGEN THERAPY in Part Three.)

❏ N-acetylcysteine and L-carnitine both show some promise in the ability to prevent and counteract the extreme weight loss common in people with AIDS.

❏ Chicoric acid, a compound found in unroasted coffee beans, has been shown to inhibit the AIDS virus by blocking an enzyme the deadly virus uses to enter human cells.

❏ Maitake extract can help T cells in cell cultures from being destroyed by HIV by as much as 97 percent in vitro (in a test tube), according to researchers. The FDA approved Phase II clinical trials of maitake in 1998.

❑ People with AIDS are almost always underweight and often have malabsorption problems that contribute to malnutrition, which is common in people with AIDS. A lack of quality protein and adequate calories is a common reason for immune deficiency. (*See* MALABSORPTION SYNDROME in Part Two.)

❑ Researchers are studying the effects of phytonutrients in the blue-green algae spirulina as potential weapons in the fight to cure AIDS. Initial studies indicate these compounds tend to prevent the AIDS virus from attaching to or penetrating cells. Spirulina is also a good supplement for maintaining energy.

❑ The only *truly* safe sex is sex between life partners who are HIV-free. Other than that, abstinence is the only way to avoid any chance of infection with a sexually transmitted disease (STD). Changing partners particularly puts one at risk, and any exchange of bodily fluids is theoretically risky. A recent report claims that HIV can even be contracted through kissing if you have gum disease.

❑ There are thousands of AIDS survivors (epidemiologists call them *long-term non-progressors*) who are free from all symptoms and lead absolutely normal lives years after being identified as HIV-positive. As reported at the World AIDS Conference in Japan in 1994, there are at least 10,000 such people worldwide, and they are being studied intensively. A key to the AIDS cure may reside in these people, some of whom have had HIV for over ten years and who nevertheless remain healthy. Many thousands will continue to be HIV-positive but not manifest full-blown AIDS. And unknown to the general public and many in the medical establishment, there are also people who are now antibody-negative once diagnosed as HIV-positive, they apparently no longer have the virus present in their bodies. The medical community is amazed by this, and doctors continue to monitor the blood of such people frequently. For more information about this, read *They Conquered AIDS! True Life Adventures* by Scott Gregory and Bianca Leonardo (True Life Publications, 1989).

❑ Standard medical approaches to treatment of HIV focus on using drugs to try to block replication of the virus and thus slow the progression of disease, plus taking aggressive measures as needed to fight opportunistic infections and cancers. Medical science has probably had more success finding ways to defeat opportunistic infections than in combating the virus directly, but research continues on both fronts and progress is being made. One currently accepted element of anti-HIV drug treatment is a combination therapy approach, or the use of two or more drugs that act in different ways. Combination therapy is often more effective than the use of any single medication or type of medication.

❑ Most of the agents now widely used to target HIV fall into one of two categories:

• *Nucleoside analogues.* These drugs work by taking the place of one of the building blocks of the virus as it attempts to replicate, in effect blocking the virus's attempts to reproduce. Most of these drugs are commonly known by initials or combinations of letters and numbers derived from their original chemical names. Examples include zidovudine (Retrovir), better known as AZT; zalcitabine (HIVID), better known as ddC; didanosine (Videx), better known as ddI; stavudine (Zerit), better known as d4T; and lamivudine (Epivir), better known as 3TC. AZT was the first drug to be approved for use against HIV and has been the primary drug used to treat HIV infection ever since. It also has shown considerable effectiveness in preventing the transmission of the virus from an infected woman to a fetus during pregnancy and birth. The other nucleoside analogues were originally conceived as alternatives to AZT, but have since been found to work well with AZT in many cases. These drugs appear to prolong survival and delay the progression from the asymptomatic stage of HIV infection to full-blown AIDS, at least in some individuals. They can be used singly or in combination with each other (usually AZT plus one or more other drugs). Drawbacks include potential toxicity (especially in the case of AZT) and unpleasant side effects. In addition, the virus eventually develops resistance to these drugs, usually after a year or more of therapy.

• *Protease inhibitors.* These are drugs that bind to and block the action of a viral enzyme, protease, that plays a central role in the replication of HIV. If protease is prevented from exerting its normal action, the virus cannot reproduce. This class of drugs has shown great promise, at least in some studies, as a treatment for HIV infection. They are often used as an adjunct to treatment with AZT or another of the nucleoside analogues. Examples of protease inhibitors include indinavir (Crixivan), ritonavir (Norvir), saquinivir (Invirase), and agenerase (Amprenavir).

❑ There are different theories and some conflicting evidence about when to initiate treatment with nucleoside analogues and/or protease inhibitors, as well as about which agents are most effective (and for whom). Individual practitioners differ in their views on these issues. In addition, because of the tremendous amount of research being done on AIDS and its potential treatments, new possibilities for drugs and approaches to different aspects of the disease are emerging all the time. It is vital to work with a health care professional whose experience and judgment you trust.

❑ Some directions of antiviral drug research now being pursued include the following:

• *Anti-sense compounds.* By locking on to strands of viral DNA or RNA, these drugs act a bit like chewing gum stuck in the teeth of a zipper—they "gum up" the zipper so that the virus's genetic instructions are blocked.

• *Cellular targets.* These compounds inhibit factors inside the immune cells that HIV needs for replication, and have shown promise in interfering with the virus's ability to reproduce. One such compound is the cancer chemotherapy drug hydroxyurea (Hydrea), which appears to be particularly effective when used in combination with ddI.

• *Cyclophilin inhibitors.* These inhibit the fusion of infected and uninfected cells.

• *Glucosidase inhibitors.* These substances disrupt the structural integrity of sugars in the viral coat.

• *Reverse transcriptase inhibitors.* Reverse transcriptase is an enzyme used by retroviruses such as HIV to create copies of its genetic material, which then are incorporated into infected cells. By this mechanism the virus in effect turns normal immune cells into "factories" that continue to produce copies of viral DNA. In theory, by inhibiting reverse transcriptase, you suppress the virus.

❏ It is hoped that as scientists develop newer and more effective means of attacking the virus at various points in its life cycle, it will become possible to combine them in such a way that long-term suppression of the virus can be achieved—in effect, turning AIDS into a chronic but manageable illness rather than a terminal one. The principal unanswered question is whether, if near-perfect viral suppression does become reality, the immune system will be capable of restoring itself. The data are not yet clear on this point, though evidence from protease inhibitor studies has been encouraging. At the very least, it is fair to say that the new generation of antiviral drugs and their combinations is bringing a new era of new hope in the fight against AIDS.

❏ In some test subjects given "AIDS cocktails" containing mixtures of two, three, or more anti-AIDS drugs, the amount of HIV present in the body was dramatically reduced. Researchers theorize that if given early enough, potent combination treatments may someday even be able to eliminate the virus and allow the immune system to recover.

❏ The FDA has joined the CDC and the American Dental Association in urging dentists to autoclave—sterilize by steam under pressure—dental hand pieces and accessories between patients to remove possible contaminants. In addition, the FDA requires that all such equipment be designed to withstand autoclaving, and the labeling must include instructions for the sterilization process. While most dentists are believed to comply with the recommendations for autoclaving, it's a good idea to ask what preventive measures a dentist follows before making an appointment. Approximately 128 Americans have been infected with HIV through a dentist or doctor.

❏ It is not possible to contract HIV by donating blood. Blood donors do not come in contact with the blood of other persons, and only sterile materials, including single-use, disposable needles, are used to collect blood donations. Persons at risk of having HIV or AIDS should not donate blood, however. Many doctors recommend autologous donation—having some of your own blood collected and stored—in advance of planned surgery that will (or may) necessitate a transfusion.

❏ *See also* SEXUALLY TRANSMITTED DISEASE in Part Two.

❏ Worldwide efforts to eradicate HIV through research, drugs, vaccines, health programs, and nutrition are unprecedented. New drug and nutrient therapies offer more hope than ever before to those living with HIV and AIDS. Current drug therapies are making progress in bringing the disease under control. For example, the number of HIV-related deaths in the United States decreased from 16,516 in 1997 to 13,210 in 1998. For the first time since 1987, AIDS dropped out of the top fifteen causes of death in America. With this increased hope come some new concerns, however. Researchers are tabulating an increase in the number of highly resistant strains of the AIDS virus that render the powerful drug "cocktail" combinations ineffective. In an alarming 10 to 50 percent of these cases, high levels of the virus return. It is estimated that 4.5 percent of the 40,000 new HIV infections each year are resistant to current drugs. Another concern is that, lulled into a false sense of security by the drugs' abilities to subdue the virus, some people either forget to take their medications regularly or quit altogether, only to have illness flare up again. And in the meantime, when they are feeling better, they may unthinkingly infect their sex partners as well. Scientists also disagree over the definition of *resistance.* One group classifies resistance as a threefold increase in HIV's ability to withstand a certain drug, while another considers a strain resistant at ten times its former ability to withstand AIDS medications. If a drug combination is not effective, even though a person has been taking his or her medication faithfully, more testing is needed to determine how the combinations can be reformulated.

❏ Chronic, recurring vaginal yeast infections should be checked by a doctor. This can be a sign of HIV infection.

❏ Findings from the Johns Hopkins University School of Medicine indicate that HIV can evade even the most powerful antiviral drugs and remain hidden until the immune system is compromised, such as with an infection. Doctors believe it may be possible to eliminate the hidden virus by tricking the body into fighting it.

❏ For information about organizations that can provide information and assistance for people with HIV and AIDS, *see* HEALTH AND MEDICAL ORGANIZATIONS in the Appendix.

Alcoholism

With an estimated 75 percent of the American population consuming alcohol, it is hardly a surprise that one out of ten people suffers adverse consequences of alcohol consumption. Alcoholism is a chronic condition marked by a dependence on ethanol (ethyl alcohol). This dependence can be physiological, psychological, or a combination of the two. There are two separate classes of alcohol-related problems: alcohol abuse, or "problem drinking," and alcohol dependence, or alcoholism. Problem drinkers use alcohol on a regular basis, and although they may need a degree of support or guidance, they are not as physically and/or emotionally dependent on the drug as chronic drinkers, or alcoholics. We will use the term *alcoholism* loosely below for practical purposes, but it is important to remember this distinction.

Alcoholism affects approximately four times as many men as women, but the incidence of alcoholism among women is on the rise, as is the use of alcohol by children, adolescents, and college students. Women are physiologically more sensitive to alcohol than men are. Because of their bodies' lower water content and higher fat content, alcohol becomes more concentrated in the bloodstream and is also retained in their bodies longer. Also, men produce more alcohol dehydrogenase, the enzyme in the stomach that breaks down alcohol before it reaches the bloodstream, than women do. Even after you adjust for body weight, women are still affected more than men by the same amount of alcohol. This may be why alcohol abuse seems to have more serious long-term consequences for women. They are subject to all the same ill effects, but at lower rates of consumption. For example, women develop liver disease at lower levels of alcohol intake than men do, and they are also at increased risk for osteoporosis due to alcohol's adverse effects on bone metabolism. The overall rate of premature death related to alcohol abuse is 50 to 100 percent higher for women than for men.

Alcoholic women are more likely than alcoholic men to suffer from other psychiatric disorders, including depression, anxiety, and eating disorders. Often, these disorders existed prior to the onset of alcoholism, which means that these problems do not go away once the drinking stops; usually, independent treatment is required. Early treatment for these disorders, however, may help prevent alcohol abuse from occurring.

Alcohol affects everyone differently. Some become intoxicated with the first drink; others may be able to consume four or five drinks before showing any effects, often because they have built up a tolerance to the drug. In alcoholics, each drink triggers a craving for another. Alcoholism is a progressive disease that usually starts with acceptable social drinking. This leads to a drink for every mood: one to calm down, one to perk up, one to celebrate, one to "drown one's sorrows," and so on. The alcoholic soon needs no excuse to drink. In time, the alcoholic is completely controlled by his or her dependence on alcohol. Overindulgence often leads to depression, anxiety, memory loss, and lack of coordination, and can exaggerate antisocial behaviors such as aggression and/or other personality disorders. Intoxication also causes blood pressure and heart rates to be higher at first and then to decrease with prolonged consumption. Irregular, inefficient beating of the heart can lead to stroke. Respiration rates are lowered, and reflexes and reaction times slowed.

Alcoholics often become ashamed and angry at their compulsive behavior, and harbor deep feelings of inadequacy inside. This usually only leads to further alcohol abuse, however, as they use alcohol to numb the pain. They may also begin taking out their frustrations on those closest to them.

The National Council on Alcoholism and Drug Dependence and the American Society of Addiction Medicine define alcoholism as "a primary, chronic disease with genetic, psychosocial, and environmental factors influencing its development and manifestations." It is a complex disorder that is unique to each individual; no two cases are alike. Some people drink moderate to heavy amounts of alcohol for years before becoming clinically dependent on it, while others may become addicted to alcohol the very first time they ever take a drink. Medical science cannot yet explain why one person doesn't drink or drinks rarely, while others drink to excess. It is known, however, that alcohol itself is not the only cause of alcoholism. There is considerable debate as to whether alcoholism is genetic, environmental, or psychological. A family history of alcoholism is common among both men and women with the disorder, and research has shown that heredity is involved in almost 50 percent of the risk of contracing the disorder. While there is considerable evidence to support all sides, the truth probably lies somewhere in between; alcoholism is probably the result of a combination of many factors.

As far as the body is concerned, alcohol is a poison. Some of the effects of chronic alcohol consumption include damage to the brain, liver, pancreas, duodenum, and central nervous system. Alcohol not only reduces the amount of oxygen going to the brain, but it also directly harms brain cells, which can result in amnesia, disorientation, hallucinations, emotional disturbances, and—in cases of extreme abuse—seizures and neurological disorders. Alcoholism causes metabolic damage to every cell in the body and depresses the immune system. It may take years before the consequences of excessive drinking become evident, but if an alcoholic continues to drink, his or her life span may be shortened by ten to fifteen years or more.

The liver processes 95 percent of alcohol ingested, at a rate of about $\frac{1}{4}$ to $\frac{1}{2}$ ounce per hour. The repeated consumption of alcohol inhibits the liver's production of digestive enzymes, impairing the body's ability to absorb proteins, fats, and the fat-soluble vitamins (vitamins A, D, E, and K), as well as B-complex vitamins (especially thiamine and folic acid) and other water-soluble vitamins. It inhibits protein uptake, leading to amino acid deficiencies, and reduces the body's storage of zinc. Furthermore, many essential nutrients are not retained for use by the body; they are rapidly eliminated through the urine. The toxic effect of alcohol on the liver is very serious. First, excessive amounts of fat accumulate in the liver, a result of alcohol's effect on the body's ability to digest fats properly. Next, the alcoholic may develop hepatitis, a condition in which liver cells become inflamed and may die. The final, usually fatal, stage of alcoholic liver damage is cirrhosis of the liver, a disease characterized by inflammation, hardening, and scarring of the liver. This prevents the normal passage of blood through the liver, inhibiting the organ's ability to filter out toxins and foreign substances. An estimated one in five chronic drinkers is affected by cirrhosis of the liver.

The liver is one of the most robust organs of the body. It is the only organ that has the ability to regenerate itself after certain types of damage. Up to 25 percent of the liver can be removed, and within a short period of time, it will grow back to its original shape and size. It continually takes abuse, but if cared for properly, it will function more than adequately for decades. Alcohol is one of the toxins that the liver doesn't handle as well as others. The liver cannot regenerate after being severely damaged by alcohol.

There are many other health consequences of alcoholism as well. Alcoholics often experience damage to their peripheral nervous systems. This damage may show up initially as a loss of sensation in the hands or feet, with an accompanying difficulty in walking. Chronic drinking also causes inflammation of the pancreas. This further hampers the body's ability to digest fats and other nutrients, and can lead to diabetes. Alcoholics face an increased risk of mouth, throat, and stomach cancer due to the direct toxicity of the alcohol. The risk of liver, colon, and breast cancer may also be heightened by alcohol abuse. Smoking, which often goes hand-in-hand with drinking, increases the risk of cancer by as much as 50 percent. Problem drinkers may also experience high blood pressure, reduced testosterone production, visible dilation of blood vessels just beneath the skin's surface, and pathological enlargement of the heart that can progress to congestive heart failure.

The social consequences of alcoholism can be very destructive as well. Alcohol abuse takes a tremendous toll on society through traffic and other accidents, poor job performance, and emotional damage to entire families.

Drinking during pregnancy is particularly dangerous. The consumption of alcohol during pregnancy can cause birth defects and increases the chance of miscarriage. Alcohol passes through the mother's placenta and into the fetal circulation. This toxic substance depresses the central nervous system of the fetus. Further, the fetal liver must try to metabolize the alcohol, but since the fetus's liver is not fully developed, the alcohol remains in the fetal circulation. Women who drink during pregnancy generally give birth to babies with lower birth weights. Their growth may be retarded or stunted; their brains may be smaller than normal, and they may be of lower than normal intelligence, or even suffer mental retardation. Limbs, joints, fingers, and facial features may be deformed. Heart and kidney defects, and abnormalities of the skin, may occur. Some children exposed to alcohol *in utero* become hyperactive at adolescence and exhibit learning disabilities. Every drink a pregnant woman consumes increases her child's risk of being born with fetal alcohol syndrome, and also increases the chance of miscarriage. Even moderate amounts of alcohol may be harmful, especially in the first three to four months of pregnancy.

Alcoholics who stop drinking often experience withdrawal symptoms, especially during the first week or so that they abstain from alcohol. Insomnia, visual and auditory hallucinations, convulsions, acute anxiety, a rapid pulse, profuse perspiration, and fever can occur. With time and appropriate supervision, these symptoms pass and the alcoholic is set free to begin the lifelong work of recovery.

Dietary supplements, while important for everyone, are especially vital for alcoholics. Alcoholics need to supplement *all* the known vitamins and minerals. Evidence has shown that some of the diseases associated with alcoholism may be avoided by improving the nutritional health of the body. The program outlined below is designed to help recovering alcoholics to improve their nutritional condition. There are also some supplements that help with the psychological aspects of recovery by decreasing the desire for alcohol. You should begin with a high-potency multivitamin and mineral complex, and then add the nutrients listed below that are not included in the complex.

Unless otherwise specified, the dosages recommended in this section are for adults. For a child between the ages of twelve and seventeen, reduce the dose to three-quarters the recommended amount.

NUTRIENTS

SUPPLEMENT	SUGGESTED DOSAGE	COMMENTS
Essential		
Free-form amino acid complex plus extra L-cysteine or N-acetylcysteine	500 mg each 3 times daily, on an empty stomach. Take with 50 mg vitamin B₆ and 100 mg vitamin C for better absorption. Start with 500 mg daily and slowly work up to 1,000 mg daily.	Aids in withdrawal; needed for brain and liver function; necessary for regeneration of liver cells. (*See* AMINO ACIDS in Part One.)
Gamma-aminobutyric acid (GABA) plus inositol and niacinamide	750 mg once or twice daily, as needed. As directed on label. 500 mg once or twice daily, as needed.	To calm the body and prevent anxiety and stress.
Glutathione and L-methionine	3,000 mg daily, on an empty stomach. 1,000 mg daily, on an empty stomach. Take with water or juice. Do not take with milk. Take with 25 mg vitamin B₆ and 100 mg vitamin C for better absorption.	Protects the liver and reduces craving for alcohol. *Note:* Do not take substitute glutamic acid for glutathione. Protects glutathione, making it available to the liver. (*See* AMINO ACIDS in Part One.)
Pantothenic acid (vitamin B₅)	100 mg 3 times daily.	Aids the body in alcohol detoxification. Needed to counteract stress.

Vitamin B complex injections or sublingual plus extra vitamin B$_6$ and vitamin B$_{12}$	As prescribed by physician. 100 mg of each major B vitamin daily (amounts of individual vitamins in a complex will vary). As directed on label. 1,000 mcg 3 times daily.	To correct deficiencies. Injections (under a doctor's supervision) are best. If injections are not available, use a sublingual form. Often deficient in alcoholics. Reduces water retention and helps to relive anxiety, fear, and tension associated with recovery.
Vitamin B$_1$ (thiamine)	200 mg 3 times daily.	Alcoholics often are deficient in B vitamins, especially B$_1$.

Very Important

Alpha-lipoic acid	100 mg 2 times daily.	Aids in protecting the liver and pancreas from alcohol damage. A powerful antioxidant.
Calcium and magnesium	2,000 mg daily, at bedtime. 1,000 mg daily, at bedtime.	A vital mineral that has a sedative effect. Works with calcium. Magnesium is depleted from the body with alcohol use.
Multienzyme complex plus proteolytic enzymes	As directed on label. Take with meals. As directed on label. Take between meals.	To aid digestion. Essential for assimilation of protein. *Caution:* Do not give these supplements to a child.
Primrose oil	1,000 mg 3 times daily, with meals.	Used successfully in Europe, this supplement is a good source of essential fatty acids. It may also help reduce withdrawal symptoms.
Pycnogenol or grape seed extract	30 mg 3 times daily. 30 mg 3 times daily.	Powerful antioxidants for the protection of the cells.
Vitamin C with bioflavonoids	3,000–10,000 mg daily, in divided doses.	Acts as a powerful antioxidant with healing potential, and promotes production of interferon, which helps the body resist infection, to which alcoholics are generally more susceptible.

Important

Acidophilus (Probiata from Wakunaga)	As directed on label. Take on an empty stomach.	Needed for proper digestion. Helps the damaged liver. Helps prevent candidiasis from developing. Probiata is a non-dairy formula requiring no refrigeration.
Coenzyme A from Coenzyme A Technologies	As directed on label.	Supports the immune system's detoxification of many dangerous substances.
Inositol hexaphos-phate (IP$_6$) (Cell Forté with IP-6 from Enzymatic Therapy)	As directed on label.	Enhances natural killer cell activity.
Lecithin granules or capsules	1 tbsp 3 times daily, before meals. 1,200 mg 3 times daily, before meals.	Good for brain function. Helps correct fatty liver degeneration. May protect against cirrhosis.
Liquid Kyolic with B$_1$ and B$_{12}$ from Wakunaga	As directed on label.	Protects liver and brain cells. Reduces stress.

Multivitamin and mineral complex with manganese and selenium	As directed on label. 200 mcg daily. Take separately from calcium. 200 mcg daily. If you are pregnant, do not exceed 40 mcg daily.	All nutrients are needed because of malabsorption problems. Important trace minerals that enhance immune function.

Helpful

Choline complex or acetylcholine complex or phosphatidyl choline	As directed on label. As directed on label. As directed on label.	Effective combinations that reduce fatty liver changes, improving liver function.
Dimethylglycine (DMG) (Aangamik DMG from FoodScience of Vermont)	125 mg 3 times daily.	Carries oxygen to the cells.
Flaxseed oil	As directed on label.	Strengthens the brain's gray matter.
L-Glutamine	500 mg twice daily, on an empty stomach. Take with water or juice. Do not take with milk. Take with 50 mg vitamin B$_6$ and 100 mg vitamin C for better absorption.	An amino acid that helps to stop cravings and balance blood sugar.
Lithium	As prescribed by physician.	A trace mineral that may help depression. Available by prescription only.
Raw liver extract and raw pancreas glandular	As directed on label. As directed on label.	A rich source of vitamins and minerals that aids in repairing the liver and in preventing anemia. (*See* GLANDULAR THERAPY in Part Three.) Helps prevent pancreatic damage; beneficial for people with diabetes associated with alcoholism.
S-adenosylmethio-nine (SAMe)	As directed on label.	Its antioxidant effects can improve the health of the liver. *Caution:* Do not use if you have manic-depressive disorder or take prescription antidepressants.
Vitamin A	25,000 IU daily. If you are pregnant, do not exceed 10,000 IU daily.	To counteract deficiencies. Vitamin A is poorly absorbed if the liver is damaged. Use emulsion forms for easier assimilation and greater safety at higher doses. Avoid capsule or tablet forms.
Vitamin E	400–1,200 IU daily.	A powerful antioxidant. Use d-alpha-tocopherol form.
Zinc	50 mg daily. Do not exceed a total of 100 mg daily from all supplements.	Deficiency can cause pathological changes in the stomach similar to those caused by alcohol.

HERBS

❑ Alfalfa is a good source of needed minerals.

❑ Burdock root and red clover cleanse the bloodstream.

❏ Dandelion root and silymarin (milk thistle extract) help to repair damage done to the liver. Silymarin acts as a powerful antioxidant.

❏ Valerian root has a calming effect. It is best taken at bedtime.

RECOMMENDATIONS

❏ Avoid all alcohol. Total abstinence is an absolute requirement for regaining control over your life and your health. Even after years of sobriety, you cannot begin drinking again and expect to maintain control over it. As little as one sip of something containing alcohol can renew the drinking pattern. You must choose *not* to drink.

❏ Seek help from a person or persons knowledgeable about this disorder. Alcoholics Anonymous has been doing wonderful work for many years in helping alcoholics achieve and maintain sobriety. Al-Anon and Alateen are similar groups that provide support for the friends and families of alcoholics. A strong support system can make behavioral changes much easier for everyone. The assistance and counseling services of these groups are available in nearly every city and town nationwide. Look in your local telephone directory for the group nearest you, or call your local mental health association for information.

❏ Some programs, such as Moderation Management, are available to help problem drinkers (not true alcoholics) reduce their drinking without completely stopping. This program entails a thirty-day abstinence period. After that, you may consume no more than four drinks a day and no more than fourteen drinks per week (three per day and nine per week for women).

❏ If possible, consult a nutritionally oriented physician to determine your specific nutritional needs.

❏ Go on a ten-day live juice and cleansing fast to remove toxins from the body quickly. *See* FASTING in Part Three.

❏ Eat a nutrient-dense diet of fresh whole foods, organically grown if possible, and follow the nutritional supplement program outlined above. Your primary foods should be raw fruits and vegetables, whole grains, and legumes.

❏ Avoid saturated fats and fried foods, which put stress on the liver. For essential fatty acids, use primrose oil supplements plus small amounts of cold-pressed organic vegetable oils.

❏ Do not consume refined sugar or anything that contains it. Alcoholics often have disorders of sugar metabolism.

❏ Get plenty of rest, especially in the early weeks of recovery, to allow your body to cleanse and repair itself.

❏ Avoid people, things, and places that are associated with drinking. Make new friendships with people who do not drink. Taking up a hobby, becoming involved in sports, and exercising promote self-esteem and provide a productive outlet for energy.

❏ As much as possible, avoid stress. Cultivate patience; this will be needed for the long, slow road to recovery.

❏ Do not take any drugs except for those prescribed by your physician.

❏ If you suspect that someone you know may be abusing alcohol, encourage the person to seek professional care.

CONSIDERATIONS

❏ Poor nutrition can enhance the adverse effects of ethanol. Alcoholics are at much greater risk of malnutrition than other people, since as much as 50 percent of their caloric intake may come from ethanol at the expense of other nutritious foods. Alcoholics are commonly deficient in folic acid, and malabsorption due to pancreatic insufficiency is often a major problem.

❏ Long-term alcohol abuse can promote a zinc-deficient state, most likely because of increased fecal and urinary losses. Zinc plays a vital role in a variety of enzyme systems in the body, as well as in DNA and RNA production. It also helps to regulate copper levels in the brain, reducing anxiousness and paranoia. A deficiency of zinc can result in anorexia, impaired senses of smell and taste, growth retardation, disorders of the reproductive system, and impaired wound healing and immune function. Pathological changes in the stomach occur due to zinc deficiency as well. Alcohol-related zinc deficiency accelerates the poisoning of cells that come into contact with alcohol by altering the metabolism of fats, carbohydrates, and nutrients. This leads to malabsorption problems and other nutritional deficiencies. Chronic alcohol intake often results in a depressed metabolism caused by zinc deficiency.

❏ A Department of Health and Human Services study showed that tobacco smokers and alcohol drinkers who regularly use high-alcohol mouthwash may be more likely than other people to get oral and pharyngeal cancers.

❏ Alcohol is one of the most damaging substances to the stomach and the small intestine. It reduces the absorption of nutrients in the small intestine, and it is one of the few substances that can penetrate the lining of the stomach and cause damage. Gastric secretions increase with alcohol consumption, causing excess acidity and diluting digestive enzymes. This can lead to gastritis.

❏ Chronic alcohol consumption alters red blood cell membranes and causes various other types of cells, including gastrointestinal cells, to lose their normal flexibility.

❏ A recovering alcoholic who resumes drinking, even after years of sobriety, will damage his or her liver as though the drinking had never stopped in the first place.

❏ The drug naltrexone (ReVia) blocks the pleasurable effects of endogenous opioids, opiate-like substances released by the brain in response to alcohol, and may help problem drinkers remain sober by reducing the craving for alcohol. In two separate studies conducted at the University of Pennsylvania and the Yale University School of Medicine, people who took this drug were three times likelier than other patients to stick with their recovery programs. However, this drug is not suitable for people with liver disease.

❑ Some physicians prescribe the drug disulfiram (Antabuse) to help alcoholics stay sober. Those on this drug experience nausea, vomiting, severe headaches, blurred vision, and sometimes an impending feeling of death if they take even a small sip of alcohol. Abstinence from alcohol often results with use of this drug.

❑ Alpha-lipoic acid, a powerful antioxidant, has been used successfully to treat alcohol-induced liver damage. It aids in protecting the liver and pancreas from alcoholic damage.

❑ In some countries, hyperbaric oxygen has been used successfully in the treatment of alcoholism. (See HYPERBARIC OXYGEN THERAPY in Part Three.)

❑ Alcoholism and substance abuse specialists sometimes recommend a supervised "intervention" to force an alcoholic into admitting the problem and entering treatment. Psychological techniques have been developed and refined over the past few years, which seem to have increased the success rate among alcoholics seeking to recover and remain sober. Such interventions are delicate matters, however, and should be undertaken only under the supervision of a trained professional.

❑ Research has shown that college students today are getting drunk more often than in the past and that they are drinking in order to become drunk. The number of students who drink to become intoxicated is two to three times as high today as it was two decades ago.

❑ Binge drinking is a sign of severe alcoholism. The binge drinker will drink to the point of intoxication and stay that way for a few days, often without consuming many solid foods. The binge may end in vomiting, which is the body's way of getting rid of the excess alcohol, and then passing out. Frequently the person does not remember the events that happened during the binge. Binge drinkers consume larger quantities of alcohol on a regular basis and also experience more intoxication and alcohol-related problems than non-binge drinkers do. Binge drinking can cause dangerous cardiac arrhythmias.

❑ Some research has indicated that the children of teetotalers are actually at higher risk of becoming alcohol abusers than children of alcoholics. This has been taken to mean that children reared in homes where alcohol is accepted as a social norm and not abused are less likely than others to become alcoholics. However, the latest research has found that children of alcoholics are more inclined than children of nonalcoholics to use drugs, including cocaine. These children are 400 times more likely to use drugs than those who do not have a family history of alcohol addiction. Studies conducted in Sweden revealed that the majority of babies of alcoholics who were adopted by nonalcoholic families eventually grew up to become alcoholics, indicating a correlation between chemical dependency and genetics.

❑ Limiting one's drinking to beer or wine does not protect against alcoholism or damage from alcohol. Twelve ounces of beer or 5 ounces of wine is comparable in alcohol content to 1.5 ounces of 80-proof liquor. Because it is more concentrated, straight liquor is absorbed into the bloodstream more quickly than beer and wine are.

❑ Alcohol enters the bloodstream relatively quickly, as it can be absorbed through both the stomach and small intestines (unlike food, which is absorbed through the intestines only). It takes nearly one hour for the body to break down one unit of alcohol in the bloodstream (for older people, it can take longer). The more drinks are consumed in an hour, the higher the alcohol content of the blood. Blood alcohol levels of 400 mg/dL can be life-threatening.

❑ Once alcohol is in the blood, there is nothing that can be done to hurry the process of removing it. The idea that cold showers, coffee, and/or eating can help you sober up is a myth.

❑ Although some people fall asleep faster when drinking, alcohol depresses REM (rapid eye movement) sleep. REM is an essential part of the healthy sleep cycle and if disturbed, the result is usually a desire to sleep longer in the morning and a sluggish feeling that lasts throughout the day.

❑ "Hangovers" are thought to be caused by a combination of several factors, including dehydration, overeating, and disturbed sleep. Even small amounts of alcohol can sometimes cause unpleasant side effects the next morning in some individuals. Usually, the best remedy includes rest and rehydration. Drinking a large glass of water before retiring and another in the morning may help take the edge off "the morning after." Taking over-the-counter pain medication such as acetaminophen, ibuprofen, naproxin, or aspirin before hangover symptoms begin sometimes helps with the headache; however, extreme caution must be used, as they are not risk-free. When combined with alcohol, these medications may irritate your stomach and can even be toxic to the liver. This is why there is now a required warning label on over-the-counter painkillers, and medications that contain them, cautioning against using them if you consume more than three alcoholic drinks per day. Mixing alcohol with any medication is not recommended.

❑ Medications such as tranquilizers, antidepressants, codeine, morphine, phenobarbital, and even some antibiotics can form toxic combinations with alcohol. Combining alcohol with antihistamines can enhance depression of the central nervous system. Combining alcohol with sleeping aids can be deadly.

❑ In recovery from alcoholism, it is best to avoid tranquilizers, as there is a danger of substituting one drug addiction for another. Sobriety should be drug-free.

❑ Pregnant women should avoid all alcohol.

❑ Alcohol has been shown to affect older adults differently than other people. It is more likely to hinder the absorption of nutrients, and it can also pose a danger if mixed with many medications taken to control age-related or chronic illnesses. Unfortunately, alcoholism among elderly people is more common than one might think, and can often go unnoticed or without intervention. Some people tend to think that older people have "earned the right to drink." The truth is, however, that elders have just as much right to recovery as anyone else.

❑ Alcoholism is currently the second major preventable cause of death in the United States, second only to cigarette smoking.

❑ Contrary to the popular myth that alcohol heightens sexual arousal, it actually has the opposite effect—depression. It can cause sexual dysfunction in men and disrupt menstrual cycles in women.

❑ Various studies have shown that, in small amounts, alcohol can have protective effects against certain cardiovascular and cancerous diseases. The amount of alcohol shown to be protective has varied slightly from study to study. The accepted definition of moderate alcoholic intake according to the U.S. Department of Agriculture is one drink or less per day for women and two drinks or less per day for men (a "drink" being defined as 12 ounces of beer, 4 ounces of wine, or 1.5 ounces of 80-proof liquor). Most doctors and health authorities, however, do not suggest that nondrinkers begin drinking to protect their hearts. Instead, they suggest less risky options such as regular light exercise, not smoking, and decreasing the amount of saturated fat in the diet.

❑ A problem in treating alcoholism is that it is difficult to define. Not all alcoholics are stumbling-down drunk in public at all times, losing their jobs and family, causing traffic accidents, or getting arrested. Some drink secretly, only on weekends or in the evenings, or even only once a month. Some drink because they are depressed and others drink because they like the sensation. They may successfully hold down jobs or pursue professional careers. But at some point, they have lost the ability to control how much alcohol they consume.

❑ Alcoholism is treatable. In order to benefit from treatment, it is essential for the drinker to realize that a problem exists and to seek the kind of treatment that fits his or her particular needs. Just as every alcoholic is different, each person responds differently to the various kinds of treatment available. Some experience withdrawal symptoms so serious that they need to be hospitalized. For some, psychotherapy can be helpful; for others, it may not be. Medications may be helpful for certain individuals. Self-help programs are a widely successful method of helping the alcoholic or chronic drinker to recover. (See below for contact information for several successful programs).

❑ *See also* CIRRHOSIS OF THE LIVER and DRUG ADDICTION, both in Part Two.

❑ For information about organizations that can provide information and assistance for people dealing with alcoholism, *see* HEALTH AND MEDICAL ORGANIZATIONS in the Appendix.

Alkalosis

See under ACID/ALKALI IMBALANCE.

Allergic Rhinitis

See HAY FEVER.

Allergies

An allergy is an inappropriate response by the body's immune system to a substance that is not normally harmful. The immune system is a highly complex defense mechanism that helps us to fight infections. It does this by identifying foreign invaders and mobilizing the body's white blood cells to fight them. In some people, the immune system wrongly identifies a nontoxic substance as an invader, and the white blood cells overreact, creating more damage to the body than the invader. Thus, the allergic response becomes a disease in itself.

Typical allergic responses are nasal congestion, coughing, wheezing, itching, shortness of breath, headache, fatigue, and hives and other skin rashes. Substances that provoke allergic responses are called *allergens*. Almost any substance can cause an allergic reaction in someone, somewhere in the world, but the most common allergens are pollen, dust, certain metals (especially nickel), some cosmetics, lanolin, dust mites, animal hair, insect venom, some common drugs (such as penicillin and aspirin), some food additives (such as benzoic acid and sulfur dioxide), animal dander, and chemicals found in soap, washing powder, cleaning supplies, and many other chemicals.

Many people are allergic to mold. Molds are microcospic living organisms, neither animal nor insect, that thrive where no other life form can. Molds live throughout the house—under the sink and in the bathroom, basement, refrigerator, and any other damp, dark place. They also flourish in the air, in soil, on dead leaves, and on other organic material. Molds can be both destructive and beneficial.

Molds help to make cheese, fertilize gardens, and speed decaying of garbage and fallen leaves. Penicillin is made from molds. Molds can also provoke allergic reactions, however. Mold spores are carried by the wind and predominate in the summer and early fall. They thrive year round in warm climates. Cutting grass, harvesting crops, or walking through tall vegetation can provoke an allergic reaction. People who repair old furniture are also at risk because old wood often harbors mold spores.

Foods also can provoke allergic reactions. Some of the most common allergenic foods are chocolate, dairy products, eggs, shellfish, strawberries, and wheat. There is a difference between food allergies and food intolerances. A person with a food intolerance is unable to digest and process that food correctly, usually due to a lack of a certain enzyme or enzymes. A food allergy, on the other hand, occurs when a person's immune system generates an antibody response to the ingested food. Food intolerance can lead to allergy, however, if particles of undigested food manage to enter the bloodstream and cause a reaction. *Leaky gut syndrome* is a term used to describe a condition in which the lining of the intestinal tract becomes perforated and irritated, and tiny particles of partially digested food enter the bloodstream, causing an allergic reaction.

Some allergic reactions to food begin as soon as one starts chewing. Highly allergenic foods are easy to identify and eliminate from the diet. Delayed reactions are harder to detect. An irritating cough or tickle in the throat can be a sign of food allergy.

For most people, allergies are no more than another frustrating fact of life. But for people with asthma, or for those who suffer severe allergic reactions, allergies can be life-threatening. In people with asthma, hypersensitivity to irritants results in mucus secretions and, in severe cases, inflammation, edema, and swelling of the bronchial tubes. (*See* ASTHMA in Part Two.) According to the National Institute of Allergy and Infectious Diseases, serious allergies affect more than 50 million Americans. Insect bites produce severe reactions in approximately 2 million Americans, and there are over 40,000 occurrences of allergic drug reactions reported each year.

Allergies affect one's quality of life and productivity at work or home, school studies, or athletic pursuits. They can also lead to secondary diseases like ear and sinus infections. To make matters worse, due to the consistently warmer and wetter winters occurring in most parts of the world in recent years, seasonal allergy sufferers can count on longer periods of misery. Hay fever (*acute seasonal allergic rhinitis*) is the most common type of seasonal allergy. Its symptoms closely resemble those of the common cold, but there are some differences. Cold symptoms generally disappear in a week to ten days, but allergic rhinitis can linger miserably for weeks, or even months. The nasal discharge caused by a cold is generally watery at the very beginning, but then turns thick and yellow, while the allergic reaction produces a consistently thin and clear discharge from the nose, in ad-

dition to itchy eyes, mouth, and skin. While it is difficult to determine the cause of the common cold, in most cases, the cause or causes of allergies can be identified. This is at least one heartening fact for allergy sufferers.

No one knows why some people are allergic to certain substances. According to the Asthma and Allergy Foundation of America, some allergies have a genetic component. If one parent has allergies, it is statistically likely that one in three of their children will have allergies. If both parents have allergies, the chance that their children will have allergies rises to seven in ten. It is also believed that babies who are not breastfed are more likely to develop allergies. Although persons between the ages of fifteen and twenty-five are the most allergy-prone, allergies can strike at any age. Emotional factors such as stress and anger may aggravate allergies, especially if the immune system is not functioning properly.

FOOD ALLERGY SELF-TEST

If you suspect that you are allergic to a certain food, a simple test can help you determine if you are correct. By recording your pulse rate after consuming the food in question, you can reveal if you are having an allergic reaction. Using a watch with a second hand, sit down and relax for a few minutes. When completely relaxed, take your pulse at the wrist. Count the number of beats in a sixty-second period. A normal pulse reading is between 52 and 70 beats per minute. After taking your pulse, consume the food that you are testing for an allergic reaction. Wait to twenty minutes and take your pulse again. If your pulse rate has increased more than ten beats per minute, omit this food from your diet for one month, and then retest yourself.

For the purposes of this test, it is best to use the purest form of the suspected food available. For example, if you are testing yourself for an allergy to wheat, it is better to use a bit of plain cream of wheat cereal than to use wheat bread, which contains other ingredients besides wheat. This way you will know that if you observe a reaction, it is the wheat that is responsible.

NUTRIENTS

SUPPLEMENT	SUGGESTED DOSAGE	COMMENTS
Very Important		
Acidophilus (Probiata from Wakunaga)	As directed on label.	Powerful immune enhancer with digestive enzymes for improved digestion.
AntiAllergy formula from Freeda Vitamins	As directed on label.	A combination of quercetin, calcium pantothenate, and calcium ascorbate (vitamin C).
Calcium and magnesium	1,500–2,000 mg daily. 750 mg daily.	Needed to help reduce stress. Use calcium chelate form. Needed to balance with calcium.
Inositol hexaphosphate (IP$_6$) (Cell Forté from Enzymatic Therapy)	As directed on label.	Supports the immune system.

Supplement	Suggested Dosage	Comments
Kyolic Super Formula 102 from Wakunaga	50 mg 3 times daily.	Powerful immune enhancer with digestive enzymes. For improved digestion.
Methylsulfonyl-methane (MSM)	As directed on label.	Has antiallergic properties equal to or better than those of antihistamines.
Multienzyme complex or pancreatin	As directed on label. Take with meals.	For improved digestion. *Caution:* If you have a history of ulcers, do not use a formula containing HCl.
Quercetin (Quercitin-C from Ecological Formulas is a good source) plus	500 mg twice daily.	Increases immunity and decreases reactions to certain foods, pollens, and other allergens.
bromelain or	100 mg twice daily.	Enhances absorption of quercetin and reduces inflammation.
Activated Quercetin (from Source Naturals)	As directed on label.	Contains quercetin plus bromelain and vitamin C.
Raw adrenal glandular and raw spleen glandular and raw thymus glandular	500 mg each twice daily.	To stimulate proper immune function. Raw adrenal is very important to prevent adrenal exhaustion.
Vitamin B complex	100 mg of each major B vitamin daily (amounts of individual vitamins in a complex will vary).	Needed for proper digestion and nerve function. Use a high-stress formula. Consider injections.
plus extra pantothenic acid (vitamin B_5) and	100 mg 3 times daily.	The anti-stress vitamin. Use a lozenge or sublingual form.
vitamin B_{12} and	300–1,000 mcg 3 times daily.	Needed for proper assimilation of nutrients. Use a lozenge or sublingual form.
Vitamin B_6	50 mg 3 times daily.	Helps to relieve wheezing and allergy attacks.
Vitamin C with bioflavonoids	5,000–20,000 mg daily, in divided doses. (*See* ASCORBIC ACID FLUSH in Part Three.)	Protects the body from allergens and moderates the inflammatory response.
Important		
Liquid Kyolic with B_1 and B_{12} from Wakunaga	As directed on label.	An excellent cell protector.
Natural carotenoid complex (Betatene)	As directed on label.	Free radical scavengers that inhibit allergic reactions.
Proteolytic enzymes	As directed on label. Take between meals on an empty stomach.	To aid digestion and destroy free radicals. *Caution:* Do not give these supplements to a child.
Helpful		
Aller Bee-Gone from CC Pollen	As directed on label.	A combination of herbs, enzymes, and nutrients designed to fight acute allergy attacks.
Bee pollen	Start with a few granules at a time and work up to 2 tsp daily.	Strengthens the immune system. Use raw crude pollen, preferably produced within 10 miles of your home. *Caution:* Bee pollen may cause an allergic reaction in some individuals. Discontinue use if a rash, wheezing, discomfort, or other symptoms occur.
Coenzyme A from Coenzyme-A Technologies.	As directed on label.	Supports the immune system's detoxification of many dangerous substances.
Coenzyme Q_{10}	100 mg daily.	Improves cellular oxygenation and immune function.
Free-form amino acid complex	As directed on label.	Supplies protein in a form that is rapidly absorbed and assimilated. Use a sublingual form.
Grape seed extract	As directed on label.	A powerful antioxidant to prevent free radical damage.
Glucosamine sulfate or N-acetylglucosamine (N-A-G from Source Naturals)	As directed on label. As directed on label.	Important for regulating the mucous secretions of respiratory system.
L-Cysteine and L-tyrosine	500 mg each daily, on empty stomach. Take with water or juice, not milk. Take with 50 mg vitamin B_6 and 100 mg vitamin C for better absorption.	Promotes healing from respiratory disorders. Helpful for stress and allergic disorders. (*See* AMINO ACIDS in Part One.)
Manganese	4 mg daily for 3 months. Take separately from calcium.	An important component in many of the body's enzyme systems. Use manganese chelate form.
Multivitamin and mineral complex with calcium and magnesium and vitamin D_3	As directed on label. 400 IU daily.	All nutrients are needed in balance. Use a hypoallergenic formula. Three nutrients necessary for proper immune function.
Potassium	100 mg daily.	Necessary for adrenal gland function. Use potassium protinate or potassium chelate form.
Proteolytic enzymes or Inflazyme Forte from American Biologics	As directed on label. Take between meals, on an empty stomach. As directed on label.	To aid digestion and destroy free radicals. *Caution:* Do not give these supplements to a child.
Vitamin A and vitamin E and zinc	10,000 IU daily. 600 IU daily. 50 mg daily. Do not exceed a total of 100 mg daily from all supplements.	Three nutrients necessary for proper immune function. Use d-alpha-tocopherol form.

HERBS

❏ Allergy Helper from Continental Vitamin Company is an herbal combination formula that is good for relieving allergy symptoms.

❏ Boswellia (*Boswellia serrata,* also known as Indian frankincense) works at the cellular level to reduce inflammatory and allergic responses.

❏ Decongest Herbal Formula from Zand is a good allergy-fighting product.

❑ Ephedra (ma huang) is good for relieving nasal and chest congestion.

Caution: Do not use this herb if you suffer from anxiety, glaucoma, heart disease, high blood pressure, or insomnia, or if you are taking a monoamine oxidase (MAO) inhibitor drug for depression.

❑ Eucalyptus and/or thyme leaves can be used to ease congestion. Soak an ounce of either one in a cup of boiling water and inhale the steam.

❑ Eyebright tea has been noted to reduce hay fever symptoms such as watery eyes and runny nose in children.

❑ Goldenseal root aids the absorption of nutrients.

Caution: Do not take goldenseal on a daily basis for more than one week at a time, and do not use it during pregnancy. If you have a history of cardiovascular disease, diabetes, or glaucoma, use it only under a doctor's supervision.

❑ Japanese researchers have found that licorice root can help allergy sufferers. It has been traditionally used in Japan to battle allergic inflammation.

Caution: If overused, licorice can elevate blood pressure. Do not use this herb for more than one month at a time. Avoid it completely if you have high blood pressure.

❑ Nettle (also known as stinging nettle) reduces inflammation in the sinus cavities. It is also a powerful antioxidant that helps prevent free radical damage and aids in preventing allergy attacks.

❑ Wild yam stimulates the production of hormones that reduce inflammation caused by allergies. Wild yam is not for everyone, however (*see* HERBS in Part One).

❑ Yerba maté helps to relieve allergic symptoms. Take 2 to 3 teaspoons of yerba maté in 16 ounces of hot water on an empty stomach.

❑ The following Chinese herbs support sinus health:

• Magnolia flower (*Magnolia liliflora,* also known as xho yi hua) has been used for centuries in traditional Chinese medicine to open nasal passages and relieve headaches associated with sinus problems.

• Scutellaria (*Scutellaria baicalensis*) root contains powerful flavonoids and antioxidants that enhance the immune system. It inhibits the contraction of tissues in allergic reactions.

• Trichosanth (*Trichosanthes kirilowii*) has been used for centuries in traditional Chinese medicine to benefit the respiratory system.

• Wild angelica (*Angelica dahurica,* also known as aka bai zhi) is particularly useful for clearing sinus problems. It has been found to help relieve discomfort around the eyes that occurs when the sinuses above the eyes are blocked. It normalizes swelling, opens nasal passages, and promotes the discharge of pus often associated with sinus infections. Another important action of this herb is the balancing of histamine levels.

❑ Ayurveda is a body of medical knowledge originating in India. (*See* AYURVEDIC REMEDIES in Part Three.) According to this system, some allergic responses are created by the presence of *ama,* or toxins in the system that are the by-product of improperly digested food. The Ayurvedic herbs picrorrhiza (*Picrorrhiza kurrooa*) and phyllanthus (*Phyllanthus acidus*) are suggested for cooling and cleaning the blood, and helping the liver detoxify the body of ama. Trifala is a traditional Ayurvedic herbal combination formula that is sometimes recommended for allergies. It is said to act on vata, one of the three vital principles that govern the body (vata controls respiration, among other functions) in the intestines and keep it from aggravating and drying the upper respiratory system. Other Ayurvedic herbs suggested for allergies include amla (*Emblica officinalis*), guggul (*Commiphora mukul*), and mulethi (*Glycyrrhiza glabra,* better known in English as licorice).

❑ Other herbs that can be beneficial for allergies include burdock, dandelion, ginkgo, and horseradish.

RECOMMENDATIONS

❑ Rotate your foods. (*See* Rotating Foods: Sample Daily Menus, at the end of this section.) Eat a different group of foods for each of four days and then repeat the cycle. You can select as many of the foods allowed on a specific day as you like but it is essential that no type of food be ingested more often than every four days.

❑ *See* Detecting Hidden Food Allergies on page 159 and fill out the Food Sensitivity Questionnaire. Then omit from your diet for thirty days any food you have listed as consumed four times per week or more.

❑ Follow a fasting program. *See* FASTING in Part Three. After a fast, you can try adding back the "foods to avoid" (listed below) in very small amounts, such as 1 teaspoon at a time. Record your reactions after eating. If you feel bloated or have a slight headache, an upset stomach, gas, diarrhea, a rapid pulse, or heart palpitations after eating certain foods, eliminate them from your diet for sixty days and try introducing them again in small amounts. If you experience a reaction again, eliminate them from your diet permanently.

❑ Avoid the following foods until it is determined you are not allergic to them: bananas, beef products, caffeine, chocolate, citrus fruits, corn, dairy products, eggs, oats, oysters, peanuts, processed and refined foods, salmon, strawberries, tomatoes, wheat, and white rice.

❑ Avoid any food products that contain artificial color, especially FD&C Yellow No. 5 dye. Many people are allergic to food colorings. Other food additives to avoid include vanillin, benzaldehyde, eucalyptol, monosodium glutamate, BHT-BHA, benzoates, and annatto. Read labels carefully.

❑ If you are allergic to ragweed, do not eat cantaloupe. It contains some of the same proteins as ragweed.

❑ Take the underarm temperature test to determine if you have an underactive thyroid. (*See* HYPOTHYROIDISM in Part Two.)

❑ Be sure to take only hypoallergenic supplements, as these do not contain potentially irritating substances.

❑ Keep rooms free from dust, keep windows shut (use the air conditioner whenever possible), and use a dehumidifier in the basement.

❑ Use mold-proof paint and a disinfectant on walls and furniture.

❑ Purchase an air filter to clean pollen, molds, and dust from your home or office.

❑ For airborne allergies, try using an air purification device. The Air Supply personal air purifier from Wein Products is a miniature unit that is worn around the neck. It sets up an invisible pure air shield against micro-organisms (such as viruses, bacteria, and mold) and microparticles (including dust, pollen, and pollutants) in the air. It also eliminates vapors, smells, and harmful volatile compounds in the air. The Living Air XL-15 unit from Alpine Industries is an ionizing unit that is good for purifying the air in the home or workplace.

❑ Depending on the severity of your allergies, be sure to wear long pants and long-sleeved shirts when spending time outside. Change your clothes and shower as soon as you return indoors. For some, using a "high-efficiency" mask (available in drugstores and medical supply stores) may be advisable.

❑ Pollen counts in late summer are highest between 5:00 A.M. and 10:00 A.M., so schedule your gardening and other outdoor activities with this in mind. You can learn what trees and plants are pollinating around you by calling a hot line set-up by the National Allergy Bureau at 800–9–POLLEN (800–976–5536).

❑ If you are a chronic allergy sufferer, avoid exercising outdoors.

❑ On windy days, when more pollen is blown through the air, try to avoid going outside if your allergies are severe. The best time for you to be outdoors is after a rainstorm, when pollen levels drop significantly.

❑ Do not smoke, and avoid secondhand smoke.

❑ Avoid taking aspirin within three hours of eating.

CONSIDERATIONS

❑ Steroid nasal sprays can be very effective for allergies and are less expensive than many prescription medications. These sprays, however, do not relieve itchiness of the eyes. They generally need up to ten days to become effective, so it is advisable to begin taking them about a week prior to hay fever season. Be sure to check first with your doctor before using them, as recent studies suggest a possible link between steroid nasal sprays and the development of glaucoma—a concern for older adults.

❑ Plants produce oxygen as a normal part of their growth and living process, and help to remove pollutants from indoor air. Some plants suggested for this purpose include areca palm, bamboo palm, Boston fern, dracaena, dwarf date palm, English ivy, ficus alii, lady palm, peace lily, rubber plant, and spider plant.

❑ Acupressure and acupuncture have had some success in relieving allergy symptoms. (*See* ACUPRESSURE and ACUPUNCTURE *under* PAIN CONTROL in Part Three.)

❑ IgE is an antibody formed by the body as part of an allergic response to a food substance. If IgE is present in your lung tissue, it frequently causes symptoms such as shortness of breath or asthma. If present in the skin, it can cause hives. If IgE is present in the wall of the intestinal tract, it can result in severe pain, gas, or bloating. IgE can be present anywhere in the body, causing severe problems. Even healthy natural foods can have an adverse effect if you are allergic to them.

❑ Cerebral allergies cause swelling of the lining of the brain. Entire food families can cause such allergic reactions in susceptible individuals. Recurrent headaches, or schizophrenic, violent, or aggressive reactions, can be an indicator of cerebral allergy. Foods such as corn, wheat, rice, milk, and chocolate, and certain food additives, are the most common offenders.

❑ *The British Medical Journal* reported that taking aspirin before consuming an allergenic food makes it possible for more of the allergy-provoking food to be absorbed. In contrast, taking Aerobic Bulk Cleanse from Aerobic Life Industries combined with aloe vera juice may slow the absorption of foods that cause a reaction. Taking oat bran or guar gum in the morning works in the same way. Wheat bran is not recommended as a source of fiber for allergy-prone individuals because wheat is highly allergenic. (*See* NATURAL FOOD SUPPLEMENTS in Part One for a discussion of fiber.)

❑ Many allergy sufferers are turning to homeopathic remedies to combat allergy symptoms. They work with the body's natural functions to shut off the allergic response instead of masking symptoms. Combination remedies are often the easiest way to use homeopathy for allergies. BioAllers has a line of homeopathic combination remedies designed for specific allergies, including Animal Hair/Dander, Grain/Dairy, Grass Pollen, Mold/Yeast/Dust, Pollen/Hayfever, Sinus & Allergy Nasal Spray, and Tree Pollen Allergy Relief formulas.

❑ Research is being conducted on the ability of coenzyme Q_{10} to counter histamine for asthma and allergy sufferers.

❑ The Allergy and Asthma Relief Catalog is a free catalog of useful products for allergy sufferers. To order, call 1–800–553–5398.

Sulfite Allergies

Sulfites are common food additives used as sanitary agents and preservatives to prevent discoloration of foods. They are usually used in restaurant salad bars and are also present in many supermarket foods, including frozen foods, dried fruits, and certain fresh fruits and vegetables.

Many people are allergic to sulfites. The types and severity of reactions to sulfites in sensitive individuals vary, and may include breathing difficulties, anaphylactic shock, severe headaches, abdominal pain, stuffy and/or runny nose, flushing of the face and a "hot flash" feeling, diarrhea, irritability, and/or feelings of anger. These symptoms tend to occur quickly, usually within twenty to thirty minutes after consuming sulfites.

Sulfites pose a greater danger to some people than to others. People with asthma, a history of allergies, or a deficiency of the liver enzyme sulfite oxidase can suffer great harm. Sulfites have been implicated in at least thirteen deaths in the United States.

It is not always easy to determine if a food product contains sulfites. Sulfiting agents appear in food ingredient lists in a variety of ways, including *sodium sulfite, sodium bisulfite, sodium metabisulfite, potassium bisulfite, potassium metabisulfite,* and *sulfur dioxide.* Any ingredient ending in *-sulfite* should be assumed to be a sulfiting agent. If you have ever suffered a reaction after ingesting a food you believe contained sulfites, you should beware of the foods and beverages listed in the table below, which often contain these substances. Sulfite-free forms of some of these foods may be found in health food stores.

FOODS AND BEVERAGES THAT OFTEN CONTAIN SULFITES

Fresh Fruits and Beverages

Avocado dip (guacamole)	Grapes	Potatoes	Prepared cut fruit or
Cole slaw	Mushrooms		vegetable salads

Fish and Shellfish

Canned seafood soups	Dried fish	Frozen, canned, or dried	Oysters
Clams	Fresh shellfish, especially	shellfish	Scallops
Crabs	shrimp	Lobster	Shrimp

Prepared Processed Foods

Beet sugars	Cornstarch	Horseradish	Sauerkraut
Breading mixes	Dietetic processed foods	Jams and jellies	Shredded coconut
Breakfast cereals	Dried or canned soups	Maraschino cherries	Trail mixes
Brown sugar	Dry salad dressing mixes	Noodle and rice mixes	Wine vinegar
Canned fruit pie fillings	Frozen, canned, or dried	Olives	
Canned mushrooms	fruits and vegetables	Onion relish	
Caramels	Frozen French fries	Pickles	
Corn, maple, and	Glazed fruits	Potato chips	
pancake syrups	Hard candies	Sauces and gravies	

Miscellaneous

Apple cider	Bottled, canned, or frozen	Cordials	Gelatin
Baked goods	vegetable juices	Cornmeal	Instant tea mixes
Beer	Cocktail mixes	Frozen doughs	Wines
Bottled, canned, or frozen	Colas	Fruit drinks	
fruit juices			
vegetable juices			

Detecting Hidden Food Allergies

The first step in discovering hidden food allergies is to develop a list of suspect foods. Using the form below, keep track of how often you consume different foods. Be careful to note each time you consume one of the foods listed below. Add up your weekly total for each food. Do this for a four-week period.

FOOD SENSITIVITY QUESTIONNAIRE

Type of Food	First Week	Second Week	Third Week	Fourth Week
Beans and Legumes				
Kidney beans	_____	_____	_____	_____
Lentils	_____	_____	_____	_____
Lima beans	_____	_____	_____	_____
Mung beans	_____	_____	_____	_____
Pinto beans	_____	_____	_____	_____
Soybeans	_____	_____	_____	_____
Soymilk	_____	_____	_____	_____
Tofu and tofu products	_____	_____	_____	_____
White beans	_____	_____	_____	_____
Condiments				
Catsup	_____	_____	_____	_____
Gravy	_____	_____	_____	_____
Jams and jellies	_____	_____	_____	_____
Mustard	_____	_____	_____	_____
Pepper	_____	_____	_____	_____
Pickles	_____	_____	_____	_____
Salsa	_____	_____	_____	_____
Salt	_____	_____	_____	_____
Soy sauce	_____	_____	_____	_____
Dairy Products				
Butter	_____	_____	_____	_____
Buttermilk	_____	_____	_____	_____
Cheese	_____	_____	_____	_____
Cottage cheese	_____	_____	_____	_____
Cow's milk	_____	_____	_____	_____
Cream cheese	_____	_____	_____	_____
Eggs	_____	_____	_____	_____
Goat's milk	_____	_____	_____	_____
Ice cream	_____	_____	_____	_____
Margarine	_____	_____	_____	_____
Milk shake	_____	_____	_____	_____
Sour cream	_____	_____	_____	_____
Yogurt	_____	_____	_____	_____

Type of Food	First Week	Second Week	Third Week	Fourth Week
Fruits and Their Juices				
Apples	_____	_____	_____	_____
Apricots	_____	_____	_____	_____
Bananas	_____	_____	_____	_____
Blackberries	_____	_____	_____	_____
Blueberries	_____	_____	_____	_____
Cherries	_____	_____	_____	_____
Coconut	_____	_____	_____	_____
Cranberries	_____	_____	_____	_____
Dates	_____	_____	_____	_____
Dried fruits (most)	_____	_____	_____	_____
Figs	_____	_____	_____	_____
Grapefruit	_____	_____	_____	_____
Grapes	_____	_____	_____	_____
Lemons	_____	_____	_____	_____
Melons	_____	_____	_____	_____
Oranges	_____	_____	_____	_____
Nectarines	_____	_____	_____	_____
Papayas	_____	_____	_____	_____
Peaches	_____	_____	_____	_____
Pears	_____	_____	_____	_____
Pineapple	_____	_____	_____	_____
Plums	_____	_____	_____	_____
Prunes	_____	_____	_____	_____
Raisins	_____	_____	_____	_____
Raspberries	_____	_____	_____	_____
Strawberries	_____	_____	_____	_____
Tangerines	_____	_____	_____	_____
Grains and Grain Products				
Brown rice	_____	_____	_____	_____
Buckwheat	_____	_____	_____	_____
Cold cereal	_____	_____	_____	_____
Cornmeal	_____	_____	_____	_____
Millet	_____	_____	_____	_____
Oats	_____	_____	_____	_____
Quinoa	_____	_____	_____	_____
Pancakes	_____	_____	_____	_____
Pasta	_____	_____	_____	_____
Rye	_____	_____	_____	_____
Spelt	_____	_____	_____	_____
Tapioca	_____	_____	_____	_____
Wheat and whole-wheat products	_____	_____	_____	_____
White flour products	_____	_____	_____	_____
White rice	_____	_____	_____	_____

Type of Food	First Week	Second Week	Third Week	Fourth Week
Meats, Poultry, and Fish				
Bacon	_____	_____	_____	_____
Beef	_____	_____	_____	_____
Bologna	_____	_____	_____	_____
Chicken	_____	_____	_____	_____
Fish	_____	_____	_____	_____
Ham	_____	_____	_____	_____
Lamb	_____	_____	_____	_____
Liver	_____	_____	_____	_____
Luncheon meat	_____	_____	_____	_____
Pork	_____	_____	_____	_____
Sausage	_____	_____	_____	_____
Shellfish	_____	_____	_____	_____
Turkey	_____	_____	_____	_____
Veal	_____	_____	_____	_____
Nuts and Seeds				
Almonds	_____	_____	_____	_____
Brazil nuts	_____	_____	_____	_____
Cashews	_____	_____	_____	_____
Chestnuts	_____	_____	_____	_____
Hazelnuts	_____	_____	_____	_____
Nut butter (other than peanut)	_____	_____	_____	_____
Nut milk	_____	_____	_____	_____
Peanut butter	_____	_____	_____	_____
Peanuts	_____	_____	_____	_____
Pecans	_____	_____	_____	_____
Pistachios	_____	_____	_____	_____
Sesame seeds	_____	_____	_____	_____
Sunflower seeds	_____	_____	_____	_____
Walnuts	_____	_____	_____	_____
Oils				
Canola oil	_____	_____	_____	_____
Corn oil	_____	_____	_____	_____
Cottonseed oil	_____	_____	_____	_____
Olive oil	_____	_____	_____	_____
Peanut oil	_____	_____	_____	_____
Safflower oil	_____	_____	_____	_____
Sesame oil	_____	_____	_____	_____
Soy oil	_____	_____	_____	_____

Type of Food	First Week	Second Week	Third Week	Fourth Week
Sweeteners				
Aspartame (NutraSweet)	_____	_____	_____	_____
Brown sugar	_____	_____	_____	_____
Corn syrup	_____	_____	_____	_____
Fructose	_____	_____	_____	_____
Honey	_____	_____	_____	_____
Maple syrup	_____	_____	_____	_____
Saccharin	_____	_____	_____	_____
White sugar	_____	_____	_____	_____
Vegetables				
Alfalfa sprouts	_____	_____	_____	_____
Artichokes	_____	_____	_____	_____
Asparagus	_____	_____	_____	_____
Avocado	_____	_____	_____	_____
Beets	_____	_____	_____	_____
Broccoli	_____	_____	_____	_____
Brussels sprouts	_____	_____	_____	_____
Cabbage	_____	_____	_____	_____
Carrots	_____	_____	_____	_____
Cauliflower	_____	_____	_____	_____
Celery	_____	_____	_____	_____
Corn	_____	_____	_____	_____
Cucumbers	_____	_____	_____	_____
Eggplant	_____	_____	_____	_____
Garlic	_____	_____	_____	_____
Green beans	_____	_____	_____	_____
Kale	_____	_____	_____	_____
Lettuce	_____	_____	_____	_____
Mushrooms	_____	_____	_____	_____
Okra	_____	_____	_____	_____
Olives	_____	_____	_____	_____
Onions	_____	_____	_____	_____
Parsley	_____	_____	_____	_____
Peas	_____	_____	_____	_____
Peppers	_____	_____	_____	_____
Potatoes	_____	_____	_____	_____
Radishes	_____	_____	_____	_____
Spinach	_____	_____	_____	_____
Summer squash	_____	_____	_____	_____
Sweet potatoes	_____	_____	_____	_____
Swiss chard	_____	_____	_____	_____
Tomatoes	_____	_____	_____	_____
Turnips	_____	_____	_____	_____
Winter squash	_____	_____	_____	_____
Zucchini	_____	_____	_____	_____

Type of Food	First Week	Second Week	Third Week	Fourth Week
Miscellaneous and Junk Foods				
Alcoholic beverages	_____	_____	_____	_____
Candy	_____	_____	_____	_____
Cheeseburger	_____	_____	_____	_____
Chewing gum	_____	_____	_____	_____
Chocolate	_____	_____	_____	_____
Coffee	_____	_____	_____	_____
Cola	_____	_____	_____	_____
Corn chips	_____	_____	_____	_____
Flavored gelatin	_____	_____	_____	_____
French fries	_____	_____	_____	_____
Fried foods	_____	_____	_____	_____
Hamburger	_____	_____	_____	_____
Pastry	_____	_____	_____	_____
Peppermint	_____	_____	_____	_____
Pizza	_____	_____	_____	_____
Popcorn	_____	_____	_____	_____
Potato chips	_____	_____	_____	_____
Pudding	_____	_____	_____	_____
Tea	_____	_____	_____	_____

Note any other snacks or other foods not listed above that you eat regularly. _____

_____

After the one-month recording period, go through the form and compile a list of all the foods you ate four times a week or more. This is your list of suspect foods.

KEEPING A FOOD DIARY

Once you have your list of suspect foods, omit these foods from your diet for a period of thirty days to give your body a rest from them. Then reintroduce the suspect foods, one at a time. Add only one new food a day. As you add foods back to your diet, keep a diary of any symptoms you experience and monitor your reaction with the Food Allergy Self-Test (see page 154), as in the following sample:

Sample Food Diary

Date	Meal	Time	Foods Consumed	Symptoms
4/12	Breakfast	8:39 a.m.	milk, toast	gas, bloating
	Lunch	12:30 p.m.	pea soup, salad	no symptoms

If you note a reaction to any of the reintroduced foods, omit that food from your diet for another two months, then try a small amount of it again. If you have a reaction after the second reintroduction, eliminate that food from your diet permanently.

Use the form that follows to record your experiences as you reintroduce the banished foods into your diet. By first eliminating foods, then slowly adding them back into your diet, you will be able to pinpoint exactly which foods are giving you trouble.

Food Diary

Date	Meal	Time	Foods Consumed	Symptoms
_____	Breakfast			
_____	Lunch			
_____	Dinner			
_____	Snack			
_____	Breakfast			
_____	Lunch			
_____	Dinner			
_____	Snack			
_____	Breakfast			
_____	Lunch			
_____	Dinner			
_____	Snack			
_____	Breakfast			
_____	Lunch			
_____	Dinner			
_____	Snack			
_____	Breakfast			
_____	Lunch			
_____	Dinner			
_____	Snack			
_____	Breakfast			
_____	Lunch			
_____	Dinner			
_____	Snack			
_____	Breakfast			
_____	Lunch			
_____	Dinner			
_____	Snack			

Medications:_____

_____

_____

Herbs: _____

_____

Miscellaneous:_____

_____

When monitoring your reactions to different foods, it is important to be aware that food allergies can manifest themselves in many ways, not all of them obvious. The following symptoms are the most common manifestations of food allergies:

- Acne, especially pimples on the chin or around the mouth.

- Arthritis.

- Asthma.

- Chest and shoulder pains.

- Colitis.

- Depression.

- Fatigue.

- Food cravings.

- Headaches.

- Hemorrhoids.

- Insomnia.

- Intestinal problems.

- Muscle disorders.

- Obesity.

- Sinus problems.

- Ulcers.

- Unexplained dramatic weight gain or loss.

Your health care provider may look also for the following signs and symptoms when trying to determine if you have an allergy:

- Acid/alkaline imbalance.

- Anemia.

- Bed-wetting.

- Conjunctivitis.

- Diarrhea.

- Dizzy spells and floating sensations.

- Excessive drooling.

- Dark circles under the eyes or puffy eyes.

- Eye pain, tearing.

- Fluid retention.

- Hearing loss.

- Hyperactivity.

- Learning disabilities.

- Nasal congestion or chronic runny nose.

- Noises in the ear.

- Periods of blurred vision.

- Phobias.

- Poor memory and concentration.

- Poor muscle coordination.

- Red circles on the cheeks (as if wearing rouge, even in children).

- Repeated colds or ear infections, especially in children.

- Sensitivity to light.

- Severe menstrual symptoms.

- Swollen fingers and cold hands.

- Unusual body odor.

- Watery, itchy, red eyes.

- Recurrence of any illness despite treatment.

THE ROTATION DIET

Although some people have a reaction soon after ingesting a particular food for the first time, food allergies often develop slowly. The reason for this is that if you consume the same foods daily, your body eventually develops an intolerance to them. Rather than nourishing the body, these foods provoke harmful reactions.

Once you have identified and avoided an allergenic food for sixty to ninety days, you can usually reintroduce it without any adverse reactions, as long as you maintain a rotation diet. The basic principle behind the rotation diet is that each type of food is to be consumed only on one out of every four days. For example, if you eat beans on Monday, you wouldn't eat beans again on Tuesday, Wednesday, or Thursday. If you eat salmon on Friday, you would wait at least until Tuesday before consuming any other fish. Rotating foods in this way will not only make you feel better, it will also help to stabilize your weight.

Before starting the rotation diet, follow a fasting program to cleanse your system of offending foods and toxins. (*See* FASTING in Part Three.) After you have finished the program, consume only the following foods for the next two weeks:

- Baked or broiled chicken or turkey.

- Broiled, boiled, or baked fish.

- Brown rice.

- Fresh, unsweetened fruit and vegetable juices.

- Fresh fruits (except oranges).

- Herbal teas.

- Raw, steamed, or broiled vegetables.

Although you may feel that this list of foods does not offer much variety, there are numerous fruits and vegetables available, in addition to a variety of fish. After two weeks on this cleansing diet, you can once again begin to eat a greater number of different foods, but on a rotating basis, eating each type of food on no more than one out of four days. Use the sample menus below as a guide to help you put together daily menus rotating among different foods. Of course, if you are sensitive to any of the foods listed, substitute a food that agrees with you. Once you start following this program, you should start seeing an increase in your energy level in a week or less.

Rotating Foods: Sample Daily Menus

Breakfast	Lunch	Dinner	Snacks
Day 1			
Glass of distilled water Papaya juice with vitamin C Fresh papaya or peach Oatmeal or oat bran cereal with 1 tbsp raw honey Skim milk Rose hip tea	Tomato stuffed with tuna salad or tuna burger on wheat-free bread with tomato, onion, alfalfa sprouts, and eggless mayonnaise Fresh lemonade	Broiled whitefish or salmon with dill Cole slaw or sprout salad with tomato, onion, celery, and eggless mayonnaise Steamed asparagus Herbal tea or lemonade *Substitutions:* Cauliflower, Brussels sprouts, or sauerkraut can be substituted for asparagus.	Celery sticks Pecans Fresh papaya or peach
Day 2			
Glass of distilled water Apple juice with vitamin C Fresh apple Cream of wheat cereal with with 2 tsp pure maple syrup and soymilk Herbal tea	Home-cooked sliced turkey or chicken on whole wheat bread with lettuce and mustard Potato soup and wheat crackers (make soup with soymilk) Herbal tea or apple juice *Substitutions:* Soy burger or eggless egg salad with eggless mayonnaise for turkey or chicken; tofu soup for potato soup.	Baked skinless turkey or chicken with lemon juice, garlic, and onion powder Baked potato with 2 tsp sesame oil, chopped chives, and a dash of onion powder Tossed salad with radishes, zucchini, yellow squash, kale, and soy oil dressing Herbal tea *Substitutions:* Cornish game hens for turkey or chicken; vinaigrette dressing for soy oil dressing.	Apple Walnuts *Substitutions:* Baked apple with pure maple syrup; wheat crackers; sugar-free applesauce topped with walnuts.
Day 3			
Glass of distilled water Cranberry juice with vitamin C Sliced banana with almond milk Cream of rice or puffed rice cereal Herbal tea	1/2 avocado filled with cooked brown rice and fresh peas, water chestnuts, and a dash of herbal seasoning and lemon juice, topped with slivered almonds Split pea soup with rice crackers (make soup with rice milk)	Stir-fried vegetables with broccoli, green peppers, leeks, pea pods, sweet red peppers, bean sprouts, bamboo shoots, and grated fresh ginger, served over cooked brown rice Rice cakes with almond butter Coffee substitute (from a health food store) or herbal tea	Raw almonds Rice crackers with almond butter Sliced bananas

---

Day 4

Glass of distilled water
Grape juice with vitamin C
2 poached or soft-boiled
    eggs or corn cereal
Rye toast with sugar-free
    grape jam
Herbal tea

Egg salad with chopped
    cucumber, green onions,
    black olives, and low-fat
    cottage cheese, topped
    with raisins
RyKrisp crackers with
    sugar-free grape jelly
    or jam
Lentil soup or cool lentil
    salad

Spinach mushroom quiche
Fresh spinach salad with
    hard-boiled eggs,
    artichoke, shredded raw
    beets, raisins, and olive
    oil and lemon dressing
Iced herbal tea flavored
    with grape juice

RyKrisp crackers with
    sugar-free grape jam
    or sesame butter and
    sesame seeds
Fresh grapes
Raisins
Hard-boiled eggs

❑ *See also* CHEMICAL ALLERGIES in Part Two and FASTING in Part Three.

❑ For information about organizations that can provide information and assistance for people with allergies, *see* HEALTH AND MEDICAL ORGANIZATIONS in the Appendix.

Alopecia

See HAIR LOSS.

Aluminum Toxicity

Aluminum is not a heavy metal, but it can be toxic if present in excessive amounts—even in small amounts, if it is deposited in the brain. Many of the symptoms of aluminum toxicity are similar to those of Alzheimer's disease and osteoporosis. Aluminum toxicity can lead to colic, rickets, gastrointestinal disturbances, poor calcium metabolism, extreme nervousness, anemia, headaches, decreased liver and kidney function, forgetfulness, speech disturbances, memory loss, softening of the bones, and weak, aching muscles.

Because aluminum is excreted through the kidneys, toxic amounts of aluminum may impair kidney function. The accumulation of aluminum salts in the brain has been implicated in seizures and reduced mental faculties. To reach the brain, aluminum must pass the blood-brain barrier, an elaborate structure that filters the blood before it reaches this vital organ. Elemental aluminum does not readily pass through this barrier, but certain aluminum compounds, such as aluminum fluoride, do. Many municipal water supplies are treated with both alum (aluminum sulfate) and fluoride, and these two chemicals readily combine with each other in the blood. Moreover, aluminum fluoride, once formed, is very poorly excreted in the urine.

Intestinal absorption of high levels of aluminum and silicon can result in the formation of compounds that accumulate in the cerebral cortex and prevent nerve impulses from being carried to and from the brain in the proper manner. Chronic calcium deficiency can aggravate the situation. People who have worked in aluminum smelting plants for long periods have been known to experience dizziness, impaired coordination, and a loss of balance and energy. The accumulation of aluminum in the brain has been cited as a possible cause for these symptoms. Perhaps most alarming, there is evidence to suggest that long-term accumulation of aluminum in the brain may contribute to the development of Alzheimer's disease.

It has been estimated that the average person ingests between 3 and 10 milligrams of aluminum a day. Aluminum is the most abundant metallic element in the earth's crust. It is absorbed into the body primarily through the digestive tract, but also through the lungs and skin, and is absorbed by and accumulates in body tissues. Because aluminum permeates our air, water, and soil, it is found naturally in varying amounts in nearly all food and water. Aluminum is also used to make cookware, cooking utensils, and foil. Many other everyday products contain aluminum as well, including over-the-counter painkillers, anti-inflammatories, and douche preparations. Aluminum is an additive in most baking powders, is used in food processing, and is present in products ranging from antiperspirants and toothpaste to dental amalgams to bleached flour, grated cheese, table salt, and beer (especially when packaged in aluminum cans). One prominent source of aluminum is our municipal water supplies.

The excessive use of antacids is probably the most common cause of aluminum toxicity in this country, especially in people who have kidney problems. Many over-the-counter antacids contain amounts of aluminum hydroxide that may be too much for the kidneys to excrete successfully. Even antacids containing a mixture of aluminum and other ingredients may pose a problem; in some people, such products may cause the same reaction as products composed entirely of aluminum compounds.

NUTRIENTS

SUPPLEMENT	SUGGESTED DOSAGE	COMMENTS
Helpful		
Apple pectin	2 tbsp twice daily.	Binds with metals in the colon and excretes them from the body.
Calcium and magnesium	1,500 mg daily. 750 mg daily.	Minerals that bind with aluminum and eliminate it from the body. Use chelate forms.
Coenzyme A from Coenzyme-A Technologies	As directed on label.	Supports the immune system's detoxification of many dangerous substances.
Garlic (Kyolic from Wakunaga)	2 capsules 3 times daily.	Acts as a detoxifier.
Kelp	2,000–3,000 mg daily.	Has a balanced mineral content. Acts as a detoxifier of excess metals.
Lecithin granules or capsules	1 tbsp 3 times daily, before meals. 1,200 mg 3 times daily, before meals.	Aids in healing of the brain and cell membranes.
L-Glutathione	As directed on label.	Aids in blocking damage from toxic metals and radiation.
Multivitamin and mineral complex	As directed on label.	Basic for stabilizing vitamin and mineral imbalances in toxic conditions. Use a hypoallergenic high-potency formula.
Oxy-Cleanse from Earth's Bounty	As directed on label.	Helps remove heavy metals, other pollutants, and anaerobic pathogens from the body.
S-Adenosylmethionine (SAMe)	As directed on label.	Helps reduce stress and nervousness caused by excess aluminum. *Caution:* Do not use if you have manic-depressive disorder or take prescription antidepressants.
Vitamin B complex plus extra vitamin B_6 and vitamin B_{12}	100 mg of each major B vitamin 3 times daily (amounts of individual vitamins in a complex will vary). 50 mg 3 times daily. 300 mcg 3 times daily.	The B vitamins, especially B_6, are important in ridding the intestinal tract of excess metals and in removing them from the body. Sublingual forms are recommended for better absorption. Injections (under a doctor's supervision) may be necessary.
Vitamin E	600 IU daily.	A powerful antioxidant. Fights cellular aging by protecting cell membranes. Also improves circulation and prolongs the life of red blood cells. Use d-alpha-tocopherol form.

HERBS

❏ Burdock root, echinacea, ginseng, ginkgo biloba, and fiber, when taken regularly, are beneficial for blocking damage to the body by toxic heavy metals and radiation.

Caution: Do not take echinacea if you have an autoimmune disorder.

RECOMMENDATIONS

❏ Maintain a diet that is high in fiber and includes apple pectin.

❏ Use only stainless steel, glass, or iron cookware. Stainless steel is best.

❏ Beware of products containing aluminum. Read labels and avoid those that contain aluminum, or dihydroxyaluminum.

CONSIDERATIONS

❏ A hair analysis can be used to determine levels of aluminum in the body. (*See* HAIR ANALYSIS in Part Three.)

❏ If you use chelation therapy, use oral chelating agents only (*see* CHELATION THERAPY in Part Three). Many researchers believe aluminum cannot be chelated out of the body, as some metals can, but *can* be displaced or moved.

❏ Some research indicates that the longer you cook food in aluminum pots, the more they corrode, and the more aluminum compounds migrate into food and are absorbed by the body. Aluminum is more readily dissolved by acid-forming foods, such as coffee, cheeses, meats, black and green tea, cabbage, cucumbers, tomatoes, turnips, spinach, and radishes.

❏ Acid rain leeches aluminum out of the soil and into drinking water.

❏ *See also* ALZHEIMER'S DISEASE in Part Two.

Alzheimer's Disease

Alzheimer's disease is a common type of dementia, or decline in intellectual function. Once thought rare, Alzheimer's disease is now known to affect more than 4.1 million people in the United States. It afflicts 10 percent of Americans over sixty-five and as many as 50 percent of those over eighty-five. However, the disease does not affect only the elderly, but may strike when a person is in his or her forties.

This disorder was first identified in 1906 by a German neurologist named Alois Alzheimer. It is characterized by progressive mental deterioration to such a degree that it interferes with one's ability to function socially and at work. Memory and abstract thought processes are impaired. Alzheimer's disease is an irreversible, progressive disorder. Deterioration in critical areas of the brain may precede symptoms by as much as twenty to forty years. As Alzheimer's disease progresses, there is severe memory loss, particularly in short-term memory. The person may recall distant events but is unable to remember a just-viewed television show. At this stage, disorientation usually begins as well. Dysphasia (the inability to find the right word) may occur, and mood swings can be unpredictable and sudden. In the final stage, Alzheimer's disease creates severe confusion and disorientation, and possibly hallucinations or delusions. Some people become violent and angry, while others may be docile and passive. It is in this later stage that people with Alzheimer's disease may wander without purpose, experience incontinence, and neglect personal hygiene. Since the behavioral symptoms of Alzheimer's disease result from changes in the brain, the person neither intends nor can control this behavior.

Once considered a psychological phenomenon, Alzheimer's disease is now known to be a degenerative disorder that is characterized by a specific set of physiological changes in the brain. Nerve fibers surrounding the hippocampus, the brain's memory center, become tangled, and information is no longer carried properly to or from the brain. New memories cannot be formed, and memories formed earlier cannot be retrieved. Characteristic plaques accumulate in the brain as well. These plaques are composed largely of a protein-containing substance called beta-amyloid. Scientists believe that the plaques accumulate in and damage nerve cells.

Many people worry that their forgetfulness is a sign of Alzheimer's disease. Most of us forget where we have put our keys or other everyday objects at one time or another, but this is not an indication of Alzheimer's disease. A good example of the difference between forgetfulness and dementia is the following: If you do not remember where you put your glasses, that is *forgetfulness*. If you do not remember that you wear glasses, that may be a sign of *dementia*.

Other disorders can cause symptoms similar to those of Alzheimer's disease. Dementia may result from arteriosclerosis (hardening of the arteries) that slowly cuts off the supply of blood to the brain. The death of brain tissue from a series of minor strokes, or from pressure exerted by an accumulation of fluid in the brain, may cause dementia. The presence of small blood clots in vessels that supply the brain, a brain tumor, hypothyroidism, and advanced syphilis all can cause symptoms similar to those of Alzheimer's disease. In addition, the average person over the age of sixty-five is likely to be taking between eight and ten different prescription and over-the-counter drugs. Drug reactions, coupled with a nutrient-poor diet, often adversely affect people not only physically, but mentally as well.

The precise cause or causes of Alzheimer's disease are unknown, but research reveals a number of interesting clues. Many of them point to nutritional deficiencies. For example, people with Alzheimer's tend to have low levels of vitamin B_{12} and zinc in their bodies. The B vitamins are important in cognitive functioning, and it is well known that the processed foods constituting so much of the modern diet have been stripped of these essential nutrients. The development of the neurofibrillary tangles and amyloid plaques in the brain that are characteristic of the disease have been associated with zinc deficiency. Malabsorption problems, which are common among elderly people, make them more prone than others to nutritional deficiencies. Alcohol and many medications further deplete crucial vitamins and minerals.

Levels of the antioxidant vitamins A and E and the carotenoids (including beta-carotene) also are low in people with Alzheimer's disease. These nutrients act as free radical scavengers; deficiencies may expose the brain cells to increased oxidative damage. In addition, deficiencies of boron, potassium, and selenium have been found in people with Alzheimer's disease.

Some research has drawn a connection between Alzheimer's disease and high concentrations of aluminum in the brain. Autopsies of people who have died of Alzheimer's disease reveal excessive amounts of aluminum in the hippocampus area and in the cerebral cortex, the external layer of gray matter responsible for higher brain functions such as abstract thinking, judgment, memory, and language. It may be that exposure to excessive amounts of aluminum, especially if combined with a lack of essential vitamins, minerals, and antioxidants predispose one to developing Alzheimer's disease. However, one recent study, published in *Archives of Neurology* in May 1998, showed no further correlation between the density of neurofibrillary tangles in the frontal and temporal lobes of the cortex and bulk aluminum concentration. This study further demonstrated that levels of aluminum are not elevated in the cerebrospinal fluid of patients with Alzheimer's disease.

Brains of people with Alzheimer's disease have been found to contain higher than normal concentrations of the toxic metal mercury. For most people, the release of mercury from dental amalgams is the primary means of mercury exposure, and a direct correlation has been demonstrated between the amount of inorganic mercury in the brain and the number of amalgam surfaces in the mouth. Mercury from dental amalgam passes into body tissues, and it accumulates in the body over time. Mercury exposure, especially from dental amalgams, cannot be excluded as a major contributor to Alzheimer's disease.

Many people who develop Alzheimer's disease have a family history of the disorder, suggesting that heredity may be involved. By age ninety, the risk is at least 50 percent for those with a first-degree relative (father, mother, brother, sister) who has (or had) Alzheimer's disease. The equivalent rate is about 50 percent for identical twins. As with other brain disorders, such as schizophrenia and manic-depressive disorder, the hereditary pattern is complicated. At least four gene variations are linked to Alzheimer's disease. All of them reduce the clearance, or increase the production, of beta-amyloid. A variation of a gene involved in the synthesis of beta-amyloid, located on chromosome 21, is associated with a rare type of Alzheimer's disease that typically begins between the ages of forty and fifty. Interestingly, people with Down syndrome, who carry an extra copy of chromosome 21, are prone to develop very early Alzheimer's disease, beginning in their thirties and forties.

Yet another possible culprit in the death of brain cells is the immune system. Many illnesses result from immune system malfunction causing it to attack the body's own tissues. Powerful immune system proteins called *complement proteins* have been found around the plaques and tangles in the brains of people who have died of Alzheimer's disease. In animals, brain injury is known to result in an alteration in the genetic "instructions" for two kinds of complement proteins. Some experts theorize that complement proteins normally help clear away dead cells, but in Alzheimer's disease, they begin to attack healthy cells as well. Cell degeneration results in accumulations of amyloid. Many researchers believe that beta-amyloid is a key player in this memory-destroying disease. This substance is not unique to the brain, but is produced in virtually every cell in the body as a result of the degeneration of tissue. Amyloid itself is not highly toxic, but it might possibly trigger dementia if a critical mass accumulates in the brain. Further evidence reveals that the presence of amyloid may trigger the release of a cascade of complement proteins, perhaps sparking a vicious cycle of inflammation and further plaque deposits. However, an immune system attack on brain cells may be a result, or may be merely one element, of Alzheimer's disease, rather than the cause. Other potential risk factors being studied are head injury, very high blood pressure, and low education levels.

Although all of these findings offer hope that Alzheimer's disease may one day be fully understood, and thereby prevented, science does not yet know what can be done to arrest the mental deterioration. Even diagnosis of the disease is not a precise science. There are tests that can suggest a diagnosis of Alzheimer's and that can dismiss other problems as the cause of symptoms, but there currently is no single laboratory procedure or biochemical marker that can definitively confirm the disorder in a living person. Physicians can, however, make a *probable* diagnosis by performing a comprehensive evaluation including a complete health history and physical examination, a mental status assessment, neurological tests, blood tests, urinalysis, an electrocardiogram (EKG), and x-rays. Additional tests may be conducted, such as a computerized tomography (CT) scan, electroencephalography (EEG, a recording of brain-wave patterns), and formal psychiatric assessment. These tests are necessary to rule out other possible causes of dementia symptoms, such as pernicious anemia, hypothyroidism, or tumors. Documenting symptoms over time, in a diary-like fashion, helps doctors to understand each individual case. Unfortunately, the diagnosis of Alzheimer's disease is often made long after the person has lost the ability to communicate and comprehend information. As more is learned about the contribution of genetic and other factors to Alzheimer's disease, the possibility of delaying the progression of disease may become more real.

NUTRIENTS

SUPPLEMENT	SUGGESTED DOSAGE	COMMENTS
Essential		
Acetylcholine	500 mg 3 times daily, on an empty stomach.	Deficiency has been implicated as possibly causing dementia.
Acetyl-L-carnitine	500 mg twice daily.	May enhance brain metabolism. Slows down deterioration of memory and reduces the production of free radicals.
Boron	3 mg daily. Do not exceed this amount.	Improves brain and memory function.
Coenzyme A from Coenzyme-A Technologies	As directed on label.	Supports the immune system's detoxification of many dangerous substances.
Coenzyme Q$_{10}$	100–200 mg daily.	Increases oxygenation of cells and is involved in the generation of cellular energy.
Folic acid	As directed on label.	To aid in controlling homocysteine levels. Studies have shown high levels of homocysteine in this disorder.
Iron	As directed by physician.	A deficiency may be present. *Caution:* Do not take iron unless prescribed by your physician.
Lecithin granules or capsules	1 tbsp 3 times daily, before meals. 1,200 mg 3 times daily, before meals.	Needed for improved memory. Contains choline.
Multivitamin and mineral complex with potassium	99 mg daily.	All nutrients are necessary in balance. Use a high-potency formula. Needed for proper electrolyte balance.
Phosphatidyl serine	300 mg 3 times daily.	Improves memory.
Pycnogenol or grape seed extract	60 mg three times daily. As directed on label.	Potent antioxidants that readily pass the blood-brain barrier to protect brain cells from free radical damage.
S-Adenosylmethionine (SAMe)	400 mg twice daily.	Lowers homocysteine levels. *Caution:* Do not use if you have manic-depressive disorder or take prescription antidepressants.
Selenium	200 mcg daily.	Powerful antioxidant for brain cell protection.
Trimethylglycine (TMG)	500–1,000 mg daily, in the morning.	Assists the body in utilizing vitamin B$_{12}$, folic acid, and vitamin B$_6$. It also helps to rid the body of toxic elements (such as homocysteine) and increases levels of the natural mood elevator S-adenosylmethionine.
Vitamin A plus carotenoids (including beta-carotene) and vitamin E	15,000 IU daily. 25,000 IU daily. Start at 400 IU daily and increase slowly to 800 IU daily.	Deficiencies of antioxidants expose the brain to oxidative damage. An antioxidant that helps in the transport of oxygen to the brain cells and protects them from free radical damage. Use d-alpha-tocopherol form. *Caution:* If you are taking blood-thinning medication, consult your physician before taking vitamin E.

Vitamin B complex injections plus extra	2 cc 3 times weekly or as prescribed by physician.	Needed for brain function; aids in the digestion of food.
vitamin B₆ (pyridoxine) and	$1/2$ cc once weekly or as prescribed by physician.	Deficiency can cause depression and mental difficulties.
vitamin B₁₂	1 cc 3 times weekly or as prescribed by physician.	Important for brain function. Deficient in people with Alzheimer's. Injections (under a doctor's supervision) are fast and produce good results. If injections are not available, use a sublingual form.
or Vitamin B complex	100 mg of each major B vitamin 3 times daily (amounts of individual vitamins in a complex will vary).	
plus extra pantothenic acid (vitamin B₅)	100 mg 3 times daily.	Plays a role in converting choline into acetylcholine, needed for memory.
Zinc	50–100 mg daily. Do not exceed this amount.	Helps stop amyloid plaque formation induced by zinc deficiency.

Important		
Apple pectin	As directed on label.	Aids in removing toxic metals such as mercury, which can contribute to dementia.
Calcium and	1,600 mg daily, at bedtime.	Has a calming effect and works with magnesium.
magnesium	800 mg daily.	Acts as a natural calcium channel blocker.
Free-form amino acid complex	1,000–2,500 mg daily, 1 hour before meals. Take with 8 oz of fluid and a small amount of vitamins B₆ and C for better assimilation.	Needed for improved brain function and tissue repair. Use free-form amino acids for best absorption.
Huperzine A	100 mcg daily.	Improves cognitive functions and may improve short-term memory.
Kelp	1,000–1,500 mg daily.	Supplies needed minerals and aids in thyroid function.
Melatonin	2–3 mg daily, taken 2 hours or less before bedtime.	Improves brain function and aids sleep. Reduces cell destruction in the brain and has antioxidant properties.
RNA and DNA	As directed on label.	These are the brain's cellular building blocks. Use a formula containing 200 mg RNA and 100 mg DNA per tablet. *Caution:* Do not take this supplement if you have gout.
Superoxide dismutase (SOD) plus	As directed on label.	A potent antioxidant that improves utilization of oxygen.
copper	3 mg daily.	SOD needs copper to function properly as an antioxidant.
Vitamin C with bioflavonoids	6,000–10,000 mg daily in divided doses.	Enhances immune function and increases energy level; a powerful antioxidant. Use a buffered form.

HERBS

❏ Butcher's broom promotes healthy circulation.

❏ Ginkgo biloba extract, taken in liquid or capsule form, acts as an antioxidant and increases blood flow to the brain.

According to a report published in the October 22, 1977, edition of the *Journal of the American Medical Association* (JAMA), ginkgo biloba extract can stabilize and, in some cases, improve the mental functioning and social behavior of people with Alzheimer's disease. Take 100 to 200 mg of ginkgo biloba extract three times daily.

❏ Kava kava and St. John's wort help calm people who anger easily.

❏ The Chinese herb qian ceng ta (*Huperzia serata*) increases memory retention. This is the same herb that is the source of huperzine A, and it is also known as club moss. Pure and standardized extracts of this herb have been shown to increase clearheadedness, language ability, and memory in a significant percentage of subjects with Alzheimer's disease. It is a potent blocker of acetylcholinesterase, an enzyme that regulates the activity of acetylcholine, which is an important chemical of the brain that maintains healthy learning and memory functions.

❏ Valerian root improves sleep patterns when taken at bedtime.

RECOMMENDATIONS

❏ Eat a well-balanced diet of natural foods and follow the supplementation program recommended above.

❏ Have a hair analysis to rule out the possibility of heavy metal intoxication as the cause of symptoms. (*See* HAIR ANALYSIS in Part Three.)

❏ Include plenty of fiber in your diet. Try oat bran or rice bran.

❏ Have allergy testing performed to rule out environmental and/or food allergies. (*See* ALLERGIES in Part Two.)

❏ Avoid alcohol, cigarette smoke, processed foods, and environmental toxins, especially metals such as aluminum and mercury. Smoking more than doubles the risk of developing dementia and Alzheimer's disease, according to a study published in the British medical journal *The Lancet*. While recent studies have not substantiated a connection between aluminum and Alzheimer's disease, it is still wise to avoid aluminum intake as much as possible. All metals in excess are toxic to the body.

❏ Do not drink tap water, as it may contain aluminum. Consume steam-distilled water only and drink at least eight glasses a day. (*See* WATER in Part One.)

❏ If you are involved in caring for someone with Alzheimer's disease, seek counseling and support from the various agencies and groups, such as the Alzheimer's Association, that are trained to help. They can teach you how to handle such things as difficult behaviors. With aggressive behaviors, for example—whether name-calling, shouting, or physical aggression towards the caregiver—understanding *why* the the behavior occurred is the key. Some tips from the Alzheimer's Association: 1) Think about what happened just before the reaction that may have "triggered" the behavior; 2) look for the *feelings* behind the words; 3) be positive, reassuring, and speak slowly, with a *soft* tone; and 4) use music, massage, and/or exercise to help soothe the person. Memory loss and confusion can cause a person with Alzheimer's disease to become suspicious of those around him or her. If this occurs, try not to take offense or argue, but rather offer a simple answer or try to divert the person's attention to another activity.

CONSIDERATIONS

❑ Using your brain, remaining busy, writing, reading and learning new things are important overall factors in staying sharp and preventing mental disorders.

❑ Carbamazepine (Tegretol), an anti-seizure medication, can ease Alzheimer's-related anger and hostility, according to a recent study. Aggression was markedly reduced in three out of four of the Alzheimer's patients in the study.

❑ Recent studies show that the progression of Alzheimer's disease can be slowed or even reversed by reducing free radical accumulation through the use of antioxidants. Tests conducted in Switzerland over a twenty-two-year period produced evidence of significantly higher memory scores associated with antioxidant therapy.

❑ The herbs balm and sage are being researched for possible beneficial effects on brain chemistry. Balm appears to simulate the neurological receptors that bind acetylcholine. Sage contains compounds that are cholinesterase inhibitors.

❑ Preliminary studies performed on rats at the University of Washington in Seattle indicate that cat's claw, when mixed with other herbal extracts (such as ginkgo, gotu kola, and rosemary) inhibit the buildup of plaques in the brain.

❑ Vitamin E can slow the advancement of Alzheimer's disease by 25 percent, according to a study published in the April 24, 1997, issue of *The New England Journal of Medicine*.

❑ Some experts distinguish between a rapidly progressing form of Alzheimer's disease that begins earlier in life (usually between the ages of thirty-six and forty-five) and a more gradual form that develops in people around the ages of sixty-five or seventy. For more information, consult *Complete Guide to Symptoms, Illness and Surgery for People Over 50* by H. Winter Griffith, M.D. (The Body Press/Perigee Books, 1992).

❑ The signs of alcohol abuse and the symptoms of Alzheimer's can be very similar. For example, actress Rita Hayworth, who had Alzheimer's disease, was at first thought to be an alcoholic.

❑ No one should accept a diagnosis of Alzheimer's disease without first undergoing a trial of intensive nutritional therapy, particularly vitamin B_{12} injections. Vitamin B_{12} functions in numerous metabolic processes affecting nerve tissue, including the synthesis of neurotransmitters and the formation of the insulating sheath surrounding many nerves, and it may play a role in the fight against Alzheimer's disease. Strange prickly or tingling sensations, loss of coordination, and dementia can be caused by B_{12} deficiency even if the person does not have pernicious anemia, the classic sign of that deficiency. If an individual responds to B_{12} treatment, Alzheimer's can be ruled out.

❑ Beta-amyloid, the protein-containing substance that makes up the characteristic senile plaques in the brain, has also been found in the spinal fluid of people with Alzheimer's disease. This finding may lead to the development of methods for earlier diagnosis of the condition. Research studies supported by the Alzheimer's Association and studies done at the Department of Research at Oakwood College in Huntsville, Alabama, found that liquid aged garlic extract (Kyolic) may prove to be useful in the improvement of Alzheimer's disease symptoms. Kyolic protected the cells from toxic effects of beta-amyloid. The journal *Science* reported in October 1999 that researchers had identified an enzyme, beta-secretase, which is responsible for the formation of beta-amyloid. However, nothing has been found yet to stop the formation of beta-amyloid.

❑ Homocysteine, an amino acid that forms as the result of the breakdown of another amino acid, methionine, is a biomarker for the development of dementia and Alzheimer's disease. Some scientists speculate that Alzheimer's disease might be avoided if people reduced the levels of homocysteine levels in their blood, although it has not yet been determined whether homocysteine itself actually contributes to Alzheimer's disease. A more likely explanation is that elevated homocysteine levels are an indication of a severe disruption of methylation (a type of biochemical process essential for the repair and maintenance of genetic material and the production of neurotransmitters, among other things) in the brains of people with Alzheimer's disease. Methylation deficiencies can result in severe damage to brain cells. Other researchers report that abnormal amino acid metabolism in Alzheimer's disease causes higher homocysteine levels. This may lead to the neurological damage that occurs as the disease advances.

❑ A test that measures electrical activity in the brain and stores the information on a computer disk for analysis can be used to help diagnose Alzheimer's disease. A skin test is also under development that may provide earlier and more rapid diagnosis.

❑ A decline in the sense of smell often occurs as much as two years prior to the beginning of mental decline in people with Alzheimer's. Scientists at the University of California—San Diego Medical Center found that people with this disorder need to be exposed to very strong concentrations of a substance before they can detect its odor. The rate at which the ability to distinguish smells is lost is a useful predictor of how rapidly an individual will lose cognitive functioning. Smoking can damage cells involved in the sense of smell, however, making this less useful as an indicator of disease in smokers.

❏ Regular exercise throughout adulthood can reduce the chances of developing Alzheimer's disease. A study reported in the April 1998 issue of *Neurology* concludes that, overall, people who developed Alzheimer's disease had led far more sedentary lives and scored much lower on activity rating scales than their healthier counterparts. Activities associated with reduced risk include biking, walking, swimming, and golf.

❏ Researchers at the University of California/Davis questioned the caregivers of eighty-eight elderly people, half of whom had either Alzheimer's or a related form of dementia, about their eating habits. Half of the people with Alzheimer's disease had such a strong desire for sweets that their access to these foods had to be restricted.

❏ The hormone dehydroepiandrosterone (DHEA) may help to prevent Alzheimer's disease. (*See* DHEA THERAPY in Part Three.)

❏ Preliminary trials suggest that nicotinamide adenine dinucleotide (NADH) may benefit those afflicted with Alzheimer's. In a study conducted by Austrian researcher and physician Dr. George Birkmayer and colleagues, seventeen patients with Alzheimer-type dementia were treated with NADH for eight to twelve weeks. The patients' cognitive function improved as measured by two standard tests, according to the Folstein Mini-Mental Status Examination and the global deterioration scale. The patients reportedly did not suffer any adverse side effects.

❏ High doses of lecithin may be helpful for people with Alzheimer's disease. However, a double-blind controlled trial of high doses of lecithin reported in the *Journal of Neurology, Neurosurgery, & Psychiatry* found that there may be a "therapeutic window" for the effects of lecithin on people with Alzheimer's disease, and that this may be more evident in older people.

❏ In his book *Beating Alzheimer's* (Avery Publishing Group, 1991), Tom Warren cites evidence that diet and chemical allergies may play an important role in Alzheimer's disease. Reactions to allergens can cause swelling in the brain. Recurring headaches are a common symptom of cerebral (brain-related) allergies. (*See* ALLERGIES in Part Two.)

❏ Research conducted at the University of Kentucky found that the brains of a group of individuals with Alzheimer's disease contained higher levels of mercury than the brains of a comparable control group, particularly in areas of the brain responsible for cognitive functioning, movement, and expression. The Alzheimer's group also had higher ratios of mercury to the trace minerals selenium and zinc, which help to protect the body against the toxic effects of mercury.

❏ Women with Alzheimer's disease have been found to have lower estrogen levels than their healthy counterparts.

❏ Researchers at the Massachusetts Institute of Technology discovered that levels of choline and ethanolamine are significantly lower than normal in people suffering from Alzheimer's disease. Both choline and ethanolamine are used for the synthesis of phospholipids that are major components of the cell membranes of neurons in the brain.

❏ There are two prescription drugs currently approved for the treatment of Alzheimer's disease—donepezil (Aricept) and tacrine (Cognex)—and a number of others are in clinical trials, including galantamine, lazabemide, and metrifonate. All of these drugs are cholinesterase inhibitors. By blocking the action of an enzyme that breaks down acetylcholine, a neurotransmitter involved in learning and memory, they increase levels of this important brain chemical and can improve cognitive functioning in some people with Alzheimer's disease. They are not a cure for the disease, however. In addition, studies have raised some concerns about liver damage as a side effect of tacrine therapy.

❏ Experts are now considering ways to attack the disease at its earliest stages through the use of anti-inflammatory drugs. One approach is to block the theorized inflammatory response to plaques. In fact, inflammation has been under suspicion as a cause of Alzheimer's disease, partly because nonsteroidal, anti-inflammatory drugs (NSAIDs) like aspirin, indomethacin (Indocin), naproxen (Naprosyn), and ibuprofen (Motrin) seem to slow the progress of the disease.

❏ Scientists at the University of Kentucky found that levels of glutamine synthetase, an enzyme that controls the production of ammonia and glutamate, were higher in a group of people with Alzheimer's disease than in a healthy control group. Glutamate is vital to the brain in small amounts, but it can be poisonous in high concentrations. Abnormally high levels of glutamate have recently been associated with amyotrophic lateral sclerosis (ALS, also known as Lou Gehrig's disease) and glaucoma as well.

❏ An estimated 2 percent of Americans have two copies of a gene for the production of a substance called apolipoprotein E4, or APO-E4. APO-E4 transports cholesterol through the bloodstream and also changes the form of amyloid in the brain. Those with two copies of the gene have a 50-percent chance of getting Alzheimer's before the age of seventy. In contrast, for those with no copies of the gene, the risk of developing the disease does not rise to 50 percent until the after age of ninety.

❏ Experts say that it is in an individual's best interest to be told as soon as there is reason to suspect a diagnosis of Alzheimer's disease. Early warning cannot prevent the disease, but it gives people time to settle their affairs and make informed judgments about future care and other matters.

❏ Anyone who cares for a person with Alzheimer's disease may eventually find the job overwhelming and need support. For many, adult day-care centers are a godsend. A good day-care center should be clean, safe (without glass doors, uneven or slippery floors, furniture with sharp corners, and so on), and have barriers at entrances and exits to protect wanderers without making them feel trapped. Food

Ten Warning Signs of Alzheimer's Disease

Everyone experiences forgetfulness or the momentary inability to pull up the proper word from time to time and, especially as we get older, we may worry that such episodes are a sign of Alzheimer's disease. The symptoms of Alzheimer's disease are distinctly different from those of everyday forgetfulness. The Alzheimer's Association gives the following ten warning signs of Alzheimer's disease:

1. Recent memory loss that affects job performance. Everyone forgets things and then recalls them later. People with Alzheimer's disease forget often, never recall, and repeatedly ask the same question, forgetting the earlier answer.

2. Difficulty performing familiar tasks. For example, a person with Alzheimer's disease might prepare a meal, forget to eat or serve it, and even forget that he or she made it.

3. Problems with language. A person with Alzheimer's disease may forget simple words or use inappropriate words, making speech incomprehensible.

4. Disorientation as to time and place. A person with Alzheimer's disease may get lost on his or her own street and forget how he or she got there or how to get home.

5. Poor or weaker judgment. For example, anyone might get distracted and fail to watch a child. A person with

Alzheimer's disease, however, might entirely forget the child under his or her care and leave the house.

6. Problems with abstract thinking. Anybody can have trouble balancing a checkbook; a person with Alzheimer's disease might completely forget what numbers are and what needs to be done with them.

7. Misplacing things. A person with Alzheimer's disease may put things in inappropriate places—an iron in the freezer or a wristwatch in the sugar bowl, for example—and not be able to retrieve them.

8. Changes in mood or behavior. Everyone has occasional mood swings, but people with Alzheimer's disease can have rapid mood swings—from calm, to tears, to anger—within a few minutes.

9. Personality changes. A person with Alzheimer's disease may experience drastic and inappropriate personality changes, becoming uncharacteristically irritable, suspicious, or fearful.

10. Loss of initiative. People with Alzheimer's disease may become passive and reluctant to get involved in activities.

If you notice several of these symptoms in yourself or a loved one, consult a doctor for a complete examination and evaluation.

---

should be nutritious and appetizing. Staff members should be friendly, compassionate, and professionally trained to work with Alzheimer's patients. There should be psychologists or social workers on the staff to help patients cope with the ordinary frustrations of daily life and to assist them in coping with anger and depression. A quiet room should be available where an agitated or ill person can be separated from others. The availability of other specific services, such as physical therapy, help with hygiene, family counseling, or support groups for caregivers, as well as the usual activities of the center, should be suited to particular needs of the individual and his or her family.

❑ The calming effect of watching fish swimming peacefully in an aquarium is found to help people with Alzheimer's disease eat better by helping them to concentrate long enough to eat well, according to Nancy Edwards, Ph.D., a professor of nursing at Purdue University.

❑ Milder signs of Alzheimer's disease may not be detected in the very old, and many people die before developing obvious symptoms. People with family members who have Alzheimer's disease are probably more able to detect the early signs.

❑ For names and addresses of organizations that can provide further information about this disorder, see HEALTH AND MEDICAL ORGANIZATIONS in the Appendix.

Amblyopia

See Dimness or Loss of Vision under EYE PROBLEMS.

Anemia

Millions of Americans suffer from anemia, a reduction in either the number of red blood cells or the amount of hemoglobin in the blood. This results in a decrease in the amount of oxygen that the blood is able to carry. Anemia reduces the amount of oxygen available to the cells of the body. As a result, they have less energy available to perform their normal functions. Important processes, such as muscular activity and cell building and repair, slow down and become less efficient. When the brain lacks oxygen, dizziness may result, and mental faculties are less sharp.

Anemia is not a disease, but rather a symptom of various diseases. Anything that causes a deficiency in the formation or production of red blood cells, or that leads to the too-rapid destruction of red blood cells, can result in anemia. It is sometimes the first detectable sign of arthritis, infection, or certain major illnesses, including cancer. Drug use, hormonal disorders, chronic inflammation in the body, surgery, infections, peptic ulcers, hemorrhoids, diverticular disease, heavy menstrual bleeding, repeated pregnancies, liver damage, thyroid disorders, rheumatoid arthritis, bone marrow disease, and dietary deficiencies (especially deficiencies of iron, folic acid, and vitamins B_6 and B_{12}) can all lead to anemia. There are also a number of hereditary disorders, such as sickle cell disease and thalassemia, that cause anemia. Sickle cell anemia affects about 31,000 people (mostly of African-American descent) in the United States. It is a rare, inherited blood disease that causes red blood cells to become brittle and crescent-shaped. Painful "crises" arise when affected cells become jammed in narrow blood vessels, producing painful swelling of the hands and feet accompanied by fever, fatigue, and pneumonia-like symptoms.

Pernicious anemia is a severe form of anemia that is due to vitamin B_{12} deficiency. Persons with this disorder cannot absorb any form of vitamin B_{12} from the gastrointestinal tract. Malabsorption can cause pernicious anemia, as can poor eating habits, gastrointestinal infection, Crohn's disease, gastric surgery, and sometimes even strict vegetarianism. If B_{12} levels fall too far, the result is lagging energy, depression, indigestion, diarrhea, and anemia. Ongoing vitamin B_{12} deficiency carries a risk of neurological damage.

The most common cause of anemia is iron deficiency. Iron is an important factor in anemia because this mineral is used to make hemoglobin, the component of red blood cells that attaches to oxygen and transports it. Red blood cells exist only to oxygenate the body, and have a life span of about 120 days. If a person lacks sufficient iron, the formation of red blood cells is impaired. Iron-deficiency anemia can be caused by insufficient iron intake and/or absorption, or by significant blood loss. The latter is commonly seen in women who suffer from menorrhagia (heavy or prolonged menstrual bleeding), which in turn may be caused by a hormonal imbalance, fibroid tumors, or uterine cancer. Women who use intrauterine devices for contraception are also at a higher risk of blood loss, as are those who overuse anti-inflammatory medications such as aspirin or ibuprofen, which can cause blood loss through irritation of the digestive tract. Excessive aspirin usage, particularly by elderly people, may cause internal bleeding.

Anemia's symptoms can easily go unrecognized. The first signs of developing anemia may be loss of appetite, constipation, headaches, irritability, and/or difficulty in concentrating. Established anemia can produce such symptoms as weakness; fatigue; coldness of the extremities; depression; dizziness; overall pallor, most noticeable in pale and brittle nails; pale lips and eyelids; soreness in the mouth; and in women, cessation of menstruation. Anemia has also been linked to a loss of libido. Of those suffering from anemia, 20 percent are women and 50 percent are children.

Anemia should always be investigated and the cause determined. If you are anemic and your diet is ironclad, your physician can run a simple test called ESR (erythrocyte sedimentation rate) to detect any inflammation lurking in the body.

Unless otherwise specified, the dosages recommended in this section are for adults. For a child between the ages of twelve and seventeen, reduce the dose to three-quarters the recommended amount. For a child between six and twelve, use one-half the recommended dose, and for a child under the age of six, use one-quarter the recommended amount.

NUTRIENTS

SUPPLEMENT	SUGGESTED DOSAGE	COMMENTS
Essential		
Raw liver extract	500 mg twice daily.	Contains all the elements needed for red blood cell production. Use liver from organically raised beef. Consider injections (under a doctor's supervision).
Very Important		
Blackstrap molasses	1 tbsp twice daily for adults; 1 tsp added to milk for children and infants.	Contains iron and essential B vitamins.
Folic acid plus biotin	800 mcg twice daily. 300 mcg twice daily.	Needed for red blood cell formation.
Iron or Floradix Iron + Herbs from Salus Haus	As prescribed by physician. Take with 100 mg vitamin C for better absorption. 2 tsp twice daily.	To restore iron. Use ferrous gluconate form. *Caution:* Do not take iron unless anemia is diagnosed. Contains a readily absorbable form of iron that is nontoxic and from a natural source.
Vitamin B_{12} injections or vitamin B_{12}	2 cc once weekly or as prescribed by physician. 2,000 mcg 3 times daily.	Essential in red blood cell production and to break down and prepare protein for cellular use. Injections (under a doctor's supervision) are best. If injections are not available, use a lozenge or sublingual form for best absorption.
Important		
Vitamin B complex	50 mg of each major B vitamin 3 times daily. (amounts of individual vitamins in a complex will vary).	B vitamins work best when taken together. A sublingual form is recommended.
plus extra pantothenic acid (vitamin B_5) and	50 mg 3 times daily.	Important in red blood cell production. Involved in cellular reproduction.
vitamin B_6 (pyridoxine)	100 mg daily.	Aids absorption of vitamin B_{12}.
Vitamin C plus bioflavonoids	3,000–10,000 mg daily.	Important in iron absorption.
Helpful		
Brewer's yeast	As directed on label.	Rich in basic nutrients and a good source of B vitamins.
Coenzyme A from Coenzyme-A Technologies	As directed on label.	Supports the immune system's detoxification of many dangerous substances.

Copper	2 mg daily.	Needed in red blood cell production. *Note:* If more zinc is used, increase copper proportionately. Needed to balance with copper.
and zinc	30 mg daily. Do not exceed this amount.	
Raw spleen glandular	As directed on label.	*See* GLANDULAR THERAPY in Part Three for its benefits.
S-Adenosylmethio-nine (SAMe)	As directed on label.	Helps reduce stress and depression. *Caution:* Do not use if you have manic-depressive disorder or take prescription antidepressants.
Vitamin A plus	10,000 IU daily.	Important antioxidants.
natural beta-carotene or	15,000 IU daily.	
carotenoid complex (Betatene)	As directed on label.	
Vitamin E	600 IU daily. Take separately from iron supplements.	Important for red blood cell survival; prolongs the life span of these cells. Use emulsion form for easier assimilation. Use d-alpha-tocopherol form.

HERBS

❏ Alfalfa, bilberry, cherry, dandelion, goldenseal, grape skins, hawthorn berry, mullein, nettle, Oregon grape root, pau d'arco, red raspberry, shepherd's purse, and yellow dock are good for anemia.

Caution: Do not take goldenseal or Oregon grape root during pregnancy. Do not take goldenseal for more than one week at a time, and use it only under a doctor's supervision if you have a history of cardiovascular disease, diabetes, or glaucoma.

❏ Herbalists consider nettle (*Urtica dioica*), a nutritious plant rich in iron, vitamin C, chlorophyll, and other minerals, an effective supplement in the treatment of iron-deficiency anemia.

RECOMMENDATIONS

❏ Include the following in your diet: apples, apricots, asparagus, bananas, broccoli, egg yolks, kelp, leafy greens, okra, parsley, peas, plums, prunes, purple grapes, raisins, rice bran, squash, turnip greens, whole grains, and yams. Also eat foods high in vitamin C to enhance iron absorption.

❏ Consume at least 1 tablespoon of blackstrap molasses twice daily (for a child, use 1 teaspoon in a glass of milk or formula twice daily). Blackstrap molasses is a good source of iron and essential B vitamins.

❏ Eat foods containing oxalic acid in moderation or omit them from the diet. Oxalic acid interferes with iron absorption. Foods high in oxalic acid include almonds, cashews, chocolate, cocoa, kale, rhubarb, soda, sorrel, spinach, Swiss chard, and most nuts and beans.

❏ Avoid beer, candy bars, dairy products, ice cream, and soft drinks. Additives in these foods interfere with iron absorption. For the same reason, avoid coffee (which contains polyphenols) and tea (which contains tannins).

❏ Have a complete blood test to determine if you have an iron deficiency before taking iron supplements. Excess iron can damage the liver, heart, pancreas, and immune cell activity, and has been linked to cancer. Use iron supplements only under the supervision of a qualified health care provider.

❏ Because iron is removed through the stool, do not eat foods high in iron and/or iron supplements at the same time as fiber. Avoid using bran as a source of fiber.

❏ If you are a strict vegetarian, watch your diet closely. Taking supplemental vitamin B_{12} is advised (*see* VITAMINS in Part One).

❏ Do not smoke. Avoid secondhand smoke.

❏ Minimize your exposure to lead and other toxic metals. (*See* ALUMINUM TOXICITY; CADMIUM TOXICITY; LEAD POISONING; and/or MERCURY TOXICITY for suggestions.)

❏ Do not take calcium, vitamin E, zinc, or antacids at the same time as iron supplements. These can interfere with iron absorption.

CONSIDERATIONS

❏ The following foods are among the highest in iron content, with over 5 milligrams of iron per average serving: kidney beans, pinto beans, liver (eat only liver from organically raised animals), blackstrap molasses, rice bran, raw beet greens (not the beets), mustard greens, lentils, dried peaches, and prune juice. Foods with a moderately high iron content (3 to 5 milligrams per average serving) include cooked dried apricots, cooked beet greens, dates, lean meat (lamb, turkey, and veal), lima beans, chili, cooked spinach, and dry and fresh peas.

❏ Eating fish at the same time as vegetables containing iron increases iron absorption. Omitting all sugar from the diet increases iron absorption as well.

❏ Iron-deficiency anemia should disappear when the underlying cause is corrected.

❏ Physicians can sometimes detect vitamin B_{12} deficiency by measuring serum B_{12} levels, taking a complete blood cell count, and doing a blood test called the Schilling test, which evaluates B_{12} absorption. Persons with pernicious anemia must take vitamin B_{12} sublingually (dissolved under the tongue), by retention enema, or by injection. This treatment must be maintained for life, unless the underlying cause of the deficiency can be corrected.

❏ Hydroxyuria (Droxia), a cancer drug, may be prescribed for people with sickle cell anemia who are over the age of eighteen and have experienced three or more crises in a one-year period. The drug eases symptoms, but is not a cure for the disease.

❏ The American Academy of Pediatrics (AAP) recommends that children under one year old *not* drink cow's milk. Milk can cause anemia by interfering with iron absorption and possibly causing internal bleeding. The AAP published the results of a University of Iowa study that found the blood content in the stool of infants fed cow's milk was five times higher than children fed infant formula. Researchers concluded the amount of iron lost was "nutritionally important."

Angina

See under CARDIOVASCULAR DISEASE.

Ankylosing Spondylitis

See under ARTHRITIS.

Anorexia Nervosa

The term *anorexia nervosa* was first coined in 1988. A doctor writing in the British medical journal *The Lancet* used the term to describe people who, although thin and weak, insisted that they needed to lose weight and would not eat a sufficient amount of food to remain alive.

Anorexia nervosa is a nervous, psychological eating disorder characterized by a refusal to eat, even to the point of starvation. Other symptoms include an intense fear of becoming fat that never goes away, no matter how thin the individual becomes; extreme overactivity and an obsession with working out; negative feelings about the way the body looks; deep feelings of shame; and problems with drug and/or alcohol abuse. Ninety-five percent of the people who suffer from this disorder are female. Anorexia typically appears during adolescence. The incidence of eating disorders, particularly among young women in the United States, has escalated dramatically during the past decade. An estimated 8 million Americans struggle with anorexia, according to the National Association of Anorexia Nervosa and Associated Diseases (ANAD). And eating disorders are not limited to teenage girls. Women aged forty and older are also susceptible. Doctors suspect that low levels of serotonin, a neurotransmitter, may be the cause, producing psychological problems linked to anorexia and bulimia.

Some people with anorexia just quit eating; some make themselves vomit immediately after eating; some take laxatives after eating; and some do all three. Most people with anorexia have normal feelings of hunger at the onset of the disease but teach themselves to ignore them. Despite their refusal to eat, people with anorexia often become obsessed with food and may spend hours fantasizing about it, reading recipes, or even preparing elaborate meals for others. Another characteristic feature of the disorder is that people with anorexia usually deny that there is anything wrong and claim that they simply "aren't hungry" and even insist that they need to lose more weight.

Many females who are anorexic are also bulimic. *Bulimia nervosa* is defined as the consumption of extremely large quantities of food in short periods of time (binging), followed by self-induced vomiting or the use of either diuretics or cathartics (purging). (*See* BULIMIA.) If anorexia and bulimia occur in the same individual, the disorder is called *bulimarexia*.

Anorexia can lead to underweight, extreme weakness, dizziness, cessation of menstruation, swelling of the neck, ulcers and erosion of the esophagus, erosion of the enamel of the back teeth from repeated vomiting, broken blood vessels in the face, and a low pulse rate and blood pressure. In some extreme cases, spoons or sticks used to induce vomiting have become stuck in the digestive tract and have had to be surgically removed. Systemic physiological changes in those suffering from anorexia include thyroid dysfunction, disturbances in the heartbeat, and irregularity in the secretion of growth hormone and the hormones cortisol, gonadotropin, and vasopressin.

Eventually, if anorexic behavior continues long enough, classic complications associated with starvation appear. Electrolyte imbalances created by insufficient potassium and sodium levels cause dehydration, muscle spasms, and, ultimately, cardiac arrest. If laxatives are used, these further deplete the body of potassium. Hypokalemia (potassium deficiency) is a major problem for people with anorexia. Chronic hypokalemia can cause an irregular heartbeat, which can lead to heart failure and death.

Initially, anorexia nervosa was thought to be strictly a psychological problem. However, in the last few years, medical scientists and nutritionists have identified several physical components as well. For example, people with eating disorders have been found to have chemical imbalances similar to those found in individuals with clinical depression. Some cases of anorexia have been found to be caused by severe zinc deficiency.

As researchers become increasingly aware of the physiological elements of anorexia, the psychological ones continue to be important. Teasing by peers or parents can play a role in making individuals obsessed with the idea that they are fat. In addition, many people who suffer from anorexia display great fear at the prospect of growing up, and girls often have difficult mother/daughter relationships. Some may try to live up to images their parents set for them, but feel inadequate—that they are not as beautiful or intelligent as their parents want them to be. A girl with anorexia may then develop an inferiority complex, seeing herself as fat and/or ugly, and no amount of common sense or persuasion can alter her distorted mental image.

Warning Signs of Anorexia Nervosa

Anorexia nervosa is a serious medical condition that requires treatment. The first step in getting help is recognizing that there is a problem. The following are characteristic warning signs of this condition:

- Self-starvation and weight loss.
- Intense, persistent fear of gaining weight.
- Continuous dieting.
- Excessive growth of facial or body hair because of inadequate protein in diet.
- Cessation of menstruation or irregular periods.
- Broken blood vessels in the face.
- Preoccupation with food.
- Refusal to eat, except tiny portions.
- Compulsive exercising.
- Abnormal weight loss.
- Sensitivity to cold.
- Hair loss.
- Erosion of the enamel of back teeth.

If you notice any of these symptoms in yourself or a loved one, consult a doctor for examination and evaluation.

About 30 percent of all people with anorexia struggle with the disorder all their lives. Another 30 percent have at least one life-threatening bout with it, while the remaining 40 percent outgrow it. Even if an individual recovers fully from the acute phase of the disorder, serious damage may have been done to the body.

Unless otherwise specified, the dosages recommended in this section are for adults. For a child between the ages of twelve and seventeen, reduce the dose to three-quarters the recommended amount.

NUTRIENTS

SUPPLEMENT	SUGGESTED DOSAGE	COMMENTS
Very Important		
Multivitamin and mineral complex with		All nutrients are needed and must be taken in extremely high doses because they are passed through the gastrointestinal tract rapidly and are poorly assimilated.
natural beta-carotene and	25,000 IU daily.	
mixed carotenoids and	Amounts in a complex will vary.	
vitamin A and	10,000 IU daily.	
calcium and	1,500 mg daily.	
magnesium and	1,000 mg daily.	
potassium and	99–200 mg daily.	
selenium	200 mcg daily. If you are pregnant, do not exceed 40 mcg daily.	
Zinc plus copper	80 mg daily. Do not exceed a total of 100 mg daily from all supplements. 3 mg daily.	All enzymes important for increased appetite and taste require zinc and copper. Zinc and copper work together to prevent copper deficiency.
Important		
Acidophilus (Probiata from Wakunaga)	As directed on label. Take on an empty stomach so that it passes quickly to the small intestine.	Needed to replace the "friendly" bacteria lost from use of laxatives and/or from vomiting.
Free-form amino acid complex (Amino Balance from Anabol Naturals)	As directed on label.	To supply easily assimilable protein, needed for tissue repair.
5-Hydroxy L-tryptophan (5-HTP)	As directed on label.	Aids in treating depression and nervousness.
Gamma-aminobutyric acid (GABA) or	As directed on label.	Low levels of this amino acid have been found in people who suffer from anxiety and depression.
S-Adenosylmethionine (SAMe)	As directed on label.	Aids in reducing stress and depression, providing a sense of well-being. *Caution:* Do not use if you have manic-depressive disorder or take prescription antidepressants.
Liquid Kyolic with B_1 and B_{12} from Wakunaga	As directed on label.	Helps reduce stress and anxiety.
Multimineral complex	As directed on label.	Needed to replace lost minerals.
Primrose oil or	As directed on label.	Important for all body functions and cell repair and reduces inflammation in nerve cells.
flaxseed oil or	As directed on label.	
Kyolic-EPA from Wakunaga	As directed on label.	To calm the nervous system.
Vitamin B complex	100 mg of each major B vitamin 3 times daily (amounts of individual vitamins in a complex will vary).	Helps to prevent anemia and replaces lost B vitamins. The B vitamins are important for proper brain functioning and help increase the appetite. Use a sublingual form.
Vitamin B12 injections	1 cc 3 times weekly or as prescribed by physician.	Increases appetite; prevents loss of hair and damage to many bodily functions. If injections are not available, use a lozenge or sublingual form.
plus liver extract injections	2 cc 3 times weekly or as prescribed by physician.	To supply B vitamins and other valuable nutrients.
Vitamin C with bioflavonoids	5,000 mg daily, in divided doses.	Needed for the impaired immune system and to alleviate stress on the adrenal glands.

Helpful		
Bio-Strath from Nature's Answer or	3 times daily.	An herbal and yeast-based tonic. A natural source of iron.
Floradix Iron + Herbs from Salus Haus	As directed on label 3 times daily.	Aids in increasing the appetite.
Brewer's yeast	Start with 1 tsp daily and work up to 1 tbsp daily.	Contains balanced amounts of the B vitamins.
Kelp	2,000–3,000 mg daily.	Needed for mineral replacement and thyroid function.
Proteolytic enzymes	As directed on label. Take between meals and with meals.	To aid in digestion and in rebuilding of tissue.
Vitamin D_3	600 IU daily.	Needed for calcium uptake and to prevent bone loss.
Vitamin E	600 IU daily.	Increases oxygen uptake in the body for healing and a powerful antioxidant. Use d-alpha-tocopherol form.

HERBS

❑ To rebuild the liver and cleanse the bloodstream, use dandelion, milk thistle, red clover, or wild yam.

❑ The following herbs are appetite stimulants: ginger root, ginseng, gotu kola, and peppermint.

Caution: Do not use ginseng if you have high blood pressure.

❑ St. John's wort and kava kava calm the nervous system and aid in preventing depression.

RECOMMENDATIONS

❑ While a normal eating pattern is being established, eat a well-balanced diet that is high in fiber. Eat plenty of fresh raw fruits and vegetables. These foods are cleansing to the system. When the body is cleansed, the appetite tends to return to normal.

❑ Be sure to eat adequate amounts of healthy protein foods, such as fish and soy protein. Quality protein is important for repairing body tissues and restoring lost muscle mass.

❑ Consume no sugar, and avoid white flour products.

❑ Avoid processed and junk foods. The additives these foods contain tend to add to the aversion to eating.

❑ Seek out a practitioner or practitioners who specialize in the treatment of eating disorders and who can address the complex of physical and psychological elements involved. Some type of specialized counseling, in addition to nutritional counseling, is usually necessary for recovery.

❑ Look at your level of self-esteem. Women with low self-esteem tend to engage in self-destructive behaviors such as entering into abusive relationships, compulsive sexual behavior, and eating disorders. Cultivate relationships with people who make you feel important—people who are admiring and encouraging of your accomplishments and interests. As much as possible, remove from your life anything and anyone who makes you feel inadequate and "put-down." Consider counseling to help you learn to cope with those negative situations you cannot avoid.

CONSIDERATIONS

❑ If an individual shows any of the signs of anorexia, he or she should be seen by a physician.

❑ In many cases, a person with anorexia must be hospitalized and given intravenous nutrient feedings of potassium and multivitamins.

❑ Starvation tends to increase feelings of depression, anxiety, irritability, and anger. It may take up to a year or more for a person recovering from anorexia to improve his or her body image, to reestablish normal eating patterns, and to reverse the effects of starvation on mood and behavior.

❑ Some researchers believe that neurotransmitters—such as dopamine, serotonin, norepinephrine, and the endogenous opioids—play a role in anorexia.

❑ Researchers have found that zinc supplementation not only decreases depression and anxiety, but that anorexic women taking zinc gain twice as much weight, on average, as anorexic women who do not take the supplement. Zinc, whether as part of the diet or in supplemental form, has been successful in helping many individuals with anorexia to regain their normal appetite and weight. Zinc deficiency by itself, however, does not result in anorexia nervosa.

❑ The self-esteem problems typical of those with anorexia often begin at an early age. A child who is told that she is stupid, worthless, and/or unlovable is likely to come to believe it. In addition, recent research has shown that many (if not most) American girls undergo a severe loss of self-esteem in early adolescence, the very time that eating disorders are most likely to occur.

❑ For information on organizations that can help you learn more about eating disorders and treatments, *see* HEALTH AND MEDICAL ORGANIZATIONS in the Appendix.

Anxiety Disorder

Anxiety disorder is a far more common problem than was once thought. It can affect people in their teenage years through middle age and later. Anxiety disorder appears to affect twice as many women as men, though there may not actually be that wide a disparity between the sexes. Psychologists believe that men are far less prone to report or even acknowledge having a problem of this nature.

Anxiety disorder can be either acute or chronic. Acute anxiety disorder manifests itself in episodes commonly known as panic attacks. A panic attack is an instance in which the body's natural "fight or flight" reaction occurs at the wrong time. This is a complex, involuntary physiological response in which the body prepares itself to deal with an emergency situation. Stress causes the body to produce more adrenal hormones, especially adrenaline. The increased production of adrenaline causes the body to step up its metabolism of proteins, fats, and carbohydrates to quickly produce energy for the body to use. In addition, the muscles tense, and heartbeat and breathing become more rapid. Even the composition of the blood changes slightly, making it more prone to clotting.

In the face of a threat such as an assault, an accident, or a natural disaster, this type of reaction is perfectly normal and helpful for survival. At other times, the symptoms caused by a surge in adrenaline can be distressing and frightening. A person having a panic attack often is overwhelmed by a sense of impending disaster or death, which makes it impossible to think clearly. Other feelings that can accompany a panic attack include shortness of breath; a smothering, claustrophobic sensation; heart palpitations; chest pain; dizziness; hot flashes and/or chills; trembling; numbness or tingling sensations in the extremities; sweating; nausea; a feeling of unreality; and a distorted perception of the passage of time. Eventually, the disorder can have other, cumulative effects, such as generalized aches and pains, muscular twitching and stiffness, depression, insomnia, nightmares and early waking, decreased libido, and abnormal feelings of tension with an accompanying inability to relax. Women may experience changes in the menstrual cycle and increased premenstrual symptoms.

Panic attacks are usually abrupt and intense. They can occur at any time of the day or night, lasting from several seconds up to half an hour. To the panic sufferer, it often feels as though they are much longer. A person having a panic attack often believes that he or she is experiencing a heart attack or a stroke. The attacks themselves are very unpredictable; some people experience one every few weeks, while others may have several a day. They are often triggered by stress (conscious or unconscious) or certain emotions, but may also occur in response to certain foods, drugs, or illness. Food allergies and hypoglycemia are both common among people with this disorder, and can promote panic attacks. An attack may follow ingestion or overindulgence in caffeine-based stimulants such as tea or coffee. Some attacks occur with no apparent cause. The unpredictability of the attacks makes them even more distressing.

Many people with acute anxiety disorder become fearful of being alone and of visiting public places because they fear having a panic attack. Of course this only adds to the level of anxiety and leads to their lives being abnormally restricted. Many psychologists believe that at least in some cases, panic attacks are self-induced; that is, the fear of a panic attack is the very thing that brings one about.

For years, panic attacks were dismissed as a psychosomatic phenomenon. However, repeated studies have shown that this disorder has a real, physical basis. Experts believe that panic attacks are caused principally by a malfunction in brain chemistry, wherein the brain sends and receives false "emergency signals." Hyperactivity in certain areas of the brain causes the release of norepinephrine, which causes the pulse, blood pressure, and breathing to become more rapid, producing the classic symptoms of a panic attack. According to Mayo Clinic researchers, between 10 and 20 percent of Americans will have a panic attack at some time in their lives. Panic attacks are now recognized as a potentially disabling, but treatable condition.

Chronic anxiety is a milder, more generalized form of this disorder. Many sufferers feel a vague sense of anxiety much of the time, but the intensity of the feeling does not reach the levels of those in an actual panic attack. They may feel chronically uneasy, especially in the presence of other people, and tend to startle easily. Headaches and chronic fatigue are common among people with this form of the disorder. Generalized anxiety disorder can begin at any age, but the onset typically occurs in one's twenties or thirties. Some people with chronic anxiety disorder also suffer from occasional panic attacks.

Anxiety disorder may be hereditary to some extent, as it seems to run in families. Some cases may be linked to a relatively harmless abnormality of heart function called mitral valve prolapse. Anxiety disorder manifests itself in different ways, but doctors agree that conflict, whether internal or interpersonal, promotes a state of anxiety.

Unless otherwise specified, the dosages recommended in this section are for adults. For a child between the ages of twelve and seventeen, reduce the dose to three-quarters the recommended amount.

NUTRIENTS

SUPPLEMENT	SUGGESTED DOSAGE	COMMENTS
Very Important		
Calcium and	2,000 mg daily.	A natural tranquilizer.
magnesium	600–1,000 mg daily.	Helps relieve anxiety, tension, nervousness, muscular spasms, and tics. Best taken in combination with calcium.
Floradix Iron + Herbs from Salus Haus	As directed on label.	Check for iron deficiency; this can increase the risk of panic attacks. Floradix is a natural source of iron.
Liquid Kyolic with B₁ and B₁₂ from Wakunaga	As directed on label.	Helps reduce stress and anxiety.
Multivitamin and mineral complex with	As directed on label.	To provide all needed nutrients in balance.
potassium and	99 mg daily.	Essential for proper functioning of the adrenal glands.
selenium	100–200 mcg daily. If you are pregnant, do not exceed 40 mcg daily.	Low levels have been found in this disorder. A powerful antioxidant that protects the heart.

S-Adenosylmethio-nine (SAMe)	400 mg twice daily.	Important physiological agent involved in over 40 biochemical reactions in the body. Is a natural anti-depressant and has a calming effect. *Caution:* Do not use if you have manic-depressive disorder or take prescription anti-depressants.
Vitamin B complex plus extra vitamin B$_1$ (thiamine) and vitamin B$_6$ (pyridoxine) and niacinamide	As directed on label. 50 mg 3 times daily, with meals. 50 mg 3 times daily, with meals. 50 mg 3 times daily. 100 mg 3 times daily.	Helps maintain normal nervous system function. Helps reduce anxiety and has a calming effect on the nerves. A known energizer that also exerts a calming effect. Important in the production of certain brain chemicals. In large doses, has a calming effect. *Caution:* Do not substitute niacin for niacinamide. Niacin can be toxic in such high doses.
Vitamin C	5,000–10,000 mg daily, in divided doses.	Necessary for proper function of adrenal glands and brain chemistry. In large doses, can have a powerful tranquilizing effect and is known to decrease anxiety. Vital for dealing with stress.
Vitamin E	As directed on label.	Helps transport oxygen to brain cells and protect them from free radical damage. Use d-alpha-tocopherol form.
Zinc	50–80 mg daily. Do not exceed a total of 100 mg daily from all supplements.	Can have a calming effect on the central nervous system.
Important		
Chromium picolinate	200 mcg daily.	Chromium deficiency can produce symptoms of anxiety.
DL-Phenylalanine (DLPA)	600–1,200 mg daily. Discontinue use if no improvement is seen in 1 week.	For chronic anxiety. Increases the brain's production of endorphins, which help relieve anxiety and stress. *Caution:* Do not take this supplement if you are pregnant or nursing, or suffer from panic attacks, diabetes, high blood pressure, or PKU.
L-Glutamine and L-tyrosine plus L-glycine	500 mg 3 times daily, on an empty stomach. Take with water or juice. Do not take with milk. Take with 50 mg vitamin B$_6$ and 100 mg vitamin C for better absorption. 500 mg 3 times daily, on an empty stomach. 500 mg 3 times daily, on an empty stomach.	Has a mild tranquilizing effect. See AMINO ACIDS in Part One. Important for anxiety and depression. *Caution:* Do not take this supplement if you are taking an MAO inhibitor drug. Necessary for central nervous system function.
Helpful		
Coenzyme A from Coenzyme-A Technologies	As directed on label.	Supports the immune system's detoxification of many dangerous substances.

Essential fatty acids (flaxseed oil and Total EFA from Health From The Sun are good sources)	As directed on label.	Important for proper brain function.
Gamma-aminobutyric acid (GABA) plus inositol	750 mg twice daily. As directed on label.	Necessary for proper brain function. See AMINO ACIDS in Part One. Combined with inositol, has a tranquilizing effect.
Melatonin	Start with 2–3 mg daily, taken 2 hours or less before bedtime. If necessary, gradually increase the dosage until an effective level is reached.	A natural sleep aid. Helpful if symptoms include insomnia.

HERBS

❑ A body under stress is more vulnerable to free radical damage. Bilberry, ginkgo biloba, and milk thistle are rich in flavonoids that neutralize free radicals. Milk thistle also proects the liver.

❑ Catnip, chamomile, cramp bark, kava kava, hops, linden flower, motherwort, passionflower, and skullcap promote relaxation and aid in preventing panic attacks.

Caution: Do not use chamomile on an ongoing basis, as ragweed allergy may result. Avoid it completely if you are allergic to ragweed. Kava kava can cause drowsiness. If this occurs, discontinue use or reduce the dosage.

❑ Fennel relieves anxiety-related gastrointestinal upsets, reduces flatulence, and abdominal tension, and relaxes the large intestine. It is most effective when taken as a tea, before or after meals, and has no known side effects. Lemon balm and willow bark also soothe stomach distress.

❑ Feverfew, used to relieve migraines, can help with anxiety-induced headaches. Drinking meadowsweet tea or extract can also relieve headaches related to anxiety and stress, with no side effects.

Caution: A few people may develop mouth sores and experience nausea after taking this herb. If that happens, stop taking it. Do not take feverfew during pregnancy.

❑ St. John's wort can ease depression and restore emotional stability. Results in mood should be noticed in approximately two to four weeks.

❑ Skullcap and valerian root can be taken at bedtime to promote sleep and aid in preventing panic attacks at night.

❑ *Avoid* ephedra *(ma huang)*, as it can aggravate anxiety.

RECOMMENDATIONS

❑ Include in the diet apricots, asparagus, avocados, bananas, broccoli, blackstrap molasses, brewer's yeast, brown rice, dried fruits, dulse, figs, fish (especially salmon), garlic, green leafy vegetables, legumes, raw nuts and seeds, soy products, whole grains, and yogurt. These foods supply valuable minerals such as calcium, magnesium, phosphorus, and potassium, which are depleted by stress.

❏ Try eating small, frequent meals rather than the traditional three meals a day.

❏ Limit your intake of animal protein. Concentrate on meals high in complex carbohydrates and vegetable protein.

❏ Avoid foods containing refined sugar or other simple carbohydrates. For a nutritional treatment plan to have maximum benefits, the diet should contain *no* simple sugars, carbonated soft drinks, tobacco, or alcohol.

❏ Do not consume coffee, black tea, cola, chocolate, or anything else that contains caffeine.

❏ Keep a food diary to detect correlations between your attacks and the foods you eat. Food allergies and sensitivities may trigger panic or anxiety attacks. (*See* ALLERGIES in Part Two.)

❏ Learn relaxation techniques. Biofeedback and meditation can be very helpful.

❏ Get regular exercise. Any type of exercise will work—a brisk walk, bicycle riding, swimming, aerobics, or whatever fits your individual lifestyle. After a few weeks of regular exercise, most people notice an improvement in anxiety symptoms.

❏ Be sure to get adequate rest. If sleep is a problem, consult INSOMNIA in Part Two for suggestions.

❏ To help manage an acute attack, use breathing techniques. Inhale slowly through the nose to a count of four, hold your breath for a count of four, exhale from the mouth slowly to a count of four, and then do nothing for a count of four. Repeat this sequence until the attack subsides. Remind yourself that panic attacks last for a limited amount of time, and that the attack will pass after a few minutes. Although it is rare, some may last up to a few hours.

❏ Call a trusted friend or family member. Talking things over can diffuse anxiety.

❏ If the self-help recommendations in this section do not help, and particularly if panic or anxiety is interfering with your life, consult your health care provider. If an underlying physical problem is ruled out, expect to be referred to a mental health professional for evaluation and treatment.

CONSIDERATIONS

❏ People with anxiety disorder, especially those who experience acute attacks, often seek medical assistance in hospital emergency rooms only to be told they are just suffering from stress and that everything will be fine with rest. In one study, up to 70 percent of people who had panic attacks were found to have seen ten or more different physicians before being correctly diagnosed.

❏ Taking tricyclic antidepressants such as imipramine hydrochloride (Janimine, Tofranil) or imipramine pamoate (Tofranil-PM) in the presence of low serum levels of iron may increase the risk of developing anxiety and jitteriness.

❏ A type of cognitive-behavioral therapy called panic control is being used with promising, long-term results for many chronic sufferers of panic attacks. Therapists coach patients into recreating the feeling of an attack and then teach them to deal with the sensations it produces. Often panic control is used in conjunction with antidepressant drugs or tranquilizers.

❏ Chromium deficiency can produce nervousness, shakiness, and other general symptoms of anxiety. Chromium deficiency is common among alcoholics and people who consume large amounts of refined sugars. Brewer's yeast is a rich source of this essential trace element.

❏ There have been numerous reports on the benefits of DL-phenylalanine (DLPA) in treating anxiety and depression. DLPA is a supplement consisting of both D-phenylalanine and L-phenylalanine, and is much more potent than either of these amino acids taken alone. This should be used under the supervision of a nutritionally oriented physician.

❏ Selenium has been shown to elevate mood and decrease anxiety. These effects were more noticeable in people who had lower levels of selenium in their diets to begin with.

❏ Biofeedback can aid in managing anxiety symptoms. (*See under* PAIN CONTROL in Part Three.)

❏ Music can be effective in reducing anxiety. (*See* MUSIC AND SOUND THERAPY in Part Three.) Color also can be used to induce relaxation and calm. (*See* COLOR THERAPY in Part Three.)

❏ A number of different drugs are used to block panic attacks. Their use must be carefully monitored by a physician. The effectiveness of any given drug varies from individual to individual, and all drugs used for this disorder can cause unpleasant side effects. Alprazolam (Xanax), one of the drugs most commonly used for this illness, has varying effectiveness and can cause drowsiness and lightheadedness. It also can be very addictive. The risk of dependence and its severity seem to be higher if this drug is taken in relatively high doses (more than 4 milligrams per day) and for more than eight weeks.

❏ Recreational drugs such as marijuana can cause anxiety attacks.

❏ A healthy diet plus appropriate nutritional supplementation can be of considerable benefit, reducing overall anxiety and even decreasing the frequency and intensity of panic attacks. If you are taking antianxiety medication, following the plan outlined in this section may make it possible to stop taking the medication, or at least to reduce the dosage. You should always consult with your physician before making any change in a prescription regimen, however.

❏ *See also* STRESS in Part Two.

Appendicitis

Appendicitis is inflammation of the appendix, a lymphoid organ that opens into the first part of the large intestine. For many years, the appendix was believed to be a vestigial organ that served no function, but that is no longer the case. In the fetus, the appendix contains endocrine cells that manufacture hormones and other important body chemicals. In young adults, the appendix is believed to play a part in the functioning of the immune system. It is involved in the maturation of B lymphocytes (a type of white blood cell) and assists in producing an antibody called immunoglobulin A.

Appendicitis is primarily caused by improper diet. It can be either acute or chronic. Most cases involve a blockage of the large intestine resulting from a fiber-deficient diet. The blockage stops the natural flow of fluids, which facilitates the growth of harmful bacteria from the intestinal tract, resulting in inflammation of the appendix. Appendicitis is rare in children under the age of two. The incidence peaks between the ages of fifteen and twenty-four. The risk of developing appendicitis increases after a recent illness, especially a gastrointestinal infection or a roundworm infestation.

Symptoms include severe abdominal pain that begins close to the navel and migrates toward the right lower abdomen. Taking deep breaths, coughing, sneezing, moving, or being touched in this area worsens the pain. Frequently, nausea and vomiting accompany these symptoms, with the pain becoming persistent and well-localized. Other symptoms may include diarrhea, abdominal swelling (in late stages), mild fever (usually less than 102°F), an elevated white blood cell count, constipation, inability to pass gas, painful urination, and blood in the urine.

Acute appendicitis is the most common reason for abdominal surgery. Without prompt treatment, the likelihood increases that the inflamed appendix will burst, contaminating the abdominal cavity with fecal matter and causing peritonitis.

Appendicitis is seldom found in older people. Since the symptoms are usually milder in this age group, however, there is a greater danger for rupture, with resulting peritonitis or the formation of abscesses. In addition, the symptoms can be difficult to diagnose because they are similar to those of bladder infections, kidney stones, and inflammations of the colon, stomach, and small bowel (and, in women, pelvic infections or ovarian cysts). Older adults should therefore be very aware of the symptoms of appendicitis.

The nutrients and herbs recommended in this section are intended to support recovery after surgery, if appropriate, has been performed. Unless otherwise stated, the dosages recommended here are for adults. For a child between the ages of twelve and seventeen, reduce the dose to three-quarters of the recommended amount. For a child between the ages of six and twelve, use one-half the recommended dose, and for a child under six, use one-quarter of the recommended amount.

NUTRIENTS

SUPPLEMENT	SUGGESTED DOSAGE	COMMENTS
Essential		
Carotenoid complex with beta-carotene	25,000 IU 4 times daily.	Enhances immunity and protects against infection.
Coenzyme A from Coenzyme-A Technologies	As directed on label.	Supports the immune system's detoxification of many dangerous substances.
Liquid chlorophyll	In water three times daily as directed on the label.	Helps speed the cleansing of the bloodstream.
Vitamin B complex	100 mg of each major B vitamin 3 times daily (amounts of individual vitamins in a complex will vary).	Necessary for proper assimilation of all nutrients.
Very Important		
Vitamin C (Ester-C, vitamin C crystals, or capsules)	1/4 tsp 4 times daily or as directed on label.	Helps detoxify the system, protects against infection, and enhances immunity.
Vitamin E	400 IU twice daily with meals.	Promotes healing. A powerful antioxidant. Use d-alpha-tocopherol form.
Important		
Zinc	30 mg daily	Strengthens immune system and accelerates healing. Use zinc picolinate form.

HERBS

❑ Alfalfa, agrimony, buckthorn, and slippery elm teas are soothing.

❑ Aloe vera juice can help reduce symptoms.

❑ Echinacea relieves discomfort and enhances the immune system.

Caution: Do not take echinacea if you have an autoimmune disorder.

RECOMMENDATIONS

❑ If you suspect appendicitis, do not take a laxative and do not use a heating pad, as these can provoke rupturing of the appendix. Also, avoid pain relievers as they can lead to a misdiagnosis. Avoid eating and drinking. See your doctor immediately.

CONSIDERATIONS

❑ There are two schools of thought on treating appendicitis. Most medical experts recommend removal of the appendix. Another group recommends attempting to save it as a lymphoid organ. In addition, it may be useful if reconstructive surgery on the bladder becomes necessary. If you should develop bladder cancer at a later time and the bladder must be removed, the appendix can be fashioned into a sphincter muscle and joined to a section of intestine that will serve as a new bladder. If the appendix is about to burst, it must be removed at once. However, this is a valuable organ, and we believe it should not be removed unless your doctor deems it absolutely necessary because he or she believes it will burst. In any case, you should not allow a doctor to remove your appendix during an operation for some other condition ("As long as we're in there. . . .").

❑ To lessen the risk of appendicitis, you should eat a diet high in soluble fiber, avoid refined and fried foods, and limit your intake of cooked animal proteins to one serving a day.

Appetite, Poor

A poor appetite is not a disorder in itself, but usually a symptom of some other problem. Emotional factors such as depression, illness, stress, and trauma may cause a person's appetite to diminish noticeably. Certain controllable factors, such as the use of alcohol, tobacco, or other drugs, can also result in poor appetite. An undetected underlying illness, heavy metal poisoning, and/or nutritional deficiencies may also be involved.

Unless otherwise specified, the dosages recommended in this section are for adults. For a child between the ages of twelve and seventeen, reduce the dose to three-quarters the recommended amount. For a child between six and twelve, use one-half the recommended dose, and for a child under the age of six, use one-quarter the recommended amount.

NUTRIENTS

SUPPLEMENT	SUGGESTED DOSAGE	COMMENTS
Very Important		
Bio-Strath from Nature's Answer	As directed on label.	A yeast and herb formula that aids in gaining back strength and energy.
Coenzyme A from Coenzyme-A Technologies	As directed on label.	Supports the immune system's detoxification of many dangerous substances.
Floradix Iron + Herbs from Salus Haus	As directed on label.	Helps digestion and stimulates appetite.
Multivitamin and mineral complex with		All nutrients are needed in large amounts. Use a high-potency formula.
vitamin A	25,000 IU daily. If you are pregnant, do not exceed 10,000 IU daily.	
and calcium	1,500 mg daily.	
and magnesium	750 mg daily.	
S-Adenosylmethio- nine (SAMe)	As directed on label.	Helps reduce stress and depression. Gives a sense of well-being. *Caution:* Do not use if you have manic-depressive disorder or take prescription antidepressants.
Vitamin B complex	100 mg or more of each major B vitamin daily, before meals (amount of individual vitamins in a complex will vary).	Increases the appetite. Use a high-stress formula. A sublingual form is recommended. Injections (under a doctor's supervision) may be necessary.
Vitamin E	600 IU daily.	To correct deficiencies. All nutrients are important for improving appetite. Use d-alpha-tocopherol form.
Zinc plus copper	80 mg daily. Do not exceed a total of 100 mg daily from all supplements. 3 mg daily.	Enhances the sense of taste. Needed to balance with zinc.
Helpful		
Brewer's yeast	Start with 1/2 tsp daily and work up to 1 tbsp daily.	Rich in nutrients, especially the B vitamins. Improves the appetite.
Spiru-tein from Nature's Plus	As directed on label. Take between meals.	To supply protein, needed to build and repair tissue. Also acts as an appetite stimulant.

HERBS

❑ To stimulate a poor appetite, try using catnip, fennel seed, ginger root, ginseng, gotu kola, papaya leaves, peppermint leaves, and/or saw palmetto berries.

Caution: Do not use ginseng if you have high blood pressure.

RECOMMENDATIONS

❑ To obtain needed protein and calories, drink 3 or more cups a day of skim milk, soymilk, Rice Dream, or almond milk. Use a soy carob drink and yogurt fruit shakes. Eat only whole-grain bread, rolls, macaroni, crackers, and hot and cold cereals. Use cream soups (made with soymilk) as desired. These are usually higher in protein than broth soups.

❑ Between meals, snack on foods such as avocados, banana soy pudding, buttermilk, cheese, chicken or tuna, custard, fruit shakes, nuts and nut butters, whole-grain breads and cereals, turkey, and yogurt. In addition to promoting weight gain, these snacks are easy to digest, are high in protein and essential fatty acids, and contain "friendly" bacteria.

❑ Do not drink liquids before or during meals.

❑ Take supplemental B vitamins as outlined under Nutrients, above. The B-complex vitamins increase appetite.

❑ Try eating small quantities of food at frequent intervals throughout the day rather than two or three large meals. The sight of large amounts of food can cause a person to lose his or her appetite. Frequent small meals may be better tolerated, with a gradual increase in the volume of food.

❑ Exercise if possible, but avoid strenuous exercise. Walking and/or moderate exercise can increase the appetite. Exercise also helps the body to assimilate nutrients better.

❑ If you smoke, quit. Smoking decreases the appetite. It is one of the main causes of loss of appetite.

❑ When trying to stimulate a poor appetite, consider whether the appearance and aroma of the foods are appealing, and whether the environment is conducive to eating.

❑ If you experience a significant loss of appetite, see your physician to rule out an underlying physical problem.

CONSIDERATIONS

❑ To stimulate a poor appetite, the diet must be individualized according to the person's tolerances and tastes.

❑ There are many products on the market that can be helpful for people with appetite and weight problems. They are often found in the "sports" sections of health food stores, but they are not only for those who are into sports.

❑ *See also* ANOREXIA NERVOSA and BULIMIA in Part Two. *See also* HYPOTHYROIDISM in Part Two for the self-test.

Arsenic Poisoning

Arsenic is a highly poisonous metallic element found at varying levels in a wide variety of sources, including pesticides, laundry aids, smog, tobacco smoke, bone meal, dolomite, kelp, table salt, beer, seafood, and even drinking water. When ingested, inorganic arsenic is deposited in the hair, skin, and nails. Once it makes its way into the hair follicles, its presence can be detected in the hair shaft for years.

Headaches, confusion, drowsiness, convulsions, and changes in fingernail pigmentation may occur with chronic arsenic poisoning. Symptoms of acute arsenic poisoning include vomiting, diarrhea, bloody urine, muscle cramps and/or weakness, fatigue, hair loss, dermatitis, gastrointestinal pain, and convulsions. Arsenic poisoning primarily affects the lungs, skin, kidneys, and liver. The accumulation of toxic levels of arsenic can result in coma and death.

Exposure to arsenic has been implicated in the development of certain types of cancer as well. Workers involved in pesticide production, agricultural insecticide spraying, copper smelting, mining, sheep dipping, and metallurgical industries are at a high risk for skin cancer, scrotal cancer, a type of liver cancer, cancer of the lymphatic system, and lung cancer due to arsenic exposure. The toxic effects of arsenic are cumulative.

Unless otherwise specified, the dosages recommended in this section are for adults. For a child between the ages of twelve and seventeen, reduce the dose to three-quarters the recommended amount. For a child between six and twelve, use one-half the recommended dose, and for a child under the age of six, use one-quarter the recommended amount.

NUTRIENTS

SUPPLEMENT	SUGGESTED DOSAGE	COMMENTS
Very Important		
Garlic (Kyolic from Wakunaga)	2 tablets 3 times daily, with meals.	A potent detoxifier.
Superoxide dismutase (SOD) or	As directed on label.	A powerful detoxifying agent.
Cell Guard from Biotec Foods	As directed on label.	An antioxidant complex that contains SOD.
Vitamin C with bioflavonoids	5,000–20,000 mg daily, in divided doses. (*See* ASCORBIC ACID FLUSH in Part Three.)	A potent detoxifier. (Use a buffered form.)
Helpful		
L-Cysteine and L-methionine	500 mg each daily, on an empty stomach. Take with water or juice. Do not take with milk. Take with 50 mg vitamin B$_6$ and 100 mg vitamin C for better absorption.	Potent detoxifiers of the liver. Cysteine contains sulfur, which eliminates arsenic. (*See* AMINO ACIDS in Part One.)
Pectin plus antioxidant complex (ACES + Zn from Carlson Labs)	As directed on label. As directed on label.	Aids in removing arsenic from the body. To protect against free radical damage.
Selenium	200 mcg daily. If you are pregnant, do not exceed 40 mcg daily.	Helps to rid the body of arsenic.

RECOMMENDATIONS

❑ Eat eggs, onions, beans, legumes, and garlic to obtain sulfur. You can also obtain sulfur from garlic supplements. Sulfur helps eliminate arsenic from the body. The amino acid cysteine also provides sulfur. Sulfur can be purchased in tablet form as well.

❑ Supplement your diet with plenty of fiber daily.

Note: Always take supplemental fiber separately from other supplements and medications.

❑ If you have symptoms of chronic arsenic poisoning, have a hair analysis performed to determine the level of toxic metals in your body. (*See* HAIR ANALYSIS in Part Three.)

❑ In case of accidental arsenic ingestion, *immediately* take 5 charcoal tablets, and take 5 more every fifteen minutes until you reach your health care provider or the emergency room of the nearest hospital. Charcoal tablets should be kept on hand in every household in case of accidental overdose of drugs.

CONSIDERATIONS

❑ Chelation therapy removes toxic metals from the body. (*See* CHELATION THERAPY in Part Three.)

❑ *See also* CHEMICAL POISONING and ENVIRONMENTAL TOXICITY in Part Two.

Arteriosclerosis/Atherosclerosis

Arteriosclerosis and atherosclerosis involve the buildup of deposits on the insides of the artery walls, which causes thickening and hardening of the arteries. In arteriosclerosis, the deposits are composed largely of calcium; in atherosclerosis, the deposits consist of fatty substances, and artery walls lose elasticity and harden. Both conditions have about the same effect on circulation, causing high blood pressure and ultimately leading to angina (chest pain brought on by exertion), heart attack, stroke, and/or sudden cardiac death.

Although arteriosclerosis causes high blood pressure, high blood pressure can also *cause* arteriosclerosis. Calcium-based and fatty deposits typically form in areas of the arteries weakened by high blood pressure or strain. The consequent narrowing of the arteries then makes blood pressure that is already high, even higher. As the arteries become less pliable and less permeable, cells may experience ischemia (oxygen starvation) due to insufficient circulation. If one of the coronary arteries becomes obstructed by accumulated deposits or by a blood clot that has either formed or snagged on the deposit, the heart muscle will be starved for oxygen and an individual will suffer a heart attack, also referred to as a myocardial infarction (MI) or coronary occlusion (a coronary). Older adults are at a greater risk for this kind of heart trouble. When arteriosclerosis occludes the arterial supply of blood to the brain, a cerebrovascular accident, or stroke, occurs.

An estimated 1 million Americans are disabled by peripheral vascular disease (diseases involving the blood vessels in the extremities) each year. Most of those affected have at least one of the major risk factors for atherosclerosis: smoking, family history, hypertension, diabetes, or abnormal cholesterol levels. Advancing age increases the likelihood of developing these diseases, as does atherosclerosis of the coronary or cerebral arteries.

Peripheral atherosclerosis, also called *arteriosclerosis obliterans*, is a type of peripheral vascular disease in which the lower limbs are affected. In the early stages, the major arteries carrying blood to the legs and the feet become narrowed by fatty deposits. Atherosclerosis of the leg or foot not only can limit a person's mobility, but can also lead to loss of a limb. People who have diseased arteries in the leg or foot are likely to have them elsewhere, mainly in the heart and brain. Early signs of peripheral atherosclerosis are aching muscles, fatigue, and cramping pains in the ankles and legs. Depending on which arteries are blocked, there may also be pain in the hips and thighs.

Pain in the legs (most often in the calf, but sometimes in the foot, thigh, hip or buttocks) brought on by walking and quickly relieved by rest is called *intermittent claudication*. This is typically the first symptom of developing peripheral atherosclerosis. Additional symptoms include numbness, weakness, and a heavy feeling in the legs. These symptoms occur because the amount of oxygenated blood passing through the plaque-clogged arteries is insufficient to meet the needs of the exercising leg muscles. The closer the problem lies to the abdominal aorta—the central artery that branches into the legs—the more tissue affected and the more dangerous the condition.

PERIPHERAL ARTERY FUNCTION SELF-TEST

A simple test can determine how well your blood flows through the arteries of your legs. There are three areas on the lower leg where a pulsating artery can be felt by lightly touching the skin covering the artery. One spot is the top of the foot, the second spot is the inner aspect of the ankle, and the third spot is behind the knee.

Apply pressure lightly to the skin on these spots. If you cannot find a pulse, this is an indication that the artery supplying the leg may be narrowed. Special studies may be needed and you should consider consulting your health care provider.

NUTRIENTS

SUPPLEMENT	SUGGESTED DOSAGE	COMMENTS
Very Important		
Calcium and	1,500 mg daily, taken at bedtime.	Needed to maintain proper muscle tone in the blood
magnesium plus	750 mg daily, taken at bedtime.	vessels. Use chelate forms.
vitamin D₃	400 mg daily.	Aids calcium uptake and enhances immune system.
Coenzyme Q₁₀	100 mg daily.	Improves tissue oxygenation.
Essential fatty acids (flaxseed oil, MaxEPA, and omega-3 and omega-6 oil complexes are good sources)	As directed on label.	Reduces blood pressure, lowers cholesterol levels, and helps to maintain proper elasticity of blood vessels. Be sure to use a product that contains vitamin E to keep the essential fatty acids from becoming rancid.
Garlic (Kyolic from Wakunaga)	As directed on label.	Has a lipid (fat) regulating effect.
Multivitamin and mineral complex	As directed on label.	All nutrients are needed for protection.
Selenium	200 mcg daily.	Promotes the action of vitamin E.
Vitamin A plus	25,000 IU daily. If you are pregnant, do not exceed 10,000 IU daily.	A potent antioxidant and free radical scavenger. Use emulsion form for easier assimilation.
natural beta-carotene or	15,000 IU daily.	An antioxidant and precursor of vitamin A.
carotenoid complex (Betatene) and	As directed on label.	
vitamin E	Start with 200 IU daily and increase by 200 IU each week until you reach 1,000 IU daily.	A powerful antioxidant that helps to block the first steps leading to the disease. Powerful antioxidant. Use d-alpha-tocopherol form. Use emulsion form for easier assimilation.
Vitamin C with bioflavonoids	5,000–20,000 mg daily, in divided doses. (*See* ASCORBIC ACID FLUSH in Part Three.)	Antioxidant that acts as a free radical scavenger. Works with Vitamin E. Use a buffered form.

Important		
Choline or lecithin granules or capsules	As directed on label. 1 tbsp 3 times daily, with meals. 2,400 mg 3 times daily, with meals.	Aids in breaking down fat and expelling it from the body. Phosphatidyl choline is best. A good source of choline.
Citrin		See under HERBS, below.
Dimethylglycine (DMG) (Aangamik DMG from FoodScience of Vermont)	125 mg 3 times daily.	Improves tissue oxygenation.
Germanium	200 mg daily.	Lowers cholesterol and improves cellular oxygenation.
Heart Science from Source Naturals	As directed on label.	Contains antioxidants, herbs, vitamins, and other nutrients that promote cardiovascular function.
Inositol hexaphosphate (Cellular Forte with IP-6 from PhytoPharmica)	As directed on label. Take on an empty stomach.	Protects the heart by preventing blood clots and reducing cholesterol and triglyceride levels.
Melatonin	2–3 mg daily, taken 2 hours or less before bedtime.	A powerful antioxidant that also improves sleep.
Multienzyme complex	As directed on label. Take with meals.	Important for proper digestion.
Proteolytic enzymes	As directed on label. Take with meals.	Aids in destroying free radicals. Improves digestive function.
Pycnogenol or grape seed extract	50 mg twice daily. As directed on label.	Possibly the most powerful free radical scavengers. Also enhances and strengthens connective tissue, including that of the cardiovascular system.
Vitamin B₁₂ and folic acid	As directed on label. As directed on label.	Vitamin B₁₂ and folic acid combine forces to reduce homocysteine levels, a risk factor for atherosclerosis. May also reduce stress, increase stamina and endurance.

Helpful		
Coenzyme A from Coenzyme-A Technologies.	As directed on label.	Supports the immune system's detoxification of many dangerous substances.
L-cysteine and L-methionine plus L-carnitine	500 mg daily, on an empty stomach. Take with water or juice. Do not take with milk. Take with 50 mg vitamin B₆ and 100 mg vitamin C for better absorption. 500 mg daily, on an empty stomach. 500 mg daily, on an empty stomach.	Promotes the burning of fat and the building of muscle. Helps to prevent fatty buildup in the arteries. Protects the heart and lowers blood triglyceride levels.

Vitamin B complex plus extra niacinamide	100 mg of each major B vitamin 3 times daily (amounts of individual vitamins in a complex will vary). 100 mg 3 times daily.	The B vitamins work together as a complex. Dilates small arteries. Caution: Do not substitute niacin for niacinamide.
Zinc plus copper	50 mg daily. Do not exceed a total of 100 mg daily from all supplements. 3 mg daily.	Aids in cleansing and in the healing process. Use chelate forms. (See also CHELATION THERAPY in Part Three.) Needed to balance with Zinc.

HERBS

❑ The following herbs are helpful if you suffer from arteriosclerosis: cayenne (capsicum), chickweed, and hawthorn berries.

❑ Citrin is an herbal extract that inhibits the synthesis of potentially dangerous fats in the body.

❑ Ginkgo biloba has been called "nature's circulation wonder." It can improve circulation, increasing oxygen and blood flow in the arms, brain, and heart.

❑ Green tea lowers cholesterol and lipid levels, thus decreasing chances of atherosclerosis. Drink green tea (we suggest one to four cups each day) or take it in extract form. A recent Japanese study recommends not only green tea but black tea as well to lower your rate of lipoprotein oxidation, a chemical reaction that makes fats in the blood more likely to be deposited in the arteries.

RECOMMENDATIONS

❑ Eat high-fiber foods that are low in fat and cholesterol. Fruits, vegetables, and grains should be your primary foods.

❑ Eat plenty of foods rich in vitamin E to improve circulation. Good choices include dark green leafy vegetables, legumes, nuts, seeds, soybeans, wheat germ, and whole grains.

❑ Use only pure cold-pressed olive oil or unrefined canola oil (in moderate amounts) as fats in the diet. These may aid in lowering cholesterol. Do not heat these oils.

❑ Drink steam-distilled water only.

❑ Do not eat any candies, chips, fried foods, gravies, high-cholesterol foods, junk foods, pies, processed foods, red meat, or saturated fats. Avoid egg yolks, ice cream, salt, and all foods containing white flour and/or sugar. Do not use stimulants such as coffee, colas, and tobacco. Also, eliminate alcohol and highly spiced foods.

❑ Maintain a healthy weight for your height. Obesity causes unfavorable changes in serum lipoprotein levels.

❑ Reduce stress and learn techniques to help you handle stress that cannot be avoided. (See STRESS in Part Two.)

❑ Get regular moderate exercise. A daily walk is good.

Caution: If you are over thirty-five and/or have been sedentary for some time, consult your health care provider before beginning any type of exercise program.

❑ Periodically monitor your blood pressure, and take steps to lower it if necessary. (*See* HIGH BLOOD PRESSURE in Part Two.) Control of high blood pressure is important.

❑ Do not smoke. Avoid exposure to secondhand smoke. Cigarette smoke contains large quantities of free radicals, many of which are known to oxidize low-density lipoproteins (LDL, the so-called "bad cholesterol"), making them more likely to be deposited on the walls of blood vessels. The free radical is one of the primary factors in the development of atherosclerosis. The effect of cigarette smoke may be due to the direct oxidation of lipids and proteins, and may also have indirect effects, such as the depletion of various antioxidant defenses, which then allows other cellular processes (inflammation, for example) to modify LDL. In addition, smoking increases levels of LDL, lowers levels of high-density lipoproteins (HDL, or "good cholesterol"), and increases the blood's tendency to form clots.

❑ Do not take any preparations containing shark cartilage unless specifically directed to do so by your health care provider. Shark cartilage may inhibit the formation of new blood vessels, the mechanism by which the body can increase circulatory capacity.

CONSIDERATIONS

❑ In the Lifestyle Heart Trial study, conducted over a period of six years at the California Pacific Medical Center, eighteen of twenty-two people (82 percent) who adopted a vegetarian diet that restricted fat intake to 10 percent of total calories showed a significant regression of advanced coronary artery disease after one year. The diet also limited dietary cholesterol to no more than 5 milligrams per day. In contrast, most Americans consume 37 percent of their total calories as fats and 300 to 500 milligrams of dietary cholesterol each day.

❑ Dehydroepiandrosterone (DHEA) is a natural hormone that has been shown to help prevent hardening of the arteries. (*See* DHEA THERAPY in Part Three.)

❑ Chelation therapy can break up arterial plaque and improve circulation. Some two to three thousand doctors perform this type of therapy in the United States. (*See* CHELATION THERAPY in Part Three.)

❑ Hyperbaric oxygen is used in some countries to treat arteriosclerosis. (*See* HYPERBARIC OXYGEN THERAPY in Part Three.)

❑ Many doctors recommend angioplasty or bypass surgery for people with hardening of the arteries, particularly for those with disabling angina. Angioplasty is a procedure in which blocked vessels are reopened by flattening cholesterol and debris against artery walls. Bypass surgery involves taking healthy blood vessels from elsewhere in the body (usually the leg) and inserting them to detour around a diseased coronary artery. Unless people undergoing these procedures make significant nutritional and lifestyle changes, however, the disease process (atherosclerosis) will continue, and it is only a matter of time before the fatty deposits begin to build up again.

❑ Anticoagulants such as aspirin are often prescribed to make the blood less prone to clotting. For this to be effective, supplemental vitamin K and foods rich in vitamin K must be avoided. (*See* CARDIOVASCULAR DISEASE in Part Two.)

❑ Impotence can result from this disease. (*See* IMPOTENCE in Part Two.)

❑ Omega-3 and omega-6 essential fatty acids (EFAs) can be beneficial for the cardiovascular system. They are precursors of prostaglandins that aid in reducing hypertension, migraine headaches, arthritis, and other conditions. Omega-3 EFAs are found in fresh deepwater fish, fish oil, canola oil, flaxseed oil, and walnut oil. Omega-6 EFAs can be obtained from raw nuts, legumes, seeds, grape seed oil, primrose oil, sesame oil, and soybean oil. Reports indicate that native Arctic peoples, whose diets are high in these oils, have very low rates of arteriosclerosis.

Arthritis

Arthritis is the inflammation of one or more joints. It is characterized by pain and stiffness (especially in the morning or after exercise), swelling, deformity, and/or a diminished range of motion. Bone growths or spurs may develop in the affected joints, increasing pain and decreasing mobility. There may be audible cracking or grating noises when the joint moves. More than 55 million Americans suffer from osteoarthritis, rheumatoid arthritis, and related conditions, including fibromyalgia, gout, lupus, Lyme disease, psoriatic arthritis, bursitis, scleroderma, Reiter's syndrome, Sjögren's syndrome, and ankylosing spondylitis. Indeed, arthritis and other diseases of the musculoskeletal system are the primary source of disability in the United States today.

Arthritis is not a modern ailment—it has been with us since the beginning of time. Archeologists have discovered evidence of the disorder in the skeletons of Neanderthals and other prehistoric mammals, and even dinosaurs. Still, as long as this disorder has plagued humankind, conventional medicine remains confounded as to why it occurs.

These conditions affect the body's movable, or *synovial*, joints at the knees, wrists, elbows, fingers, toes, hips, and shoulders. The neck and back also have joints between the bones of the spine. There are six different types of synovial joints (hinge, ball-and-socket, and so on), but although the types of motion they allow are different, their underlying physiological structure is essentially the same: two or more adjoining movable bones, whose adjacent surfaces are covered with a layer of cartilage, surrounded by a fluid-filled capsule made up of ligaments (tough, fibrous tissue). Fluid is secreted by a thin membrane, the synovial membrane, that lines the inside of the joint capsule. Thanks to this viscous fluid, and to the smooth, rubbery, blue-white cartilage covering the ends of the bones, the bones within the joint normally glide smoothly past one another.

In healthy joints, the synovial membrane is thin, the cartilage that covers the bones is smooth, and a thin layer of synovial fluid covers the bone surfaces. A problem in any of these areas can result in arthritis. Arthritis may appear suddenly or come on gradually. Some people feel a sharp burning or grinding pain. Others compare the pain to that of a toothache. Moving the joint usually hurts, although sometimes there is only stiffness. The swelling and deformity that takes place in arthritic joints can result from a thickening of the synovial membrane, an increase in the secretion of synovial fluid, enlargement of the bones, or some combination of these factors.

There are many different types of arthritis. Here we primarily discuss the most common forms: osteoarthritis and rheumatoid arthritis (RA). *Osteoarthritis,* also called degenerative joint disease, involves deterioration of the cartilage protecting the ends of the bones. It is sometimes caused by injury or an inherited defect in the protein that forms cartilage. More commonly, it is a result of the wear and tear of aging, diet, and lifestyle. The once-smooth surface of cartilage becomes rough, resulting in friction. The cartilage begins to break down, and the normally smooth sliding surfaces of the bones become pitted and irregular. Osteoarthritis affects the weight-bearing joints—the knees, hips, and back—most severely, but it also commonly affects the hands and the knuckles. The tendons, ligaments, and muscles holding the joint together become weaker, and the joint becomes deformed, painful, and stiff. There is usually some stiffness and pain (more stiffness than pain at first), but little or no swelling. Any resulting disability is most often minor. However, fractures become an increasing risk because osteoarthritis makes the bones brittle. As osteoarthritis advances, bony outgrowths called osteophytes tend to develop. Often referred to as "spurs," osteophytes can be detected by x-ray and develop near degenerated cartilage in the neck or in the lower back. This condition does not change a person's appearance.

Osteoarthritis rarely develops before the age of forty, but it affects nearly everyone past the age of sixty. It may be so mild that a person is unaware of it until it appears on an x-ray. Nearly three times as many women as men have osteoarthritis.

Rheumatoid arthritis (RA), a type of inflammatory arthritis, is an autoimmune disorder. An overactive immune system can be just as harmful as a weak one. As with other autoimmune disorders, rheumatoid arthritis is a "self-attacking-self" disease. In this case, the body's immune system improperly identifies the synovial membrane as *foreign.* Inflammation results, damaging cartilage and tissues in and around the joints. Often, the bone surfaces are destroyed as well because inflammation in the joints triggers the production of enzymes that slowly digest adjacent tissue. The body replaces this damaged tissue with scar tissue, forcing normal spaces within the joints to become narrow and the bones to fuse together. Rheumatoid arthritis creates stiffness, swelling, fatigue, anemia, weight loss, fever, and, often, crippling pain.

Rheumatoid arthritis frequently occurs in people under forty years of age. Currently, 2.1 million Americans have this disabling disorder, 75 percent of them female. Juvenile arthritis is a form of rheumatoid arthritis that strikes children under the age of sixteen. It affects 71,000 young Americans, again, most of them female. The onset of rheumatoid arthritis is associated with physical or emotional stress, poor nutrition, and bacterial infection. Rheumatologists have discovered that the blood of many people with rheumatoid arthritis contains antibodies called "rheumatoid factors," a finding that can aid in the diagnosis of the condition. While osteoarthritis affects individual joints, rheumatoid arthritis affects all of the body's synovial joints. Joints affected by rheumatoid arthritis tend to make a sound like crinkling cellophane, whereas osteoarthritic joints make popping, clicking, and banging noises.

Arthritis can also be caused by bacterial, viral, or fungal infection of a joint. The microorganisms most commonly involved in this type of the disorder are streptococci, staphylococci, gonococci, hemophilus or tubercle bacilli, and fungi such as *Candida albicans.* Usually the infecting organism travels to the joint through the bloodstream from an infection elsewhere in the body, but injury or even surgery can result in joint infection as well. Symptoms include redness, swelling, pain, and tenderness in the affected joint, often accompanied by systemic symptoms of infection such as fever, chills, and body aches.

The *spondyloarthropathies* are a group of rheumatic disorders that tend to affect the spine. Ankylosing spondylitis (AS) is the most common of these. In this disorder, certain joints of the spine become inflamed, then stiffen and become rigid. If confined to the lower back, AS causes virtually no limitation of movement. In some cases, however, the entire spine may become rigid and bent. If the joints between the ribs and spine are affected, breathing problems may result as the chest wall's ability to expand becomes limited. Postural deformities are common. More than 400,000 Americans suffer from AS. Twice as many men as women have this disorder.

Gout, an acute form of inflammatory arthritis, occurs most often in people who are overweight and/or who indulge regularly in rich foods and alcohol. It typically attacks the smaller joints of the feet and hands, especially the big toe. Deposits of crystallized uric acid salt in the joint cause swelling, redness, and a sensation of heat and extreme pain. Approximately 1 million Americans suffer from gout, and unlike most forms of arthritis, gout overwhelmingly affects men. Ninety percent of those who suffer from gout are male. (*See* GOUT in Part Two.)

Arthritis can be reversible and, in some cases, curable with proper diet and lifestyle changes. These simple changes can not only relieve the inflammation and pain but stop degeneration and rejuvenate the affected joints. Most of the supplements listed below can be found in multinutrient complexes.

NUTRIENTS

SUPPLEMENT	SUGGESTED DOSAGE	COMMENTS
Essential		
Bromelain	As directed on label 3 times daily.	An enzyme that helps to stimulate production of prostaglandins. Reduces inflammation when taken between meals. Helps digestion of protein when taken with meals.
Chondroitin sulfate	500–1,000 mg daily.	Nutritional support for strengthening joints, ligaments, and tendons.
Essential fatty acids (Total EFA and EFA Joint Formula from Health From The Sun, omega-3 and omega-6 oil complexes, salmon oil from Carlson Labs, flaxseed oil, Kyolic-EPA from Wakunaga, and Lyprinol are good sources)	As directed on label twice daily. Take with meals.	To supply essential fatty acids that increase production and activity of anti-inflammatory prostaglandins. Helps to control arthritis pain and inflammation.
Glucosamine sulfate (GS-500 from Enzymatic Therapy) or N-Acetylglucosamine (N-A-G from Source Naturals)	As directed on label. 500–1,000 mg daily.	Very important for the formation of bones, tendons, ligaments, cartilage, and synovial (joint) fluid.
Methylsulfonyl-methane (MSM)	500–1,000 mg 3 times daily.	A sulfur compound needed for reducing inflammation and for joint and tissue repair.
S-Adenosylmethio-nine (SAMe) (SAMe Rx-Mood from Nature's Plus)	400 mg twice daily.	A deficiency results in the inability to maintain cartilage properly. Aids in reducing pain and inflammation. *Caution:* Do not use if you have manic-depressive disorder or take prescription antidepressants.
Sea cucumber (bêche-de-mer)	As directed on label.	A rich source of specific lubricating compounds found abundantly in all connective tissues, especially the joints and joint fluid. It may take 3 to 6 weeks to note an improvement.
Silica	As directed on label.	Supplies silicon, important for formation of apatite crystal, the primary constituent in bone.
Superoxide dismutase (SOD) or Cell Guard from Biotec Foods	As directed on label. As directed on label.	An antioxidant that protects fluid in the joints from destruction by free radicals. A sublingual form is recommended. Consider injections (under a doctor's supervision). An antioxidant complex that contains SOD.
Trimethylglycine (TMG)	500–1,000 mg in the morning.	Reduces homocysteine levels.
Vitamin E	400–800 IU daily.	A powerful antioxidant that protects the joints from damage by free radicals. Increases joint mobility. Low levels of vitamin E have been found in people people with arthritis and lupus. Use d-alpha-tocopherol form. *Caution:* If you are taking blood-thinning medication, consult your physician before taking this supplement.
Very Important		
Boron	3 mg with each meal.	A trace mineral required for healthy bones and uptake of calcium.
Calcium and magnesium plus copper and vitamin D$_3$ and zinc	2,000 mg daily. 1,000 mg daily. 3 mg daily. 800 IU daily. 50 mg daily. Do not exceed a total of 100 mg daily from all supplements.	Needed to prevent bone loss. Use calcium chelate form. Needed to balance with calcium. A cofactor for lysyl oxidase, which strengthens connective tissue and bone formation. Needed for calcium uptake and bone formation. Needed for bone growth. Often deficient in those with arthritis. Use zinc picolinate form.
Cerasomal-cis-9-cetylmyristoleate (CMO)	300 mg morning and night daily.	An anti-inflammatory that reduces inflammation in the joints. *Caution:* Do not take this supplement if you are pregnant or nursing, or if you have liver problems.
Dimethylglycine (DMG) (Aangamik DMG from FoodScience of Vermont)	125 mg 3 times daily.	Helps to prevent further damage to joints.
Free-form amino acid complex (Amino Balance from Anabol Naturals)	As directed on label.	To supply protein, needed for tissue repair. Protein is a major component of bone tissue.
Glucosamine/ Chondroitin MSM Ultra Rx-Joint Cream from Nature's Plus	As directed on label.	Topical cream for relief of inflamed joints.
Kelp or alfalfa	As directed on label.	A rich source of minerals needed for good skeletal health. *See under* Herbs, below.
Multienzyme complex	As directed on label. Take with meals.	To aid digestion. *Caution:* If you have a history of ulcers, do not use a product containing HCl.

Selenium	200 mcg daily. If you are pregnant, do not exceed 40 mcg daily.	A powerful antioxidant.
Vitamin B complex with para-aminobenzoic acid (PABA)	50 mg of each major B vitamin 3 times daily (amounts of individual vitamins in a complex will vary).	B vitamins work best when taken together. Use a hypoallergenic formula. Good for swelling.
plus extra vitamin B$_3$ (niacin) or niacinamide	100 mg 3 times daily. Do not exceed this amount. Good for knee pain.	Increases blood flow by dilating small arteries. *Caution:* Do not take niacin if you have a liver disorder, gout, or high blood pressure. Especially for rheumatoid
plus pantothenic acid (vitamin B$_5$) and	500–1,000 mg daily.	arthritis; vital for the production of steroids in the adrenal gland.
vitamin B$_6$ (pyridoxine)	50 mg daily.	Reduces swelling in tissue.
Vitamin B$_{12}$ and folic acid	1,000 mcg daily. 400 mcg daily.	Needed for proper digestion, the formation of cells, production of myelin and the protective coating surrounding the nerves. Prevents nerve damage.
Vitamin C plus bioflavonoids	3,000–10,000 mg daily, in divided doses. 500 mg daily.	Powerful free radical destroyer that also aids in pain relief because of its anti-inflammatory effect. Use a buffered form. Boosts the activity of vitamin C.
Vitamin K	As directed on label.	Helps deposit minerals into the bone matrix.

Helpful

Bone Defense from KAL	As directed on label.	Contains calcium, magnesium, phosphorus and other valuable bone-reinforcing nutrients.
DL-Phenylalanine (DLPA)	500 mg daily every other week.	Good for pain relief. *Caution:* Do not take this supplement if you are pregnant or nursing, or if you suffer from panic attacks, diabetes, high blood pressure, or PKU.
EPA Joint Formula from Health From The Sun	As directed on label.	Contains essential fatty acids and other important nutrients that help to maintain healthy cartilage, connective tissue, and bones.
Garlic (Kyolic from Wakunaga)	2 capsules 3 times daily, with meals.	Inhibits the formation of free radicals, which can damage the joints.
Healthy Joint Image from Coenzyme-A Technologies	As directed on label.	Contains pantothenic acid, glucosamine sulfate, chondroitin sulfate, cerasomal-cis-9-cetylmyristoleate, methylfsulfonylmethane (MSM), and other nutrients to support healthy bone, joint, ligament, and cartilage function.
L-Cysteine	500 mg twice daily, on an empty stomach. Take with water or juice. Do not take with milk. Take with 50 mg vitamin B$_6$ and 100 mg vitamin C for better absorption.	A detoxifier essential for immune function; a source of sulfur and component of collagenous tissue. (*See* AMINO ACIDS in Part One.)
L-Histidine	As directed on label.	Aids in building joints and connective tissue.

MSM Lotion from Aerobic Life Industries and emu oil or Arthritic Pain Relief Cream from Wakunaga	Apply topically as directed on label. As directed on label.	Good for stiffness and pain. A cooling, fast-acting arthritis cream. It can also be used on animals.
Multivitamin complex with vitamin A and natural beta-carotene	10,000 IU daily. 15,000 IU daily.	All nutrients are needed to aid in repairing tissues and cartilage.
Pregnenolone	As directed on label.	Good for pain and inflammation.
Proteolytic enzymes or Inflazyme Forte from American Biologics	As directed on label. Take between meals. As directed on label.	To protect the joints from free radical damage.
Pycnogenol or grape seed extract	As directed on label. As directed on label.	Improves joint flexibility, repairs connective tissue by reducing the prostaglandins that cause inflammation, and inhibits histamine release responsible for tissue damage.
Shark cartilage (BeneFin from Lane Labs) or VitaCarte from Phoenix BioLabs	Start with 1 gram per 15 lbs of body weight daily, divided into 3 doses. When relief is achieved, reduce the dosage to 1 gm per 40 lbs of body weight daily. As directed on label.	Treats pain and inflammation. Aids in repairing joints and bones. Contains bovine cartilage, shown to be effective in improving rheumatoid arthritis.

HERBS

❑ Alfalfa contains all the minerals essential for bone formation, and may be helpful for arthritis. It can be taken in capsules or in whole, natural form. Kelp also contains essential minerals and is good for thyroid function.

❑ Boswellia, an Ayurvedic herb, is important for reducing inflammation. It also helps restore blood vessels around inflamed connective tissue. Choose a product standardized to contain 150 milligrams of boswellic acids per tablet or capsule. Boswellia can also be used topically, in cream form, to relieve pain. Boswellin Cream from Nature's Herbs is a good source.

❑ Cat's claw is helpful for relieving arthritis pain. Feverfew and ginger also are good for pain and soreness. Ginger is a powerful antioxidant that has anti-inflammatory effects. The active component is gingerol.

Caution: Do not use cat's claw or feverfew during pregnancy.

❑ The hot peppers known as cayenne (capsicum) contain a compound called capsaicin that relieves pain, apparently by inhibiting the release of substance P, a neurotransmitter responsible for communicating pain sensations. Capsaicin can be absorbed through the skin. Mix cayenne powder with enough wintergreen oil to make a paste and apply it to painful joints, or use cayenne peppers in a poultice. (*See* USING A POULTICE in Part Three). This may cause a stinging sensation at first, but with repeated use, pain should diminish markedly. Cayenne can also be taken in capsule form (Cool Cayenne from Solaray is a good source).

❏ Du Huo Jisheng Wan is an herbal Chinese patent medicine that has proven to be beneficial for arthritis sufferers.

❏ Joint Care from Himalaya USA is an Ayurvedic herbal combination formula designed to support joint health.

❏ Nettle leaf is used in Germany for its anti-inflammatory properties.

❏ Noni, known as "the sacred plant" to Polynesian peoples in the South Pacific, has been used for over 2,000 years for pain, arthritis, and other health problems.

❏ Olive leaf extract is good for infectious arthritis. Used for thousands of years by people living in the Mediterranean, it is said to be nature's safe and effective antibiotic. Natural compounds such as oleuropein in the leaf act as powerful germ-killers capable of destroying microbes that can cause arthritis. There are reportedly no adverse side effects.

❏ Phytodolor from either PhytoPharmica or Enzymatic Therapy is a patented blend of ash bark, aspen bark, and goldenrod. It has been used in Germany for both osteoarthritis and rheumatoid arthritis for more than thirty years. Research has found it to be safe and easy on the stomach.

Caution: Do not use this formula if you are sensitive to salicylates.

❏ Turmeric contains curcumin, which has anti-inflammatory and pain-relieving properties. It is good for inflammatory conditions such as arthritis. The recommended dose is 600 milligrams daily.

❏ Willow bark is also good for pain and inflammation.

❏ Other beneficial herbs include brigham tea, buchu leaves, burdock root, celery seed, corn silk, devil's claw tea, horsetail, nettle, parsley tea, willow bark, and yucca.

RECOMMENDATIONS

❏ Eat more sulfur-containing foods, such as asparagus, eggs, garlic, and onions. Sulfur is needed for the repair and rebuilding of bone, cartilage, and connective tissue, and it also aids in the absorption of calcium. Other beneficial foods include fresh vegetables (especially green leafy vegetables, which supply vitamin K), nonacidic fresh fruits, whole grains, oatmeal, brown rice, fish, soybean products, and avocados. Be sure to include these foods in your diet. Also, tart red cherries can relieve pain and inflammation. Eat about 20 cherries each day. If you can't find fresh cherries, the frozen variety is fine.

❏ Consume foods containing the amino acid histidine, including rice, wheat, and rye. Histidine is good for removing excess metals from the body. Many people with arthritis have high levels of copper and iron in their bodies.

❏ Eat fresh pineapple frequently. Bromelain, an enzyme found in pineapple, is excellent for reducing inflammation. To be effective, the pineapple must be fresh, as freezing and canning destroy enzymes.

❏ Eat some form of fiber, such as ground flaxseeds, oat bran, or rice bran, daily.

❏ Reduce the amount of fat in your diet. Do not consume milk, dairy products, or red meat. Also avoid caffeine, citrus fruits, paprika, salt, tobacco, and everything containing sugar.

❏ Avoid the nightshade vegetables (peppers, eggplant, tomatoes, white potatoes). These foods contain a substance called solanine, to which some people, particularly those suffering from arthritis, are highly sensitive. Solanine interferes with enzymes in the muscles, and may cause pain and discomfort.

❏ If you use ibuprofen or other nonsteroidal anti-inflammatory drugs (NSAIDs), avoid sodium (salt), which causes water retention. Spread doses of these medications throughout the day, take them only after eating, and take an antacid an hour after taking the drug. Ask your health care provider about a protective agent to take along with the NSAID especially if you are over sixty-five or have had previous gastrointestinal bleeding.

❏ Do not take iron supplements, or a multivitamin containing iron. Iron is suspected of being involved in pain, swelling, and joint destruction. Consume iron in foods instead. Good sources include blackstrap molasses, broccoli, Brussels sprouts, cauliflower, fish, lima beans, and peas.

❏ For relief of pain, try using cold gel packs. These retain cold for long periods when frozen. Place them on inflamed joints. Alternate with applications of heat.

❏ Hot tubs and baths may provide relief. Raw lemon rubs and hot castor oil packs are also extremely beneficial. To make a hot castor oil pack: place castor oil in a pan and heat but do not boil it. Dip a piece of cheesecloth or other white cotton material into the oil until the cloth is saturated. Apply the cloth to the affected area and cover it with a piece of plastic that is larger in size than the cotton cloth. Place a heating pad over the plastic and use it to keep the pack warm. Keep the pack in place for one-half to two hours, as needed.

❏ In the morning, take a hot shower or a bath to help relieve morning stiffness.

❏ Take a free-form amino acid complex regularly to help repair tissue.

❏ Check for possible food allergies. Many sufferers of neck and shoulder pain have found relief when they eliminate certain foods. Allergies trigger inflammation and can aggravate arthritic symptoms, especially those of rheumatoid arthritis.

❏ Consider having a hair analysis to determine the levels

of toxic metals in your body. Lead levels have been found to be higher than normal in some arthritis sufferers. (*See* HAIR ANALYSIS in Part Three.)

❏ Spend time outdoors for fresh air and sunshine. Exposure to the sun prompts the synthesis of vitamin D_3, which is needed for proper bone formation.

❏ Get regular moderate exercise. Exercise is essential for reducing pain and retarding joint deterioration. Regular activity that does not put stress on affected joints, but that strengthens surrounding bones, muscles, and ligaments, is valuable for many types of arthritis. Bicycle riding, walking, and water exercises are good choices. Avoid weight-bearing or impact exercises.

❏ If you are overweight, lose the excess pounds. Being overweight can cause and aggravate osteoarthritis.

CONSIDERATIONS

❏ If the blood is too acidic, the cartilage in the joints may dissolve. The joints lose their normal smooth sliding motion, bones rub together, and the joints become inflamed, causing pain. (*See* Acidosis in Part Two.)

❏ Etanercept (Enbrel) is a relatively new drug used to treat rheumatoid arthritis. It apparently blocks the action of tumor necrosis factor, an infection-fighting protein linked to inflammation. This drug has been tied to a number of cases of serious infection and several deaths. The drug's manufacturer, a Seattle-based company called Immunex, now adds a warning to the packaging label informing doctors about the infections.

❏ Celecoxib (Celebrex) is an anti-inflammatory drug sometimes prescribed for both osteoarthritis and rheumatoid arthritis. It works by inhibiting the enzyme cyclo-oxygenase-2 (COX-2). COX-2 inhibitors fight inflammation without causing as many stomach problems as nonsteroidal anti-inflammatory drugs (NSAIDs).

❏ Researchers at Jefferson Medical College in Philadelphia have identified a possible genetic component of osteoarthritis. They found that some individuals have a defect in the gene that instructs cartilage cells to manufacture collagen, an important protein in connective tissue. As a result, the collagen in these individuals' joints is more prone to wear down, depriving the bones of their protective cushion.

❏ In one study, people with rheumatoid arthritis were found to have lower blood levels of folic acid, protein, and zinc than healthy persons. The researchers concluded that drugs prescribed for arthritis had brought about biochemical changes in the subjects' bodies, increasing their a need for certain nutrients.

❏ Eating deep-sea fish, which are rich in eicosapentaenoic acid (EPA) and docosahexaenoic acid (DHA), helped relieve the symptoms of rheumatoid arthritis in a study conducted by Charles Dinarello, M.D., of the Tufts University

School of Medicine. Albany Medical College researcher Joel M. Kremer conducted a study in which twenty people with rheumatoid arthritis were given daily doses of 15 capsules of MaxEPA, a fish oil concentrate, and twenty were given a placebo. After fourteen weeks, the groups were switched. The people taking the fish oil reported only about half as many tender joints as the placebo group. The fish oil also slowed the onset of fatigue.

❏ Omega-3 essential fatty acids found in fish may alleviate symptoms of rheumatoid arthritis by suppressing the immune system reaction that causes joint inflammation. Over a dozen studies have shown that people with rheumatoid arthritis have fewer tender and swollen joints and less morning stiffness after several months of taking large doses of fish oil supplements (2.5 to 5 grams a day) with meals. A limited amount of people have even been able to reduce or discontinue use of anti-inflammatory drugs.

❏ Gamma-linolenic acid (GLA), an omega-6 fatty acid, may ease symptoms of rheumatoid arthritis by suppressing the production of prostaglandins that trigger inflammation. Evening primrose oil and borage seed oil contain GLA.

❏ Researchers are currently looking at an ointment containing the immunosuppressant drug cyclosporine, which is used in transplant patients to prevent rejection of the transplanted organ, as a treatment for a variety of autoimmune diseases, including rheumatoid arthritis. Using the ointment form of cyclosporine apparently lessens the potentially hazardous side effects this drug has when administered by mouth or by injection, such as kidney damage and reduced resistance to infection.

❏ Chlamydia, the organism responsible for many cases of urethritis, has been linked to a form of arthritis that affects young women. In nearly half of the women with unexplained arthritis tested in one study, chlamydia was found in the joints. Seventy-five percent had elevated levels of antibodies to chlamydia in their blood.

❏ Most chiropractors and osteopaths advise women to avoid high-heeled shoes because they place a 30-percent greater compressive pressure on the knees than flat or low-heeled shoes, which may eventually lead to arthritis of the knees. The higher the heel, the greater the force.

❏ Silicone gel breast implants and other silicone prostheses may cause arthritis-like symptoms, such as swelling of joints, contractures, fever, chronic fatigue, and pain. Silicone has also been known to trigger such severe autoimmune diseases as scleroderma and lupus. In a study at the University of California in Davis, sixteen of forty-six women with implants had antibodies that attacked collagen, whereas in a group of forty-five women without implants, only four had the antibodies. Some women have seen arthritic symptoms disappear after having the implants removed but this is not true in all cases.

❏ In one laboratory study, injections of a protein called anti-TGF-B banished painful joint swelling in 75 percent of

Types of Arthritis

Swollen, painful joints can have a variety of causes. The particular symptoms involved make different arthritic conditions distinguishable from one another.

The following table gives an overview of different types of arthritic disorders, their relative incidence, and characteristic features.

Cause of Arthritis	Incidence in U.S.	Typical Age at Onset	Symptoms
Osteoarthritis	15.8 million.	Over 40.	Stiffness and pain on joint motion. Most often comes on gradually, over a period of years. Inflammation is not usually present at first, but in the later stages, inflammation, enlargement of the joint, and muscle contractures may occur. Joint mobility may become limited, and movement may be accompanied by a grating sensation.
Rheumatoid arthritis	2.9 million.	25–50.	Joint stiffness upon awakening that lasts an hour or longer; swelling in specific finger or wrist joints; swelling in the soft tissue around the joints; swelling on both sides of the joint. Swelling can occur with or without pain, and can worsen progressively or remain the same for years before progressing.
Spondyloartho-pathies (including psoriatic arthritis, ankylosing spondylitis, Reiter's syndrome)	2.5 million.	20–40.	A group of disorders that tend to affect the spine, causing pain, stiffness, inflammation, and changes in posture.
Gout	1.6 million (85 percent male).	40.	Sudden onset of extreme pain and swelling of a large joint (usually a big toe, but occasionally other joints).
Systemic lupus erythematosus	300,000 (90 percent female).	18–50.	Fever, weakness, upper body and facial pain, joint pain.
Juvenile rheumatoid arthritis	250,000.	Under 18.	Joint stiffness, often in knee, wrist, and hand. Can also involve kidneys, heart, lungs, and nervous system.
Infectious arthritis	100,000.	Any age.	Body aches, chills, and fever; confusion, dizziness, low blood pressure, pneumonia, and shock; redness, swelling, tenderness, and throbbing pain in the affected joint. Pain sometimes spreads to other joints and worsens with movement.
Kawasaki syndrome	Hundreds of cases in local outbreaks.	6 months– 11 years.	Fever, joint pain, red rash on palms and soles, heart complications.

the subjects, according to Dr. David Pisetsky of the National Arthritis Foundation. This protein destroys TGF-B, a chemical produced by the body in response to infection that causes inflammation and triggers swelling in the hands and feet.

❑ Mobility from Parametric Associates and Cosamin from Nutramax Laboratories are two formulas that may help the joints and ligaments. They are not generally available in health food stores, however. They may be ordered directly from the manufacturers. (*See* MANUFACTURER AND DISTRIBUTOR INFORMATION in the Appendix.)

❑ Dimethylsulfoxide (DMSO), a byproduct of wood processing, is a liquid that can be applied topically to relieve pain, reduce swelling, and promote healing.

Note: Only DMSO from a health food store should be used for the treatment of arthritis. Commercial-grade DMSO such as that found in hardware stores is not suitable for healing purposes. The use of DMSO may result in a garlicky body odor. This is temporary, and is not a cause for concern.

❑ Arthritic pain and inflammation may respond to treatment with honeybee venom. The venom contains a powerful anti-inflammatory substance and also acts as an immune system stimulant. It is administered by injection, either with a hypodermic needle or by the bees themselves. It is believed to be effective for both osteoarthritis and rheumatoid arthritis, although the latter generally takes longer to respond. Further information is available from the American Apitherapy Society (*see* HEALTH AND MEDICAL ORGANIZATIONS in the Appendix). Bee venom is also available in cream form as Bee Venom Balm from Aerobic Life Industries. You should not use this product if you are allergic to bee stings.

❑ Nonsteroidal anti-inflammatory drugs (NSAIDs) such as ibuprofen (found in Advil, Nuprin, and numerous other products), indomethacin (Indocin), and piroxicam (Feldene) are commonly prescribed for relief of arthritis pain. Unfortunately, these drugs also can have side effects. At least 1 in 100 people who take NSAIDs on a regular basis for arthritis develops stomach ulcers or experiences severe gastrointestinal bleeding—effects that are potentially very dangerous. The U.S. Food and Drug Administration recently estimated that as many as 200,000 cases of gastrointestinal bleeding, including 10,000 to 20,000 deaths, occur each year in the United States as a result of nonsteroidal anti-inflammatory drugs prescribed for arthritis. These drugs can also cause kidney or liver damage. According to a study reported in *Annals of Internal Medicine*, the use of NSAIDs can lead to serious health problems if you have even mild kidney dysfunction.

❑ Misoprostol (Cytotec) and ulcer drugs like ranitidine (Zantac) and sucralfate (Carafate) can prevent the development of ulcers associated with NSAIDs. However, these drugs have their own side effects and double the cost of treatment.

❑ Diclofenac sodium (Voltaren), a drug often prescribed for arthritis, may cause serious liver problems in some cases. People who take it should be monitored very closely. If this medication is prescribed, the physician should perform a blood liver enzyme study to determine whether there is a risk of side effects. This test should be done within eight weeks after the beginning of treatment.

❑ For some forms of arthritis, drugs such as hydroxychloroquine (Plaquenil) and gold compound (Ridaura) may be prescribed.

❑ For some individuals, the ulcer drug sucralfate (Carafate) may give the same relief as aspirin and other anti-inflammatory drugs without damaging the stomach lining.

❑ Acetaminophen (sold as Tylenol, Datril, and others) may be a better medication for osteoarthritis than NSAIDs. In many cases, it may be able to relieve the pain of osteoarthritis as well as ibuprofen. Acetaminophen is relatively safe and inexpensive. However, it is important not to exceed the recommended dose of acetaminophen, and it should not be used by persons who consume alcohol. If taken in excessive amounts or in combination with alcohol, this drug can cause liver damage.

❑ Drugs do not always help everyone. Some people who use drugs obtain only partial relief.

❑ Kawasaki syndrome is an infectious disease that can cause symptoms of arthritis in children, accompanied by conjunctivitis; fever; a red rash on the body; a swollen, red tongue; and/or red or purplish-red discoloration and swelling of the palms of the hands and the soles of the feet. The cause of this disorder is not known. It primarily affects children under five years of age. Most children recover, but some, unfortunately, suffer permanent heart damage.

❑ Lyme disease can mimic arthritis, causing many of the same symptoms. (*See* LYME DISEASE in Part Two.)

❑ Systemic lupus erythematosus (SLE) is an autoimmune disease that often manifests itself as arthritis. For reasons unknown, the body produces antibodies that act against its own tissues. (*See* LUPUS in Part Two.)

❑ In its early stages, ulcerative colitis can cause symptoms like those of arthritis. Because this may occur before there are any abdominal symptoms, it can lead to misdiagnosis and delayed treatment. (*See* COLITIS in Part Two.)

❑ More information about arthritis is available from the Arthritis Foundation (*see* HEALTH AND MEDICAL ORGANIZATIONS in the Appendix).

❑ *See also* GOUT in Part Two and PAIN CONTROL in Part Three.

Asthma

Asthma is a lung disease that causes obstruction of the airways. During an asthma attack, spasms in the muscles surrounding the bronchi (small airways in the lungs) constrict, impeding the outward passage of air. Asthma sufferers often describe this plight as "starving for air." Typical symptoms of an asthma attack are coughing, wheezing, a feeling of tightness in the chest, and difficulty breathing. An attack can last for a few minutes or several hours.

The spasms characterizing an acute attack are not the cause of the disorder, but a result of chronic inflammation and hypersensitivity of the airways to certain stimuli. An attack can be triggered if a susceptible individual is exposed to an allergen or irritants. There are two forms of asthma: allergic and nonallergic, although the two often occur together. Common asthma-provoking allergens include animal dander, chemicals, drugs, dust mites, environmental pollutants, feathers, food additives (such as sulfites), fumes, mold, and tobacco smoke. But any kind of allergen can precipitate an asthma attack. Factors that can trigger nonallergic asthma attacks include adrenal disorders, anxiety, temperature changes, exercise, extremes of dryness or humidity, fear, laughing, low blood sugar, and stress. A respiratory infection such as bronchitis can also provoke an attack. Whatever the particular instigator, the bronchial tubes swell and become plugged with mucus. This inflammation further irritates the airways, resulting in even greater sensitivity. The attacks become more frequent and the inflammation more severe.

Asthma can be difficult to diagnose conclusively. Its symptoms may resemble those of other diseases, such as emphysema, bronchitis, and lower respiratory infections. To distinguish asthma from other conditions, a physician may recommend blood tests, chest x-rays, and spirometry (a procedure that measures air breathed into and out of the lungs). If not treated properly, bronchial asthma can lead to pulmonary emphysema. However, with prompt diagnosis and appropriate treatment, serious danger from asthma should be preventable.

Cardiac asthma is a condition that causes the same symptoms as other types of asthma, but is caused by heart failure. Intrinsic asthma, a less common form of the disease, which generally appears during adulthood, is often associated with other respiratory diseases such as bronchitis or sinusitis, and tends to appear during upper respiratory viral infections. People who suffer from intrinsic asthma are usually vulnerable to changes in weather, exercise, emotional stress, and other factors related to inner feelings.

A hereditary link to asthma was discovered in late 1999 by two Berkeley, California, researchers who spliced human genes into mice and determined that asthmatic activity could be diminished by slowing the activity of two particular genes. The value of the research, they said, centered on the fact that scientists now have an opportunity to develop a medicine to prevent asthma, rather than merely treat its symptoms.

This genetic-based research milestone in asthma prevention arrived at an important juncture. Medical scientists are growing increasingly alarmed over what they consider to be an epidemic rise in the number of new asthma cases each year. In the past fifteen years, the number of Americans with asthma has doubled. Currently, asthma affects more than 14 million people (5 million children and 9 million adults). Children under age sixteen, particularly those living in urban areas, and adults over the age of sixty-five are most likely to suffer from asthma. It is the number-one cause of hospitalization for children, and the number-one cause of school absenteeism. The incidence of asthma has shot up 75 percent since 1980 and, unfortunately, the rate among children has increased 160 percent. The cause of asthma's continued rise over the years has researchers scratching their heads and looking at a wide spectrum of possible causes, including pollution, global warming, food additives, genetics, toxins, and allergens. Asthma specialists speculate that rising levels of environmental pollution lead to higher incidences of asthma. Asthma epidemics re-

lated to atmospheric contamination—situations in which dust and chemical particles are abundant, especially in enclosed environments—are well known. Occupational exposure to certain substances, such as urethane and polyurethane, used in the adhesives and plastics industry; rubber epoxy resins from paint; textile cleaners fumes; dry-cleaning chemicals; and others may also be a major risk factor.

The dosages recommended here are for adults. For a child between the ages of twelve and seventeen, reduce the dose to three-quarters the recommended amount. For a child between the ages of six and twelve years old, reduce the dose to one-half the recommended amount. For a child under six years old, use one-third the recommended amount.

NUTRIENTS

SUPPLEMENT	SUGGESTED DOSAGE	COMMENTS
Essential		
Flaxseed oil or primrose oil	1,000 mg twice daily, before meals.	Sources of essential fatty acids needed for production of anti-inflammatory prostaglandins.
Pantothenic acid (vitamin B$_5$)	50 mg 3 times daily.	The anti-stress vitamin.
Quercitin-C from Ecological Formulas plus bromelain	500 mg 3 times daily. 100 mg 3 times daily.	Powerful immunostimulants. Quercetin-C has an antihistaminic effect. Stabilizes cells to stop inflammation. Take these supplements together for best results.
or Activated Quercetin from Source Naturals	As directed on label.	Contains quercetin plus bromelain and vitamin C.
Vitamin A plus	15,000 IU daily. If you are pregnant, do not exceed 10,000 IU daily.	Needed for tissue repair and immunity.
natural beta-carotene or	10,000 IU daily.	An antioxidant and precursor of vitamin A.
carotenoid complex (Betatene)	As directed on label.	
Vitamin B complex plus extra	50 mg of each major B vitamin 4 times daily (amounts of individual vitamins in a complex will vary).	Stimulates the immune system.
vitamin B$_6$ (pyridoxine) injections or	$^1/_2$ cc weekly or as prescribed by physician.	Helpful in the treatment of allergies and asthma. Injections (under a doctor's supervision) are best.
capsules plus	50 mg 3 times daily.	
vitamin B$_{12}$	1,000 mcg twice daily, between meals.	Decreases inflammation that occurs in the lungs during an attack. Use a lozenge or sublingual form.
Vitamin C with bioflavonoids	1,500 mg 3 times daily. *Caution:* If you have a history of kidney stones or hemochromatosis, do not take vitamin C at this dosage level.	Needed to protect lung tissue and keep down infection. Also increases air flow and fights inflammation.
Vitamin E	600 IU and up daily.	A potent antioxidant. Use d-alpha-tocopherol form.

Very Important		
Betaine hydrochloride with pepsin	As directed on label, or as prescribed by physician.	Combats malabsorption problems leading to "leaky gut syndrome."
Coenzyme Q$_{10}$	100 mg daily.	Has the ability to counter histamine.
Magnesium plus calcium	750 mg daily. 1,500 mg daily.	May stop the acute asthmatic episode by increasing the vital capacity of the lungs. Has a dilating effect on the bronchial muscles. Use chelate or asporotate forms.
Multivitamin and mineral complex with selenium	As directed on label. 200 mcg daily. If you are pregnant, do not exceed 40 mcg daily.	Necessary for enhanced immune function. Use a high-potency formula. A powerful destroyer of free radicals created from air pollutants.
Helpful		
Bee pollen	Start with a few granules at a time and slowly work up to 2 tsp daily.	Strengthens the immune system. Use raw crude pollen, preferably produced within 10 miles of your home. Caution: Bee pollen may cause an allergic reaction in some individuals. Discontinue use if a rash, wheezing, discomfort, or other symptom occurs.
Coenzyme A from Coenzyme-A Technologies	As directed on label.	Promotes detoxification of dangerous substances from the immune system.
Dimethylglycine (DMG) (Aangamik DMG from FoodScience of Vermont)	As directed on label twice daily.	Improves oxygenation in lung tissue.
Glucosamine sulfate or N-Acetylglucosamine (N-A-G from Source Naturals)	As directed on label. As directed on label.	Important for regulation of mucous secretions of the respiratory tract.
Kelp	2,000–3,000 mg daily for 21 days, then reduce to 1,000–1,500 mg daily.	For minerals in balanced amounts.
L-Cysteine and L-methionine	500 mg twice daily, on an empty stomach. Take with water or juice. Do not take with milk. Take with 50 mg vitamin B$_6$ and 100 mg vitamin C for better absorption. 500 mg twice daily, on an empty stomach.	Repairs lung tissue and reduces inflammation. (See AMINO ACIDS in Part One.) An important antioxidant.
Pycnogenol or grape seed extract	As directed on label. As directed on label.	Powerful antioxidants and anti-inflammatories.
S-Adenosylmethio-nine (SAMe)	As directed on label.	Reduces stress and eases depression. Promotes a sense of well-being. Caution: Do not use if you have manic-depressive disorder or take prescription antidepressants.
Urban Air Defense from Source Naturals	2 tablets daily.	Contains many of the necessary nutrients listed in this table.
Vitamin D$_3$	600 IU daily.	Needed for repair of tissues.

HERBS

❑ Asthma-X$_5$ from Olympian Labs is an herbal combination formula containing coleus forskohlii, feverfew, ginger, green tea, licorice root, lobelia, Mormon tea, schisandra berries, and skullcap. The recommended dosage is 500 to 1,000 milligrams, three times daily. For best results, use for about eight weeks.

❑ ClearLungs from RidgeCrest Herbals is a Chinese herbal formula designed to reduce inflammation and mucus, opening up the airways to the lungs and promoting free breathing. Take 2 capsules twice daily.

❑ Ginkgo biloba, an herb containing the active ingredient ginkgolide B, has shown good results in many studies.

❑ Lobelia extract is helpful during an asthma attack; it is a bronchial soothing muscle relaxant and expectorant.

Caution: Do not take lobelia internally on an ongoing basis.

❑ Mullein oil is said to be a powerful remedy for bronchial congestion. The oil stops coughs, unclogs bronchial tubes, and helps clear up asthma attacks. Users say that when they take it in tea or fruit juice, the effect is almost immediate.

❑ Nettle can be helpful in relieving respiratory problems caused by asthma. It is rich in butyric acid, necessary for a healthy metabolism, as well as other vitamins and minerals.

❑ Pau d'arco acts as a natural antibiotic and reduces inflammation. Drink 3 cups of pau d'arco tea daily.

❑ Shuan Huang Lian is a Chinese herbal combination remedy made up of at least twenty-nine components, including shuang hua (*Lonicera japonica* flower bud), lian qiao (*Forsythia suspensa* fruit), and huang qin (*Scutellaria baicalensis* root). It has long been used by the Chinese to treat infections of the respiratory tract. According to a study published in the June 1999 issue of *Complementary Medicine for the Physician,* Chinese doctors and researchers tested Shuan Huang Lian on infants hospitalized with acute bronchitis and saw a quick reduction of the symptoms and a shorter duration of illness. It is not classified as an antibiotic, and researchers are still delving into how it relieves acute bronchial suffering in infants.

❑ Proponents of the East Indian mind-body-earth philosophy called Ayurveda recommend the following herbs for people with asthma: vasaka (*Adhatoda vasica*) relieves cough, bronchitis, and other asthmatic symptoms; boswellia (*Boswellia serrata*), to relieve pain and inflammation; and tylophora (*Tylophora indica*) for respiratory relief. Sabinsa Corporation is a good source of these Ayurvedic herbs.

❑ Other herbs beneficial for asthma include echinacea, ephedra (ma huang), goldenseal, horsetail, juniper berries, licorice root, and slippery elm bark tablets.

Caution: Do not take echinacea if you have an autoimmune disorder. Do not use ephedra if you suffer from anxiety, glaucoma, heart disease, high blood pressure, or insomnia, or if you are taking a monoamine oxidase (MAO) inhibitor drug for depression. Do not take goldenseal on a daily basis for more than one week at a time and do not use it during pregnancy. If you have a history of cardiovascular disease, diabetes, or glaucoma, use it only under supervision. Do not use licorice on a daily basis for more than seven days in a row, and avoid it completely if you have high blood pressure.

RECOMMENDATIONS

❑ Eat a diet consisting primarily of fresh fruits and vegetables, nuts, oatmeal, brown rice, and whole grains. The diet should be relatively high in protein, low in carbohydrates, and contain no sugar. (*See* HYPOGLYCEMIA in Part Two for suggestions.)

❑ Include garlic and onions in your diet. These foods contain quercetin and mustard oils, which have been shown to inhibit an enzyme that aids in releasing inflammatory chemicals.

❑ Include "green drinks" in your program. Kyo-Green from Wakunaga is excellent. Take it three times a day, one-half hour before meals.

❑ Avoid gas-producing foods, such as beans, brassicas (broccoli, cauliflower, and cabbage) and large amounts of bran, or take an enzyme complex such as Be Sure from Wakunaga of America. Gas can irritate an asthmatic condition by putting pressure on the diaphragm.

❑ Do not eat ice cream or drink extremely cold liquids. Cold can shock the bronchial tubes into spasms.

❑ Use a juice fast, a fast using distilled water and lemon juice, or a combination of both for three days each month to help rid the body of toxins and mucus. (*See* FASTING in Part Three.)

❑ Try using bee propolis, which is soothing to the mucous membranes.

❑ Eat lightly—a large meal can cause shortness of breath by making the stomach put pressure on the diaphragm.

❑ Use an elimination diet to see if certain foods aggravate the asthmatic condition. Common culprits include alfalfa, corn, peanuts, soy, eggs, beets, carrots, colas, cold beverages (which may cause bronchial spasm), dairy products (including milk and ice cream), fish, red meat (especially pork), processed foods, salt, spinach, chicken and turkey, white flour, and white sugar. (*See* ALLERGIES in Part Two.)

❑ We all need exercise to become and remain healthy. If you find exercise can induce an asthma attack, try taking 2,000 milligrams of vitamin C one hour before your workout. Recent studies showed that those who took vitamin C prior to their workouts suffered no coughing, wheezing, or shortness of breath. However, people at risk for kidney stones or hemochromatosis (an iron-absorption disorder) should not take vitamin C at this dosage level.

❑ If exercise produces an asthmatic response, check your salt intake. According to one report, people with asthma who eat high-sodium diets (4,000 milligrams daily) have more difficulty breathing while exercising and immediately afterwards than those who habitually consume far less sodium (1,500 milligrams daily). Ask your doctor what sodium level is right for you.

❑ If you use aspirin or other nonsteroidal anti-inflammatory drugs (NSAIDs), do so with caution. Painkillers such as aspirin, ibuprofen (Advil, Nuprin, and others), naproxen (Naprosyn), and piroxicam (Feldene) account for over two-thirds of drug-related asthmatic reactions, with aspirin causing over half of these. Chemotherapeutic agents and antibiotics also can induce asthma reactions.

❑ Keep an ongoing list of things that trigger your asthmatic responses and then avoid them as best as you can. Also, try keeping a diary of your symptoms, medications, and so on. It can be very helpful to you and your doctor in creating and maintaining your best asthma management program.

❑ Apply castor oil packs to the back and around the lung and kidney areas. To make a castor oil pack, place castor oil in a pan and heat but do not boil it. Dip a piece of cheesecloth or other white cotton material into the oil until the cloth is saturated. Apply the cloth to the affected area and cover it with a piece of plastic that is larger in size than the cotton cloth. Place a heating pad over the plastic and use it to keep the pack warm. Keep the pack in place for one-half to two hours, as needed.

❑ Practice methods to relieve stress. Stress and strong emotions like worry and fear can trigger an asthma attack. (*See* STRESS in Part Two.)

❑ Avoid furry animals; the food additives BHA and BHT; FD&C Yellow No. 5 food dye; tobacco and other types of smoke; and the amino acid tryptophan.

❑ If you suspect that dust mites are causing your asthma symptoms, try to get rid of the microscopic bugs. There are vacuum cleaners on the market that destroy these mites. An application of benzyl benzoate powder (such as X-MITE from Allersearch) will eliminate mites for two to three months. One pound of this powder treats approximately 150 square feet of carpeting or fabric. If local pharmacies don't carry the powder, you can order it from Aller-Guard Corporation of Ocean, New Jersey; telephone 800-234-0816.

❑ Consider removing carpeting, at least in the bedroom, to help keep dust mites, germs, and bacteria from aggravating asthma. Covering mattresses in plastic casings and washing sheets in hot water at least once a week can be helpful, too.

CONSIDERATIONS

❑ Life-threatening cases of asthma diagnosed as *status*

asthmaticus require immediate hospitalization, and sufferers may have to remain hospitalized for days.

❏ People with asthma may be deficient in certain nutrients, such as vitamin B_6 (pyridoxine), vitamin C, magnesium, manganese, and selenium, as well as in the enzyme glutathione peroxidase. People with asthma often have lower than normal levels of gastric hydrochloric acid, which is needed for proper digestion. Dr. Jonathan Wright, a noted nutritionist, claims excellent results using a combination of gastric acid replacement therapy (usually in the form of betaine hydrochloride) and supplementation with vitamin B_6, vitamin B_{12}, and magnesium for treatment of asthma.

❏ According to *Nutrition Health Review,* strong feelings of anger, anxiety, and depression may be an important cause of asthma attacks. Unfortunately, many of the drugs used to control and alleviate asthma cause jittery nerves, mood swings, and insomnia.

❏ Many people with asthma are sensitive to food additives known sulfites. Some people have had severe attacks after consuming foods containing sulfites. Many restaurants use sulfiting agents—including sodium bisulfite, potassium metabisulfite, potassium bisulfite, and sulfur dioxide—to prevent discoloration and bacterial growth in green salads, cut and sliced fruit, frozen shellfish, and other foods. Although most common in these foods, sulfites can be found in any type of food. (*See* Sulfite Allergies on page 158 for additional information.)

❏ Beta-blocking medications, used to treat high blood pressure, can constrict the bronchial muscles and cause life-threatening problems for a person with asthma.

❏ Ozone, sulfur dioxide, nitrogen dioxide, cigarette smoke, carbon monoxide, hydrocarbons, nitrogen oxide, and photochemical substances are air pollutants that can trigger asthma attacks.

❏ Inhaling a muscle-relaxing medication such as albuterol (Proventil, Ventolin) from a bronchodilator can relieve an acute asthma attack immediately by opening the bronchial tubes. Bronchodilators do not treat the underlying problem, however.

❏ A sustained-release form of the drug theophylline, sold under the brand name Theo-Dur Sprinkle, has been used with good results. For children, this medication can be administered by opening a capsule and sprinkling the contents on a soft food such as applesauce. Theophylline has side effects, such as producing a rapid heart beat and/or insomnia in some users. Some doctors believe that inhaled drugs or topical treatments are safer than asthma pills because they are drawn directly into the bronchial tubes and lungs.

❏ Researchers at Harvard and the U.S. Environmental Protection Agency (EPA) have shown that people with asthma who drink coffee and other caffeine-containing drinks generally have one-third fewer symptoms than those who do not. This is most likely due to the action of the caffeine, which has a dilating effect on the bronchial airways.

❏ A study reported in the *Journal of Allergy and Clinical Immunology* suggested that taking 2 salmon oil capsules before each meal and eating fish three times weekly may be beneficial for asthma.

❏ The Air Supply personal air purifier from Wein Products is a miniature unit that is worn around the neck. It sets up an invisible pure air shield against microorganisms (such as viruses, bacteria, and mold) and microparticles (including dust, pollen, and pollutants) in the air. It also eliminates vapors, smells, and harmful volatile compounds in the air. The Living Air XL-15 unit from Alpine Air of America is an ionizing unit that is good for purifying the air in the home or workplace.

❏ Regular exercise is beneficial, but exercise can also trigger an acute attack in some individuals. No one is sure why this is, but it has been speculated that inhaling lots of cool, dry air while working out aggravates the respiratory system. Running, for example, induces many more asthma attacks than swimming. One way to control exercise-induced asthma is to wear a mask that retains heat and moisture and limits the effects of breathing cold, dry air.

❏ Zanamivir (Relenza), a relatively new antiviral drug used for the treatment of influenza, can have a detrimental side effect on asthma sufferers. The U.S. Food and Drug Administration (FDA) notes that it should be used with caution by anyone with asthma or chronic lung disease, and if a person with asthma does take this drug, he or she should have emergency bronchodilator therapy readily available. Interestingly, although the FDA granted clearance for the drug to be marketed, an FDA advisory panel voted against approval, noting that it considered the drug's overall effectiveness as negligible.

❏ A study conducted by North Dakota State University found that people with asthma and arthritis markedly improved their health simply by setting aside time—from twenty minutes a day to three days a week—to write. Of the seventy patients participating in the one-month study, 47 percent showed definite improvement, as opposed to only 24 percent who showed improvement without writing. The researchers concluded that putting your thoughts and observations on paper relieves stress and eases the mind.

❏ Children with asthma experience much more successful treatment through mind and body control training, according to numerous recent studies. Asthma specialist Richard Firshein, D.O., based in New York City, uses a technique in which children are taught not to panic when they realize an asthma attack is approaching. He calmly guides their thought processes into focuses on images and smells that please them; like the warm sun, hot dogs, or a favorite pet. At the same time, he helps them bring their breathing under control. This helps them feel less helpless and afraid. Adults too can benefit from this calming technique.

❑ Goose feathers may cause and aggravate lung ailments.

❑ Air-duct cleaning, sometimes touted as beneficial for people with asthma, may actually swirl even more allergens into the air in your home. According to the American Academy of Allergy and Immunology in Milwaukee, there is no scientific evidence of its effectiveness.

❑ For names and addresses of organizations that can provide further information about this disorder, *see* HEALTH AND MEDICAL ORGANIZATIONS in the Appendix.

Atherosclerosis

See ARTERIOSCLEROSIS/ATHEROSCLEROSIS.

Athlete's Foot

Athlete's foot (tinea pedis) is a fungal infection that thrives in an environment of warmth and dampness. It is the most common fungal infection of the skin and affects about 4 percent of Americans, mostly men. The fungi live off the dead skin cells and calluses of the feet, especially on the skin between the toes. Symptoms include inflammation, burning, itching, scaling, cracking, and blistering.

The fungus that causes athlete's foot spreads rapidly when beneficial bacteria are destroyed by antibiotics, drugs, or radiation. It is especially prevalent and highly contagious in warm, damp places such as gyms and swimming pool locker rooms.

NUTRIENTS

SUPPLEMENT	SUGGESTED DOSAGE	COMMENTS
Essential		
Colloidal silver	Apply topically as directed on label.	A natural antibiotic and disinfectant. Destroys fungi, viruses, and bacteria. Promotes healing.
Kyo-Dophilus from Wakunaga	As directed on label.	Contains acidophilus and aged garlic extract. Both are beneficial in treating fungal disease.
Very Important		
Garlic (Kyolic from Wakunaga)	2 capsules 3 times daily.	Aids in destroying fungus.
Important		
Vitamin B complex	As directed on label.	Needed for healthy skin. Use a yeast-free, high-potency formula. A sublingual form is best.
Vitamin C plus bioflavonoids	3,000–10,000 mg 3 times daily, in divided doses.	Reduces stress and promotes immune function. Use a buffered form.
Zinc	50 mg daily. Do not exceed a total of 100 mg daily from all supplements.	Inhibits fungus and stimulates the immune system.
Helpful		
Aerobic 07 from Aerobic Life Industries	9 drops in a glass of water twice daily. Also apply a few drops directly on affected areas and let dry.	Supplies oxygen to the cells, killing germs and harmful bacteria.
Essential fatty acids (fish oil from Omega-Life and Ultimate Oil from Nature's Secret are good sources)	As directed on label.	Promotes healing of skin disorders.
Vitamin A plus beta-carotene	25,000 IU daily for month, then reduce to 25,000 IU. If you are pregnant, do not exceed 10,000 IU daily.	Needed for healing of tissues and stimulation of the immune system.
Vitamin E	Start with 400 IU daily and increase slowly to 1,000 IU daily.	An antioxidant that promotes healthy skin. Use d-alpha-tocopherol form.

HERBS

❑ Drink 3 cups of pau d'arco tea daily. Pau d'arco tea can also be used topically. Prepare a strong pau d'arco tea, using 6 teabags to 2 quarts of warm water. Add 20 drops of Aerobic 07 from Aerobic Life Industries. Soak your feet in this mixture for fifteen minutes three times daily for quick relief.

❑ As an alternative footbath, add 20 drops of tea tree oil to a small tub of water, and use this to soak your feet for fifteen minutes three times daily. After soaking your feet, dry them thoroughly and dab a few drops of undiluted tea tree oil on the affected area. Tea tree oil is a powerful natural antifungal.

❑ To help ease the redness, cracking, and itching of athlete's foot, rub the oils of myrrh and lavender into your feet at bedtime.

❑ Olive leaf extract is an excellent, safe natural healer of microbial infections.

RECOMMENDATIONS

❑ Eat a balanced diet that includes plenty of raw fruits and vegetables, broiled fish, broiled skinless chicken, whole grains, and yogurt and other acidophilus-containing foods.

❑ Avoid cola drinks, processed foods, refined grains, and all forms of sugar. Do not eat fried or greasy foods.

❑ Take supplements of vitamins A, B, and C as outlined under Nutrients, above.

❑ Keep your feet dry. After bathing, dry carefully between your toes. Make sure to use each towel only once before laundering. Wear absorbent socks made of cotton.

Air your shoes out and change socks daily. Wash socks, towels, and anything that comes into contact with the infected area in very hot water, with chlorine bleach added if possible.

❑ Cut raw garlic into tiny pieces (or into slivers, wrapped in gauze) and wear them in your shoes for a few days. The garlic will be absorbed into the skin. Also dust your feet with garlic powder. Though there are nonprescription antifungal drugs available, we believe garlic works better.

❑ Bathe your feet daily in a half-and-half mixture of vinegar and water. Dry them thoroughly and apply pure, unprocessed oil, such as olive oil, to the infected area. Or soak your feet in a solution of 2 teaspoons of salt in a pint of warm water for ten minutes. Repeat this treatment daily until the condition clears up.

❑ To ease pain and itching, use cold compresses. Soak a white cotton cloth in Burow's solution (available in drugstores) dissolved in 1 pint of cold water. Apply compresses several times a day for fifteen to twenty minutes at a time.

❑ Take care to protect your feet from direct contact with floors in communal areas such as locker rooms. Wear shoes or slippers in such places. Do not share shoes, socks, towels, or anything else that comes into contact with the feet.

❑ Wear well-ventilated shoes such as sandals, leather shoes, or sneakers with holes that allow your feet to breathe. Do not wear shoes made of rubber of vinyl material. Try not to wear the same shoes every day, and be sure to change wet shoes immediately.

❑ If the condition doesn't clear up in four weeks, if there is pus in the blisters or in the cracked skin, if a fever develops, or if there is swelling in the foot or leg, see your health care provider. Severe cases may require medical attention.

CONSIDERATIONS

❑ Several over-the-counter antifungal drugs called known as *azoles* are considered among the best treatments for athlete's foot. These include clotrimazole (in Lotrimin AF), miconazole (Micatin, Zeabsorb-AF), and undecylenic acid (Cruex, Desenex). A newer antifungal medication called terbinafine (Lamisil) cream is also available.

❑ Athlete's foot can become complicated by a fungal toenail infection (*See* NAIL PROBLEMS in Part Two). Keep the toenails clean, but do not use a metal file that can damage the nail and give the fungus a place to grow. If the toenails become thick and discolored, see a podiatrist.

❑ Those with recurrent fungal infections of the feet often have a fungal infection in the groin area. Both areas must be treated simultaneously. To prevent transmission of the foot fungus to the groin area, put clean socks on before putting on your underwear when dressing.

❑ *See also* CANDIDIASIS and FUNGAL INFECTION in Part Two.

Attention Deficit Disorder (ADD)/ Attention Deficit Hyperactivity Disorder (ADHD)

Attention deficit hyperactivity disorder (ADHD), or attention deficit disorder (ADD) with hyperactivity, is the newest name given to a group of disorders of certain mechanisms in the central nervous system. With the long list of names this disorder has been given over the years, it can be confusing as to exactly what the criteria are for a diagnosis of ADHD or ADD. In the fourth edition of its *Diagnostic and Statistical Manual of Mental Disorders* (DSM-IV), the American Psychiatric Association describes three different categories of ADHD—ADHD inattentive, ADHD hyperactive-impulse, and a third category that is a combination of the two. For the sake of simplicity, we will use the term ADD when referring to the inattentive form without hyperactivity, and ADHD for the hyperactive-impulsive and combined forms.

ADD/ADHD is the fastest growing childhood disorder in the United States, reportedly affecting an astounding 9 to 10 percent of all school-aged children. Ten times more boys than girls are diagnosed with ADD or ADHD. Although primarily thought of as a childhood disorder, ADD/ADHD can be found in adults as well. It causes a variety of learning and behavioral problems, often making it difficult not only for the affected individual, but for the entire family. Although the ADD/ADHD child is often labeled as having a learning disability, the child usually is of average or above-average intelligence and is also highly creative.

Factors that have been linked to the development of ADD/ADHD include heredity, anxiety, allergies, smoking during pregnancy, hyperinsulinemia, oxygen deprivation at birth, environmental stress or pollutants, artificial food additives, injury, infection, lead poisoning, allergies, and prenatal trauma. In recent years, more emphasis has been placed on the role of diet in ADD/ADHD. Many people with these conditions react to certain preservatives, dyes, and salicylates in foods. These items can throw off the balance in the chemistry of the brains, often producing undesirable changes in behavior. A low-protein diet may be a contributing factor. Though the topic has been hotly debated for decades, studies have definitively shown that food additives do play a major role in hyperactivity.

ADHD/ADD may be characterized by one or a combination of some the following. Note that any of these symptoms can be present in a person suffering from ADD either with or without hyperactivity; however, symptoms marked with an asterisk (*) are most strongly associated with the headings under which they are listed.

Symptoms of ADD

- Difficulty solving problems or managing time*
- Extreme distractibility*
- Procrastination*
- Forgetfulness; a tendency to lose things frequently*
- Disorders of speech and hearing*
- Difficulty in organizing or finishing tasks*
- Absentmindedness; inability to remember sequences or events*
- Sloppy and/or impulsively done schoolwork that contains obvious mistakes*
- Lack of concentration*
- Continuous "brain chatter"*
- Learning disabilities
- Emotional instability; daily or hourly mood swings
- Sleep disturbances
- Lack of goals
- In adulthood, failure in career or relationships

Symptoms of ADHD

- Problems adapting to new things*
- A tendency to disturb other children*
- Self-destructive behavior*
- Difficulty doing assignments or chores on one's own*
- Temper tantrums*
- Impatience; difficulty waiting*
- Low tolerance for stress and otherwise ordinary problems*
- A tendency to become frustrated quickly*
- Inability to sit still for any length of time*
- Impulsive, unpredictable, or daring behavior*
- Clumsiness or awkwardness*
- A tendency to talk too much*
- Disruptiveness in the classroom*
- A tendency to blurt out answers without having heard the entire question*
- Failure in school despite average or above-average intelligence

The ADD child may be harder to diagnose than the ADHD child because the hyperactivity is more obvious than the inattentiveness. However, the procrastination, difficulty in concentrating, and inability to start or finish projects that is charactistic of the disorder can have damaging effects that can last through adulthood. ADHD produces hyperactive, restless, impatient, and impulsive behavior. Despite this, children with ADHD can have the ability to pay attention and complete assignments, often spending hours doing things that interest them. Adults with ADHD seem to constantly be going and getting things done, but they often grow impatient easily and have a tendency to lose their tempers quickly. The combined form of ADD/ADHD can be the most debilitating. Children with this type of the disorder often have low self-esteem, are impatient, do not follow rules or act responsibly, are often clumsy, think that they are always right, do not want to accept change, and do not adapt well.

With the enormous increase in the number of recently diagnosed cases of ADD and ADHD, many researchers feel that it is being overdiagnosed. It is difficult to diagnose accurately because many of the symptoms appear in normal, healthy children at many times during childhood. In fact, over 60 percent of parents suspect that their child has ADD or ADHD at some point during the child's upbringing. What may merely be creativity or a high energy level can be misdiagnosed as ADD or ADHD. A diagnosis of ADD/ADHD should made by a team of specialists who are experts in the disorder, and it is wise to get a second opinion if your child is diagnosed as having ADD or ADHD.

Unless otherwise specified, the dosages recommended here are for adults. For a child between the ages of twelve and seventeen, reduce the dose to three-quarters of the recommended amount. For a child between six and twelve, use one-half of the recommended dose, and for a child under the age of six, use one-quarter of the recommended amount.

NUTRIENTS

SUPPLEMENT	SUGGESTED DOSAGE	COMMENTS
Essential		
Calcium and magnesium	As directed on label, at bedtime.	Has a calming effect.
Coenzyme A from Coenzyme-A Technologies and	As directed on label.	Supports the immune system's detoxification of many dangerous substances.
Coenzyme Q$_{10}$	As directed on label.	Can streamline metabolism, ease depression and fatigue, supports adrenal glands, processes fats, improves overall physical and mental processes. Coenzyme A is more effective when combined with coenzyme Q$_{10}$.
Efalex Focus from Efamol or Kyolic-EPA by Wakunaga	As directed on label. As directed on label.	Provides essential fatty acids and helps to maintain eye and brain function. Restores proper fatty acid balance.
Gamma-amino-butyric acid (GABA)	750 mg daily.	Calms the body much in the same way as some tranquilizers, without side effects or danger of addiction. (*See* AMINO ACIDS in Part One.)
Multivitamin and mineral complex	As directed on label.	All nutrients are needed for equilibrium within the body.

Supplement	Suggested Dosage	Comments
Pycnogenol or grape seed extract	As directed on label. / As directed on label.	Powerful antioxidants offering cellular protection for the body and brain.
Quercetin	As directed on label.	Prevents allergies from aggravating symptoms.
S-Adenosylmethionine (SAMe)	As directed on label.	Aids in relieving stress and depression. *Caution:* Do not use if you have manic-depressive disorder or take prescription antidepressants. Do not give to a child under 12.
Vitamin B complex	50 mg of each major B vitamin 3 times daily (amounts of individual vitamins in a complex will vary).	B vitamins are needed for correct brain function and digestion. Also enhance adrenal gland function, regulate neurotransmitters, and aid in processing carbohydrates for energy.
plus extra vitamin B_3 (niacin)	100 mg daily. Do not exceed a total of 300 mg daily from all supplements.	*Caution:* Do not take niacin if you have a liver disorder, gout, or high blood pressure. The anti-stress vitamin.
and pantothenic acid (vitamin B_5)	100 mg daily.	
and vitamin B_6 (pyridoxine)	50 mg daily.	Important for proper brain function.

Helpful

Supplement	Suggested Dosage	Comments
Acetylcholine	As directed on label.	Can improve memory and ability to pay attention.
Attend from Växa International	As directed on label.	A nutritional combination designed to address the specific dietary and neurochemical deficiencies thought to occur in people with ADD/ADHD. Can be used by both children and adults.
Bio-Strath from Bioforce	As directed on label.	Contains yeast, herbs, and all B vitamins that have a calming effect.
Chromium	As directed on label.	Needed for metabolism of glucose and production of energy. It is also vital in the synthesis of cholesterol, fats, and protein. Maintains stable blood sugar levels through proper insulin utilization.
Dimethylaminoethanol (DMAE)	As directed on label.	Aids in concentration by improving nerve impulse transmission in the brain. May also produce antidepressant effects.
EFA Attention Formula from Health From The Sun	As directed on label.	Contains essential fatty acids, vitamins, minerals, and Ayurvedic herbs that support normal brain, nerve, and eye function. Suitable for both children and adults.
Essential fatty acids (borage oil, flaxseed oil, and primrose oil are good sources)	As directed on label.	Often deficient in those with ADD or ADHD.
L-Cysteine	As directed on label, on an empty stomach. Take with water or juice. Do not take with milk. Take with 50 mg vitamin B_6 and 100 mg vitamin C for better absorption.	Take this amino acid if a hair analysis reveals high levels of metals. (*See* AMINO ACIDS in Part One.)
Pedia-Calm from Olympian Labs	As directed on label.	A combination formula for hyperactive children that includes phoshatidyl serine, phosphatidyl choline, cephalin, phosphoinositides, DMAE, and GABA. It can be taken in capsule form or sprinkled on food.
Phosphatidyl serine	As directed on label.	May aid in balancing neurotransmitters in the brain; also may alleviate depression.
Taurine Plus from American Biologics	As directed on label.	The most important antioxidant and immune regulator, necessary for white blood cell activation and neurological function.
Vitamin C with bioflavonoids	1,000 mg 3 times daily.	An anti-stress vitamin.
Vitamin E	600 IU daily.	A powerful antioxidant. Protects cell membranes and improves circulation. Use d-alpha-tocopherol form.
Zinc	As directed on label. Do not exceed a total of 100 mg (or, for children, the appropriate fraction of 100 mg) daily from all supplements.	Many ADHD children are zinc-deficient. Take in addition to the multivitamin and mineral complex.

HERBS

If you are giving herbs to a child, be sure to adjust the dosage for age as recommended by the manufacturer.

❏ Bacopin from Sabinsa Corporation, an extract of the Ayurvedic herb bacopa (*Bacopa monniera*), is a good memory enhancer.

❏ Ginkgo biloba is helpful for brain function and concentration.

❏ Ginseng or mullein oil may be helpful for memory.

❏ Valerian root extract has been used for this disorder with dramatic results and no side effects. Mix the alcohol-free extract in juice (as directed on the product label according to age) and drink the mixture two to three times a day.

❏ Other herbs that may be beneficial for hyperactivity include catnip, chamomile, gotu kola, hops, kava kava, lemon balm, licorice, lobelia, oats, passionflower, skullcap, St. John's wort, thyme, and wood betony.

Caution: Do not use chamomile or lobelia on an ongoing basis. Avoid chamomile completely if you are allergic to ragweed.

RECOMMENDATIONS

❏ Include in the diet all fruits and vegetables (except for those containing salicylates, listed below), plus breads, cereals, and crackers that contain only rice and oats.

❏ Include cold-water fish such as tuna, salmon, and herring in your diet. These are all good sources of docosahexaenoic acid (DHA), an essential fatty acid that is thought to be vital for brain development and is often deficient in those with ADD/ADHD.

❑ Follow a high-protein diet, similar to the one prescribed for hypoglycemia. (*See* HYPOGLYCEMIA in Part Two.) Proteins are needed to supply the body with amino acids. Some researchers are studying a possible connection between hypoglycemia and ADD/ADHD.

❑ Be sure that your child is getting his or her carbohydrates from foods that contain *complex* carbohydrates and cut down on *simple* carbohydrates. Complex carbohydrates can be found in fresh vegetables, fresh fruits, beans, and natural whole grains. They provide dietary fiber and have only a third of the calories found in fats and simple carbohydrates. Simple carbohydrates, such as glucose, fructose, and galactose, are found in all forms of sugars, some juices, and in processed and refined grains (not whole grains).

❑ Limit dairy products if you notice behavioral changes after they are consumed. Dairy foods have been known to cause behavioral problems in some ADHD/ADD sufferers.

❑ Remove from the diet all forms of refined sugar (simple carbohydrates) and any products that contain it. Also eliminate junk food and all foods that contain artificial colors, flavorings, monosodium glutamate (MSG), yeast, or preservatives; processed and manufactured foods; and foods that contain salicylates. Certain foods naturally contain salicylates. These include almonds, apples, apricots, all berries, cherries, cucumbers, currants, oranges, peaches, peppers, plums, prunes, and tomatoes.

❑ Do not consume any of the following: apple cider vinegar, bacon, butter, candy, catsup, chocolate, colored cheeses, chili sauce, corn, ham, hot dogs, luncheon meat, margarine, meat loaf, milk, mustard, pork, salami, salt, soy sauce, sausage, tea, and wheat.

❑ Do not use antacid tablets, cough drops, perfume, throat lozenges, or commercial toothpaste. Use a natural toothpaste from a health food store.

❑ Avoid carbonated beverages, which contain large amounts of phosphates. Phosphate additives may be responsible for hyperkinesis (exaggerated muscle activity). High levels of phosphorus and very low calcium and magnesium levels (which can be revealed through a hair analysis) can indicate a potential for hyperactivity and seizures. Meat and fat also are high in phosphorus.

❑ Limit exposure to television, video and electronic games, and loud music. Instead, encourage outdoor physical activity or activities to expand creativity.

❑ Consider trying cognitive-behavioral therapy. This can often alleviate or eliminate many of the behavior problems caused by ADHD/ADD.

❑ Use an elimination diet to identify foods that may be causing or aggravating symptoms. (*See* ALLERGIES in Part Two.)

CONSIDERATIONS

❑ When you are dealing with this disorder, it is best to think of the diet as feeding the brain rather than the stomach. Many researchers believe that if the contributors are removed from the diets of the patients and the right nutritional supplements are added, numerous symptoms often disappear, and medications used to treat ADD/ADHD (some of which can cause serious side effects) can often be eliminated.

❑ A hair analysis to rule out heavy metal intoxication is important. Lead and copper have both been linked to behavioral problems. (*See* HAIR ANALYSIS in Part Three.)

❑ Family- or allergy-related problems can elicit ADD/ADHD-related behaviors. It is important to explore this possibility with your specialist.

❑ A strong link has been established between learning disabilities and juvenile crime.

❑ The prescription medication methylphenidate (Ritalin) has become the most commonly prescribed medication to ease hyperactivity. Researchers are discovering, however, that this medication has many potentially serious, long-term side effects including decreased appetite, weight loss, insomnia, slowed growth, increased heart rate, increased blood pressure, a period of increased irritability and intolerance at the onset of use, and the possibility of developing Parkinson's disease. Increasing adverse reports have been released in recent years, warning parents of the possible side effects of Ritalin—with some reports even comparing it to cocaine.

❑ Other prescription medications often prescribed include detroamphetamine (Dexadrine, a stimulant that produces calming effects equivalent to Ritalin), pemoline (Cylert, a stimulant that has been restricted by the FDA to use as a secondary medication because it can cause liver failure), methamphetamine (Desoxyn), amphetamine-dextroamphetamine combination (Adderall), and tricyclic antidepressants (if depression is suspected). For periods of extreme anger and aggression, a tranquilizer called thiordazine (Mellaril) may be prescribed, but it should be used only as a last resort. Various side effects, some of them serious, have been reported with all of these medications.

❑ Due to the many potentially harmful side effects of the medications available for ADD/ADHD sufferers, a growing number of parents and health professionals are turning to all or a combination of the following as a way to reduce, and even possibly eliminate the symptoms of ADD/ADHD: alteration of diet; vitamin and mineral supplementation; herbal remedies; counseling; and the love and support of family, teachers, and friends. Many believe that medicating the problem is merely masking the symptoms without getting to the root of the problem.

❑ Homeopathic remedies, taken in small doses, may be helpful in relieving certain symptoms of ADD/ADHD.

Gelsemium can help to relieve anticipatory anxiety, and *Ignatia* can help to alleviate anger or temper tantrums.

❏ Researchers who performed five-hour oral glucose tolerance tests on 261 hyperactive children found that 74 percent displayed abnormal glucose tolerance curves, suggesting a connection between hyperactive behavior and the consumption of sugar.

❏ Some studies have found that many children with ADD/ADHD have high levels of toxic byproducts of yeast and other harmful bacteria in their urine. The use of probiotics (supplements that add beneficial bacteria to the body, such as acidophilus) can help to alleviate this problem.

❏ Studies indicate that administration of gamma-amino butyric acid (GABA) decreases hyperactivity, as well as tendencies toward violence, epilepsy, mental retardation, and learning disabilities.

❏ More and more evidence is showing that those with ADD/ADHD are at greater risk for depression, alcoholism, restlessness, difficulties with careers and relationships, and antisocial behavior as adults.

❏ Parents of children with ADD or ADHD often have a very difficult time dealing with the behavioral problems of their children. These parents deserve a lot of credit. It is important to remember, though, that the children deserve a lot of credit, too. When things seem as though they are getting out of control, it can be helpful to remember that a child with ADD or ADHD is dealing with a physiological disability. Although they desire to please and want to be good, their minds can go in and out of overload without their control. Because of this, they often feel confused and ashamed, and they can eventually develop low self-esteem. When problems arise, it is important to explain to them what they did wrong, and why it was wrong, in a calm, one-on-one fashion whenever possible. These children need a great deal of love, support, and encouragement from everyone around them—but *most of all,* from their parents.

❏ You can ask your health care provider to help you find a professional who specializes in treating people with attention deficit disorders, or seek a referral through one of the the resource organizations that deal with these disorders (*see* HEALTH AND MEDICAL ORGANIZATIONS in the Appendix).

Autism

Autism is not a disease. It is a little-understood developmental brain disorder affecting approximately 4 out of every 10,000 people. Researchers estimate that over 400,000 individuals in the United States are autistic. In spite of over fifty years of research into the varying manifestations of autism and the families affected by it, the disorder continues to mystify doctors, psychologists, and scientists. According to the Autism Society of America, autism is the third most common developmental disability, more common than Down syndrome.

How autistic individuals are affected by the disorder varies widely. People with severe cases display self-injurious, aggressive, and unusual behaviors. The mildest forms may appear, at least to the layperson, to be a personality disorder, possibly associated with a learning disability. Males are three times more likely to have the disorder than females. Recent studies suggest that some people have a genetic predisposition to autism. Scientists estimate that families with one autistic child have a 5-percent (one in twenty) chance of having a second autistic child.

An autistic adult or child might at first appear to be mentally retarded or hard of hearing. But autism caregivers stress that it is important to distinguish autism from other conditions. Physically, autistic individuals do not appear different from others but exhibit marked differences in behavior from a very early age. Autism is usually diagnosed in early childhood (before the age of three) and is characterized by a marked unresponsiveness to other people and to the surrounding environment. While most babies love to be held and cuddled, autistic infants appear indifferent to love and affection, or may be overly agitated, crying most of the time they are awake. Autistic children cannot form attachments to others in the way most children do and seem to withdraw into themselves. Many exhibit various unpredictable and unusual behaviors that can range from constant rocking, feet-pounding, or sitting for long periods of time in total silence. Some experience bursts of hyperactivity that include biting and pounding on their bodies.

According to the National Institute of Neurological Disorders and Stroke, the criteria used to diagnose autism include the following:

- Absence or impairment of imaginative and social play.

- Impaired ability to make friends with peers.

- Impaired ability to initiate or sustain a conversation.

- Stereotyped, repetitive, or unusual use of language.

- Restricted patterns of interests that are abnormal in intensity or focus.

- Apparent inflexibility with regard to changes in routine or rituals.

- Preoccupation with parts of objects.

Autistic children have learning disabilities and are often mentally disabled. Speech development is usually delayed and in many cases is absent or limited to nonsensical rhyming or babbling. Some autistic children appear to have lower than normal intelligence, while others seem to fall into the normal range. About half of the people with autism score below 50 on IQ tests, 20 percent between 50 and 70, and 30 percent score higher than 70. To be accurately diagnosed with autism, a child must be observed by a skilled professional, because diagnosis is difficult for a practitioner with limited training or exposure to autism. Specialists suggest a multidisciplinary team that would include, for example, a neurologist, a psychologist, a developmental pediatrician, a speech/language therapist, and a learning consultant.

Individuals diagnosed as *autistic savants* attract a great deal of attention from the media and general public. Many movies, television reports, and newspaper articles highlight the extraordinary skills of these individuals, most particularly in the areas of mathematics, art, music, and memory. Such an individual might, for example, be able to multiply and divide large numbers or calculate square roots with little hesitation, paint like Rembrandt without ever having a drawing lesson, memorize an entire phone book, or be capable of reciting the birth date of every person he or she has ever met. Less than 1 percent of the general population is capable of such feats, but the incidence of such abilities is 10 percent in individuals who are autistic. No one knows why this occurs. One speculation is that autistic people have incredible concentration abilities and can focus complete attention on a specific area of interest.

The cause of autism is unknown. Some experts believe that it is a result of a neurological imbalance or malfunction that renders the autistic individual painfully oversensitive to external stimuli. Many researchers believe that autism may be the result of genetics and/or some environmental factors, such as certain viruses or chemicals. Researchers are also studying how brain function differs in autistic individuals. Some theories suggest that brain development may have been interrupted in the early fetal stages in people who become autistic. Other studies reveal a possible signaling problem within the brain. It is known that autism is not caused by parental neglect or actions as was once believed.

Unless otherwise specified, the following recommended dosages are for persons over the age of eighteen. For a child between twelve and seventeen years old, reduce the dose to three-quarters the recommended amount. For a child between six and twelve, use one-half the recommended dose, and for a child under six years old, use one-quarter the recommended amount.

NUTRIENTS

SUPPLEMENT	SUGGESTED DOSAGE	COMMENTS
Very Important		
Calcium and magnesium	1,500 mg daily. 1,000 mg daily.	Essential for normal brain and nervous system function.
Choline	500–2,000 mg daily.	Improves brain function and circulation to the brain. Use under professional supervision.
Coenzyme Q$_{10}$	As directed on label.	Improves brain function.
Dimethylglycine (DMG) (Aangamik DMG from FoodScience of Vermont)	100 mg daily.	An oxygen carrier to the brain. Important for normal brain and nervous system function.
Neuro Logic from Wakunaga	As directed on label.	Contains elements essential for quick assimilation of brain nutrients. Enhances neuron function.
S-Adenosylmethionine (SAMe) (SAMe Rx-Mood from Nature's Plus)	As directed on label.	Critical in the manufacture of many body components, especially brain chemicals. A natural antidepressant. *Caution:* Do not use if you have manic-depressive disorder or take prescription antidepressants.
Vitamin B complex	50 mg of each major B vitamin 3 times daily, with meals (amounts of individual vitamins in a complex will vary.	Essential for normal brain and nervous system function. A sublingual form is recommended.
plus extra vitamin B$_3$ (niacin)	50 mg 3 times daily. Do not exceed this amount.	Improves circulation. Helpful for many psychological disorders. *Caution:* Do not take niacin if you have a liver disorder, gout, or high blood pressure.
and niacinamide	300 mg daily.	Aids circulation.
and pantothenic acid (vitamin B$_5$)	500 mg daily.	Helps reduce stress.
and vitamin B$_6$ (pyridoxine)	50 mg 3 times daily. Do not exceed this amount except at the direction of a physician.	Deficiencies have been linked to autism.
Vitamin C with bioflavonoids	5,000–20,000 mg daily, in divided doses. *See* ASCORBIC ACID FLUSH in Part Three.	A powerful free radical scavenger.
Helpful		
L-Glutamine and L-phenylalanine and L-tyrosine and taurine	500 mg each daily, on an empty stomach. Take with water or juice. Do not take with milk. Take with 50 mg vitamin B$_6$ and 100 mg vitamin C for better absorption.	Amino acids needed for normal brain function. (*See* AMINO ACIDS in Part One.) *Caution:* Do not take phenylalanine if you are pregnant or nursing, or suffer from panic attacks, diabetes, high blood pressure, or PKU.
Melatonin	2–3 mg daily for adults, 1 mg or less daily for children, taken 2 hours or less before bedtime. If this is not effective, gradually increase the dosage until an effective level is reached.	Helpful if symptoms include insomnia.
Methylsulfonylmethane (MSM)	As directed on label.	Increases alertness, mental calmness, the ability to concentrate, and energy.
Multivitamin and mineral complex with vitamin A	As directed on label. 15,000 IU daily. If you are pregnant, do not exceed 10,000 IU daily.	All nutrients are needed in balance. Use a high-potency formula.
and natural beta-carotene	25,000 IU daily.	
and selenium	200 mcg daily.	
and zinc	50 mg daily. Do not exceed a total of 100 mg daily from all supplements.	

RNA and	200 mg daily.	To aid in repairing and building of new brain tissues.
DNA	100 mg daily.	*Caution:* Do not take this supplement if you have gout.
Vitamin D$_3$	400 IU daily	Protects against muscle weakness and is involved in regulation of heartbeat.
Vitamin E	200–600 IU daily.	Improves circulation and brain function. Use d-alpha- tocopherol form.

HERBS

❏ Ginkgo biloba is a powerful free radical destroyer that protects the brain. It also improves brain function by increasing circulation to the brain. Take it in capsule or extract form as directed on the product label, three times daily.

RECOMMENDATIONS

❏ Eat a high-fiber diet consisting of 50 to 75 percent raw foods, including large amounts of fruits and vegetables plus brown rice, lentils, and potatoes. For protein, eat beans and legumes, fish, raw nuts and seeds, skinless white turkey or white chicken breast, tofu, and low-fat yogurt.

❏ Eliminate alcohol, caffeine, canned and packaged foods, carbonated beverages, chocolate, all junk foods, refined and processed foods, salt, sugar, sweets, saturated fats, soft drinks, and white flour from the diet. Avoid foods that contain artificial colors or preservatives. Avoid fried and fatty foods such as bacon, cold cuts, gravies, ham, luncheon meats, sausage, and all dairy products except for low-fat soured products.

❏ Omit wheat and wheat products from the diet.

❏ Drink steam-distilled water.

❏ Get regular moderate exercise.

❏ Use an elimination diet to test for food allergies, which can aggravate the condition. (*See* ALLERGIES in Part Two.)

❏ Have a hair analysis test to rule out heavy metal poisoning. (*See* HAIR ANALYSIS in Part Three.)

❏ Try to improve blood oxygen supply to the brain with deep breathing exercises. Hold your breath for thirty seconds each half hour for a thirty-day period. This promotes deeper breathing and helps to increase oxygen levels in the tissues of the brain.

❏ Do not go without food. Eating frequent small meals daily is better than eating two or three large meals.

CONSIDERATIONS

❏ In the medical sense, there is no cure for the differences in the brain that result in autism. However, researchers are finding better ways to understand the disorder and help people cope with the various symptoms. Some symptoms can lessen as the child ages and others disappear altogether. With appropriate intervention, many autistic behaviors can be changed for the better, even to the point that the affected individual may, to the untrained eye, seem perfectly normal. The majority of autistic people continue to display some symptoms throughout their lives, however.

❏ The onset of puberty can be a difficult time for autistic children. Many experience more frequent and severe behavioral problems, and nearly 20 percent of those afflicted begin to experience seizures during puberty. This is believed to be the result of hormonal changes.

❏ During adulthood, appropriate living arrangements for autistic people vary depending on the severity of each individual case. While those who are only mildly affected may be able to live on their own, other options can include living in a group home or residential home, or living with parents. For those who are severely affected individuals, an institutional setting may be the only choice. While some autistic adults are unable to adapt to a regular lifestyle, others graduate from college, have careers, form relationships, and marry.

❏ The Center for the Study of Autism cites a Utah study of eleven families in which the father had autism. Twenty-five (over half) of the forty-four total offspring produced by these men were autistic. Allergies and food sensitivities are beginning to receive more attention than ever before, because research and case studies are beginning to suggest that they contribute to autistic behaviors. Researchers have also recently detected the presence of abnormal protein levels in the urine of autistic individuals. It is thought this protein may be due to the body's inability to break down certain dietary proteins into amino acids. These proteins are gluten (found in wheat, barley, oats, and other foods) and casein (found in human and cow's milk). Many parents of autistic children have removed these foods from their children's diets and have, in many cases, observed positive changes in health and behavior.

❏ Research strongly suggests that many autistic people are sensitive to dairy products and certain foods eaten most often in the spring and summer. These foods include strawberries and citrus fruits, which can affect an autistic individual's sensitive immune system. Doctors have noted that a variety of problems—including headaches, nausea, bed-wetting, appearing "spaced out," stuttering, excessive whining and crying, aggression, and depression—can be magnified by these food products. Such a reaction can be almost immediate or appear up to thirty-six hours after the suspect food is eaten. Besides eliminating problem foods, increasing the amount of vitamins such as vitamin C may reduce allergy and sensitivity symptoms (*see* ALLERGIES in Part Two).

❏ Secretin, a hormone found in the pancreas, liver, and upper intestinal tract that has been used for years as a test injection in the evaluation of intestinal problems, has reportedly produced marked improvements in approximately 200 autistic individuals in the United States, according to the Center for the Study of Autism. Following infusions of secretin, many appeared to improve within a few days, with sudden improvement in speech/language, sleep, eye contact, and attentiveness. Some suffering from chronic diarrhea formed stool for the first time. The center emphasizes that the use of secretin to treat autism is still under study, however.

❑ Autistic children may benefit from taking vitamin B$_6$ and magnesium, as well as other nutrients vital to biochemical reactions in the body. One theory is that these children may have leaky gut syndrome and are unable to absorb nutrients from their diets efficiently. In studies of autistic children, a significant number have been found to have gastrointestinal disorders, including celiac disease and other food intolerances. Allergy induced Autism (AiA), a British support group and charity for autism, notes that some children with autism in England are taking enzymes to help them digest food more easily.

❑ Elevated serum and tissue copper levels may be a factor in autism and other mental problems, as may excessive exposure to lead and mercury. Excessive copper also seems to contribute to autism. Even low-level lead exposure in young children has been associated with impaired intellectual development and behavior problems.

❑ Infants and toddlers whose diets consist largely of processed baby foods need supplemental vitamins and minerals to ensure that all of their nutritional needs are met. Nutritional deficiencies are a factor in many psychological disorders.

❑ The prognosis for autistic children is difficult to predict. There have been documented cases of apparent recovery from autism, usually after adolescence. Some children seem to progress well only to inexplicably regress. Many become marginally self-sufficient and independent. However, most autistic individuals ultimately need lifelong care of some type.

❑ *See also* HYPOGLYCEMIA and HYPERACTIVITY in Part Two.

❑ For names and addresses of organizations that can provide further information about autism, *see* HEALTH AND MEDICAL ORGANIZATIONS in the Appendix.

Backache

Nearly 80 percent of adults are affected by back pain at some point in their lives, most often in the lower back. It can be either acute or chronic. Acute pain starts suddenly and is usually the result of misusing the body in some way. Chronic backache keeps recurring and can be brought on by almost any movement, for no particular reason. It is one of the most common reasons for hospitalization. A variety of problems in the muscles, tendons, bones, ligaments, or an underlying organ, such as the kidneys, may also cause

backaches. Attempting to move or lift heavy objects is said to be the primary cause of back problems in the United States, sometimes because of damage done to a spinal disk.

For many years, it was assumed that most back pain was the result of spinal degeneration or injury, especially damage to the intervertebral disks. These structures are located between the vertebrae and act as cushions. Each disk consists of a tough, fibrous outer layer surrounding the soft interior, which provides the cushioning. With the ordinary wear and tear of living, the disks show signs of aging and may be injured. When a disk begins to degenerate, a strain—even something as small as a sneeze—can cause the disk to rupture, or herniate, allowing the soft interior material to protrude out of the disk and press against the spinal cord. This situation is sometimes erroneously referred to as a *slipped disk.*

Herniated disk, prolapsed disk, and *slipped disk* are all names for the same problem, and are usually found in the lumbar region of the back (the lower back). A herniated disk can result in severe intermittent or constant back pain, particularly if it presses on the sciatic nerves and causes a condition known as *sciatica.* The sciatic nerves are responsible for transmitting all signals from the lower body. They are the longest nerves in the body and any pressure on them, typically by a disk protruding from the vertebrae, results in a shooting pain, usually in the leg and foot. Some people experience a debilitating numbness that renders them almost incapable of walking; others experience only a tingling sensation in the toes or numbness in the foot or leg. Infrequently, if the lower part of the spinal cord is inflamed, people may experience loss of bladder or bowel control.

It is difficult to pinpoint disk disease as the cause of most cases of back pain. That is because many adults past the age of forty—whether they experience back pain or not—can be shown to have some degree of disk degeneration. Further, in many instances, disk degeneration and even herniation do not produce any symptoms.

Simple muscle strain is another leading cause of back pain. Although symptoms may come on suddenly and can be acutely painful, this is actually a problem that develops over a long period of time. When muscles contract, lactic and pyruvic acids are produced as byproducts of muscular activity. It is the presence of lactic acid in the muscles that produces the familiar sensation of muscle fatigue following strenuous activity. If high levels of these acidic byproducts accumulate in the muscles, they cause irritation that can eventually turn into pain and interfere with the normal conduction of electrical impulses in the muscle tissue. This results in a phenomenon called *delayed-onset muscle soreness* (DOMS).

Fibrositis, a rather ill-defined soreness of the neck, trunk, and shoulders caused by inflammation of connective tissue, may also account for a number of backaches. This usually happens in older people and is thought more likely to occur because of stress, tension, allergies, or fibromyalgia rather than from any particular injury.

Lumbago is a folk term for muscle pain in the lower back, near the pelvis.

Backaches during pregnancy are commonplace. The abdominal muscles stretch because the uterus is getting bigger and the back muscles are becoming shorter and tighter. Coupled with this, your spine has to support additional weight, so your posture may change and backaches can result.

Most cases of back pain also have an important psychological component, usually a deep-seated emotional or stress-related problem. Other contributors to back pain can include poor posture, improper footwear and walking habits, improper lifting, straining, calcium deficiency, slouching when sitting, and sleeping on a mattress that is too soft. Kidney, bladder, and prostate problems, female pelvic disorders, and even constipation may produce back pain. Chronic conditions that can cause back pain include arthritis, rheumatism, bone disease, and abnormal curvature of the spine. Fractures are rarely the cause of back pain.

Although the great majority of back pain cannot be explained, and is not due to protruding disks, arthritis, osteoporosis, poor posture, or any other discernable illness, it is always advisable to take back problems seriously and have them checked out.

NUTRIENTS

SUPPLEMENT	SUGGESTED DOSAGE	COMMENTS
Very Important		
Calcium	1,500–2,000 mg daily.	Needed for strong bones. To assure absorption, use a mixture of 3 different forms: calcium carbonate, calcium chelate, and calcium asporotato.
and magnesium	700–1,000 mg daily.	Works with calcium. Use magnesium chelate form.
and vitamin D	400 IU daily.	Aids absorption of calcium and magnesium.
DL-Phenylalanine (DLPA)	Take daily every other week, as directed on label.	This natural amino acid, helps to alleviate pain. *Caution:* Do not take this supplement if you are pregnant or nursing, or suffer from panic attacks, diabetes, high blood pressure, or PKU.
Multivitamin and mineral complex with vitamin A	15,000 IU daily. If you are pregnant, do not exceed 10,000 IU daily.	To supply a balance of nutrients important in formation and metabolism of bone and connective tissue, and needed for healing.
and natural beta-carotene	15,000 IU daily.	
and vitamin E	400–800 IU daily.	
Silica or horsetail	3 times daily, as directed on label.	Supplies silicon, which improves calcium uptake. *See under* Herbs, below.
Vitamin B₁₂	2,000 mcg daily.	Aids in calcium absorption and digestion. Use a lozenge or sublingual form. Requires visit to doctor.
or vitamin B₁₂ injections	As prescribed by physician.	
Zinc	50 mg daily. Do not exceed a total of 100 mg daily from all supplements.	Required for protein synthesis and collagen formation. Promotes a healthy immune system.
plus copper	3 mg daily.	Works in balance with zinc and vitamin C to form elastin, and is needed for healthy nerves.
Important		
Boron	3 mg daily. Do not exceed this amount.	Improves calcium uptake. Take boron only until healed, unless you are over age 50.
Chondroitin sulfate (CS) and	As directed on label.	Studies have shown these are important components of many body tissues, including bones and connective tissue.
bovine cartilage or	As directed on label.	
shark cartilage and	As directed on label.	
glucosamine sulfate	As directed on label.	
Free-form amino acid complex	As directed on label.	Essential in bone and tissue repair.
L-Proline	500 mg daily, on an empty stomach. Take with water or juice. Do not take with milk. Take with 50 mg vitamin B₆ and 100 mg vitamin C for better absorption.	Heals cartilage and strengthens muscles and tissues. (*See* AMINO ACIDS in Part One.)
Manganese	2–5 mg daily. Take separately from calcium.	Aids in healing cartilage and tissue in the neck and back. Use manganese gluconate form.
Methylsulfonyl-methane (MSM)	As directed on label.	Aids with inflammation.
S-Adenosylmethio-nine (SAMe)	As directed on label.	Methionine derivative. Eases arthritic pain. *Caution:* Do not use if you have manic-depressive disorder or take prescription antidepressants.
Helpful		
Essential fatty acids (flaxseed oil is a good source)	As directed on label. Take with meals.	Needed for repair and flexibility of muscles.
Glucosalage S04 (Extra Strength) from Olympian Labs	As directed on label.	To supply glucosamine, an important component of many body tissues, including bones and connective tissue. Contains several nutrients listed in this table plus enzymes.
Glucosamine & Chondroitin from Amerifit	As directed on label.	A chewable formula that provides joint health. It also contains MSM.
Multienzyme complex with bromelain and pancreatin	As directed on label. Take with meals.	To aid digestion and relieve muscle tension and inflammation.
Vitamin B complex	As directed on label 3 times daily.	Needed for repair and to relieve stress in the back muscles. Use a high-stress formula high in vitamin B₆ (pyridoxine) and vitamin B₁₂.

Vitamin C with bioflavonoids	3,000–10,000 mg daily.	Essential for formation of collagen, which holds the tissues together. Needed for repair of tissues. Relieves tension in the back area.

HERBS

❑ Arth-X from Trace Minerals Research is a formula containing herbs, sea minerals, calcium, and other nutrients for the bones and joints.

❑ Horsetail is a good source of silica, which is necessary for bones and connective tissue.

❑ Other herbs recommended for backache include alfalfa, burdock, oat straw, slippery elm, and white willow bark. They can be taken in capsule, extract, or tea form.

RECOMMENDATIONS

❑ Avoid all meats and animal protein products until you are healed. Animal foods contain uric acid, which puts undue strain on the kidneys that can contribute to back pain. Eat no gravies, oils, fats, sugar, or rich or highly processed foods.

❑ Follow a fasting program. (*See* FASTING in Part Three.)

❑ When pain hits, immediately drink two large glasses of quality water. This often gives relief within minutes. Muscle aches and back pain are frequently connected to dehydration. The body needs a minimum of eight 8-ounce glasses of water daily to keep acidic wastes from building up in muscles and other tissues.

❑ If pain follows an injury or sudden movement, apply ice for the first forty-eight hours, and then apply heat. Rest on a firm bed. When getting up, roll to your side, draw your knees up, push up to a sitting position, and stand by pushing up with your legs.

❑ To relieve back muscle pain, soak in a very warm bath or apply a heating pad directly to your back. Be careful not to set the heat too high, however.

❑ *Rhus toxicodendron*, a homeopathic remedy, is helpful in relieving stiffness. Take it as directed.

❑ Once the acute pain has subsided, doing exercises to strengthen the abdominal muscles may help to prevent recurrences; these muscles help to support the back. Sit-ups are good for this purpose. Always do sit-ups with your knees bent, not with your legs flat on the floor.

❑ When sitting, keep your knees a little higher than your hips and keep your feet flat on the floor.

❑ When carrying things on your shoulder, switch the weight to the other side from time to time. Carrying heavy shoulder bags may produce neck, back, and shoulder pain.

❑ Learn to recognize and reduce stress. Relaxation techniques can be very helpful.

❑ Always push large objects; never pull them.

❑ Wear comfortable, well-made shoes. The higher the heels of your shoes, the greater the risk of backache.

❑ Move around. Do not sit in the same position for long periods of time.

❑ Never lean forward without bending your knees. Lift with your legs, arms, and abdomen—not with the muscles of the small of your back. Avoid lifting anything heavier than twenty pounds. If you must work close to the ground, squat down so that you avoid bending at the waist.

❑ Do not sleep on your stomach with your head raised on a pillow. Instead, rest your back by lying on your side with your legs bent, so that your knees are about an inch higher than your hips. Sleep on a firm mattress with your head supported on a pillow. If your mattress is not firm enough, place a board between the box spring and the mattress.

❑ Maintain a healthy weight and get regular moderate exercise. A lack of exercise can cause back pain. Activities that are good for the back include swimming, cycling, walking, and rowing. *Avoid* the following activities:

• *Baseball, basketball, football.* The quick responses needed for these sports involve sudden twisting and jumping motions.

• *Bowling.* Lifting a heavy weight while bending and twisting puts strain on the back.

• *Golf.* The twisting motion involved in the swing, and the body's tendency to bend forward at the waist, are stressful to the lower back.

• *Tennis.* Playing tennis puts strain on the back due to the quick "stop-and-go" action of the game.

• *Weightlifting.* This sport is potentially the most damaging because it places great strain on the lower portion of the spine and back.

❑ If pain lasts longer than seventy-two hours, if the pain radiates into the legs, or if other symptoms such as unexplained weight loss occur, consult your health care provider. If your backaches are chronic, look for a physician who specializes in backs—and who does not rush to recommend surgery.

❑ If your back pain also involves a high temperature or weight loss, or if you have a past history of cancer, bowel or bladder control problems, any numbness in the groin or lower back, or loss of feeling in the legs or feet, see your doctor.

❑ If you have pain in one side of the small of your back, feel sick, and have a fever, see your physician immediately. You may have a kidney infection.

❑ If pain follows an injury and is accompanied by sudden loss of bladder or bowel control, if you have difficulty moving any limb, or if you feel numbness, pain, or tingling in a limb, do not move, but call for medical help immediately. You may have hurt your spinal cord.

CONSIDERATIONS

❑ People seeking professional advice about back pain face a bewildering array of generalists and specialists to choose from. Complex back problems are rapidly becoming a subspecialty. True specialists now focus on people with back problems only. For treatment of back pain, you can try any of the following types of therapies:

• *Acupuncture* has the backing of the World Health Organization for the treatment of back pain. (*See* PAIN CONTROL in Part Three.)

• *Chiropractors* are licensed to perform spinal manipulation and may recommend nutritional and/or lifestyle changes. They primarily use high-velocity manipulations of the neck and back to correct problems. According to a 1994 report issued by the U.S. Agency for Health Care Policy and Research, spinal manipulation may be the most effective treatment for acute back pain. Chiropractors are not medical doctors and therefore cannot prescribe drugs or perform surgery. A good chiropractor should be willing to recommend a medical doctor if necessary.

• *Kinesiology* can sometimes alleviate back problems. By testing muscle response, practitioners can pinpoint the origin of the pain and use various methods, including gentle manipulation, to treat it.

• *Magnet therapy* is gaining ground in some quarters. A magnetic mattress pad has been developed and some people have found relief from chronic back pain after sleeping on it for only a short time. Experiments have shown that magnet back support has proven useful for golfers.

• *Massage therapists* work with muscles and tendons, using different techniques like muscle kneading and compression to lessen tension in the muscles. This increases circulation and helps the body flush out cellular debris, which speeds tissue repair and aids in healing back problems. (*See* MASSAGE THERAPY *under* PAIN CONTROL in Part Three.)

• *Orthopedic surgeons* are medical doctors who prescribe medication (painkillers, muscle relaxers, anti-inflammatory drugs), bed rest, and physical therapy for some cases of back pain. Since these doctors can perform surgery, they may be more likely to recommend it than other practitioners. *Vertebroplasty,* for vertebral compression fractures, has offered relief for some people, although it is still considered a new and experimental treatment. In this outpatient procedure, a needle injected through the skin into the affected vertebra fills the vertebra with a cement-like substance called methylmethacrylate, and when this substance hardens (in about fifteen to twenty minutes), it offers support to an otherwise weak part of the backbone.

• *Osteopaths* can prescribe drugs and perform surgery, but because of their philosophy of treatment, they often try manipulation or physical therapy first.

• *Physiatrists,* also known as doctors of physical rehabilitation medicine, are medical doctors who treat back pain by the use of various physical therapies, lifestyle changes, and back braces, which promote healing by reducing the load on the spine. Physiatrists are not licensed to perform surgery, and are less likely than other doctors to hospitalize their patients. They have a good record for treating back problems, including low back pain and herniated disks.

• *Physical therapists* specialize in improving joint and spine mobility and muscle strength. They are not medical doctors and are strictly limited to physical therapy.

❑ There is a theory that backache may be caused by repressed rage. This may be something to consider pursuing with a psychiatrist or other mental health professional.

❑ Bed rest makes little difference with sciatica. Both the long-term and short-term consequences of sciatica remain the same whether you observe complete rest or continue your usual routine.

❑ With signs of rapidly progressive nerve damage (increasing weakness in a leg, or loss of bladder or bowel function), back surgery moves high on the list of options. It must also be considered when pain is unremitting or getting worse. Surgery always entails a degree of risk; there is always the chance of permanent damage and impaired mobility. According to U.S. government data, only 1 percent of those who suffer from back pain appear to benefit from surgery. Back surgery is useful only for problems in four broad categories:

1. Disk displacement (a protruded or "slipped" disk).

2. Painful (and abnormal) motion of one vertebra in relation to another.

3. Narrowing of the spine around the spinal cord itself from overgrowth of bone (spinal stenosis).

4. Some cases in which misalignment of one vertebra with another (spondylolisthesis) leads to pain.

❑ X-rays are often considered a routine part of back pain diagnosis, yet only a few back conditions show up on x-rays. If the pain is caused by muscle strain or a herniated disk, an x-ray will do little to aid the diagnosis, since disks, muscles, and ligaments are all soft tissues. X-ray exposure bears special hazards for pregnant women.

❑ With imaging procedures such as computerized tomography (CT) and magnetic resonance imaging (MRI), disks can be seen. However, Dr. Richard A. Deyo, a professor of medicine and health services at the University of Washington School of Medicine and School of Public Health, notes that 20 to 30 percent of people with back pain have herniated disks that are not the source of their discomfort. If these disks show up during imaging procedures, a perscn may end up having surgery for a condition that, while present, is not really the cause of his or her pain.

❑ If pain comes after lifting something heavy, after

coughing, or after unusually heavy exercise, and the pain prevents you from moving or shoots down one leg, you may have a herniated disk.

❏ Epidemiological studies in the United States, as well as studies of smoking and nonsmoking pairs of twins in Scandinavia, have shown that smoking aggravates problems in the disks.

❏ Numerous studies have shown that people with lower back pain who are treated at chiropractic clinics recover faster, and at less cost, and end up with less pain and more mobility than those treated in hospitals.

❏ *See also under* PREGNANCY-RELATED PROBLEMS in Part Two.

❏ *See also* PAIN CONTROL in Part Three.

Bad Breath

See HALITOSIS.

Baldness

See HAIR LOSS.

Bedsores

Bedsores, also known as pressure sores, are deep ulcers that form when pressure is exerted over bony areas of the body for long periods of time, restricting circulation and leading to the death of cells in the underlying tissue. They are most commonly found on the heels, buttocks, hips, sacrum, and shoulder blades.

As their name implies, they tend to occur during periods of prolonged bed rest, although wheelchair users also may develop bedsores. People who suffer from bedsores are usually deficient in many nutrients, especially zinc and vitamins A, E, B$_2$ (riboflavin), and C, and they often have a high bodily pH (*see* ACID/ALKALI IMBALANCE in Part Two).

Anyone who is confined to a bed, chair, or wheelchair due to illness is at risk for developing bedsores, which can range from mild to severe. An area of reddening skin that doesn't go away, even after pressure is relieved, is an indication of a developing bedsore, as is local swelling and/or hardening of the tissue. Severe bedsores can require surgery for removal of dead tissue.

NUTRIENTS

SUPPLEMENT	SUGGESTED DOSAGE	COMMENTS
Very Important		
Essential fatty acids (flaxseed oil, primrose oil, and salmon oil are good sources)	As directed on label.	Needed for proper cell reproduction.
or		
Ultra Omega-3 Fish Oil from Health From The Sun	One or two capsules with each meal daily.	Prevents moisture loss and promotes healing.
Vitamin E	400 IU daily and up.	Improves circulation.
Zinc	50–80 mg daily. Do not exceed a total of 100 mg daily from all supplements.	Important in healing of tissues.
plus copper	3 mg daily.	Needed to balance with zinc.
Important		
Free-form amino acid complex	As directed on label.	To supply protein needed for healing.
Vitamin B complex	100 mg of each major B vitamin twice daily, with meals (amounts of individual vitamins in a complex will vary).	Needed to reduce stress and for healing.
plus extra vitamin B$_{12}$	2,000 mcg twice daily.	Use a lozenge or sublingual form.
Vitamin C	3,000–10,000 mg daily, in divided doses.	Aids in healing, improves circulation, and enhances immune function.
Vitamin D	400–1,000 IU daily.	Essential for healing. Lack of exposure to sunshine increases the need for this nutrient.
Helpful		
All-Purpose Bactericide Spray from Aerobic Life Industries	Apply topically to irritated areas as directed on label.	Destroys harmful bacteria.
or colloidal silver	Apply topically as directed on label.	A natural antibiotic. Destroys bacteria, viruses, and fungi. Protects against infection and promotes healing.
Calcium and	2,000 mg daily.	Needed for the central nervous system and to keep bones from softening through disuse.
magnesium	1,000 mg daily.	
Carotenoid complex	As directed on label.	Repairs bedsores by improving skin tissue.
Garlic (Kyolic from Wakunaga)	2 capsules 3 times daily, with meals.	Has a natural antibiotic effect; protects against infection.
Kelp	500–1,000 mg daily.	Provides necessary minerals.
Panoderm I from American Biologics	Apply topically as directed on label.	A natural antioxidant skin moisturizer and cleanser that contains squalene.
Vitamin A	50,000 IU daily for 1 month, then reduce to 15,000 IU daily. If you are pregnant, do not exceed 10,000 IU daily.	Needed for healing of skin tissue. Use emulsion form for easier assimilation.

HERBS

❑ Herbal ointments should be applied to closed wounds only. Open wounds should always be treated by a qualified health care practitioner or physician.

❑ Aloe vera gel, ointment, or cream can be applied topically to the bedsores.

❑ Calendula cream, gel, or ointment can be applied topically to the affected area. Use as directed on the label.

❑ Comfrey ointment or Calendula Ointment from NatureWorks can be used externally.

Note: Comfrey is recommended for external use only.

❑ Goldenseal, myrrh gum, pau d'arco, and suma, taken in tea or extract form, are beneficial for bedsores. Buckwheat tea and lime flower tea are also helpful.

Caution: Do not take goldenseal for more than one week at a time; do not use it during pregnancy; and use it under supervision if you have heart disease, diabetes, or glaucoma.

❑ Mix equal amounts of goldenseal powder or extract and vitamin E oil with a small amount of honey to make paste, and apply the mixture to the sores often. This mixture gives fast relief and helps the healing process. Alternate this with raw honey, vitamin E cream, and aloe vera gel.

RECOMMENDATIONS

❑ Eat a simple, well-balanced diet with plenty of raw, fresh fruits and green and yellow vegetables to ensure a good supply of vitamins, minerals, and phytonutrients.

❑ Essential fatty acids (EFAs) have been shown to play an integral role in the health of the skin. Taken internally or applied externally as a lotion, they help maintain the integrity and elasticity of the skin, as well as preventing a loss of moisture, which leads to dry and scaly skin. Excellent sources of EFAs are natural vegetable oils such as canola, corn, olive, safflower, and soy oils; wheat germ; edible seeds, such as pumpkin, sesame, and sunflower; and fish oils—especially cod-liver oil.

❑ Consume liquids around the clock, even if you are not thirsty. Use steam-distilled water, herbal teas, and sugar-free juices. Liquids are important in keeping the colon clean and the bladder functioning properly.

❑ Eliminate animal fats, fried foods, junk foods, processed foods, and sugar from the diet.

❑ Use ground flaxseeds, oat bran, psyllium husks, or Aerobic Bulk Cleanse (ABC) from Aerobic Life Industries to provide fiber. Fiber absorbs dangerous toxins and helps prevent constipation.

Note: Always take supplemental fiber separately from other supplements and medications.

❑ Make sure that the bowels move every day. On days when the bowels do not move, use an enema. (*See* ENEMAS in Part Three.)

❑ Give immediate attention to lowering the body's pH level to 5.5 or lower to prevent bacteria in the sores from multiplying. Place 2 to 3 teaspoons of apple cider vinegar in glass of water, add a little honey, and sip this with meals. *See* Alkalosis under ACID/ALKALI IMBALANCE in Part Two for additional suggestions.

❑ Try applying essential oils and/or aloe vera with a little tea tree oil added to the affected area. This is very good for the skin, and helps existing bedsores to heal as well as preventing new ones from forming. (Keep these oils away from the eyes, however, because they burn.)

❑ Take the following measures to prevent bedsores from developing:

• Prevention of bedsores is based on limiting the time an area of the body is subjected to pressure. Therefore, do not let an immobilized individual stay in one position for long—move him or her to alternate positions every two hours.

• Keep the skin dry; include thorough drying after bathing.

• Inspect pressure points daily for reddening or other signs that a sore may be developing.

• If the person can sit up, have him or her do so three to four times daily, or use pillows as a prop.

• Give a sponge bath daily using warm water and a mild herbal or vitamin E soap. Do not use harsh soaps.

• Gently but firmly massage pressure points and other affected areas once daily to increase circulation.

• Give frequent alcohol rubs to stimulate circulation and prevent blood vessels from closing up. Use isopropyl (rubbing) alcohol and cotton balls or sterile gauze to apply the alcohol. As an alternative, witch hazel can be used instead.

• Allow as much light and fresh air into the bedridden person's room as he or she can tolerate.

• Have the individual wear loose-fitting clothing made from all-natural materials. Cotton is best because it allows air to penetrate to the skin. Pay attention to clothing construction as well. Avoid items with seams, gathers, or other features that may press on sensitive areas.

• Keep the bed clean, dry, and tidy. Lying on wrinkled bed linens can lead to bedsores.

CONSIDERATIONS

❑ A good diet is very important and makes bedsores less likely to develop.

❑ People who suffer from bedsores are usually seriously deficient in many nutrients, especially zinc and vitamins A, E, B$_2$ (riboflavin), and C. A good multivitamin and mineral supplement should be taken every day. A simple diet with plenty of fresh fruits is recommended. Vitamins A and E are useful in healing bedsores. Vitamin C acts as an anti-inflammatory and is generally good for the health of the skin and blood vessels.

❑ Although most bedsores can be prevented, once formed, they can be kept in check if you regularly examine the affected areas, keep the skin clean and dry, and relieve any pressure on sensitive areas. If mobility is limited, you can use special foam, gel, or air cushions to relieve this pressure. Also, make sure that anyone with limited mobility gets turned on a regular basis.

❑ Special air mattresses are available that help to decrease the pressure on sensitive areas when a person has to lie in one position for long periods of time. Anatomically shaped cushions can be used to help distribute the weight more evenly, along with special pads designed specifically for heels and elbows.

❑ Special absorbent foam-like bandages can be used for persistent bedsores to reduce the pressure on sensitive areas and help promote healing.

❑ Dimethylsulfoxide (DMSO) is also helpful for promoting healing. It is applied topically directly to the affected area.

Note: Only DMSO from a health food store should be used for therapeutic purposes. Commercial-grade DMSO found in hardware stores is not suitable. The use of DMSO may result in a garlicky body odor. This is temporary and is not a cause for concern.

Bed-Wetting

Bed-wetting, known in the medical community as *enuresis*, is the act of urinating in bed habitually and, especially, involuntarily at night when asleep. Bed-wetting is common in early childhood. It also occurs sometimes in early adulthood and frequently among the aging. The causes are often unknown. The most popular theories center on the roles of behavioral disturbances, very sound sleeping, the consumption of too much liquid before bedtime, dreaming about using the rest room, food allergies, heredity, stress, nutritional deficiencies, and psychological problems (one of the most common factors in young adults).

In children under the age of five or so, the most common cause of bed-wetting is simply the size of the bladder; it is often too small to hold enough urine to last through the night every single night. This type of bed-wetting is usually outgrown. Occasional bed-wetting by older children usually stops spontaneously by the teenage years. An underlying illness such as a urinary tract infection or diabetes may also result in bed-wetting. It is wise to rule out the possibility of underlying medical problems before proceeding with any other form of treatment.

Unless otherwise specified, the following recommended doses are for those over the age of eighteen. For a child be-

tween twelve and seventeen years old, reduce the dose to three-quarters the recommended amount. For a child between six and twelve years old, use one-half the recommended dose, and for a child under six, use one-quarter the recommended amount.

NUTRIENTS

SUPPLEMENT	SUGGESTED DOSAGE	COMMENTS
Very Important		
Free-form amino acid complex	As directed on label.	Helps to strengthen bladder muscle. Use a product made from a vegetable source.
Important		
Calcium and magnesium	1,500 mg daily. 350 mg daily.	To aid in controlling bladder spasms.
Helpful		
Multivitamin and mineral complex with vitamin B complex	As directed on label.	Aids in relieving stress and supplies all needed nutrients.
Potassium	99 mg daily.	Aids in balancing sodium and potassium in the body.
Vitamin A or cod liver oil and vitamin E	As directed on label. If you are pregnant, do not exceed 10,000 IU daily. As directed on label. 600 IU daily.	To aid in normalizing bladder muscle function. Use d-alpha-tocopherol form.
Zinc	10 mg daily for children; 80 mg daily for adults. Do not exceed these amounts.	For improved bladder function. Also enhances the immune system.

HERBS

❑ For bed-wetting, try using buchu, corn silk, oat straw, parsley, and/or plantain. Take these herbs before 3:00 p.m. so that they have time to work before bedtime.

RECOMMENDATIONS

❑ Consume more foods that are high in vitamin B_2 (riboflavin) and pantothenic acid (vitamin B_5), including bee pollen, brewer's yeast, soaked nuts, and spirulina.

Caution: Both bee pollen and brewer's yeast can cause an allergic reaction in some individuals. Start with a small amount at first, and discontinue use if any allergic symptoms occur.

❑ Do not drink liquids within thirty minutes of bedtime.

❑ See your health care provider for food allergy testing. Bed-wetting is often caused by food allergies. Omit cow's milk, which is highly allergenic, from your diet. Also eliminate from the diet carbonated beverages, chocolate, cocoa, cooked spinach, refined carbohydrates (including junk food), rhubarb, and products containing caffeine or food coloring.

❑ Bed-wetting in children has been shown to cause low

self-esteem, attention deficit, or behavioral problems and is best treated with sympathy and understanding. Do not spank or scold a child for bed-wetting. This only complicates the problem. Instead, give rewards for *not* wetting the bed.

CONSIDERATIONS

❏ We know of several cases of bed-wetting (among children and adults) that were relieved within a matter of days when supplements of certain nutrients were supplied. Among these were magnesium, vitamin B_2, and pantothenic acid. In addition, all allergy-causing foods were removed from the diet, and a protein supplement was added. Bee pollen, brewer's yeast, and spirulina, are excellent sources of protein.

❏ Supplemental magnesium is especially helpful for certain people. Magnesium citrate is one of the better forms to use, since the body can readily assimilate it.

❏ Behavior modification techniques have proved useful in some cases, especially with children. One technique involves the use of an alarm that goes off as soon as the individual starts to wet the bed. Over time, this is believed to help a child respond to the body's cues and wake up when he or she needs to urinate during the night.

❏ The National Kidney Foundation hotline (800–622–9010) can provide information and a list of physicians in your area who are experienced in treating this condition.

Bee Sting

There are numerous stinging insects in the United States, and not all of them are bees. Hornets, yellow jackets, wasps, spiders, and some species of ants can also inflict painful stings. In some people, honeybee and yellow jacket stings can cause more serious reactions than the stings of hornets and wasps. When an insect stings, it injects venom through a stinger into the victim. Bees generally leave their stingers behind at the sting site; wasps most often do not. Usually, a stinging insect attacks because it is trying to protect itself, or its territory, from danger. This is why a person who stumbles on a beehive may end up receiving multiple stings from the hive's residents. Most stings cause localized swelling, redness, and acute pain that may throb or burn. This is a reaction to the insect's venom. However, some people are highly allergic to insect venom, and if they are stung, a very severe reaction can occur. Symptoms of an allergic reaction include difficulty swallowing, hoarseness, labored breathing, weakness, confusion, severe swelling, and a feeling of impending disaster. People who are highly allergic to insect stings can experience anaphylactic shock, which can lead to unconsciousness and, in extreme circumstances,

death. Anaphylactic shock can cause symptoms such as bluish skin, coughing, difficulty breathing, dizziness, hives, nausea, severely swollen eyes, lips or tongue, stomach cramps, and wheezing.

Unless otherwise indicated, the following recommended dosages are for people over the age of eighteen. For a child between twelve and seventeen years old, reduce the dose to three-quarters of the recommended amount. For a child between six and twelve, use half the recommended dose. Children under six years old should receive only one-quarter of the recommended amount.

NUTRIENTS

SUPPLEMENT	SUGGESTED DOSAGE	COMMENTS
Helpful		
Calcium	1,500 mg daily.	Helps relieve pain. Use calcium gluconate form.
Oxy-Mist from Earth's Bounty	As directed on label.	Helps the healing process.
Pantothenic acid (vitamin B_5)	500 mg daily.	Acts to inhibit allergic response.
Vitamin C with bioflavonoids	10,000 mg within the first hour. Then 5,000–25,000 mg daily in divided doses. *See* ASCORBIC ACID FLUSH in Part Three.	Protects the body from allergens and moderates the inflammatory response.
Vitamin E	Slit capsule and apply oil topically to the sting site.	Promotes healing. Use d-alpha-tocopherol form.

HERBS

❏ Poultices made from comfrey, slippery elm, and white oak bark and leaves can ease pain and promote healing. Lobelia poultices and plantain poultices or salve are also beneficial.

Note: Comfrey is recommended for external use only.

❏ Take echinacea and/or goldenseal in tea or capsule form to boost immune function. Goldenseal is a natural antibiotic and functions well as a poultice. It reduces inflammation and prevents infection.

❏ Juniper tea cleanses the venom from your internal system and can also make an excellent external poultice when the berries are crushed and applied to the sting.

❏ Drink as much yellow dock tea as you can, or take 2 capsules of yellow dock every hour until symptoms are relieved.

RECOMMENDATIONS

❏ If you are stung, immediately and carefully remove any stinger left in the skin. Do not pull the stinger out with your fingers or tweezers. Instead, gently scrape it out. A sterilized knife is best for this purpose, but you can use your fingernail or the edge of a credit card if nothing else is available. Be careful not to squeeze the stinger or the attached venom sac as this may inject more poison into the skin. Afterward, wash the area and rinse thoroughly. If you have *ever* had an allergic reaction to a sting in the past, seek emergency medical attention immediately. Life-threatening allergic reactions can come on suddenly and progress very quickly, so you do not want to waste time. If you have no history of insect allergy, no medical treatment is needed, but do remain alert for symptoms of a developing allergic reaction. Reactions can occur within minutes or hours, and they can happen the first time or the thousandth time you are stung by a bee.

❏ If you are aware that you are highly allergic and prone to anaphylactic shock, carry an emergency kit containing a pre-measured dose of *epinephrine*. You must obtain the kit by prescription, and your doctor should show you how to administer the epinephrine. Any allergic reaction to a sting should be taken seriously because, no matter how slight, the reaction may prove to be more serious in a second incident.

❏ Once the stinger has been removed and the area cleansed, try one or more of the following home remedies to ease pain and swelling:

• Make a paste by adding a bit of cool water to baking soda, a crushed aspirin, or a crushed papaya enzyme tablet, and apply the mixture to the sting.

• Charcoal tablets, available in health food stores, can be used as a poultice. Empty 2 capsules, add 6 drops of liquid alcohol-free goldenseal extract to make a paste, then smooth on a sterile gauze pad and place on the sting area. This will absorb the poisons and prevent infection. Use only charcoal recommended for internal use.

• Apply an ice compress to the sting area a few minutes every two hours for the first day after you've been stung. Not only will you reduce the swelling and pain from the sting, but you will be stopping the spread of venom.

• Apply lavender oil to the sting area to reduce inflammation and pain.

• Crush plantain leaves and squeeze out the juice. Apply this extract directly to the sting. Within 30 minutes, the pain and swelling should be greatly reduced.

• Other remedies to consider include: Rubbing toothpaste on the sting (Its cooling effect can make the sting area feel better); applying calamine lotion to the area, or rubbing a meat tenderizer containing papain (an enzyme) on the sting can also ease the pain.

If you have been stung on the foot or leg, elevate it for about half an hour after removing the stinger.

❏ Use *Apis mellifica*, a homeopathic remedy, to reduce inflammation and pain if the sting area is very swollen and red. *Ledum palustre*, a homeopathic remedy, reduces inflammation from stings and is the most commonly used medication for insect stings and snakebite.

CONSIDERATIONS

❏ Aspirin or ibuprofen, taken every four hours, is helpful for pain and inflammation.

❏ Itching caused by the sting can be relieved by taking an oral antihistamine and/or anti-itch medication such as cortisone cream or Benadryl tablets (or cream).

❏ A venom extractor called Lil Sucker fits inside a pocket or purse. If you get stung, it produces a vacuum that sucks the venom out within two minutes. The end of the extractor can also be used to remove a honeybee stinger. For more information on this, call International Reforestation Suppliers at 800–321–1037.

❏ Taking large doses of vitamin C has been known to reduce the severity of bee stings.

❏ To avoid bee stings, wear plain, light-colored clothing. Also avoid wearing clothing that is flowered or dark-colored; perfume, suntan lotion, hair spray, or anything scented; shiny jewelry; and open sandals or loose-fitting clothes.

❏ To protect yourself if you are highly allergic to bee stings, wear long-sleeved shirts and long pants when you are outdoors and near bees and wasps.

❏ When a yellow jacket is squashed, its body releases a chemical that causes other yellow jackets in the area to attack. It is better to leave the area than to swat at these insects.

❏ *See also* INSECT ALLERGY and INSECT BITE in Part Two.

Benign Prostatic Hypertrophy

See under PROSTATITIS/ENLARGED PROSTATE.

Bite

See BEE STING; DOG BITE; INSECT ALLERGY; SNAKEBITE; SPIDER BITE.

Bitot's Spots

See under EYE PROBLEMS.

Bladder Infection (Cystitis)

Both women and men suffer from bladder infections. The kidneys, ureters, bladder, penis, and urethra all play a part in filtering and expelling waste material (urine) from the body. *Cystitis* (an infection of the bladder), *urethritis* (an infection of the urethra), and acute *pyelonephritis* (a kidney infection) are more common in women. But all of these conditions can also occur in men and may be a sign of serious underlying conditions such as problems with the prostate gland. *Urethritis* in the male is most often contracted as a result of sexual contact. Many conditions affecting the kidneys, bladder, or urethra are described as urinary tract infections, or UTIs, and most UTIs are concentrated in the bladder and urethra.

Nearly 85 percent of urinary tract infections are caused by *Escherichia coli,* a bacterium that is normally found in the intestines. Chlamydia may also cause bladder problems. In women, bacteria introduced by means of fecal contamination or from vaginal secretions can gain access to the bladder by traveling up through the urethra. Cystitis, pyelonephritis, and urethritis occur much more frequently in women than in men because of the close proximity of the anus, vagina, and urethra in females, and also because of the short length of the female urethra. This allows for relatively easy transmission of bacteria from the anus to the vagina and urethra, and thus to the bladder. In males, bacteria can reach the bladder either by ascending through the urethra or by migrating from an infected prostate gland. While bladder infections are relatively common in women, in men they may signal a more serious problem, such as prostatitis.

Bladder infections are characterized by an urgent desire to empty the bladder. Urination is typically frequent and painful; even after the bladder has been emptied, there may be a desire to urinate again. The urine often has a strong, unpleasant odor, and may appear cloudy. Children suffering from bladder infections often complain of lower abdominal pain and a painful burning sensation while urinating. There may be blood in the urine. While cystitis itself is usually more of an annoyance than a serious health problem, it can lead to kidney infection if left untreated.

The possibility of developing a bladder infection can be increased by many factors, including pregnancy, sexual intercourse, the use of a diaphragm, and systemic disorders such as diabetes. The risk of cystitis is also increased if there is a structural abnormality or obstruction of the urinary tract resulting in restriction of the free flow of urine, or if past infections have resulted in a narrowing of the urethra. Bladder cancer is more common in men than women, and can often cause bladder infections. (*See under* CANCER in Part Two.)

Unless otherwise specified, the dosages recommended in this section are for adults. For a child between the ages of twelve and seventeen, reduce the dose to three-quarters the recommended amount. For a child between six and twelve, use one-half the recommended dose, and for a child under the age of six, use one-quarter the recommended amount.

URINARY TRACT INFECTION SELF-TEST

An FDA-approved home testing kit is available to help determine if you have a urinary infection. Bayer N-Multistix reagent strips are available in drugstores. The pharmacist may have to order them if they are not in stock.

NUTRIENTS

SUPPLEMENT	SUGGESTED DOSAGE	COMMENTS
Very Important		
Colloidal silver	As directed on label.	A natural antibiotic. Destroys bacteria, viruses, and fungi. Promotes healing.
Garlic (Kyolic from Wakunaga)	2 capsules 3 times daily.	A natural antibiotic and immune enhancer.
Vitamin C plus bioflavonoids	4,000–5,000 mg daily, in divided doses. 1,000 mg daily.	Produces antibacterial effect through acidification of urine. Important in immune function.
Important		
Acidophilus (Kyo-Dophilus from Wakunaga is a good source)	As directed on label. Take on an empty stomach. Also use 1 tbsp in 1 qt warm water as a douche.	Needed to restore "friendly" bacteria. Especially important if antibiotics are prescribed.
Calcium and magnesium	1,500 mg daily. 750–1,000 mg daily.	Reduces bladder irritability. Aids in the stress response and works best when balanced with calcium. Use magnesium chelate form.
Dioxychlor from American Biologics	10 drops twice daily. Also use 30 drops in 1 qt warm water as a douche.	An important antibacterial, antifungal, and antiviral agent.
Multivitamin and mineral complex with vitamin A with carotenoids	10,000 IU daily. 15,000 IU daily.	Needed for essential balanced vitamins and minerals. Use a high-potency, hypoallergenic form.
N-Acetylcysteine	500 mg twice daily, on an empty stomach.	A potent detoxifier that neutralizes free radicals.
Potassium	99 mg daily.	Replaces potassium lost as a result of frequent urination.
Vitamin B complex	50–100 mg of each major B vitamin twice daily, with meals (amounts of individual vitamins in a complex will vary).	Necessary for proper digestion. High doses are necessary if antibiotics are used.
Vitamin E	600 IU daily.	Combats infecting bacteria. Use d-alpha-tocopherol form.
Zinc plus copper	50 mg daily. Do not exceed a total of 100 mg daily from all supplements. 3 mg daily.	Important in tissue repair and immunity. Needed to balance with zinc.

HERBS

❑ Cranberry is one of the best herbal remedies for bladder infections. Quality cranberry juice produces hippuric acid in the urine, which acidifies the urine and inhibits bacterial growth. Other components in cranberry juice prevent bacteria from adhering to the lining of the bladder. Drink 1 quart of cranberry juice daily. Purchase pure, unsweetened juice from a health food store. If pure cranberry juice is not available, cranberry capsules can be substituted. Always take these with a large glass of water. Avoid commercial cranberry juice cocktail products. These contain relatively little pure cranberry juice (less than 30 percent in some cases) and have high-fructose corn syrup or other sweeteners added.

❏ Birch leaves are a natural diuretic and reduce some of the pain associated with bladder infections; dandelion tea or extract acts as a diuretic and liver cleanser, and aids in relieving bladder discomfort; hydrangea is good for stimulating the kidneys and flushing them clean. Diuretics help to cleanse the system. By promoting the release of fluids from the tissues, diuretics also help to relieve the false sensations of urgency that are characteristic of cystitis. Combinations of these herbs are often most effective in flushing the kidneys and helping to reduce the urgent need to urinate.

❏ Fresh blueberries are a very effective antioxidant. Anthocyanidins are present in the blue pigment, and may prove as useful as cranberries in preventing urinary tract infections. The herb bilberry, a type of blueberry, is also good.

❏ Buchu is good for a bladder infection with a burning sensation upon urination.

❏ Goldenseal is good for bladder infections if there is bleeding, and is most effective as an herbal antimicrobial agent.

Caution: Do not take goldenseal on a daily basis for more than one week at a time, and do not use it during pregnancy. If you have a history of cardiovascular disease, diabetes, or glaucoma, use it only under a doctor's supervision.

❏ Kidney Bladder formula from Nature's Way and SP-6 Cornsilk Blend from Solaray are herbal formulas that have a diuretic effect and reduce bladder spasms. Take 2 capsules twice daily.

❏ Marshmallow root increases the acidity of urine, inhibiting bacterial growth. Drink 1 quart of marshmallow root tea daily. It helps to strengthen and cleanse the bladder.

❏ Uva ursi (bearberry, a type of cranberry), used in small amounts and diluted with other herbal teas, acts as a mild diuretic and antiseptic. It is effective against *E. coli.*

❏ Other beneficial herbs include burdock root, juniper berries, kava kava, and rose hips.

Caution: Kava kava may cause drowsiness. If this occurs, discontinue use or decrease the dosage.

RECOMMENDATIONS

❏ Drink plenty of liquids, especially cranberry juice (*see under* Herbs, above). Drink at least one 8-ounce glass of quality water every hour. This is extremely beneficial for urinary tract infections. Steam-distilled water is preferable to tap water.

❏ Include celery, parsley, and watermelon in your diet. These foods act as natural diuretics and cleansers. Celery and parsley juice or extract can be purchased at a health food store or made fresh at home if you have a juicer.

❏ Avoid citrus fruits; these produce alkaline urine that encourages bacterial growth. Increasing the acid content in urine inhibits the growth of bacteria. *See* Acidosis *under* ACID/ALKALI IMBALANCE in Part Two for a list of acid-forming foods.

❏ Stay away from alcohol, caffeine, carbonated beverages, coffee, chocolate, refined or processed foods, and simple sugars. Chemicals in food, drugs, and impure water have an adverse effect on the bladder.

❏ Perform a one- to three-day cleansing fast.

❏ Take 2 teaspoonfuls of whey powder or 2 acidophilus tablets or capsules with each meal. This is especially important if antibiotic therapy is required.

❏ Take a twenty-minute hot sitz bath twice daily. Hot sitz baths help to relieve the pain associated with cystitis. Batherapy, a product that can be found in health food stores, is excellent. Or you can add one cup of vinegar to a sitz bath (or to shallow bath water) once a day. A woman should position her knees up and apart so that the water can enter the vagina. Alternate this with a bath made with two cloves of crushed garlic or an equivalent amount of garlic juice. (*See* SITZ BATH in Part Three.)

❏ Use acidophilus douches as recommended under Nutrients, above. If cystitis is associated with vaginitis, alternate this with apple cider vinegar douches.

❏ Avoid taking excess zinc and iron supplements until healed. Taking over 100 mg of zinc daily can depress the immune system; bacteria require iron for growth. If a bacterial infection is present, the body stores iron in the liver, spleen, and bone marrow in order to prevent further growth of the bacteria.

❏ Do not delay emptying the bladder. Making sure that you urinate every two to three waking hours—"voiding by the clock"—can help.

❏ Keep the genital and anal areas clean and dry. Women should wipe from front to back after emptying the bladder or bowels, should empty the bladder before and after exercise and sexual intercourse, and should wash the vagina after intercourse.

❏ Wear white cotton underwear; nylon underwear should be avoided.

❏ Change into dry clothes as soon as possible after swimming; avoid sitting around in a wet bathing suit.

❏ Do not use "feminine hygiene sprays," packaged douches, bubble baths, tampons, sanitary pads, or toilet paper containing fragrance. The chemicals these products contain are potentially irritating.

❏ If you suffer from frequent urinary tract infections, use sanitary pads rather than tampons.

❏ If urination is painful but harmful bacteria cannot be found, discontinue use of all types of soaps and use only water to cleanse the vaginal area. Some people are sensitive to soap; an all-natural soap from a health food store is recommended.

❏ If there is blood in the urine, consult your health care provider. This can be a sign of a more serious problem that warrants medical attention.

CONSIDERATIONS

❏ Optimal immune function is important in both fighting and preventing all bacterial disorders.

❏ Caffeine causes the muscles around the bladder neck to contract, and can produce painful bladder spasms.

❏ Habitually retaining the urine in the bladder for long periods increases a woman's risk of urinary tract infection, and may increase the risk of bladder cancer.

❏ Shrinkage of urethral and vaginal membranes, which most commonly occurs after menopause as a result of a reduction in the amount of estrogen in the body, can increase the tendency to develop bladder infections. Urethral dilation helps stretch a contracted urethra.

❏ Food allergies often cause symptoms that mimic bladder infections. Food allergy testing can determine which foods are causing the allergic reaction. (*See* ALLERGIES in Part Two.)

❏ Using aluminum cookware may cause cystitis symptoms. Cadmium, a toxic metal, may cause urinary problems as well.

❏ Colloidal silver is a natural broad-spectrum antiseptic that fights infection, subdues inflammation, and promotes healing. It is a clear golden liquid composed of 99.9-percent pure silver particles approximately 0.001 to 0.01 micron ($1/1,000,000$ to $1/100,000$ millimeter) in diameter that are suspended in pure water. It can be taken by mouth, administered intravenously, or applied topically. Colloidal silver is available in health food stores.

❏ Antibiotics and analgesics may be necessary treatments for cystitis, especially for persistent and/or painful infections. Beware of resorting to them too often, however. Antibiotics disturb the normal internal flora and may actually promote recurrent infections by promoting the development of antibiotic-resistant strains of bacteria. In fact, because antibiotics have been widely overprescribed over the years, many of the bacteria in our bodies (estimates run from 50 to 80 percent) are now resistant to common antibiotics, such as sulfa drugs and tetracycline. This forces doctors to resort to more powerful and potentially more dangerous antibiotics that pose a greater risk of adverse reactions and side effects. For most bladder infections, a natural approach to treatment appears to be best.

❏ Recurrent cystitis may be a sign of a more serious problem, such as bladder cancer, an anatomical anomaly, or immune deficiency. Cystoscopy, a simple visual examination of the bladder, is indicated.

❏ *See also* KIDNEY DISEASE, PROSTATITIS, and VAGINITIS in Part Two.

❏ For sources of additional information about bladder infections, *see* HEALTH AND MEDICAL ORGANIZATIONS in the Appendix.

Blepharitis

See under EYE PROBLEMS.

Blood Pressure Problems

See HIGH BLOOD PRESSURE.

Blood Sugar Problems

See DIABETES; HYPOGLYCEMIA.

Boil

Boils, referred to as *furuncles* by medical professionals, are round pus-filled nodules on the skin that result from infection with *Staphylococcus aureus* bacteria. The infection begins in the deepest portion of a hair follicle, or in an oil-producing sebaceous gland, and works its way up to the skin's surface. Poor nutrition, illness that has depressed immune function, diabetes mellitus, poor hygiene, and the use of immunosuppressive drugs are common contributing factors.

This disorder is common, especially among children and adolescents. Boils often appear on the scalp, buttocks, face, or underarms. They are tender, red, and painful, and they appear suddenly. Symptoms that a boil may be forming include itching, mild pain, and localized swelling. Within twenty-four hours, the boil becomes red and filled with pus. Fever and swelling of the lymph glands nearest the boil may occur.

Boils are contagious. The pus that drains when a boil opens can contaminate nearby skin, causing new boils, or can enter the bloodstream and spread to other body parts. A *carbuncle* is a cluster of boils that occurs when the infection spreads and other boils are formed. The formation of a carbuncle may be an indication of immune depression.

Without treatment, a boil usually comes to a head, opens, drains, and heals in ten to twenty-five days. With treatment, symptoms are less severe and new boils should not appear.

Unless otherwise specified, the following recommended doses are for those over the age of eighteen. For a child between twelve and seventeen years old, reduce the dose to three-quarters the recommended amount. For a child between six and twelve, use one-half the recommended dose, and for a child under six years old, use one-quarter the recommended amount.

NUTRIENTS

SUPPLEMENT	SUGGESTED DOSAGE	COMMENTS
Essential		
Colloidal silver	Apply topically as directed on label.	A natural antibiotic and disinfectant. Destroys bacteria, viruses, and fungi. Promotes healing.
Garlic (Kyolic from Wakunaga)	2 capsules 3 times daily.	A natural antibiotic that potentiates immune function.
Kyo-Green from Wakunaga	As directed on label.	To aid in cleansing the bloodstream and reducing infection.
Very Important		
Proteolytic enzymes	As directed on label. Take on an empty stomach.	Speeds up cleansing process at infection sites.
Vitamin A and carotenoid complex	75,000 IU daily for 1 month, then reduce to 25,000 IU daily. If you are pregnant, do not exceed 10,000 IU daily. As directed on label.	Antioxidants necessary for proper immune system function. Use emulsion forms for easier assimilation and greater safety at high doses. *Caution:* Do not take this supplement if you are pregnant or nursing.
Vitamin E	600 IU daily.	A powerful antioxidant. Use d-alpha-tocopherol form.
Vitamin C with bioflavonoids	3,000–8,000 mg daily, in divided doses.	Powerful anti-inflammatory and immune system stimulant.
Zinc	50 mg daily	Aids in healing and enhances the immune system.
Helpful		
Coenzyme Q10 plus	60 mg daily.	Important for oxygen utilization and immune function.
Coenzyme A from Coenzyme-A Technologies	As directed on label.	Works well with coenzyme Q10 in ridding the body of impurities.
Kelp plus multimineral complex	2,000–3,000 mg daily, in divided doses. As directed on label.	To supply balanced minerals. Use a high-potency formula.
Raw thymus glandular	500 mg daily.	Stimulates the immune system. (*See* GLANDULAR THERAPY in Part Three.)
Silica or oat straw	As directed on label.	Supplies silicon, which reduces inflammatory reaction. *See under* Herbs, below.

HERBS

❑ Burdock root, goldenseal, olive oil extract, and pau d'arco are all natural antibiotics that help to rid the body of infections and toxins.

❑ Dandelion, burdock root, and milk thistle cleanse the bloodstream and the liver.

❑ Echinacea and goldenseal help to cleanse the lymph glands.

Caution: Do not take goldenseal on a daily basis for more than one week at a time, and do not use it during pregnancy. If you have a history of cardiovascular disease, diabetes, or glaucoma, use it only under a doctor's supervision.

❑ Flax and fenugreek, simmered together and mashed into a pulp, can be used as a compress.

❑ Oat straw, taken in tea form, supplies silica, which has an anti-inflammatory effect.

❑ Onion poultices are good for boils. Apply pieces of onion wrapped in a piece of cloth—not directly to the area. (*See* USING A POULTICE in Part Three.)

❑ Propolis is made by bees and is a natural antibiotic. It can be taken in tincture form.

❑ Red clover acts as a natural antibiotic and is good for bacterial infections. It cleanses the liver and the bloodstream.

❑ Suma boosts the immune system.

❑ Tea tree oil compresses act as an antiseptic. Add 9 to 10 drops of the oil to 1 quart of warm water. Soak a clean cloth in the warm liquid and apply to the boil. The tea tree oil can be left on the boil for thirty minutes or more, and may be applied three or four times a day.

RECOMMENDATIONS

❑ Use a cleansing fast to clear the system and rid the body of toxins that may cause boils. *See* FASTING in Part Three.

❑ To relieve pain and help to bring the boil to a head, apply moist heat three or four times a day. Wet a clean towel or sterile gauze pad with warm water and apply it to the boil. Place a heating pad or a hot water bottle on top. Do this for twenty minutes three or four times a day. Use a clean towel or fresh piece of gauze each time to prevent spreading the infection. Warm Epsom salts baths are also good.

❑ Do not cover a boil with an adhesive bandage, but do avoid irritation, injury, or trauma to the affected area. To avoid sweating, do not exercise or engage in strenuous activity until the boil heals.

❑ Keep the skin clean. Wash the infected area several times a day and swab it with antiseptic. You can also apply honey directly to the boil. Vitamin A and E emulsion, applied directly on boils, is helpful. Clay packs and/or chlorophyll are also good. Both of these can be found in health food stores. Apply them directly to the boil with a sterile gauze pad.

❑ Charcoal capsules made into a paste and applied to the boil will help draw out the infection. Break open 2 capsules of charcoal and mix with just enough water to make the paste.

❑ *Belladonna,* a homeopathic remedy, helps reduce swelling and inflammation. Another homeopathic remedy, Calcarea sulphurica, is useful if a boil has opened and is draining, but is not healing properly.

❑ If a boil is very large, persistent, or recurrent, consult your physician. Surgical incision and drainage may be necessary. Severe cases may require bed rest.

CONSIDERATIONS

❑ Boils may be symptomatic of a more serious infection within the body. They should always be treated with care, especially if they are accompanied by other symptoms, such as a fever or a poor appetite.

❑ Boils should not be squeezed or punctured prematurely. In very serious cases, boils may need to be incised by a doctor.

❑ A doctor may prescribe an oral antibiotic. These drugs have side effects, however. It is best not to use them unless other measures fail.

❑ The area around a draining boil (especially on the face) may be protected with a prescribed antibiotic cream to help prevent complications such as septicemia or meningitis.

❑ Over-the-counter antibiotic ointments are ineffective for boils and should be avoided.

Breast Cancer

Cancer of the breast is the most common cancer among women (alongside skin cancer), and is the second leading cause of cancer death (following lung cancer) for women in the United States. The American Cancer Society estimates that every year, about 175,000 people are diagnosed as having breast cancer, and about 43,300 deaths occur from the disease. The lifetime risk of developing breast cancer for American women is one in eight. Surveys suggest that it is the health problem most feared by women—but the good news is that, since 1990, the number of new cases of breast cancer has stopped increasing. And if breast cancer is detected early, the five-year-and-beyond survival rate is very high—about 95 percent.

The human breast is a gland that contains milk ducts, lobes, fatty tissue, and a network of lymphatic vessels. Cancerous tumors can arise in virtually any part of the breast and are most often detected when a woman feels a lump. In general, cancerous lumps are firm, never go away, and are usually (though not always) pain-free. The vast majority of breast lumps are not cancerous (many are cysts or fibroid masses), but there is no way to tell without a professional's examination. A lump that seems to be growing or does not move when pushed may be cancerous or may simply be caused by normal fibrocystic changes during the menstrual cycle. A biopsy is required to identify the lump. Breast cancer can also cause a yellow, bloody, or clear discharge from the nipple.

People tend to think of breast cancer as a single entity, but there are actually different types of the disease. Some types of breast cancer include the following:

• *Adenoid cystic carcinoma, malignant cytosarcoma phylliodes, medullary carcinoma, and tubular carcinoma.* These and several other relatively uncommon types of breast cancer tend to be less aggressive than the other forms.

• *Ductal carcinoma in situ (DCIS).* This is a condition that most doctors consider to be breast cancer at its earliest stage. DCIS is a cancer contained within the milk ducts. The rate of this type of cancer has increased dramatically over the past twenty-five years. Fortunately, the survival rate for DCIS is nearly 100 percent.

• *Infiltrating ductal carcinoma.* This is a cancer that arises in the lining of the milk ducts and infiltrates (invades) the surrounding breast tissue. Approximately 80 percent of all cases of breast cancer are infiltrating ductal carcinomas.

• *Inflammatory carcinoma.* In this type of cancer, a tumor arises in the lining of the milk ducts and, as it grows, it plugs the lymphatic and blood vessels. The skin thickens and turns red, and the breast becomes extremely tender and looks infected. This type of cancer spreads very quickly due to the rich blood and lymph vessel supply associated with the inflammatory reaction.

• *Intraductal carcinoma in situ.* This is a localized type of cancer in which cancerous cells grow within the ducts. This type of cancer may not invade other tissues.

• *Lobular carcinoma.* A less common form of breast cancer, lobular carcinoma—breast cancer that arises in the lobes— accounts for about 9 percent of breast cancers. Lobular carcinomas occasionally occur in both breasts simultaneously.

• *Paget's disease of the nipple.* This form of cancer occurs when cells from an underlying cancerous tumor migrate to the nipple. The symptoms are itching, redness, and soreness of the nipple. Paget's disease always signals the presence of primary ductal carcinoma elsewhere in the breast tissue.

There is probably no single answer as to what causes breast cancer, and it is reported that as many as 60 percent of breast cancers develop without any known risk factors. Researchers believe, however, that the female sex hormone estrogen is the most likely culprit in many cases of breast cancer. Estrogen promotes cellular growth in the tissues of the breasts and reproductive organs, and cancer is a disorder of unrestrained cellular growth. Moreover, some of the known risk factors for breast cancer include onset of menstruation before age nine, menopause after age fifty-five, having a first child after age forty, and having no or few children. One thing all of these risk factors have in common is that they result in the breasts being exposed to more estrogen for longer periods. Currently, research does not point clearly to environmental factors (such as exposure to pesticides and other pollutants) as a possible factor in the development of breast cancer. However, research on the effects of pesticides is ongoing, and there are many health care professionals that advise avoiding these substances as much as possible, as they may mimic estrogen in the body.

There may be a link between obesity and an increased risk of developing breast cancer, especially for women over fifty years of age. However, this is a complex issue. The risk appears to vary depending on whether a woman has been obese since childhood, or if she gained the excess weight during adulthood. A study reported in the journal *Cancer* found that women who gained more than twenty-two pounds since their teenage years doubled their chances of getting breast cancer. Interestingly, the increased risk posed by obesity may also be linked to estrogen. Obese women tend to have higher levels of estrogen in their bodies than thin women. There are conflicting reports as to whether eating a high-fat diet is linked to an increased risk of breast cancer. However, many physicians believe that it is among the highest risk factors. When a woman eats a diet high in fat and low in fiber, her body produces more estrogen.

Heredity is a factor in breast cancer as well; there are certain types of the disease that clearly run in families. Researchers estimate that only 5 to 10 percent of breast cancers occur in women with a clearly defined genetic predisposition for the disease. Hereditary cancers usually develop before the age of fifty.

Although it is possible for a woman to get breast cancer at any age, the disease is most common in women over forty, especially postmenopausal women. Estrogen replacement therapy (ERT), often used in the treatment of menopause, may slightly increase the risk of breast cancer

after long-term use (ten years or more). This risk applies to those who are still using (or have recently stopped using) ERT. Five years after stopping ERT, the breast cancer risk returns to normal. A recent report from the Iowa Women's Health Study has reported that ERT may not increase risk for most common types of breast cancer, but it may increase risk for certain rare forms of the disease. This is the first report of its kind to come out pinpointing risk for specific tumor types.

Men also can get breast cancer, but they account for fewer than 1 percent of breast cancer cases. However, while it occurs less frequently, breast cancer in men usually is diagnosed at a later, and therefore more serious, stage because neither physicians nor their patients tend to suspect it. Cure rates are, in general, the same for men as they are for women.

It is important to detect breast cancer in its earliest and most curable stage. Making healthy changes in diet and lifestyle, examining your breasts regularly (*See* Breast Self-Examination, below), and having regular mammograms can increase your chances of avoiding or, if need be, overcoming breast cancer.

BREAST SELF-EXAMINATION

It is important to examine your breasts each month past age twenty, at the same point in your menstrual cycle, preferably the first week after your menstrual period ends. Do not examine them during your menstrual period. Before the period, a woman's breasts may swell and become tender or lumpy. This usually decreases after the period. The breasts also become larger and firmer during pregnancy, in preparation for breastfeeding. Familiarize yourself with the normal feel of your breasts so that you can detect any changes such as enlargement of a lump. A woman who is accustomed to the way her breasts feels is better able to notice subtle changes. Any changes in your breasts should be reported to your health care provider, and you should be rechecked by a professional if you have any doubt concerning your examination. Since men also can get breast cancer, they can benefit from self-examination as well. The

Breast Implants and Breast Cancer

Although the use of silicone/polyurethane implants—silicone-filled implants coated with polyurethane—has been banned since 1992 because of concerns about their safety, an estimated 200,000 American women still have these implants in their bodies. Polyurethane releases a human carcinogen known as toluene diisocyanate, or TDA, which was banned for use in hair dye long before the controversy over breast implants arose. Silicone occasionally leaks from its envelope and can sometimes enter the bloodstream. It is not known if leaking silicone causes cancer in humans.

There is also great debate over whether breast implants make it harder to detect breast cancer in the earlier stages. Many researchers believe that implants may hide some breast tissue, interfering with the ability to take and interpret mammograms properly. Saline is currently the FDA-approved substance now being used for implant fillings in the United States. Trilucent implants, or implants filled with a soybean-oil derivative, are currently under evaluation. Not only may these implants prove to be a safer alternative to silicone and saline, but the substance also allows for better mammography readings.

following is the recommended procedure for breast self-examination:

1. While standing and looking in the mirror, raise your hands over your head and press them together. Notice the shape of your breasts. Place your hands on your hips, apply pressure, and look for irritation or dimpling of the skin, nipples that seem to be out of position, one breast that looks different from the other, swelling in a portion of the breast, nipple pain, an inward curve of the nipple, a discharge from the nipple (other than breast milk), or red scaling or thickening of the skin and nipples.

2. Raise one arm above your head. With the other hand, firmly explore your breast. Beginning at the outer edge, using a circular motion, gradually work toward the nipple. Take your time when examining the area between the nipple and the armpit, and feel the armpit as well. You have lymph nodes in the armpit; they move freely and feel soft, and are not painful to the touch. Look for lumps that are hard and not mobile. Cancers are often attached to underlying muscle or the skin. When you have finished examining one breast, repeat this on the other side.

3. Lie down on your back and repeat step 2. Lumps may be more easily detected in this position. Also, squeeze each nipple gently to check for blood or a watery yellow or pink discharge.

In addition to monthly self-examination, the American Cancer Society recommends that women between the ages of twenty and thirty-nine have their breasts examined by a physician every one to three years. After age forty, the exam should be performed every year. Women should get their first mammogram by age forty, then have one every year along with their yearly exam.

The program recommended below is designed for women who have been diagnosed with breast cancer as well as for women who want to increase their odds of avoiding breast cancer.

NUTRIENTS

SUPPLEMENT	SUGGESTED DOSAGE	COMMENTS
Essential		
Coenzyme Q₁₀	100 mg daily.	Improves cellular oxygenation. There is mounting evidence supporting the theory that coenzyme Q₁₀ reduces the risk of breast cancer.
Colostrum (New Life Colostrum from Symbiotics [original and high-Ig formulas] or Colostrum Specific from Jarrow Formulas)	As directed on label.	Promotes accelerated healing and boosts the immune system.
Dimethylglycine (DMG) (Aangamik DMG from FoodScience of Vermont)	As directed on label.	Improves cellular oxygenation.
Essential fatty acids (Kyolic-EPA from Wakunaga, black currant seed oil, borage oil, flaxseed oil are good sources)	As directed on label.	Needed for proper cell reproduction.
Garlic (Kyolic from Wakunaga)	2 capsules 3 times daily.	Enhances immune function.
Germanium	200 mg daily.	A powerful immunostimulant that improves cellular oxygenation, deterring cancer growth.
Melatonin	3–50 mg at bedtime.	Blocks estrogen-receptor sites on breast cancer cells.
Multimineral complex with calcium and magnesium and potassium and zinc	2,000 mg daily. 1,000 mg daily. 99 mg daily. 50 mg daily.	Essential for normal cell division and function. Use a comprehensive formula that contains all major minerals and trace elements but that is iron-free. Good for strengthening immunity.
Multivitamin complex	As directed on label. Take with meals.	All nutrients are needed for nutritional balance. Do not use a sustained-release formula or a formula that contains iron.
Natural beta-carotene or carotenoid complex (Betatene)	10,000 IU daily. As directed on label.	A powerful antioxidant that destroys free radicals.
Proteolytic enzymes (Wobenzym N from Marlyn Nutraceuticals or Inflazyme Forte from American Biologics) plus multienzyme complex	2 tablets between meals (to reduce inflammation) and 2 tablets with meals (to aid digestion). When taking them with meals, it is best to take them with protein foods. As directed on label.	Powerful free radical scavengers. Reduce inflammation. To aid in digestion.
Selenium	200–400 mcg daily. If you are pregnant, do not exceed 40 mcg daily.	Protects the immune system by preventing the formation of free radicals, which can damage the body. It has also been found to function as a preventive against the formation of certain types of tumors, including breast tumors.
Shark cartilage (BeneFin)	For cancer treatment, 1 gm per 2 lbs of body weight daily, divided into 3 doses. If you cannot tolerate taking it orally, it can be administered in a retention enema. (*See under* ENEMAS in Part Three.) For cancer prevention, 2,000–4,500 mg 3 times daily.	Inhibits tumor growth and stimulates the immune system.
Superoxide dismutase (SOD)	As directed on label.	Destroys free radicals. Consider injections (under a doctor's supervision).
Vitamin B complex plus extra vitamin B₃ (niacin) and choline	100 mg of each major B vitamin 3 times daily (amounts of individual vitamins in a complex will vary). 100 mg daily. Do not exceed this amount.	To improve circulation, build red blood cells, and aid liver function; necessary for normal cell division and function. Involved in the regulation of enzyme and hormone production.

plus vitamin B$_{12}$ and folic acid	2,000 mcg daily. 400–800 mcg daily.	Caution: Do not take niacin if you have a liver disorder, gout, or high blood pressure. To prevent anemia and aid in proper digestion and absorption of nutrients. Consider injections (under a doctor's supervision). If injections are not available, use a sublingual form such as Superior Source supplements from Continental Vitamin.
plus brewer's yeast	100 mg 3 times daily. As directed on label.	Aids in reducing estrogen production. A source of B vitamins.
Vitamin C with bioflavonoids plus extra quercetin	5,000–20,000 mg daily, in divided doses. See ASCORBIC ACID FLUSH in Part Three. 400 mg 3 times daily or as directed on label.	Powerful anticancer agent.
Vitamin E	Start with 400 IU daily and increase slowly to 1,000 IU daily.	Deficiency has been linked to breast cancer. Also aids in hormone production and immune function. Use emulsion form for easier assimilation and greater safety at higher doses. Blocks free-radical damage in fatty breast cells. Use d-alpha-tocopherol form.
Important		
Maitake	4,000–8,000 mg daily.	Inhibits the growth and spread of cancerous tumors. Also boosts immune response.
Vitamin D$_3$	As directed on label.	Inhibits cell division and growth. Low levels of vitamin D have been linked to higher breast cancer rates.
Helpful		
Acidophilus (Kyo-Dophilus or Probiata from Wakunaga)	As directed on label.	To replenish "friendly" bacteria in the colon. Contains powerful anti-carcinogenic compounds. Breaks down metabolites of estrogen. Use a nondairy formula.
Aerobic 07 from Aerobic Life Industries or Dioxychlor from American Biologics	As directed on label. As directed on label.	Antimicrobial agents.
Kelp or seaweed	1,000–1,500 mg daily. As directed on label.	For mineral balance.
L-Carnitine	As directed on label.	Protects the skin after mastectomy and/or radiation treatment. Use a form derived from fish liver (squalene).
plus L-cysteine and L-methionine and glutathione	As directed on label. Take with water or juice. Do not take with milk. Take with 50 mg vitamin B$_6$ and 100 mg vitamin C for better absorption.	To detoxify harmful substances. (See AMINO ACIDS in Part One.)
plus Taurine Plus from American Biologics	As directed on label.	Functions as foundation for tissue and organ repair. Use the sublingual form.
Pycnogenol	As directed on label.	A powerful antioxidant.
Raw glandular complex plus raw thymus and raw adrenal glandulars	As directed on label. As directed on label. As directed on label.	To stimulate glandular function, especially the thymus, the site of T lymphocyte production. (See GLANDULAR THERAPY in Part Three.)
S-Adenosylmethio- nine (SAMe)	As directed on label.	Aids in stress-relief, relieves depression, eases pain, and produces anti-oxidant effects. Has been found to inhibit growth of breast cancer cells in laboratory tests. Caution: Do not use if you have manic-depressive disorder or take prescription antidepressants.

HERBS

❏ Astragalus root and echinacea enhance immune function. These herbs are best used in a rotating fashion, for no more than seven to ten days in a row.

Caution: Do not use astragalus in the presence of a fever.

❏ Drink herbal teas such as bilberry, burdock root, ginger, green tea, peppermint, and red clover instead of regular tea.

❏ Black cohosh, chasteberry, red clover, and turmeric are herbs that are high in phytoestrogens. Phytoestrogens are forms of estrogen that are much weaker than the body's estrogens, but that are capable of blocking the stronger, more damaging estrogens (they can fit into the same receptors in breast cells that estrogens can, thus preventing the estrogen's ability to dock there). Phytoestrogens also expand the length of the menstrual cycle, possibly lowering the lifetime exposure to estrogen.

❏ Burdock root, dandelion root, milk thistle, and red clover all protect the liver and aid in cleansing the bloodstream.

❏ Chaste tree berry (also known as vitex), ginseng, and soy extracts may inhibit the growth of breast cancer cells.

❏ Ongoing research is finding that curcumin (found in turmeric), genistein (in soy), and green tea have cancer-fighting abilities.

❏ Garlic is known to be a cancer-preventing nutrient.

❏ Ginkgo biloba enhances circulation and brain function.

❏ Licorice root aids in maintaining proper organ function.

Caution: If overused, licorice can elevate blood pressure. Do not use this herb on a daily basis for more than seven days in a row. Avoid it completely if you have high blood pressure.

❏ Silymarin, an antioxidant extract of milk thistle, has shown promise for fighting breast cancer. It also protects the liver.

❏ An herbal preparation known as Spes, produced by BotanicLab, has shown good results in treating breast cancer when combined with a high dose of genistein (soy extract), curcumin, and 83-percent green tea extract.

RECOMMENDATIONS

❑ Eat a high-fiber diet based on fresh fruits and vegetables, plus grains, legumes, raw nuts (except peanuts) and seeds, and soured products such as low-fat yogurt. Very important are the cruciferous vegetables, such as broccoli, Brussels sprouts, cabbage, and cauliflower, and yellow/orange vegetables, such as carrots, pumpkin, squash, sweet potatoes, and yams. Eat vegetables raw or lightly steamed. For grains, use unpolished brown rice, millet, oats, and wheat. Eat whole grains only. If at all possible, consume only organically grown foods. Pesticides and other chemicals have been linked to breast cancer (they may mimic the effect of estrogen on the body).

❑ Include soy foods in your diet. Diets high in fiber and soy foods are associated with a lowered risk of breast cancer. Some good sources of soy include fresh soybeans, tempeh, soymilk, soy nuts, tofu, and soy powder.

❑ Include in your diet fresh apples, cherries, grapes, plums, and all types of berries.

❑ Eat onions and garlic, or take garlic in supplement form.

❑ Make sure your diet provides adequate amounts of essential fatty acids (EFAs). Omega-3 EFAs (found in fish and flaxseed) and omega-9 fatty acids (found in olive oil) lower cancer risk. Eating salmon weekly and tuna three times a week will provide a good amount of fatty acids. Processed fish oil supplements are also a good idea, but avoid cod liver oil, as its levels of vitamin A and D are too high. Fish oil has been reported to possibly slow tumor growth. Flaxseed oil can be sprinkled onto food.

❑ Make a daily juice using a combination of fresh organic broccoli, cauliflower, carrots, kale, dark leafy greens, and an apple. These are high in phytochemicals and help to combat breast cancer.

❑ Limit your intake of fatty, charred, or grilled foods, which have been linked with a higher risk of cancer.

❑ Drink spring or steam-distilled water only, never tap water. Also drink fresh homemade vegetable and fruit juices. Drink fruit juices in the morning and vegetable juices in the afternoon.

❑ If you consume meat, poultry, and dairy products, select organic, hormone-free products. Otherwise, these foods often contain residues of estrogenic hormones that are given to animals in order to promote growth. Well-done red meat has been linked to a higher risk for breast cancer in some studies. Unsweetened low-fat yogurt is an acceptable source of protein.

❑ Do not consume any alcohol, caffeine, junk foods, processed refined foods, saturated fats, salt, sugar, or white flour.

❑ Take extra fiber daily. Fiber keeps toxic wastes from being absorbed into the bloodstream. Psyllium husks are a recommended source. The colon must be kept clean and the bowels must move daily for healing. *See* COLON CLEANSING, ENEMAS, and FASTING in Part Three.

Note: Always take supplemental fiber separately from other supplements and medications.

❑ Do not take supplements containing iron. Iron may be used by tumors to promote their growth.

❑ If you experience itching, redness, and soreness of the nipples, especially if you are not currently breastfeeding a baby, seek evaluation by a physician. These can be symptoms of Paget's disease.

❑ If you are undergoing treatment for breast cancer and find yourself feeling depressed or frightened, try to keep in mind that when medications (especially chemotherapy drugs) are stopped, you will probably start to feel better and to look at things in a different light. Think about all the women, including many celebrities and public figures, who have had breast cancer and have gone on to have fulfilling lives and careers. Thousands of women who have had breast cancer are living happy, normal lives.

CONSIDERATIONS

❑ Mammograms can detect small tumors and breast abnormalities up to two years before they can be felt, when they are most treatable. A mammogram should be scheduled within the first fourteen days of your menstrual cycle, when the breasts are less likely to be swollen. You should not use any antiperspirant, deodorant, or powder on the day of the test, as it can interfere with the reading.

❑ The Bosom Buddies breast self-examination kit from Jason Natural Cosmetics includes a moisturizing cream, a "how-to" breast self-exam chart, a breast self-examination recording booklet, and a bottle of breast comforting cream. The kit is available in health food stores.

❑ When breast cancer is caught in the very early stages—when it has not invaded nearby tissues—the cure rate is near 100 percent with surgery alone. Tumors of 1 centimeter or less in size carry a particularly good prognosis—less than a 10-percent likelihood of recurrence within ten years. In general, the risk of recurrence rises with increasing tumor size and lymph node involvement.

❑ The connection between exercise and cancer is a fairly new area of research. Some studies suggest that getting regular exercise in youth might give life-long protection against breast cancer. Even moderate physical activity as an adult may lower breast cancer risk. More research is underway to confirm these findings. Outdoor exercise where you are getting some (but not too much) sun exposure also raises vitamin D levels (low levels have been associated with a greater risk of cancer).

❑ Relaxation techniques such as writing, meditation, yoga, or massage therapy can aid in battling breast cancer.

❑ There is a clear link between alcohol consumption and an increased risk of breast cancer. *The New England Journal of Medicine* has stated that consuming as few as three alcoholic drinks a week increases the potential for breast cancer by 50 percent. The American Cancer Society (ACS) estimates that those who have two to five drinks daily increase their risk to about 1.5 times that of women who drink no alcohol. The ACS recommends that you limit the amount you drink to two drinks, two times weekly.

❏ There is great debate about whether or not fat intake has an effect on the risk of developing breast cancer. The National Women's Health Network urges all women to cut their total fat intake to 20 percent of total calories. Saturated fats should account for no more than 5 percent of calories.

❏ It is still not clear what part birth control pills might play in breast cancer risk. It may be that women using birth control pills have a slightly greater risk of breast cancer. Women should discuss the risks and benefits of birth control pills with their doctors.

❏ Frequent exposure to medical x-rays has been linked to an increased risk for breast cancer.

❏ Early or prolonged use of permanent dark hair dyes have been linked to breast cancer.

❏ New methods of testing for breast cancer are increasing the likelihood of catching it early. *Minimally invasive breast biopsies* (MIBB) can be performed with virtually no recovery time. *Ultrasounds* and *high-resolution ultrasounds* offer a safer alternative to x-rays and can provide sharp digital pictures. *Magnetic resonance imaging* can create a three-dimensional image and can be useful in detecting ruptures in silicone breast implants.

❏ A computerized mammogram scanner may increase the likelihood that a woman's cancer can be cured by calling a radiologist's attention to a suspicious area on a mammogram. The M1000 ImageChecker analyzes the content of mammograms and highlights suspicious areas on the images after the radiologist has done the initial evaluation. The device has been shown to improve a radiologist's detection rate from about 80 cancers out of 100 to 88 out of 100.

❏ The use of digital x-rays is predicted to reduce the number of undetected breast cancers significantly.

❏ A new method of detecting if cancer has spread to the lymph nodes, called sentinel node biopsy, allows doctors to pinpoint the first lymph node into which a tumor drains (the sentinel node), and remove only the nodes most likely to contain cancer cells.

❏ If you have a personal family history of breast cancer, you may want to consider genetic testing. Over half of women with certain genetic mutations develop breast cancer by the age of 70. Genetic testing can determine whether you have a genetic mutation, but it cannot predict whether you will develop breast cancer. Talk to your doctor if you are considering genetic testing. It is expensive, it is not always covered by insurance companies, and if your results are positive, insurance companies may choose to deny you coverage.

❏ People with breast cancer have been found to have lower than normal levels of vitamin E and the mineral selenium, two important antioxidants that work together to neutralize free radicals. Selenium has been shown in lab studies to kill tumors and protect healthy tissue. Research has shown that people with cancer of the lung, bladder, breast, colon, and skin all have levels of vitamin A that are lower than normal.

❏ It has been difficult to evaluate whether or not DHEA may prevent breast cancer because studies have yielded conflicting evidence on this point. 7-keto DHEA is a stronger, natural descendant of DHEA. Unlike DHEA itself, 7-keto DHEA is not converted into testosterone or estrogens in the body. It may be a safer alternative to DHEA in combating breast cancer.

❏ Low levels of vitamin B_{12} have been linked to an increased risk of breast cancer.

❏ Glucaric acid is currently under study with women at high risk for breast cancer. Numerous studies have found it to help eliminate toxic, carcinogenic substances from the body. It also lowers levels of estradiol, a form of estrogen linked to breast cancer. Glucaric acid occurs naturally in apples, grapefruit, and sprouts.

❏ Some studies have found tocotrienols to be effective in inhibiting the growth of breast cancer cells. Tocotrienols are substances that are members of the vitamin E family of compounds. D-alpha-tocopherol, the natural supplement form of vitamin E, is most readily absorbed by the body.

❏ Studies have shown that genistein, found in soy, inhibits new tumor growth, slowing the growth of existing cancer.

❏ Pro Fem progesterone cream is a natural progesterone cream that can be applied to the breast for direct absorption through the fat under the skin. Progesterone may help reduce the risk of breast cancer.

❏ Breast Health from NaturalMax is a supplement designed to act as defense against breast cancer. It contains a variety of herbal extracts, phytochemicals, and nutrients, including genistein, black currant blend, freeze-dried broccoli, gotu kola, indole-3-carbinol, saw palmetto, and lycopene. It should not be taken by pregnant women or nursing mothers.

❏ Treatment for breast cancer may include surgery, radiotherapy (or radiation therapy), chemotherapy, hormone therapy, or a combination of these to control the breast tumor. Hormone therapy may be used, in the form of selective estrogen receptor modulators (SERMs) such as tamoxifen (Nolvadex). Tamoxifen has been found to reduce the risk of breast cancer by about 45 percent, but it also has been linked to an increased risk of uterine cancer, blood clots in major veins and the lungs, cataracts, and, possibly, stroke. The long-term effects still remain to be discovered. It may be wise to consider this drug if you are at low risk for the possible side effects and at high risk for breast cancer. An evaluation from your health care provider, including the discussion of your risk factors, will help you to determine if tamoxifen would be an appropriate consideration for you.

❏ Raloxifene (Evista), a newer drug similar to tamoxifen, has been found in two clinical trials to be at least as effective in the prevention of breast cancer, without the increased risk of uterine cancer linked to tamoxifen. These findings are preliminary, however, because they were secondary findings in studies that were not focused on breast cancer prevention, and the studies were not run as long as the tamoxifen studies. The drug appears to also pose the same risk factors for blood clotting that tamoxifen does. The FDA has not yet approved the drug for the prevention of breast cancer; however, it has been approved for the prevention of osteoporosis in menopausal women.

❏ Epirubicin (Ellence) is a chemotherapy drug that can be used to combat early-stage breast cancer that has spread to the lymph nodes.

❏ Capecitabine (Xeloda) is a drug approved for use in women with advanced breast cancer for which no acceptable alternative treatments are available. It was given accelerated approval, an early approval process applied to some drugs that are used to treat life-threatening conditions. This drug is specifically for patients whose tumors are resistant to other treatments. In studies, the drug measurably shrank some patients' tumors. Possible side effects include diarrhea, nausea, vomiting, fatigue, painful inflammation of the mouth, and painful rash and swelling of the hands and feet.

❏ Doctors once believed that extensive surgery could control the spread of breast cancer. However, they now believe that cancer cells may break away from the primary tumor during surgery and spread through the bloodstream, even in the earliest stages of the disease. These cells cannot be felt by examination or seen on x-rays or other imaging methods, and they produce no symptoms. Adjuvant therapy—the use of drug treatment after surgery—can be used to kill these hidden cells. Your health care provider can make recommendations as to whether or not adjuvant therapy is needed in your individual situation. Drugs approved by the FDA to improve the chances of successfully treating breast cancer include: capecitabine (Xeloda); docetaxel (Taxotere), which may be used if locally advanced or metastasized breast cancer has progressed despite treatment with other drugs; paclitaxel (Taxol), which is used for both treatment of metastatic or advanced breast cancer and prevention of relapses; tamoxifen (Nolvadex); and trastuzumab (Herceptin), an immunotherapy regimen that can be used alone if other drugs have been unsuccessful, or as a first-line treatment in combination with other drugs. In addition to these new drugs, cyclophosphamide (Cytoxan) and doxorubicin (Adriamycin), with or without fluorouracil (Adrucil), may be used to treat breast cancer. Chemotherapy treatment is given in cycles, followed by recovery periods.

Depending on how far the cancer has spread, treatments can last from three to six months.

❏ Fentanyl (Actiq) is a drug that may be prescribed for people in severe pain. It is a narcotic drug that is more potent than morphine and comes in a flavored sugar lozenge form.

❏ After surgery, analysis of the tumor is done to determine the type of cancer and to test for the presence of a substance called estrogen-receptor protein, to determine whether the cancer is estrogen-dependent. If the tumor is found to be estrogen-dependent, tamoxifen may be an alternative to conventional chemotherapy.

❏ Most women with breast cancer have some type of surgery, depending on the stage of the breast cancer. Options for the surgical treatment of breast cancer have expanded greatly in the past couple of decades. Surgical treatment now emphasizes breast conservation—preserving the breast when possible. Some of the treatment options in breast surgery include:

• Lumpectomy, also known as *segmental mastectomy* or *tylectomy*. The tumor and a small amount of surrounding tissue are removed. This is the least extensive type of breast cancer surgery. In most cases, a lumpectomy is followed by several weeks of radiation, which is an integral part of breast-conserving treatment.

• Quadrantectomy, also known as *partial mastectomy*. The quadrant of the breast in which the tumor was found is removed, including some skin and the lining of the chest muscle below the tumor.

• Simple mastectomy. The entire breast is removed and a sample of the underarm lymph nodes is taken.

• Modified radical mastectomy, also known as *total mastectomy*. The entire breast and all underarm lymph nodes are removed. The lining over the chest muscles may also be removed.

• Radical mastectomy, also known as the *Halsted radical mastectomy*. The entire breast, all the axillary (underarm) lymph nodes, and the underlying chest muscle are removed. This procedure was once the standard in breast cancer surgery, but today, women with breast cancer rarely undergo this type of surgery because doctors believe that a modified radical mastectomy is just as effective.

• Bilateral prophylactic mastectomy. This type of surgery is done in a small percentage of women who are at particularly high risk for breast cancer. In this procedure, both healthy breasts are removed to prevent breast cancer from forming. This is most often performed on women who have an inherited genetic defect that increases their risk of getting breast cancer to 85 percent by the age of 70. Researchers at the Mayo Clinic have found that this procedure may reduce the risk of developing the disease by almost 90 percent, and deaths due to breast cancer by over 80 percent.

No single procedure can be recommended as ideal for all

individuals. A woman and her surgeon must base their decision on the patient's medical status and her particular concerns. Her choice may be influenced by emotional considerations, finances, access to care, body image, and personal beliefs. Depending on the type of surgery that is done, there is the option of having breast reconstruction later.

❏ A new form of reconstructive surgery may soon be an option for women who have had a mastectomy. The procedure involves growing their own tissue from a sample of fat and blood vessel cells taken from the thigh or buttocks. Growth hormones are then added, actually causing the tissue to grow. This method, developed by ReproGenesis with the help from researchers at the University of Michigan and the University of North Carolina, may be a better option for women who are considering breast reconstruction.

❏ A technique called rotating delivery of excitation off-resonance (RODEO) MRI-guided laser lumpectomy soon may be available to treat breast cancer without surgery, radiation, or chemotherapy. The outpatient procedure uses magnetic resonance imaging with lasers that destroy early-stage cancers.

❏ A relatively new approach to breast cancer treatment involves a combination of high-dose chemotherapy and a bone marrow transplant. Doctors first extract and freeze a small amount of marrow, then administer extremely high doses of chemotherapy to eradicate the cancer cells. The marrow is then reinjected into the patient to replace the marrow destroyed by chemotherapy. This treatment was tested at Duke University on women with advanced breast cancer that had spread to the lymph nodes in the armpits. After two years, 72 percent of the treated women were free of cancer, compared with 38 percent of those who received standard chemotherapy treatment. This treatment is very expensive, however; it can cost more than $100,000, and many insurance companies are reluctant to pay for it because they consider it experimental. It is also extremely difficult physically for the woman who undergoes it. This is a risky procedure, and it is still widely considered experimental, although many women with late-stage breast cancer are hoping that it will be able to help them in their battle. Researchers at Duke University Medical Center have identified some characteristics that may help doctors and patients decide if a bone marrow transplant may be an option. The best candidates are:

• Those who begin the treatment before the cancer has metastasized past the chest wall and lymph nodes.

• Those who have never had chemotherapy in their lifetime.

• Those whose cancer is slowly metastasizing.

• Those who have metastasized tumors with estrogen-positive receptors and have been treated with tamoxifen.

• Those whose metastasized tumors are still small.

❏ In any type of breast cancer surgery, some or all of the underarm lymph nodes may be removed. This is done to check for possible spread of the cancer. If the cancer has spread to the lymph nodes, postoperative therapy may include radiation, chemotherapy, or hormonal therapy. Radiation is always required after a lumpectomy or quadrantectomy to ensure that no more cancer cells remain.

❏ After surgery, women are usually advised to avoid moving or carrying heavy objects, to wear loose-fitting clothes and gloves, and to avoid overexposure to the sun. Some women whose lymph nodes are removed during breast cancer surgery have a problem with swelling of the arm, or lymphedema, on that side due to an accumulation of lymphatic fluid. This is not unusual. It can develop just after surgery, or months or even years later, and can be brought on by an injury to (or overuse of) the arm or an infection. To reduce the risk of developing lymphedema, do not have any blood work, chemotherapy, or blood pressure work done on the affected arm. Certain arm exercises are usually prescribed to keep the arm from becoming stiff and to assist in healing. If there is any unusual swelling, redness, or pain in the hand or arm, this should be evaluated by a physician.

❏ The Johns Hopkins Breast Center offers an outpatient mastectomy option for cancer patients. Here, the patients and their families are put through a trial run of the operation, from what the operating room looks like to how the wounds will appear after the surgery.

❏ In the near future, it is expected that more treatments that include biologically and hormonally based regimens will be used to treat breast cancer. They are less likely to show the harsh side effects than some chemotherapy treatments.

❏ With the recent discovery of two "breast cancer genes" (BRCA1 and BRCA2), gene therapy is receiving more attention; however, this research is still in its infancy and much more investigation in this area needs to be done.

❏ Less invasive techniques are being developed in the detection and treatment of breast cancer. Biopsies may soon be able to be done by physicians using a fine needle aspiration (removing cells from a breast lump) and stereotactic core biopsies (which uses a bigger needle that a computer guides to remove suspicious tissue seen on a mammogram). Surgery may soon be replaced using microwave radiation or therapeutic ultrasound to destroy small tumors without opening up the breast.

❏ Family support is necessary for the person with breast cancer. Depression, anxiety, and fear are not uncommon. *See also* CANCER in Part Two.

❏ Even when treatment is initially successful, the American Cancer Society (ACS) says that breast cancer will return in about 50 percent of cases. However, new drugs, treatment regimens, and better diagnostic techniques have improved the outlook for many, and are responsible, according to the ACS, for a decline in breast cancer death rates.

❏ For agencies and organizations that can provide more information and services for people with breast cancer, *see* HEALTH AND MEDICAL ORGANIZATIONS in the Appendix.

Breastfeeding-Related Problems

Breastfeeding, or lactation, is the natural way in which the mother of a newborn can feed her child instead of relying on cow's milk or artificial formula preparations. A woman's breasts are ideally suited for the task of feeding a baby, and nursing provides many benefits to both mother and baby that bottles and formulas do not. For example, mother's milk is much easier to digest, prevents constipation, lowers the incidence of food allergies, and protects the baby from many infectious diseases. Nursing also promotes healthy oral development, satisfies suckling needs, and enhances bonding and skin-to-skin contact between mother and child. Breastfeeding is beneficial to the mother in that it reduces the chance of hemorrhaging from the placental site, gives the mother an opportunity to rest, and encourages the uterus to contract, returning it to its pre-pregnant size.

Besides giving an infant more resistance to bacteria and illness and creating a closer bond between the mother and child, the benefits of breastfeeding include higher brain development. Breastfed infants have been found to be more intelligent than formula-fed infants and to achieve higher academic levels in adult life. In an eighteen-year study conducted on 1,000 children, it was shown that polyunsaturated fatty acids, particularly the docosahexaenoic acid (DHA) contained in mother's milk, boosted intellectual (neural) development. DHA is considered essential for a baby's development. Formula-fed babies do not receive DHA, and while the mother passes a large amount of DHA on to the infant in the last trimester of pregnancy, a baby fed with formula does not continue to ingest this most important developmental nutrient.

A study of 2,200 Australian children shows that infants who are breastfed for at least the first four months of life are significantly less likely to develop asthma, wheezing, or respiratory allergies by the age of six. A mother's milk also prevents *Clostridium difficile*, the intestinal bacteria that causes serious colon inflammation and diarrhea in adults, from binding to the cells of the baby's intestinal walls.

Many infants are fed formulas, either for medical reasons or because the mother cannot or chooses not to breastfeed. A debate continues over breastfeeding versus formula feeding. One controversy centers on soy-based infant formulas. If a baby is allergic to milk protein or lactose (milk sugar), a doctor may prescribe a soy-based formula. Twenty-five percent of the infant formulas on the U.S. market are soy-based. But concern has risen over the effect that isoflavones (phytochemicals present in soy) have on the endocrine functions of test animals and in cultured cells. Isoflavones, present in varying degrees in soy-based infant formulas, can create problems in the endocrine system. But proponents of soy-based formulas maintain that the reports present no evidence of endocrine effects on humans who were fed soy formulas as infants.

In breastfeeding, as with anything else that is new and unfamiliar, problems may occur. This section offers explanations and solutions to the most common breastfeeding problems.

ENGORGEMENT

This is a temporary problem that most commonly occurs between two to five days after childbirth. It is caused by a combination of the increased blood supply to the breast and the pressure of the newly produced milk, resulting in the swelling of the tissues in the breast. A low-grade fever may be present; the breasts feel full, hard, tender, and tight; and the skin of the breasts is hot, shiny, and distended. You do not need engorgement in order to nurse.

Recommendations

❏ Give your baby short, frequent feedings. A feeding schedule of every one and a half to two hours day and night should be maintained while engorgement lasts.

❏ Express milk between feedings to relieve pressure.

❏ Apply moist heat for thirty minutes preceding each feeding, and massage the breast during feedings to help get the milk flowing.

❏ Do not use nipple shields, as they can confuse the baby's sucking pattern, damage nipples, reduce stimulation of the breast, and decrease the milk supply.

❏ To prevent engorgement, feed your baby on demand and without delay, and allow unrestricted suckling time. Do not skip or delay feedings during the day or night. Do not give your baby any formula or sugar water, and allow the baby to empty each breast completely at each feeding. The American Academy of Pediatrics (AAP) recommends that newborns nurse eight to twelve times every twenty-four hours until the baby is satisfied, usually ten to fifteen minutes on each side.

MASTITIS (BREAST INFECTION)

If a plugged duct is not taken care of, mastitis can result. *Acute mastitis* is an infection and swelling of the breast, usually occurring as a result of bacteria (most often *Staphylococcus aureus*) entering the nursing mother's breast through cracks or fissures in the nipple. Mothers are most vulnerable to acute mastitis in the first few weeks of nursing because cracks in the nipple develop more often during this time. Soreness and redness in the breast, fever, yellow, pus-like secretions from the nipple, general tiredness, and flulike symptoms are indicators of this problem. In fact, in a nursing mother, all flulike symptoms should be considered a breast infection until proven otherwise. A mother who has a high fever, in addition to the aforementioned symptoms, should see a doctor.

Recommendations

❏ Drink plenty of fluids.

❏ Get plenty of rest.

❏ Air-dry the nipples after nursing to prevent cracking. If the nipples do crack, you can coat them with breast milk, or apply aloe vera juice after they dry to help them heal. You can also apply heat with a hot water bottle or heating pad before and after nursing, or use a heat lamp with a regular 100-watt bulb for a few minutes after nursing in order to heal cracks and prevent infections. Place the light bulb twelve to eighteen inches from the breast—not so close as to cause discomfort.

❏ Your doctor may advise you to stop breastfeeding until the infected breast heals. If so, use a breast pump to prevent the breast from becoming engorged.

❏ Remember to always wash your hands before and after breastfeeding to remove germs, and always wash the breast and nipple area afterwards.

Considerations

❏ Most of the minor infections will heal by themselves in a few days. More severe ones can heal in about a week if treated with antibiotics.

❏ Your health care provider may prescribe antibiotics that can be taken by a nursing mother.

❏ In rare cases, a breast infection results in a breast abscess, in which the sore breast fills with pus. An abscess may have to be incised to allow drainage. This procedure is performed in a physician's office. If an abscess develops, milk should be hand-expressed (massaged) from the infected breast and discarded. Breastfeeding should continue on the uninfected breast until the abscess is healed.

PLUGGED DUCT

Incomplete emptying of the milk ducts by the baby, or wearing a tight bra, can cause a plugged duct. Soreness and a lump in one area of a breast is an indication of this problem.

Recommendations

❏ Check the nipple very carefully for any tiny dots of dried milk, and remove them by gentle cleansing. Together with frequent nursing on the affected breast, this should allow the duct to clear itself within twenty-four hours.

❏ Massage the breasts with firm pressure, from the chest wall toward the nipple, to stimulate milk flow.

❏ Alter the position of the baby on the nipple so all the ducts are drained.

❏ Make sure you offer the affected breast first, when the baby's sucking is strongest.

SORE NIPPLES

Sore nipples are usually caused by improper nursing positions and nursing schedules, or incorrect sucking by the baby. They can also be caused by infection, most commonly with the fungus *Candida albicans*.

Recommendations

❏ Nurse on the least sore side first. However, if both breasts are sore, hand-express (massage the breast) until let-down occurs and milk is readily available to the baby.

❏ Make sure that the baby's jaws exert pressure on the least tender spots. Do not pull away when the baby is about to begin feeding. Learn to relax.

❏ Massage your breasts from base to tip to prevent engorgement. Do this during the final weeks of your pregnancy and continue through postpartum.

❏ If cracked nipples accompany soreness, apply aloe vera gel to the nipples to alleviate pain and promote healing. Also, aloe vera (fresh), calendula, marshmallow, and slippery elm are soothing when used in paste form as a poultice, or as wet tea bags, and applied to sore nipples.

❏ Apply avocado oil, calendula ointment, lanolin, and olive oil (separately or in combination) to the breasts to help prevent soreness during pregnancy and while breastfeeding.

❏ To prevent sore nipples, feed your baby frequently to avoid having a baby who is overly hungry bite down roughly on the nipple. Be sure your baby's mouth takes in as much of the areola (the dark area of the nipple) as possible. The baby shouldn't make slurping noises when feeding. Change nursing positions often to rotate the pressure of the baby's mouth on the breast, and learn to break suction correctly. Between feedings, keep the nipples dry. Expose them to sunlight and air. Do not wash them with soap, alcohol, or petroleum-based products, which can wash away their natural protection. Instead, you can apply a little colostrum on the nipple and let it air dry

❏ If the pain is severe and persists despite these measures, it may be a sign of a candida infection (*see* FUNGAL INFECTION in Part Two). Consult your health care provider.

NUTRITIONAL HEALTH WHILE NURSING

The following supplements are beneficial for nursing mothers. After a discussion with your health care provider, you may decide to supplement your diet with these vitamins and minerals.

NUTRIENTS

SUPPLEMENT	SUGGESTED DOSAGE	COMMENTS
Essential		
Free-form amino acid complex (Amino Balance from Anabol Naturals)	As directed on label.	To supply needed protein. Soy protein and free-form amino acids are better sources than animal protein.
Helpful		
Bifido Factor from Natren and	1/2 tsp daily, between meals.	For mother. Boosts immune system and provides necessary "friendly" bacteria. Use only unchilled water in preparation.
LifeStart from Natren	1/4 tsp daily, added to water or juice.	For baby. Use only unchilled water in preparation.
Calcium and magnesium	1,000–1,500 mg daily. 500–750 mg daily.	Needed by both mother and baby. Use chelate forms. Do not use bone meal or dolomite, as these may contain lead.
Multivitamin and mineral complex with vitamin B complex plus extra folic acid and vitamin C and vitamin D and iron and manganese	As directed on label. 400 mcg daily. 3,000 mg daily. 400 IU daily. As directed by physician. 2 mg daily. *Note:* Do not take calcium and manganese together, as they compete for absorption.	All nutrients are needed by both mother and baby. Use a high-potency formula. Needed for production of milk and to relieve stress.

Herbs

❏ Any of the following herbs can be beneficial for the nursing mother: alfalfa, blessed thistle, dandelion, fennel, horsetail, and raspberry.

❏ Nettle leaf has a tonic effect and contains iron, in addition to many other nutrients.

❏ The following herbs *decrease* milk supply, and should be avoided until a woman is no longer nursing: black walnut, sage, and yarrow.

Recommendations

❏ Eat plenty of brewer's yeast, eggs, nuts and seeds, and whole grains. Raw foods should be plentiful in the diet.

❏ A mother's milk is a nearly perfect food. However, it is low in vitamins C and D and iron. A nursing mother should maintain a balanced diet, but can also benefit from taking multivitamins and nutritional supplements. Discuss the need for supplements with your health care provider.

❏ If you need to supplement mother's milk, try almond milk, Rice Dream (made from brown rice), or a soymilk formula with a small amount of papaya (put through a blender). This resembles mother's milk. You can add a small amount of blackstrap molasses and brewer's yeast after the baby is a few months old. Always consult your health care provider before making any changes in your baby's diet.

Considerations

❏ The UCLA Medical School reported that mother's milk kills a tiny parasite (*Giardia lamblia*) that can cause intestinal disease in children.

❏ In recent studies, mothers who consumed garlic increased their babies' desire for milk, and the babies nursed longer. Garlic is good for both the mother and the infant. *Kyolic* from Wakunaga is an ideal way to consume garlic since it is odorless and therefore more "sociable."

❏ Since breast milk is produced from protein drawn from either your diet or the protein stored in your body, you should consider increasing your protein intake, especially during postpartum weight loss. Studies show you will lose body fat, but not muscle.

❏ In 1998, the AAP published broad new guidelines urging women to breastfeed their infants, stating that *breast milk is the foundation of good infant nutrition.* They recommend that newborns receive nothing other than breastmilk for the first six months, meaning no juices, fluorides, iron, or vitamins.

❏ Dr. Ruth Lawrence, author of *Breastfeeding: A Guide for the Medical Profession,* says that, depending on the mother's wishes, breastfeeding should continue for at least a year, along with other foods as they are introduced, and even longer if the mother feels it is best for her and her child.

❏ Almost all drugs have been found to enter a nursing mother's milk, including acetaminophen (Tylenol and others), alcohol, amphetamines, antibiotics, antihistamines, aspirin, barbiturates, caffeine, cimetidine (Tagamet), cocaine, decongestants, diazepam (Valium), ergotamine, chlordiazepoxide (Librium), marijuana, nicotine, and opiates (codeine, meperidine [Demerol], morphine). Some of the effects these drugs can have on an infant include diarrhea, rapid heart rate, restlessness, irritability, crying, poor sleeping, vomiting, and convulsions. In addition, some of these drugs may accumulate in an infant's body and cause addiction.

❏ In a study of new mothers, those who were trained and sent home from the hospital with a breast pump were found to breastfeed their infants longer than those who were given no pumps.

❏ Breastfed babies run a very low risk of ever developing meningitis or severe blood infections. They also have a 500- to 600-percent lower risk of developing childhood lymphoma and suffer from 50 percent fewer middle ear infections than bottlefed babies.

❏ Breast milk contains high amounts of inositol, a B vitamin that plays a crucial role in survival and infant development.

❏ Women who undergo reduction mammoplasty (breast

reduction surgery) and subsequently become pregnant can retain the ability to lactate and nurse. However, in one study, only 35 percent of such women breastfed successfully, whereas 65 percent either did not breastfeed or discontinued nursing for various reasons. It was not disclosed whether any of these women were actually unable to secrete sufficient amounts of milk to nurse their babies. Women who are considering breast reduction surgery should nevertheless consider this if they wish to have children later on and hope to breastfeed.

❑ Included among AAP recommendations to hospitals, pediatricians, and mothers are the following: 1) Even if the baby and mother are hospitalized, breastfeeding should continue unless the mother is required to take a medication that could be harmful to the breastfeeding infant. If so, breastfeeding should only be stopped temporarily, until the mother's body no longer contains traces of the medication(s). 2) Private areas for breastfeeding mothers should be provided by all hospitals. 3) Breast pumps should be provided to breastfeeding mothers in hospitals. 4) Insurance companies will be encouraged to provide breastfeeding services and supplies as part of coverage policies.

❑ There are resources available to help women learn to breastfeed successfully and overcome any problems that arise. Certified lactation consultants are practitioners who specialize in this area. Your health care provider or the facility where you give birth should be able to give you a referral. La Leche League is another valuable resource for the breastfeeding mother. This is an organization of nursing women that can serve as both an educational resource and a support group. Consult your local telephone directory for the chapter nearest you, or contact La Leche League International (see HEALTH AND MEDICAL ORGANIZATIONS in the Appendix).

Bronchitis

The lungs are among the body's largest organs. The air we breathe enters our bodies through the trachea (windpipe), which connects with the bronchi, the breathing tubes that lead into the alveoli (air sacs) in the lungs. In the lungs, air is exchanged for carbon dioxide.

Bronchitis is an inflammation or obstruction in the bronchial tubes. This inflammation results in a buildup of mucus, along with coughing, fever, pain in the chest and/or back, fatigue, sore throat, difficulty breathing, and, often, sudden chills and shaking. Bronchospasm, a contraction of the smooth muscle in the walls of the bronchi, may also occur. Swelling of the mucous membranes and hypersecretion by the bronchial glands frequently accompany bronchospasm.

Bronchitis can be either acute or chronic. Acute bronchitis is usually caused by an infection, which can be bacterial, viral, chlamydial, mycoplasmal, or caused by a combination of agents. It typically follows an upper respiratory tract infection, such as a cold or influenza. In acute bronchitis, bronchospasm is more often associated with viral (rather than bacterial) infection. Most cases of acute bronchitis are self-limiting, with full recovery in a matter of weeks. In some cases, however, the condition can lead to pneumonia. This is more likely to occur in those who also have a chronic respiratory disease or other debilitating health problem.

Chronic bronchitis results from frequent irritation of the lungs, such as from exposure to cigarette smoke, air pollutants, or other noxious fumes, rather than from infection. Allergies may also be the cause of chronic bronchitis. As chronic bronchitis diminishes the exchange of oxygen and carbon dioxide in the lungs, the heart works harder in an attempt to compensate. Over time, this can lead to pulmonary hypertension, enlargement of the heart, and, ultimately, heart failure.

Chronic bronchitis is one of the most common diseases seen by allergists, otolaryngologists, and primary care physicians. Specialists in occupational medicine have long known that an adverse environment produces a vulnerability to respiratory infections. Climatic factors and epidemics of viral infections also increase the risk. Among people who live or work in unhealthy environments, shortness of breath is frequently aggravated by dampness and cold, exposure to dust, or even minor respiratory infections.

Unless otherwise specified, the following recommended doses are for those over the age of eighteen. For a child between twelve and seventeen years old, reduce the dose to three-quarters the recommended amount. For a child between six and twelve years old, use one-half the recommended dose, and for a child under six, use one-quarter the recommended amount.

NUTRIENTS

SUPPLEMENT	SUGGESTED DOSAGE	COMMENTS
Essential		
Colloidal silver	As directed on label. For one week on and one week off, alternating until you find relief.	A natural antibiotic that destroys bacteria, viruses, and fungi. Promotes healing.
Pycnogenol	As directed on label.	Removes dangerous substances and protects the lungs. A powerful antioxidant.
Quercitin-C from Ecological Formulas or	500 mg 3 times daily.	For allergic bronchitis. Has an antihistaminic effect.
Activated Quercetin from Source Naturals	As directed on label.	Contains quercetin plus bromelain and vitamin C for increased absorption.
Vitamin A	20,000 IU twice daily for 1 month; then reduce to 15,000 IU daily. If you are pregnant, do not exceed 10,000 IU daily.	For healing and protection of all tissues.
plus natural beta-carotene or	50,000 IU daily.	Needed for protection and repair of lung tissue.
carotenoid complex (Betatene)	As directed on label.	

Vitamin C with bioflavonoids (including rutin)	3,000–10,000 mg daily, in divided doses.	Enhances immune function and reduces histamine levels. Use a buffered powder form.

Very Important		
Coenzyme Q10 plus	60 mg daily.	For improved circulation and breathing.
Coenzme A from Coenzyme-A Technologies	As directed on the label.	Works well with coenzyme Q10 and removes dangerous substances from the body.
Methylsulfonyl-methane (MSM)	As directed on label.	Clinical tests have shown that this improves lung problems such as bronchitis, pneumonia, emphysema, cysts, or damage due to heavy smoking.
Proteolytic enzymes with bromelain	As directed on label. Take between meals.	Helps reduce inflammation.
Vitamin E	400 IU and up twice daily. Take with 50–100 mg vitamin C.	Powerful free-radical scavenger and oxygen carrier. Needed for healing of tissues and improved breathing. Use d-alpha-tocopherol form.
Zinc lozenges	1 15-mg lozenge 5 times daily. Do not exceed a total of 100 mg daily from all supplements.	Needed for repair of all tissues.

Important		
Chlorophyll or "green drinks" (fresh wheatgrass juice or Kyo-Green from Wakunaga)	As directed on label, 3 times daily. As directed on label.	To improve circulation, and to keep tissues free of toxic substances. Use liquid or tablet form. To supply chlorophyll and important nutrients.
Garlic (Kyolic from Wakunaga)	2 tablets 3 times daily, with meals.	A natural antibiotic that reduces infection and detoxifies the body.
Vitamin B complex	100 mg of each major B vitamin 3 times daily (amounts of individual vitamins in a complex will vary).	Activates many enzymes needed for healing.

Helpful		
Magnesium plus calcium	500 mg daily. 1,000 mg daily.	Acts as a bronchodilator. Use chelate or asporotate form. Needed to balance with magnesium.
Maitake extract or shiitake extract or reishi extract	As directed on label. As directed on label. As directed on label.	Mushroom extracts that boost immunity and fight viral infection.
Multivitamin complex	As directed on label.	All nutrients are needed in balance for healing.
N-Acetylcysteine (NAC) plus L-arginine and L-lysine and	500 mg twice daily, on an empty stomach. Take with water or juice. Do not take with milk. Take with 50 mg vitamin B6 and 100 mg vitamin C for better absorption. 500 mg twice daily, on an empty stomach. 500 mg twice daily, on an empty stomach.	Protects and preserves the cells. A sulfur-bearing amino acid that lessens the viscosity of bronchial mucus, making it easier to expel. *See* AMINO ACIDS in Part One. Aids in liver detoxification. Needed for protein synthesis to aid in healing. Also aids in destroying serious viruses.

L-ornithine	500 mg twice daily, on an empty stomach.	Lowers blood ammonia levels, which can be increased by respiratory illness.
Raw thymus glandular	500 mg twice daily.	Needed to protect and enhance immune function. (*See* GLANDULAR THERAPY in Part Three.)
Silica or horsetail	As directed on label.	Acts as an anti-inflammatory, reduces mucus flow, and reduces coughing. *See under* Herbs, below.

HERBS

Herbal medicine has proven to be very effective in the treatment of bronchitis. The following treatment plans may be helpful in alleviating some of the symptoms common to bronchitis. Rather than using only one of the herbs listed below, alternate among several to get all of their healing benefits.

❑ American and Siberian ginseng are especially good for the lungs. They clear bronchial passages and reduce inflammation.

Caution: Do not use American ginseng if you have high blood pressure. Do not use Siberian ginseng if you have hypoglycemia, high blood pressure, or a heart disorder.

❑ Astragalus, myrrh, olive oil extract, and pau d'arco are natural antibiotics.

Caution: Do not use astragalus in the presence of a fever.

❑ Black radish, chickweed, elderberry, ginkgo biloba, lobelia, and mullein improve lung and bronchial congestion and circulation.

❑ Boneset contains immunostimulatory polysaccharides that are good for inflammation of the mucous membranes.

Caution: Do not use boneset on a daily basis for more than one week, as long-term use can lead to toxicity.

❑ Boswellia, bromelain, cayenne, ginger, and peppermint can aid in reducing inflammation.

❑ Bronc-Ease from Nature's Herbs is an excellent herbal formula. It relieves congestion, coughing, and irritation.

❑ Expectorant herbs such as cayenne, elecampane, horehound, hyssop, and mullein have been effective in clearing congestion.

❑ ClearLungs from RidgeCrest Herbals is a Chinese herbal formula that helps provide relief from shortness of breath, tightness in the chest, and wheezing due to bronchial congestion. It is available in two formulas: one with ephedra and the other without. Both have been found to be equally effective. Take 2 capsules three times daily.

❑ Coltsfoot, slippery elm bark, and wild cherry bark soothe the throat and are good for a cough.

❑ Cordyceps is an herb used in Chinese medicine to restore the yin and yang connection between the lungs and the kidneys. It is said to contain inhibitor substances that attack damaged lung cells and may slow down the degeneration of the lung. Bai qian (*Cynanchum stautoni*), another Chinese herb, aids in coughing up the sputum obstructing the bronchial passageways.

❏ Echinacea, licorice, and Siberian ginseng are good for building up the immune system.

Caution: If overused, licorice can elevate blood pressure. Do not use this herb on a daily basis for more than seven days in a row. Avoid it completely if you have high blood pressure. Do not use Siberian ginseng if you have hypoglycemia, high blood pressure, or a heart disorder.

❏ Echinacea and goldenseal help to fight viruses and bacteria and boost the immune system. At the first sign of illness, put ½ dropperful in your mouth. Hold it there for ten minutes, then swallow. Do this every three hours until symptoms are relieved (but not for longer than one week at a time). Be sure to use the alcohol-free extracts.

❏ Ephedra (ma huang) is good for relieving nasal and chest congestion, as well as bronchial spasms. This botanical acts like epinephrine.

Caution: Do not use this herb if you suffer from anxiety, glaucoma, heart disease, high blood pressure, or insomnia, or if you are taking a monoamine oxidase (MAO) inhibitor drug for depression.

❏ Inhaling the vapors of eucalyptus leaves helps to relieve respiratory problems. To use eucalyptus as a steam inhaler, boil a quart of water, remove the boiling water from the stove and add 6 to 8 drops of eucalyptus extract. Place a towel over your head and breathe in deeply through the nose, holding your breath in for as long as is comfortable.

❏ Fenugreek is good for reducing the flow of mucus.

❏ Ginkgo biloba leaf is a free-radical fighter that is especially good for the lungs.

❏ Goldenseal has antibiotic properties and is good for all conditions involving inflammation of the mucous membranes of the bronchial tubes, throat, nasal passages, and sinuses. In addition to taking goldenseal orally, you can place a cloth soaked with a strong goldenseal tea under a hot water bottle. Place 3 wet goldenseal tea bags on each lung under the soaked cloth.

Caution: Do not take goldenseal internally on a daily basis for more than one week at a time, and do not use it during pregnancy or if you are breastfeeding. If you have a history of cardiovascular disease, diabetes, or glaucoma, use it only under a doctor's supervision.

❏ Gumplant (*Grindelia squarrosa*) is an expectorant and antispasmodic.

❏ Horsetail, taken in extract form, is a good source of silica, which has anti-inflammatory and expectorant properties, and also reduces coughing.

❏ Iceland moss is good for mucous congestion.

❏ A massage with essential oil of lavender is good for bronchitis. Also, to relieve congestion, put 4 drops of lavender oil, alone or combined with eucalyptus and lemon oils, in a pot of steaming water. Hold your head, covered with a towel, over the steaming pot and inhale the vapors.

Caution: Lavender oil is not to be taken internally.

❏ Lobelia may be rubbed directly on the chest to aid in breathing. It can also be used as an expectorant; however, use it with caution, as too much may induce vomiting, and do not take it on an ongoing basis.

❏ Lomatium (*Lomatium dissectum*) has been used by Native Americans to treat bronchitis. Lomatium acts in reducing mucus in the lungs and has an antibacterial effect.

❏ Lung Tonic from Herbs, Etc. is a combination of many organic herbs designed to support the lungs.

❏ Lungwort leaves are rich in vitamin C and quercetin and make an effective treatment for coughs and mucus.

❏ Thyme strengthens the lung tissue. It can be used for children with lung ailments.

RECOMMENDATIONS

❏ Include garlic and onions in your diet. These foods contain quercetin and mustard oils, which have been shown to inhibit lipoxygenase, an enzyme that aids in releasing an inflammatory chemical in the body. Garlic is also a natural antibiotic.

❏ Drink plenty of fluids. Pure water, herbal teas, and soups are all good choices.

❏ Avoid mucus-forming foods such as dairy products, processed foods, sugar, sweet fruits, and white flour; also avoid gas-producing foods such as beans, cabbage, cauliflower, and so on. A vegetarian diet is best.

❏ Do not smoke, and avoid secondhand smoke. Cigarette smoke is very harmful. If you have chronic bronchitis, little improvement can be expected unless the irritating substances that cause the mucus to clog the air passages are eliminated.

❏ Add moisture to the air. Use a humidifier, a vaporizer, or even a pan of water placed on a radiator. Clean the equipment frequently to prevent the growth of bacteria.

❏ Rest in bed in the early stages, when fever is present. Once fever subsides and you are feeling better, alternate periods of rest with periods of moderate activity to prevent secretions from settling in the lungs.

❏ Apply warm, moist heat, or a hot water bottle over the chest and back before bedtime to aid in sleeping and reduce inflammation. It is also good to rub eucalyptus oil on your chest first.

❏ To aid recovery, blow up a balloon a few times daily. One research study showed that after eight weeks of this therapy, people with bronchitis were much less breathless.

❏ Supplement your diet with vitamin C. Vitamin C is essential for all infectious disorders because the white blood cells use up large amounts of this vitamin fighting infection.

❑ Do not use a cough suppressant if you have bronchitis. Coughing is essential for eliminating mucous secretions.

❑ Do not swallow mucus. Dispose of it in a tissue.

❑ If persistent and/or severe coughing, difficulty breathing, high fever, lethargy, weakness, wheezing sounds, and/ or chest pains develop, consult your health care provider. These may be signs of developing pneumonia. (See PNEUMONIA in Part Two.)

CONSIDERATIONS

❑ Diet, nutrition, and environment all play important roles in any respiratory disease. A healthy household environment can make respiratory problems easier to control.

❑ Scientists have found many nutrients that make the lungs and bronchioles stronger and, therefore, better able to fight off infections. Many of these nutrients also make the lungs less sensitive to the air particles that can sometimes trigger bronchitis.

❑ For people who are unable to cough up sputum, bronchoscopy may be recommended. This is a procedure in which a flexible tube is inserted to examine the bronchial tree. It can be done simply for the sake of a visual examination, to suction out congestion, to remove foreign bodies, or even to biopsy (sample) tissue from the bronchial tubes for the purpose of identifying the infecting organism.

❑ If bronchitis does not clear up in a reasonable amount of time, a chest x-ray may be recommended to rule out lung cancer, emphysema, tuberculosis, or other conditions that can cause similar symptoms.

❑ It is not unusual for people with chronic respiratory disorders to be taking a variety of medications—inhalers, antianxiety medications, even diuretics—to help them breathe. Exercise is important; it helps one to breathe more efficiently and to tolerate daily activities.

❑ If bacteria are the cause of acute bronchitis, treatment with antibiotics may be necessary to cure the infection and to prevent pneumonia from developing.

❑ In recent years a newer type of bronchitis, probably viral in origin, has afflicted many women. It is very difficult to treat and often lasts three weeks to five months. Antibiotics, especially doxycycline hyclate (Doryx, Vibramycin), and the newer drug, azithromycin (Zithromax), are good for chronic bronchitis.

❑ A common treatment for bronchitis is a bronchodilator. If you use a bronchodilator, do not inhale more than the prescribed dose, as larger doses may cause side effects, including nervousness, restlessness, and trembling. Before using an inhaler, discuss with your doctor possible side effects and warning signs of dangerous reactions. Your doctor should be aware of any personal health concerns you have, such as a possible pregnancy; a medical problem, such as diabetes, hypothyroidism, or a seizure disorder; a history of drug use; adverse reactions to drugs; or current use of other over-the-counter or prescription drugs.

❑ The Air Supply personal air purifier from Wein Products is a small unit worn around the neck. It sets up an invisible pure air shield against microorganisms (such as viruses, bacteria, and mold) and microparticles (including dust, pollen, and pollutants) in the air. It also eliminates vapors, smells, and harmful volatile compounds in the air. The Air Supply is a very useful item when traveling, especially on a long flight when the air becomes stale. The Living Air XL-15 unit from Alpine Air of America is an ionizing unit that is good for purifying the air in the home or workplace.

❑ See also ASTHMA; EMPHYSEMA; HAY FEVER; PNEUMONIA; and SINUSITIS in Part Two.

Bruising

A bruise occurs when the tissues underlying the skin become injured. The skin is not broken, but the delicate capillaries (small blood vessels) below the skin's surface rupture, and blood drains out into the surrounding area. The blood seeps into the layers of the skin, resulting in pain, swelling, and "black-and-blue marks"—discoloration that starts out red, then turns dark and bluish, and finally may become a yellowish color as the blood under the skin is absorbed.

Body parts often become bruised after banging into hard objects; this is normal. However, there are other factors that do not involve a trauma to the skin that can cause bruising. People who do not eat enough fresh, uncooked foods to supply the body with needed nutrients are prone to easy bruising. Nutritional deficiencies, especially in vitamin C, or blood-clotting disorders can make the blood-vessel walls very thin and delicate, causing them to rupture with even the slightest amount of pressure, such as leaning against a table or having someone grab you firmly with his or her hand. Unexplained or easy bruising can be related to heavy smoking or menstruation, or it can be an indication of an underlying health condition, including AIDS (AIDS-related bruises do not go away), allergies, anemia, cancer, hemophilia, infections, obesity, myelocytic leukemia, and abnormal platelet function caused by a liver or kidney disorder.

Unless otherwise specified, the following recommended doses are for those over the age of eighteen. For a child between twelve and seventeen years old, reduce the dose to three-quarters the recommended amount. For a child between six and twelve years old, use one-half the recommended dose, and for a child under six, use one-quarter the recommended amount.

NUTRIENTS

SUPPLEMENT	SUGGESTED DOSAGE	COMMENTS
Very Important		
Multivitamin and mineral complex with zinc	As directed on label.	Needed to strengthen skin and reduce bruising.
Vitamin C with bioflavonoids	3,000–10,000 mg daily, in divided doses.	Helps to prevent bruising by supplying oxygen to the injured cells and strengthening capillary walls.
Vitamin K or alfalfa	As directed on label.	Necessary for blood clotting and healing. *See under* Herbs, below.
Important		
Inositol hexaphosphate (IP₆) (Cell Forté with IP-6 from Enzymatic Therapy or IP6 from Jarrow Formulas)	As directed on label.	A powerful antioxidant. Prevents blood clots.
Vitamin E	Start with 400 IU daily and increase slowly to 800 IU daily. Do not exceed 400 IU daily if you take anticoagulant medication.	Powerful antioxidant. Also improves circulation in body tissues and prolongs the life of red blood cells. Fights cellular aging by protecting cell membranes. Use d-alpha-tocopherol form.
Helpful		
Coenzyme Q₁₀	60 mg daily.	Essential for construction and reconstruction of body cells.
Dimethylglycine (DMG) (Aangamik DMG from FoodScience of Vermont)	100 mg daily.	Improves oxygen metabolism in the cells and tissues.
Iron (ferrous fumarate from Freeda Vitamins) or	As directed by physician. Take with 100 mg vitamin C for better absorption.	To correct deficiencies. *Caution:* Do not take iron unless anemia is diagnosed.
Floradix Iron + Herbs from Salus Haus	As directed on label.	A natural iron supplement.
Multienzyme complex plus	As directed on label. Take with meals.	To prevent inflammation in bruised areas.
proteolytic enzymes	As directed on label. Take between meals.	
Pycnogenol or	As directed on label.	Potent antioxidants for protecting skin tissue.
grape seed extract	As directed on label.	
Vitamin B complex	100 mg of each major B vitamin twice daily (amounts of individual vitamins in a complex will vary).	Aids in protecting the tissues.
Vitamin D plus	400–800 IU daily.	To help protect the skin. Needed for blood cell formation.
calcium and	2,000 mg daily.	
magnesium	1,000 mg daily.	

HERBS

❑ Alfalfa supplies beneficial minerals and vitamin K, which is needed for healing. Take it in tablet form as directed on the product label.

❑ Bluebottle, buchu, and comfrey root have all been known to reduce the swelling, pain, and discoloration of bruising in some people. Make a tea from them and place a terry cloth towel that has been soaked in the tea over the bruised area for twenty minutes at a time, two or three times daily.

❑ An ointment made by adding one part ground cayenne pepper to five parts melted Vaseline has been used successfully in China and Taiwan for treating bruises. Mix the combination well and cool. Apply it once every one or two days.

❑ Dandelion and yellow dock are good sources of iron.

❑ Oil of oregano, applied topically, has had some positive effects on healing bruises.

❑ Fresh parsley leaves, crushed and applied directly to the bruise, are known to ease discoloration within a few days.

❑ Wild pansy can be applied externally to treat a bruise.

❑ Other beneficial herbs include bilberry, black walnut, garlic extract, horsetail, and rose hips.

RECOMMENDATIONS

❑ To minimize bruising, as soon as possible after an injury, place an ice pack on the bruised area and keep it in place for twenty to thirty minutes. This stops the bleeding by constricting the blood vessels. If the bruise is severe, you may wish to further treat the injured area with an ice pack every two to three waking hours for twenty-four to forty-eight hours, and then switch to fifteen minutes of heat, three times daily. The injured area should also be elevated above heart level, if possible, to allow blood to flow away from the injured area and minimize the bruise.

❑ If you have a bruise in an area of the body that requires a moldable ice pack, fill a plastic bag or a rubber surgical glove with a solution of two parts water and one part rubbing alcohol and put it in the freezer. The bag will be pliable and conform to your body, and it won't "sweat" like most ice packs do. This would be an ideal ice pack for a black eye. Another excellent ice pack for the eye, or any area, is a bag of frozen peas! They conform to any injured area and can be used over and over again. Be sure to set this bag of peas aside for use as an ice pack only; you should not consume the peas after they have been thawed and refrozen.

❑ To reduce the pain, swelling, and discoloration of a black eye, immediately apply cold compresses and an ice pack to the injury. Unfortunately, if the discoloration has set in before the ice bag has been applied, there will be little hope of lightening the bruise.

❑ Rub a sterile cotton ball soaked with distilled witch hazel on an injury to stop the swelling.

❑ To reduce discoloration and soreness, try applying shredded raw potato directly to the injury for about an hour.

❑ Eat a lot of fresh, uncooked foods—people who do not eat enough of these can be prone to easy bruising.

❑ Eat an abundance of dark green leafy vegetables, buckwheat, and fresh fruits. These foods are high in vitamin C and bioflavonoids, which help to prevent bruising. Dark leafy greens such as broccoli, Brussels sprouts, cabbage, kale, and spinach are also good sources of vitamin K, which is necessary for blood clotting and healing.

❑ Eat plenty of products rich in zinc, such as chicken, eggs, soybeans, and wheat germ. Zinc is important for strengthening blood-vessel walls and aids in blood clotting.

❑ Try taking vitamin C with bioflavonoids if you find you are bruising very easily, as a deficiency in these often causes easy or unexplained bruising.

❑ Do not take aspirin or ibuprofen (Advil, Nuprin, and others) for pain, as these can worsen the discoloration due to their blood-thinning qualities. Instead, take acetaminophen (such as Tylenol) as directed on the label.

❑ Do not take any nonsteroidal anti-inflammatory drugs (NSAIDs). If bruising is frequent, consult your health care provider.

CONSIDERATIONS

❑ Bruising that is accompanied by swollen and/or bleeding gums can be an indication of a deficiency in vitamin C, folic acid, or riboflavin.

❑ Studies show that people with vitamin C deficiencies bruise more easily than others, probably because their blood vessels are generally weaker. Other studies have shown that vitamin C can actually reduce the time it takes for the discoloration to fade.

❑ A "black eye" is actually a bruise in the cheek, eyebrow, and/or eyelid area. An impact hard enough to cause a black eye can also cause damage to the eye itself. If your eye has swollen shut, it should not be forced open or pressed on in any way. Blurry vision or "seeing double" should prompt you to see an ophthalmologist, who may prescribe an antibiotic and/or an eye patch to protect the eye while healing.

❑ It generally takes from several days to about a week for a bruise to go through the healing process. If a bruise does not begin to heal within a week, you may want to have your doctor examine it.

❑ Some people can bruise as a result of taking medications that can interfere with normal blood clotting, including local anesthetics, prescription anticoagulants, antidepressants, antihistamines, aspirin, cortisone, and penicillin. If you are taking any of these medications and find that bruises are appearing without any reason, you should contact your doctor, who may change or discontinue your medication.

❑ If you have bruising underneath the fingernails, this may be an early indication of skin melanoma. Consult your doctor.

Bruxism

Bruxism, or bruxomania, is the medical term for tooth-grinding. This usually occurs during sleep, often without the person being aware of it (although family members may be). It can also occur when a person is awake, as a way of releasing tension. Over time, chronic tooth-grinding can result in loosened teeth, with damage to the supporting bones in the jaw and receding gums. The teeth may be pushed out of line, and the bite may need adjusting. Eventually, tooth loss can occur. Long-term tooth-grinding can cause temporomandibular joint (TMJ) syndrome. This usually occurs in the muscles, joints, and discs of the jaw, and may cause pain while chewing. (See TMJ SYNDROME in Part Two.)

Bruxism can develop if the teeth are sensitive to heat and cold. Stress, allergies, and nutrient deficiencies are often the cause of tooth-grinding, which can also involve blood-sugar levels.

NUTRIENTS

SUPPLEMENT	SUGGESTED DOSAGE	COMMENTS
Essential		
Calcium and magnesium	1,500–2,000 mg daily. 750 mg daily.	Deficiencies have been linked to tooth-grinding.
Pantothenic acid (vitamin B₅)	500 mg twice daily.	Reduces stress.
Vitamin B complex	100 mg of each major B vitamin twice daily (amounts of individual vitamins in a complex will vary).	Necessary for proper nerve function. Use a high-stress formula.
Very Important		
Vitamin C with bioflavonoids	3,000–5,000 mg daily.	Potentiates adrenal function; acts as an anti-stress vitamin.
Helpful		
Chromium	200–400 mcg daily.	Helps to normalize blood sugar levels. Use chromium picolinate form. Hypoglycemia is often linked to this disorder.
L-Tryosine	As directed on label.	An amino acid that reduces stress.
Melatonin	As directed on label.	Aids restful sleep and may reduce tooth-grinding. Not recommended for anyone under 30, or for long-term use.

Multivitamin and mineral complex plus	As directed on label.	All nutrients are needed to reduce stress.
raw adrenal glandular	As directed on label.	To support adrenal function. *See* GLANDULAR THERAPY in Part Three.
S-adenosylmethio-nine (SAMe)	As directed on label.	Reduces stress and acts as an antidepressant. *Caution:* Do not use if you have manic-depressive disorder or take prescription antidepressants.
Zinc	50 mg daily. Do not exceed a total of 100 mg daily from all supplements.	Helps to support the immune system and reduce stress.

RECOMMENDATIONS

❏ Adopt a hypoglycemic diet that is high in fiber and protein and includes plenty of fresh vegetables and high-fiber fruits, plus legumes, raw nuts and seeds, skinless white turkey or chicken, broiled fish, and whole grains. Consume starchy vegetables and very sweet fruits in moderation only. Eat six to eight small meals spread evenly throughout the day rather than two or three large meals. Hypoglycemia, related to low adrenal function, is often the cause of bruxism. (*See* HYPOGLYCEMIA in Part Two.)

❏ Do not consume alcoholic beverages. Alcohol often makes the problem worse.

❏ Avoid fast foods, fried foods, processed foods, red meat, refined sugar, saturated fats, and all dairy products except for yogurt, kefir, and raw cheese. Also avoid all foods with artificial flavors, colors, preservatives, and other chemicals.

❏ Do not eat anything sweet within six hours of going to bed. If you are hungry, have a light protein-and-fiber snack.

❏ As much as possible, avoid stress. Learn stress management and relaxation techniques. *See* STRESS in Part Two.

❏ Take supplemental calcium and pantothenic acid as directed under Nutrients, above. Calcium is often effective for treating involuntary movement of muscles.

❏ Consider having a hair analysis done to determine if you have any mineral imbalances, such as abnormal levels of sodium and potassium. *See* HAIR ANALYSIS in Part Three.

❏ *See* ALLERGIES in Part Two to rule out any food allergies that may be the problem.

CONSIDERATIONS

❏ Dentists sometimes recommend a type of splint that is worn over the teeth for people with bruxism. This does not cure the problem, but it can help to prevent tooth damage.

❏ *Belladonna*, a homeopathic remedy, is known to be an effective treatment for this condition.

❏ Biofeedback is helpful for overcoming bruxism in some cases. (*See* Biofeedback *under* PAIN CONTROL in Part Three.)

Bulimia

Bulimia nervosa is an eating disorder characterized by episodes of uncontrolled binge eating, often involving extremely large amounts of high-calorie foods, followed by one or more of the following: induced vomiting or the use of laxatives, diuretics, or enemas; and/or obsessive exercising to "purge" the body of the food eaten during the binge. The binge/purge episodes vary in frequency, from a few times a week to several times daily. The length of the binging can range from several minutes to an hour or two. Usually the person doing the binging feels out of control—a sense of not being able to stop eating until he or she is completely full—then is so immediately overwhelmed and shamed by the sense of fullness that he or she feels the need to get rid of the food just consumed. The binge eating and purging are usually carried out in secret—an indication of a serious medical and psychological problem with potentially dangerous complications.

Some of the many serious problems bulimia can lead to include anemia, depletion of fluid balance, electrolyte imbalances, erratic heartbeat, hypoglycemia, infertility, internal bleeding, kidney or liver damage, malnutrition, cessation of the menstrual cycles, mental fuzziness, loss of muscle and bone mass, a low pulse rate and blood pressure, a ruptured stomach or esophagus, stones in the salivary glands, tooth and/or gum erosion, ulcers, and a weakened immune system. Also, if the fat content in a woman's body drops to too low a level, the body will not produce enough estrogen, which can result in destruction of bone tissue and an increased risk of osteoporosis. Due to extreme weight loss, extreme exercise, starvation, and/or lack of needed vitamins and minerals, the body can turn to using muscle mass as an energy source—a very serious side effect that few with eating disorders are aware of. Eventually, life-threatening problems can result, including cancers of the breast, bowel, esophagus, or reproductive organs; kidney or liver damage; and finally, cardiac arrest.

According to the National Association of Anorexia Nervosa and Associated Disorders, there are 8,000,000 men and women with eating disorders in the United States, and this number is on the rise. Bulimia affects many more women than men (although the number of men with this disorder is increasing), and it does not discriminate on the basis of age, sex, or social status. In today's society, we are constantly bombarded with the message that the thinner you are, the better you look. Our role models are mostly actors/actresses, music artists, and models who set standards of beauty that are difficult or impossible for some to attain. Although people may develop an eating disorder because they want to look and feel better about themselves, the opposite is usually the result. People with bulimia can become consumed with their weight, have a distorted image of their figures, and feel disgusted with themselves for not having what they think of as the "perfect body." Other typical psychological implications can include extreme anger at anyone they believe is trying to interfere, anxiety, depression, fear of being found out, isolation, loneliness, and obsessive-compulsive behavior. People with bulimia may also exhibit other extreme behavior, such as alcohol or drug abuse, credit card abuse, or shoplifting. They usually spend an exorbitant amount of money on food, sometimes using money meant for paying bills or other necessities to buy certain foods, and they may also bypass social or work-related obligations for an opportunity to binge.

Although there is no known cause of eating disorders, many believe that bulimia may result from one or a combination of psychological, biological, and societal factors. Some studies of families and twins suggest that heredity may also play a role. Psychologically, food has offered us pleasure, comfort, solace, and security from the moment we are born. Episodes of binging are commonly stress related, and they may be an attempt to manage emotions by focusing attention away from unpleasant or uncomfortable emotional problems. Many individuals who suffer from this disorder come from families in which they were subjected to physical or sexual abuse. In some families, substance abuse is also a factor. Many women started their first binge because of real or imagined male rejection. Others are perfectionists and overachievers with high standards, but low self-esteem. In particular, if a woman's basic, emotional needs were not met in childhood, she may come to believe that her problems would be resolved if only she were attractive (that is, thin) enough, and this obsession leads to bulimia.

There are indications of possible physiological elements in this disorder, as well. For example, people with eating disorders tend to have a type of chemical imbalance similar to one found in people with clinical depression. Both have high levels of adrenocorticotropic hormone (ACTH), a hormone produced by the pituitary gland that inhibits T-cell function and thereby depresses immunity. People who suffer from bulimia may also have low levels of the neurotransmitter serotonin, which can lead to cravings for simple carbohydrates—common binge foods. Some researchers have found bulimia to be associated with right temporal disturbance in the brain.

Unlike people with anorexia, whose self-starvation eventually becomes obvious, those with bulimia can hide the disorder for long periods, even years, because their weight is usually in the normal range (some are even overweight, depending on the frequency and length of the binging episodes) and the binging and purging are done in secret. Physical signs of bulimia may be swollen glands in the face (resulting in a "chipmunk" appearance) and neck; erosion of the enamel of back teeth; broken blood vessels in the eyes or face; constant sore throat; inflammation of the esophagus; and hiatal hernia. All of these are the consequences of induced vomiting. Sometimes emboweled spoons or sticks used to induce vomiting have to be surgically removed. If laxative abuse is part of the picture, damage to the bowel,

rectal bleeding, and perpetual diarrhea may result. Laxative use also washes potassium and sodium from the body, which can result in electrolyte imbalances that may lead to dehydration, muscle spasms, and, eventually, cardiac arrest. Other signs of bulimia can include bad dreams, bad breath, constantly cold feet and hands, dizziness, excess facial and body hair, fainting, hair loss, mental fuzziness, muscle fatigue, dry skin, yellowish or grayish skin, extreme weakness, and premature wrinkles.

People with bulimia often feel extremely guilty about their behavior, which is why they may successfully hide the disorder for years, even from their spouses and children. Trips to the bathroom after meals, the sudden disappearance of large quantities of food, frequent dental visits, scrapes and abrasions on the hands and knuckles, and mood changes may be hints that something is wrong.

Unless otherwise specified, the following recommended doses are for those over the age of eighteen. For a child between twelve and seventeen years old, reduce the dose to three-quarters the recommended amount.

NUTRIENTS

SUPPLEMENT	SUGGESTED DOSAGE	COMMENTS
Very Important		
Multivitamin and mineral complex with carotenoids and	As recommended by physician. Take with meals.	The bulimic syndrome results in severe vitamin and mineral deficiencies. Extremely high doses are needed because nutrients pass rapidly through the gastrointestinal system and are poorly assimilated. Do not use a sustained-release formula.
potassium and	99 mg daily.	
selenium	200 mcg daily. If you are pregnant, do not exceed 40 mcg daily.	
Zinc	50–100 mg daily. Do not exceed a total of 100 mg daily from all supplements.	Necessary in protein metabolism; aids the sense of taste and increases the appetite. May aid in easing depression and anxiety, and facilitating weight gain. Deficiencies are common in people with this disorder.
plus copper	3 mg daily.	Needed to balance with zinc.
Important		
Acidophilus (Probiata from Wakunaga)	As directed on label. Take on an empty stomach so it can pass quickly to the small intestine.	Stabilizes intestinal bacteria. Protects the liver.
Calcium and magnesium	1,500 mg daily, at bedtime. 750 mg daily.	Has a calming effect and replaces lost calcium stores. Relaxes smooth muscles and has a bronchodilating effect.
Coenzyme A from Coenzyme-A Technologies and coenzyme Q10	As directed on label. 60–100 mg daily.	Can streamline metabolism, ease depression and fatigue, and increase energy. Supports adrenal glands, processes fats, and removes toxins from the body. Can also boost the immune system and improve overall physical and mental processes. Protects the heart muscle and aids in circulation.

Efalex Focus from Efamol **or** Attention Focus from Nature's Way **or** Kyolic-EPA from Wakunaga	As directed on label.	Provides essential fatty acids and helps to maintain eye and brain function.
	As directed on label.	Restores proper fatty acid balance. Needed by all bodily cells.
5-Hydroxy L-tryptophan (5-HTP from Solaray)	As directed on label.	Improves low levels of serotonin commonly associated with bulimia.
Free-form amino acid complex (Amino Balance from Anabol Naturals)	As directed on label.	To counteract protein deficiency, a serious problem in bulimia. Free-form amino acids are morereadily available for use by the body than other protein forms.
Gamma-amino-butyric acid (GABA) compound **plus**	As directed on label.	Relieves stress and aids in nerve building.
Ester-C with bioflavonoids	3,000 mg daily.	Promotes healthy tissues and collagen growth.
Gamma-oryzonol (GO)	60 mg daily.	Aids in calorie use and muscle growth.
S-adenosylmethio-nine (SAMe)	As directed on label.	Aids in stress-relief, depression, eases pain, and produces antioxidant effects. Do not use if you have manic-depressive disorder or take prescription antidepressants.
Vitamin B complex	100 mg of each major B vitamin 3 times daily (amounts of individual vitamins in a complex will vary).	Essential for all cellular functions.
Vitamin B$_{12}$ injections **or** vitamin B$_{12}$	1 cc 3 times weekly or as prescribed by physician. As directed on label.	Needed for the digestion of foods and the assimilation of all nutrients, including iron. Injections (under a doctor's supervision) are best. If injections are not available, use a lozenge or sublingual form.
Vitamin C with bioflavonoids	5,000 mg daily, in divided doses.	Necessary for all cellular and glandular functions.
Helpful		
Bio-Strath from Nature's Answer **or** brewer's yeast	As directed on label 3 times daily. Start with 1 tsp daily and work up to the amount recommended on label.	For increased strength and energy. Aids in tissue repair and increases the appetite. Contains the B vitamins and other necessary nutrients. A good source of B vitamins. *Caution:* Discontinue use if any allergic reactions occur.
Iron (ferrous fumarate from Freeda Vitamins) **or** Floradix Iron + Herbs from Salus Haus	As directed by physician. Take with 100 mg vitamin C for better absorption. As directed on label, 3 times daily.	To correct deficiencies and increase appetite. *Caution:* Do not take iron unless anemia is diagnosed. A natural source of iron that is easily assimilated.
Kelp	2,000–3,000 mg daily.	Supplies essential minerals, especially iodine.
Proteolytic enzymes **or** Inflazyme Forte from American Biologics	As directed on label. Take with meals and between meals.	Important for proper digestion and absorption of nutrients.
Silica	As directed on label.	Aids in the growth of collagen and new body tissue.
Vitamin D$_3$ (cholecalciferol)	600 IU daily.	Needed to aid in calcium uptake and prevent bone loss, which can lead to tooth loss.
Vitamin E **or** ACES + Zn from Carlson Labs	600 IU daily. As directed on label.	Necessary for tissue repair and a powerful antioxidant. Use d-alpha-tocopherol form. To supply a combination of antioxidants.

HERBS

❑ Burdock root, milk thistle, and red clover are good for cleansing the bloodstream and protecting the liver.

❑ Ginger Dry Extract from Sabinsa Corporation helps in digestion.

❑ Licorice is good for glandular function.
Caution: If overused, licorice can elevate blood pressure. Do not use this herb on a daily basis for more than seven days in a row. Avoid it completely if you have high blood pressure.

❑ A combination of high-potency royal jelly and angelica tea, taken once daily, has shown good results.

❑ St. John's wort is a good antidepressant and helps to reduce cravings.

RECOMMENDATIONS

❑ While healthier eating behaviors are being established, a well-balanced, high-fiber diet is essential. Eat as many vegetable proteins and complex carbohydrates as possible.

❑ Consume no sugar in any form. Avoid junk foods, heavy starches, and white flour products. Be aware that you may experience withdrawal symptoms such as anxiety, depression, fatigue, headache, insomnia, and/or irritability for a time after you eliminate sugar from the diet.

❑ Instead of the standard three meals a day, eat smaller, more frequent portions. It may help to control both feelings of fullness and hunger pains. Above all, don't go hungry. This only adds to your craving for food. Breakfast is especially important.

❑ Keep a variety of healthy snacks around you, both at work (or school) and at home, and make them readily available for when you feel a hunger pang.

❑ Chew your food slowly and well. Stop eating as soon as you feel uncomfortable or as if you might have to purge.

❑ Try keeping an eating journal with a price list of the foods you eat in it. This can sometimes help to break the bulimic chain. While seeing on paper what you have actually consumed will, no doubt, be overwhelming, it may make you realize exactly what you are doing and how much it is costing you financially. It can also help to note your surrounding circumstances (if you are alone, with someone, what you are doing at the time, and so forth) and how you feel before, during, and after you eat and/or purge. This will let you see how it happened, and how it made you feel. It can also help you to identify things that may trigger the pattern, such as certain foods, situations, or even people. Once these "trigger" elements have been identified, avoid them as much as possible.

❏ Taking 5-hydroxy L-tryptophan (5-HTP) improves serotonin levels and can be helpful if low serotonin levels are associated with bulimia. Several studies have also shown it can reduce caloric intake and curb hunger. Blood testing for eosinophil levels every three months is suggested if taking high doses of 5-HTP (greater than 300 mg per day). HTP.Calm from Natural Balance and L-5-HTP from Solaray are good sources of 5-HTP.

❏ Cravings can often trigger a binge. The first thing to remember is that cravings do not last long—from several seconds to ten or twenty minutes. When a craving hits you, you can do one of three things: grab a small, light snack (such as a carrot or grapefruit), distract yourself, or meet and defeat the craving head-on. To distract yourself, drink a full glass of water and then remove yourself from the area by taking a walk, going out somewhere, working on a hobby, or attacking a task that needs accomplished. After the task, reward yourself with a healthy snack.

❏ Practice control with other things you do in excess, whether it is alcohol consumption, exercising, shopping, or anything else. The key to a higher self-esteem is for *you* to be in control of your life, not for something else to be in control of you.

❏ Develop and maintain relationships with positive people who make you feel good about yourself and who you admire. Anyone bad for your mental health is a waste of your time and feelings.

❏ Practicing stress management can greatly assist anyone fighting bulimia. Regular, moderate exercise, deep breathing, meditation, visualization, and yoga are all excellent ways to relieve stress. They are also good for easing depression.

CONSIDERATIONS

❏ It is wrong to categorize bulimia as "just a food addiction," as its roots are tied to many other factors that vary from case to case, including low self-esteem, psychological, biological, and societal factors.

❏ The most successful treatment plans for bulimia include a psychologist (who can help assess the psychological implications of the person's disorder) and a physician (to evaluate and monitor his or her physical state). Long-term treatment may be needed to improve self-esteem and ensure that the person is mentally and physically able to recover.

❏ According to researchers at the National Institute of Mental Health (NIMH) and Duke University, lack of a hormone that controls appetite may be the reason those with bulimia fail to feel full. For these people, eating a meal apparently does not stimulate adequate production of the hormone cholecystokinin-pancreozymin (CCK), which is found in the small intestine and the brain. They have to keep eating, and binging, in order to feel satisfied. However, more research is needed to determine whether this is the cause behind the majority of cases of binge eating.

❏ According to an article published in the October 1997 issue of *The Harvard Mental Health Letter*, women with diabetes who are bulimic often lose weight after a binge by reducing their doses of insulin. This can damage eye tissue and raise the risk of diabetic retinopathy, which can lead to blindness.

❏ A study conducted at the University of Iowa College of Medicine and the University of Wisconsin found that reducing weight as part of athletic training may lead to bulimia. A survey of 700 high-school wrestlers found that 2 percent were involved with binge eating followed by vomiting, fasting, excessive exercise, or the use of laxatives to avoid weight gain.

❏ For sources of additional information about eating disorders and treatments, *see* HEALTH AND MEDICAL ORGANIZATIONS in the Appendix.

Burns

A serious burn on the skin is one of the most traumatic injuries that the body can sustain. The skin is the body's largest organ, and one of its most complex. Among other things, it helps to regulate temperature and it serves as the first line of defense against infection.

There are three basic classifications of burns on the skin, each varying in severity. First-degree burns affect only the outer layer of the skin, causing redness and sensitivity to the touch. Sunburn is usually a first-degree burn. Second-degree burns extend somewhat into underlying skin layers, and are characterized by redness, blistering, and acute pain. In third-degree burns, the entire thickness of the skin and possibly underlying tissues, such as muscle, are destroyed. The skin may be red, or it may be white or yellowish, or leathery and black. There is usually little or no pain because the nerves in the skin are severely damaged.

About 51,000 Americans are hospitalized for burn treatment each year, and 5,500 of these people die, according to the American Burn Association. As large as they are, these figures represent a significant decline in the number of incidents, and the severity of burn injuries in the past twenty years, partly due to advances in treatment that lessen the initial shock and prevent fluid loss and infection. Doctors have also improved their techniques for surgically removing burned tissues from the wound as soon as possible and for subsequently transferring new skin grafts to the damaged area(s). In addition, specialized nutrition, focusing on specific nutrients, has been developed and shown to improve recovery and speed the healing process for both minor and serious burns.

The following nutrients are important for healing once appropriate local treatment has been administered. Unless otherwise specified, the following recommended doses are for those over the age of eighteen. For a child between twelve and seventeen years old, reduce the dose to three-quarters the recommended amount. For a child between six and twelve years old, use one-half the recommended dose, and for a child under six, use one-quarter the recommended amount.

NUTRIENTS

SUPPLEMENT	SUGGESTED DOSAGE	COMMENTS
Very Important		
Colloidal silver	Apply topically as directed on label.	A natural antibiotic and disinfectant. Promotes healing. For severe burns, use spray form.
Free-form amino acid complex	As directed on label.	Important in the healing of tissues.
Liquid Kyolic with B_1 and B_{12} from Wakunaga	As directed on label.	Important for tissue repair. Promotes healing. Natural antibiotic.
Potassium	99 mg daily.	Needed to replace potassium lost from burns.
Vitamin A	100,000 IU daily for 1 month, then reduce to 50,000 IU daily. If you are pregnant, do not exceed 10,000 IU daily.	Needed for tissue repair. Use emulsion form for easier assimilation and greater safety at high doses.
plus natural beta-carotene or carotenoid complex (Betatene)	25,000 IU daily. As directed on label.	An antioxidant and precursor of vitamin A.
Vitamin B complex	100 mg of each major B vitamin daily, with meals (amounts of individual vitamins in a complex will vary).	Important in the healing of skin tissue.
plus extra vitamin B_{12}	1,000 mcg twice daily.	Needed for protein synthesis and cell formation. Use a lozenge or sublingual form.
Vitamin C with bioflavonoids	10,000 mg immediately after a burn; 2,000 mg 3 times a day thereafter until healed.	An antioxidant that is essential in the formation of collagen; promotes the healing of burns.
Vitamin E	Start with 600 IU daily and increase slowly to 1,600 IU daily. Also, open a capsule and apply the oil directly to the scar once healing has begun.	Needed for healing and to prevent scarring. Use d-alpha-tocopherol form.
Zinc	30 mg 3 times daily. Do not exceed a total of 100 mg daily from all supplements.	Needed for healing of tissues.

Important		
Essential fatty acids (Kyolic-EPA from Wakunaga, flaxseed oil, and primrose oil are good sources)	As directed on label.	Speeds healing.
Selenium	200 mcg daily. If you are pregnant, do not exceed 40 mcg daily.	Needed for tissue elasticity. Provides antioxidant protection at the cellular level. Speeds healing.
Helpful		
All-Purpose Bactericide Spray from Aerobic Life Industries	Apply topically as directed on label.	Kills bacteria and prevents infection.
Calcium and	1,500 mg daily.	Promotes healthy skin.
magnesium and	750 mg daily.	Loss of body fluids increases the need for magnesium.
vitamin D	400 IU daily.	Needed for calcium uptake.
Coenzyme Q_{10}	100 mg daily.	Helps circulation and healing of tissue.
Germanium	200 mg daily.	Enhances circulation and healing of tissue.
Inflazyme Forte from American Biologics	As directed on label. Take between meals.	Reduces inflammation.

HERBS

❏ Aloe vera pulp, gel, or liquid can be applied to the burn as needed to relieve pain and to speed healing.

❏ Bayberry, black or green tea, blackberry leaves, sumac leaves, sweet gum, and white oak bark contain tannic acid, which has been used in clinics for surface burns that have begun to heal. These herbs can be used as teas and as wet compresses.

❏ Calendula, applied topically to the burned area as a gel or ointment, is effective as an anti-inflammatory agent and antiseptic.

❏ An herbal compress made with comfrey leaf and wheat germ oil can be applied to the burn to help soothe the pain.
   Caution: Comfrey is recommended for external use only.

❏ Apply fresh ginger juice or strong black tea to the burned area, using cotton balls or a compress.

❏ Goldenseal can be taken in pill or extract form, or used in a poultice and applied to the burned area. It is a natural antibiotic that helps to prevent infection.
   Caution: Do not take goldenseal internally on a daily basis for more than one week at a time, and do not use it during pregnancy. If you have a history of cardiovascular disease, diabetes, or glaucoma, use it only under a doctor's supervision.

❏ Horsetail and slippery elm help skin tissues to heal.

❏ Tea tree oil is effective for minor burns, primarily as an antiseptic and to help soothe the burned area. It is safe for both children and adults. Apply topically to the burned area.

RECOMMENDATIONS

❏ If you suspect a third-degree burn, see your physician at once or go to the emergency room of the nearest hospital. Do not attempt to treat the injury, do not remove clothing that is stuck to the burned area, and do not put ice or water on the burn. A third-degree burn requires professional treatment.

❏ Cool a first- or second-degree burn at once to reduce pain and swelling. Immerse the area in cool running water, or use cool compresses for a minimum of ten minutes. *Do not* use ice water or ice cubes, and do not stop prematurely. While cooling the burn, remove rings, wristwatches, belts, or anything else that could constrict the injured area once it begins to swell. Also take away any loose clothing that has not adhered to the burned area.

❏ To remove hot tar, wax, or melted plastic from the skin, use ice water to harden the heated substance.

❏ After the burn has been cooled, apply aloe vera gel or a product such as Burn Gel from Aerobic Life Industries, which contains aloe vera, to ease pain and promote healing. Do not put oils, greasy ointments, or butter on burns. Do not break blisters.

❏ While your body is recovering from a burn—especially a second- or third-degree burn—change your diet to provide a high intake of protein- and mineral-rich foods, up to 5,000 or 6,000 calories per day. These are needed for tissue repair and healing.

❏ Watch for signs of infection, odor, pus, or extreme redness in the area of the burn. Protect the injury from exposure to sun.

❏ Drink plenty of fluids throughout the healing phase. Potassium juice and green drinks (*see* JUICING in Part Three) are recommended for fast tissue repair.

❏ For acid or chemical burns, use baking soda or apple cider vinegar added to warm water. Apply the mixture to the affected area using a thoroughly clean cloth. If possible, soak the burned area in this liquid. With either method—covering or soaking—apply the mixture for five minutes once a day.

❏ Keep burn injuries elevated to minimize swelling and promote healing. This is especially important for burns on the hands, legs, or feet.

❏ Keep the burn *lightly* covered to minimize the chance of bacterial infection.

❏ Try adding 1 tablespoon of powdered vitamin C to 1 quart of cool water and spraying it on the burn site. This has been found to enhance healing. Or try using cool clay poultices. *See* USING A POULTICE in Part Three.

❏ If infection starts to set in, apply honey three times a day after gently washing the area with hydrogen peroxide.

CONSIDERATIONS

❏ Hygiene is very important when dealing with any type of burn.

❏ For third-degree burns, your doctor may prescribe silver sulfadiazine cream (Silvadene). Reactions to silver sulfadiazine are rare, but they can occur.

❏ A medically supervised program for a more serious burn or for a burn in a sensitive location may include the use of antibiotics, debridement to remove dead tissue, hydrotherapy to loosen dead skin, and physical therapy or splinting to prevent contractures (permanent muscular contractions).

❏ In cases of severe burns, hyperbaric oxygen therapy may be employed to reduce edema (swellings), scarring, and contractures. This treatment also improves the chances that a skin graft will take. (*See* HYPERBARIC OXYGEN THERAPY in Part Three.)

❏ Severe burns often need to be treated with skin grafts to help restore the damaged skin. Healthy upper-layer skin from another part of the body can be transplanted to the burned area, but people with large burns often do not have enough of their own skin for transplanting. There are several biotechnological companies that make an artificial skin from collagen, a fibrous protein, and this serves as a scaffold to help promote growth of new skin cells and blood vessels, and also to temporarily protect the wounded area.

❏ A study on the effects of high-dose vitamin-C therapy for third-degree burns that was reported in the *Journal of Burn Care and Rehabilitation* concluded that people with serious burns should immediately begin taking vitamin C (*See under* Nutrients, above).

❏ Applied topically to burned skin, dimethylsulfoxide (DMSO), a byproduct of wood processing, has been reported to have a remarkable ability to relieve pain and promote healing.

Note: Only DMSO from a health food store should be used for healing purposes. Commercial-grade DMSO found in hardware stores is not suitable. The use of DMSO may result in a garlicky body odor. This is temporary and is not a cause for concern.

❏ *See also* SUNBURN in Part Two.

❏ *See also* PAIN CONTROL in Part Three.

Bursitis

Bursitis is an inflammation of a bursa. The bursae are small sacs filled with lubricating fluid that are located between tendons and bones in various places in the body. They help to promote muscular movement by cushioning against friction between bones and other tissues. An inflamed bursa causes pain, tenderness to the touch of the affected body part, and limitation of motion. There may be redness and swelling as well.

Bursitis can be caused by injury, chronic overuse, reactions to certain foods, airborne allergies, or calcium deposits. Tight muscles also may lead to bursitis. *Calcified bursitis* occurs when scar tissue develops in the bursa because an original injury was left untreated. The bursae in the hip and shoulder joints are most often affected. *Epicondylitis* or *epitrochlear bursitis,* affecting the arm, is often called "tennis elbow" or "frozen shoulder." Tennis elbow may start as a small tear in the tendon, and is more likely to occur in people whose jobs require repeated tight gripping of an object. Occupational bursitis is not uncommon and is known by old, familiar names such as "housemaid's knee," "policeman's heel," or the "beat knee" or "beat shoulder" of coal miners. *Trochanteric bursitis* is inflammation of the bursa in the hip. This may be caused by continual physical activity, by standing for a long time, or by a displacement of the hip. It is normally accompanied by an aching pain that may radiate down the leg. One of the most common foot ailments, the bunion, is actually a form of bursitis caused by friction; a tight-fitting shoe causes a sac on the joint of the big toe to become inflamed.

Tendinitis is closely related to bursitis, and the two are often confused. Tendinitis is the inflammation of the tendons, usually caused by strain. It is found most commonly in the shoulders, hips, Achilles tendons, or hamstrings.

Bursitis can affect anyone, at any age. However, older people, especially athletes, are more likely than others to get this ailment. Bursitis is usually characterized by a dull, persistent ache that increases with movement, whereas tendinitis typically causes sharp pain on movement, and rotation of the arm may be difficult if it is in the shoulder. This condition is often worse at night, and the pain usually extends from the top of the shoulder to just under the large shoulder muscle in the back. Tendinitis often affects people who routinely have to reach to perform certain activities, such as domestic workers and painters. Tendon inflammation may also result from calcium deposits that press against a tendon. Unlike tendinitis, bursitis is often accompanied by swelling and fluid accumulation.

NUTRIENTS

SUPPLEMENT	SUGGESTED DOSAGE	COMMENTS
Very Important		
Calcium and magnesium	1,500 mg daily. 750 mg daily.	Needed for repair of connective tissue. Needed to balance with calcium and for proper muscular function.
Free-form amino acid complex	As directed on label. Take on an empty stomach.	Needed for healing of tendons and tissues.
Multienzyme complex with pancreatin	As directed on label. Take with meals.	To aid digestion. Use a formula with high amounts of pancreatin.
Proteolytic enzymes or Inflazyme Forte from American Biologics	As directed on label. Take between meals. 2 tablets 2–3 times daily, between meals.	Contains a powerful anti-inflammatory substance.
Vitamin A plus natural beta-carotene or carotenoid complex (Betatene) plus selenium	15,000 IU daily. If you are pregnant, do not exceed 10,000 IU daily. 25,000 IU daily. As directed on label. 200 mcg daily. If you are pregnant, do not exceed 40 mcg daily.	Needed for tissue repair and immune function. Potent antioxidant and precursor of vitamin A.
Vitamin C with bioflavonoids	3,000–8,000 mg daily, in divided doses.	Reduces inflammation and potentiates immune function. Essential for the formation of collagen, a protein in connective tissue.
Vitamin E	Start with 400 IU daily and increase slowly to 1,000 IU daily.	An anti-inflammatory free-radical scavenger. Use d-alpha-tocopherol form.
Zinc plus copper	50 mg daily. Do not exceed a total of 100 mg daily from all supplements. 3 mg daily.	Important in all enzyme systems and tissue repair. Needed to balance with zinc.
Helpful		
Boron	3 mg daily. Do not exceed this amount.	For better calcium absorption.
Coenzyme Q_{10}	60 mg daily.	Good for circulation.
Glucosamine sulfate or N-Acetylglucosamine (N-A-G from Source Naturals)	As directed on label. As directed on label.	Important for the formation of connective tissues.
Methylsulfonyl-methane (MSM)	As directed on label.	Has therapeutic properties. Aids in pain relief and immune function.
Multivitamin and mineral complex	As directed on label.	Needed for tissue repair.
Pycnogenol or grape seed extract	As directed on label. As directed on label.	Powerful antioxidants and anti-inflammatories.
Silica or horsetail	As directed on label.	Supplies silicon, necessary for repair of connective tissues. *See under* Herbs, below.
Vitamin B complex	100 mg of each major B vitamin twice daily (amounts of individual vitamins in a complex will vary).	Important in cellular repair.
Vitamin B_{12} injections or vitamin B complex	As prescribed by physician. As directed on label.	Needed for proper digestion and absorption of foods and for the repair of nerve damage. Injections (under a doctor's supervision) are best. If injections are not available, use a lozenge or sublingual form.

HERBS

❑ Boswellia and bromelain both reduce inflammation.

❑ Horsetail, meadowsweet, and willow bark, combined in equal measure and taken three times daily, help with inflammation. Horsetail extract supplies silica, a form of the trace mineral silicon, which is necessary for tissue repair and healing.

RECOMMENDATIONS

❑ Go on a seven-day raw-food diet, followed by a three-day cleansing fast. (*See* FASTING in Part Three.)

❑ Eat no processed foods or any form of sugar.

❑ To relieve pain, use hot castor oil packs. Place castor oil in a pan and heat but do not boil it. Dip a piece of cheesecloth or other white cotton material into the oil until the cloth is saturated. Apply the cloth to the affected area and cover it with a piece of plastic that is larger in size than the cotton cloth. Place a heating pad over the plastic and use it to keep the pack warm. Keep the pack in place for one-half to two hours, as needed. Some physicians recommend ice packs.

❑ You may need to abstain from activity and get plenty of rest. When engaging in physical activity, do not push yourself too hard or too long. If you are in pain, stop.

CONSIDERATIONS

❑ Treatment for bursitis involves removing the cause of the injury (controlled exercise of the affected area and/or immobilization and rest may be recommended for this), clearing up any underlying infection, and possibly surgically removing calcium deposits.

❑ Applied topically, dimethylsulfoxide (DMSO), a by-product of wood processing, can relieve pain and reduce swelling.

Note: Only DMSO from a health food store should be used for healing purposes. Commercial-grade DMSO found in hardware stores is not suitable. The use of DMSO may result in a garlicky body odor. This is temporary, and is not a cause for concern.

❑ An alternative treatment for bursitis involves injecting honeybee venom directly at the site. The venom contains a powerful anti-inflammatory and can provide rapid relief. It can be injected either with a hypodermic needle or by the bees themselves. Further information is available from the American Apitherapy Society (*see* HEALTH AND MEDICAL ORGANIZATIONS in the Appendix). Bee venom is also available in cream form as Bee Venom Balm from Aerobic Life Industries. You should not use this product if you are allergic to bee stings.

❑ *See also* PAIN CONTROL in Part Three.

Cadmium Toxicity

Cadmium is an inorganic metal that is naturally present in the environment. Like lead, cadmium accumulates in the body and has varying degrees of toxicity. Cadmium replaces the body's stores of the essential mineral zinc in the liver and kidneys. Not surprisingly, therefore, cadmium levels rise in people who have zinc deficiencies.

Cadmium is present in the environment in different chemical forms, such as cadmium sulfide, cadmium oxide, cadmium sulfate, cadmium carbonate, and cadmium chloride. It is used in the production of colored inks and dyes, as well as in many industrial applications, such as metal-plating, engraving, and soldering. Cadmium is also used in plastics and in the production of nickel-cadmium (Ni-Cad) batteries, which are in widespread use in cell phones, portable computers, and in many toys. Trace amounts of cadmium are found in most foods. In shellfish, however, cadmium accumulates at a significantly higher level. Cadmium exposure from eating shellfish varies, depending on where the shellfish come from. Other common sources of cadmium include drinking water, fertilizer, fungicides, pesticides, soil, air pollution, refined grains, rice, coffee, tea, and soft drinks. Daily intake of cadmium should not exceed 60 grams per day, according to the World Health Organization.

Tobacco smoke contains cadmium, and studies have shown that cigarette smokers have higher levels of cadmium in their bodies than nonsmokers. You can also accumulate cadmium from secondhand smoke. Dangerous exposure to cadmium usually occurs through inhalation of fumes and dust. Cadmium in this form is extremely irritating to the lungs and can lead to such symptoms as headaches, chills, muscle aches, nausea, vomiting, and diarrhea.

The human body can tolerate low levels of cadmium, but long-term chronic exposure can lead to serious health problems. Elevated levels of cadmium may result in hypertension (high blood pressure); a dulled sense of smell; anemia; yellow discoloration of the teeth; inflammation of the mucous membrane of the nose (rhinitis); joint soreness; hair loss; dry, scaly skin; and loss of appetite. Cadmium toxicity threatens the health of the body by weakening the immune system. It causes a decreased production of T lymphocytes (T cells), key white blood cells that protect the body by destroying foreign invaders and cancer cells. Because cadmium is retained in the kidneys and liver (50 to 70 percent of accumulated cadmium is deposited in those organs), excessive exposure can lead to kidney disease and serious liver damage. Possible effects of intense cadmium exposure include emphysema, bone disorders such as osteoporosis and osteomalacia, cancer, and a shortened life span.

A blood test is the best method of determining acute cadmium toxicity. A urine test helps to determine the total body burden of cadmium.

Unless otherwise specified, the dosages recommended here are for adults. For a child between the ages of twelve and seventeen, reduce the dose to three-quarters the recommended amount. For a child between six and twelve, use one-half the recommended dose, and for a child under the age of six, use one-quarter the recommended amount.

NUTRIENTS

SUPPLEMENT	SUGGESTED DOSAGE	COMMENTS
Important		
Alfalfa		*See under* Herbs, below.
Calcium and magnesium	2,000 mg daily. 1,000 mg daily.	Minerals that help rid the body of cadmium.
Coenzyme A from Coenzyme-A Technologies	As directed on label.	Aids in removing toxic substances from the body.
Garlic (Kyolic)	2 capsules 3 times daily.	Helps to rid the body of cadmium. A potent detoxifier.
L-Cysteine and L-lysine and L-methionine	500 mg each daily, on an empty stomach. Take with water or juice. Do not take with milk. Take with 50 mg vitamin B$_6$ and 100 mg vitamin C for better absorption.	These amino acids act as antioxidants; they protect the organs, especially the liver. (*See* AMINO ACIDS in Part One.)
Lecithin granules or capsules	2 tbsp 3 times daily, with meals. 2,400 mg 3 times daily, with meals. Take with vitamin E (see below) for better assimilation.	Protects all cells.
Rutin	200 mg 3 times daily. Take with 100 mg vitamin C.	Aids in removing high amounts of metals from the body.
Vitamin E	600–1,000 IU daily.	An antioxidant. Use d-alpha-tocopherol form, and use emulsion form for easier assimilation.
Zinc	50–80 mg daily. Do not exceed a total of 100 mg daily from all supplements.	Needed to restore zinc displaced by cadmium and to prevent cadmium levels from rising.
Helpful		
Copper	3 mg daily.	Works with zinc to remove cadmium deposits.
Iron or Floradix Iron + Herbs from Salus Haus	As directed by physician. Take with 100 mg vitamin C for better absorption As directed on label.	To correct deficiency. Use ferrous fumarate form. *Caution:* Do not take iron unless anemia is diagnosed. Contains nontoxic, natural iron from food sources that is easily assimilated into the body.

HERBS

❏ Alfalfa contains chlorophyll and vitamin K, and helps to remove cadmium from the body. Take 2,000 to 3,000 milligrams in tablet form daily.

❏ Burdock root and red clover help to purify the bloodstream and stimulate the immune system.

❏ Milk thistle is very effective in protecting the liver. It also stimulates the production of new liver cells

RECOMMENDATIONS

❏ Make sure that you include plenty of fiber and apple pectin in your diet. Also eat pumpkin seeds and other foods that are high in zinc.

CONSIDERATIONS

❏ Chelation removes toxic metals from the body. (*See* CHELATION THERAPY in Part Three.)

❏ *See also* ENVIRONMENTAL TOXICITY in Part Two.

Cancer

The entire human body is made up of cells, each of which contains its own genetic material, or DNA—a long string of molecules that tells the cell what to do. In a healthy body, cells divide at a controlled rate so as to grow and repair damaged tissues and replace dying cells. This predetermined rate of cell division is what keeps our bodies healthy. If cells keep multiplying when new ones are not necessary, a mass of tissue called a growth, or tumor, is formed.

A tumor can be either benign or malignant. Benign tumors are not cancerous. They can occur anywhere in the body and generally do not pose a threat to health, do not *metastasize* (spread to other parts of the body), and do not grow back if removed. Malignant tumors are cancerous. They are usually serious and can be life-threatening. Malignant tumors grow uncontrollably, interfere with normal metabolic and organ functioning, and have the ability to metastasize and invade other tissues.

If a portion of a cell's DNA is damaged, the cell can become abnormal. When the abnormal cell divides, it forms new cells that contain a photocopy of the damaged genetic material. This is an ongoing process occurring constantly within our bodies. Most of the time, our bodies have the ability to destroy these abnormal cells and maintain a sort of cellular equilibrium. If a crucial portion of the DNA is destroyed, however, and the abnormal cells cannot be controlled any longer, cancer forms. All cancer cells have two things in common: they grow uncontrollably and they have the ability to metastasize. They can spread through the lymphatic system, the bloodstream, or avenues such as the cerebrospinal fluid (the watery cushion that protects the brain and spinal chord).

It is not known exactly what causes the cell damage that initiates the cancer process. The chain of events that leads to cancer is very complex, and each individual body reacts differently. A combination of genetic, behavioral, environmental, and lifestyle factors are believed to be involved in turning normal cells into abnormal cells, and abnormal cells into cancer. There are also factors called *inhibitors* (such as certain vitamins and nutrients found in fruits and vegetables) that are believed to slow the process, while other factors, called *promoters* (such as smoking or eating a high-fat diet), can speed up the process.

Possible contributors to the development and growth of cancer can be divided into three categories—external, internal, and lifestyle. External factors include unhealthy workplace environments and exposure to air and water pollution, chemicals, pesticides, and herbicides. Internal factors include both genetics and infections. Lifestyle factors are those we personally can most readily control. These are also the factors scientists believe account for the largest proportion of cancers. They include diet, smoking, drinking, and sun exposure. Persons exposed to cigarette smoke have significantly higher rates of lung cancer than other people. Regular alcohol consumption increases the risk of mouth and throat cancers. A diet that is high in fat and low in fiber is associated with a greater risk of colorectal cancer and is a factor in breast and prostate cancer as well. According to a study released by the Harvard University School of Public Health, poor diet, lack of exercise, and unhealthy lifestyle elements are responsible for about 65 percent of cancer deaths. The following is a breakdown of the overall percentages of cancers many researchers and health care professionals attribute to different lifestyle factors:

Poor diet and obesity	30 percent
Smoking	30 percent
Genetics	10 percent
Carcinogens in the workplace	5 percent
Family history	5 percent
Lack of exercise	5 percent
Viruses	5 percent
Alcohol	3 percent
Reproductive factors	3 percent
Socioeconomic status	3 percent
Environmental pollution	2 percent

Many experts believe that what these risk factors have in common is that they increase the body's exposure to free radicals. They theorize that damage from free radicals is an important factor in causing the uncontrolled cellular growth that is characteristic of cancer (*see* Free Radicals on page 54). Others believe that factors such as cigarette smoking and poor dietary habits increase the risk of cancer because they impair the immune system. While most researchers do not think stress brings on cancer directly, they do believe that it weakens the immune system, impairing the body's ability to destroy precancerous cells before they develop into cancer. By making ourselves aware of all of the factors that may promote or inhibit the development and growth of cancer, and by taking appropriate action, we can reduce our cancer risk.

There are more than 100 different varieties of cancer. They have different causes, cause different symptoms, and vary in aggressiveness (the speed at which they spread). However, most types of cancer fall into one of four broad categories:

1. Carcinomas—cancers that affect the skin, mucous membranes, glands, and internal organs.

2. Leukemias—cancers of blood-forming tissues.

3. Sarcomas—cancers that affect muscles, connective tissue, and bones.

4. Lymphomas—cancers that affect the lymphatic system.

The seven classic early warning signs of cancer, which can be remembered by the acronym *CAUTION*, are the following:

- Change in bowel or bladder habits.
- A sore that does not heal.
- Unusual bleeding or discharge.
- Thickening or lump in breast or elsewhere.
- Indigestion or difficulty in swallowing.
- Obvious change in a wart or mole.
- Nagging cough or hoarseness.

According to the American Cancer Society, 50 percent of all men and 33 percent of all women in the United States will develop some form of cancer at some point in their lives. The good news is that with the increasing information and treatment methods available today, millions of people are either living with, or have been cured of, cancer, and the risk of developing most types of cancer can be reduced by adopting a healthy lifestyle.

The nutritional program and other recommendations outlined in this section are designed for persons who have been diagnosed with cancer, as well as for those who wish to enhance their chances of avoiding this disease. Vitamins should be taken in injection form whenever possible. If you must use oral supplements, take them daily with meals (except for vitamin E, which should be taken before meals). Use only *natural* vitamin supplements.

Unless otherwise specified, the doses recommended here are for persons over the age of eighteen. For a child between twelve and seventeen years old, reduce the dose to three-quarters the recommended amount. For a child between six and twelve, use one-half the recommended dose, and for a child under six years old, use one-quarter the recommended amount.

SELF-TESTS

Breast Cancer Self-Test

See under BREAST CANCER in Part Two.

Colon Cancer Self-Test

A test kit can be purchased at most drugstores for detecting blood in the stool (an early sign of colon cancer). In one test,

Alternative Cancer Therapies

A growing number of people with cancer are now turning to alternative means of cancer treatment. Some of the available alternative therapies provide help by strengthening the body and controlling the side effects of conventional treatments. Other approaches, because of their gentle, noninvasive nature, may in some cases be preferred over, or used in tandem with, more orthodox treatments.

Although there are a large number of different alternative therapies, most of them do have common themes. For instance, many of them are based on the belief that a truly healthy body is less vulnerable to cancer. They emphasize that cancer develops as the result of a problem with the immune system or an imbalance in the body, either or both of which may allow the cancer to develop. Thus, they try to reduce or eliminate the underlying problem that allowed the cancer to take hold, and to activate the body's own inherent healing processes so that the body can heal itself.

Usually, alternative treatments are holistic in approach. This means that the goal is to treat the whole body, rather than just the area seemingly affected by the cancer. Cancer is seen as a systemic disease and treatment is individualized, depending on the particular person. Many alternative approaches also aim to treat the individual on a number of different levels, including physical, mental, spiritual, and emotional.

TYPES OF ALTERNATIVE TREATMENTS

Most of the alternative treatments used in cancer therapy fall into one of the following categories: biologic and pharmacologic therapies, immunologic therapies, herbal therapies, metabolic therapies, mind-body therapies, and nutritional therapies. Although there is a certain amount of overlapping between categories—an immunologic therapy, for instance, may have nutritional components—these categories do serve to highlight the central focus of the many treatments and regimens that fall within them. Be aware though, that the following discussion by no means mentions all of the individual therapies available. It is meant to familiarize you with the various approaches that may be used. Nor should this be seen as a recommendation for any of the following methods of treatment. The choice to seek alternative approaches of treatment for any illness must be made by the individual after a great deal of research and soul-searching.

Biologic and Pharmacologic Therapies

These therapies use biologic substances or nontoxic pharmacologic agents—nontoxic medications usually derived from biological sources, such as plants or human cells. Each of these treatments works in a different way. Antineoplaston therapy, for instance, uses amino acid derivatives to inhibit the growth of cancer cells. Dr. Stanislaw Burzynski maintains that antineoplastons are part of the body's defense system and appear to be absent in people with cancer. He has been able to construct synthetic antineoplastons and administer them to cancer patients. Another such treatment, shark cartilage therapy, is thought to work by blocking angiogenesis, the creation of new blood vessels required for tumor growth, and thus starve the tumor of needed nourishment.

Russian immunologist Dr. Valentin Govallo's VG–1000 theory, developed in the 1960s, is based on the belief that cancer results when a tumor evades and suppresses the immune system. Dr. Govallo believes that placenta extracts allow the immune system to readjust and attack the tumor that had escaped its attention in the first place. This method of treatment is called immuno-placental therapy.

The Revici method, developed by Dr. Emanuel Revici, is based on the premise that tumors are a result of an imbalance of lipids in the cells. After analysis of the tumor, the doctor delivers a compound into the tumor to establish the proper balance within the cells.

French physician Dr. Gaston Naessens developed a system of treatment known as 714-X treatment, which consists of injections of nitrogen-rich camphor and organic salts directly into the lymphatic system. The theory behind this treatment is that cancer cells excrete a poisonous compound that shuts down the immune system. The 714-X allows the immune system to reestablish itself and fight the cancer.

Herbal Therapies

In these therapies, herbal remedies—probably the oldest form of treatment in the world—are used to strengthen the body's ability to eliminate cancer cells. Hoxsey therapy, for instance, first tested in the 1920s employs internal and external herbal preparations, along with diet, vitamin and mineral supplements, and psychological counseling, to strengthen the body and fight the cancer. Hoxsey's treatment proved to be too controversial for America however, and the Hoxsley formula is now continuing in Mexico.

Immunologic Therapies

Immunologic therapies are based on the belief that cancer develops because of a breakdown of the immune system. The aim of these therapies is to bolster those parts of the immune system that combat and destroy cancer cells. An example of the treatments in this category is Dr. Josef Issels' whole-body programs, which use detoxifying diets, uncontaminated water, and vitamins.

Metabolic Therapies

These therapies are based on the idea that many factors cause the occurrence of cancer and that a multifaceted healing approach is required to eliminate the disorder. The therapies use detoxification, including colon cleansing, to flush out toxins; anticancer diets based on whole foods; and vitamins, minerals, and enzymes, which further cleanse the body, repair damaged tissues, and stimulate immune function. Dr. Max Gerson's therapy—which is based on a diet of organically grown fresh fruits and vegetables, as well as nutritional supplements—is one such regimen. Gerson's treatment was developed in the 1940s and is based on a theory of detoxification. William B. Coley developed Coley toxins in the 1890s. This treatment uses bacterial vaccines to enhance the immune system. This system is still being used today but with some adaptations. It is normally used as an adjunct to conventional treatment.

Mind-Body Therapies

These treatments focus on the role that emotions, behavior, and faith play in recovery from illness. In the case of some therapies, counseling, hypnosis, biofeedback, or other techniques are used to promote greater emotional and spiritual well-being. In other therapies, the aim is to use mind-body techniques to actually change the course of the illness, possibly bringing the person into remission. For instance, Dr. O. Carl Simonton and Stephanie Matthews-Simonton, based in California, have developed an imagery and visualization technique to help patients increase the effectiveness of their immune systems. Yoga has become popular as part of this type of treatment. Dr. Barrie Cassileth of Memorial Sloan-Kettering Cancer Center in New York has designed a series of complementary treatments for cancer patients. These include massage therapy, meditation, music therapy, imagery, and relaxation techniques.

Nutritional Therapies

Therapies that focus on nutrition are perhaps the most popular alternative approach to cancer, especially since research began showing the link between diet and health. Almost every alternative therapy includes an emphasis on diet as an important component of both prevention and, possibly, cure. For instance, studies have indicated that a high-fat diet increases the risk of cancer, while a low-fat diet that is rich in fiber, fresh fruits and vegetables, and whole grains actually helps the body to fight cancer. Three of the therapies that fall into this category are wheatgrass therapy, a diet based on wheatgrass and other raw foods; the macrobiotic diet, a traditional Japanese diet high in whole grains and vegetables; and the Moerman regimen, a meatless high-fiber diet that includes nutritional supplements.

CHOOSING AN ALTERNATIVE THERAPY

Unless you already have a specific therapy in mind, the first step in choosing one is to learn more about those that are available. By visiting libraries and bookstores and contacting health organizations that focus on cancer, you should be able to find a number of comprehensive, up-to-date books that provide additional information about alternative treatments.

Once you have a better idea of the therapy or therapies that would best serve your needs, contact educational organizations and patient-referral services that provide information on these treatments. *See* Part Three, REMEDIES AND THERAPIES, for further information about alternative treatments.

When researching a particular therapy, try to get information from other people who have used that treatment. Some information organizations and some alternative clinics will provide lists of recovered patients whom you can call or write to. Focus on those people who have the same kind of cancer you have, and ask them what specific treatments they found helpful.

When screening alternative practitioners and clinics, ask what their success has been in treating your specific form of cancer. Keep in mind that a therapy that is effective against one type of cancer will not necessarily be effective against another. Ask to see supportive studies, documented cases, and patients' testimonials, and view all information with a healthy dose of skepticism. As much as possible, pin the practitioner down regarding what you can expect from the treatment—short-term improvement or long-term survival, for instance. Finally, consider whether the therapy fits in with your lifestyle, personality, and belief system. Be honest with yourself. Some therapies require a degree of commitment that you may not be willing to make. Others may require too much time, too much travel, or too much money to truly be feasible. However, if you have the fortitude and resources to follow an alternative method of treatment to overcome an illness, the rewards are priceless. It is worth checking to see if your health insurance will cover any part of your alternative medicine. Conventional and alternative (or secondary) treatments may be used together—one method of treatment does not necessarily preclude the other.

---

you simply drop a strip of chemically treated paper into the commode after a bowel movement. The paper will change to the color blue if blood is present in the stool.

If your test result is positive, take a second test in three days. If the second test is also positive, see your physician immediately. The presence of blood in the stool does *not* necessarily mean that you have cancer. The consumption of red meat or the presence of diverticulitis, hemorrhoids, polyps, ulcers, or an inflamed colon can all cause a positive test result. Only about 10 percent of those who test positive for blood in the stool have cancer.

Testicular Cancer Self-Test

With the fingers of both hands, gently roll each testicle between the thumb and the fingers, checking for hard lumps or nodules. Be sure to include the epididymis (the rope-like portion) in your examination. Normally, testicles feel smooth and a little spongy. A mass will feel firm but not painful when pressed, unless there is bleeding inside the tumor. If you find a suspicious lump, see your physician. You will be better able to feel for lumps if you check for them after a warm bath or shower, when the scrotal skin is relaxed.

NUTRIENTS

SUPPLEMENT	SUGGESTED DOSAGE	COMMENTS
Essential		
Coenzyme Q₁₀ plus	90 mg daily.	Improves cellular oxygenation.
Coenzyme A from Coenzyme-A Technologies	As directed on label.	Facilitates the repair of RNA and DNA. Supports the immune system's detoxification of many dangerous substances. Can streamline metabolism, ease depression and fatigue, and increase energy.
Colostrum (New Life Colostrum from Symbiotics [original and high-Ig formulas] and Colostrum Specific from Jarrow Formulas are good sources)	As directed on label.	Promotes accelerated healing and boosts the immune system.
Dimethylglycine (DMG) (Aangamik DMG from FoodScience of Vermont)	As directed on label.	Enhances oxygen utilization.
Garlic (Kyolic from Wakunaga)	2 capsules 3 times daily.	Enhances immune function.
Inositol hexaphosphate (IP₆)	As directed on label.	Has powerful anticancer properties; possesses natural killer cell activity.
Melatonin	2–3 mg daily, taken 2 hours or less before bedtime.	A powerful antioxidant that also aids sleep.
Methylsulfonyl-methane (MSM)	As directed on label.	A powerful cancer prevention agent.
Proteolytic enzymes or Wobenzym N from Marlyn Nutraceuticals	As directed on label. Take with meals (to aid in digestion of proteins) and between meals (to reduce inflammation). 2–6 tablets 2–3 times daily, between meals.	Powerful free radical scavengers.
Selenium	200 mcg daily. Do not exceed a total daily intake of 800 mcg daily from all sources, including diet. If you are pregnant, do not exceed 40 mcg daily.	Powerful free radical scavenger and protector against cancer. Aids in protein digestion. *Caution:* Do not take supplemental selenium if you are pregnant or have heart, kidney, or liver disease.
7-Keto DHEA	As directed on label.	A metabolite of DHEA that possesses anticancer properties without being converted into testosterone or estrogens.
Shark cartilage (BeneFin)	For cancer treatment, 1 gm per 2 lbs of body weight daily, divided into 3 doses. If you cannot tolerate taking it orally, it can be administered in a retention enema. For cancer prevention, 2,000–4,500 mg 3 times daily.	Has been shown to inhibit and even reverse the growth of some types of tumors. Also stimulates the immune system.
Superoxide dismutase (SOD)	As directed on label.	Destroys free radicals. Consider injections (under a doctor's supervision).
Vitamin A (Micellized Vitamin A emulsion from American Biologics)	50,000 IU daily for 10 days, then reduce to 25,000 IU daily. If you are pregnant, do not exceed 10,000 IU daily.	People with cancer require higher than normal amounts of this antioxidant. Use emulsion form for easier assimilation and greater safety at higher doses. Capsule forms put more stress on the liver.
plus carotenoid complex with beta-carotene	As directed on label.	Enhances natural killer cell activity. Low beta-carotene levels have been especially associated with lung, bronchial, and stomach cancer.
plus vitamin E	Up to 1,000 IU daily.	A powerful antioxidant and cancer-fighter. Use d-alpha-tocopherol emulsion form for easier assimilation and greater safety at high doses.
Vitamin C with bioflavonoids	5,000–20,000 mg daily, in divided doses. (*See* ASCORBIC ACID FLUSH in Part Three.)	Powerful anticancer agent that promotes the production of interferon in the body.
Important		
Grifron Maitake D-fraction from Maitake Products	As directed on label.	A mushroom extract that contains D-fraction form of isolated beta-1,6-glucan, a substance that prevents carcinogenesis and inhibits the growth of cancerous tumors. Also helps the body adapt to the stress of cancer treatments such as chemotherapy.
Shiitake extract or reishi extract	As directed on label. As directed on label.	Mushroom extracts with valuable immune-boosting and anti-tumor properties.
Helpful		
Acidophilus (Probiata from Wakunaga)	As directed on label. Take on an empty stomach.	Has an antibacterial effect on the body. Use a nondairy formula.
Aerobic 07 from Aerobic Life Industries or Dioxychlor from American Biologics	As directed on label. As directed on label.	Contain antimicrobial agents.
Chromium picolinate	At least 600 mcg daily.	Helps to build and maintain muscle mass. Useful if muscle atrophy exists.
Flaxseed oil or Kyolic-EPA from Wakunaga	As directed on label. As directed on label.	Has antioxidant properties and may protect against, and prevent the spread of, cancer. Speeds healing.
Grape seed extract	As directed on label.	A powerful antioxidant.
Kelp or seaweed	1,000–1,500 mg daily. As directed on label.	For mineral balance and to help the body avoid damage resulting from radiation therapy.
L-Carnitine	As directed on label.	Protects against damage from free radicals and toxins. Use a form derived from fish liver (squalene).
Multienzyme complex	As directed on label, with meals.	To aid digestion. *Caution:* Do not give this supplement to a child.

Multimineral complex with		Essential for normal cell division and function. Use a comprehensive formula that contains all major minerals and trace elements except iron.
calcium and	2,000 mg daily.	
magnesium and	1,000 mg daily.	
potassium plus	99 mg daily.	
vitamin D₃	400–600 IU daily.	Important for the prevention and/or treatment of several forms of cancer.
Multivitamin complex	As directed on label, with meals.	Do not use a sustained-release formula. Use a formula without iron.
N-Acetylcysteine (NAC)	As directed on label, on an empty stomach. Take with water or juice. Do not take with milk. Take with 50 mg vitamin B₆ and 100 mg vitamin C for better absorption.	To detoxify harmful substances and protect the liver and other organs. Has shown preventive effects against cancer. (See AMINO ACIDS in Part One.)
plus glutathione	As directed on label.	Essential for the functioning of the immune system. Found deficient in cancer patients.
and lipoic acid	As directed on label.	Can boost glutathione levels.
Raw glandular complex plus	As directed on label.	Stimulates glandular function, especially the thymus (site of T lymphocyte production).
raw thymus glandular and	As directed on label.	(See GLANDULAR THERAPY in Part Three.)
raw spleen glandular	As directed on label.	
Taurine Plus from American Biologies	As directed on label.	Functions as foundation for tissue and organ repair. Necessary for white blood cell activation. Use the liquid or sublingual form.
Vitamin B complex	50 mg of each major B vitamin 3 times daily vitamins in a complex will vary).	B vitamins that improve circulation, build red blood cells, and aid liver function.
plus extra vitamin B₃ (niacin)	100 mg daily. Do not exceed this amount.	Caution: Do not take niacin if you have a liver disorder, gout, or high blood pressure.
and choline plus	500–1,000 mg daily.	
vitamin B₁₂ and	1,000–2,000 mcg daily.	To prevent anemia. Use a lozenge or sublingual form.
folic acid	400–600 mcg daily.	Affects the repair of DNA. Has been linked to cancer protection.

HERBS

❑ Alternate the following in your cancer prevention or cancer therapy program: astragalus, birch, burdock root, cat's claw, chaparral, chuchuhuasi (a rainforest herb), cranberry, dandelion, echinacea, fennel, green tea, licorice, macela, milk thistle, parsley, pau d'arco, red clover, and suma.

❑ Spices such as cardamom, cayenne pepper, ginger, rosemary, sage, thyme, and turmeric have anti-cancer properties.

❑ Cat's claw enhances immune function and has anti-tumor properties. Cat's Claw Defense Complex from Source Naturals is a combination of cat's claw and other herbs, plus antioxidant nutrients such as beta-carotene, N-acetylcysteine, vitamin C, and zinc.

Caution: Do not use cat's claw during pregnancy.

❑ Many people with external cancers, such as skin cancers, have responded well to poultices made from comfrey, pau d'arco, ragwort, and wood sage. (*See* USING A POULTICE in Part Three.)

❑ Curcumin, an extract from the spice turmeric, is gaining attention for its antioxidant properties and its ability to protect against cancer. Laboratory studies indicate that curcumin has the ability to guard against many carcinogenic substances, and that it may inhibit the rapid cell division characteristic of cancer cells.

❑ Essiac herbal tea from Resperin Corporation has a long tradition of use for many types of cancer..

❑ Green tea, which has gained a lot of attention for its cancer-fighting properties, contains a substance known as epigallocatechin-3-gallate (or EGCg), which has been found by a Swedish research team to cut off blood vessels that feed cancerous tumors.

❑ Modified citrus pectin has been shown to substantially inhibit the growth of cancer cells and is especially effective in combating skin and prostate cancers.

❑ Noni is a fruit resembling the pineapple. Research suggests it may be effective not only in blocking tumor growth, but also in inducing cancer cells to return to normal.

❑ Ojibwa Herbal Tea, a Native American Indian herbal tea composed of sheep sorrell, burdock root, slippery elm bark, and turkey rhubarb root, reportedly has healing powers for battling cancer.

❑ Olive leaf extract enhances the immune system and has shown good results in fighting cancer.

Note: Comfrey is recommended for external use only.

❑ Rosemary is currently being studied as a form of cancer therapy due to its antioxidant, anti-inflammatory, and carcinogen-blocking effects.

❑ Ayurvedic herbs said to protect against cancer include boswellia (*Boswellia serrata*), green tea (*Camellia sinensis*), and haldi (*Curcuma longa,* known in English as turmeric).

❑ The Chinese patent medicine Dang Gui Longhui Wan (a traditional mixture of eleven herbs that is customarily prescribed for chronic myelocytic leukemia) contains indirubin, which is currently under study for its possible ability to control the division of cancer cells.

RECOMMENDATIONS

❑ Eat a diet that includes grains, nuts, seeds, and unpolished brown rice. Millet cereal is a good source of protein. Eat wheat, oat, and bran.

❑ Eat plenty of cruciferous vegetables, such as broccoli, Brussels sprouts, cabbage, cauliflower, and spinach. Also consume yellow and deep-orange vegetables such as carrots, pumpkin, squash, and yams. Apples, berries (including blueberries, raspberries, and strawberries), Brazil nuts, cantaloupes, cherries, grapes, legumes (including chickpeas, lentils, and red beans), oranges, and plums all help to fight cancer. Berries protect DNA from damage. Many of the plant pigments in red, yellow, orange, and blue fruits and vegetables are good sources of antioxidants. Green plants contain chlorophyll, which has been studied as a cancer fighter.

❑ Cook all sprouts slightly (except for alfalfa sprouts, which should be washed thoroughly and eaten raw).

❑ Eat onions and use garlic liberally, as it enhances the immune system and is a good cancer-fighter. Crushing garlic and then leaving it to rest for ten minutes before use seems to raise the levels of its cancer-fighting component, allyl sulfide. If you do not like the taste of garlic, take it in supplement form.

❑ Try to eat seven servings of whole-grain foods a day. Include at least five different types of grain foods in your diet each week.

❑ Eat ten raw almonds every day. They contain laetrile, which has anticancer properties.

❑ Eat as many tomatoes and tomato-based products as you can. Lycopene, an antioxidant agent in tomatoes, protects cells from oxidants associated with cancer. Eating a diet that includes plenty of tomatoes cuts the risk of cervical, lung, stomach, and prostate cancers. Preliminary reports suggest it may also prevent breast, colorectal, esophagus, mouth, and pancreatic cancers.

❑ Eat a lot of tart cherries, both fresh and in pies, jams, and sugar-free juice. They contain anthocyanins, antioxidants that may help prevent cancer and heart disease.

❑ Drink beet juice (from roots and greens), carrot juice (a source of beta-carotene), fresh cabbage juice, and asparagus juice often. Grape, black cherry, and all dark-colored juices are good, as are black currants. Also beneficial is apple juice, if it is fresh. Fruit juices are best taken in the morning, vegetable juices in the afternoon.

❑ Drink spring or steam-distilled water only, *not* tap water. Increased levels of radium in public water has been associated with an increased rate of lung, bladder, and breast cancers, as well as leukemia. Also, soaking in a bath of chlorinated water exposes you to as much chlorine as drinking two quarts of chlorinated water does due to the rate at which this chemical is absorbed through the skin. If possible, filter your water, and take showers instead of baths.

❑ Limit your consumption of dairy products; a little yogurt, kefir, or raw cheese occasionally is sufficient.

❑ *Do not* consume any of the following: peanuts, junk foods, processed refined foods, saturated fats, salt, sugar, or white flour. Instead of salt, use sea salt, kelp, or a potassium substitute. If necessary, a small amount of blackstrap molasses or pure maple syrup can be used as a natural sweetener in place of sugar. Use whole wheat or rye instead of white flour. Do not consume anything containing alcohol or caffeine. Avoid all teas except for herbal teas.

❑ Do not eat any animal protein—*never* eat luncheon meat, hot dogs, or smoked or cured meats. As your condition improves, eat broiled fish three times a week.

❑ *See* FASTING in Part Three, and follow the program.

❑ A green drink that is a good master cleanser combines the juice of 2 organic lemons, 2 tablespoons pure grade-C maple syrup, ¼ teaspoon cayenne pepper, 1 ounce fresh wheatgrass juice, and 1 quart of distilled water. If fresh wheatgrass is not available, powdered Sweet Wheat from Sweet Wheat, Inc. is a good substitute.

❑ Take coffee enemas alternated with enemas made by adding 1 ounce of fresh wheatgrass juice to 1 cup of water. Do this daily to help the body eliminate toxins. Wheatgrass enemas contain many nutrients and enzymes, and are used in many alternative clinics for cancer treatment. Also use cleansing enemas with lemon and water or garlic (Kyolic liquid) and water two or three times weekly. (*See* ENEMAS in Part Three.)

❑ *Do not* take supplemental iron. The body naturally withholds iron from cancer cells to inhibit their growth. People with excessive iron in their blood have an increased risk of developing cancer. Excess iron may suppress the cancer-killing action of macrophages (cells that engulf and devour bacteria and other foreign invaders) and interfere with the activity of lymphocytes.

❑ Use only glass or stainless steel cookware and wooden cooking utensils.

❑ Get regular exercise. Cancer is less prevalent in physically active people. Exercise also helps to stave off depression and promotes oxygenation of the tissues.

❑ Check the radon level in your home. Radon is a radioactive gas that occurs naturally within the earth's crust that has been classified by the Environmental Protection Agency (EPA) as a known carcinogen. Radon test kits are easy to find at hardware stores and are relatively inexpensive. If radon is found, sealing cracks and improving ventilation in the basement will usually improve the situation.

❑ Because of potential low-level radiation leakage, avoid microwave ovens. Do not sit close to television sets—sit at least eight feet away. Also avoid x-rays.

❑ Avoid chemicals such as hair sprays, cleaning compounds, waxes, fresh paints, and garden pesticides. Many chemicals promote the formation of free radicals in the body, which may lead to cancer. People with cancer can further weaken their immune systems by coming into contact with chemicals. The body then must expend energy trying to protect itself from the damaging chemicals instead of fighting the cancer.

❑ Use a shower head that removes the chlorine from your water. A product called Showerwise from Waterwise will do this. (*See* MANUFACTURER AND DISTRIBUTOR INFORMATION in the Appendix.)

❑ Remove known and suspected carcinogens from your life and from your home. *The Safe Shoppers Bible* by David

Steinman and Samuel S. Epstein, M.D. (Macmillan, 1995) provides information on the safety of many different types of products, including cleaning products, paints, pesticides, pet supplies, auto products, art and craft supplies, cosmetics, personal care products, as well as foods and beverages. Another good source of information is Mary Kerney Levenstein's *Everyday Cancer Risks and How to Avoid Them* (Avery Publishing Group, 1992).

❏ Do not take any drugs except for those prescribed by your physician.

❏ As much as possible, avoid stress. Learn relaxation and stress management techniques (such as meditation, visualization, deep breathing, and support groups) to help you deal with those stresses you cannot avoid. *See* STRESS in Part Two.

CONSIDERATIONS

❏ Many people with cancer have achieved good results with a macrobiotic diet.

❏ German physician and cancer specialist Dr. Hans Nieper used fresh raw cabbage and carrot juice with excellent results. Dr. Nieper also used Carnivora, a substance derived from a South American plant, to fight cancer.

❏ New York–based immunologist Dr. Nicholas Gonzalez has developed a cancer treatment regimen under study by the National Institutes of Health that incorporates changes in diet, nutritional supplementation, and toxin-removal systems, including coffee enemas.

❏ Various types of mushrooms can be good sources of vitamin D, B$_1$ (thiamine), B$_2$ (riboflavin), B$_3$ (niacin), minerals, and amino acids. They have the ability to enhance the body's immune system T cells that seek and destroy cancer cells. Shiitake, zhu ling, enoki, reishi, and maitake mushrooms have all been reported to have anti-cancer properties.

❏ Exceptionally low cholesterol levels have been associated with an increased risk of dying from cancer, possibly because people with lower cholesterol levels tend to consume more polyunsaturated fats, which may increase cancer risk.

❏ People in Japan and Iceland have low rates of both goiter and breast cancer. In fact, breast cancer is almost nonexistent in Japanese women. Colon cancer rates in Japan are also low. Breast cancer has been linked to iodine deficiency, and the soil in both Japan and Iceland is rich in both iodine and selenium. Japanese people also consume large amounts of fish, vegetables, and green tea, which may be a factor. The Cancer Control Convention in Japan has reported that germanium may be important in the prevention and cure of cancer.

❏ A daily dose of seven to ten servings of fruits and vegetables can reduce cancer risk by about 30 percent. Many phytochemicals found in plant foods are currently being studied for anticancer properties, including:

• Lutein, one of the carotenoids, is under investigation as a possible anticancer nutrient. Good sources of lutein include dark, leafy greens and broccoli.

• Genistein and diadzein, two isoflavones found in soy, act as antioxidants and may protect against most forms of cancer, especially prostate cancer, breast cancer, leukemia, glioblastoma multiforme, and bladder cancer. Mega Soy Formula from Prolongevity is a good supplement that contains a substantial amount of genistein and other isoflavones that help to fight cancer.

• D-glucaric acid, a phytochemical found in broccoli, Brussels sprouts, and cauliflower, has shown evidence in several clinical studies of reducing the incidence of cancers of the breast, lung, liver, and skin. D-glucaric acid is also available in supplement form combined with calcium (calcium d-glucarate).

❏ A four-year study conducted at the University of Illinois College of Medicine showed that high levels of antioxidants have a protective effect against cancerous tumors.

❏ Calcium may prevent precancerous cells from becoming cancerous.

❏ Inositol hexaphosphate (IP$_6$), a form of the B vitamin inositol, is gaining attention for its ability to aid in the prevention and treatment of cancer. It is found naturally in whole grains, beans, lentils, pork, veal, citrus fruits, and nuts. Evidence has shown that it may not only shrink tumors, but also prevent tumor growth.

❏ Niacin may play a major role in the prevention and treatment of cancer.

❏ Low levels of selenium have been associated with greater risk of several types of cancer, including leukemia, esophageal, lung, colorectal, prostate, breast, and ovarian cancers. However, a total daily intake of over 800 micrograms is toxic to the body. Selenium supplementation should be discussed with a physician. Dietary sources of selenium include brazil nuts, tuna, flounder, pork, turkey, pasta, bagels, pinto beans, and navy beans.

❏ Studies have shown that supplementation of vitamins A, C, and E can decrease the effect of lipid peroxidation, or the oxidation of body fats, which leads to the creation of free radicals in the body.

❏ Research is underway to determine the effects of vitamin D on cancer. Early findings suggest that daily exposure to a limited amount of sunlight (a good source of vitamin D) may reduce the risk of breast, colon, and prostate cancers.

❏ Gamma E Tocopherol Formula from Prolongevity is a vitamin E supplement containing gamma-tocopherol, delta-tocopherol, alpha-tocopherol, and beta-tocopherol—all natural forms of vitamin E. This product offers powerful protection against dangerous free radicals.

❏ Nutritional supplements and better dietary habits offer great support to cancer patients who are receiving chemo-

Types and Warning Signs of Cancer

Knowing the warning signs and factors that increase the risk of developing different forms of cancer can save your life. The American Cancer Society estimates that of the 500,000 cancer deaths that occur in the United States, about one-third can be attributed to dietary factors, with another third being caused by cigarette smoking. Healthy lifestyle choices at any stage of life are a major step toward cancer prevention. Following are descriptions of some of the major types of cancer, including information about who is affected, what the symptoms are, how these diseases can be detected and diagnosed, and what you can do to reduce your risk of contracting them.

BLADDER CANCER

Bladder cancer is the fourth most common cancer in males, eighth most common in females, and fifth leading cause of cancer deaths in the United States. It is four times more common in men than women, twice as common in Caucasians as in African-Americans, and is usually diagnosed later in life.

Causes and Risk Factors

The cause of bladder cancer is not known. Smoking is the number-one factor associated with bladder cancer. Also linked to bladder cancer are exposure to certain chemicals, such as benzidines, aniline dyes, naphthalenes; radiation exposure; heredity; possibly extremely high consumption of saccharin; a history of schistosomiasis (a tropical disease); chronic urinary tract infections or inflammation; and working in the dye, chemical, rubber, and leather industries.

Signs and Symptoms

Often symptoms do not appear in the early stages. The first warning sign is usually blood in the urine. Other symptoms can be pain and burning with urination, increased frequency of urination, and difficulty urininating.

Detection and Diagnosis

Bladder cancer can be detected by examining the bladder through a cytoscope, examining cells in the urine, or having intravenous pyelography (IVP, a special kidney x-ray) performed. Sometimes a large tumor can be detected through a rectal or vaginal exam. Researchers are studying a new screening test that detects telomerase, an enzyme produced by bladder tumors.

Dietary and Nutritional Factors

Cruciferous vegetables such as broccoli, Brussels sprouts, cabbage, cauliflower, and kale have been credited with lowering the risk of bladder cancer due to their antioxidant and other cancer-fighting compounds. Eating the USDA-recommended number of servings of fruits such as apples, berries, cherries, oranges, pears, and tomatoes can reduce the risk by 45 percent. Drinking a lot of liquids, especially *pure* water, helps to dilute carcinogens and increase urination, lessening the time any carcinogens in the bladder have to do any damage.

Taking vitamin A, beta-carotene, vitamin C, and a multi-vitamin have shown reductions in the risk of getting bladder cancer. Dimethylsulfoxide (DMSO) is an FDA-approved, nontoxic solvent that has been shown to aid in treatment.

BREAST CANCER

See BREAST CANCER in Part Two.

CERVICAL CANCER

Invasive cervical cancer is the second most common type of cancer in women and accounts for over 11 percent of all cancers around the world. The majority of cervical cancers grow gradually over several years with precancerous cells (dysplasia) existing previous to the cancer cells. If dysplasia is detected early enough and removed, cervical cancer can often be prevented.

Causes and Risk Factors

Most cervical cancers are associated with infection with human papillomaviruses (HPV), which can be transmitted sexually. Associated risk factors include having had more than five complete pregnancies; first intercourse before age eighteen; unprotected sex; sexually transmitted infections, including HIV, HPV, and genital herpes; early childbearing; multiple sex partners; infertility; low socioeconomic status; smoking; and nutritional deficiencies.

Signs and Symptoms

Cervical cancer usually causes no symptoms until it is advanced, which is why it is essential for women to have regular pelvic exams and Pap tests. It can cause bleeding between menstrual periods, bleeding after intercourse or douching, unusual discharge, painful menstrual periods, and heavy periods.

Detection and Diagnosis

The presence of abnormal cells can be detected by a Pap test, followed up with a biopsy. Women should begin having annual pelvic exams and Pap tests when sexual activity begins, or at age eighteen (after three or more normal exams, your doctor may recommend decreasing the frequency of the exams unless you have had dysplasia or are at increased risk for other reasons). Researchers are exploring the idea of screening for HPV as a method of early detection.

Dietary and Nutritional Factors

A diet low in fatty meats (especially pork), red meat, cheeses, and white bread, and high in soy products, fruits, dark green vegetables, tomatoes, whole grains, and yogurt offers the best dietary protection. Shiitake mushrooms are also a good source of protection.

If you do not consume 3–5 servings of fruits and vegetables daily, you should take vitamin C (500–1,000 milligrams daily), E, A, and beta-carotene (25,000–50,000 international units daily) in supplemental form. Folic acid, one of the B vitamins (400–800 micrograms daily), can not only aid in prevention, but it has been known to reverse precancerous changes in cervical cells. Shark cartilage may also be helpful in fighting or preventing cervical cancer.

COLORECTAL CANCER

The large intestine is made up of the colon (the upper five to six feet) and the rectum (the last six to eight inches). This is where the last stage of digestion occurs and where solid waste is held until it is released. Colorectal cancer is second only to lung cancer among cancers that kill both men and women. Mostly credited to an increase in screening for and removal of polyps, the incidence has been declining during the past decade.

Most colon cancers occur in people over fifty. It strikes men and women nearly equally. Colorectal cancer develops over a ten- to fifteen-year period and produces no symptoms until it is advanced. If the disease is detected early enough and the tumor has not metastasized, the survival rate is quite high.

Causes and Risk Factors

A genetic defect is connected with some forms of familial colon cancer. Other causes are not known. Risk factors associated with colorectal cancer include calcium deficiency; colorectal polyps; family history of colon cancer (Lynch syndrome); continued constipation and/or diarrhea; personal history of colon-related diseases or uterine or ovarian cancer, such as polyps, non-polyposis colon cancer, or inflammatory bowel disease; buildup of toxins in the colon; possibly diabetes; a diet high in saturated animal fat and low in fiber; high intake of charbroiled, burned, wood-smoked, or fried foods; obesity; smoking; alcohol consumption; and cancer in another part of the body. Many studies have shown that active people are not as likely to develop colon tumors as those who do not regularly engage in physical activity.

Signs and Symptoms

Symptoms of colorectal cancer can include rectal bleeding; blood in the stool; changes in bowel habits (persistent diarrhea, gas pains, and/or constipation); persistent abdominal pain or bloating; anemia or significant weight loss; unusual paleness or fatigue; and ulcerative colitis.

Detection and Diagnosis

Screening for colon cancer is the best way to detect polyps before they turn cancerous. During regular checkups (and annually after age forty), men and women should have a rectal exam. Beginning at age fifty, one of the following tests should be performed along with a rectal exam:

1. Fecal occult blood test (FOBT) and flexible sigmoidoscopy (if normal, repeat the FOBT yearly and the flexible sigmoidoscopy at 5-year intervals).

2. Colonoscopy (if normal, repeat at 10-year intervals).

3. Double contrast barium enema or colon x-ray (if normal, repeat at 5–10-year intervals).

If you have a personal history of inflammatory bowel disease, you should have a colonoscopy every one to two years. If you have a family history of colorectal cancer, you may have an inherited genetic mutation that can lead to polyps and/or cancers developing at an early age, even in the teenage years. Investigate any family history of colon cancer and discuss proper screening guidelines with your physician.

In addition, a test kit for detecting blood in the stool can be purchased at most drugstores (*See* Colon Cancer Self Test in this section).

Dietary and Nutritional Factors

It was once believed that a high-fiber diet protects the colon by reducing the time any harmful carcinogens that are present in the stool are in contact with the intestinal wall. There have since been conflicting reports on this, but most health professionals still recommend a high-fiber, low-fat diet. A high-fat diet has a strong link with colon cancer. Either a vegetarian diet or a diet low in red meat, alcohol, and refined foods and high in vegetables, fruits, soy, fish, whole-grain breads, and cereals, as well as low- or nonfat dairy products and lots of fruit and vegetable juices offers optimum dietary protection. Garlic, broccoli, cabbage, cauliflower, brussels sprouts, citrus fruits, melons, and dark green, red, and yellow vegetables are recommended for their antioxidant and sulfur compounds. Tomatoes may lower risk. Consumption of chlorinated water has been linked to a greater incidence of colon cancer. Coffee has been reported to have positive effects on reducing colon cancer risk.

Beta-carotene, calcium (1,200 milligrams daily), selenium, and vitamins C and E, and the long-term use of a multivitamin containing folic acid (above 400 micrograms daily) have been linked to a reduced risk of colon cancer. Probiotics (which can be found in yogurt and supplements) may inhibit colon cancer. Low levels of vitamin D and, possibly, excessive iron intake, have been associated with an increased risk of colon cancer. Quercetin has been shown to have anticancer properties with respect to colon cancer.

ENDOMETRIAL CANCER

See under ENDOMETRIOSIS in Part Two.

ESOPHAGEAL CANCER

Esophageal cancers are more common in men than in women, and in African-Americans than in whites. Tumors in the esophagus usually occur in the middle or lower half of the esophagus. Esophageal cancer is one of the fastest-growing and deadliest forms of cancer in the United States because symptoms usually do not occur before it is in advanced stages when there is little chance of recovery.

Causes and Risk Factors

The cause or causes of esophageal cancer are not well understood. Risk factors include the use of tobacco and/or alcohol; age; personal history of Barrett's esophagus (a precancerous condition resulting from the reflux of stomach fluid into the bottom portion of the esophagus over an extended period of time), achalasia (constriction of the lower portion of the esophagus), tylosis (a very rare inherited disease that causes the overgrowth of skin on the palms of the hands and soles of the feet), or esophageal webs (small portions of tissue that stick out into the esophagus, often making it difficult to swallow); a high-fat diet; consumption of wood-smoked foods; previous ingestion of lye; and frequent heartburn. The risk generally rises with age. Those who smoke or drink heavily (or both) are at greatest risk. People with tylosis have nearly a 100-percent chance of developing esophageal cancer. Screening must begin at an early age for people with tylosis.

Signs and Symptoms

Usually there are no symptoms until the cancer is in the advanced stages. When they develop, symptoms may include progressive dysphagia (difficulty swallowing), often with a feeling of something being stuck in the throat or chest; vomiting and vomiting of blood; bringing up excess mucus; and unintended weight loss.

Detection and Diagnosis

See your doctor without delay if swallowing becomes even the slightest problem. Your doctor may use a barium x-ray and an endoscopic exam, or request a biopsy. A computerized tomography (CT) scan or a newer procedure called an endoscopic ultrasound (an endoscope with an ultrasound probe) may also be ordered.

Dietary and Nutritional Factors

A diet high in fruits (including tomatoes) and vegetables may decrease the risk of this form of cancer. Fish, berries, mushrooms, and Brussels sprouts are all good sources of omega-3 fatty acids, which offer protection. The consumption of salted, pickled, or moldy foods has been associated with an increased risk. Another risk factor may the consumption of extremely hot or cold foods that cause physical damage to the esophagus.

Vitamins A and C, selenium, and riboflavin may help protect against esophageal cancer. Spirulina has been found in several studies to inhibit the growth of oral tumors.

LARYNGEAL CANCER

The larynx (also known as the voice box) is the part of the respiratory tract between the pharynx and the trachea, containing the vocal chords. Cancer of the larynx affects more men than women. It usually strikes after the age of 50. Most laryngeal cancers develop from squamous cells, the thin layer of cells that make up the lining of the larynx. This type of laryngeal cancer usually begins as dysplasia and forms over a period of time—in fact, most of the precancerous cells go away on their own without treatment. However, some of them form *carcinoma in situ* (CIS), the earliest form of cancer. Tumors located on the true vocal chords rarely spread because the connective tissues underneath do not contain lymph nodes, but tumors on other parts of the larynx are apt to spread early. Laryngeal cancer can be treated by radiation therapy, especially if diagnosed early, and by surgery to remove part or all of the larynx. If the larynx is completely removed, you must learn a new method of speech that involves the swallowing of air and bringing it up again. Some surgical techniques have been developed to reconstruct larynx tissue so that speaking can be returned to almost normal. One method that has worked for many people is the insertion of a prosthetic device.

Causes and Risk Factors

Most cases of laryngeal cancer are associated with the prolonged use of tobacco and/or alcohol. Associated risk factors include chronic inhalation of fumes; frequent laryngitis or vocal straining; and an inherited predisposition.

Signs and Symptoms

Possible symptoms of laryngeal cancer include a persistent cough; hoarse throat; swallowing difficulties, sometimes with a pain that radiates to the ear; persistent ear pain; chronic sore throat, sometimes so mild that it is hardly noticed; blood in saliva or sputum; unintended weight loss; and difficulty breathing.

Detection and Diagnosis

Persistent symptoms such as those listed above should be evaluated by a doctor who specializes in the head and neck area, or an otolaryngologist. Most voice changes are not a sign of cancer, but it is better to be safe and see a doctor if you are hoarse for more than two weeks. Diagnosis is made by laryngoscopy (visual examination of the larynx by means of a scope) plus biopsy.

Dietary and Nutritional Factors

The diet should be rich in fruits, vegetables, and foods containing vitamin A, the B vitamins, and retinoids. It is best to avoid alcohol.

If you are unable to acquire proper amounts of the above nutrients through diet alone, you should take supplements. Be sure that your total daily intake of vitamin A does not exceed 25,000 international units.

LEUKEMIA

Leukemia is any of a variety of diseases of the blood-forming tissues (bone marrow, lymph system, or spleen). Leukemia involves the production of abnormal white blood cells that do not function like normal cells, do not mature properly, and do not die off in a normal fashion. Leukemia affects both children and adults, although certain forms are most common in particular age groups. It is somewhat more common in Causasians than in African-Americans.

There are many different types of leukemia. Leukemias are categorized by type (named after the type of cell infected) and by whether they are chronic (in which the growth rate is slow) or acute (in which the onset is sudden). While there is no known cure, transfusions, chemotherapy, and bone marrow transplants are often effective treatments. Newer treatments include stem cell transplant, umbilical cord blood cell transplant, infusion of cell-specific antibodies, and biological therapy.

Causes and Risk Factors

No one knows exactly what causes leukemia, but suspected causal factors include genetics, viruses, and exposure to certain toxic chemicals. Known risk factors include heredity, radiation exposure, chronic viral infections, age, Down Syndrome, having a sibling with leukemia, exposure to human T-cell lymphotropic virus 1 (HTVL-1), use of commercial hair dyes, alkylating agents, certain cancer therapies, and environmental exposure to benzene (found in unleaded gasoline) or radon.

Signs and Symptoms

Signs and symptoms of leukemia can include paleness; fatigue; shortness of breath when active; weight loss; repeated infections; excessive sweating; fever; easy bruising; slow-healing cuts; bone and joint pain; nosebleeds; swollen lymph nodes; and an enlarged liver or spleen.

Detection and Diagnosis

Leukemia is usually diagnosed by means of blood tests and, possibly, bone marrow biopsy.

Dietary and Nutritional Factors

Soy products, which contain genistein and other isoflavones, may offer protecton against leukemia. Good soy foods include tempeh, roasted soy nuts, soy powder protein, and miso.

The bioflavonoid quercetin has been found in numerous studies to have anti-leukemia properties. Genistein has shown positive effects in destroying leukemia cells in laboratory tests. Low selenium levels have been associated with a greater risk.

LUNG CANCER

Lung cancer is the most common cause of cancer-related death in both men and women. The average age at diagnosis is sixty. There are two general types of lung cancer: small cell (or oat cell) lung cancer, which accounts

for approximately 25 percent of all lung cancers, and non-small cell lung cancer, which acccounts for approximately 75 percent of lung cancers. Small cell lung cancer grows very rapidly and has a tendency to spread early to other parts of the body. This type of lung cancer is commonly found in smokers. There are three main types of non-small cell lung cancer: squamous cell carcinoma (the most common form of lung cancer), adenocarcinoma, and large cell carcinoma.

About 170,000 new cases of lung cancer are diagnosed each year, and nearly 160,000 people die of the disease. If caught before it has spread to the lymph nodes or other organs, lung cancer has about a 50-percent survival rate. However, most cancers (about 85 percent) are not caught at an early stage because they do not generally produce early symptoms, making the all-around survival rate relatively low—only about 12 percent—although it has been improving thanks to new diagnostics and drugs.

Causes and Risk Factors

Smoking is the leading cause of lung cancer, and is thought to be responsible for over 80 percent of cases. Associated risk factors include marijuana use; exposure to secondary smoke; exposure to asbestos, nickel, chromates, radon, or radioactive materials; alcohol consumption; chronic bronchitis; history of tuberculosis; exposure to certain carcinogenic chemicals in the workplace, such as pesticides and herbicides; pollution; radon exposure; having had previous lung cancer; personal history of lung diseases caused by breathing certain minerals; tuberculosis; arsenic compounds; lung scarring from certain types of pneumonia; exposure to raw forms of talcum powders (not those found in household powders such as baby and facial powders); and deficiency (or excess) of vitamin A.

Signs and Symptoms

Lung cancer can cause a persistent cough; sputum with blood; chest pain; shortness of breath; fatigue; hoarseness; unintended weight loss; loss of appetite; recurring bronchitis or pneumonia; fever for an unknown reason; new onset of wheezing; swelling of neck and face.

Detection and Diagnosis

If you have any persistent symptoms, see your doctor. Although many of these symptoms are often caused by other conditions, an examination is a crucial step in early detection. If your doctor does suspect lung cancer, he or she may order a series of imaging screenings, a study of a phlegm culture, a biopsy, a mediastinoscopy, a bronchoscopy, a bonemarrow biopsy, and/or blood tests. There are also two diagnostic imaging tools that may be used in place of a biopsy: The Xillix LIFE-Lung Fluorescence Endoscopy System and Nofetumomab. Another imaging test, called NeoTect, may also aid in diagnosing cancer—possibly eliminating the need to have a biopsy done on a suspicious growth. A new chest scanning technique called low-dose computed tomography (CT) may be a screening option if you are at high risk for lung cancer. Researchers are looking into the possibility of using routine CAT scans as a screening method for lung cancer, in the hope that this might substantially improve the survival rate for the disease. This type of screening is able to detect tumors smaller than the size of a kernel of corn, rather than the size of an orange.

Dietary and Nutritional Factors

A diet high in fruits (including tomatoes) and vegetables is associated with a greatly reduced risk of lung cancer. Shiitake mushrooms contain lentinan, which may also offer protection.

Genistein, an antioxidant found in soybeans, may have an inhibiting effect on the growth of lung cancer cells. Alpha-carotene, beta-carotene, and other carotenoids are believed by many researchers to aid in reducing the risk of lung cancer, although there is some evidence that beta-carotene may be linked to a higher rate of lung cancer and mortality in smokers, former smokers, and those subjected to exposure to asbestos in their working environments. Vitamins C and E and beta-carotene all work together, and when taken together, the potential adverse side effects are counteracted. Selenium, lycopene, lutein, and glutathione have been associated with a reduced risk of lung cancer. Vitamins E and C, beta-carotene, selenium, and the B vitamins have also been associated with a decreased risk of lung cancer.

LYMPHOMA (NON-HODGKIN'S)

A key player in the body's immune system, the lymphatic system. is made up of a circuitry of vessels that branch out and spread to all of the body's tissues—much like blood vessels do. Lymph nodes, found in the abdomen, chest, groin, neck, and underarms, are located along these vessels. Other parts of the lymph system include adenoids, bone marrow, the spleen, tonsils, and thymus gland. The intestines, skin, and stomach also contain lymphatic tissue. Lymph is a colorless fluid that contains lymphocytes, which fight infection.

Cancer that develops within the lymphatic system is categorized as either Hodgkin's disease or non-Hodgkin's lymphoma (all other forms of cancers in the lymph system). In non-Hodgkin's lymphoma (NHL), the body's ability to fight off infection is significantly decreased because fewer than normal white blood cells are produced. In addition, the cancer can spread through the lymphatic vessels to other parts of the body. NHL can be low-grade (slow-growing), intermediate-grade, or high-grade. Both intermediate-grade and high-grade NHL are fast-growing and can be deadly within 1 to 2 years if left untreated.

Non-Hodgkin's lymphoma is the fifth most common cancer in the United States, and the number of cases diagnosed has increased by nearly 50 percent in the past fifteen years. The actual number of new cases has increased, but the increase is also due in part to better methods of detection. Although this type of cancer can develop at any age, older adults are at highest risk.

Causes and Risk Factors

At least some cases of lymphoma are linked to a viral cause. In other cases, the cause is unknown. Risk factors include heredity; immune-system dysfunction; exposure to herbicides, pesticides, or black hair dye; a diet high in red meat; AIDS; immune-depressing therapies; previous organ transplantation; benzene; and HTVL-1.

Signs and Symptoms

Symptoms of non-Hodgkin's lymphoma vary, depending on the area of cancer growth. If cancer is in the abdomen, it can cause nausea, vomiting, and abdominal pain or enlargement; in the chest—shortness of breath and cough; in the brain—headaches, vision changes, and seizures; in the bone marrow—anemia; in the thymus—shortness of breath or feeling of suffocation, and coughing.

Detection and Diagnosis

A biopsy can be done on lymphatic tissue to detect if there is any cancer present, and if so, what type. If any symptoms of non-Hodgkin's lymphoma are persistent, you should see your doctor for proper evaluation.

Dietary and Nutritional Factors

The diet should be low in fat and high in fiber. Alcohol should be avoided.

MOUTH (ORAL) CANCER

Ten thousand Americans each year die from oral cancer. It is twice as common in men as in women, although the incidence is rising in women and falling in men.

Tumors in the oral cavity are not always malignant, however, some tumors can be precancerous. *Oral leukoplakia* is a precancerous condition of the mouth to which smokers and drinkers are particularly prone. People who have had cancer in the oral cavity are at greater risk of developing cancer in nearby areas and should have follow-up exams regularly throughout their lives.

Causes and Risk Factors

Smoking and the use of chewing tobacco are the primary causes of oral cancer. According to the American Cancer Society, 90 percent of people with mouth and throat cancers use tobacco, and the risk of developing these cancers increases with the amount smoked or chewed and the duration of the habit. Other risk factors include irritants inside the mouth, such as a broken tooth, or ill-fitting or broken dentures; excessive alcohol intake; chronic use of a mouthwash with high alcohol content; poor oral and dental hygiene; ultraviolet light exposure to the lips; vitamin deficiency; Plummer-Vinson syndrome; HPV; immune system depression.

Signs and Symptoms

While some oral cancers produce early symptoms, others

do not until it is advanced. Symptoms may include a chronic sore of the mouth, tongue, or throat that does not heal; loss of feeling in the mouth or tongue; discolored patches in the mouth or throat area; swallowing difficulty or a feeling that something is stuck in the throat; mass in the cheek or neck; swelling or motion difficulty of the jaw; changes in the voice; and unintended weight loss. Cancer in the mouth has been known to disguise itself as another condition—even as a toothache.

Detection and Diagnosis

Cancer in the mouth can be found early through recommended regular exams by the dentist or doctor. If cancer is suspected, your doctor will refer you to an otolaryngologist (head and neck specialist). The doctor may perform a complete head and neck exam, which may or may not include a biopsy. If it is likely that cancer is present, a panendoscopy will be done, which includes a complete, thorough exam performed under anesthesia. A mouthwash containing a blue dye that helps dentists to see very small suspicious sores and ulcers is undergoing testing.

Dietary and Nutritional Factors

A diet low in fat and high in fruits (including tomatoes) and vegetables, with little or no alcohol consumption, is recommended. Omega-3 fatty acids, found in fish, berries, mushrooms, and Brussels sprouts, offer protection against oral cancer. Fiber-containing foods, soy, and other legumes may also reduce the risk. A study published in the *Archives of Otalaryngology—Head and Neck Surgery* suggests that taking beta-carotene supplements may reverse oral leukoplakia.

Vitamin deficiencies have been associated with oral cancer. Spirulina has been found in several studies to inhibit the growth of oral tumors.

OVARIAN CANCER

Ovarian cancer is a deadly form of cancer—it kills more women than any other type of cancer of the reproductive system. If diagnosed and treated early, however, the survival rate is quite high. Unfortunately, ovarian cancer is known as a *silent* disease—it produces no symptoms until it is in its later stages, so the death rate is also quite high.

Ovarian cancer is the second most common cancer of the female reproductive system. It affects approximately 1 in 70 American women at some point in their lives. The risk of developing ovarian cancer heightens past the age of 40 and menopause further increases the risk.

Causes and Risk Factors

The cause or causes of ovarian cancer are not known. Risk factors include not having gone through pregnancy and childbirth; exposure to asbestos or radiation; high dietary fat intake; the use of talcum powder in the genital area; personal history of breast, uterine, colon, or nonpolyposis colon cancers; family history of breast or ovarian cancer; HPV infection; early onset and/or late cessation of menstruation; obesity; and a diet high in saturated animal fat and low in fiber. Taking birth control pills has been known to *reduce* the risk of ovarian cancer by 50 to 60 percent.

Signs and Symptoms

Often there are no obvious symptoms until the cancer is in its later stages of development. These symptoms may include enlargement of the abdomen, diarrhea or constipation, frequent urination, or in rare cases, vaginal bleeding.

Detection and Diagnosis

Any enlargement of the abdomen or persistent digestive disturbances that cannot be explained by any other condition should prompt you to see a gynecologist for an exam. Women who have a family history of ovarian cancer may want to be tested for genes with which it has been associated. Routine pelvic exams can detect a hardened or enlarged ovary or an ovarian growth, while Pap smears are not very useful in detecting this. A tumor may also show up on a transvaginal ultrasound. A biopsy is needed to confirm any suspicions. Researchers are studying the possibility of developing a blood test to detect ovarian and other gynecological cancers. Levels of lysophosphatidic acid (LPA), a substance found in the blood, seem to rise consistently in women who have ovarian cancer. This may provide a basis for a blood test in the future.

Dietary and Nutritional Factors

A diet that is high in fiber and low in saturated animal fats is a good defense against ovarian cancer.

Quercetin has been found to have properties that protect against ovarian cancer. Low levels of selenium have been associated with a greater risk of ovarian cancer.

PROSTATE CANCER

See PROSTATE CANCER in Part Two.

SKIN CANCER

See SKIN CANCER in Part Two.

STOMACH CANCER

Stomach cancer affects approximately 8 in 100,000 Americans. It is nearly twice as common in men as in women, and is more common among lower income people. The risk of stomach cancer increases past the age of forty. Stomach cancer is more common in foreign countries such as Japan, Chile, and Austria, while stomach cancer in the United States is on the decline, probably due to healthier diets and lifestyles, and to an increased use of refrigeration.

The stomach is divided into five portions, and cancer can develop in any of them. Depending on the location where the cancer develops, stomach cancer can produce different symptoms and different outcomes. Most researchers agree that stomach cancer develops gradually and is often preceded by the development of precancerous cells. Stomach cancer has the ability to spread in several ways: through the stomach lining to surrounding organs, through the blood or lymphatic system, or by extending into the esophagus or small intestine.

Causes and Risk Factors

Some cases are probably a result of *Helicobacter pylori* (*H. pylori*) infection. In other cases, the cause is unknown. Risk factors for stomach cancer include pernicious anemia; lack of hydrochloric acid and dietary fiber; high-fat diet; diet high in smoked, salted, or pickled foods; foods high in starch and low in fiber; tobacco and/or alcohol use; previous stomach surgery; chronic gastritis; stomach polyps; heredity; having type A blood; and a personal history of pernicious anemia or atrophic gastritis (a condition resulting in a reduction of gastric acid secretions).

Signs and Symptoms

There are often no symptoms in the early stages. When they develop, symptoms can include indigestion, pain, and bloating after eating; pain in the stomach that cannot be relieved by antacids; vomiting after eating or vomiting blood; black or tarry stools; anemia; fatigue; and unintended weight loss.

Detection and Diagnosis

If you are experiencing any of the symptoms listed above, it is important to see your doctor (especially if you are in a higher risk category), even though many of the symptoms can be caused by other less threatening conditions. If your doctor suspects stomach cancer, he or she may run several tests, including laboratory blood and fecal occult blood tests, an endoscopy, or a barium upper GI radiograph. A biopsy is needed for formal diagnosis. An endoscopic ultrasound is a newer method that can be used to see how far along the cancer is.

Dietary and Nutritional Factors

A diet high in fruits (including tomatoes), vegetables, rice, pasta, and beans, with limited amounts of meat products, is a good defense. Broccoli, onions, garlic, and pineapple are high in sulfur compounds, which offer protection against stomach cancer. Also, you should keep your consumption of smoked, barbecued, pickled, or salt-cured foods to a minimum, and avoid alcohol and tobacco products.

Antioxidants are a strong defense against free radicals that can damage cells and, possibly, make them turn cancerous. Vitamins C and E, alpha-carotene, beta-carotene, selenium, and lycopene are good sources of protection.

TESTICULAR CANCER

Testicular cancer generally strikes men of younger ages—usually between the ages of twenty and thirty-five—and the chance of developing testicular cancer declines with age. It is more likely to occur in Caucasians than in African-Americans. The incidence of testicular cancer has been rising in recent years.

Tumors in the testicle tend to grow very rapidly—they can double in size in only 20 to 30 days. They can also spread quickly through the lymph nodes. For this reason, testicular cancer often spreads before diagnosis. The cure rate for testicular cancer is very high—over 95 percent—if it is detected early. Thankfully, new treatment methods can destroy even testicular cancers that have spread.

Causes and Risk Factors

The cause of testicular cancer is not known. It is known that cryptorchidism (undescended testicles) substantially increases the risk, even if the condition is corrected by surgery. Other risk factors include inguinal hernea during childhood and a personal history of mumps orchitis.

Signs and Symptoms

Symptoms of testicular cancer include a lump or lumps in the testicle; enlargement of a testicle; thickening of the scrotum; sudden collection of fluid in the scrotum; pain or discomfort in a testicle or in the scrotum; mild ache in the lower abdomen, back, or groin; enlargement or tenderness of the breasts; blood in the semen; and breast enlargement.

Detection and Diagnosis

A monthly self exam is the best way to detect testicular cancer early (*See* Testicular Cancer Self-Test on page 249), especially for boys and men between the ages of fifteen and forty. Yearly examinations by a physician are suggested as well. If cancer is suspected after examination of a mass, your physician will request a testicular ultrasound. Ultimately, a biopsy is needed for complete diagnosis.

Dietary and Nutritional Factors

A low-fat diet that includes generous helpings of fruits, vegetables, and grains is recommended. Tomatoes and watermelon are good sources of lycopene, which may protect against testicular cancer. Avoid high-fat foods and alcohol.

Vitamin E and other antioxidants may help reduce the risk. Some studies have suggested that vitamin A supplements may raise the risk.

therapy and/or radiation, or who are in remission. Taking shark liver oil prior to radiation therapy has been shown to protect healthy tissue against injury from the procedure. Shark liver oil contains alkylglycerols (AKGs), vitamins A and E, omega-3 fatty acids, trace minerals, and squalene. A study published in the *European Journal of Cancer* in 1997 reported that glutamine can reduce adverse side effects associated with chemotherapy.

❑ Some types of cancer are treated with chemotherapy, which can apparently cause cancer to go into remission. Cancer chemotherapy is the administration of highly toxic medications meant to kill cancer cells. Most chemotherapy medications destroy normal cells in the process, causing adverse side effects including hair loss, extreme nausea, vomiting, fatigue, weakness, sterility, and damage to the kidneys and heart. Certain nutrients may help the body avoid some of the damage done by this treatment, among them vitamin B_6 (pyridoxine), coenzyme Q_{10}, glutathione, and vitamin C.

❑ In some cases, radiation therapy may be recommended. This involves aiming concentrated x-rays directly at a tumor to kill the cancerous cells. Radiation therapy too has unpleasant side effects, including fever, headache, nausea and vomiting, and loss of appetite.

❑ There is a wide variety of drugs employed to fight cancer, and new drugs and therapies are being studied and developed on an ongoing basis, with many new treatments being approved by the FDA. Taxotere is a drug recently approved for battling cancer.

❑ Non-small cell lung cancers, which account for most cases of lung cancer in the United States, may be treated with porfimer (Photofrin), paclitaxel (Taxol) in combination with the commonly used cancer drug cisplatin (Platinol), and gemcitabine (Gemzar) in combination with cisplatin. Docetaxel (Taxotere) is another drug approved for treating non-small cell lung cancer that does not respond to cisplatin-based chemotherapy.

❑ Doxorubicin (Adriamycin) is a potent chemotherapeutic drug used for treating many forms of cancer. However, irreversible heart damage can occur with use of this drug. Supplementation with vitamins A and E and selenium are suggested to alleviate some of the side effects of this drug.

❑ ONYX-015 is a genetically engineered virus that is designed to infect and kill cancer cells without harming healthy ones. It is under study at the University of Texas and the University of Glasgow in Scotland. Other drugs undergoing testing as cancer therapies include:

• Antiostatin and endostatin, promising anticancer agents that stop the growth of new blood vessels to feed tumors.

• BR96-DOX, a drug that zeroes in on cancer cells, leaving the healthy cells alone. Its active ingredient is doxorubicin, a proven chemotherapy cancer-killing substance.

• Hydrazine sulfate is a monoamine oxidase (MAO) inhibitor available as a dietary supplement that may help offset the inability to eat, fatigue, weight loss, and muscle deterioration often associated with cancer. It also has been studied for over three decades as a treatment for cancer itself. Possible side effects include nausea and vomiting, tingling, loss of feeling, and inflammation of the nerves in the hands and feet, and irregularities in glucose level, alkaline phosphatase, and liver function tests have been reported. Dizziness, weakness, drowsiness, and itching may also occur.

• Interleukin-2 (IL-2), an immune system chemical that is currently used for kidney and skin cancer, is under study for potential use against other forms of cancer, including leukemia. Since its discovery, IL-2 has decreased the rate of death from kidney cancer by more than 30 percent.

❑ Hyperthermia, a procedure in which body tissue is exposed to extremely high temperatures (up to 106°F), may be effective against tumor cells and can be used alone or in combination with radiation therapy and other therapies. Researchers believe that the heat may damage tumor cells or deprive them of the nutrients they need to live. It is important that hyperthermia is applied in a safe way under a physician's care.

❑ Conventional therapies (chemotherapy, radiation, and surgery) may not be as effective at fighting cancers of the lung, pancreas, liver, and bone, and advanced colon and breast cancers, as they are at fighting other types of cancer.

❑ Evidence is growing that bee products may contain anti-cancer properties. Propolis, a substance bees produce to seal their hives, is rich in polyphenolic antioxidants and has been shown to combat the disease in laboratory tests.

❑ The hormone dehydroepiandrosterone (DHEA) is believed to help prevent cancer by blocking an enzyme that promotes cancer cell growth. 7-keto DHEA is a form of DHEA that, unlike DHEA itself, is not converted into testosterone or estrogens, and it may be a better option for those at high risk for breast, endometrial, uterine, and prostate cancers. (*See* DHEA THERAPY in Part Three.)

❑ Some physicians use dimethylsulfoxide (DMSO), either alone or in combination with other therapies, to treat certain forms of cancer.

❑ Studies have shown grape seed extract to not only enhance the development of normal cells, but also inhibit abnormal cell growth.

❑ Hyperbaric oxygen therapy has been effective in reducing the death of healthy tissue due to radiation treatment for cancer (*see* HYPERBARIC OXYGEN THERAPY in Part Three).

❑ Studies are underway on an Investigational New Drug (IND) application that contains an extract of maitake for use on patients with advanced breast and prostate cancer.

❑ Research is ongoing regarding the anticancerous effects of melatonin, a hormone involved in regulating the production of estrogen and testosterone, among other things. It may also regulate other hormones that promote certain types of tumor growth. It is particularly effective in fighting cancers of the male and female reproductive system, breast, and prostate. Studies are needed to determine the effects of long-term use of melatonin in supplement form.

❑ Shark cartilage has been shown to be helpful for certain types of cancer, including cancer of the breast, cervix, pancreas, and prostate, as well as Kaposi's sarcoma, a type of skin cancer. It suppresses angiogenesis (the development of new blood vessels), depriving cancerous tumors of nourishment and, often, causing them to shrink and die. Squalamine, a substance present in shark tissue (especially in the liver), is currently being studied by Georgetown University and the Cancer and Therapy Research Center for its effectiveness in slowing the growth of tumors.

❑ The single most avoidable cancer risk is smoking. Cigarette smoke is made up of over 4,000 chemicals, including 43 that are known to cause cancer. It also contains the poisonous gases nitrogen oxide and carbon monoxide. Lung cancer was a rare disease until the twentieth century, when cigarette smoking became widespread. The American Cancer Society estimated that in 1999, tobacco use caused about 173,000 cancer deaths and alcohol caused an additional 20,000 cancer deaths. The cancerous effects of smoking are multiplied by alcohol consumption, and the two are frequently used in combination. Research suggests that if you quit smoking when precancerous signs are found, damaged lung tissue may return to normal, oftentimes within five years. There has been some debate on this subject, however.

❑ Recent evidence has shown that women who smoke are at greater risk of developing lung cancer than male smokers.

❑ Regular exposure to secondhand smoke can increase a nonsmoker's chance of getting cancer by 30 percent.

❑ There have been some claims that dairy products increase the risk of cancer. However, it is more likely that it is fat that is the problem, not milk. Almond, rice, and soy milk are good low-fat alternatives.

❑ A study published by the *American Journal of Epidemiology* has disproved suggestions that there is a link between lactose and/or galactose (sugars found in milk) and ovarian cancer.

❑ Obesity in men may cause or contribute to colon and rectal cancer; in women, it has been linked to gallbladder, cervical, uterine, and breast cancer. Overweight women are more likely to develop cancer of the uterine lining than other women and tend to do poorly if they develop breast cancer. Fat affects the level of sex hormones in the body. Hormones produced by the adrenal glands are converted into estrogen in fat tissue, so the greater the amount of fat present, the higher a woman's estrogen levels are likely to be. Estrogen stimulates cells in the breast and reproductive system to divide.

❑ Fluoride (which is in toothpaste, tap water, and every product made with tap water) may be a risk factor for cancer.

❑ The incidence of leukemia among children who were breastfed has been found to be significantly lower than that among bottlefed children.

❑ A group of seventy-five Environmental Protection Agency (EPA) experts ranked pesticide residues among the top three environmental cancer risks.

❑ The risk of prostate cancer for men who have undergone vasectomies may be as much as three times greater than that of men who have not had vasectomies.

❑ Urinating frequently may reduce your risk of bladder cancer by releasing dangerous substances from the body.

❑ According to the American Cancer Society, estrogen replacement therapy lowers the risk of osteoporosis and Alzheimer's disease in postmenopausal women, but it may increase breast and uterine cancer risk. Estriol can be used in place of synthetic estrogens in post-menopausal women. It is a natural form of estrogen that is better to reduce cancer risk.

❑ High-voltage power lines have been under study as a possible contributor to cancer. Researchers at the National Institute of Environmental Health Sciences (NIEHS) have reported that, while it is a possibility, it is not likely. Many researchers believe that further evaluation is needed, however.

❑ Since women have been having Pap smears, the mortality rate for cervical cancer has dropped by about 70 percent; however, Pap smears are not always accurate—5 to 10 percent of the results can show a false-negative reading. The most common cause of false-negative results is sampling error. This can occur as a result of either improper preparation (women should not have intercourse, douche, or use any type of vaginal creams, medicines, foams, or jellies for two days prior to the test, and the test should be done between ten and twenty days after the first day of the menstrual period) or inadequate cell collection (there must be enough cells from the entire cervical surface collected, placed on the slide, and preserved immediately).

❑ Some tests show promise for improving the accuracy of Pap tests. Papnet and AutoPap are two different computerized screening tests designed to improve the Pap test's accuracy. ThinPrep is another variation on the Pap test. It utilizes a different method of collecting the cells that can make it easier to detect cell abnormalities. Another test, the Hybrid Capture HPV DNA test, can detect the presence of human papillomavirus (HPV), which is associated with cervical cancer. Women at higher risk for cervical cancer may want to discuss these tests with their doctors. Research on other types of tests to detect cervical cancer is ongoing. For example, testing is underway on an at-home test that uses a tampon-like probe designed to measure cervical cells.

❏ Irritable bowel syndrome does not increase the risk of colon cancer.

❏ A gene linked to the development of colon cancer (when it becomes defective and shuts off in individuals who do not seem to have a family history of the disease) has been identified by researchers at the Ireland Cancer Center at University Hospitals of Cleveland and Case Western Reserve University School of Medicine. The gene, called hMLH1, normally acts to correct errors in cell replication. If it becomes defective and "shuts off," colon cancer may be the result. It is known that this gene can be "turned on" again by an experimental drug called 5-azacytidine. This drug, however, is toxic to humans, so researchers are working to develop a safe form. They say that if the gene can be turned back on again in people with tumors of the colon, their cancers might be more responsive to chemotherapy, and new tumors might possibly be prevented.

❏ Cancer has been reported to be badly underdiagnosed. In one autopsy review, of those found with malignancies, over half of the deaths were caused by undiagnosed cancer.

❏ Just as each of us looks different, each of our bodies has its own unique composition. What some of us react well to may cause an adverse reaction in others—which is why some treatments prove to be successful for some, but not for others. This is why dietary wellness and prevention are so important. If we can keep our bodies healthy and avoid known cancer-causing agents, we have a good defense against ever getting cancer in the first place. And if you have cancer, it is imperative to maintain optimum health: If you go into battle unarmed, you don't stand much chance of winning; but if you go in with a full coat of armor, through the healthiest diet and nutrition, you have the best fighting chance to successfully conquer cancer.

❏ There are many hospitals, research centers, and treatment centers that specialize in cancer treatment. For a list of organizations that may be of assistance in obtaining information and/or treatment options, *see* HEALTH AND MEDICAL ORGANIZATIONS in the Appendix.

❏ *See also* BREAST CANCER; PROSTATE CANCER; SKIN CANCER; and TUMORS, all in Part Two.

❏ *See also* PAIN CONTROL in Part Three.

Candidiasis

Candida albicans, a single-celled fungus, is always present in the genital and intestinal tracts. If it is present in dispro-

portionate quantities, however, it can cause infection. Diaper rash, vaginitis, and thrush are some of the possible manifestations of candida infection.

Because candidiasis can affect various parts of the body—the most common being the mouth, ears, nose, toenails, fingernails, gastrointestinal tract, and vagina—it can be characterized by a wide array of symptoms. These include constipation, diarrhea, colitis, abdominal pain, headaches, bad breath, rectal itching, impotence, memory loss, mood swings, prostatitis, canker sores, persistent heartburn, muscle and joint pain, sore throat, congestion, nagging cough, numbness in the face or extremities, tingling sensations, acne, night sweats, severe itching, clogged sinuses, PMS, burning tongue, white spots on the tongue and in the mouth, extreme fatigue, vaginitis, kidney and bladder infections, arthritis, depression, hyperactivity, hypothyroidism, adrenal problems, and even diabetes. Symptoms often worsen in damp or moldy places, or after consumption of foods containing sugar and/or yeast. Because of its many and varied symptoms, this disorder is often misdiagnosed.

When the candida fungus infects the mouth, it is called *thrush.* White sores form on the tongue, gums, and inside the cheeks. In a baby, the white spots of oral thrush may resemble milk spots. Oral thrush in an infant can spread to the mother's nipples by breastfeeding, and can lead to a situation in which mother and baby continually reinfect each other. Thrush may also infect a baby's buttocks, appearing as a diaper rash. Candida infection may also take the form of athlete's foot or jock itch. *Systemic candidiasis* is an overgrowth of candida everywhere, throughout the body. In the most severe cases, candida can travel through the bloodstream to invade every organ system in the body, causing a type of blood poisoning called *candida septicemia.* This condition almost always occurs in persons with serious underlying illnesses, such as advanced cancer or AIDS.

Candidiasis may affect both men and women; however, it is rarely transmitted sexually. It is most common in babies (an infected mother may pass the fungal infection to her newborn) and in persons with compromised immune systems—and as it proliferates, the fungus releases toxins that weaken the immune system further. Other factors that increase the chances of contracting a yeast infection include pregnancy and the use of corticosteroid drugs.

Very often, people with candida infections also have food allergies. Oral thrush, athlete's foot, ringworm, jock itch, fingernail or toenail fungus, and even diaper rash can develop as a result of the combination of food allergies and *C. albicans.* The symptoms of a food allergy or environmental sensitivity can also mimic those of candidiasis. To further complicate matters, some people with candidiasis go on to develop environmental sensitivities as well. Many cannot tolerate contact with rubber, petroleum products, tobacco, exhaust fumes, and chemical odors.

Yeasts, including candida, feed on sugar. If the body's pH balance is upset for any reason, the friendly bacteria (such as lactobacilli) that normally metabolize sugars cannot thrive and do their job properly, and there is a risk of *Candida albicans* flourishing in this sugar-rich environment. Some women find they suffer more yeast infections when using oral contraceptives or during pregnancy. This is most probably due to an increase in the amount of sugar (glycogen) in the vagina induced by changing hormone levels. Antibiotics, which kill beneficial bacteria along with the harmful ones, are another common cause of yeast infections. Anything that depresses immune function, including HIV and AIDS, also often leads to these types of infections. In fact, it is said that infections such as candidiasis rarely occur in people with robust immune systems who eat a healthy diet that is low in sugar and yeast. The debate continues as to whether candidiasis exists in the body as the result, or the cause, of some immunologic diseases.

Unless otherwise specified, the dosages recommended here are for adults. For a child between the ages of twelve and seventeen, reduce the dose to three-quarters of the recommended amount. For a child between six and twelve, use one-half of the recommended dose, and for a child under the age of six, use one-quarter of the recommended amount.

NUTRIENTS

SUPPLEMENT	SUGGESTED DOSAGE	COMMENTS
Very Important		
Acidophilus (Kyo-Dophilus from Wakunaga) or	As directed on label. Take on an empty stomach.	Fights candida infection. Use a nondairy formula.
Bio-Bifidus from American Biologics or	As directed on label.	Enhances cell function to destroy candida.
Eugalan Forte from Bio Nutritional	As directed on label.	
Caprylic acid (Caprystatin from Ecological Formulas, Capralin from Synergy Plus)	As directed on label.	An antifungal agent that destroys the candida organism.
Dioxychlor from American Biologics	5 drops in water twice daily.	A stabilized oxygen product that destroys the fungus while preserving the "good" bacteria.
Essential fatty acids (black currant seed oil and flaxseed oil are good sources)	As directed on label.	Important in healing and preventing the fungus from destroying cells.
Garlic (Kyolic from Wakunaga)	2 capsules 3 times daily. For candida vaginitis, use Kyolic vaginal suppositories as directed on label.	Inhibits the infecting organism.
Quercetin plus	500 mg twice daily, 30 minutes before meals.	Speeds healing and reduces the effects of food allergies and inflammation.
bromelain or	100 mg twice daily, 30 minutes before meals.	Improves absorption of quercetin.
Activated Quercetin from Source Naturals	As directed on label.	Contains quercetin plus bromelain and vitamin C for increased absorption.

Vitamin B complex	100 mg 3 times daily.	B vitamins are required for all bodily functions, resistance to infection, and all enzyme systems. Important for brain function. Use a yeast-free formula. Consider injections (under a doctor's supervision). Needed for healthy skin.
plus extra biotin and	50 mg 3 times daily.	
vitamin B$_{12}$	1,000–2,000 mcg daily.	Important for digestion. Needed for metabolism of carbohydrates, fats, and proteins. Use a lozenge or sublingual form.
Important		
Calcium and	1,500 mg daily.	Often deficient in people with this disorder. Use calcium citrate form.
magnesium and	750–1,000 mg daily.	Needed to balance with calcium.
vitamin D$_3$	400 IU daily.	Enhances calcium absorption.
Helpful		
Coenzyme A from Coenzyme-A Technologies and	As directed on label.	Removes toxins from the body.
Coenzyme Q$_{10}$	100 mg daily.	Improves tissue oxygenation.
Colloidal silver	As directed on label.	Can aid in healing.
Free-form amino acid complex (Amino Balance from Anabol Naturals)	As directed on label. Take between meals, on an empty stomach.	Rebuilds damaged tissue. Use a sublingual form for best absorption.
Glutathione	500 mg twice daily.	Needed for brain function. Candida may impair brain function.
Grapefruit seed extract	As directed on label. Always dilute before use.	Rids the body of potentially harmful microorganisms.
L-Cysteine	500 mg twice daily, on an empty stomach. Take with water or juice. Do not take with milk. Take with 50 mg vitamin B$_6$ and 100 mg vitamin C for better absorption.	A potent antioxidant and free radical destroyer. (*See* AMINO ACIDS in Part One.)
Multivitamin and mineral complex with vitamin A and	25,000 IU daily. If you are pregnant, do not exceed 10,000 IU daily.	All nutrients are needed for proper immune function and for repair of intestinal lining and all tissues; build resistance to infection. Choose a yeast-free formula that includes zinc and iron.
mixed carotenoids and	15,000 IU daily.	
selenium	200 mcg daily. If you are pregnant, do not exceed 40 mcg daily.	
New Life Colostrum from Symbiotics	As directed on label	Powerful immune enhancer.
Orithrush from Ecological Formulas	Use as a mouth rinse or as a douche.	Aids in destroying candida.
Vitamin C with bioflavonoids	1,000 mg 3 times daily.	Builds up immunity and protects the body tissues from damage by the toxins released from candida. Use an esterified form.
Vitamin K	As directed on label.	To replace vitamin K balance upset by antibiotic use or overgrowth of bad candida.

HERBS

❑ Aloe vera juice has been shown to boost the white blood cells' ability to kill yeast cells.

❑ Kolorex is a patented herbal formula containing extracts of the New Zealand herb horopito (*Pseudowintera colorata*) and aniseed. Horopito contains a strong antifungal agent called polygodial. Kolorex has been shown in laboratory experiments to be effective in controlling *Candida albicans*.

❑ Olive leaf extract with oleuropein is a powerful healer of microbial infections.

❑ Pau d'arco (also known as lapacho or taheebo) contains an antibacterial and antifungal agent, although it does have an alkaloid base and a small percentage of people may not benefit from its use. If you do not benefit from this tea, try clove tea instead. It is a good idea to alternate between the two, because clove tea has some benefits that pau d'arco does not have and vice versa. To make pau d'arco tea, boil 1 quart of distilled water with 2 tablespoons of herb for five minutes. Cool and store it in the refrigerator with the tea leaves in. Strain before drinking, if needed. Drink 3 to 6 cups daily.

❑ Some people who no longer respond to pau d'arco can benefit from maitake tea. It is a good alternative. While pau d'arco must be boiled, maitake is prepared as a regular tea. Resistant strains of candida develop rapidly due to genetic mutation. Rotating treatment programs is beneficial.

❑ Wild oregano oil is a potent antiseptic, powerful in killing a range of fungi.

RECOMMENDATIONS

❑ Eat vegetables, fish, and gluten-free grains such as brown rice and millet.

❑ Eat plain yogurt that contains live yogurt cultures. For vaginal candidiasis, apply natural unprocessed and unsweetened yogurt directly into the vagina or mix one small container of plain yogurt with an equal amount of water and use it as a douche once or twice daily until you see an improvement. You can also open two capsules of acidophilus and add the contents to a douche. This helps to inhibit the growth of the fungus.

❑ Take supplemental acidophilus or bifidus to help to restore the normal balance of flora in the bowel and vagina.

❑ Take some type of fiber daily. Oat bran or flax seed is a good source.

❑ Drink distilled water only.

❑ Make sure your diet is fruit-free, sugar-free, and yeast-free. Candida thrives in a sugary environment, so your diet should be low in carbohydrates and contain no yeast products or sugar in any form.

❑ Avoid aged cheeses, alcohol, baked goods, chocolate, dried fruits, fermented foods, all grains containing gluten (wheat, oats, rye, and barley), ham, honey, nut butters, pickles, potatoes, raw mushrooms, soy sauce, sprouts, and vinegar.

❑ Eliminate citrus and acidic fruits such as oranges, grapefruit, lemons, tomatoes, pineapple, and limes from your diet for one month; then add back only a few twice weekly. Although they seem acidic, these fruits are actually alkaline-forming in the body and candida thrives on them.

❑ Once a month, to replace "friendly" intestinal bacteria, use an *L. bifidus* retention enema until the infection is better. (*See* ENEMAS in Part Three.)

❑ Take only hypoallergenic supplements.

❑ To prevent reinfection, replace your toothbrush every thirty days. This is a good preventive measure against both fungal and bacterial infections of the mouth.

❑ Wear white cotton underwear. Synthetic fibers lead to increased perspiration, which creates a hospitable environment for candida, and also traps bacteria, which can cause a secondary infection. Change underclothing daily.

❑ Do not use corticosteroids or oral contraceptives until your condition improves. Oral contraceptives can upset the balance of microorganisms in the body, leading to proliferation of *C. albicans*.

❑ Avoid household chemical products and cleaners, chlorinated water, mothballs, synthetic textiles, and damp and moldy places, such as basements.

❑ If you have chronic and/or unusually persistent candida infections, consult your health care provider. This may be a sign of an underlying illness such as diabetes or immune system dysfunction, which makes for an environment more conducive to the growth of yeast.

CONSIDERATIONS

❑ All persons on long-term antibiotics or chemotherapy are at high risk for severe cases of candidiasis. Taking antibiotics also can cause a deficiency of vitamin K, which is manufactured by the "good bacteria" in the intestines. Eating plenty of leafy greens, alfalfa, strawberries, whole grains, and yogurt can restore the vitamin K balance.

❑ If a breastfed baby develops oral thrush or a nursing mother develops a thrush infection of the nipples, both mother and baby should be treated to eradicate the infection, even if only one of them seems to be affected.

❑ Because there is no simple, accurate test for candida, it is difficult to determine if it is the cause of a baby's diaper rash.

❑ Allergy testing is advised for anyone with symptoms of candida infection. (*See* ALLERGIES in Part Two.)

❑ Medical treatment for vulvovaginal candidiasis may involve the use of antifungal medications such as butoconazole cream, clotrimazole vaginal tablets, miconazole cream or suppositories, nystatin vaginal tablets, tioconazole ointment or cream, or fluconazole oral tablets. Most of these preparations are now available over the counter under various brand names. We recommend that only women who have been diagnosed with candidiasis use these preparations. Unfortunately, the use of these agents, especially if chronic or repeated, can lead to the development of stronger strains of yeast that are drug resistant. Higher dosages are then required, which in turn further weaken the immune system. Many doctors no longer use nystatin or antibiotics because they weaken the immune system and can damage certain organs. Others prescribe them for short-term treatment only. If you treat yourself with over-the-counter medications and symptoms continue or recur within two months, it would be wise to seek medical advice.

❏ Colloidal silver is a natural broad-spectrum antiseptic that fights infection, subdues inflammation, and promotes healing. It is a clear golden liquid composed of 99.9-percent pure silver particles approximately 0.001 to 0.01 microns ($\frac{1}{1,000,000}$ to $\frac{1}{100,000}$ millimeter) in diameter that are suspended in pure water. Colloidal silver can be taken by mouth, administered intravenously, or applied topically.

❏ High levels of mercury in the body can result in candidiasis. Mercury salts inhibit the growth of the necessary "friendly" bacteria in the intestines. You may want to have a hair analysis done to determine the levels of toxic metals. (See HAIR ANALYSIS in Part Three.)

❏ Systemic yeast infection (candidiasis) and AIDS both cause immunosuppressive symptoms. Because they can mimic each other, misdiagnosis is common. Severe yeast infections are common in people with AIDS.

❏ Candida Forte from Nature's Plus is good for mild cases.

❏ Candidiasis may be related to hypoglycemia. (See HYPOGLYCEMIA in Part Two.)

❏ See also FUNGAL INFECTION and YEAST INFECTION in Part Two.

Canker Sores (Aphthous Ulcers)

Canker sores are small, white swellings that develop into ulcers. They can appear on the tongue, the lips, the gums, or the insides of the cheeks. The ulcers then become covered by a coagulated yellowish mixture of fluids, bacteria, and white blood cells. The development of a canker sore may be preceded by a burning and tingling sensation. Canker sores do not form blisters as cold sores (fever blisters) do. The cold sore, commonly confused with the canker sore, is caused by the herpes simplex virus type 1. The canker sore, on the other hand, is an inflammation, rather than an infection.

Canker sores range in size from as small as a pinhead to as large as a quarter. They appear suddenly and often leave suddenly, usually lasting from four to twenty days. Some experts believe that these painful mouth ulcerations are contagious, but others disagree. Canker sores occur most often in females. They can be triggered by any of a number of factors, including poor dental hygiene, irritation from dental work, food allergies, nutritional deficiencies, hormonal imbalances, viral infection, an underlying immunologic disease (such as HIV infection), trauma (such as that caused by biting the inside of the cheek or using a hard-bristled toothbrush), stress, and/or fatigue. They may result from an abnormal immune response to normal bacteria in the mouth. Canker sores are occasionally associated with Crohn's disease, which affects the bowels. Deficiencies of iron, lysine, vitamin B$_{12}$, and folic acid have been linked to this disorder in some people.

Unless otherwise specified, the dosages recommended here are for adults. For a child between the ages of twelve and seventeen, reduce the dose to three-quarters the recommended amount. For a child between six and twelve, use one-half the recommended dose, and for a child under the age of six, use one-quarter the recommended amount.

NUTRIENTS

SUPPLEMENT	SUGGESTED DOSAGE	COMMENTS
Very Important		
Acidophilus (Probiata from Wakunaga)	As directed on label. Take on an empty stomach.	Aids in maintaining healthy balance of intestinal flora ("friendly" bacteria). Use a high-potency powdered form.
L-Lysine	500 mg 3 times daily, on an empty stomach. Take with water or juice. Do not take with milk. Take with 50 mg vitamin B$_6$ and 100 mg vitamin C for better absorption.	A deficiency may cause an outbreak of sores in and around the mouth. *See* AMINO ACIDS in Part One. *Caution:* Do not take lysine for longer than 6 months at a time.
Vitamin B complex	50 mg of each major B vitamin 3 times daily (amounts of individual vitamins in a complex will vary).	B vitamins are basic for immune function and healing.
plus extra vitamin B$_3$ (niacin)	50–100 mg 3 times daily. Do not exceed this amount.	Deficiencies have been linked to mouth sores. *Caution:* Do not take niacin if you have a liver disorder, gout, or high blood pressure.
and pantothenic acid (vitamin B$_5$)	50–100 mg 3 times daily.	An anti-stress vitamin necessary for adrenal function.
and vitamin B$_{12}$	1,000–2,000 mcg daily, on an empty stomach.	Use a lozenge or sublingual form.
and folic acid	400 mcg daily.	Use a lozenge or sublingual form.
Vitamin C with bioflavonoids	3,000–8,000 mg daily, in divided doses.	Fights infection and boosts the immune system. Use a buffered form.

Important		
Zinc lozenges	1 15-mg lozenge every 3 waking hours for 2 days. Do not exceed a total of 100 mg daily.	Enhances immune function and aids healing.

Helpful		
Garlic (Kyolic from Wakunaga)	3 capsules 3 times daily.	Acts as a natural antibiotic and immunostimulant.
Iron	As prescribed by physician.	May be helpful if canker sores are related to iron deficiency. *Caution:* Do not take an iron supplement unless your physician finds that you are iron-deficient.
Multivitamin and mineral complex	As directed on label.	A balance of minerals is always important.
Vitamin A with mixed carotenoids	50,000 IU daily for 10 days, then reduce to 25,000 IU daily. If you are pregnant, do not exceed 10,000 IU daily. Also put a few drops of vitamin A oil directly on the affected area.	Speeds healing, especially of the mucous membranes. Use emulsion form for easier assimilation.

HERBS

❏ Alfalfa, calendula, capsicum, comfrey, garlic, and peppermint are useful in the treatment of canker sores.

Note: Comfrey is recommended for external use only. Do not take it internally.

❏ Use burdock, goldenseal, pau d'arco tea, and red clover to cleanse the bloodstream and decrease infection.

Caution: Do not take goldenseal on a daily basis for more than one week at a time, and do not use it during pregnancy. If you have a history of cardiovascular disease, diabetes, or glaucoma, use it only under a doctor's supervision.

❏ Goldenseal extract or tea tree oil, applied gently on the sore twice during the day and again at bedtime, helps to speed healing. To use these as mouthwashes, add 3 drops to 4 ounces of water. Add a drop or two to your toothpaste before brushing. Use alcohol-free goldenseal extract.

❏ Red raspberry tea contains valuable flavonoids and is very helpful.

❏ Rockrose, also known as sun rose, used as a mouthwash, both heals and eases the pain of mouth sores.

❏ Wintergreen mouthwash is a good antiseptic. Wintergreen oil can be rubbed into the sores for temporary relief.

RECOMMENDATIONS

❏ Eat plenty of salad with raw onions. Onions contain sulfur and have healing properties.

❏ Include in the diet yogurt and other soured products, such as kefir, cottage cheese, and buttermilk.

❏ Avoid sugar, citrus fruits, and processed and refined foods.

❏ Do not eat fish or meat of any kind for two weeks. The consumption of animal protein increases the body's acidity, which slows healing.

❏ Avoid chewing gum, lozenges, mouthwashes, tobacco, coffee, citrus fruits, and any other foods that you know trigger these sores.

❏ Consider trying the homeopathic remedies *Belladonna*, *Echinacea*, and *Borax*. These agents are commonly used in the treatment of canker sores.

❏ If you have repeated attacks of canker sores, check for nutritional deficiencies.

❏ To avoid getting canker sores, it is important to maintain a proper balance of minerals, acidity, and alkalinity in the body. (*See* ACID/ALKALI IMBALANCE in Part Two for the acid and alkaline self-test.) Have a hair analysis done to test for mineral levels. (*See* HAIR ANALYSIS in Part Three.)

❏ Do not take iron supplements unless your doctor prescribes them. Obtain iron from natural food sources.

❏ Consult your dentist if you have a mouth sore that does not heal.

CONSIDERATIONS

❏ Stress and allergies are probably the most common cause of open sores in the mouth.

❏ Some doctors prescribe mouthwashes that contain tetracycline, an antibiotic, for canker sores.

❏ If you get recurrent canker sores, your toothpaste may be the culprit. Try a toothpaste that does not contain the detergent sodium lauryl sulfate. This is a detergent that may cause the mucous surfaces in the mouth to dry out, leaving them vunerable to attack from acidic foods. Also, do not use the same toothbrush for longer than one month. When canker sores on the gum are healing, it is best to use a very soft toothbrush.

❏ The drug Zilactin is a gel-like ointment that is applied directly to the ulcer. It sticks to the canker sore and gives relief from irritating foods.

❏ *See also* COLD SORES in Part Two.

Cardiovascular Disease

Cardiovascular disease is a general term encompassing heart attack, stroke, and other disorders of the heart and blood vessel system. Cardiovascular disease is the leading health problem in the Western world. It is the number one cause of death in the United States, claiming more than 1 million lives annually. An estimated 50 million Americans have heart and blood vessel disease, although many do not know it because they have no symptoms. Traditionally thought of a disease primarily affecting men, cardiovascular disease is also and increasingly a problem for women. It is responsible for the deaths of 250,000 women a year in the United States. In fact, more women die from heart disease than from breast cancer and uterine cancer combined. African-American woman are at greater risk than women of other ethnic backgrounds.

The arteries that supply blood to the heart are called the *coronary arteries*. If the heart's blood vessels narrow, the amount of blood they supply to the heart may be insufficient to provide the oxygen the heart needs. This oxygen deprivation is what causes a type of chest pain known as *angina pectoris*. Angina is characterized by a heavy, tight pain in the chest area, usually after some type of exertion. The pain usually recedes with rest.

If the coronary arteries that carry oxygen and nutrients to the heart muscle become obstructed, the flow of blood is cut off completely, and a *heart attack*, or *myocardial infarction*, can occur, resulting in damage to the heart muscle. Arteriosclerosis, or hardening of the arteries, and the presence of a thrombus, or clot, in a blood vessel are the most common causes of obstruction. Arteriosclerosis is responsible for most of the deaths resulting from heart attacks. Spasms of the coronary arteries can also result in a heart attack. A heart attack may feel as if someone is applying intense pressure to the chest. This pain may last for several minutes, often extending to the shoulder, arm, neck, or jaw. Other signs of heart attack include sweating, nausea, vomiting, shortness of breath, dizziness, fainting, feelings of anxiety, difficulty swallowing, sudden ringing in the ears, and loss of speech. The amount and type of chest pain vary from one person to another. Some people have intense pain, while others feel only mild discomfort. Many mistake the signs of a heart attack for indigestion. Some have no symptoms at all, a situation referred to as a "silent" heart attack.

Hypertension (high blood pressure) is often a precursor to heart problems. Hypertension is an extremely common form of cardiovascular disease. It usually results from a decrease in the elasticity or a reduction in the interior diameter of the arteries (or both), which may be caused by arteriosclerosis, defects in sodium metabolism, stress, nutritional deficiencies, and enzyme imbalances. Kidney disease, hyperthyroidism, disorders of the pituitary or adrenal glands, and heredity may be contributing factors. It was once thought that the use of oral contraceptives increased the risk of heart disease in women. Now, however, with pills that contain a much lower dose of estrogen—35 milligrams or less—it is thought that only certain high-risk people are in danger. People considered to be at high risk are those with diabetes, those who smoke, or those who already have had a heart attack or stroke.

Because it is essentially painless, especially in the early stages, many people don't even know they have it—hence the term "silent killer." By the time hypertension causes complications that result in symptoms (such as rapid pulse,

Healthy Cholesterol and Blood Pressure Levels

Two important measurements used in assessing cardiovascular health are blood fat (including cholesterol and triglycerides) levels and blood pressure. The tables below are approximate guides to both cholesterol and blood pressure levels. Keep in mind that both levels vary from person to person, so it is always wise to have your blood pressure and cholesterol level checked by your physician on a regular basis.

Cholesterol and Triglyceride Levels for People without Heart Disease (mg/dL)

Blood Lipid	Good	Borderline	High
Total cholesterol	200 or less	200–239	240 and above
LDL cholesterol ("bad cholesterol")	130 or less	130–159	160 and above
Triglycerides	200 or less	200–399	400 and above

The desirable level of HDL cholesterol ("good cholesterol") is 60 mg/dL or *above*.

Blood Pressure Levels for People without Heart Disease

Blood Pressure	Good	Normal	Borderline	High
Systolic (when the heart contracts and pumps blood out.)	120 or less	120–130	131–140	141 and higher
Diastolic (between beats, as your heart fills with blood again.)	80 or less	80–85	86–90	91 and higher

shortness of breath, dizziness, headaches, and sweating), the disorder is more difficult to treat. Untreated hypertension is the leading cause of stroke and also greatly increases the risk of heart attack, heart failure, and kidney failure.

Other types of cardiovascular disease include heart failure, arrhythmias, and valvular disease. While a heart attack occurs because of an interruption in blood flow *to* the heart, *heart failure* is characterized by inadequate blood flow *from* the heart—the heart fails to pump enough blood to meet the body's needs. Symptoms include fatigue, poor color, shortness of breath, and edema (swelling due to the accumulation of fluid in the body's tissues), especially around the ankles.

Arrhythmias are disturbances in the normal rhythm of the heartbeat. There are different kinds of arrhythmias. Some are quite dangerous—even immediately life threatening—while others may be merely annoying (or scarcely noticeable), and pose no particular danger.

Valvular disease is a term for disorders that impair the functioning of one or more of the heart's valves. It may be caused by congenital defect, or it may be the consequence of illness such as rheumatic fever or endocarditis (infection of the heart muscle). *Mitral valve proplapse* (MVP) is a condition in which the mitral valve, which controls blood flow from the left atrium to the left ventricle (the heart's main pumping chamber), protrudes too far into the left atrium while it is pumping. In many cases, this causes no symptoms at all, although some people experience occasional fatigue, dizziness, palpitations, and/or vague chest pain. Mitral valve prolapse also causes a distinctive sound that a skilled physician can identify by means of a stethoscope. This condition is now known to be rarer than was once thought. And for most of those who do have MVP, it is not thought to lead to severe complications.

Unfortunately, despite remarkable new technology for both diagnosis and treatment of heart conditions, the first sign of cardiovascular disease may be a life-threatening calamity. Disorders of the cardiovascular system are often far advanced before they become symptomatic. An estimated 25 percent of people who have heart attacks have no previous symptoms of heart trouble.

Cardiovascular disease is not an inevitable result of aging. Many preventive measures can be taken to avoid heart disease. Controllable factors that can contribute to heart disease include smoking, high blood pressure, excessive alcohol consumption, elevated serum cholesterol, a type-A personality, stress, obesity, a sedentary lifestyle, and diabetes. You *can* alter your lifestyle to keep your heart healthy.

HEART FUNCTION SELF-TEST

Your heart is the most important muscle in your body. A simple pulse test can help you determine how well your heart is functioning. The best time to check your pulse is first thing in the morning. The heart rate should be between 60 and 100 beats per minute. To take your pulse, place the first two fingers of your right hand between the bone and tendon of your left wrist. Count the beats for fifteen seconds, and then multiply by four to find the beats per minute. If your pulse remains rapid, consult your health care provider to rule out problems. A chronically high pulse rate is often a precursor of hypertension. Taken daily, this pulse test can forewarn you of oncoming illness.

As the most active muscle in the body, the heart requires proper nutrition. Poor nourishment has a profound effect on the heart, and research has shown that as people age, their eating habits get worse, thus increasing their risk of cardiovascular disease.

NUTRIENTS

SUPPLEMENT	SUGGESTED DOSAGE	COMMENTS
Essential		
Coenzyme Q$_{10}$	50–100 mg 3 times daily.	Increases oxygenation of heart tissue. Has been shown to prevent recurrences in individuals who have had a heart attack.
plus Coenzyme A from Coenzyme-A Technologies	As directed on label.	Can streamline metabolism, increase energy, support adrenal glands, process fats, remove toxins from the body, boost the immune system, and improve overall physical and mental processes.
Kyolic-EPA from Wakunaga or	As directed on label.	Reduces triglyceride levels in the blood.
essential fatty acids (black currant seed oil, flaxseed oil, primrose oil, and salmon oil are good sources)	As directed on label.	Helps prevent hardening of the arteries. If you use a fish oil, use a product with vitamin E added to prevent rancidity.
L-Arginine	As directed on label. Take with carbohydrates rather than protein, which inhibits absorption.	Improves blood flow.
Vitamin C with bioflavonoids and L-lysine	1,000 mg 3 times daily.	Extremely important as a regulator of high blood pressure.
Very Important		
Bio-Cardiozyme Forte from Biotics Research or	1 tablet 3 times daily, on an empty stomach.	A complex that strengthens the heart muscle.
Heart Science from Source Naturals	As directed on label.	Contains antioxidants, cholesterol-fighters, herbs, and vitamins that work together to protect the heart and promote cardiovascular function.
Calcium and magnesium	1,500–2,000 mg daily, in divided doses, after meals and at bedtime. 750–1,000 mg daily, in divided doses, after meals and at bedtime. Take with 50 mg vitamin B$_6$.	Important in the proper functioning of the cardiac muscle. Use chelate forms. Vital for a healthy heart. Connected to over 300 enzyme actions controlling glucose, proteins, and fats.
Cardio Logic from Wakunaga	As directed on label.	Increases the oxygenation of heart tissue.

Supplement	Suggested Dosage	Comments
L-Carnitine	500 mg twice daily, on an empty stomach. Take with 50 mg vitamin B$_6$ and 100 mg vitamin C for better absorption.	Reduces fat and triglyceride levels in the blood. Increases oxygen uptake and stress tolerance.
Lecithin granules or capsules	1 tbsp 3 times daily, before meals. 2,400 mg 3 times daily, with meals. Take with vitamin E (see below).	Acts as a fat emulsifier.
Liquid Kyolic with B$_1$ and B$_{12}$ from Wakunaga and	2 capsules 3 times daily.	Lowers blood pressure and thins the blood.
Kyo-Green from Wakunaga	As directed on label.	Concentrated barley and wheat-grass juice; contains nutrients needed for healing and prevention of heart disease.
Lycopene plus lutein	As directed on label. As directed on label.	Carotenoids that lower LDL cholesterol ("bad cholesterol").
Pantethine	As directed on label.	A derivative of pantothenic acid that reduces LDL cholesterol.
Phosphatidyl choline or lipotropic factors	As directed on label. As directed on label.	Reduces fat and triglyceride levels in the blood.
Pycnogenol	As directed on label.	Found to be more effective than aspirin in reducing buildup of platelets in the arteries, a major risk factor in heart disease.

Important

Supplement	Suggested Dosage	Comments
Aerobic Heart from Aerobic Life Industries	As directed on label.	Contains vitamins B$_6$ and B$_{12}$, folic acid, and trimethylglycine, all of which help to reduce homocysteine levels.
Chitosan	As directed on label.	A polysaccharide derived from shellfish that has been shown to reduce blood cholesterol levels.
Dimethylglycine (DMG) (Aangamik DMG from FoodScience of Vermont)	50 mg 4 times daily.	Promotes the utilization of oxygen.
Niacin plus chromium picolinate	As directed on label. As directed on label.	Lower LDL cholesterol.
Potassium	99 mg daily.	Needed for electrolyte balance, especially if taking cortisone or blood pressure medication.
Red yeast rice (Cholestin from Pharmanex)	As directed on label.	Contains lovastatin, which has been proven to reduce cholesterol levels (synthetic lovastatin is often prescribed for this purpose).
Selenium	200 mcg daily. If you are pregnant, do not exceed 40 mcg daily.	Deficiency has been linked with heart disease. Destroys free radicals in the heart.
Superoxide dismutase (SOD)	As directed on label.	A powerful antioxidant.
Taurine Plus from American Biologics	1,000 mg daily. Take with 50 mg vitamin B$_6$ and 100 mg vitamin C for better absorption.	Helps stabilize the heartbeat and correct cardiac arrhythmias. An important antioxidant and immune regulator, necessary for white blood cell activation and neurological function. Use the sublingual form.

Supplement	Suggested Dosage	Comments
Vitamin E	Start with 100–200 IU daily and increase slowly, adding 100 IU each week until daily dosage is 800–1,000 IU. If you take an anticoagulant drug, do not exceed 400 IU daily.	Strengthens the immune system and heart muscle, improves circulation, and destroys free radicals. Use d-alpha-tocopherol form. *Caution:* Use this supplement only under the supervision of a physician.

Helpful

Supplement	Suggested Dosage	Comments
Copper	As directed by physician.	Deficiency may be linked to some heart problems.
Kelp	1,000–1,500 mg daily, with meals.	A rich source of important vitamins, minerals, and trace elements.
Melatonin	2–3 mg daily, taken 2 hours or less before bedtime.	A powerful antioxidant that may help prevent stroke and also aids sleep.
Multienzyme complex (Inflazyme Forte from American Biologics) plus bromelain	As directed on label. Take between meals. 300 mg daily.	To aid digestion.
Octacosanol and/or wheat germ	As directed on label. As directed on label.	Improves endurance; relieves muscle pain.
Sea mussel	As directed on label.	A source of protein that aids in the functioning of the cardiovascular system.
Trimethylglycine (TMG)	As directed on label.	TMG converts homocysteine into methionine. SAMe is a byproduct of this conversion.
Vitamin B complex plus extra vitamin B$_1$ (thiamine) and vitamin B$_3$ (niacin) and vitamin B$_6$ (pyridoxine) and folic acid	50 mg of each major B vitamin 3 times daily, with meals (amounts of individual vitamins in a complex will vary). 50 mg daily. 50 mg daily. Do not exceed a total of 200 mg daily if you have a history of rheumatic heart disease or other valvular heart problem. 50 mg daily. 400 mcg daily.	B vitamins work best when taken together. Lowers cholesterol and improves circulation. *Caution:* Do not take niacin if you have a liver disorder, gout, or high blood pressure. Deficiency has been linked to heart disease. Extremely important for formation of red blood cells and neurotransmitters. Studies have shown that deficiencies of B$_6$ and folic acid may lead to an increase in levels of homocysteine levels, an amino acid that has been linked to heart disease.

HERBS

❏ Citrin, an extract from the plant *Garcinia cambogia*, inhibits the synthesis of fatty acids in the liver, thus helping to prevent the accumulation of potentially dangerous fats in the body.

❏ Cordyceps, a Chinese herb, can slow the heart rate, increase blood supply to the arteries and heart, and lower blood pressure.

❑ Ginkgo biloba can benefit the cardiovascular system by preventing the formation of free radicals. Take a ginkgo extract containing 24-percent ginkgo flavone glycosides.

❑ Grape seed extract with oligomeric proanthocyanidins (OPCs) may lower high blood pressure, which can cause heart disease.

❑ Hawthorn increases blood flow and lowers blood pressure.

❑ Sanhelio's Circu Caps from Health From The Sun is an herbal combination formula that has given good results.

❑ People with cardiovascular disease may benefit from suma tea. Take 3 cups of this herbal tea daily with ginkgo biloba extract as directed on the product label.

❑ Other herbs and herbal products beneficial for cardiovascular disorders include barberry, black cohosh, butcher's broom, cayenne (capsicum), dandelion, ginseng, SP-8 Hawthorn Motherwort Blend from Solaray, and valerian root.

Caution: Do not use barberry or black cohosh during pregnancy. Do not use ginseng if you have high blood pressure.

❑ *Avoid* the herbs ephedra (ma huang) and licorice; they can cause a rise in blood pressure.

RECOMMENDATIONS

❑ If you experience any of the symptoms of a heart attack, contact your doctor or go *immediately* to the emergency room of the nearest hospital, even if symptoms last only a few minutes. Half of all heart attack deaths occur within three to four hours of the onset of the attack, so a person suffering from a heart attack requires immediate medical attention.

❑ Make sure your diet is well balanced and contains plenty of fiber. Some studies have found that among the sources of dietary fiber—cereal, vegetables, and fruits—that fiber from breakfast cereals appears to be the most beneficial.

❑ Eat plenty of raw foods. For protein, eat broiled fish and skinless turkey and chicken, which are low in fat.

❑ Include garlic and onions in your diet. They contain compounds that help to reduce serum cholesterol levels.

❑ Eat plenty of fresh fruits and vegetables. An eight-year study of almost 40,000 men found that men who ate five or more servings of fruits and vegetables each day had a 39-percent lower risk of stroke than those who did not.

❑ Add raw nuts (except peanuts), olive oil, pink salmon, trout, tuna, Atlantic herring, and mackerel to your diet. These foods contain essential fatty acids.

❑ Do not consume stimulants, such as coffee and black tea, that contain caffeine. Studies show that coffee increases stress hormones in the body, putting coffee drinkers at greater risk of heart disease. Also avoid tobacco, alcohol, chocolate, sugar, butter, red meat, fats (particularly animal fats and hydrogenated oils), fried foods, processed and refined foods, soft drinks, spicy foods, and white flour products, such as white bread.

❑ Drink steam-distilled water only, and get at least eight 8-ounce glasses every day. It is recommended that you drink at least 64 ounces of water a day. One study found that men who drank at least five glasses of water every day had a 51-percent lower risk of heart disease than those who did not. For women, the risk of heart disease was 35 percent lower.

❑ Eliminate *all* sources of sodium from your diet. Read all labels and avoid those food products that have "soda," "sodium," or the symbol "Na" on the label. These indicate that the product contains sodium. Some foods and food additives that should be avoided on a salt-free diet include:

• Monosodium glutamate or MSG (Accent flavor enhancer).

• Baking soda.

• Canned vegetables.

• Commercially prepared foods.

• Diet soft drinks.

• Foods with mold inhibitors.

• Foods with preservatives.

• Meat tenderizers.

• Saccharin (found in Sweet'n Low) and products containing saccharin.

• Some medicines and dentifrices (tooth care products).

• Softened water.

❑ If you take an anticoagulant (blood thinner) such as warfarin (Coumadin) or heparin, or even aspirin, limit your intake of foods high in vitamin K. Eating foods containing vitamin K increases the blood's tendency to clot, so they should be eaten only in small quantities. Foods that are rich in vitamin K include alfalfa, broccoli, cauliflower, egg yolks, liver, spinach, and all dark green vegetables. To enhance the effect of anticoagulants, eat more of the following: wheat germ, vitamin E, soybeans, and sunflower seeds.

❑ Learn all about any drugs that have been prescribed for you. Know what to do in case of an emergency. Keep emergency and ambulance numbers easily accessible. If you have a heart condition, someone close to you should know what to do if cardiac arrest occurs. Make sure your loved one knows how to do cardiac massage and mouth-to-mouth breathing. The American Red Cross and many local hospitals offer training in these techniques.

❑ Keep your weight down. Obesity is a risk factor for heart attacks and high blood pressure. Get regular moderate exercise.

Caution: If you are over thirty-five and/or have been

271

Common Heart Problems and Procedures

If either you or a loved one has heart trouble, you can better understand and participate in treatment if you familiarize yourself with the following medical terms that may be used by your physician:

- **Aneurysm.** A spot in a blood vessel where the wall becomes thin and bulges outward as blood presses against it. If it ruptures, circulation is disrupted. Depending on the location of the aneurysm, the consequences of this can be grave. If detected in time, aneurysms can be repaired surgically in many cases.

- **Angina pectoris.** Pain or heavy pressure in the chest that is caused by an insufficient supply of oxygen to the heart tissue. This chest pain may be severe or mild and is usually associated with physical exertion and relieved by rest. It can be a warning sign of impending heart attack.

- **Angiogram.** A diagnostic picture produced by injecting into the heart and/or blood vessels a type of dye that is visible on x-ray. It may be done to diagnose valvular disease, blood vessel blockage, and other conditions.

- **Angioplasty.** A procedure in which a small balloon is inserted into a blocked or partially blocked artery and then inflated. This compresses the plaque on the vessel wall, widening the artery and allowing more blood to flow through it.

- **Aorta.** The main channel for arterial circulation; the large artery into which oxygenated blood is pumped by the heart.

- **Aortic stenosis (AS).** A condition in which the aortic valve is narrowed, restricting blood flow from the heart into the aorta. It can result from congenital malformation of the valve or from damage, such as from rheumatic fever. Symptoms, which may begin in early childhood, include fainting, chest pain, and shortness of breath, especially with exertion.

- **Arrhythmia.** Disruption in the natural rhythm of the heartbeat caused by improper functioning of electrical system cells in the heart. There are different kinds of arrhythmias. *Palpitations* is a term that refers to the feeling of a pounding heartbeat, whether regular or irregular. *Tachycardia* is an abnormal increase in the resting heart rate; *bradycardia* is the opposite, an abnormally slow heart rate. *Ectopic beats* are premature beats (often felt as "skipped" beats). *Flutter* and *fibrillation* are situations in which the normal steady beating of the heart are converted by electrical error into a rapid twitching of the heart muscle. This ineffective functioning results in an insufficient supply of blood being carried to the body's tissues.

- **Cardiac arrest.** Cardiac arrest occurs when the heart stops beating. When this happens, the blood supply to the brain is cut off and the person loses consciousness. A person in apparent good health who experiences cardiac arrest usually has unsuspected coronary artery disease.

- **Cardiomegaly.** The medical term for enlargement of the heart. If the heart is unable to function effectively, as in heart failure, or if there is too much resistance to the normal pumping of blood through the blood vessels, as in high blood pressure, the body attempts to increase the strength of the heart by increasing its size. Cardiomegaly is characteristic of a number of different heart disorders. It is also known as *cardiac hypertrophy.*

- **Cardiomyopathy.** Any of a group of diseases of the heart muscle that result in impaired heart function and, ultimately, heart failure. Cardiomyopathies are classified according to characteristic physical changes in the heart, such as enlargement of the heart, dilation of one or more of the heart's chambers, or rigidity of the heart muscle. These disorders may be related to inherited defects or may be caused by any of a number of different diseases. Often, the cause is unknown.

- **Cardioversion.** A procedure used to correct arrythmia, in which electrical current is applied to the heart to restore normal rhythm.

- **Carditis.** Inflammation of the heart muscle. This can result from infection or from an inflammatory response, as in rheumatic fever, and it can lead to permanent heart damage if not treated.

- **Carotid artery.** The major artery to the brain.

- **Catheterization.** A procedure sometimes used to diagnose the condition of the heart and/or circulatory system and, in some cases, to treat cardiovascular disease. A hollow, flexible tube called a catheter is inserted by means of a very fine flexible wire into a blood vessel somewhere in the body (usually the arm, neck, or leg), and from there is threaded through the blood vessel to the heart or other location being investigated. Catheterization can be used to detect (and in some cases to treat) arterial blockage, to discover malformations of the heart, and to study electrical conduction in the heart, among other things.

- **Claudication.** Cramplike pains in the legs as a result of poor circulation to the leg muscle. This usually occurs as a result of atherosclerosis.

- **Congenital heart defect.** A heart defect that is present at birth, though not necessarily inherited.

- **Congestive heart failure.** A condition of chronic heart failure that results in fluid accumulation in the lungs, labored breathing after even mild exertion, and edema (swelling) in the ankles and feet.

- **Coronary arteries.** The arteries that supply blood to the heart.

- **Coronary artery disease (CAD).** Atherosclerosis of the coronary arteries.

- **Echocardiogram.** A procedure in which ultrasound technology is used to form an image of the heart. It is used to detect structural and functional abnormalities, enlargement or inflammation of the heart, and other conditions.

- **Electrocardiogram (ECG or EKG).** A diagnostic test that tracks electrical impulses in the heart.

- **Embolism.** A circulatory condition in which a foreign object such as air, tissue, gas, or a piece of a tumor is transported around the body and becomes trapped in a blood vessel, obstructing the flow of blood.

- **Endoarteritis obliterans.** Inflammation of the arterial walls that narrows the passage and obstructs the flow of blood.

- **Endocarditis.** Inflammation of the endocardium, the membrane surrounding the heart muscle, usually as a result of bacterial infection. Endocarditis is not uncommon in persons with compromised immune systems, such as those with HIV and AIDS. It also can occur as a complication of surgery to replace defective heart valves. This disorder can result in permanent heart damage.

- **Fibrillation.** An irregular heartbeat characterized by a rapid twitching or vibrating of heart muscle rather than slow, steady beats. Atrial fibrillation can be episodic or chronic, even constant. Symptoms may include dizziness, light-headedness, and general weakness. Ventricular fibrillation is a medical emergency that can lead rapidly to loss of consciousness and death. It most often is a complication of heart attack.

- **Gated blood pool scan.** A diagnostic test in which a small amount of radioactive tracer is injected to "tag" red blood cells, which are then tracked as they progress through the heart, creating a series of pictures that show the size and shape of the heart, the motion of the heart wall, and the heart's pumping efficiently. The test can be done while you are resting or during exercise. It is also known as multi-unit gated analysis (MUGA).

- **Heart attack.** The medical term for a heart attack is *myocardial infarction* (MI). This refers to the formation of *infarcts* (areas of local tissue death or decay) in the *myocardium* (heart muscle). Infarction occurs when the blood supply to an area of the heart is cut off, usually as a result of a blood clot that blocks a narrowed coronary artery. Depending on the size and location of the areas affected, a heart attack may be described as mild or severe, but it always involves some irreparable damage to the heart.

- **Heart failure.** This disorder occurs when a damaged heart becomes unable to pump effectively, depriving the body's tissues of adequate oxygen and nutrients to function properly. Heart failure can be either acute (short-term) or chronic, and has a variety of different causes.

- **Heart murmur.** A sound made by the heart that may or may not point to the existence of a heart condition. A diastolic murmur occurs between beats. A systolic murmur occurs during heart contractions.

- **Hematoma.** A collection of blood trapped in the skin, or in an organ, after a trauma or surgery.

- **Holter monitor.** A small device worn on the body that monitors the heart on a twenty-four-hour-hour basis.

- **Hypertension.** High blood pressure

- **Hypotension.** Low blood pressure

- **Ischemic heart disease.** Ischemic heart disease is caused by obstruction of the blood flow to the heart, usually as a result of atherosclerosis. Ischemia (lack of sufficient oxygen) can lead to angina, cardiac arrhythmias, congestive heart failure, or a heart attack.

- **Magnetic resonance spectroscopy (MRS).** Used in conjunction with magnetic resonance imaging (MRI), an imaging test that can show areas of damaged heart muscle. It does this by measuring levels of creatine kinase MB, an enzyme that is severely depleted after a heart attack.

- **Mitral valve prolapse (MVP).** A condition in which the mitral valve, which controls blood flow from the left atrium and left ventricle, protrudes too far into the left atrium between beats. It may or may not cause symptoms, such as dizziness or palpitations. It is not considered dangerous. It may also be called Barlow's syndrome.

- **Pericarditis.** Inflammation of the sac that surrounds the heart.

- **Phlebitis (or thrombophlebitis).** Inflammation of a vein, most often accompanied by a clot. This condition may be caused by trauma to the vessel wall, clots forming in the blood, infection, or long periods of immobility.

- **Positron emission tomography (PET) scan.** A diagnostic test that can be used to assess blood flow through the arteries to the heart.

- **Pulmonary stenosis (PS).** A condition in which the pulmonic valve is narrowed, restricting the flow of blood from the heart to the pulmonary artery, which carries blood from the heart to the lungs. This is most often a congenital defect. It causes a distinctive murmur and may or may not cause symptoms.

- **Rheumatic heart disease.** Damage to the heart caused by rheumatic fever, a complication of infection with group A streptococcus bacteria, the bacteria that cause strep throat. It causes scarring and contracture of heart valves, and can lead to arrhythmias and heart failure.

- **Stress test.** A diagnostic test used to assess blood flow to the heart. The first part of the test involves the injection of a radioactive imaging agent into the arm. About an hour later, the heart is photographed. In the second part of the test, an intravenous line is placed in the arm and an EKG reading is taken as the patient walks on a treadmill. When the heart is working at its hardest, the first part of the test is repeated. Also known as a myocardial perfusion stress test.

- **Stroke.** Interruption of blood flow to the brain. A *hemorrhagic stroke* occurs when there is bleeding in the brain; an *ischemic stroke,* which is more common, is caused by a clot that forms in a blood vessel that supplies the brain, or a clot that moves from another part of the body to the brain.

- **Thrombosis.** The formation of a clot in a blood vessel.

- **Troponin T test.** A blood test that can detect damage to heart muscle from a heart attack. It assesses levels of the protein troponin T, which is released into the bloodstream after a heart attack. This test can detect even the mildest "silent" heart attack.

sedentary for some time, consult with your health care provider before beginning an exercise program.

❏ Avoid stress, and learn stress-management techniques. (*See* STRESS in Part Two.)

CONSIDERATIONS

❏ Defibrillators are devices used to restore a normal rhythm to the heart during a heart attack. Portable defibrillators are available, and are commonly used in aircraft and police cars during emergencies. They are not issued for use at home, however, unless someone in the household is properly trained and unless it is authorized by a physician. Training on the proper use of defibrillators is conducted by both the American Red Cross and the American Heart Association.

❏ The use of a test called cardiokymography (CKG) together with electrocardiograms (ECGs) may help to detect "silent" heart disease. A comparison study revealed that electrocardiograms alone missed 39 percent of heart disease cases. When CKG was used with ECGs, only 8 percent of cases were undetected.

❏ Nitroglycerin, which is sold in sublingual tablet, patch, and lingual spray form, is commonly prescribed to relieve chest pain and to improve the oxygen supply to the heart. This drug is taken at the first sign of chest pain. If dry mouth prevents sublingual nitroglycerin tablets from dissolving, the spray form may be a better choice. Nitroglycerin has some side effects, including headache, weakness, and dizziness. These usually disappear with continued use.

❏ Studies suggest that the hormone dehydroepiandrosterone (DHEA) may help to prevent cardiovascular disease. DHEA therapy has been linked with a 48-percent reduction in death from heart disease in research populations. (*See* DHEA THERAPY in Part Three.)

❏ Controlling high blood pressure, either with drugs or lifestyle changes (or a combination of the two), can prevent, or at least delay, dangerous complications.

❏ It is not recommended that people take up drinking to prevent heart disease, but research has shown that having a small amount of beer, wine, or liquor occasionally may make it more likely that you will avoid heart disease.

❏ Current research indicates that soy isoflavones may enhance coronary blood flow and prevent blocked arteries.

❏ According to some studies, magnesium supplementation can correct some types of irregular heartbeat, and could save the lives of many people with heart trouble.

❏ *Arnica montana, Arsenicum album, Magnesia phosphorica,* and *Spongia tosta* are homeopathic remedies often recommended for angina. They should be used under the direction of a qualified homeopathic physician.

❏ The risks of coronary bypass surgery can be lessened by correcting potassium deficiencies before surgery.

❏ Recent studies have shown a connection between heart disease and infection with *Chlamydia pneumoniae, Helicobacter pylori,* herpesviruses, and, possibly (but not conclusively) bacteria in dental plaque. The inflammatory response, which is associated with the body's defense mechanisms triggered by infection, may affect the arteries and ultimately lead to the deposition of plaque there. More alarming, researchers have found that some adenoviruses, which cause respiratory infections, may cause left ventricular dysfunction that can lead to sudden death. Because of the connection between infection and heart disease, research is being conducted on the use of antibiotics and prevention of heart attacks. Data published in the *Journal of the American Medical Association* indicate that people who had taken either tetracycline or quinolones in the three years preceding this research proved to be at a lower risk for heart attacks.

❏ Research is being conducted into the role of nitric oxide (NO) in the cardiovascular system. NO keeps the surface of blood vessels smooth so that platelets cannot bind together and form potentially dangerous clots. As researchers are aware that too much NO is toxic to the body, studies are being conducted into controlling NO levels.

❏ Transmyocardial laser revascularization is a method of treating refractory angina. In this technique, a laser is used to create holes in the heart in order to increase the flow of blood to deprived areas of the heart.

❏ Substances known as thrombolytic agents, including streptokinase (Streptase) and alteplase (Activase, also known as tissue plasminogen activator [TPA]) have the ability to break up clots. When injected intravenously, they circulate through the arteries, locating and disintegrating blood clots. Studies have shown that thrombolytic therapy within the first six hours of the onset of a heart attack increases the chances of survival. However, this treatment may be contraindicated in people who have peptic ulcers, extremely high blood pressure, a history of stroke, or recent head injury or abdominal surgery.

❏ It is important for women over the age of fifty-five, and women of any age who have gone through menopause, to consider heart disease as a possible cause of chest pain or discomfort. The chest pain may even be mild and less prominent than upper abdominal pain, shortness of breath, or nausea. Studies have shown that women are not as likely as men to receive drugs protecting them against heart disease; that they are less likely to undergo bypass surgery or angioplasty if they have cardiovascular disease; and that, when symptoms of heart trouble occur, they do not go to the hospital for treatment as quickly as men do. Because of these factors, women with cardiovascular disease are more likely to die from it than are men in comparable health.

❏ Research has shown that women with hypothyroidism (underactive thyroid) have a sharply increased risk of developing blockages in the aorta.

❏ The FDA asserts that taking one baby aspirin a day can reduce the risk of heart attack and/or stroke without side effects, although this is disputed by some experts who believe that there is insufficient evidence to support it. If you do use aspirin, keep in mind that it can cause internal bleeding and stomach ulceration.

❏ Allergies may be linked to some heart attacks. When a reaction in the walls of the arteries triggers a spasm in the coronary arteries, a heart attack may result. Allergies can also cause a temporarily rapid pulse. Your pulse rate may increase after you eat certain foods or when you come into contact with particular allergens. Allergy testing is recommended to determine whether you react to certain foods or other allergens. (*See* ALLERGIES in Part Two.)

❏ Women who gain weight around the midsection in their late forties may be experiencing insulin resistance (the beginnings of diabetes), which can lead to heart disease. Your physician can administer a binding protein (BP-1) test to check for insulin resistance.

❏ Being exposed to excessive noise for more than thirty minutes can increase blood pressure considerably.

❏ People who have had a heart attack that resulted in damage to the left ventricle have been shown to have a longer expectancy if given the angiotensin-converting enzyme (ACE) inhibitor trandolapril (Mavik) for at least two years. ACE inhibitors are a type of drug most often used to treat high blood pressure. Other ACE inhibitors include enalapril (Vasotec) and ramipril (Altace). These drugs stop the formation of a natural chemical, angiotensin II, that narrows the blood vessels. (Angiotensin II inhibitors block the action, rather than the formation, of the same chemical.) Possible side effects are constipation, dry mouth, decreased sexual desire or impotence, and a decrease in mental function.

❏ Other drugs often prescribed for people with high blood pressure include beta-blockers, calcium channel blockers, central-acting agents, and diuretics. Beta-blockers allow the heart to beat more slowly and with less force. Side effects can include a decrease in left ventricular function, a decrease in sexual desire in women, and impotence in men. Calcium channel blockers, also known as calcium antagonists, relax the blood vessel muscle. Possible side effects are sexual dysfunction, dryness of the mouth, muscle pain, and heart arrhythmia. Central-acting agents (central adrenergic inhibitors) act on the brain, preventing the nervous system from increasing the heart rate and narrowing the blood vessels. Diuretics, also known as water pills, help the kidneys get rid of sodium and water, thus reducing the volume of blood coursing around the body. Possible side effects of diuretics include dehydration, diabetes, fainting spells, and possible heart and kidney malfunctions.

❏ Anticoagulant (blood-thinning) drugs, such as warfarin (Coumadin), are often prescribed for those in particular danger of developing blood clots, such as people who are bedridden, cancer patients (the formation of blood clots containing cancer cells that may colonize other parts of the body is a concern), and people with certain types of cardiac arrhythmias. Studies show that, for those in peril of recurring clots, blood-thinning drugs should be taken for at least two years. Vitamin E and aspirin also make an effective blood-thinning combination. All three of these kinds of agents should *not* be taken at the same time, however, as this might cause severe bleeding.

❏ Men taking medication for hypertension can suffer from erectile dysfunction (ED) as a side effect. The anti-impotence drug sildenafil (Viagra), once thought to be dangerous for such individuals, may in fact be a viable option for those with high blood pressure, researchers say. It is advisable to consult your physician to determine if your medication for high blood pressure has lowered your blood pressure too much, and if any of your medications contain nitrates. The combination of nitrates and sildenafil can cause dangerously low blood pressure. Your doctor may also suggest a stress test before he or she makes a decision about prescribing sildenafil.

❏ For further information on cardiovascular disease, you can consult the American Heart Association or the National Heart, Lung, and Blood Institute (*see* HEALTH AND MEDICAL ORGANIZATIONS in the Appendix).

❏ *See also* ARTERIOSCLEROSIS; CIRCULATORY PROBLEMS; HEART ATTACK; and HIGH BLOOD PRESSURE, all in Part Two, and CHELATION THERAPY in Part Three.

Carpal Tunnel Syndrome

Almost unheard of only a generation ago, carpal tunnel syndrome (CTS) has rapidly become a bane of modern existence. It is one of many injuries called repetitive strain injuries (RSIs), which include trigger finger, nerve spasms, and carpal tunnel syndrome. CTS is the term used to describe a set of symptoms that occur when the median nerve in the wrist is compressed or damaged. The median nerve controls the thumb muscles, and is also responsible for sensation felt in the thumb, the palm, and the first three fingers of the hand. The carpal (from the Greek word *karpos*, meaning "wrist") tunnel is a very small opening about one-quarter inch below the surface of the wrist through which the median nerve passes. The median nerve is vulnerable to compression or injury from a number of sources—swelling due to pregnancy or water retention, pressure from bone spurs, diabetes, bone dislocation or fracture, inflammatory arthritis, or even tendinitis.

CTS is associated with repetitive wrist motion injury, which is linked to continuous rapid use of the fingers. Once considered an occupational hazard affecting only supermarket checkout clerks and bookkeepers, CTS did not become widely known until the 1980s, when personal computers came to dominate the workplace. Today, CTS is commonplace among people who use computers extensively. Carpal tunnel syndrome can also be caused by strong, steady vibrations that shake the wrist for long periods (such as using a jackhammer or chain saw). Other people whose occupations have been linked to CTS include assembly line workers, athletes, drivers, hairstylists, musicians, restaurant servers, and writers. Although CTS affects both sexes, women between the ages of twenty-nine and sixty-two seem to be affected more than any other segment of the population. People with square wrists (wrists that are roughly as deep as they are wide) are said to be more disposed to getting CTS than people whose wrists are wider than they are deep. Whatever the cause, an estimated 1.2 million people a year consult a physician about this injury. Factors that increase the risk of CTS include menopause, obesity, Raynaud's disease, pregnancy, hypothyroidism, and diabetes mellitus.

Symptoms of CTS can range from mild numbness and faint tingling to excruciating pain accompanied by a crippling atrophy of the muscles in the thumb. Most commonly, it is experienced as burning, tingling, or numbness in the thumb and the first three fingers. (The little finger is spared because it receives its nerve impulses from outside the carpal tunnel.) The tingling is often referred to as feeling similar to the "pins and needles" associated with a limb "falling asleep," and it also involves a gradual weakening of the thumb. In the beginning, symptoms are often intermittent, but they become persistent as the condition worsens. CTS can affect one or both hands. Symptoms are often worse at night or in the morning, when circulation slows down. Pain may spread to the forearm and, in severe cases, to the shoulder. Carpal tunnel syndrome may have its genesis in either the neck, upper back, and/or shoulders. A visit to a chiropractor or osteopath may help in determining whether this is the case.

Not all nerve entrapment problems are in the carpal tunnel area. Though far less common, entrapment of the ulnar nerve, located in the elbow, produces symptoms almost identical to those of CTS. This condition can be very painful and disabling. It can also be misdiagnosed as myofascial dysfunction. Myofascial dysfunction stems from the overuse or misuse of muscles. It is not connected with nerve damage.

CTS SELF-TEST

A simple self-test can help you determine whether you have carpal tunnel syndrome.

Place the backs of your hands together, with the fingers pointing straight down and the wrists at a 90-degree angle, so that your elbows point straight out to the sides. If holding this position for over a minute brings on symptoms, you probably have CTS. If your job or hobby causes you to develop a burning sensation, numbness, or clumsiness affecting the first three fingers of one or both hands, chances are that CTS is the culprit

This self-test is not foolproof, however. The only truly conclusive tests for CTS is *electromyography* (EMG), which involves transmitting electrical impulses through the arm. The nerve impulses that direct motion are nothing more than a very low voltage current. Normal nerve impulse transmission occurs at a speed of approximately 136 meters per second, which is fast enough to appear instantaneous to us. If nerves are damaged or entrapped by swollen tissue, however, they cannot transmit electrical neural impulses at the normal rate of speed. If you are found to have a neuro-transmission speed of only 90 to 95 meters per second, nerve damage or compression is strongly suggested.

NUTRIENTS

SUPPLEMENT	SUGGESTED DOSAGE	COMMENTS
Essential		
Coenzyme Q$_{10}$ plus Coenzyme A from Coenzyme-A Technologies	30–90 mg daily.	Improves tissue oxygenation.
Lecithin granules or capsules	1 tbsp 3 times daily, before meals. 1,200 mg 3 times daily, before meals.	Supplies choline and inositol for nerve function. A fat emulsifier.
Vitamin B complex	100 mg of each major B vitamin 3 times daily (amounts of individual vitamins in a complex will vary).	B vitamins are essential in nerve function.
plus extra vitamin B$_1$ (thiamine) and	50 mg 3 times daily for 12 weeks.	Increases the uptake of vitamin B$_6$ and improves tissue oxygenation.
vitamin B$_6$ (pyridoxine)	100 mg twice daily for 12 weeks. Do not exceed this amount, or nerve damage may result.	A potent diuretic.
Zinc	50 mg daily. Do not exceed a total of 100 mg daily from all supplements.	Enhances healing. Use zinc gluconate lozenges or OptiZinc for best absorption.
Helpful		
Grape seed extract	As directed on label.	A powerful antioxidant and anti-inflammatory.
Kelp	As directed on label.	Beneficial to nerves.
Manganese	As directed on label. Take separately from calcium.	Helpful for nerve problems.
Multivitamin and mineral complex	As directed on label.	For general nutritional supplementation. Use a formula without iron.
Primrose oil or Kyolic-EPA from Wakunaga	As directed on label. As directed on label.	Contain essential fatty acids necessary for nerve function.
Vitamin A with mixed carotenoids	25,000 IU daily. If you are pregnant, do not exceed 10,000 IU daily.	Important antioxidants.
Vitamin C with bioflavonoids	1,000 mg 4 times daily.	Important in healing. A potent antioxidant. Aids in reducing swelling.
Vitamin E	400 IU daily.	An important antioxidant. Use d-alpha-tocopherol form.

HERBS

❏ Aloe vera, devil's claw, yarrow, and yucca are helpful for restoring flexibility and reducing inflammation.

❏ Bromelain and boswella both reduce inflammation and swelling.

❏ Butcher's broom helps to relieve inflammation.

❏ Capsicum relieves pain and is a catalyst for other herbs.

❏ Corn silk and parsley are natural diuretics that help keep swelling down.

❏ CT Cream from Biomax Laboratories contains both herbal and pharmacological agents, including arnica extract, camphor, vitamin B_6, and choline bitartrate. It is said to reduce inflammation and improve the health of the nerves.

❏ Ginkgo biloba, taken in either tea or capsule form, is beneficial for improving circulation and also aids nerve function.

❏ Gravel root tightens and soothes tissues and acts as an antiseptic.

❏ Marshmallow root soothes and softens tissues and promotes healing.

❏ Rhus toxicodendron, a homeopathic remedy, helps in any conditions where stiffness exists in a joint when it is first used. This substance is also helpful in soothing restlessness at night and in injuries caused by overuse of the joints.

❏ St. John's wort stimulates circulation and helps to restore local nerve impulse transmission.

❏ Skullcap relieves muscle spasms and pain.

❏ Venaforce from Bioforce, which contains standardized extract of horse chestnut, helps improve circulation.

Minimizing the Risk of Carpal Tunnel Syndrome

Carpal tunnel syndrome is an occupational hazard for anyone whose job involves making repetitive movements with the hands and/or fingers. In this age of computers, that means virtually anyone who works in an office, as well as assembly line workers, bookkeepers, cashiers, jackhammer operators, musicians, and many others. Spending a great deal of time engaging in a hobby such as knitting and needlework can also cause problems. No matter what your occupation, the following measures are recommended to help you reduce the risk of developing this painful and disabling condition:

• Use your whole hand and all of your fingers when you grip an object.

• Whenever possible, use a tool instead of flexing your wrists forcibly.

• Make sure your posture is correct. For keyboard tasks, sit straight in your chair with your body tilted slightly back. Raise or lower your chair so that your knees are bent at a right angle and your feet are flat on the floor. Your wrists and hands should be straight and your forearms parallel to the floor. Keep your wrists and hands consistently in a straight line.

• Keep your elbows bent. This lessens the load close to your body and reduces the amount of force required to do your job. Give yourself elbow room to allow you to use as much of your arm as you can while keeping your wrist straight. Use your whole arm while performing tasks in order to minimize the stress on your elbow.

• Adjust your computer screen so that it is about two feet away from you and just below your line of sight.

• Use arm rests that attach to the chair to keep your wrists from flexing too much.

• If the relative positions of your desk, chair, and keyboard do not allow you to keep your wrists straight while keyboarding, the use of a "wrist rest" pad in front of the keyboard is highly recommended to alleviate pressure on the carpal tunnel.

• Slow your rhythm while varying wrist and hand movements.

• Take a break from handwork for a few minutes every hour.

• Shake out your hands periodically throughout the day.

• Perform simple stretching exercises before your daily tasks to improve overall circulation and aid in warming up the muscles. The American Physical Therapy Association recommends these exercises:

1. Resting one forearm on a table, grasp the fingertips of that hand and pull back gently. Hold this position for five seconds, then repeat the exercise with the other hand.

2. Press the palms flat on a table, as if doing a push-up. Lean forward to stretch the forearm muscles and the wrists.

• Another recommended gentle exercise is done by rotating the wrist. Move your hands around in a circle for about two minutes, thoroughly stretching the muscles of the hand. This helps to restore circulation and improve the posture of the wrist.

• Do strengthening exercises. Place a rubber band around the fingers to provide resistance, and then open and close the fingers. Three times a day, do a set of ten repetitions with each hand.

❏ Wintergreen oil aids in pain relief and circulation to the muscles.

❏ Zhen Gu Shi, a potent Chinese liniment for inflamed joints, is good for easing CTS symptoms. It is also sold in many Asian markets.

RECOMMENDATIONS

❏ Consume foods that contain or lead to the production of oxalic acid in moderation only. These include asparagus, beets, beet greens, eggs, fish, parsley, rhubarb, sorrel, spinach, Swiss chard, and vegetables of the cabbage family. Large amounts of oxalic acid can promote joint problems.

❏ Eat half of a fresh pineapple daily for one to three weeks, until relief is achieved. Pineapple contains bromelain, which reduces pain and swelling. Only fresh pineapple is effective. Bromelain is also available in supplement form.

❏ Eat foods high in vitamin B_6, such as bananas, avocados, potatoes, nuts, bluefin tuna, Atlantic salmon, chicken, whole grains, and sweet potatoes.

❏ Avoid salt and all foods containing sodium. They promote water retention and may aggravate carpal tunnel syndrome. They will also counteract any diuretics that your physician may prescribe.

❏ If you engage in repetitive mechanical tasks, try to reduce the impact on your wrists and hands. *See* Minimizing the Risk of Carpal Tunnel Syndrome, on page 277.

❏ If possible, stop all repetitive finger movements for several days and see if any improvement occurs. If it does, try to rearrange your schedule so that you spend less time in CTS-stimulating activities. If possible, alternate tasks rather than performing a single task for long periods. Fortunately, employers have become more mindful of the possibility of repetitive motion injuries and are often more understanding than they might have been only a few years ago. Many now try to have their employees rotate the tasks they perform so that the risk of injury is reduced.

❏ Maintain ideal weight, and lose weight if necessary. Excess weight results in extra pressure on the carpal tunnel. Losing weight has brought relief to many people with CTS.

❏ Try using *Rhus toxicodendron*, a homeopathic remedy that helps in any conditions in which there is stiffness in a joint when it is first used. This substance is also helpful in soothing restlessness at night and in injuries caused by overuse of the joints.

❏ Use a splint to help prevent flare-ups. Splints are cloth-covered metal or plastic braces that attach to the forearm with an elastic bandage (an Ace bandage or the equivalent) or hook and loop fasteners (Velcro). These devices are available at medical supply houses and many pharmacies. If you cannot find one that fits properly, have one custom-made. Be sure to apply and wear the splint properly; if you don't,

its effectiveness may be reduced or it may even aggravate the problem. Cock your wrist back slightly so that your thumb is parallel to your forearm. Your hand should be in approximately the same position as if it were holding a pen. This position keeps the carpal tunnel as open as possible. Wear the splint as much as possible for several days to see if your symptoms are reduced. Splinting is often very helpful for those who have suffered a repetitive motion injury that results in CTS.

❏ Keep your workplace warm and dry. Cool and/or damp conditions tend to aggravate CTS.

❏ Avoid taking supplements that contain iron. They are suspected of aggravating pain and swelling in joints.

CONSIDERATIONS

❏ If CTS develops as a result of the edema of pregnancy, it usually clears up of its own accord once the baby arrives and the excess fluid of pregnancy disappears.

❏ Physicians treat CTS in a variety of ways, most often with a combination of anti-inflammatory medications, splints, and the recommendation that you avoid any aggravating activity. Sometimes corticosteroid injections in the wrist are used. This treatment is controversial, however, and should not be used unless the pain from CTS is debilitating, since the injections themselves are a source of considerable discomfort.

❏ If weakness develops in the thumb, it is an indication that the median nerve has sustained some amount of damage, and surgical treatment may be recommended. This surgery involves cutting the transverse carpal ligament, a thick, fibrous band that covers part of the carpal tunnel. The surgeon can make either a small incision or a relatively large one. A small incision causes minimal scarring, but it affords the surgeon a very limited area view, which increases the risk of damage to other important structures in the wrist. A larger incision reduces the risk of peripheral damage, but a more prominent scar is usually the result, and the scarring itself may cause some pain and disability. A splint or cast must be worn for two to four weeks following surgery. A less invasive type of surgery, called the *endoscopic technique,* has become popular. This procedure takes only ten minutes and the incision, made in the palm, is tiny. Most people return to work within a few days.

❏ Many doctors maintain that surgery for CTS is too often performed unnecessarily. A second opinion should always be obtained before surgery is agreed to. However, if the second doctor's opinion confirms that surgery is unavoidable, it is best not to put the operation off for too long, as delay may result in permanent nerve damage.

❏ The numbness, tingling, and pain of CTS usually subside within a few days after surgery, but some people find that it takes as much as two years for the symptoms to resolve. When this happens, it is often because the median nerve has sustained some damage and a long time is needed for any nerve regeneration to occur. If surgery is necessary and is put off for too long, the thumb may be left permanently weakened and the mobility of the affected hand may be diminished.

❑ A new treatment for CTS involves the use of a low-energy ("cold") laser to penetrate tissues, stimulate nerves, and increase microcirculation in the affected area.

❑ Additional information about repetitive strain injuries is available from the National Institute for Occupational Safety and Health (*see* HEALTH AND MEDICAL ORGANIZATIONS in the Appendix).

❑ *See also* PAIN CONTROL in Part Three.

Cataracts

See under EYE PROBLEMS.

Cavities

See TOOTH DECAY.

Celiac Disease

Celiac disease (also called celiac sprue) is a chronic digestive disorder that is caused by a hereditary intolerance to gluten. Gluten is a component of wheat (including durum, semolina, and spelt), rye, oats, barley, and related grain hybrids such as triticale and kamut. The cause of celiac disease is unknown, although it is known to affect mostly Caucasians of European descent.

When a person with celiac disease consumes gluten, damage to the small intestine results. It is believed that the body responds to gluten as if it were an antigen, and launches an immune-system attack when it is absorbed by the intestine. This, in turn, causes the lining of the small intestine to swell. As a result, tiny hairlike projections called villi suffer damage and destruction, which impairs the body's ability to absorb vital nutrients. Malabsorption becomes a serious problem, and the loss of vitamins, minerals, and calories results in malnutrition despite an adequate diet. Diarrhea compounds the problem. Because celiac disease impairs digestion, food allergies may also appear.

Celiac disease affects both adults and children, and it can appear at any age. It often appears when a child is first introduced to cereal foods, at around three or four months of age. In others, the disease can be triggered by emotional stress or physical trauma, such as a surgery or pregnancy. The first signs are usually diarrhea, weight loss, and nutritional deficiencies. Other symptoms include nausea; abdominal swelling; large, and, frequently, pale and/or light-yellow-colored, foul-smelling stools that float; depression; fatigue; irritability; muscle cramps and wasting; and joint and/or bone pain. Infants and children may exhibit stunted growth, vomiting, an intense burning sensation in the skin, and a red, itchy skin rash called *dermatitis herpetiformis*. A baby with celiac disease may gain weight more slowly than normal or may lose weight. The infant may have a poor appetite, gas, and offensive-smelling bowel movements. The child is likely to have an anemic, undernourished appearance. Ulcers may develop in the mouth.

If left untreated, celiac disease can be quite serious, even life-threatening. Bone disease, such as osteoporosis, central and peripheral nervous system impairment, seizures caused by inadequate absorption of folic acid, internal hemorrhaging, pancreatic disease, infertility, miscarriages and birth defects, and gynecological disorders are just some of the long-term maladies that can affect those with celiac disease. There is also a risk of developing intestinal lymphoma and other intestinal malignancies. Certain autoimmune disorders also can be associated with celiac disease, including kidney disease (nephrosis), sarcoidosis (the formation of lesions in the lungs, bones, skin, and other places), insulin-dependent diabetes mellitus, systemic lupus erythematosus, thyroid disease, and, rarely, chronic active hepatitis, scleroderma, myasthenia gravis, Addison's disease, rheumatoid arthritis, and Sjögren's syndrome.

Celiac disease is often difficult to diagnose because the symptoms are similar to those of other diseases, such as irritable bowel syndrome, gastric ulcers, and anemia. Advances in blood testing have made it easier to detect celiac disease. A diagnosis based on a blood test should be followed up with a biopsy of intestinal tissue, which is usually an outpatient procedure. However, due to the fact that symptoms are so diverse, and that some people with celiac disease do not show obvious symptoms, many people go a long time before being diagnosed correctly. Because celiac disease is hereditary, if one family member is diagnosed with it, other family members should also be tested.

Celiac disease is much more prevalent than was once believed. Recent studies suggest that as many as 1 in 500 persons in the United States is affected. The incidence may be even higher in many areas of Europe. There is no known cure for celiac disease, but it can be controlled by lifelong adherence to a gluten-free diet.

Unless otherwise specified, the dosages recommended here are for adults. For a child between the ages of twelve and seventeen, reduce the dose to three-quarters of the recommended amount. For a child between six and twelve, use one-half of the recommended dose, and for a child under the age of six, use one-quarter of the recommended amount.

NUTRIENTS

SUPPLEMENT	SUGGESTED DOSAGE	COMMENTS
Essential		
Essential fatty acids (Kyolic-EPA from Wakunaga, flaxseed oil, and primrose oil are good sources)	As directed on label.	Needed for the villi in the intestines.
Free-form amino acid complex	As directed on label.	To supply protein in a form readily available for use by the body.
Glutathione	500 mg 3 times daily.	An amino acid needed for repair of the intestional tract.
Kyo-Dophilus from Wakunaga	As directed on label.	A dairy- and yeast-free probiotic formula to replace the friendly bacteria.
Liquid Kyolic with B_1 and B_{12} from Wakunaga	As directed on label.	Dramatically increases levels of vitamins B_1 and B_{12} for immune enhancement.
Multivitamin and mineral complex with		All nutrients are necessary in balance. Use a wheat- and yeast-free product only.
vitamin A	15,000 IU daily. If you are pregnant, do not exceed 10,000 IU daily.	
and mixed carotenoids	10,000 IU daily.	
and vitamin E	400 IU daily.	
Vitamin B complex injections plus extra	2 cc weekly, or as prescribed by physician.	Necessary for proper digestion. Injections (under a doctor's supervision) are best because they bypass the digestive system. If injections are not available, a sublingual form is recommended. Use a wheat- and yeast-free product.
vitamin B_6 (pyridoxine) or	$1/2$ cc weekly, or as prescribed by physician.	
vitamin B complex	As directed on label.	
Vitamin B_{12} and	1,000–2,000 mcg daily.	Malabsorption of vitamin B_{12} results from celiac disease. Injections may be necessary. If injections are not available, use a lozenge or sublingual form.
folic acid	400–800 mcg daily.	
Important		
N-acetylglucosamine (N-A-G from Source Naturals)	As directed on label.	Forms the basis of complex molecular structures of the mucous membranes of the intestinal lining.
Vitamin K or alfalfa	As directed on label.	Fat-soluble vitamins are not absorbed well in this disorder. See under Herbs, below.
Zinc lozenges	1 15-mg lozenge 5 times daily. Do not exceed a total of 100 mg daily from all supplements.	Needed for immunity and healing.
plus copper	3 mg daily.	Needed to balance with zinc.
Helpful		
Magnesium	750 mg daily.	Helps maintain the body's normal pH balance. Deficiency is common in people with celiac disease.
plus calcium	1,500 mg daily.	Works with magnesium.
Proteolytic enzymes	As directed on label, 3 times daily. Take between meals, on an empty stomach.	Additional digestive enzymes may be needed to aid in breakdown and absorption of foods.
Psyllium seed or flaxseeds or Aerobic Bulk Cleanse (ABC) from Aerobic Life Industries	As directed on label. Take separately from other supplements and medications.	Fiber products not absorbed by the intestines. Drink large amounts of water because the fiber expands to several times its dry volume.
Vitamin C plus bioflavonoids	2,000–5,000 mg daily, in divided doses.	Boosts immune function.
Vitamin D_3	As directed on label.	Stimulates absorption of calcium. People with celiac disease frequently have calcium deficiencies.

HERBS

❏ Alfalfa supplies vitamin K, which is often deficient in those with celiac disease. Take 2,000 to 3,000 milligrams in tablet form daily.

❏ Olive leaf extract and/or goldenseal is helpful for keeping infection down.

Caution: Do not take goldenseal on a daily basis for more than one week at a time, and do not use it during pregnancy. If you have a history of heart disease, diabetes, or glaucoma, use it only under a doctor's supervision.

RECOMMENDATIONS

❏ Avoid any and all foods that contain gluten. Do not eat any products that contain barley, oats, rye, or wheat. Rice and corn can be eaten. Substitute rice, potato, cornmeal, and soy flour for wheat flour. Read all labels carefully. Watch for "hidden" sources of gluten, such as hydrolyzed vegetable protein, textured vegetable protein, hydrolyzed plant protein, and all derivatives of wheat, rye, oats, and barley, including malt, modified food starch, some soy sauces, grain vinegars, binders, fillers, excipients, and "natural flavorings." Do not consume hot dogs, gravies, luncheon meat, beer, mustard, catsup, non-dairy creamer, white vinegar, curry powder, or seasonings. Gluten-free products are available at health food stores.

❏ Eat fresh vegetables, legumes (such as lentils, beans, and peas), rice bran, nuts, sunflower seeds, raisins, figs, and "seedy" fruits, such as strawberries, raspberries, and blackberries. Include in the diet blackstrap molasses, which is high in iron and the B vitamins. People with celiac disease need fiber and foods rich in iron and the B vitamins.

❏ Be sure to chew your foods thoroughly before swallowing. This will improve the intake of nutrients.

❏ Do not eat sugary products, processed foods, dairy products, bouillon cubes, chocolate, and bottled salad dressings.

❏ Celiac disease causes malabsorption of the B vitamins and the fat-soluble vitamins (vitamins A, D, E, and K), so take these nutrients. Note that gluten is found in many nutritional supplements. Read labels carefully, and use supplements that are hypoallergenic, wheat-free, and yeast-free.

❏ If a child develops any of the symptoms of celiac disease, omit all gluten-containing foods from the child's diet and see if the problem clears up. Also eliminate milk, as lactose intolerance can occur with celiac disease. The disease can begin in the first few months of life, depending on the child's diet.

CONSIDERATIONS

❏ Any child who is not thriving could have celiac disease. The disease manifests itself differently with each person. Symptoms can include irritability, fatigue, and/or behavior changes; they do not always involve obvious digestive problems.

❏ A child who gets blisters and sores all over his or her body should be checked for celiac disease.

❏ If celiac disease is suspected, an intestinal biopsy should be performed to make a definitive diagnosis.

❏ Starting a gluten-free diet is challenging because gluten is present in so many foods, including most grains, pasta, cereals, and processed foods. However, people with celiac disease can still eat a varied, well-balanced diet that includes breads and pastas made from potato, rice, soy, or bean flour. Gluten-free products are available from many health food stores and specialty food companies. There are also many cookbooks available for those on a gluten-free diet.

❏ Several studies suggest that people with celiac disease can safely eat oats. However, since oats are frequently processed with other grains, it is difficult to determine whether oats are completely gluten-free. Follow your physician's or dietician's advice about including oats in a gluten-free diet.

❏ It may be necessary to remove milk and milk products from the diet because of a secondary lactase deficiency (see LACTOSE INTOLERANCE in Part Two).

❏ Vitamin K deficiency caused by celiac disease may lead to a hypoprothrombinemia (a lack of clotting factors in the blood). One form of vitamin K is manufactured by "friendly" bacteria in the intestines; another is present in certain foods, especially leafy greens, alfalfa, tomatoes, strawberries, whole grains, and yogurt. Bacteria such as those found in yogurt and acidophilus can also help to restore the intestinal flora necessary for vitamin K production.

❏ Martin F. Kagnoff, M.D., of the University of California at San Diego says that heredity is a vital factor in the development of this disease. He also says that celiac disease often develops in childhood but may trail off in adolescence; in some cases, reappearing in adults in their thirties and forties. Factors that may trigger the onset of celiac disease are emotional stress, physical trauma, a viral infection, pregnancy, or surgery.

❏ A report published in the British medical journal *The Lancet* pointed to a possible connection between celiac disease and epilepsy. Theories as to how the two might be linked include the possibility that endorphin-like substances may be created from wheat gluten and may affect brain metabolism; another possibility is that celiac disease increases intestinal permeability, which in turn allows the absorption of substances that may affect brain chemistry.

❏ Schizophrenia has been observed to occur more often in those with celiac disease. (*See* SCHIZOPHRENIA in Part Two.)

❏ For more information about celiac disease, you can contact the Celiac Disease Foundation (*see* HEALTH AND MEDICAL ORGANIZATIONS in the Appendix). There are also good books available on this subject.

❏ *See also* ALLERGIES and MALABSORPTION SYNDROME in Part Two.

Chemical Allergies

When the body is exposed to certain foreign chemicals, it may respond by producing antibodies to defend itself against the foreign invaders. Virtually any substance can provoke a reaction in some individuals. Some of the environmental contaminants that most frequently cause problems include air pollution; gas, oil, or coal fumes; formaldehyde; chlorine; phenol; carbolic acid; insecticides; disinfectants; paint; hair sprays; household cleaning products; and metals such as nickel, mercury, chrome, and beryllium. Chemical allergies often manifest themselves as skin reactions. Other possible allergic responses to foreign chemicals include watery eyes, ringing in the ears, stuffy nose, diarrhea, nausea, upset stomach, asthma, bronchitis, arthritis, fatigue, eczema, intestinal disorders, depression, and headache. Some people may have a reaction immediately after encountering a chemical allergen; others may not develop a rash for twenty-four hours after coming in contact with the irritant.

The following supplement program is designed to protect you from, and help you cope with, the effects of chemical allergies. Unless otherwise specified, the dosages recommended here are for adults. For a child between the ages of twelve and seventeen, reduce the dose to three-quarters the recommended amount. For a child between six and twelve, use one-half the recommended dose, and for a child under the age of six, use one-quarter the recommended amount.

NUTRIENTS

SUPPLEMENT	SUGGESTED DOSAGE	COMMENTS
Very Important		
Vitamin A plus carotenoid complex with beta-carotene	50,000 IU daily for 10 days, then reduce to 25,000 IU daily. If you are pregnant, do not exceed 10,000 IU daily. 5,000–10,000 IU daily.	Powerful free radical scavengers and immune enhancers. Use emulsion forms for easier assimilation.
plus vitamin E	400–800 IU daily.	A powerful antioxidant. Use d-alpha-tocopherol form.
Vitamin B complex	100–200 mg of each major B vitamin daily (amounts of individual vitamins in a complex will vary).	Allergies hinder absorption of B vitamins. Consider injections (under a doctor's supervision).
plus extra vitamin B$_6$ (pyridoxine)	100 mg 3 times daily.	A natural antihistamine. Also aids in detoxifying foreign substances and eliminating them through the kidneys.
plus niacinamide	500 mg 3 times daily.	Aids circulation. *Caution:* Do not substitute niacin for niacinamide, or toxicity may result.
Vitamin C with bioflavonoids	5,000–20,000 mg daily, in divided doses. *See* ASCORBIC ACID FLUSH in Part Three.	Protects the body from allergens and moderates the inflammatory response.
Important		
Coenzyme Q$_{10}$	60 mg daily.	Helps to counter histamine, a body chemical involved in allergic reactions.
plus Coenzyme A from Coenzyme-A Technologies		Supports the immune system's detoxification of many dangerous substances. Removes toxins from the body.
Pycnogenol or grape seed extract	As directed on label. As directed on label.	Serves as a free radical scavenger and aids in protecting bodily cells from damage.
Selenium	200 mcg daily. If you are pregnant, do not exceed 40 mcg daily.	Essential in immune function and protection of cells.
Superoxide dismutase (SOD) or Cell Guard from Biotec Foods	As directed on label. As directed on label.	A potent free radical scavenger. An antioxidant complex that contains SOD.
Zinc plus copper	50 mg daily. Do not exceed a total of 100 mg daily from all supplements. 3 mg daily.	Important in proper immune function. Use zinc gluconate lozenges or OptiZinc for best absorption. Needed to balance with zinc. Copper is lost when high doses of vitamin C are taken.
Helpful		
Aller Bee-Gone from CC Pollen	As directed on label.	A combination of herbs, enzymes, and nutrients that fight allergic outbreaks.
Dioxychlor from American Biologics	5 drops in water twice daily.	A potent detoxifier.
Garlic (Kyolic from Wakunaga)	2 capsules 3 times daily.	A powerful immunostimulant.

L-Cysteine and L-methionine plus L-glutamic acid	500 mg each daily. Take on an empty stomach with juice or water. Do not take with milk. Take with 50 mg vitamin C for better absorption.	Excellent detoxifiers, especially of the liver. (*See* AMINO ACIDS in Part One.)
Manganese	As directed on label. Take separately from calcium.	Interacts with zinc and copper. Use manganese chelate form.
Pancreatic enzymes and proteolytic enzymes	As directed on label 3 times daily, with meals. As directed on label 3 times daily, between meals.	Both pancreatic and proteolytic enzymes are needed for proper digestion and assimilation of necessary nutrients. Proteolytic enzymes also control inflammation.
Raw thymus glandular	As directed on label.	Important for immune function.
Taurine Plus from American Biologics	500 mg daily.	The most important antioxidant and immune regulator, necessary for white blood cell activitation and neurological function. Use the sublingual form.

HERBS

❑ If you develop a skin rash from exposure to metal in watchbands, earrings, snaps, or other items that come in contact with the skin, try using Calendula Ointment from NatureWorks. Calendula, chamomile, elder flower, and tea tree oil also can be used as a soothing wash on rashes.

RECOMMENDATIONS

❑ The first step in managing chemical allergies is to determine which chemicals are provoking the allergic reaction, then to avoid coming in contact with these chemicals. If the source of the problem is not obvious, see an allergy specialist.

❑ Avoid foods that have been sprayed or that contain artificial colorings (found in some apples and oranges), ripening agents, or protective waxes (found on some apples, cucumbers, and other items). Avoid things containing FD&C Yellow No. 5 dye. Read all food product labels carefully.

❑ Supplement your diet with plenty of fiber. Oat bran is a good source of fiber. Apple pectin also can be a useful addition to your diet. It removes unwanted metals that may trigger allergic reactions.

Note: Always take supplemental fiber separately from other supplements and medications.

CONSIDERATIONS

❑ Mercury and silver in dental fillings can cause allergic reactions as well as heavy metal poisoning. *See* MERCURY TOXICITY in Part Two.

❑ *See also* CHEMICAL POISONING in Part Two.

Chemical Poisoning

Like toxic metals, poisonous chemicals such as chlorine, disinfectants, heavy metals, herbicides, insecticides, petroleum products, and solvents can enter the body and decrease the functioning capacity of its organs. This is chemical poisoning. Some chemicals are absorbed through the skin; others may be inhaled or ingested. The body's immune system is threatened by these chemicals and tries to cleanse the body of the poisons. Damage to internal organs, especially the liver, may occur.

Chronic chemical poisoning occurs most often in people who use or who are exposed to chemicals in their work environments, or who use excessive amounts of chemical sprays. People who live near landfills or certain industrial installations may also be chronically exposed to toxic chemicals. Acute chemical poisoning can result from accidental ingestion of household chemicals (particularly among children) or taking improper or excessive medications.

Unless otherwise specified, the dosages recommended here are for adults. For a child between the ages of twelve and seventeen, reduce the dose to three-quarters the recommended amount. For a child between six and twelve, use one-half the recommended dose, and for a child under the age of six, use one-quarter the recommended amount.

NUTRIENTS

SUPPLEMENT	SUGGESTED DOSAGE	COMMENTS
Very Important		
Free-form amino acid complex	As directed on label twice daily, on an empty stomach.	Helps liver function. Use a sublingual form.
Garlic (Kyolic from Wakunaga)	As directed on label.	Helps to detoxify and cleanse the bloodstream; chelates heavy metals.
Raw liver extract	As directed on label or as prescribed by physician.	Supplies needed B vitamins and iron, and detoxifies chemicals. For severe chemical poisoning, injections (under a doctor's supervision) are best.
Superoxide dismutase (SOD) or	As directed on label.	A powerful free radical destroyer.
Cell Guard from Biotec Foods	As directed on label.	An antioxidant complex that contains SOD.
Vitamin B complex injections	As prescribed by physician.	Protects the liver and bodily functions. Injections (under a doctor's supervision) are best. If injections are not available, use a sublingual form.
plus choline and inositol	50 mg 3 times daily, with meals. 50 mg 3 times daily, with meals.	
Vitamin C with bioflavonoids	5,000–20,000 mg daily, in divided doses. *See* ASCORBIC ACID FLUSH in Part Three.	Protects the body from pollutants and aids in the elimination of toxic substances.
Important		
Grape seed extract	As directed on label.	A powerful antioxidant.
L-Cysteine and L-methionine	500 mg each daily, on an empty stomach. Take with water or juice. Do not take with milk. Take with 50 mg vitamin B_6 and 100 mg vitamin C for better absorption.	To remove toxins and rebuild the body. (*See* AMINO ACIDS in Part One.)
Selenium	200 mcg daily. If you are pregnant, do not exceed 40 mcg daily.	Works with vitamins C and E to detoxify the body.
Vitamin E	400–800 IU daily.	A powerful antioxidant. Use d-alpha-tocopherol form.
Helpful		
Coenzyme Q_{10}	30–60 mg daily.	Aids in rebuilding the immune system and providing oxygen to the tissues.
Dioxychlor from American Biologics	5 drops in water twice daily.	Delivers oxygen to the tissues.
Multivitamin and mineral complex	As directed on label.	All nutrients are needed to aid in strengthening the immune system and lessening toxicity.

RECOMMENDATIONS

❏ To aid recovery, eat a well-balanced diet that is high in fiber. Fiber helps to cleanse the system. Recommended foods include almonds, apricots, bananas, barley, beans, beets, Brazil nuts, brown rice, carrots, dates, fish, garlic, grapes, hazelnuts, lemons, lentils, oatmeal, onions, spinach, and yogurt.

❏ If at all possible, eat only organically grown foods.

❏ Always wear protective clothing and gloves when handling chemicals. Carefully follow the directions on the label of any product that contains chemicals.

❏ Avoid being outside during any aerial application of insecticides or pesticides.

❏ Drink steam-distilled water only. (*See* WATER in Part One.)

❏ Perform a cleansing fast for three days each month to help the body get rid of toxins. (*See* FASTING in Part Three.)

❏ Avoid chemicals whenever possible.

CONSIDERATIONS

❏ *See also* CHEMICAL ALLERGIES and POISONING in Part Two.

Chickenpox

Chickenpox is a very common and highly contagious disease. The symptoms are usually mild, with a low-grade fever, general fatigue, and a characteristic itchy rash. The same virus that causes chickenpox—*Varicella zoster*—can lie dormant for years, then resurface as shingles in adulthood. (*See* SHINGLES in Part Two.)

The chickenpox virus is transmitted by direct contact with an infected person or through the air when an infected person coughs or sneezes. A person can also contract chickenpox (but not shingles) from direct contact with a person with the shingles rash. Outbreaks are common within families and in schools and day-care facilities. Symptoms do not appear until after a person reaches the infectious stage, so it is difficult to isolate those who are contagious. Repeated exposures to the virus during the incubation period can result in worse symptoms. One bout with chickenpox generally affords lifetime immunity against the illness. Second attacks are possible, but rare.

Most children contract chickenpox before the age of ten. It first manifests itself as a fever and headache, usually starting between seven and twenty-one days after exposure to the virus. Twenty-four to thirty-six hours later, small round "pimples" appear on the face and body. They are filled with fluid and look like water blisters. The fluid leaks from the swollen areas of the skin, forming a crust. These eruptions continue in cycles, lasting from three days to one week. The blisters and crusts are infectious and itchy, and scratching them can lead to bacterial infection and scarring. Once the scabs are gone, the individual is no longer infectious. Adults who contract the infection tend to have more severe cases than children do.

Chickenpox usually runs its course in two weeks or less for otherwise healthy children. Potentially serious complications can arise for some people, especially for newborns, adults, and those with weakened immune systems. Anyone with an impaired immune system, such as a person whose immune system is suppressed by drugs or who has a disorder such as AIDS can develop pneumonia or encephalitis, an infection of the brain. A newborn baby also can develop complications from chickenpox, especially if infected prenatally or soon after birth.

About 3.5 to 4 million people, mostly children, get chickenpox every year. The Centers for Disease Control and Prevention (CDC) report that about 9,300 people are hospitalized and about 100 people die in the United States each year due to complications from the disease.

Unless otherwise specified, the dosages recommended here are for adults. For a child between the ages of twelve and seventeen, reduce the dose to three-quarters the recommended amount. For a child between six and twelve, use one-half the recommended dose, and for a child under the age of six, use one-quarter the recommended amount.

NUTRIENTS

SUPPLEMENT	SUGGESTED DOSAGE	COMMENTS
Essential		
Carotenoid complex with beta-carotene	15,000 IU daily.	Heals tissues and stimulates the immune system.
Vitamin A capsules or emulsion	20,000 IU daily for 1 month, then 15,000 IU daily for 1 week. 100,000 IU daily for 1 week, then 75,000 IU daily for 1 week. If you are pregnant, do not exceed 10,000 IU daily.	An immunostimulant that aids healing of tissues. Emulsion form is recommended for easier assimilation and greater safety at higher doses.
Vitamin C with bioflavonoids	1,000 mg 4 times daily.	Powerful immune stimulant that aids in keeping down fever.
Very Important		
Potassium and zinc	99 mg daily. 80 mg daily. Do not exceed a total of 100 mg daily from all supplements.	Helps reduce fever and speed healing. Enhances immune function. Use zinc gluconate lozenges or OptiZinc for best absorption.
Vitamin E	400–600 IU daily.	A powerful free radical scavenger that increases oxygenation and promotes healing. Use d-alpha-tocopherol form.
Helpful		
Maitake extract or shiitake extract or reishi extract	As directed on label. As directed on label. As directed on label.	Mushroom extracts with immune-stimulating and antiviral properties.
Multivitamin and mineral complex	As directed on label.	All nutrients help to speed the healing process.
Raw thymus glandular	As directed on label.	Stimulates the production of T lymphocytes by the thymus gland. Needed for immune function. (*See* GLANDULAR THERAPY in Part Three.)

HERBS

❑ Catnip tea sweetened with molasses is good for fever and can be given to infants and children as well as to adults. For a child over age two, catnip tea enemas can reduce fever.

❑ Other recommended herbs include burdock root, echinacea, ginger, goldenseal, pau d'arco, and St. John's wort.

RECOMMENDATIONS

❑ Drink freshly made juices with protein powder and brewer's yeast added. Also drink pure vegetable broth.

❑ When the fever drops and the appetite returns, use a "starter diet" consisting of only mashed bananas, avocados, fresh raw applesauce, and/or yogurt. Do not use cooked or processed foods.

❑ Do not give any cow's milk or formula to a feverish infant. Instead, use pure, freshly made juices that have been diluted with a combination of 4 ounces of steam-distilled water and 100 to 1,000 milligrams of vitamin C for each 4 ounces of juice. Infants who are six months old or older can have almond, rice, or soy milk, available in health food stores. Give a sick infant lots of water to prevent dehydration.

❏ Consult a doctor immediately if symptoms include dizziness, a fever higher than 103°F, rapid heartbeat, shortness of breath, loss of muscle coordination, tremors, vomiting, and/or a stiff neck.

❏ Take warm baths with uncooked oatmeal or cornstarch added to the water to help relieve some of the itching caused by chickenpox.

❏ Stay out of bright sunlight and keep interior areas dimly lit. Do not use bright lights until completely healed.

❏ Take care not to scratch the pocks. Keep a child's nails short and clean, and bathe the child often. Put mittens on a young child's hands if necessary. Use warm baths made with tea prepared with the recommended herbs, or ginger baths using cool water. Sponge the affected area with the tea. Wet compresses help to control the itching; use these often.

❏ Family members who have not had chickenpox should have limited contact with other family members who are known to be infected. Repeated exposure to the virus can worsen the effects. Keep an infected child away from elderly people, newborn babies, and pregnant women who have not had chickenpox.

❏ Never give aspirin to a child who has a fever. Studies have shown an increased risk of Reye's syndrome, a rare and potentially fatal disorder, in children given aspirin for fever. (See REYE'S SYNDROME in Part Two.)

❏ If you are unlucky enough to contract chickenpox in adulthood, contact your health care provider. Use a fasting program to help speed healing. See FASTING in Part Three.

CONSIDERATIONS

❏ Fetal exposure to chickenpox has been associated with an increased risk of birth defects.

❏ If the sores become infected, an antibiotic ointment is usually prescribed.

❏ Acyclovir (Zovirax) is an antiviral medication that lessens the severity of symptoms and shortens the duration of rash formation. It is most often recommended for those at risk for severe chickenpox: premature babies, adolescents, and adults.

❏ A chickenpox vaccine called Varivax was approved by the FDA in 1995. The American Academy of Pediatrics recommends a single dose of the vaccine for all children between twelve months and twelve years of age who have not yet had the disease, and who have not had the vaccine. Children older than thirteen who have not had chickenpox and have never been vaccinated should receive two doses of the vaccine, four to eight weeks apart. The vaccine is 70 to 90 percent effective in preventing chickenpox, however, its long-term effectiveness is not yet known. A booster shot may be recommended later in life.

❏ See also SHINGLES in Part Two.

Chlamydia

According to the U.S. Centers for Disease Control and Prevention (CDC), sexually transmitted chlamydia infection accounts for the bulk of the sexually transmitted disease (STD) epidemic in the United States. *Chlamydia trachomatis* is believed to be twice as common as gonorrhea. This infection can be transmitted or contracted during anal, oral, or vaginal sex with an infected partner. Each year, some 4 million new cases are diagnosed and an estimated 50,000 women are rendered sterile by the disease. About 18 percent of American adolescents have had a chlamydial infection, and one recent study found that 50 percent of the women on one college campus had been infected. The group most affected is people between the ages of fifteen and nineteen, with twenty- to twenty-four-year-old people coming in second.

Symptoms of chlamydia include genital inflammation, vaginal or urethral discharge, difficulty in urinating, a burning sensation during urination, painful intercourse, and itching around the inflamed area. The symptoms appear within one to three weeks of contact with an infected partner. These symptoms can appear in both men and women. However, as many as 50 percent of the men and 75 percent of the women who have chlamydia experience no symptoms at all, or symptoms so mild that they do not seek treatment. This is unfortunate, as untreated chlamydial infection in women leads to sterility in an estimated 30 percent of cases. Pelvic inflammatory disease and irreparable damage to the reproductive system can occur, and hysterectomy may be required. Also, women who have been infected with chlamydia may have three to five times the risk of becoming infected with HIV if they are exposed to it. Babies born to mothers with chlamydia may suffer from pneumonia or conjunctivitis (an eye infection). Both of those ailments require treatment with antibiotics.

In males, prostatitis and inflammation of the seminal vesicles may be caused by chlamydia. Symptoms of prostatitis include pain when urinating and a watery mucous discharge from the penis. Men may also notice pain and swelling in the testicles. Diagnosis of chlamydia infection is made on the basis of bacteriologic examination of urine or vaginal or urethral discharge. There are also a number of tests available today that can supplement or even replace the traditional culture.

NUTRIENTS

SUPPLEMENT	SUGGESTED DOSAGE	COMMENTS
Important		
Garlic (Kyolic from Wakunaga)	2 capsules 3 times daily.	Acts as a natural antibiotic and aids in healing.

Vitamin B complex	50–100 mg of each major B vitamin 3 times daily, with meals (amounts of individual vitamins in a complex will vary).	Needed for proper functioning of the liver and gastrointestinal tract.
Vitamin C	1,500 mg 4 times daily.	Immunostimulant that aids healing. Use a buffered form.
Vitamin E	600 IU daily. Can also be used directly on the inflamed site; cut open a capsule and apply.	Needed to protect red blood cells. Immune enhancer. Use d-alpha-tocopherol form.
Helpful		
Acidophilus (Probiata from Wakunaga)	As directed on label. Take on an empty stomach.	Replenishes "friendly" bacteria destroyed by antibiotics. Use a nondairy formula.
Bio-Bifidus from American Biologics	Use as a vaginal douche as directed on label.	Replaces normal vaginal and bowel flora.
Coenzyme Q$_{10}$	60 mg daily.	Aids in healing and is a powerful antioxidant and immune stimulant.
plus Coenzyme A from Coenzyme-A Technologies	As directed on label.	Works with coenzyme Q$_{10}$ and aids in the detoxification of many dangerous substances.
Dioxychlor from American Biologics	As directed on label.	An important antibacterial, antifungal, and antiviral agent.
Kelp	2,000–3,000 mg daily.	A rich source of minerals.
Multivitamin complex with mixed carotenoids	As directed on label.	Necessary for healing of all bodily tissues. Use a high-potency formula.
Zinc	50 mg daily. Do not exceed a total of 100 mg daily from all supplements.	Important for immune function and healing. Use zinc gluconate lozenges or OptiZinc for best absorption.
plus copper	3 mg daily.	Needed to balance with zinc.

HERBS

❑ Astragalus, echinacea, goldenseal, pau d'arco, and red clover aid in healing.

Caution: Do not take goldenseal on a daily basis for more than one week at a time, and do not use it during pregnancy. If you have a history of cardiovascular disease, diabetes, or glaucoma, use it only under a doctor's supervision.

RECOMMENDATIONS

❑ Eat a diet consisting mainly of fresh vegetables and fruits, plus brown rice, raw seeds and nuts, turkey, white fish, and whole grains.

❑ Avoid highly processed, fried, and junk foods, as well as chicken. Approximately one-third of all chickens sold in this country contain pathogenic bacteria such as salmonella. Turkey is acceptable; such bacteria are not found in turkey.

❑ Drink only steam-distilled water, sugar-free juices, and herbal teas.

❑ Take acidophilus to replenish the "friendly" bacteria destroyed by antibiotics.

❑ If you have symptoms of chlamydia infection, do not delay seeking treatment. The danger of complications increases as time passes.

CONSIDERATIONS

❑ If you are under thirty-five and have more than one sexual partner, you should be tested for infection yearly.

❑ Both partners must be treated for this disorder so that the disease is not transmitted back and forth. (Both sexes have similar discharges, and it is through this discharge that the disease is transmitted during sexual contact.) Antibiotics such as tetracycline and doxycycline (Doryx, Vibramycin, and others) kill chlamydia. Alternatively, a single 1-gram oral dose of azithromycin (Zithromax) may be used. This is relatively expensive (a single dose costs as much as a one-week regimen of doxycycline), but the convenience of single-dose treatment may be worth it.

❑ Chlamydia has been linked to a form of arthritis in young women. In one study, the microorganism was found in the joints of nearly half those with unexplained arthritis.

❑ There are currently three FDA-approved methods of testing for chlamydia:

• *Direct fluorescent antibody test.* In this method, a scientific method technique called *staining* makes chlamydia easier to detect under the microscope. A culture can be taken from the eye, cervix or penis.

• *Enzyme immunoassay.* This test can be performed without specialized laboratory equipment. The results are processed more quickly than with the traditional culture.

• *Urine sample.* This test is very accurate and much less invasive than genital sampling.

❑ For further information about this disease, you can call the Centers for Disease Control and Prevention (CDC) National STD Hotline (*see* HEALTH AND MEDICAL ORGANIZATIONS in the Appendix).

❑ *See also* SEXUALLY TRANSMITTED DISEASE (STD) in Part Two.

Cholesterol Problems

See HIGH CHOLESTEROL.

Chronic Fatigue Syndrome

Chronic fatigue syndrome (CFS) is is not a disease as such, but a characteristic and complex array of symptoms that may mimic other illnesses. The symptoms of CFS may include aching muscles and joints, anxiety, depression, difficulty concentrating, poor memory, fever, headaches, low blood pressure, intestinal problems and pain, irritability, environmental sensitivities, jaundice, loss of appetite, mood swings, muscle spasms, recurrent upper respiratory tract infections, nasal congestion, candidiasis, sensitivity to light and heat, sleep disturbances, night sweats, sore throat, swollen glands (lymph nodes)—and most of all, extreme and often disabling fatigue. Immunologic abnormalities that show up on various diagnostic tests are common as well.

CFS is often difficult to diagnose. The symptoms of this syndrome resemble those of flu and other viral infections, so it is often mistaken for other disorders. It is often misdiagnosed as hypochondria, psychosomatic illness, or depression because routine medical tests do not detect any problems. The syndrome is three times more prevalent in women than in men, and primarily affects young adults between the ages of twenty and fifty.

The cause or causes of chronic fatigue syndrome are not well understood. Some experts believe it is linked to infection with the Epstein-Barr virus (EBV) and/or cytomegalovirus (CMV), members of the herpesvirus family that also cause mononucleosis and retinal and gastrointestinal infections. This belief is based in large part on the fact that many people with chronic fatigue syndrome have been found to have high levels of EBV antibodies in their blood, and that many people date the onset of symptoms to a prolonged bout with a viral infection. However, no connection between EBV and chronic fatigue syndrome has ever been conclusively proved. Moreover, it is now known that many people have high EBV antibody levels without any apparent ill effects on their health, and that many cases of chronic fatigue occur without any known preceding infection. This has led researchers to look for other possible causes. Some suspect an as-yet-unidentified immune system problem or a defect in the mechanisms that regulate blood pressure. Other proposed causes of chronic fatigue syndrome include anemia, arthritis, chronic mercury poisoning from amalgam dental fillings, hypoglycemia, hypothyroidism, infection with the fungus *Candida albicans,* and sleep problems. Fibromyalgia, a muscle disorder that causes muscle weakness and fatigue, has been found in many people with chronic fatigue syndrome. Intestinal parasites are also comparatively common in people with this condition. It is likely that there are different combinations of factors that can result in chronic fatigue in susceptible individuals. A poor diet, nutritional deficiencies, allergies, thyroid dysfunction, candida, anemia, and stress all compromise the immune system, and can contribute to CFS.

Even though chronic fatigue syndrome is not life-threatening, it cannot be cured, and it can result in serious damage to the immune system. Some people appear to recover spontaneously, but once you have had this condition, it can recur at any time, usually following a bout with another illness or during times of stress.

The major criteria used to distinguish chronic fatigue syndrome are:

1. Persistent fatigue that does not resolve with bed rest and that is severe enough to reduce average daily activity by at least 50 percent for at least six months.

2. The presence of other chronic clinical conditions, including psychiatric disorders, should be ruled out.

Jesse A. Stoff, M.D., coauthor of the book *Chronic Fatigue Syndrome,* believes that CFS is a hidden epidemic, affecting more than 4 million people in the United States alone. Chronic fatigue syndrome should not be confused with the results of overwork and stress. With CFS, a normal, active level of life is impossible to maintain and the symptoms exceed, by far, the normal lethargy or tiredness associated with a stressful and hardworking lifestyle.

NUTRIENTS

SUPPLEMENT	SUGGESTED DOSAGE	COMMENTS
Essential		
Acidophilus (Kyo-Dophilus from Wakunaga)	As directed on label.	To replace necessary "friendly" bacteria. Also fights candida infection. Chronic fatigue and candidiasis often occur together. Use a nondairy formula.
Chromium polynicotinate	200–300 mg daily.	Aids in controlling hypoglycemia.
Coenzyme Q$_{10}$ plus Coenzyme A from Coenzyme-A Technologies	75 mg daily. As directed on label.	Enhances the effectiveness of the immune system and protects the heart. Works with coenzyme Q$_{10}$ and aids in the removal of toxic substances from the body.
Kyolic-EPA from Wakunaga	As directed on label.	Supplies essential fatty acids.
L-Carnitine	1,000 mg daily, on an empty stomach. Take with 50 mg vitamin B$_6$ and 100 mg vitamin C for better absorption.	Transports fatty acids into the mitochondria where it is used to make ATP, thus increasing energy levels.
Lecithin granules or capsules	1 tbsp 3 times daily, with meals. 1,200 mg 3 times daily, with meals.	Promotes energy and enhances immunity.
Malic acid and magnesium	As directed on label. 500–1,000 mg daily.	Involved in energy production in many cells of the body, including including muscle cells. Needed for sugar metabolism. Deficiency has been linked to CFS. Often deficient in people with CFS, magnesium is needed for ATP synthesis.
Manganese	5 mg daily.	Influences the metabolic rate by its involvement in endocrine function.
Nicotinamide adenine dinucleotide (NADH) (Enada NADH from Kal)	10–20 mg with water first thing in the morning, on an empty stomach.	Studies have shown that it increases energy levels and aids in preventing depression. May take 2–3 weeks to work.
Proteolytic enzymes or Inflazyme Forte from American Biologics or Wobenzym N from Marlyn Nutraceuticals	As directed on label, 6 times daily, on an empty stomach. Take with meals, between meals, and at bedtime.	Reduces inflammation and improves absorption of nutrients, especially protein, which is needed for tissue repair.

Vitamin A with mixed carotenoids and vitamin E	25,000 IU daily for 1 month, then slowly reduce to 10,000 IU daily. If you are pregnant, do not exceed 10,000 IU daily. 800 IU daily for 1 month, then slowly reduce to 400 IU daily.	Powerful free radical scavengers that protect the cells and enhance immune function to fight viruses. Use emulsion forms for easier assimilation and greater safety at high doses. Use d-alpha-tocopherol form of vitamin E.
Vitamin C with bioflavonoids	5,000–10,000 mg daily.	Has a powerful antiviral effect and increases the energy level. Use a buffered form.
Very Important		
Dimethylglycine (DMG) (Aangamik DMG from FoodScience of Vermont)	50 mg 3 times daily.	Enhances oxygen utilization and destroys free radicals.
Free-form amino acid complex (Amino Balance from Anabol Naturals)	As directed on label.	For tissue and organ repair. Use a formula containing all the essential amino acids.
Kyo-Green from Wakunaga	As directed on label.	To improve digestion and cleanse the bloodstream.
Liquid Kyolic with B$_1$ and B$_{12}$ from Wakunaga	As directed on label.	Provides energy and builds red blood cells.
Vitamin B complex injections	2 cc twice weekly or as prescribed by physician.	B vitamins are essential for increased energy levels and normal brain function. Injections (under a doctor's supervision) are best. All injectables can be combined in a single syringe. Aids in absorption of vitamin B$_{12}$.
plus extra vitamin B$_6$ (pyridoxine) and	$1/2$ cc twice weekly or as prescribed by physician.	
vitamin B$_{12}$ plus liver extract injections or	1 cc twice weekly or as prescribed by physician. 2 cc twice weekly or as prescribed by physician.	A natural energy booster needed to prevent anemia. A good source of B vitamins plus other valuable nutrients.
vitamin B complex	100 mg of each major B vitamin 3 times daily (amounts of individual vitamins in a complex will vary).	If injections are not available, a sublingual form is recommended for best results.
plus pantothenic acid	100 mg 3 times daily.	Needed for proper adrenal function.
Important		
Gamma-amino-butyric acid (GABA)	As directed on label, on an empty stomach. Take with water or juice. Do not take with milk. Take with 50 mg vitamin B$_6$ and 100 mg vitamin C for better absorption.	To maintain proper control of brain activity and to control anxiety. (See AMINO ACIDS in Part One.)
Multivitamin and mineral complex with		All nutrients are necessary in balance. Use a high-potency, hypoallergenic product.
calcium and	1,500 mg daily.	
potassium and	99 mg daily.	
selenium	200 mcg daily. If you are pregnant, do not exceed 40 mcg daily.	
and zinc	50 mg daily.	

Raw thymus glandular and	As directed on label.	To boost the immune system. (See GLANDULAR THERAPY in Part Three.)
spleen glandular plus	As directed on label.	
raw glandular complex	As directed on label.	
Shiitake extract or	As directed on label.	Help to combat fatigue, boost immunity, and fight viral infection.
reishi extract or	As directed on label.	
maitake extract	As directed on label.	
Helpful		
Melatonin	As directed on label, taken 2 hours or less before bedtime.	A natural sleep-regulating hormone that is helpful for promoting sound, restful sleep.

HERBS

❏ Astragalus and echinacea enhance immune function and are good for cold and flu symptoms. *Caution:* Do not use astragalus in the presence of a fever.

❏ Fresh black walnut hulls, garlic, gentian root, fresh ginger root, neem leaves, quassia bark, and fresh wormwood all help to rid the body of parasites, a common problem for people with CFS.

❏ Teas brewed from burdock root, dandelion, and red clover promote healing by cleansing the blood and lymphatic system, as well as enhancing immune function. Combine or alternate these herbal teas, and drink 4 to 6 cups daily.

❏ China Gold from Aerobic Life Industries is an herbal formula containing thirty-six different herbal extracts, including ten varieties of ginseng. It helps to enhance adrenal function and overcome fatigue.

❏ Use goldenseal to control infection. At the first signs of a sore throat, take a few drops of alcohol-free goldenseal extract, hold it in your mouth for a moment, then swallow.

Caution: Do not take goldenseal on a daily basis for more than one week at a time, and do not use it during pregnancy. If you have a history of cardiovascular disease, diabetes, or glaucoma, use it only under a doctor's supervision.

❏ Ginkgo biloba improves circulation and brain function.

❏ Kava kava, skullcap, and valerian root improve sleep.

❏ Licorice root supports the endocrine system and increases cortisol levels by blocking the action of an enzyme that breaks it down. Since adrenal exhaustion leads to low production of cortisol, licorice may prove to be beneficial for CFS sufferers.

Caution: Do not use this herb on a daily basis for more than seven days in a row. Avoid it completely if you have high blood pressure.

❏ Milk thistle protects the liver.

❏ Olive leaf extract has antibiotic and antiviral properties, and helps fight infections.

❏ Pau d'arco, taken in capsule or tea form, is good for treating candida infection.

❏ St. John's wort has antiviral properties and is a good antidepressant.

RECOMMENDATIONS

❏ Eat a well-balanced diet of 50 percent raw foods and fresh "live" juices. The diet should consist mostly of fruits, vegetables, and whole grains, plus raw nuts, seeds, skinless turkey, and some deep-water fish. These quality foods supply nutrients that renew energy and build immunity.

❏ Add some form of acidophilus to your diet, and regularly consume soured products such as yogurt and kefir. Many people with chronic fatigue syndrome also are infected with candida. Acidophilus helps to keep candida under control.

❏ Consume plenty of water—at least eight 8-ounce glasses a day—plus juices, preferably freshly made vegetable juices. Drink a full glass of water every two to three waking hours. Water flushes out toxins and aids in reducing muscle pain.

❏ Do not eat shellfish, fried foods, junk foods, processed foods; stimulants such as coffee, tea, and soft drinks; sugar; and products containing yeasts and/or white flour, such as bread and pasta. You may find this difficult—people with CFS generally have cravings for sugar and carbohydrate products, and may also develop a craving for alcohol—but it is important.

❏ Make sure that the bowels move daily, and add fiber to the diet. Give yourself occasional cleansing enemas. *See* ENEMAS in Part Three.

❏ Take chlorophyll in tablet form or obtain it from the liquid of vegetables, such as a "green drink" from leafy vegetables, wheatgrass, or Kyo-Green from Wakunaga. Take a protein supplement from a vegetable source—Spirutein from Nature's Plus is a good protein drink to take between meals.

❏ Get plenty of rest, and make sure that you do not overexert yourself. Moderate exercise may be helpful, however. Deep breathing exercises in particular are recommended. People with CFS tend to take shallow breaths, which can cause sleeping problems. (*See* Breathing Exercises *under* PAIN CONTROL in Part Three.)

❏ Avoid chocolate, soft drinks, caffeine, and highly processed foods. These foods deplete the body of magnesium, which leads to fatigue. Magnesium is important for people with CFS.

❏ Do not smoke, and avoid secondhand smoke. This can make symptoms worse.

❏ Do not take aspirin. If a viral infection is present, Reye's syndrome may result.

CONSIDERATIONS

❏ Colloidal silver may keep bacteria in check because of its antibiotic and antiviral properties.

❏ There are other health problems that can cause symptoms of chronic fatigue, including anemia, cardiovascular disease (especially in women), depression, fibromyalgia, hepatitis, and Lyme disease, among others. Anyone who experiences extreme fatigue that persists for longer than a week or two should consult a health care provider. There may be an underlying medical disorder that requires treatment.

❏ Some researchers believe that CFS may be hormone related. Pregnenolone is a steroid hormone that the body can metabolize into a variety of other vital hormones. It can bring about greatly improved resistance to stress and reduced adrenal exhaustion, which in turn, reduces fatigue.

❏ If you are diagnosed as having chronic fatigue syndrome, it is wise to seek out a health care provider who has specific experience in the management and treatment of this complex condition.

❏ Taking regular cold showers may produce an improvement in CFS symptoms. Many also find improvement with taking hot baths or showers. However, people with heart or circulatory disorders or other serious health problems should not attempt cold or hot water treatment without first consulting their health care providers.

❏ Certain of the amino acids may be beneficial to people with chronic fatigue. These include tyrosine, leucine, isoleucine, and valine, as well as lysine and taurine. (*See* AMINO ACIDS in Part One.)

❏ A study at Johns Hopkins University Hospital in Baltimore identified a link between chronic fatigue and a problem in the body's mechanisms for regulating blood pressure. In this study, twenty-two out of twenty-three subjects with chronic fatigue were found to have a syndrome in which the body responds inappropriately to periods of prolonged standing—the heart rate slows and blood pressure drops, resulting in lightheadedness, followed by a feeling of weakness and exhaustion that can persist for days afterward. A significant percentage of those in the study experienced an improvement when they were treated for the blood pressure problem.

❏ Some research points to chemical and/or food sensitivities and hypoglycemia as possible causes of chronic fatigue. People living in the past fifty years have been exposed to more different chemicals than all of the rest of humankind combined. It is no wonder that some people have become sensitive to chemicals. (*See* CHEMICAL ALLERGIES in Part Two.)

❏ Evidence is pointing to exhausted adrenal glands and a disturbance in the hypothalmic-pituitary-adrenal axis (HPA axis, a complex of biochemical controls that coordinate certain basic metabolic activities) as a possible cause of this disorder.

❑ Parasites are common in people with chronic fatigue. Parasitin+ from Växa International and ParasiVeda from Solaray are supplements designed to rid the body of parasites.

❑ Family members, friends, and coworkers must understand the nature of the disorder and realize that the person suffering from it is not exaggerating or faking symptoms.

❑ Depression can be a major feature of this illness. To combat it, your physician may prescribe an antidepressant. Antidepressants commonly recommended for people with CFS include the following:

• Doxepin (Sinequan) is a tricyclic antidepressant that may relieve symptoms of general fatigue, nasal congestion, gastritis, muscle tension and tightness, and insomnia. Other tricyclic antidepressants such as amitriptyline (Elavil) may also be prescribed for people with CFS.

• Fluoxetine (Prozac) increases the amount of serotonin in the brain. Serotonin is a neurotransmitter, a natural chemical that transmits messages from one part of the brain to another. Prozac may help to give people more energy, but will not help with sleeplessness.

• Gamma-globulin treatment uses a transfusion of a blood product to provide protective antibodies that may be absent in the person suffering from CFS.

However, many people with CFS suffer from disturbing side effects from prescription drugs. If this is the case, S-adenosylmethionine (SAMe) and 5-hydroxy L-tryptophan (5-HTP) both work well as antidepressants, help to relax muscle tension, and prevent insomnia.

❑ The National Institute of Allergy and Infectious Diseases (NIAID), a part of the National Institutes of Health, provides current information on chronic fatigue syndrome (See HEALTH AND MEDICAL ORGANIZATIONS in the Appendix).

❑ See also CANDIDIASIS; FIBROMYALGIA; HYPOTHYROIDISM; and MONONUCLEOSIS, all in Part Two.

Circulatory Problems

There are many disorders associated with circulatory problems, which exist when oxygenated blood cannot make the complete circuit of the body without restriction. There are many reasons why blood flow around the body may be inhibited. Clots may form in the larger veins in the leg or pelvic area, travel to the lung, and become trapped in a pulmonary artery. This results in diminished blood flow and less oxygen getting pumped to the rest of the body. *Pulmonary embolism*, as this condition is called, is difficult to detect, but is usually accompanied by a sudden shortness of breath and can be life-threatening.

When plaque or fatty deposits form along the walls of the arteries, it causes them to harden and constrict. *Hypertension,* or high blood pressure, results because the blood exerts greater force against the walls of the narrowed and/or more rigid blood vessels. Hypertension can lead to stroke, angina pectoris (chest pain), kidney damage, and heart attack.

A circulatory disease that is brought on by chronic inflammation of the blood vessels in the extremities is *thromboangiitis obliterans (Buerger's disease)*. This disease is most prevalent among people who smoke. It usually affects the foot or lower leg, but it can occur in the hand, arm, or thigh as well. Early signs of Buerger's disease are a tingling sensation (commonly referred to as "pins and needles") and a burning sensation in the fingers and toes. It can lead to ulceration and gangrene; in severe cases, amputation may be required.

Another serious circulatory condition is *Raynaud's disease,* which is characterized by constriction and spasm of the blood vessels in the extremities, such as in the fingers, toes, and tip of the nose. Cold, stress, smoking, and other factors may cause fingers and toes to become numb; extremities may appear colorless or bluish due to lack of circulation and arterial spasm. This disorder most commonly affects women between fifteen and fifty, and, although it is extremely rare, it can lead to dry gangrene if tissue dies because of a lack of oxygen. *Raynaud's phenomenon* is a condition with the same symptoms as Raynaud's disease, but it is brought on by another condition, such as surgery, injury, or frostbite. Raynaud's may be provoked or aggravated by some heart medications and drugs taken for migraine, lupus, and rheumatoid arthritis. (*See* RAYNAUD'S PHENOMENON in Part Two.)

Marfan's syndrome, a very rare condition, can also lead to serious circulatory problems. This syndrome is characterized by defects of the connective tissue in areas such as the skeletal system, eyes, and blood vessels, as well as such anatomical anomalies as unusually long toes and/or fingers, a high palate, an enlarged aorta, and/or taller than average height. This condition is usually hereditary.

Poor circulation can also result from *varicose veins,* which develop because of a loss of elasticity in the walls of the veins.

NUTRIENTS

SUPPLEMENT	SUGGESTED DOSAGE	COMMENTS
Essential		
L-Carnitine	500 mg twice daily.	Helps to strengthen the heart muscle and to promote circulation by transporting long fatty acid chains.
Very Important		
Chlorophyll (Kyo-Green from Wakunaga and wheatgrass are good sources)	As directed on label.	Enhances circulation and helps build healthy cells. Use liquid or tablet form. Also prepare fresh "green drinks" from green leafy vegetables.

Coenzyme Q10 plus	100 mg daily.	Improves tissue oxygenation.
Coenzyme A from Coenzyme-A Technologies	As directed on label.	Removes toxic substances from the body.
Lecithin granules or capsules	1 tbsp 3 times daily, before meals. 2,400 mg 3 times daily, before meals.	Emulsifies (breaks up) fats.
Liquid Kyolic with B1 and B12 from Wakunaga	As directed on label.	Helps to build red blood cells and lower blood pressure.
Multienzyme complex	As directed on label. Take with meals.	To aid digestion and circulation and enhance oxygen use in all body tissues.
Vitamin B complex	50–100 mg of each major B vitamin 3 times daily (amounts of individual vitamins in a complex will vary)	Needed for metabolism of fat and cholesterol. Consider injections (under a doctor's supervision). If injections are not available, use a sublingual form.
plus extra vitamin B1 (thiamine) and	50 mg daily.	Enhances circulation and brain function.
vitamin B6 (pyridoxine) and	50 mg daily.	A natural diuretic that protects the heart.
vitamin B12 and	1,000–2,000 mcg daily.	Prevents anemia and acts as a natural energy booster.
folic acid and	300 mcg daily.	Needed for the formation of oxygen-carrying red blood cells.
para-aminobenzoic acid (PABA)	25 mg daily.	Assists in the formation of red blood cells.
Vitamin C with bioflavonoids	5,000–10,000 mg daily, in divided doses.	Helps prevent blood clotting.

Important

Calcium and	1,500–2,000 mg daily, in divided doses, after meals and at bedtime.	Essential in normal blood viscosity.
magnesium and	750–1,000 mg daily, in divided doses, after meals and at bedtime.	Strengthens the heartbeat. Calcium and magnesium work together.
vitamin D3	400 IU daily.	Important for utilization of calcium.
Dimethylglycine (DMG) (Aangamik DMG from FoodScience of Vermont)	50 mg twice daily.	Enhances tissue oxygenation.
Multivitamin and mineral complex	As directed on label.	To provide a balance of nutrients basic to good circulatory function.
Vinpocetine	As directed on label.	A derivative of vincamine, (an extract of periwinkle) that helps with cerebral circulatory disorders.
Vitamin A with mixed carotenoids	25,000 IU daily. If you are pregnant, do not exceed 10,000 IU daily.	Aids in storage of fat and acts as an antioxidant. Use emulsion form for easier assimilation and greater safety at high doses.
and vitamin E	Start with 200 IU daily and increase slowly to 1,000 IU daily.	Inhibits the formation of free radicals. Use d-alpha-tocopherol form; use emulsion form for best absorption.

Helpful

Choline and inositol plus	100 mg each 3 times daily, with meals.	Helps to remove fat deposits and improve circulation. Helps to lower cholesterol.
vitamin B3 (niacin)	50 mg 3 times daily. Do not exceed a total of 300 mg daily from all supplements.	Helps to lower cholesterol. *Caution:* Do not take niacin if you have a liver disorder, gout, or high blood pressure.
L-cysteine and	500 mg each daily, on an empty stomach. Take with juice or water. Do not take with milk. Take with 50 mg vitamin B6 and 100 mg vitamin C for better absorption.	Protects and preserves cells by detoxifying harmful toxins.
L-methionine		Prevents accumulation of fat both in the liver and in the arteries, where it may obstruct blood flow. (*See* AMINO ACIDS in Part One.)
Proteolytic enzymes	As directed on label. Take between meals.	To combat leaky gut syndrome.
Pycnogenol or grape seed extract	As directed on label. As directed on label.	Neutralize free radicals, enhance the action of vitamin C, and strengthen connective tissue, including that of the cardio-vascular system.
Selenium	200 mcg daily. If you are pregnant, do not exceed 40 mcg daily.	Deficiency has been linked to heart disorders.
Shiitake extract or reishi extract	As directed on label. As directed on label.	Helps to prevent high blood pressure and heart disease; lowers cholesterol levels.
Zinc plus copper	50 mg daily. Do not exceed a total of 100 mg daily from all supplements. 3 mg daily.	Needed for immune function. Use zinc chelate form. Needed to balance with zinc.

HERBS

❏ The following herbs support the heart and circulatory system: black cohosh, butcher's broom, cayenne (capsicum), chickweed, gentian root, ginkgo biloba, goldenseal, hawthorn berries, horseradish, horsetail, hyssop, licorice root, pleurisy root, rose hips, and wormwood. Cayenne increases the pulse rate, while black cohosh slows it. Ginkgo is being used for circulatory disorders in many clinics.

Caution: Do not use black cohosh if you are pregnant or have any type of chronic disease. Do not use licorice on a daily basis for more than seven days in a row, and avoid it completely if you have high blood pressure. Do not use wormwood during pregnancy. It is not recommended for long-term use, as it can be habit-forming.

❏ Sanhelio's Circu Caps from Health From The Sun is an herbal combination formula beneficial for circulatory disorders.

RECOMMENDATIONS

❏ Make sure that your diet is high in fiber. Oat bran can help lower cholesterol levels.

❏ Include the following in your diet: bananas, brown rice, endive, garlic, lima beans, onions, pears, peas, and spinach.

❏ Drink steam-distilled water only.

❑ Eliminate animal protein and fatty foods (such as red meat), sugar, and white flour from your diet. Do not use stimulants such as coffee, colas, or tobacco, or eat foods with a lot of spices.

❑ Get regular exercise to help blood flow and to keep the arteries soft and unclogged.

Caution: If you are over thirty-five and/or have been sedentary for some time, consult your health care provider before beginning any type of exercise program.

❑ Keep your weight down.

❑ To boost circulation, give yourself a dry massage over your entire body using a loofah sponge or natural bath brush. Always massage towards the heart, even when massaging your legs. Also dip a towel in cold water and rub it briskly over parts of the body.

❑ If you have circulatory problems, *do not* take any preparations containing shark cartilage unless specifically directed to do so by your physician. Shark cartilage inhibits the formation of new blood vessels, the mechanism by which the body can increase circulatory capacity.

CONSIDERATIONS

❑ Blood-thinning drugs, such as warfarin (Coumadin), may be prescribed for people deemed to be in particular danger of developing blood clots, such as people who are bedridden or cancer patients. Studies show that, for those in peril of recurring clots, blood-thinning drugs should be taken for at least two years.

❑ Because sluggish circulation can have a variety of different causes, you should see your health care provider if it is persistent.

❑ Chelation therapy is helpful for improving circulation. (*See* CHELATION THERAPY in Part Three.)

❑ The simple fact of being pregnant places great strain on the circulatory system. Blood volume increases by up to 50 percent by the time a woman is nine months pregnant, and although most women with heart disease can safely have children, any such pregnancy should be closely monitored by both a cardiologist and an obstetrician.

❑ *See also* ARTERIOSCLEROSIS/ATHEROSCLEROSIS; CARDIOVASCULAR DISEASE; HIGH BLOOD PRESSURE; HIGH CHOLESTEROL; HYPOTHYROIDISM; RAYNAUD'S PHENOMENON; and VARICOSE VEINS, all in Part Two.

Cirrhosis of the Liver

Cirrhosis of the liver is a degenerative inflammatory disease that results in hardening and scarring of liver cells. The liver becomes unable to function properly due to the scarred tissue, which prevents the normal passage of blood through the liver.

The most common cause of cirrhosis of the liver is excessive alcohol consumption. Liver disease resulting from alcohol intake is the fourth leading cause of death among people aged twenty-five to sixty-four in urban areas of the United States. A less frequent cause of cirrhosis is the hepatitis C virus (HCV). It is estimated that 4 million people in the United States have hepatitis C, and about 85 percent of those will go on to develop chronic liver disease, including cirrhosis. Blood transfusions given before routine testing for HCV are presumed to be the main cause of the rising number of people infected with HCV. Malnutrition and chronic inflammation can also lead to liver malfunction.

In the early stages, symptoms of cirrhosis of the liver may include constipation or diarrhea, fever, upset stomach, fatigue, weakness, poor appetite, generalized itching, weight loss, enlarged liver, vomiting, red palms, and swelling of the abdomen and legs. Those in the later stages of the disease may develop anemia, bruising due to bleeding under the skin, jaundice, and edema. People with alcoholic cirrhosis may experience no symptoms, or they may develop very slowly.

NUTRIENTS

SUPPLEMENT	SUGGESTED DOSAGE	COMMENTS
Essential		
Liquid Kyolic with B₁ and B₁₂ from Wakunaga	As directed on label.	An excellent liver detoxifier.
Phosphatidyl choline plus choline and inositol	As directed on label. As directed on label.	For fatty liver.
Primrose oil or Total EFA from Health From The Sun	500 mg twice daily, with meals.	To prevent an imbalance of fatty acids, found in cirrhosis of the liver.
Vitamin B complex	100 mg of each major B vitamin 3 times daily (amounts of individual vitamins in a complex will vary).	The B vitamins are necessary for proper digestion, absorption of nutrients, and formation of red blood cells. Use a high-potency formula. Injections (under a doctor's supervision) may be necessary.
plus extra vitamin B₁₂	1,000–2,000 mcg daily.	To prevent anemia and protect against nerve damage. Use a lozenge or sublingual form.
and folic acid	200 mcg daily.	To correct deficiencies.
Very Important		
Bifido Factor from Natren or	As directed on label. Take on an empty stomach.	Repairs liver cells and aids in healing.
Kyo-Dophilus from Wakunaga	2 to 3 capsules 3 times daily.	Human-cultured flora from the small intestine, primarily to improve assimilation of nutrients. Detoxifies ammonia.
Garlic (Kyolic from Wakunaga)	2 capsules 3 times daily, with meals.	Detoxifies the liver and bloodstream.
Inflazyme Forte from American Biologics	As directed on label.	Balanced potent enzymes that act to inhibit inflammation.

L-Arginine plus L-cysteine	500 mg each daily, on an empty stomach. Take with water or juice. Do not take with milk. Take with 50 mg vitamin B$_6$ and 100 mg vitamin C for better absorption.	Helps to detoxify ammonia, a byproduct of protein digestion that can accumulate when the liver isn't functioning properly. Helps detoxify harmful toxins.
and L-methionine plus		
L-carnitine plus	500 mg daily, on an empty stomach.	Helps prevent accumulation of fat in the liver.
glutathione	500 mg daily, on an empty stomach.	A powerful antioxidant that protects against liver cancer.
Lecithin granules or capsules	1 tbsp 3 times daily, with meals. 2,400 mg 3 times daily, with meals.	A powerful fat emulsifier.
Multienzyme complex with betaine and hydrochloric acid (HCl) plus	As directed on label. Take with each meal.	Needed for digestion to lessen the strain on the liver.
ox bile extract	As directed on label.	Replaces the digestive enzymes normally produced by the gallbladder.
New Life Colostrum from Symbiotics	As directed on label.	Improves immune function and protects the liver.
Probiata from Wakunaga	As directed on label.	A nondairy, unrefrigerated acidophilus formula that acts as a detoxifier.
Raw liver extract	As directed on label.	Prevents anemia and aids in building the liver. (See GLANDULAR THERAPY in Part Three.)
S-Adenosylmethio- nine (SAMe)	As directed on label.	Provides antioxidant effects that improve the health of the liver. Caution: Do not use if you have manic-depressive disorder or take prescription antidepressants.
Taurine Plus from American Biologics	20 drops 3 times daily.	The most important antioxidant for health and stress from free radical damage. Use the sublingual form.
Important		
Alfalfa		See under Herbs, below.
Calcium and magnesium	1,500 mg daily, in divided doses, after meals and at bedtime. 750 mg daily.	To promote healing of tissue. Beneficial for the nervous system. Use chelate forms.
Dimethylglycine (DMG) (Aangamik DMG from FoodScience of Vermont)	As directed on label.	Supplies oxygen for healing.
Vitamin C with bioflavonoids	3,000–8,000 mg daily, in divided doses.	An important antioxidant. Use a buffered form.
Helpful		
Alpha-lipoic acid	400 mg daily	Acts as a powerful antioxidant and balances blood sugar levels.
Coenzyme Q$_{10}$ plus	100 mg daily.	Promotes tissue oxygenation.
Coenzyme A from Coenzyme-A Technologies	As directed on label.	Works with coenzyme Q$_{10}$ and removes toxic substances from the body.

Free-form amino acid complex	As directed on label.	A good source of protein that is easy on the liver.
Grape seed extract or Pycnogenol	As directed on label.	Powerful antioxidant. Aids the liver in removing toxic substances from the body.
Inositol hexaphos- phate (IP$_6$) (Cell Forté with IP-6 and Inositol from Enzymatic Therapy)	As directed on label.	Aids in reducing the buildup of fats in the liver.
Selenium	200 mcg daily. If you are pregnant, do not exceed 40 mcg daily.	A good detoxifier.
Vitamin A (Micellized Vitamin A emulsion from American Biologics is a good source) plus	As directed on label. Do not exceed 10,000 IU daily.	Needed for healing. Use emulsion form for easier assimilation and greater safety at higher doses. Caution: Do not substitute pill forms of vitamin A for emulsion. Pills put extra stress on liver. To correct deficiencies.
vitamin D and	As directed on label.	
vitamin E	As directed on label.	A potent antioxidant that aids circulation. Use d-alpha-tocopherol form.
Zinc	50 mg daily. Do not exceed a total of 100 mg daily from supplements.	Needed for the immune system and the healing process. Use zinc gluconate lozenges or OptiZinc for best absorption.

HERBS

❑ Alfalfa helps to build a healthy digestive tract and is a good source of vitamin K. It helps to prevent bleeding as a result of vitamin K deficiency, which is common with cirrhosis. It can be taken in tablet or liquid form.

❑ Aloe vera helps to cleanse and heal the digestive tract. Drink $1/4$ cup of aloe vera juice every morning and evening. George's Aloe Vera Juice from Warren Laboratories is a good product. It can be taken in a cup of herbal tea if you wish.

❑ Burdock root, dandelion, and red clover aid in liver repair by cleansing the blood stream.

❑ Silymarin (milk thistle extract) has been shown in scientific studies to repair and rejuvenate the liver. Take 200 milligrams of silymarin three times daily. Liv-R-Actin from Nature's Plus is also a good source of milk thistle.

❑ Other herbs that can be beneficial for people with cirrhosis include barberry, black radish, celandine, echinacea, fennel, fringe tree, goldenseal, hops, horsetail, Irish moss, rose hips, suma, thyme, and wild Oregon grape.

Caution: Do not use barberry, celandine, goldenseal, or wild Oregon grape during pregnancy. Do not take goldenseal on a daily basis for more than one week at a time, and use it only under supervision if you have a history of cardiovascular disease, diabetes, or glaucoma.

RECOMMENDATIONS

❑ Obtain protein from vegetable sources; do not eat foods containing animal protein.

The Liver

Weighing about four pounds, the liver is the largest gland of the body and the only internal organ that will regenerate itself if part of it is damaged. Up to 25 percent of the liver can be removed, and within a short period of time, it will grow back to its original shape and size.

The liver has many functions, perhaps the most important of which is the secretion of bile. This fluid is stored in the gallbladder and released as needed for digestion. Bile is necessary for the digestion of fats; it breaks fat down into small globules. Bile also assists in the absorption of the fat-soluble vitamins (A, D, E, and K) and helps to assimilate calcium. In addition, bile converts beta-carotene into vitamin A. It promotes intestinal peristalsis as well, which helps prevent constipation.

After nutrients have been absorbed into the bloodstream through the intestinal wall, they are transported by way of the hepatic portal system to the liver. In the liver, nutrients such as iron and vitamins A, B_{12}, and D are extracted from the bloodstream and stored for future use. These stored substances are utilized for everyday activities and in times of physical stress. The liver plays an important role in fat metabolism; in the synthesis of fatty acids from amino acids and sugars; in the production of lipoproteins, cholesterol, and phospholipids; and in the oxidation of fat to produce energy. The liver creates a substance called glucose tolerance factor (GTF) from chromium and glutathione. GTF acts with insulin to regulate blood sugar levels. Sugars not required for immediate energy production are converted into glycogen in the liver; the glycogen is stored in the liver and the muscles, and is converted back into sugar when needed for energy. Excess food is converted to fat in the liver, and the fat is then transported to the fatty tissues of the body for storage.

In addition to its important functions in digestion and energy production, the liver acts as a detoxifier. Protein digestion and bacterial fermentation of food in the intestines produce ammonia as a byproduct; this ammonia is detoxified by the liver. The liver combines toxic substances (including metabolic waste products, insecticide residues, drugs, alcohol, and other harmful chemicals) with substances that are less toxic. These substances are then excreted via the kidneys and bowels. Thus, in order for the liver to function properly, you must also have proper kidney and bowel function.

Finally, the liver is responsible for regulating thyroid function by converting thyroxine (T_4), a thyroid hormone, into its more active form, triiodothyronine (T_3). Inadequate conversion of T_4 into T_3 by the liver may lead to hypothyroidism. The liver also breaks down hormones like adrenaline, aldosterone, estrogen, and insulin after they have performed their needed functions.

❑ Eat a diet consisting of 75 percent raw foods. If cirrhosis is severe, consume only fresh vegetables and fruits and their juices for two weeks.

❑ Include the following in your diet: almonds, brewer's yeast, grains and seeds, raw goat's milk, and products derived from goat's milk. Nuts must be raw and from tightly sealed packages.

❑ Increase your consumption of foods high in potassium, such as bananas, blackstrap molasses, brewer's yeast, dulse, kelp, prunes, raisins, and rice and wheat bran.

❑ Eat plenty of foods high in vitamin K. Persons with cirrhosis of the liver are often deficient in vitamin K. Good sources of vitamin K include alfalfa sprouts and green leafy vegetables.

❑ Include legumes (kidney beans, peas, and soybeans) and seeds in your diet. These foods contain the amino acid arginine, which helps to detoxify ammonia, a byproduct of protein digestion.

❑ Drink fresh vegetable juices, such as beet, carrot, dandelion extract, and "green drinks."

❑ Drink steam-distilled water or sip barley water (see THERAPEUTIC LIQUIDS in Part Three) throughout the day. When taking supplements, always take them with a full glass of water.

❑ Use only cold-pressed vegetable oils as sources of dietary fats. Consume oils in uncooked form only, such as in salad dressings.

❑ Limit your intake of fish—haddock, bluefish, salmon, and sardines—to a maximum of two servings a week, and *do not* eat raw or undercooked seafood. A damaged liver cannot handle the amount of vitamin A contained in these foods. Avoid cod liver oil.

❑ Keep the colon clean. Toxins accumulate in the liver and must be excreted via the colon and kidneys. (*See* COLON CLEANSING in Part Three.)

❑ Avoid constipating foods. The liver has to work twice as hard if you are constipated. Be sure your diet contains sufficient amounts of choline, inositol, and lecithin, as well as bulk and fiber.

❑ Do not use harsh laxatives to cleanse the system. Lemon enemas are preferred; take these twice weekly. You can also alternate wheatgrass enemas with coffee enemas for two weeks. Both of these detoxify the system. (*See* ENEMAS in Part Three.)

❑ Do not take any drugs (over-the-counter or prescription) except for those prescribed by your doctor. Some over-the-counter products, including some medicines for children, contain alcohol in the form of propylene glycol. This product may cause liver problems and a mild form of drunkeness.

❑ Consume no alcohol in any form. Also eliminate the following from your diet: animal products, candies, milk, pastries, pepper, salt, spices, stimulants of any kind (including caffeine and colas), white rice, products containing sugar and/or white flour, and spicy or fried foods. Virtually all commercially prepared foods contain some of the above.

❑ Read all food labels carefully, and avoid most fats. Do not eat any of the following: butter, margarine, vegetable shortening, and any other hardened fats; fried or fatty foods; melted or hard cheeses; nuts or oils that have been subjected to heat (either in processing or in cooking); potato chips; and all refined and processed foods. These overwork and damage the liver.

❑ Do not smoke, and avoid secondhand smoke.

CONSIDERATIONS

❑ If alcoholic cirrhosis is detected in the early stages and the individual stops consuming alcohol, it may be possible to halt the damage to the liver.

❑ In one study, people with cirrhosis of the liver were found to have an imbalance of essential fatty acids, which are needed for cell protection. After taking 10 capsules of primrose oil daily for three weeks, these individuals showed a marked improvement in the balance of their fatty acids.

❑ Animal studies indicate that the typical American diet is damaging to the liver. Improper diet results in allergies, digestive disorders, a low energy level, and an inability to detoxify harmful substances.

❑ The four basic reasons for poor liver function are:

1. *The presence of cumulative poisons.* Insecticides, preservatives, and other toxins can build up in and impair the liver. Even though a particular toxin may not accumulate in the liver, liver function may suffer if the functioning of other organs, especially the pancreas and/or kidneys, is adversely affected by the toxin.

2. *An improper diet.* A diet that is low in protein and high in carbohydrates and fats, especially saturated fats, fried foods, and hydrogenated fats, is hard on the liver and may not provide sufficient protein building blocks necessary for repair. Poor food choices include processed foods, junk foods, refined white flour products, white sugar products, and imitation foods that are designed to appear and taste like an original product but that have been robbed of natural vitamins, minerals, and enzymes.

3. *Overeating.* Overeating is probably the most common cause of liver malfunction. Overeating creates excess work for the liver, resulting in liver fatigue. In addition, the liver must detoxify all of the various chemicals present in our food supply today. When the liver is overworked, it may not detoxify harmful substances properly.

4. *Drugs.* Drugs put a great strain on the liver. Drugs are substances that are foreign and unnatural to the body. These foreign substances cause the liver to work overtime in excreting these toxins. The liver neutralizes the effects of drugs on the body. Alcohol is particularly toxic to the liver. When excessive amounts of alcohol enter the liver, the liver begins to lose its functioning capacity. Other substances that can contribute to liver malfunction include oral contraceptives and caffeine.

❑ *See also* ALCOHOLISM and HEPATITIS, both in Part Two.

Cold

See COMMON COLD.

Cold Sores (Fever Blisters)

Cold sores, or fever blisters, are caused by herpes simplex virus 1 (HSV-1), which is related to but different from the virus that causes genital herpes. Cold sores first appear three to ten days after exposure to the virus and may last up to three weeks. The virus then remains permanently in the body, and moves into the nervous system close to the lips. It will lie dormant there until triggered by fever, a cold or other viral infection, exposure to sun and wind, stress, menstruation, high levels of amino acid arginine, or depression of the immune system. These sores are very contagious and very common. Studies have shown that between 30 and 60 percent of children carry the virus by the age of ten.

There are said to be six stages of the development of the average cold sore. First comes the prodrome, or stage one. In this first stage, no sore is visible but there is a feeling of prickling or itchiness around the affected area. In stage two, swelling may start and the area may be slightly red. Stage three brings with it the first signs of a blister or blisters. Stage four is the most painful, and generally comes on the fourth day. A soft crust or ulcer forms, and from this the cold sore moves into stage five, when a hard crust forms on the ulcer. This stage usually lasts for four days. The sixth and last stage, coming on or around the tenth day, leaves the sore red and slightly swollen, but without the hard scab. An outbreak of cold sores may last more or less than ten days, depending on its severity.

Unless otherwise specified, the dosages recommended here are for adults. For a child between the ages of twelve and seventeen, reduce the dose to three-quarters the recommended amount. For a child between six and twelve, use one-half the recommended dose, and for a child under the age of six, use one-quarter the recommended amount.

NUTRIENTS

SUPPLEMENT	SUGGESTED DOSAGE	COMMENTS
Essential		
Herpanacine from Diamond-Herpancine Associates	As directed on label.	Proven effective in treating and stopping the outbreak of herpes. It contains many of the nutrients listed in this table.
L-Lysine	500 mg twice daily.	Fights the virus that causes cold sores. *Caution:* Do not take lysine for longer than 6 months at a time. Do not take lysine pills if you are pregnant or nursing.
L-Lysine cream	Apply topically as directed on label.	This amino acid fights herpes viruses. (*See* AMINO ACIDS in Part One.)
Vitamin B complex	100–150 mg of each major B vitamin twice daily (amounts of individual vitamins in a complex will vary).	Important for healing and immune function. Use a high-stress formula.
Zinc lozenges	1 15-mg lozenge every 3 waking hours for 2 days, then 2 lozenges daily until healed. Do not exceed a total of 100 mg daily from all supplements.	Stimulates immune function to fight the virus. Zinc is absorbed quickly in lozenge form.
Very Important		
Acidophilus or Kyo-Dophilus from Wakunaga	As directed on label. Take on an empty stomach.	Inhibits pathogenic organisms.
Colloidal silver	Take orally or apply topically as directed on label.	An antiseptic and antibiotic that destroys bacteria, viruses, and fungi, and promotes healing.
Garlic (Kyolic from Wakunaga)	2 capsules 3 times daily.	Acts as a natural antibiotic and immunity enhancer.
Vitamin C	3,000–6,000 mg daily, in divided doses.	Fights the virus and boosts immune function. Use a buffered form.
Important		
Calcium and magnesium	1,500 mg daily. 750–1,000 mg daily.	To help relieve stress.
Essential fatty acids	As directed on label.	Aids skin in healing.
Helpful		
Herp-Eeze from Olympian Labs	As directed on label.	Contains lignans, nordihydro-gualaretic acid (NGDA), and other phytonutrients. Has antioxidant, anti-inflammatory, antiviral, and antimicrobal properties.
Maitake extract or shiitake extract or reishi extract	As directed on label. As directed on label. As directed on label.	To fight viruses and build resistance to disease.
Multivitamin and mineral complex	As directed on label.	All nutrients are necessary in balance.

Vitamin A plus carotenoid complex and vitamin E	25,000 IU daily. If you are pregnant, do not exceed 10,000 IU daily. 400 IU daily.	Needed for healing of tissue in mouth and lip area. Use emulsion forms for easier assimilation and greater safety at higher doses. Use d-alpha-tocopherol form.

HERBS

❏ For cold sores, use echinacea, goldenseal, pau d'arco, and red clover. Echinacea stimulates the immune system and may also aid in preventing an outbreak.

Caution: Do not take goldenseal on a daily basis for more than one week at a time, and do not use it during pregnancy. If you have a history of cardiovascular disease, diabetes, or glaucoma, use it only under a doctor's supervision.

❏ Lemon balm contains a high concentration of polyphenols and appears to minimize herpes outbreaks. It can be applied topically in cream form. Or brew lemon balm tea and apply it directly to the sore. Taken internally, lemon balm tea has antiviral qualities.

❏ Olive leaf extract is good as a natural antibiotic for viral infections.

RECOMMENDATIONS

❏ Eat plenty of raw vegetables, as well as yogurt and other soured products.

❏ If cold sore outbreaks occur often, check for low thyroid function. *See* HYPOTHYROIDISM in Part Two.

CONSIDERATIONS

❏ The drug acyclovir (Zovirax), in capsule, liquid, or ointment form, is sometimes prescribed for cold sores.

❏ In studies, penciclovir (Denavir) cream has shown to reduce the duration of the infection by one day, on average.

❏ Relaxation and visualization techniques (imagining the virus being destroyed by healing white blood cells, for example) may reduce the seriousness of cold sore outbreaks.

❏ If you are prone to allergies, you most likely have a malfunctioning immune system and may be susceptible to cold sores. *See* ALLERGIES in Part Two.

❏ *See also* HERPESVIRUS INFECTION in Part Two.

Colitis

See ULCERATIVE COLITIS.

Colorblindness

See under EYE PROBLEMS.

Common Cold

The common cold is an infection of the upper respiratory tract caused by a virus. Cold weather does not cause colds, although most colds are caught in the fall and winter. This is because most cold viruses thrive better in colder temperatures, when there is less humidity in the atmosphere. There are over 200 viruses that can cause the common cold, an infection of the upper respiratory tract, but the most common ones are rhinoviruses. The well-known symptoms include head congestion, nasal congestion, sore throat, coughing, headache, sneezing, and watery eyes. Children may develop a low-grade fever, but this is rare in adults. Colds usually strike eighteen to twenty-four hours after the virus enters the body. Most colds clear up on their own in a week to ten days, but occasionally a cold can lead to a more serious illness, such as bronchitis, a middle ear infection, or sinus infection. There is often confusion between the symptoms of the common cold, influenza, and allergies. Influenza, also a viral respiratory infection but caused by different types of viruses, is by far the most serious complaint of the three and can lead to life-threatening complications, particularly in older or frail people. (*See* INFLUENZA in Part Two.) For an outline of the symptoms of colds as opposed to those of influenza and allergies, see the inset below.

It is estimated that healthy adults get an average of two colds per year. Children generally get many more because their immune systems are immature, and they have not yet developed immunity to many of the viruses that cause colds.

Unless otherwise stated, the dosages here are for adults. For a child between the ages of twelve and seventeen, reduce the dose to three-quarters of the recommended amount. For a child between six and twelve, use one-half of the recommended dose, and for a child under the age of six, use one-quarter of the recommended amount.

NUTRIENTS

SUPPLEMENT	SUGGESTED DOSAGE	COMMENTS
Essential		
ACES + Zn from Carlson Labs	As directed on label.	Contains vitamins A, C, and E, plus the minerals selenium and zinc.
Vitamin A plus carotenoid complex (Betatene)	15,000 IU daily. If you are pregnant, do not exceed 10,000 IU daily. As directed on label.	Helps heal inflamed mucous membranes and strengthens the immune system. Antioxidants and precursors of vitamin A.

Cold, Flu, or Allergy?

Since the common cold, influenza, and seasonal allergies all cause upper respiratory symptoms, it can sometimes be difficult to distinguish among them. There are certain notable differences, however. The following is a summary of the characteristic signs and symptoms of each.

Characteristic	Cold	Influenza	Seasonal Allergies
Chest infection/cough	Common. Mild to moderate.	Common. Can become severe. Pneumonia is a common complication.	Rare.
Fever	Rare (except in young children).	Usually high (102°–104°F). May last for 3–4 days.	Not present.
General aches and pains	Mild.	Usual. Can be severe.	Rare.
Headache	Rare.	Common.	Rare.
Sneezing/red, watery, itchy eyes	Usual, but more prevalent in allergies.	Rare.	Usual, especially sneezing. These symptoms come on quickly, without the warning signs of a cold, and can last longer.
Sore throat	Usual.	Occasional.	Occasional.
Stuffy nose	Usual.	Occasional.	Occasional.
Tiredness	Mild.	Severe.	Rare.
Primary season	Late August–April.	Winter.	March–September.
Duration	7–10 days.	Up to a month.	As long as the allergen is present.

Vitamin C with bioflavonoids	5,000–20,000 mg daily, in divided doses. *See* ASCORBIC ACID FLUSH in Part Three.	Fights cold viruses. For children, use buffered vitamin C or calcium ascorbate.
Zinc lozenges	For adults and children, 1 15-mg lozenge every 3 waking hours for 3 days, then 1 lozenge every 4 hours for 1 week. Do not exceed a total of 100 mg daily from all supplements.	Boosts the immune system. Keep these on hand and use them at the first sign of a cold. *Note:* Avoid lozenges containing citric acid, sorbitol, or mannitol. These ingredients inhibit absorbtion.
Important		
Free-form amino acid complex plus	As directed on label.	To supply needed protein for healing.
N-acetylcysteine	As directed on label.	A powerful antioxidant.
Garlic (Kyolic from Wakunaga)	2 capsules 3 times daily.	A natural antibiotic and immune system enhancer.
L-Lysine	500 mg daily, on an empty stomach. Take with water or juice. Do not take with milk. Take with 50 mg vitamin B$_6$ and 100 mg vitamin C for better absorption.	Aids in destroying viruses and preventing cold sores in and around the mouth. (*See* AMINO ACIDS in Part One.) *Caution:* Do not take lysine for longer than 6 months at a time.
Helpful		
Acidophilus (Kyo-Dophilus from Wakunaga is a good source)	As directed on label. Take on an empty stomach. As directed on label.	To replace "friendly" bacteria. For adults.
Cold-X10 from Olympian Labs	As directed on label.	A combination of nutrients, herbal extracts, and enzymes that boost the immune system and fight viral and bacterial infection.
Maitake extract or shiitake extract or reishi extract	As directed on label. As directed on label. As directed on label.	Mushrooms with immune-boosting and antiviral properties.
Multimineral complex or kelp	As directed on label. 1,800–3,600 mg daily.	Minerals are needed for healing and for immune response. A rich source of necessary minerals.
Multivitamin complex with vitamin B complex	50–100 mg 3 times daily (amounts of individual vitamins in a complex will vary).	For healing and to reduce stress.
Olive leaf extract or colloidal silver	As directed on label. As directed on label.	Supplements with antibiotic and antiviral properties.

HERBS

❑ Astragalus, native to Mongolia and China, helps promotes the multiplication of the white blood cells that are vital for fighting infection.

❑ Boneset, a Native American herb, may be used to treat a fever.

❑ For fever, take catnip tea enemas and 1/4 to 1/2 teaspoon

of lobelia tincture every three to four hours until fever drops. This dosage can be used for children also.

Caution: Do not take lobelia internally on an ongoing basis.

❑ Cat's claw is useful for easing the symptoms of a cold.

❑ Chuan xin lian, a Chinese herbal remedy also known as Andrographis Anti-Inflammatory Tablets, clears the mucus from the respiratory tract.

❑ Ephedra (ma huang) is helpful for congestion and coughing.

Caution: Do not use this herb if you suffer from anxiety, glaucoma, heart disease, high blood pressure, or insomnia, or if you are taking a monoamine oxidase (MAO) inhibitor drug for depression.

❑ At the first sign of a cold, use an alcohol-free echinacea and goldenseal combination extract to boost your immune system and keep the virus from multiplying. For adults, place 1 dropperful in the mouth, hold it for five minutes, then swallow. Do this every three hours for three days. For children, place 8 to 10 drops in the mouth, hold it for a few minutes (or as long as the child can manage), then swallow. Do this every two hours for three days. Then take 8 to 10 drops in liquid daily until symptoms are gone. Besides beating colds, flu, bronchitis, and other upper respiratory infections, echinacea is good for clearing up strep throat.

Caution: Do not take goldenseal on a daily basis for more than one week at a time, and do not use it if you are pregnant or nursing. If you have a history of cardiovascular disease, diabetes, or glaucoma, use it only under a doctor's supervision.

❑ Elderberry is recommended for upper respiratory infections and headaches associated with colds. It promotes sweating and can help to break a fever. Research has found that elderberry is effective against colds because it contains antioxidant flavonoids that protect cell walls against foreign substances.

❑ Eucalyptus oil is helpful for relieving congestion. Put 5 drops in a hot bath, or put 6 drops in 2 cups of boiling water and inhale the steam. It is best to remove the boiling water from the stove, then place a towel over your head and inhale deeply through your nose for three to five minutes (be careful not to get too close to the source of the hot steam—it can cause burns). Rosemary and sage oils can be added to the eucalyptus oil to aid in breaking up decongestion.

❑ Fenu-Thyme from Nature's Way is an herbal formula that helps rid nasal passages of mucus. Take 2 capsules three times daily.

❑ Ginger, pau d'arco, slippery elm, and yarrow tea can help the common cold.

❑ Hyssop, an evergreen that can be taken as a tea, acts as an expectorant and has antiviral properties.

❑ Mullein is useful for coughs and congestion.

❑ Red clover helps clear accumulated toxins in the lymphatic system that may cause congestion and inflammation.

❑ For a sore throat, add 3 to 6 drops of pure tea tree oil to warm water and gargle. Repeat this up to three times daily. Take up to 2 tea tree oil lozenges and allow them to dissolve slowly in your mouth. Repeat this treatment as often as required, alternating it with goldenseal extract. These products can be found in most health food stores.

❑ Wild cherry bark soothes a cough.

RECOMMENDATIONS

❑ Take vitamin C and zinc lozenges at the first sign of a sore throat or stuffiness in the head or nose. This can shorten the duration of a cold, and may even stop it altogether. Take the lozenges every three hours for the first day of cold symptoms.

❑ Sip hot liquids such as turkey or chicken broth. Drink Potato Peeling Broth twice a day—make it fresh daily. You can add a carrot, a stalk of celery, garlic, and/or onions to your drink. Chicken soup is very effective in relieving the worst of the symptoms and in shortening the duration of a cold. (*See* THERAPEUTIC LIQUIDS in Part Three for both recipes.)

❑ Remain as active as possible. Not only is staying in bed for ordinary sniffles unnecessary, but it will probably make you feel worse. Moving around helps to loosen built-up mucus and fluids. Unless you have a fever, a brisk walk or any other type of moderate exercise should make you feel better.

❑ Consider using homeopathic remedies for cold symptoms. *Calcarea carbonica* is excellent for sore throats, colds, or bronchitis. *Anas barbariae* (also available as Oscillococcinum from Boiron), *Ferrum phosphoricum* (if there is a fever), and HP2 from Metagenics (a liquid homeopathic combination remedy) are also good for treating the common cold.

❑ Flush facial tissues after they have been used. Because they harbor the virus, tissues can pass on the virus or cause you to reinfect yourself.

❑ Wash your hands often. Cold viruses can survive for several hours on hands, tissues, or hard surfaces. A healthy person can contract the virus by touching a contaminated surface, then touching his or her own mouth or nose. Using an antibiotic soap may prevent you from reinfecting yourself, but these soaps can also contribute to the development of antibiotic-resistant bacteria, so it is best to use them only when necessary.

❑ Try not to spread the cold to your family or colleagues. Refrain from close contact with loved ones. Even shaking hands is out; hand contact can spread the virus.

Common Cold Remedies

Americans spend more than $1 billion every year on nonprescription treatments for coughs and colds. At best, these products can offer only temporary relief. The following is a list of some of the most common types of cold remedies, and what they can and cannot do:

• Analgesics, such as acetaminophen, aspirin, and ibuprofen, help to relieve aches and pains and reduce fever. By themselves, colds do not usually cause significant fever. Allowing a low-grade fever to run its course may actually be beneficial; an elevated temperature is one of the body's ways of fighting infection. If you have a fever that reaches 102°F or higher, chances are something other than the cold is causing it. It may be a sign of a developing bacterial infection somewhere in the body that requires treatment. By reducing fever, analgesics may mask this sign.

• Antihistamines decrease nasal secretions by blocking the action of histamine, a body chemical that causes swelling of small blood vessels, which results in sneezing and runny nose. These products may make you drowsy. In addition, it is better to allow the secretions that contain the virus to flow out of the body rather than trying to block them.

• Cough medicines come in two basic types: expectorants and antitussives. Expectorants make coughs more productive by increasing the amount of phlegm and decreasing its thickness. This helps remove irritants from respiratory airways. Guaifenesin, an expectorant found in many popular over-the-counter cough medicines, can be effective. The effectiveness of other over-the-counter expectorants is questionable. Antitussives reduce the frequency of coughing. An antitussive called dextromethorphan is generally considered reasonably safe and effective. It is often denoted by the initials "DM" on product labels. However, because coughing is the body's mechanism for clearing secretions from the lungs, it is probably best not to suppress it unless coughing is unusually severe or persistent, or it is interfering with sleep.

• Decongestants shrink nasal blood vessels to relieve swelling and congestion. These medications can cause side effects including jitteriness, insomnia, and fatigue.

Most over-the-counter cold remedies contain some combination of acetaminophen and various decongestants, antihistamines, and cough suppressants. Some experts believe that these ingredients may work against one another. For example, acetaminophen may increase nasal congestion, while the decongestant decreases it. If a cold is making you extremely uncomfortable and you feel you must take something for it, it is better to take a single-ingredient product appropriate for the particular symptom you are treating.

❏ Do not give aspirin, or any product containing aspirin, to a child with symptoms of any viral infection, including a cold. (*See* REYE'S SYNDROME in Part Two). Taking large doses of aspirin also depletes the body of Vitamin C.

CONSIDERATIONS

❏ Since there is no cure for the common cold, the best approach is prevention. Once a cold has a firm grip on you, it is hard to stop it.

❏ Bovine colostrum, taken in the cold and flu season, may help to ward off infection.

❏ There are many over-the-counter cold medications available. None of them can actually cure a cold, although they may sometimes be helpful for alleviating symptoms.

❏ It is unlikely that a vaccine will ever be developed to prevent the common cold because the viruses responsible have the ability to change in size and shape, and have hundreds of different forms. However, research being conducted in Britain may provide hope for cold sufferers. An experimental drug, tremacamra, appears to block cold viruses from finding a docking site in the nasal passages. So far, the drug's success rate has been impressive, cutting the risk of infection by 33 percent and symptoms by 45 percent.

❏ The possibility for real cold relief may lie in substances such as interferons, natural proteins that the body produces in response to viral infection. Interferons seem to improve the respiratory tract's ability to ward off viruses. Vitamin C promotes interferon production.

❏ Antibiotics are ineffective against viral infections, but many people still ask their doctors to prescribe them. It is important to understand that penicillin and most other antibiotics work only against bacterial infections, such as strep throat—not viral infections. Viruses and bacteria may produce similar symptoms, but they are very different kinds of microbes and do not respond to the same treatment. In fact, because antibiotics kill off "good" bacteria together with the bad, antibiotics actually inhibit the body's efforts to defend itself against viral invasion.

❏ You can, in a sense, catch a cold from yourself. When your immune system weakens from factors such as stress and/or a poor diet, viruses can take hold. These viruses are opportunistic and lie dormant in the body, taking hold when the immune system is at its weakest. Stress is often a factor.

❏ A five-week study of seventy-nine young adults deliberately infected with a cold virus revealed that those given the drug naproxen (Naprosyn), which is commonly prescribed for arthritis, suffered almost a third fewer cold symptoms, such as headache and coughing, than those given a placebo.

❏ Medical researchers at Dartmouth College gave a group of thirty-five cold sufferers zinc lozenges, and told these individuals to take a lozenge as often as every two hours. Another thirty-five cold sufferers were given placebos. The zinc-takers' colds subsided in an average of four days, while the control group struggled with their colds for another nine days.

❏ Under experimental conditions, polysaccharides found in the herb echinacea have been shown to enhance the immune response.

❏ Allergies can cause symptoms that mimic those of colds and flu. Allergy testing is recommended. (*See* ALLERGIES in Part Two.)

❏ Anyone who has frequent colds or bouts with the flu should be checked for thyroid malfunction. When you are well, perform the thyroid function self-test (*See under* HYPOTHYROIDISM in Part Two). If your temperature is low, consult your health care provider.

❏ Congestion, cough, and/or sore throat are signs of a cold, but if these symptoms occur together with fever or fatigue, you may have the flu. (*See* INFLUENZA in Part Two.) If congestion develops in the chest, it is best to consult a physician, as chest (lung) infections can be serious. Also contact your health care provider if your fever goes above 102°F for more than three days, if yellow or white spots appear in the throat, if the lymph nodes under the jaw and in the neck become enlarged, and/or if chills and shortness of breath occur.

Complexion Problems

See ACNE; DRY SKIN; OILY SKIN; PSORIASIS; ROSACEA; WRINKLES.

Conjunctivitis

See under EYE PROBLEMS.

Constipation

Constipation is difficulty in passing stools or the infrequent passage of hard, dry stools as a result of food moving slowly through the large intestine. Most people experience constipation from time to time, but usually lifestyle changes and better eating habits can help relieve the symptoms and prevent recurrences.

In most cases, constipation arises from insufficient amounts of fiber and fluids in the diet. Fiber is found in plant foods, such as whole grains, fruits, and vegetables. Fiber that is soluble in water takes on a soft texture and helps soften the stools. Insoluble fiber passes through the intestine largely unchanged and adds bulk to stools, which in turn helps to stimulate bowel contractions. Other factors that can cause constipation include inadequate exercise, advanced age, muscle disorders, structural abnormalities, bowel diseases, neurogenic disorders, and a poor diet, especially heavy consumption of junk food. Constipation may be a side effect of iron supplements and some drugs, such as painkillers and antidepressants. It is also common during pregnancy.

High levels of calcium and low levels of thyroid hormone are two metabolic disturbances that can lead to constipation. People with kidney failure or diabetes also tend to have problems with constipation. In older individuals, constipation is often caused by dehydration; in people of any age, depression can be a factor. Some medications can cause constipation, including cough syrups, pain medications that contain codeine, some antidepressants, iron supplements, blood pressure and heart medicines, calcium supplements, and some antihistamines.

A small percentage of people, such as persons with spinal injuries, have problems with constipation because the nerves that usually regulate bowel movement have been damaged or destroyed. In a condition called *Hirschsprung's disease*, normal excretion of feces is impossible because the nerves inside the bowel are missing. The nerve cells in the wall of the colon can also be damaged by long-term, habitual use of laxatives. When this happens, constipation is inevitable. A thrombosed hemorrhoid, anal fissure, or a pocket of infection at the anus can create a spasm of pain strong enough to contract the muscles and hinder the evacuation of stools.

Constipation can give rise to many different ailments, including appendicitis, bad breath, body odor, coated tongue, depression, diverticulitis, fatigue, gas, headaches, hemorrhoids (piles), hernia, indigestion, insomnia, malabsorption syndrome, obesity, and varicose veins. It may even be involved in the development of serious diseases such as bowel cancer.

Regular bowel movements are an important mechanism for removing toxins from the body. The colon serves as a holding tank for waste matter. Antigens and toxins from bowel bacteria and undigested food particles may play a role in the development of diabetes mellitus, meningitis, myasthenia gravis, thyroid disease, candidiasis, chronic gas and bloating, migraines, fatigue and ulcerative colitis. People can have bowel movements as infrequently as three times a week and still not be constipated, although there are some health practitioners who maintain that it is important to have a bowel movement every day.

Unless otherwise specified, the dosages recommended here are for adults. For a child between the ages of twelve and seventeen, reduce the dose to three-quarters the recommended amount. For a child between six and twelve, use one-half the recommended dose, and for a child under the age of six, use one-quarter the recommended amount.

NUTRIENTS

SUPPLEMENT	SUGGESTED DOSAGE	COMMENTS
Important		
Garlic (Kyolic from Wakunaga)	2 capsules twice daily, with meals.	Destroys harmful bacteria in the colon.
Vitamin C with bioflavonoids	5,000–20,000 mg daily, in divided doses. (*See* ASCORBIC ACID FLUSH in Part Three.)	Has a cleansing and healing effect. Use a buffered form.
Helpful		
Apple pectin	500 mg daily. Take separately from other supplements and medications.	A source of fiber that aids in correcting constipation.
Bio-Bifidus from American Biologics	As directed on label. For fast results, use it in an enema.	For bowel flora replacement to improve assimilation of nutrients from foods.
Chlorophyll liquid or alfalfa	1 tbsp daily, before meals.	Eliminates toxins and bad breath. *See under* Herbs, below.
Essential fatty acids (Kyolic-EPA from Wakunaga, flaxseed oil, and primrose oil are good sources)	As directed on label.	Restores proper fatty acid balance to aid in proper bowel movements.
Kyo-Dophilus from Wakunaga	As directed on label.	Aids in normal bowel function. Allows survival and rapid passage of "friendly" bacteria through the stomach into the small intestine.
Multienzyme complex	As directed on label. Take after meals.	To aid digestion.
Multivitamin and mineral complex with vitamin A and mixed carotenoids	As directed on label. If you are pregnant, do not exceed 10,000 IU daily.	Constipation blocks proper absorption of nutrients, resulting in vitamin and mineral deficiencies. Use a formula without iron.
Oxy-Cleanse from Earth's Bounty	As directed on label.	Removes harmful anaerobic pathogens from digestive tract.
Vitamin B complex plus extra vitamin B$_{12}$ and folic acid	50 mg of each major B vitamin 3 times daily, before meals (amounts of individual vitamins in a complex will vary). 1,000–2,000 mcg daily. 200 mcg daily.	Aids in proper digestion of fats, carbohydrates, and protein. Use a high-potency formula. A sublingual form is best. To aid in digestion and prevent anemia. Deficiency may result in constipation.
Vitamin D$_3$ plus calcium and magnesium	400 mg daily. 1,500 mg daily. 750 mg daily.	Aids in preventing colon cancer. Needed for proper muscular contraction. May also help prevent colon cancer. Works with calcium to regulate muscle tone.
Vitamin E	600 IU daily. Take before meals.	Aids in healing of the colon. Use d-alpha-tocopherol form.

HERBS

❑ Alfalfa extract contains chlorophyll, which aids in

Types of Laxatives

Laxatives are substances that are used to promote bowel movement. There are four basic types of laxatives: bulk-forming agents, stool softeners, osmotic agents, and stimulants. The following are basic descriptions of the way the different laxatives work to achieve their effects:

• **Bulk-forming agents** increase the bulk and water content of the stools. They are the only type of laxatives that can be safe to take on a daily basis. Examples include bran (both in foods and in supplement form), psyllium, and methylcellulose.

• **Stool softeners,** such as mineral oil and docusate sodium, soften fecal matter so that it passes through the intestines more easily. They should not be used on a regular basis, because they can have other effects on the body. Mineral oil can damage the lungs if inhaled, and it reduces the absorption of fat-soluble vitamins. Docusate sodium (found in Colace and Dialose) may increase the

toxicity of other drugs taken at the same time, and may cause liver damage to occur.

• **Osmotic agents** contain salts or carbohydrates that promote secretion of water into the colon, initiating bowel movement. They are among the safest laxatives for occasional use, but if they are used more than occasionally, dependency can result. Examples include lactulose (a prescription medication sold under the brand names Cephulac and Chronulac), sorbitol (which is cheaper than lactulose but just as effective), milk of magnesia, citrate of magnesia, and Epsom salts.

• **Stimulant laxatives** irritate the intestinal wall, stimulating peristalsis. They can damage the bowels with habitual use, and can lead to dependency. Examples include bisacodyl (found in Dulcolax), casanthranol (Peri-Colace), cascara sagrada, castor oil, phenolphthalein (Dialose Plus), and senna (Perdiem, Senokot).

detoxifying the body and cleansing the breath. Fennel seed tea also is good for freshening the breath.

❏ Aloe vera has a healing and cleansing effect on the digestive tract and aids in forming soft stools. Drink ½ cup of aloe vera juice in the morning and at night. It can be mixed with a cup of herbal tea if you wish.

❏ Ginger stimulates the digestive system and eases passage of foods through the intestines. Try Ginger Dry Extract and Ginger Soft Extract from Sabinsa Corporation.

❏ Use milk thistle to aid liver function and to enhance bile output to soften stools.

❏ Naturalax 2 from Nature's Way is an herbal formula that is good for constipation.

❏ Triphala Internal Cleanser from Planetary Formulas is an herbal product that aids in the formation of odor-free, firm, and healthy stools.

❏ Other herbs that are helpful for constipation include cascara sagrada, goldenseal, rhubarb root, senna leaves, and yerba maté. If you take yerba maté, take 2 to 3 teaspoons in 16 ounces of hot water on an empty stomach.

Caution: Do not take goldenseal on a daily basis for more than one week at a time, and do not use it during pregnancy. If you have a history of cardiovascular disease, diabetes, or glaucoma, use it only under a doctor's supervision.

RECOMMENDATIONS

❏ Eat high-fiber foods such as fresh fruits, raw green leafy vegetables, whole-grain oatmeal, and brown rice daily. Also eat asparagus, beans, Brussels sprouts, cabbage, carrots, garlic, kale, okra, peas, sweet potatoes, and whole grains.

Foods that contain high levels of soluble fiber are adzuki beans, barley, dried beans, oats, and some fruits, especially apples, apricots, bananas, blackberries, blueberries, cranberries, figs, grapes, peaches, and prunes. Foods high in insoluble fiber are cereals, seeds, wheat bran, whole grains, and the skins of many fruits and vegetables.

❏ Drink more water. This is important when adding fiber to the diet. Drink at least eight to ten 8-ounce glasses of water every day, whether you are thirsty or not.

❏ Consume plenty of foods that are high in pectin, such as apples, carrots, beets, bananas, cabbage, citrus fruits, dried peas, and okra. Pectin is also available in supplement form.

❏ Follow a low-fat diet. Eat no fried foods.

❏ Avoid foods that stimulate secretions by the mucous membranes, such as dairy products, fats, and spicy foods.

❏ Do not consume dairy products, soft drinks, meat, white flour, highly processed foods, salt, coffee, alcohol, or sugar. These foods are difficult to digest and have little or no fiber.

❏ For quick relief of constipation, drink a large glass of quality water every ten minutes for half an hour. This can work wonders to flush out toxins and relieve constipation.

❏ Eat prunes or figs. These are the best natural laxatives.

❏ Eat smaller portions—no large, heavy meals or high-fat foods.

❏ Consume barley juice, Green Magma from Green Foods Corporation, Kyo-Green from Wakunaga, or wheatgrass for chlorophyll.

❏ Get some exercise. Physical activity speeds the movement of waste through the intestines. A twenty-minute walk can often relieve constipation. Regular exercise is also important for preventing constipation in the first place.

❏ Go to the toilet at the same time each day, even if the urge does not exist, and relax. Stress tightens the muscles and can cause constipation. Many people find reading helpful as a way to relax. Never repress the urge to defecate.

❏ Keep the bowel clean. (*See* COLON CLEANSING in Part Three.)

❏ If constipation is persistent, take cleansing enemas. (*See* ENEMAS in Part Three.)

❏ Do not consume products containing mineral oil, which can interfere with the absorption of fat-soluble vitamins. Also avoid taking Epsom salts, milk of magnesia, and citrate of magnesia, which draw volumes of fluid into the intestines and wash out minerals from the body.

❏ If you use laxatives, take acidophilus to replace the "friendly" bacteria. The continued use of laxatives cleans out the intestinal bacteria and leads to chronic constipation.

CONSIDERATIONS

❏ Psyllium seed is helpful for constipation. If you take psyllium seed, be sure to take it with a full glass of water.

❏ Flaxseed oil or freshly ground flaxseeds help to soften stools. Freshly ground flaxseeds have a pleasant, nutty taste and can be sprinkled over cereals, salads, and other foods.

❏ It can help to fast periodically. (*See* FASTING in Part Three.)

❏ Laxatives can be used occasionally to relieve constipation, but if used regularly they can cause serious problems, including diarrhea, abdominal cramping, bloating, dehydration, and, ultimately, damage to the colon. Using laxatives too often also promotes dependence. Lifestyle changes, including getting regular exercise and eating a high-fiber diet, are better ways to avoid constipation.

❏ If added natural fiber and herbal laxatives do not improve constipation, you may have a problem with muscle coordination. Normally, the upper muscles in the bowel contract as the lower ones relax. Problems occur if the lower muscle tightens and goes into a spasm instead of relaxing.

❏ If constipation is more than an occasional problem, the possibility of a cancer or another obstruction in the lower bowel should not be dismissed unless a proctoscopic examination or a barium enema has shown that there is no blockage. Other symptoms of colon cancer include the presence of blood in the feces; severe cramping; a tender, distended abdomen; and markedly narrowed stools. However, cancer may be present even without these symptoms.

❏ Foul-smelling stools and a burning feeling in the anus may be signs of acidosis. (*See* Acidosis *under* ACID/ALKALI IMBALANCE in Part Two.)

❏ Alternating constipation and diarrhea may be a sign of irritable bowel syndrome. While this disorder is chronic and unpleasant, it is not dangerous. Other common symptoms are crampy pains, gassiness, and variation in the consistency of the stool. The cause of irritable bowel syndrome is not known, but many experts believe it is stress related. (*See* IRRITABLE BOWEL SYNDROME in Part Two.)

❏ *See also* DIVERTICULITIS and ULCERATIVE COLITIS, both in Part Two.

❏ *See also under* PREGNANCY-RELATED PROBLEMS in Part Two.

Copper Deficiency

Copper is an essential trace mineral. Even a mild copper deficiency impairs the ability of white blood cells to fight infection. Copper is necessary for proper absorption of iron in the body, and it is found primarily in foods containing iron. If the body does not get a sufficient amount of copper, hemoglobin production decreases and copper-deficiency anemia can result.

Various enzyme reactions require copper as well. Copper is needed as a cross-linking agent for elastin and collagen, as a catalyst for protein reactions, and for oxygen transport. It is also used for the metabolism of essential fatty acids. Copper deficiency can produce various symptoms, including diarrhea, inefficient utilization of iron and protein, and stunted growth. In babies, the development of nerve, bone, and lung tissue can be impaired, and the structure of these body parts may be altered.

Since copper is not manufactured by the body, it must be taken in through the diet. Too much copper produces a condition called copper toxicity or copper overload (*see* COPPER TOXICITY in Part Two). For the body to work properly, it must have a proper balance of copper and zinc; an imbalance can lead to thyroid problems. In addition, low (or high) copper levels may contribute to mental and emotional problems. Copper deficiency may be a factor in anorexia nervosa, for example.

The FDA has never published a Recommended Daily Allowance for copper, but the National Research Council recommends that adults get from 1.5 to 3.0 mg per day, 1.5 to 2.5 milligrams for children, and 0.4 to 0.6 milligrams for infants less than six months old. A normal healthy diet will provide the correct amount of copper for most people.

Copper deficiency is most likely to occur in babies who are fed only cow's milk, persons suffering from sprue (a malabsorption syndrome) or kidney disease, and those who chronically take megadoses of zinc. Long-term use of oral contraceptives can upset the balance of copper in the body, causing either excessively high or excessively low copper levels. Copper levels can be determined through a blood test, urine samples, and hair analysis. Determining mineral levels and ratios is the basis for a nutritional program to balance body chemistry.

Unless otherwise specified, the dosages recommended here are for adults. For a child between the ages of twelve and seventeen, reduce the dose to three-quarters the recommended amount. For a child between six and twelve, use one-half the recommended dose, and for a child under the age of six, use one-quarter the recommended amount.

NUTRIENTS

SUPPLEMENT	SUGGESTED DOSAGE	COMMENTS
Important		
Copper	5 mg daily for 1 month, then reduce to 3 mg daily.	To restore copper in the body. Use copper amino acid chelate.
Zinc	30 mg daily. Do not exceed this amount.	Needed to balance with copper. Use zinc chelate form.
Helpful		
Iron	As directed by physician. Take with 100 mg vitamin C for better absorption.	Copper deficiency may cause anemia. Use a chelate form. *Caution:* Do not take iron unless anemia is diagnosed.
Multivitamin and mineral complex	As directed on label.	All nutrients are necessary in balance.

RECOMMENDATIONS

❑ If you suspect that you may have a copper deficiency, increase your intake of foods rich in copper, such as legumes (especially soybeans), nuts, cocoa, black pepper, seafood, egg yolks, raisins, molasses, avocados, whole grains, oats, and cauliflower. Pregnant women in particular should be sure to eat a well-balanced diet that includes these foods.

❑ Copper deficiency can be confirmed through hair analysis. (*See* HAIR ANALYSIS in Part Three.) If deficiency is confirmed, follow the supplementation plan above to restore proper mineral balance.

CONSIDERATIONS

❑ Copper deficiencies are thought to be linked to living in, and eating foods grown in, areas where the soil has been depleted of this mineral. In 1984, Leslie M. Klevay, now Supervisory Research Medical Officer and Research Leader at the U.S. Agricultural Research Service's Trace Elements and Cardiovascular Health Laboratory in Grand Forks, North Dakota, found that about one-third of 849 people studied had copper intake of less than 1 milligram per day.

❑ *Patent ductus arteriosus* is a congenital defect in which the ductus arteriosus, or fetal blood vessel, fails to close properly shortly after birth. It results in blood flow between the pulmonary artery, which goes to the lungs, and the aorta, which brings oxygenated blood to the rest of the heart. In a laboratory experiment reported in *Developmental Pharmacology and Therapy,* the ductus arteriosus remained open in 100 percent of offspring of a copper-deficient group of rats, but in only 20 percent of the offspring of a control group not suffering from copper deficiency.

Copper Toxicity

Trace amounts of copper are essential for the human body. Since copper is not manufactured by the body, it must be taken in through the diet. A number of biochemical processes depend on copper to function normally, plus copper is involved in the function of the nervous system (*see* COPPER DEFICIENCY in Part Two). However, as with all trace minerals, excess amounts of copper in the body can be toxic.

Too much copper in the system can cause a variety of ailments, including diarrhea, eczema, hemolytic anemia, high blood pressure, kidney disease, nausea, premenstrual syndrome, sickle cell anemia, stomach pain, and severe damage to the central nervous system. As with mercury and lead, high levels of copper are also associated with mental and emotional disorders, including autism, behavioral problems, childhood hyperactivity, clinical depression, anxiety, postpartum psychological problems, hallucinatory and paranoid schizophrenia, insomnia, mood swings, stuttering, and senile dementia (senility).

Sources of copper include beer, copper cookware, copper plumbing, industrial wastes, insecticides, pasteurized milk, tap water, and various foods, as well as swimming pool chemicals and permanent-wave solutions.

The U.S. Food and Drug Administration (FDA) has never published a Recommended Daily Allowance for copper, but the National Academy of Sciences' National Research Council recommends a daily intake of 1.5 to 3.0 milligrams per day for adults, 1.5 to 2.5 milligrams for children, and 0.4 to 0.6 milligrams for infants less than six months old.

Copper levels can be determined through blood tests, urine samples, and hair analysis. Normal urine samples collected over a twenty-four-hour period contain 15 to 40 micrograms of copper. In people with diseases such as arthritis, heart disease, hypertension, schizophrenia, or cancer, serum copper levels tend to be high. During illness, copper is released from the tissues into the blood to promote tissue repair. High serum copper readings during illness should not be taken to mean that the copper is a cause of the illness; rather, it is an indication that the body's natural repair processes have been activated.

The use of oral contraceptives and/or tobacco can cause a rise in the amount of copper in the body. Excess serum copper is also characteristic of anemia, cirrhosis of the liver, leukemia, hypoproteinemia, and vitamin B_3 (niacin) deficiency. Serum copper levels tend to be higher than normal during pregnancy as well. Wilson's disease is a rare hereditary disorder in which the body is unable to metabolize copper properly, so the metal accumulates in the body. People with diminished adrenal gland function or abnormally slow metabolisms can develop high copper levels. Zinc, another mineral, plays an important role in how much copper is stored in the tissues. A deficiency of zinc, especially when combined with a high copper intake, can cause too much copper to build up in the tissues. In addition, stress can cause a decrease in the amount of zinc available to the body, which can lead to copper overload.

With knowledge of how minerals interact in the body, it is possible to lower the amount of copper in the body and maintain a proper mineral balance. Unless otherwise specified, the dosages recommended here are for adults. For a child between the ages of twelve and seventeen, reduce the dose to three-quarters the recommended amount. For a child between six and twelve, use one-half the recommended dose, and for a child under the age of six, use one-quarter the recommended amount.

NUTRIENTS

SUPPLEMENT	SUGGESTED DOSAGE	COMMENTS
Important		
Vitamin C with bioflavonoids plus extra	1,000 mg 4 times daily.	Copper chelators. Use ascorbic acid form.
rutin	60 mg daily.	A bioflavonoid that is a byproduct of buckwheat and lowers serum copper.
Zinc	50–80 mg daily. Do not exceed a total of 100 mg daily from all supplements.	Zinc deficiency predisposes one to excessive copper levels. Use zinc chelate form.
Helpful		
Calcium chelate or	1,500 mg daily.	Binds with metallic ions in the body.
calcium disodium edetate plus	As prescribed by physician.	Used by doctors to treat heavy metal poisoning. Available by prescription only.
magnesium	750 mg daily, at bedtime.	Works with calcium.
L-Cysteine and L-cystine and L-methionine	As directed on label, on an empty stomach. Take with water or juice. Do not take with milk. Take with 50 mg vitamin B_6 and 100 mg vitamin C for better absorption.	Aids in elimination of copper from the body and protects the liver. (*See* AMINO ACIDS in Part One.)
Manganese	2–4 mg daily. Take separately from calcium.	Aids in excretion of excess copper.
Molybdenum	30 mcg daily.	Prevents accumulation of excess copper in the body.

HERBS

❏ Grape seed extract serves as a free radical scavenger and aids in protecting cells from damage.

RECOMMENDATIONS

❏ Have your drinking water tested. Drinking water can be a source of copper. The level of copper and other minerals in household drinking water can be tested by special labs. If there is more than 1 part per million of copper in your drinking water, an alternate source of water, such as bottled steam-distilled water, is advisable. If this is not fea-

sible, always run the water for at least two minutes before using it to clear out some of the impurities.

❏ Increase your intake of sulfur, found in such foods as eggs, onions, and garlic. These help to rid the body of copper. In addition, supplement your diet with pectin, which can be found in apples.

❏ Do not take a multivitamin and/or mineral supplement that contains copper.

❏ Do not use copper pots or other cooking utensils.

CONSIDERATIONS

❏ Hair analysis has been shown to be a reliable test of the copper level in body tissues. (*See* HAIR ANALYSIS in Part Three.)

❏ If you have an extremely high level of copper, you may require medical treatment with chelation to remove the excess copper. Chelation therapy removes toxic metals from the body. (*See* CHELATION THERAPY in Part Three.) If the copper levels are higher than normal, but not extreme, this can often be managed with supplements.

❏ The trace minerals manganese, molybdenum, and zinc can prevent excess copper from accumulating in the body.

❏ Many people with schizophrenia have been found to have high levels of copper and iron, combined with deficiencies of zinc and manganese, probably as a result of lower than normal excretion of copper. Increasing the intake of zinc and manganese, whether through the diet or supplementation, increases elimination of copper and helps to return copper levels to normal.

❏ *See also* ENVIRONMENTAL TOXICITY and WILSON'S DISEASE, both in Part Two.

Corneal Ulcer

See under EYE PROBLEMS.

Corns and Calluses

Corns and calluses are areas of *hyperkeratosis*, or overgrowth of skin tissue. The skin thickens and hardens. Calluses most commonly form on the soles of the feet and sometimes on the hands or knees. Corns are small cone-shaped areas of skin overgrowth that most often form on or between the toes. They can be either soft or hard. If they form between the toes, the moisture of the area keeps them soft; corns that form on top of the toes are typically hard. Having a hammertoe or mallet toe may lead to a more severe form of callus called intractable plantar keratosis (IPK). This callous forms as a result of a serious imbalance in weight-bearing, with considerably more pressure being placed on one area of the foot than on others.

These growths can cause inflammation and pain. Corns especially may ache and be tender to the touch. Both corns and calluses usually form in response to repeated friction or pressure, such as from wearing ill-fitting shoes or performing certain tasks repeatedly. Other factors that may be involved include staphylococcus- or streptococcus-type infection, and an acid/alkaline imbalance in the body.

HERBS

❑ Use alternate applications of alcohol-free goldenseal extract and tea tree oil to keep down infection and speed healing.

RECOMMENDATIONS

❑ Consume raw vegetables and juices for three days to aid in balancing the acidity/alkalinity of your system. Umeboshi (Japanese salt plum) can quickly balance the body's pH. These are available in health food stores and Asian markets. Take one every three hours for two days.

❑ Avoid fried foods, meats, caffeine, sugar, and highly processed foods.

❑ To treat corns and calluses, soften the thickened skin by adding 2 tablespoons of Dr. Bronner's liquid soap (available in health food stores) or a mild dish soap to ½ gallon of warm water. Soak your feet in this mixture for fifteen minutes. Afterwards, dry your feet with a soft towel and rub a couple of drops of vitamin E oil into the affected area. Then, using a pumice stone or a special callus file, *gently* file down the top layer of the corn or callus. Clean the area with mild soap and water, using a gauze pad or cotton ball, and apply a moisturizer to the area. Do this twice a day. Wear clean white cotton socks after treatment. This is effective only if the callus is not too thick.

❑ Apply a nonmedicated corn pad (a small round or oval-shaped foam pad with a hole in the center) around a corn to help to relieve the pressure. Stretch the pad so that it clears the corn by at least one-eighth inch on all sides. Then apply vitamin E oil to the corn, cover with a gauze square, and wrap the toe with adhesive tape. Alternate between using vitamin E oil and tea tree oil.

❑ For corns between the toes, dab on vitamin E oil and place a clean piece of cotton or a cotton ball over it. Make sure to use 100-percent cotton, not synthetic cosmetic puffs. Put on clean white cotton socks and leave them on overnight after treatment. Vitamin E oil mixed with a crushed garlic clove is good for softening corns and calluses.

❑ Never use a knife or any sharp instrument to cut the hardened area away, as infection can result.

❑ Always wear properly fitting shoes.

CONSIDERATIONS

❑ Compresses made from hot Epsom salts or Footherapy solution from Para Laboratories/Queen Helene are good.

❑ Medicated pads are available that are supposed to treat corns and calluses. Most of these products are fairly aggressive, however, and may attack good tissue as well, provoking an allergic reaction.

❑ If you suffer from diabetes, you may need to consult a doctor or podiatrist. In people with diabetes, poor circulation can lead to problems with the feet. You should also consult a professional if the area becomes infected.

❑ If the problem is persistent, a physician may suggest an x-ray to rule out an underlying bone spur.

❑ *See also* ACID/ALKALI IMBALANCE, both in Part Two.

Cramps

See MUSCLE CRAMPS; PREMENSTRUAL SYNDROME.

Crohn's Disease

Crohn's disease is an inflammatory bowel disorder of unknown origin. It usually affects the lowest portion of the small intestine, but it can occur in other parts of the digestive tract, from the mouth to the anus. Crohn's disease causes inflammation that extends deep into the lining of the intestinal wall, frequently causing crampy abdominal pain, diarrhea, rectal bleeding, loss of appetite, and weight loss. A common complication of the disease is blockage of the intestine caused by scar tissue that narrows the passageway. The disease may also cause sores, or ulcers, that break through to the surrounding tissues. People with Crohn's disease also suffer from nutritional deficiencies.

A relatively small percentage of people (1.2 to 15 cases per 100,000 people in the United States) is affected by Crohn's disease. It affects men and women equally and tends to run in families. According to the Crohn's and Colitis Foundation of America (CCFA), people who have a relative with the disease have at least ten times the risk of developing Crohn's disease compared with the general population. This disorder affects people in all age groups, but the onset usually occurs either between ages fifteen and thirty or between ages sixty and eighty. Children with Crohn's disease may suffer delayed development and stunted growth due to nutritional deficiencies.

Crohn's disease can be difficult to diagnose because its symptoms are similar to those of other intestinal disorders, particularly ulcerative colitis—another inflammatory bowel disease which affects only the colon. Crohn's symptoms can also appear intermittently, occurring every few months to every few years for some people. In rare cases, the symptoms may appear once or twice and not return. If the disease continues for many years, bowel function gradually deteriorates. Left untreated, it can become extremely serious, even life threatening, and it may increase the risk of cancer by as much as twenty times.

Doctors believe that Crohn's disease has a genetic basis, but that it does not appear until triggered by the presence of bacteria or virus that provokes an abnormal activation of the immune system. The onset of Crohn's disease can be dramatic, with alarming symptoms such as sudden high fever, sudden weight loss of more than five pounds in a few days, significant rectal bleeding, severe abdominal pain that persists for more than an hour at a time, and persistent vomiting accompanied by a cessation of bowel movements. A series of tests may be required to confirm Crohn's disease. Blood tests may be done to check for anemia and/or a high white blood count. A doctor may do an upper gastrointestinal x-ray series to look at the small intestine, or a colonoscopy, in which the doctor inspects the interior of the large intestine using a long, flexible lighted tube linked to a computer and monitor. If the tests show the presence of Crohn's disease, the doctor may do more x-rays of both the upper and lower digestive tract to find out how much is affected by the disease.

Since there is no cure for Crohn's disease, the goals of treatment are to control inflammation, relieve symptoms, and correct nutritional deficiencies—all of which can help keep Crohn's disease in remission.

Unless otherwise specified, the dosages recommended here are for adults. For a child between the ages of twelve and seventeen, reduce the dose to three-quarters of the recommended amount. For a child between six and twelve, use one-half of the recommended dose, and for a child under the age of six, use one-quarter of the recommended amount.

NUTRIENTS

SUPPLEMENT	SUGGESTED DOSAGE	COMMENTS
Essential		
Duodenal glandular	As directed on label.	Aids in healing gastrointestinal ulcers.
L-Glutamine	500 mg twice daily, on an empty stomach. Take with water or juice. Do not take with milk. Take with 50 mg vitamin B_6 and 100 mg vitamin C for better absorption.	A major metabolic fuel for the intestinal cells; maintains the villi, the absorption surfaces of the gut. (*See* AMINO ACIDS in Part One.)
Liver extract injections plus	2 cc once weekly or as prescribed by physician.	Needed for proper digestion.
vitamin B complex and	1 cc once weekly or as prescribed by physician.	Helps to prevent anemia.
vitamin B_{12} and	1 cc twice weekly or as prescribed by physician.	Important for proper digestion and to prevent anemia. Deficiency aggravates malabsorption.
folic acid or	$^1/_4$ cc twice weekly or as prescribed by physician.	Needed for constant supply of new cells. Injections (under a doctor's supervision) are best. If injections are not available, use a lozenge or sublingual form.
vitamin B complex plus extra	100 mg 3 times daily.	
vitamin B_{12} and	1,000–2,000 mcg daily.	
folic acid	200 mcg daily.	
N-Acetylglucosamine (N-A-G from Source Naturals)	As directed on label.	A major constituent of the barrier layer that protects the intestinal lining from digestive enzymes and other potentially damaging intestinal contents.
Omega-3 essential fatty acids (Kyolic-EPA from Wakunaga, Intestamend from Health From The Sun, flaxseed oil, primrose oil, and salmon oil are good sources)	As directed on label.	Needed for repair of the digestive tract; reduces inflammatory processes. Studies show essential fatty acids may reduce Crohn's symptoms and aid in maintaining remission.
Pancreatin plus bromelain	As directed on label. Take with meals. As directed on label.	To break down protein and assist digestion.
Taurine Plus from American Biologics	500 mg daily, on an empty stomach. Take with 50 mg vitamin B_6 and 100 mg vitamin C for better absorption.	An important antioxidant and immune regulator. Use the sublingual form.
Vitamin C with bioflavonoids	1,000 mg 3 times daily.	Prevents inflammation and improves immunity. Use a buffered type.
Vitamin K	As directed on label.	Vital to colon health. Deficiency is common in people with this disorder due to malabsorption and diarrhea.
Zinc	50 mg daily. Do not exceed a total of 100 mg daily from all supplements.	Needed for the immune system and for healing. Use zinc gluconate lozenges or OptiZinc for best absorption.
Important		
Free-form amino acid complex (Amino Balance from Anabol Naturals)	$^1/_4$ tsp twice daily.	Protein is essential in the healing of the intestine. Use a sublingual form.
Garlic (Kyolic)	2 capsules 3 times daily, with meals.	Combats free radicals in Crohn's disease. Aids healing.
Lactobacilli (Kyo-Dophilus from Wakunaga) or Capricin from Probiologic	As directed on label. As directed on label.	Aids in digestion. Use a nondairy formula. A product containing both *L. acidophilus* and *L. bifidus* is best. Works in conjunction with butyric acid to reduce inflammation and seepage of undigested food particles.
Spiru-tein from Nature's Plus	2 capsules 3 times daily.	Supplies necessary protein. Helps stabilize blood sugar between meals.
Helpful		
Calcium and magnesium	2,000 mg daily. 1,500 mg daily.	Aids in preventing colon cancer.

Floradix Iron + Herbs from Salus Haus	2 tsp daily.	To prevent anemia. Floradix is a readily absorbable form of iron that is nontoxic and derived from food sources.
Gastro-Calm from Olympian Labs	As directed on label.	A combination of herbs and digestive enzymes to help relieve indigestion and reduce gastrointestinal inflammation.
Multivitamin and mineral complex with copper and manganese and selenium plus extra	As directed on label.	Malabsorption is often a result of this disorder. Copper, selenium, and manganese are important for treating this disorder and are often deficient because of absorption problems. Use a liquid, powder, or capsule formula.
potassium	99 mg daily.	May reduce surgical complications and also the need for surgery.
Oxy-Caps from Earth's Bounty	As directed on label.	An oxygen supplement to counter nutritional deficiencies caused by Crohn's disease.
Quercetin plus bromelain or Activated Quercetin from Source Naturals	500 mg twice daily, before meals. 100 mg twice daily, before meals. As directed on label.	Slows histamine release; helps control food allergies. Needed for a variety of enzyme functions. Improves absorption of quercetin. Contains quercetin plus bromelain and vitamin C.
Shark cartilage (BeneFin)	As directed on label. If you cannot tolerate taking it orally, it can be administered rectally in a retention enema.	Fights metastasis of cancerous tumors.
Vitamin A and vitamin E	25,000 IU daily. If you are pregnant, do not exceed 10,000 IU daily. Up to 800 IU daily.	Antioxidants that aid in controlling infection and in repair of the intestinal tract. Use emulsion forms for easier assimilation. Use d-alpha-tocopherol form of vitamin E.
Vitamin D_3	400 IU daily.	Prevents metabolic bone disease from developing as a result of malabsorption.

HERBS

❏ Aloe vera is beneficial for Crohn's disease because it softens stools and has a healing effect on the digestive tract. Drink $\frac{1}{2}$ cup of aloe vera juice three times daily.

❏ There are many combination herbal products designed to offer gastrointestinal relief. Enzymatic Therapy, Olympian Labs, and Solaray are recommended sources.

❏ Other herbs that are good for this disorder include burdock root, echinacea, fenugreek, goldenseal, licorice, marshmallow root, pau d'arco, enteric-coated peppermint (do not use any other form), red clover, rose hips, silymarin (milk thistle extract), slippery elm, and yerba maté. These herbs support digestion, cleanse the bloodstream, and reduce inflammation and infection. For best results, use them on an alternating basis.

Caution: Do not use licorice on a daily basis for more

than seven days in a row, and avoid it completely if you have high blood pressure. Do not take goldenseal on a daily basis for more than one week at a time, and do not use it during pregnancy. If you have a history of cardiovascular disease, diabetes, or glaucoma, use it only under a doctor's supervision.

RECOMMENDATIONS

❏ Eat a diet consisting mainly of non-acidic fresh or cooked vegetables such as broccoli, Brussels sprouts, cabbage, carrots, celery, garlic, kale, spinach, and turnips. Steam, broil, boil, or bake your food.

❏ Drink plenty of liquids, such as steam-distilled water, herbal teas, and fresh juices. Fresh cabbage juice is very beneficial.

❏ Add papaya to your diet. Chew a couple of the seeds to aid digestion.

❏ During an acute attack, eat organic baby foods, steamed vegetables, and well-cooked brown rice, millet, and oatmeal.

❏ Try eliminating all dairy foods (including cheese), fish, hard sausage, pickled cabbage, and yeast products from your diet, and see if symptoms improve. These foods are high in histamine. Many people with Crohn's disease are histamine-intolerant. Milk and other dairy products also contain carrageenan, a compound extracted from red seaweed. Carrageenan, which is widely used in the food industry for its ability to stabilize milk proteins, has been shown to induce ulcerative colitis in laboratory animals.

❏ Avoid alcohol, caffeine, carbonated beverages, chocolate, corn, nuts, popcorn, eggs, foods with artificial additives or preservatives, fried and greasy foods, margarine, meat, dairy products such as milk and cheese, pepper, spicy foods, tobacco, white flour, and all animal products, with the exception of white fish from clear waters. These foods are irritating to the digestive tract. Mucus-forming foods such as processed refined foods and dairy products should also be avoided. Limit your intake of barley, rye, and wheat.

❏ Avoid refined carbohydrates. Do not consume such foods as boxed dry cereals or anything containing any form of sugar. Diets high in refined carbohydrates have been associated with Crohn's disease. These foods must be eliminated from the diet.

❏ Check stools daily for bleeding.

❏ As much as possible, avoid stress. Our thoughts, nervous systems, and bodily functions are deeply interconnected. Our thoughts and moods affect our bodies. During an attack, rest is important.

❏ Make sure the bowels move daily, but do not use harsh laxatives (*see* CONSTIPATION and/or DIARRHEA in Part Two). Gentle enemas made by adding a dropperful of alcohol-free herbal extract and 1 teaspoon of nondairy acidophilus powder to 2 quarts of lukewarm water are good. Accumulations of toxic body wastes often become breeding grounds for parasitic infestation. Toxins can also be absorbed into the bloodstream through the colon wall. Psyllium husks should be used daily for fiber; this aids in removing toxins before they are absorbed.

Note: Always take supplemental fiber separately from other supplements and medications.

❏ Do not use rectal suppositories that contain hydrogenated chemically prepared fats.

❏ If you are constipated, use a cleansing enema. (*See* ENEMAS in Part Three.)

❏ Use a heating pad to reduce abdominal pain.

CONSIDERATIONS

❏ There are no consistent dietary rules that apply to everyone, but people with Crohn's disease are generally encouraged to eat a healthy diet to help the body replace lost nutrients. Moreover, some nutrients, such as essential fatty acids and the amino acid glutamine, have been shown to help maintain a state of remission.

❏ It is important that nutritional deficiencies be corrected for healing. Persons with inflammatory bowel disorders require as much as 30 percent more protein than normal. If chronic diarrhea is present, electrolyte and trace mineral deficiencies should be considered. Chronic steatorrhea (fatty stools resulting from improper digestion of fats) may result in deficiencies of calcium and magnesium.

❏ Drugs such as corticosteroids and sulfasalazine (Azulfidine), which are prescribed for inflammatory bowel diseases, and cholestyramine (Questran), which is prescribed to lower cholesterol levels, increase the need for nutritional supplements. Corticosteroids depress protein synthesis and inhibit normal calcium absorption by increasing excretion of vitamin C in the urine. Deficiencies of other nutrients, such as zinc, potassium, vitamin B_6 (pyridoxine), folic acid, and vitamin D, decrease bone formation and slow healing. Sulfasalazine inhibits the transport of folic acid and iron, causing anemia.

❏ Antioxidants have been shown to decrease the risk of developing Crohn's disease. The intestinal walls normally contain small amounts of the antioxidant enzymes superoxide dismutase (SOD), catalase, and glutathione peroxidase, but their ability to fight free radicals may be overwhelmed during periods of active inflammation, resulting in tissue damage.

❏ To reestablish a proper healing environment, it is necessary to maintain a generally alkaline bodily pH.

❏ Adhering to an allergen-free diet, replacing lost nutrients, and using selected herbs can speed healing and may prevent future disturbances. Studies have proven that when a person who has achieved remission goes back to his or her former diet, Crohn's disease returns. Other things that have been implicated in this disorder include prolonged stress, trauma, and psychosomatic and vascular factors.

❏ Nutritional deficiencies resulting from malabsorption may weaken the immune system, in turn prolonging the time required for the inflammation and ulcers to heal.

❏ Many microorganisms have been considered as possible causes of Crohn's disease, including fungi, bacteria, viruses, mycobacteria, pseudomonas-like organisms, and chlamydia. However, the cause of Crohn's disease has not yet been established. It is likely that multiple factors are involved.

❏ Antigenic reactions may result from "leaky gut syndrome," in which minute particles of undigested or partially digested food pass through the swollen and inflamed mucosal wall into the bloodstream, where they cause reactions. The mucosal wall must be repaired to avoid this. Avoiding foods that cause a reaction is important. (*See* ALLERGIES in Part Two.) Treatment with butyric acid, a monounsaturated fatty acid, reduces inflammatory conditions, reduces seepage of undigested food particles, and aids in repair of the mucosal wall. N-acetylglucosamine (NAG) prevents leaky gut syndrome.

❏ A study done in Italy found that people with Crohn's disease who took sustained-release fish oil supplements were less likely to suffer relapses than those who did not. Of the subjects in the one-year study who took fish oil, over half remained symptom-free, compared with only a quarter of those who took a placebo.

❏ Researchers have not been able to find a specific genetic marker for Crohn's disease, but they have found that the illness is four times more common in Caucasians and Jewish people than in people of other ethnic backgrounds. In 20 to 40 percent of reported cases, multiple family members have suffered either from Crohn's disease or ulcerative colitis.

❏ Most people with Crohn's disease are initially treated with drugs such as corticosteroids to help control inflammation. Drugs that suppress the immune system are also used, but they can increase susceptibility to infection. The Food and Drug Administration (FDA) has now approved a genetically engineered product called infliximab (Remicade) for people with moderate-to-severe Crohn's disease who have not responded to traditional treatments. Remicade is made from human and mouse cells, and works specifically against a protein that promotes inflammation in the body. In drug trials, one dose relieved many of the symptoms for two to four weeks, after which the benefits waned. Scientists are still studying the long-term effects.

❏ If Crohn's disease continues for many years, bowel function gradually deteriorates. Surgery may be required to remove the diseased portion of the intestine. While this surgery doesn't cure the disease, it can relieve symptoms, and five years later at least 50 percent of people who undergo it are in good health, can work full time, and enjoy life without being restricted by diarrhea or pain.

❑ People with Crohn's disease have a significantly higher than normal risk of developing colon cancer. If you have this disorder, you should undergo a colonoscopy at least once every two years, starting eight to ten years after diagnosis.

Croup

Croup or laryngotracheobronchitis, is a viral infection that causes the larynx or trachea (the upper part of the windpipe, near the vocal cords) to narrow due to swelling. The larynx goes into spasms, and the sufferer experiences difficulty breathing; a harsh, barking cough; hoarseness; tightness in the lungs; and feelings of suffocation. Mucus production may also increase, further clogging the airway.

At the beginning, croup has all the hallmarks of the common cold. It starts off with congestion, a runny nose, and a cough that develops into the distinctive barking cough associated with croup. Another trademark of croup is a harsh, wheezing noise that is made when air is breathed in through the constricted windpipe and over the inflamed vocal cords.

Croup most commonly occurs in young children and babies between the age of three months and three years whose airways are much narrower than those of adults. Attacks frequently occur at night. In the past, this illness was often caused by the measles virus, but now that children are immunized against measles, croup has become much less common than it once was. The virus usually runs its course in five to six days.

NUTRIENTS

SUPPLEMENT	SUGGESTED DOSAGE	COMMENTS
Essential		
Vitamin C with bioflavonoids	60 mg 4 times daily for children 6–12 months old; 100 mg 4 times daily for ages 1–4; 500 mg 4 times daily for children over 4.	Helps control infection and fever by boosting the immune system.
Zinc	5 mg once daily for 3 days for children 6–12 months old; 5 mg twice daily for 3 days for ages 1–3; 5 mg 3 times daily for 3 days for children over 3.	Promotes immune function and is necessary in healing. Use lozenges for faster absorption.
Very Important		
Vitamin A with mixed carotenoids	2,000 IU daily.	Needed for healing of the mucous membranes. Use an emulsion form.
Vitamin E	10 mg daily for children under 3; 20 mg daily for ages 3–6; 50 mg daily for children over 6.	Destroys free radicals and carries oxygen to all cells. Use an emulsion form for best absorption. Use d-alpha-tocopherol form.
Important		
Cod liver oil	1 tbsp twice daily in juice.	Can be used for children in place of vitamin A.

HERBS

❑ The following herbs are recommended for croup: echinacea, fenugreek, goldenseal, and thyme. Echinacea tincture should be taken if a fever is present. Take 15 drops in liquid every three to four hours.

Caution: Do not take goldenseal on a daily basis for more than one week at a time, and do not use it during pregnancy. If you have a history of cardiovascular disease, diabetes, or glaucoma, use it only under a doctor's supervision.

❑ Put a few drops of eucalyptus oil in a vaporizer and inhale the steam. It makes it easier for the child to breathe if the air is kept humidified.

❑ Fenu-Thyme combination from Nature's Way is good for congestion.

❑ Give a child with croup very warm ginger herb baths; then immediately wrap the child in a heavy towel or blanket, and put him or her to bed to perspire. This helps loosen mucus and rid the body of toxins. You can also let your child stay in a steam-filled bathroom for ten or fifteen minutes. The moisture makes it easier to breathe.

RECOMMENDATIONS

❑ Give a child with croup plenty of fluids to help to thin mucus. Steam-distilled water, herbal teas, and homemade soups are good choices.

❑ Apply hot onion packs over the chest and back three times a day. Slice onions and place them between cloths, and then apply the pack and cover it with a heating pad. Onion packs open the pores and relieve congestion.

❑ If a child with croup is having difficulty breathing, take him or her to the emergency room of the nearest hospital for treatment and for x-rays of the larynx. Oxygen may be needed. Milder cases of croup can be treated at home, but parents should be alert for signs of increasing breathing difficulty.

CONSIDERATIONS

❑ Croup is a viral infection, so antibiotics will not help.

❑ Fresh cold air may also help the child to breathe by reducing the swelling of the trachea and larynx.

Cushing's Syndrome

See under ADRENAL DISORDERS.

Cystic Fibrosis

Cystic fibrosis (CF) is the most common inherited illness among Americans of northern and western European ancestry. It occurs in people of all ethnic backgrounds and is most common in Caucasians. It occurs with approximately equal frequency in men and women.

One in every 3,000 children in the United States is born with the disorder. It is estimated that 8 million Americans are silent carriers of the defective gene that leads to this disease. The gene responsible for CF was identified in 1989 on human chromosome 7, and it encodes instructions for a protein that regulates the passage of salt in and out of the cells of the body's exocrine glands. This defective gene transforms the protein (called the cystic fibrosis transmembrane conductance regulator (CFTR) and causes it to produce a mucus too thick and too abundant for the body to excrete. In most people with CF, the genetic instructions omit just one of the protein's 1,480 constituent amino acids—a tiny glitch, but a devastating one that affects many different glands in the body, including the pancreas, sweat glands, and glands of the digestive and respiratory systems.

All human cells (except red blood cells, eggs, and sperm) contain two copies of this gene, one inherited from each parent. CF results when both copies of the "CF gene" are abnormal. If one copy is abnormal and the other normal, an individual is said to be a carrier; he or she will show no signs of CF, but is capable of passing a defective gene on to offspring. Statistically, a child of two carrier parents has a 1-in-4 chance of inheriting CF; a 1-in-4 chance of being completely free of the mutant gene; and a 1-in-2 chance of being a carrier, like the parents.

The airway, gastrointestinal tract, bile ducts of the liver, ducts of the pancreas, and the male genitourinary tract all produce mucus. Cystic fibrosis alters this normally protective mucus and transforms it into a thick, abnormal excretion that obstructs airways and damages tissue. Symptoms of CF begin early in life. Glands in the lungs and bronchial tubes secrete large quantities of thick, sticky mucus that blocks lung passages and provides the perfect place for harmful bacteria to thrive. *Pseudomonas aeruginosa* (also common in cancer and burn patients) is the bacteria that most commonly colonizes the lungs, resulting in chronic coughing and wheezing, difficulty breathing, and recurrent lung infections. Once established, the bacteria remain in the lungs and are responsible for repeated outbreaks of infection. They form their own dense structure, called a biofilm,

and are immune to most current treatments. They also produce toxic proteins that can cause tissue damage and weaken the immune system. The lungs of many children with CF are inhabited or colonized by the *Pseudomonas aeruginosa* bacteria before they are ten years of age.

Thick secretions also often obstruct the release of pancreatic enzymes, resulting in digestive difficulties and malabsorption problems, particularly problems with the metabolism of fats. Malnutrition may result because a lack of necessary digestive enzymes means that nutrients from foods are not properly absorbed. This in turn can cause pain after eating and, especially in young children, a failure to gain weight normally. Pancreatic enzymes need to be replaced to counter this.

Persons with this disease also lose excessive amounts of salt through their sweat glands. Sweating may be profuse, and the sweat itself contains abnormally high concentrations of sodium, potassium, and chloride salts. Other signs suggestive of CF include clubbing of the fingers and toes (a result of poor circulation); greasy, bulky, foul-smelling stools; and salty-tasting skin. The reproductive organs may be affected, causing infertility in almost all men and some women.

The identification of the CF gene has enabled researchers to begin developing new approaches to diagnosis and treatment of the disease. A test is now available in which cells are swabbed from the inside of the cheek and then examined for the presence of defective genes. The presence of both normal and mutant CF genes indicates that the individual is a carrier. If only mutant genes are there, CF is indicated.

The most widely used test for CF is the electrolyte sweat test. Developed over forty years ago, the sweat test detects the excessive amounts of electrolytes (charged mineral salts) found on the skin of many people with CF. A physician would likely recommend that a sweat test be performed on a child who failed to gain weight despite adequate feeding, or who suffered from very frequent respiratory infections. CF testing is currently recommended only for those individuals with symptoms highly suggestive of the disease, or with a family history of the disorder. However, if there is doubt about the diagnosis, the sweat test can be confirmed by performing a genetic test.

Unless otherwise specified, the dosages recommended here are for adults. For a child between the ages of twelve and seventeen, reduce the dose to three-quarters the recommended amount. For a child between six and twelve, use one-half the recommended dose, and for a child under the age of six, use one-quarter the recommended amount.

NUTRIENTS

SUPPLEMENT	SUGGESTED DOSAGE	COMMENTS
Very Important		
Pancreatin	As directed on label. Take with meals.	Needed for protein digestion.

Proteolytic enzymes	As directed on label, on an empty stomach. Take between meals.	Aids in controlling infection, helps digestion, and thins the mucous secretions of the lungs.
Vitamin A plus carotenoid complex with beta-carotene	As directed on label. As directed on label.	Aids in the maintenance and repair of epithelial tissue, which makes up the mucous membranes. Use emulsion form for better absorption and greater safety at higher doses.
Vitamin B complex plus extra vitamin B$_2$ (riboflavin)	100 mg of each major B vitamin 3 times daily, with meals (amounts of individual vitamins in a complex will vary). 50 mg 3 times daily.	Aids in digestion, healing, and tissue repair.
Vitamin B$_{12}$	1,000–2,000 mcg daily, on an empty stomach.	Needed for proper digestion and assimilation of nutrients, including iron. Use a lozenge, sublingual, or spray form.
Vitamin C with bioflavonoids	3,000–6,000 mg daily, in divided doses.	For tissue repair and immune function.
Vitamin E	As directed on label.	Repairs tissue and prevents cell damage. Also helps in the utilization of vitamin A. Use d-alpha-tocopherol form.
Vitamin K or alfalfa	100 mcg twice daily.	Deficiency is common in those with this disorder. Needed for proper digestion. *See under* Herbs, below.

Important		
Essential fatty acids (primrose oil is a good source)	As directed on label.	Relieves inflammation.
Protein supplement or free-form amino acid complex (Amino Balance from Anabol Naturals)	As directed on label.	Needed for healing. Use protein from a vegetable source or a free-form amino acid complex.
Zinc	50 mg daily. Do not exceed a total of 100 mg daily from all supplements.	Important in immune function and healing of tissue. Use zinc gluconate lozenges or OptiZinc for best absorption.

Helpful		
Coenzyme Q$_{10}$ plus	100 mg daily.	Acts as an immunostimulant.
Coenzyme A from Coenzyme-A Technologies	As directed on label.	Supports the immune system's detoxification of many dangerous substances.
Copper and selenium	3 mg daily. 200 mcg daily. If you are pregnant, do not exceed 40 mcg daily.	Low levels of copper and selenium have been linked to cystic fibrosis.
Kyo-Green from Wakunaga or chlorophyll	As directed on label. As directed on label.	To supply minerals and chlorophyll needed to control infection.
L-Cysteine and L-methionine	500 mg each twice daily, on an empty stomach. Take with water or juice. Do not take with milk. Take with 50 mg vitamin B$_6$ and 100 mg vitamin C for better absorption.	Needed for repair of lung tissue and to protect the liver. (*See* AMINO ACIDS in Part One.)

Lipoic acid	As directed on label.	Helps the pancreas to function properly and controls the metabolism of sugar.
Methylsulfonyl-methane (MSM)	As directed on label.	Clinical tests have proven that this supplement combats lung damage.
Pycnogenol	As directed on label.	A powerful antioxidant that also protects the lungs.
Raw pancreas glandular and raw spleen glandular and raw thymus glandular	As directed on label. As directed on label. As directed on label.	To relieve inflammation. (*See* GLANDULAR THERAPY in Part Three.)
Vitamin D	400 IU daily.	Aids in protecting the lungs.

HERBS

❏ Alfalfa extract supplies vitamin K and necessary minerals, which are often deficient in those with cystic fibrosis due to absorption problems. It is also a good source of chlorophyll.

❏ Boswella, bromelain, cayenne, ginger, and peppermint can aid in reducing inflammation.

❏ Expectorant herbs such as cayenne, elecampane, garlic, horehound, hyssop, and mullein may be effective in helping to clear some of the congestion.

❏ ClearLungs from RidgeCrest Herbals is a Chinese herbal formula that is highly recommended for this condition.

❏ Eucalyptus, garlic, onion, tea tree oil, and thyme have natural antiseptic properties and fight infection.

❏ Echinacea, licorice, and Siberian ginseng are good for building up the immune system.

Caution: If overused, licorice can elevate blood pressure. Do not use this herb on a daily basis for more than seven days in a row. Avoid it completely if you have high blood pressure. Do not use Siberian ginseng if you have hypoglycemia, high blood pressure, or a heart disorder.

❏ Lung Tonic from Herbs Etc. is a combination of many organic herbs designed to support the lungs.

❏ Other herbs beneficial for cystic fibrosis include echinacea, ginger, goldenseal, and yarrow tea.

RECOMMENDATIONS

❏ Eat a diet consisting of 75 percent raw fruits and vegetables, and raw nuts and seeds.

❏ Make sure your intake of calories, protein, and other nutrients is adequate. People with CF require as much as 50 percent more of many nutrients than normal. Take supplements to provide required enzymes, vitamins, and minerals.

❏ Include in the diet foods that are high in germanium,

such as garlic, shiitake mushrooms, and onions. Germanium helps to improve tissue oxygenation at the cellular level.

❑ During hot weather, drink plenty of fluids and increase your salt intake.

❑ Do not eat foods that stimulate secretions by the mucous membranes. Cooked and processed foods cause excess mucus buildup and drain the body of energy. These foods are harder to digest. Do not eat animal products, dairy products, processed foods, sugar, or white flour products.

❑ When you must take antibiotics, take acidophilus to replace "friendly" bacteria.

CONSIDERATIONS

❑ The symptoms of cystic fibrosis are normally controlled with a number of different drugs. Antibiotics are used to combat the infections to which people with CF are prone, especially infection with *Pseudomonas aeruginosa,* a type of microbe that is attracted to the sticky mucus in the lungs. Pancrelipase (also sold under a variety of brand names, including Viokase) is a prescription product containing a combination of digestive enzymes that is often prescribed for people with CF and other pancreatic insufficiencies. Many people also take anti-inflammatory drugs such as ibuprofen (Advil, Nuprin, and others), naproxen (Naprosyn), or prednisone (Deltasone and others).

❑ A small hand-held device called the Flutter helps people with CF to dislodge mucus from the airways. It can replace conventional physiotherapy.

❑ The future of CF treatment may lie in gene therapy. In the laboratory, normal CF genes have been successfully introduced into cells from people with CF. Experiments in rats have indicated that replacing the defective CF genes with normal ones in just 10 percent of the lung lining cells improves lung function. However, because the genes in the cells of the reproductive system are unaffected by this procedure, the defect can still be passed on to offspring. As part of this gene therapy, work is proceeding with vector aerosols. A vector is like a shuttle that can deliver a good copy of the defective gene to the appropriate place in the body.

❑ The drug amiloride (Midamor, Moduretic), which is used as an adjunct to treatment with some diuretic drugs, is being tested as a treatment for CF. It is believed to thin lung secretions by blocking sodium uptake by lung cells.

❑ DNAase (Dornase) is a naturally occurring enzyme that breaks down DNA molecules. Part of the reason the mucus that clogs the airways of people with CF is so thick and sticky is that it contains large molecules of DNA released by white blood cells as they die fighting chronic bacterial infection. This makes the mucus even denser and more difficult to expel. Breaking down the DNA molecules helps to thin the mucus.

❑ Levels of two fatty acids—arachidonic acid (AA) and docosahexaenoic acid (DHA)—have been found to be out of balance in people with CF. This lipid imbalance is most noticeable in the lungs, pancreas, and intestine—all of the areas most affected by cystic fibrosis. Research in this area seems promising.

❑ When the antibiotic tobramycin (Nebcin) is administered by aerosol spray, it has proved to be more effective in reaching infected lung tissue than when administered through the traditional intravenous route.

❑ Low levels of selenium and vitamin E have been linked to cystic fibrosis and cancer.

❑ Further information about cystic fibrosis is available from the Cystic Fibrosis Foundation (*see* HEALTH AND MEDICAL ORGANIZATIONS in the Appendix).

Cystitis

See BLADDER INFECTION.

Dandruff

Dandruff is a common scalp condition that occurs when dead skin is shed, producing irritating white flakes. It is usually a condition of oily, rather than dry, skin, and occurs as skin cells renew themselves and the old cells are shed. Some people tend to generate and discard skin cells at a faster rate than others. Recent research shows that severe cases of flaking scalp, usually associated with seborrhea (a type of dermatitis), may be caused by an overgrowth of the yeast *Pityrosporum ovale,* which lives naturally on the skin.

Dandruff can be triggered by trauma, illness, hormonal imbalances, improper carbohydrate consumption, and the consumption of sugar. Deficiencies of nutrients such as the B-complex vitamins, essential fatty acids, and selenium have been linked to dandruff as well. Dandruff is normally worse in the winter months.

Dandruff is an annoying and embarrassing problem, but is rarely serious. There is no cure for dandruff, but the condition can be minimized.

NUTRIENTS

SUPPLEMENT	SUGGESTED DOSAGE	COMMENTS
Very Important		
Essential fatty acids (flaxseed oil, primrose oil, and salmon oil are good sources)	As directed on label.	Helps to relieve itching and inflammation; essential for healthy skin and scalp.

Kelp	1,000–1,500 mg daily.	Supplies needed minerals, especially iodine, for better hair growth and healing of the scalp.
Selenium	200 mcg daily. If you are pregnant, do not exceed 40 mcg daily.	An important antioxidant to aid in controlling dry scalp.
Vitamin B complex plus extra vitamin B₆ (pyridoxine) and vitamin B₁₂	100 mg of each major B vitamin twice daily, with meals (amounts of individual vitamins in a complex will vary). 50 mg twice daily. 1,000–2,000 mcg daily.	B vitamins are needed for healthy skin and hair. Use a high-stress formula. Sublingual forms are best for absorption.
Vitamin E	400 IU and up.	For improved circulation. Use d-alpha-tocopherol form.
Zinc lozenges	1 15-mg lozenge 5 times daily for 1 week. Do not exceed a total of 100 mg daily from all supplements.	Protein metabolism depends on zinc. The skin is composed primarily of protein.
Important		
Free-form amino acid complex (Amino Balance from Anabol Naturals)	As directed on label.	Needed for repair of all tissues and for proper hair growth. Use a formula containing both essential and nonessential amino acids.
L-Cystine	500 mg daily, on an empty stomach. Take with water or juice. Do not take with milk. Take with 50 mg vitamin B₆ and 100 mg vitamin C for better absorption.	Needed for flexibility of the skin and for hair texture. (*See* AMINO ACIDS in Part One.)
Vitamin A plus mixed carotenoids	Up to 20,000 IU daily. If you are pregnant, do not exceed 10,000 IU daily. 15,000 IU daily.	Helps prevent dry skin. Aids in healing of tissue. Antioxidants and precursors of vitamin A.
Vitamin C with bioflavonoids	3,000–6,000 mg daily, in divided doses.	An important antioxidant to prevent tissue damage to the scalp and to aid in healing.
Helpful		
Lecithin granules or capsules	1 tbsp 3 times daily, before meals. 1,200 mg 3 times daily, before meals.	Protects the scalp and strengthens cell membranes of the scalp and hair.

HERBS

❏ An infusion of chaparral or thyme may be used as a hair rinse.

❏ Those with dandruff can benefit from taking dandelion, goldenseal, and red clover.

Caution: Do not take goldenseal on a daily basis for more than one week at a time, and do not use it during pregnancy. If you have a history of cardiovascular disease, diabetes, or glaucoma, use it only under a doctor's supervision.

RECOMMENDATIONS

❏ Eat a diet consisting of 50 to 75 percent raw foods. Eat soured products such as yogurt.

❏ Avoid fried foods, dairy products, sugar, flour, chocolate, nuts, and seafood.

❏ *See* FASTING in Part Three, and follow the program once a month.

❏ Before washing your hair, add about 8 tablespoons of pure organic peanut oil to the juice of half a lemon and rub the mixture into your scalp. Leave it on for five to ten minutes, then shampoo.

❏ Try rinsing your hair with vinegar and water instead of plain water after shampooing. Use 1/4 cup vinegar to 1 quart of water.

❏ If antibiotics are prescribed, take extra B-complex vitamins. Also take an acidophilus supplement to replace the "friendly" bacteria that are destroyed by antibiotics.

❏ Do not pick or scratch the scalp. Make sure to wash your hair frequently, and use a non-oily shampoo. Use natural hair products that do not contain chemicals. Avoid using irritating soaps and greasy ointments and creams. Massage your scalp first before washing your hair.

❏ Do not use a shampoo containing selenium on a daily basis, even if it aids in controlling dandruff.

❏ If dandruff is persistent or symptoms seem to be getting worse, or if it appears in areas other than the scalp, consult your health care provider.

CONSIDERATIONS

❏ Some people have found that sun exposure helps clear up dandruff, but others find that it seems to make the problem worse.

❏ It is best not to use over-the-counter ointments for dandruff. They can often do more harm than good.

❏ Nizoral A-D is an antifungal dandruff shampoo.

❏ Dermatologists usually prescribe a cleansing lotion containing a drying agent with sulfur and resorcinol, or a medicated product called Diprosone from Schering-Plough, to clear up dandruff.

❏ *See also* SEBORRHEA in Part Two.

Deafness

See HEARING LOSS.

Depression

Depression affects an estimated 17 million Americans every year, making it one of the most common medical problems in the United States. It affects young and old, and is twice as common in women as in men.

Depression is a whole-body illness, one that affects the body, nervous system, moods, thoughts, and behavior. It affects the way you eat and sleep, the way you feel about yourself, and the way you react to and think about the people and things around you. Symptoms can last for weeks, months, or years. There are many types of depression, with variations in the number of symptoms, their severity, and persistence.

People with depression typically withdraw and hide from society. They lose interest in things around them and become incapable of experiencing pleasure. Symptoms of depression include chronic fatigue, sleep disturbances (either insomnia or excessive sleeping), changes in appetite, headaches, backaches, digestive disorders, restlessness, irritability, quickness to anger, loss of interest or pleasure in hobbies, and feelings of worthlessness and inadequacy. Many think of death and consider suicide. Things appear bleak and time seems to pass slowly. A person with depression may be chronically angry and irritable, sad and despairing, or display little or no emotion at all. Some try to "sleep off" depression, or do nothing but sit or lie around.

The two major classifications of depressive disorders are *unipolar* and *bipolar*. Unipolar disorders are characterized by depressive episodes that most often recur at least several times in the course of a person's life. Bipolar disorders usually begin as depression, but as they progress, they involve alternating episodes of depression and mania. As a result, bipolar depression is commonly known as *manic depression*. (*See* MANIC-DEPRESSIVE DISORDER in Part Two.) This section focuses primarily on various types of unipolar depression.

The causes of depression are not fully understood, but they are probably many and varied. Depression may be triggered by tension, stress, a traumatic life event, chemical imbalances in the brain, thyroid disorders, nutritional deficiencies, poor diet, the consumption of sugar, mononucleosis, lack of exercise, endometriosis, any serious physical disorder, or allergies. One of the most common causes of depression is food allergies. Hypoglycemia (low blood sugar) is another common cause of depression.

Heredity is a significant factor in this disorder. In up to 50 percent of people suffering from recurrent episodes of depression, one or both of the parents also experienced depression.

Whatever the factors that trigger it, depression begins with a disturbance in the part of the brain that governs moods. Most people can handle everyday stresses; their bodies readjust to these pressures. When stress is too great for a person and his or her adjustment mechanism is unresponsive, depression may be triggered.

Perhaps the most common type of depression is a chronic low-grade depression called *dysthymia*. This condition involves long-term and/or recurring depressive symptoms that are not necessarily disabling but keep a person from functioning normally and interfere with social interactions and enjoyment of life. Research has found that this type of depression often results from (unconscious) negative thinking habits. *Double depression* is a variation of dysthymia in which a person with chronic, low-grade depression periodically experiences major depressive episodes, then returns to his or her "normal," mildly depressed state.

Some people become more depressed in the winter months, when the days are shorter and darker. This type of disorder is known as *seasonal affective disorder (SAD)*. Women are more likely to suffer from SAD than men are. People who suffer this type of depression in the winter months lose their energy, suffer anxiety attacks, gain weight as a result of craving the wrong foods, sleep too much, and have a reduced sex drive. Many people get depressed around the December holidays; while most of them probably just have the "holiday blues," some of them may be suffering from seasonal affective disorder. Suicides seem to be highest during this time of year.

Foods greatly influence the brain's behavior. A poor diet, especially one with a lot of junk foods, is a common cause of depression. The levels of brain chemicals called neurotransmitters, which regulate our behavior, are controlled by what we eat, and neurotransmitters are closely linked to mood. The neurotransmitters most commonly associated with mood are dopamine, serotonin, and norepinephrine. When the brain produces serotonin, tension is eased. When it produces dopamine or norepinephrine, we tend to think and act more quickly and are generally more alert.

At the neurochemical and physiological level, neurotransmitters are extremely important. These substances carry impulses between nerve cells. Serotonin, for example, plays a role in mood, sleep, and appetite. Low levels of serotonin can lead to depression, anxiety, and sleep disorders. The substance that processes serotonin is the amino acid tryptophan. The consumption of tryptophan increases the amount of serotonin made by the brain. Thus, eating complex carbohydrates (not simple carbohydrates such as fructose, sucrose, and lactose), which raise the level of tryptophan in the brain (thereby increasing serotonin production), has a calming effect. High-protein foods, on the other hand, promote the production of dopamine and norepinephrine, which promote alertness.

The American Psychiatric Society estimates that 80 to 90 percent of cases of depression can be treated effectively, but that two-thirds of people who suffer from depression do not get the help they need. Many people do not seek treatment because they are ashamed, or they feel lethargic and despondent. In many cases, people with major depression only seek help when they are at the point of breakdown, or when they are hospitalized following a suicide attempt (an estimated 15 percent of chronic depression cases result in suicide). A good support system from friends and family members is often crucial in getting a depressed person to seek help for his or her illness.

The following nutrients are helpful for those suffering from depression. Unless otherwise specified, the dosages recommended here are for adults. For a child between the ages of twelve and seventeen, reduce the dose to three-quarters of the recommended amount. For a child between six and twelve, use one-half of the recommended dose, and for a child under the age of six, use one-quarter of the recommended amount.

NUTRIENTS

SUPPLEMENT	SUGGESTED DOSAGE	COMMENTS
Essential		
Essential fatty acids (Kyolic-EPA from Wakunaga, salmon oil, flaxseed oil, and primrose oil are good sources)	As directed on label. Take with meals.	Aid in the transmission of nerve impulses; needed for normal brain function.
5 Hydroxytryptophan (5-HTP)	As directed on label.	Increases the body's production of serotonin. It should not be used with other antidepressants.
L-Tyrosine	Up to 50 mg per pound of body weight daily. Take on an empty stomach with 50 mg vitamin B6 and 100–500 mg vitamin C for better absorption. Best taken at bedtime.	Alleviates stress by boosting production of adrenaline. It also raises dopamine levels, which influence moods. (*See* AMINO ACIDS in Part One.) *Caution:* Do not take tyrosine if you are taking an MAO inhibitor drug.
S-adenosylmethionine (SAMe) (SAMe Rx-Mood from Nature's Plus)	As directed on label.	Works as an antidepressant. *Caution:* Do not use if you have manic-depressive disorder or take prescription antidepressants.
Sub-Adrene from American Biologics	As directed on label.	A dietary supplement for adrenal support.
Taurine Plus from American Biologics	As directed on label.	An important antioxidant and immune regulator, necessary for white blood cell activation and neurological function. Use the sublingual form.
Vitamin B complex injections	2 cc once weekly or as prescribed by physician.	B vitamins are necessary for the normal functioning of the brain and nervous system. If depression is severe, injections (under a doctor's supervision) are recommended. All injectables can be combined in a single shot.
plus extra vitamin B6 (pyridoxine) and	½ cc once weekly or as prescribed by physician.	Needed for normal brain function. May help lift depression.
vitamin B12 or	1 cc once weekly or as prescribed by physician.	Linked to the production of the neurotransmitter acetylcholine.
vitamin B complex	As directed on label.	If injections are not available, a sublingual form of B complex is recommended.
plus extra pantothenic acid (vitamin B5) and	500 mg daily.	The most potent anti-stress vitamin.
vitamin B6 (pyridoxine) plus	50 mg 3 times daily.	
vitamin B3 (niacin)	50 mg 3 times daily. Do not exceed this amount.	Improves cerebral circulation. *Caution:* Do not take niacin if you have a liver disorder, gout, or high blood pressure.
plus vitamin B12 and	1,000–2,000 mcg daily.	
folic acid	400 mcg daily.	Found to be deficient in people with depression.
Zinc	50 mg daily. Do not exceed a total of 100 mg daily from all supplements.	Found to be deficient in people with depression. Use zinc gluconate lozenges or OptiZinc for best absorption.
Important		
Choline and inositol or	100 mg each twice daily.	Important in brain function and neurotransmission. *Caution:* Do not take these supplements if you suffer from manic (bipolar) depression.
lecithin	As directed on label.	
Helpful		
Calcium and	1,500–2,000 mg daily.	Has a calming effect. Needed for the nervous system.
magnesium	1,000 mg daily.	Works with calcium. Use magnesium asporotate or magnesium chelate form.
Chromium	300 mcg daily.	Aids in mobilizing fats for energy.
Gamma-amino-butyric acid (GABA)	750 mg daily. Take with 200 mg niacinamide for best results.	Has a tranquilizing effect, much as diazepam (Valium) and other tranquilizers do. *See* AMINO ACIDS in Part One.
Lithium	As prescribed by physician.	A trace mineral used to treat bipolar (manic) depression. Available by prescription only.
Megavital Forte from Futurebiotics or	As directed on label.	A balanced vitamin and mineral formula that increases energy and sense of well-being.
multivitamin and mineral complex	As directed on label.	To correct vitamin and mineral deficiencies, often associated with depression.
Nicotinamide adenine dinucleotide (NADH)	5–15 mg daily.	Enhances production of dopamine, serotonin, and noradrenaline, which are key neurotransmitters.
Vitamin C with bioflavonoids plus extra	2,000–5,000 mg daily, in divided doses.	Needed for immune function. Aids in preventing depression.
rutin	200–300 mg daily.	Buckwheat-derived bioflavonoid. Enhances vitamin C absorption.

HERBS

❏ Balm, also known as lemon balm, is good for the stomach and digestive organs during stressful situations.

❏ Ephedra (ma huang) may be helpful for lethargic depression.

Caution: Do not use this herb if you suffer from anxiety disorder, glaucoma, heart disease, high blood pressure, or insomnia, or if you are taking a monoamine oxidase (MAO) inhibitor drug.

❏ Ginger, ginkgo biloba, licorice root, oat straw, peppermint, and Siberian ginseng may be helpful.

Caution: Do not use licorice on a daily basis for more than seven days in a row. Avoid it completely if you have high blood pressure. Do not use Siberian ginseng if you have hypoglycemia, high blood pressure, or a heart disorder.

❏ Kava kava helps to induce calm and relieve depression.

Caution: This herb can cause drowsiness. If this occurs,

discontinue use or reduce the dosage. Do not use kava kava if you are pregnant or nursing, or if you are taking antidepressants. Long-term use of kava kava may result in dry, scaly skin and yellowish discoloration of the hair and nails.

❏ St. John's wort acts in the same way as monoamine oxidase (MAO) inhibitors do, but less harshly.

Caution: Do not use this herb if you take prescription antidepressants or any medication that interacts with monoamine oxidase (MAO) inhibitor drugs. Use it with caution during pregnancy.

RECOMMENDATIONS

❏ Eat a diet that includes plenty of raw fruits and vegetables, with soybeans and soy products, whole grains, seeds, nuts, brown rice, millet, and legumes. A diet too low in complex carbohydrates can cause serotonin depletion and depression.

❏ If you are nervous and wish to become more relaxed, consume more complex carbohydrates. For increased alertness, eat protein meals containing essential fatty acids. Salmon and white fish are good choices. If you need your spirits lifted, you will benefit from eating foods like turkey and salmon, which are high in tryptophan and protein.

❏ Omit wheat products from the diet. Wheat gluten has been linked to depressive disorders.

❏ Avoid diet sodas and other products containing the artificial sweetener aspartame (NutraSweet, Equal). This additive can block the formation of serotonin and cause headaches, insomnia, and depression in individuals who are already serotonin-deprived.

❏ Limit your intake of supplements that contain the amino acid phenylalanine. It contains the chemical phenol, which is highly allergenic. Most depressed people are allergic to certain substances. If you take a combination free-form amino acid supplement, look for a product that does not contain phenylalanine, such as that made by Ecological Formulas. Phenylalanine is one of the major components of aspartame.

❏ Avoid foods high in saturated fats; the consumption of meat or fried foods, such as hamburgers and French fries, leads to sluggishness, slow thinking, and fatigue. They interfere with blood flow by causing the arteries and small blood vessels to become blocked and the blood cells to become sticky and tend to clump together, resulting in poor circulation, especially to the brain.

❏ Avoid all forms of sugar, including normally "good" sweeteners such as honey, molasses, and fruit juice. The body reacts more quickly to the presence of sugar than it does to the presence of complex carbohydrates. The increase in energy supplied by the simple carbohydrates (sugars) is quickly followed by fatigue and depression. Stevia, a concentrated natural sweetener derived from a South American shrub, does not have the same effect on the body

as sugar, and does not have the side effects of artificial sugar substitutes.

❏ Avoid alcohol, caffeine, and processed foods.

❏ Investigate the possibility that food allergies are causing or contributing to depression. *See* ALLERGIES in Part Two.

❏ Have a hair analysis to rule out heavy metal intoxication as the cause of depression. *See* HAIR ANALYSIS in Part Three.

❏ Keep your mind active, and get plenty of rest and regular exercise. Studies have shown that exercise—walking, swimming, or any activity that you enjoy—is most important for all types of depression. Avoid stressful situations.

❏ Learn to recognize, and then to "reroute," negative thinking patterns. Working with a qualified professional to change ingrained habits can be rewarding (cognitive-behavioral therapists specialize in this type of work). Keeping a daily log also can help you to recognize distorted thoughts and develop a more positive way of thinking.

❏ If you are suffering from situational depression—depression that occurs in response to an event such as in the death of a loved one or the breakup of a relationship—try using *Ignatia amara.* This is a homeopathic remedy derived from a plant, Saint Ignatius bean, that helps control emotions during periods of extreme grief and hysteria.

❏ If depression is seasonal, light therapy may help. Exposure to the sun and bright light seem to regulate the body's production of melatonin, a hormone produced by the pineal gland that is, in part, responsible for preventing the blues. Stay in brightly lit rooms on dark days. Keep all draperies, curtains, and blinds open and use full-spectrum fluorescent lights in your home. The normal room has about 500 to 800 lux of light. Choose one room and light it with about 10,000 lux of full-spectrum light and spend at least half an hour there each day. For information about devices for this type of light treatment, contact either The SunBox Company or Apollo Light Systems (*see* MANUFACTURER AND DISTRIBUTOR INFORMATION in the Appendix).

❏ *See* HYPOTHYROIDISM in Part Two and take the underarm test to detect an underactive thyroid. If your temperature is low, consult your physician. Thyroid dysfunction is behind many depressive disorders.

❏ Try using color to alleviate depression. *See* COLOR THERAPY in Part Three.

CONSIDERATIONS

❏ Depression is not a natural part of aging, but it is frequently linked to age-related nutritional problems, such as B-vitamin deficiencies or poor eating habits. Older people who suffer from depression are as likely to benefit from treatment as a person in any other age bracket.

❏ Tyrosine is needed for brain function. This amino acid is directly involved in the production of norepinephrine and dopamine, two vital neurotransmitters that are synthesized in the brain and the adrenal medulla. A lack of tyrosine can result in a deficiency of norepinephrine in certain sites in the brain, resulting in mood disorders such as depression. The effects of stress may be prevented or reversed if this essential amino acid is obtained in the diet or by means of supplements. Mustard greens, beans, and spinach are good sources of tyrosine.

Caution: If you are taking an MAO inhibitor drug for depression, *do not* take tyrosine supplements, and avoid foods containing tyrosine, as drug and dietary interactions can cause a sudden, dangerous rise in blood pressure. Discuss food and medicine limitations thoroughly with your health care provider or a qualified dietitian.

❏ Some preliminary studies show promise in using dehydroepiandrosterone (DHEA)—a hormone naturally produced by the body—in the treatment of depression. In one study, nearly all patients taking DHEA for six weeks significantly improved, and about half of those were no longer considered clinically depressed.

❏ Selenium has been shown to elevate mood and decrease anxiety. These effects were more noticeable in people who had lower levels of selenium in their diets to begin with.

❏ Vigorous exercise can be an effective antidote to bouts of depression. During exercise, the brain produces pain-killing chemicals called endorphins and enkephalins. Certain endorphins and other brain chemicals released in response to exercise also produce a natural "high." Most of those who exercise regularly say that they feel really good afterward. This may explain why exercise is the best way to get rid of depression.

❏ Music can have powerful effects on mood and may be useful in alleviating depression. (*See* MUSIC AND SOUND THERAPY in Part Three.)

❏ In one study, people suffering from depression were found to have lower than normal levels of folic acid in their blood than non-depressed individuals. Other studies have shown that zinc levels tend to be significantly lower than normal when people suffer from depression.

❏ It may be possible to diagnose depression by using a computerized tomography (CT) scan to measure a person's adrenal glands. Researchers at Duke University found that people suffering from clinical depression have larger adrenal glands than non-depressed people.

❏ A variety of different drugs are commonly prescribed to treat depression. Antidepressant drugs fight depression by changing the balance of neurotransmitters in the body. These medications include the following:

• *Monoamine oxidase (MAO) inhibitors.* These drugs increase the amounts of mood-enhancing neurotransmitters in the brain by blocking the action of the enzyme monoamine oxidase, which normally breaks them down. Examples of MAO inhibitors include isocarboxazid (Marplan), phenelzine (Nardil), and tranylcypromine (Parnate). Possi-

ble side effects include agitation, elevated blood pressure, overstimulation, and changes in heart rate and rhythm. MAO inhibitors also have a high potential for dangerous interactions with other substances, including drugs and foods. Persons taking these drugs must adhere strictly to a diet that includes no foods containing the chemical tyramine, such as almonds, avocados, bananas, beef or chicken liver, beer, cheese (including cottage cheese), chocolate, coffee, fava beans, herring, meat tenderizer, peanuts, pickles, pineapples, pumpkin seeds, raisins, sausage, sesame seeds, sour cream, soy sauce, wine, yeast extracts (including brewer's yeast), yogurt, and other foods. In general, any high-protein food that has undergone aging, pickling, fermentation, or similar processes should be avoided. Over-the-counter cold and allergy remedies should also be avoided.

• *Tetracyclics.* These drugs have an action similar to that of the tricyclics, but have a slightly different chemical structure and appear to cause fewer side effects. Maprotiline (Ludiomil) is in this category.

• *Tricyclics.* These drugs work by inhibiting the uptake of the neurotransmitters serotonin, norepinephrine, and dopamine, making more of the mood-enhancing chemical messengers available to nerve cells. Examples include amitriptyline (Elavil, Endep), desipramine (Norpramin, Pertofrane), imipramine (Janimine, Tofranil), and nortriptyline (Aventyl, Pamelor). Possible side effects include blurred vision, constipation, dry mouth, irregular heartbeat, urine retention, and orthostatic hypotension, a severe drop in blood pressure upon sitting up or standing, which can lead to dizziness, falls, and fractures.

• *Other drugs.* Several drugs known as "second-generation" antidepressants have become available in the past few years. These new drugs have not been shown to be more effective than the others, but they tend to have fewer serious side effects. They include the newer tricyclic amoxapine (Asendin); fluoxetine (Prozac), paroxetine (Paxil), and sertraline (Zoloft), which specifically block the uptake of the neurotransmitter serotonin but, unlike tricyclics, not that of norepinephrine or dopamine; buproprion (Wellbutrin), which is believed to act by inhibiting the uptake of dopamine but not serotonin or norepinephrine; and trazodone (Desyrel), an antidepressant with stimulant properties that also inhibits the uptake of dopamine. One study done in Madrid, Spain, found that people who took fluoxetine, paroxetine and sertraline were three times more likely to develop gastrointestinal bleeding than those who did not.

❏ Steroid drugs and oral contraceptives may cause serotonin levels in the brain to drop.

❏ Prozac and other "selective serotonin uptake inhibitors" work to increase the activity of serotonin, while 5-hydroxytryptophan (5-HTP) works to boost the body's production of serotonin.

❏ A study published in *The British Medical Journal* indicates that extracts of St. John's wort may be as effective as prescription antidepressants for mild and moderate depression. St. John's wort is the most-prescribed antidepressant in Germany, but is treated as a dietary supplement in the United States (it is not approved as a safe and effective drug by the FDA). Many studies are underway to determine the effectiveness and safety of long-term use of St. John's wort, including a major study by the National Institutes of Health started in 1997.

❏ People who smoke are more likely than nonsmokers to be depressed. Smokers and non-smokers alike may benefit from Zyban (a sustained-release preparation of buproprion, also sold as Wellbutrin SR), an antidepressant also approved to help people quit smoking. Bupropion elevates levels of dopamine and norepinephrine, substances that are also elevated by nicotine in tobacco products. It allows patients to obtain the same feeling while weaning themselves off nicotine.

❏ Allergies, hypoglycemia, hypothyroidism, and/or malabsorption problems can cause or contribute to depression. In people with these conditions, vitamin B_{12} and folic acid are blocked from entering the system, which can lead to depression.

❏ Individuals with depression are more likely than other people to have various disturbances in calcium metabolism.

❏ There is no doubt that attitude affects health. Study after study has shown that optimistic people are not only happier but healthier. They suffer less illness, recover better from illness and surgery, and have stronger immune defenses.

❏ Many groups and organizations offer more information on depression (see HEALTH AND MEDICAL ORGANIZATIONS in Part Three).

Dermatitis

Dermatitis is a general term for any type of inflammation of the skin. Types of dermatitis include atopic dermatitis, nummular dermatitis, seborrheic dermatitis, irritant contact dermatitis, and allergic contact dermatitis. The distinction between the use of *dermatitis* and *eczema* to describe skin disorders can be confusing. Often, the terms are used interchangeably, although many people use the term *eczema* to refer specifically to atopic dermatitis. The inflammation of the skin that accompanies dermatitis (or eczema) produces scaling, flaking, thickening, weeping, crusting, color changes, and, often, itching.

Several underlying problems can lead to eczema. Hypochlorhydria (low levels of hydrochloric acid in the stomach) has been cited, as has a condition known as "leaky gut syndrome," in which the intestines become porous and allow tiny particles of undigested food to enter the bloodstream,

provoking allergic reactions. Candidiasis (an overgrowth of yeast in the system), food allergies, and a genetically-based weakness in the enzyme delta-6-desaturase (which converts essential fatty acids into anti-inflammatory prostaglandins) are other possible causes of this condition.

Many cases of dermatitis are simply the result of allergies. This type of condition is called *allergic* or *contact dermatitis*. Skin inflammation may be linked to contact with perfumes, cosmetics, rubber, medicated creams and ointments, latex, plants such as poison ivy, and/or metals or metal alloys such as gold, silver, and nickel found in jewelry or zippers. Some people with dermatitis are sensitive to sunlight. Whatever the irritant, if the skin remains in constant contact with it, the dermatitis is likely to spread and become more severe. Stress, especially chronic tension, can cause or exacerbate dermatitis.

Atopic dermatitis (AD; also known as atopic eczema or, in children, infantile eczema) is a condition known to affect allergy-prone individuals. It typically appears on the face, in the bends of the elbows, and behind the knees, and is very itchy. In children, it usually appears in the first year of life, and almost always in the first five years. Over half of the infants who have this condition get better by the age of eighteen months. Triggers vary from person to person, but tend to include cold or hot weather, a dry atmosphere, exposure to allergens, stress, and infections such as colds. If other family members have histories of hay fever, asthma, or atopic dermatitis, it is more likely that a child will be diagnosed with AD.

Nummular ("coin-shaped") *dermatitis* is a chronic condition in which round, scaling lesions appear on the limbs. It may be caused by an allergy to nickel and is often associated with dry skin. *Dermatitis herpetiformis* is a very itchy type of dermatitis associated with intestinal and immune disorders. This form of dermatitis may be triggered by the consumption of dairy products and/or gluten. *Seborrhea* is a form of dermatitis that most commonly affects the scalp and/or face.

Unless otherwise specified, the dosages recommended here are for adults. For a child between the ages of twelve and seventeen, reduce the dose to three-quarters of the recommended amount. For a child between six and twelve, use one-half of the recommended dose, and for a child under the age of six, use one-quarter of the recommended amount.

NUTRIENTS

SUPPLEMENT	SUGGESTED DOSAGE	COMMENTS
Essential		
Betaine HCl	As directed on label.	A form of hydrochloric acid. People with dermatitis often have low levels of hydrochloric acid. *Caution:* Do not take this supplement if you suffer from stomach acidity.

OptiMSM	As directed on label.	A patented form of methylsulfonylmethane. Reduces inflammation and contains a natural analgesic.
Vitamin B complex	50–100 mg of each major B vitamin 3 times daily, with meals (amounts of individual vitamins in a complex will vary).	Needed for healthy skin and proper circulation. Aids in reproduction of all cells. Use a high-stress, yeast-free formula. A sublingual form is recommended.
plus extra vitamin B$_3$ (niacin)	100 mg 3 times daily. Do not exceed this amount.	Important for proper circulation and healthy skin. *Caution:* Do not take niacin if you have a liver disorder, gout, or high blood pressure.
and vitamin B$_6$ (pyridoxine)	50 mg 3 times daily.	Deficiency has been linked to skin disorders.
and vitamin B$_{12}$	1,000–2,000 mcg daily.	Aids in cell formation and cellular longevity. Use a lozenge or sublingual form.
and biotin	300 mg daily.	Deficiency has been linked to dermatitis.

Important

Essential fatty acids (black currant seed oil, flaxseed oil, primrose oil, and salmon oil are good sources)	As directed on label.	Promotes lubrication of the skin.
Kelp	1,000 mg daily or as directed on label.	Contains iodine and other minerals needed for healing of tissues.
Vitamin C with bioflavonoids	As directed on label.	Inhibits inflammation and stabilizes cell membranes.
Vitamin E	400 IU daily and up.	Relieves itching and dryness. Use d-alpha-tocopherol form.
Zinc	100 mg daily. Do not exceed this amount.	Aids healing and enhances immune function. Use zinc gluconate lozenges or OptiZinc for best absorption.

Helpful

Aller Bee-Gone from CC Pollen	As directed on label.	For allergic dermatitis. A combination of herbs, enzymes, and nutrients designed to fight allergic flare-ups.
Borage oil and flaxseed oil (EFA Derma-Skin Formula from Health From The Sun is a good source)	As directed on label.	Contain omega-6 and omega-3 essential fatty acids, which help skin retain its moisture and suppleness.
Coenzyme Q$_{10}$ plus Coenzyme A from Coenzyme-A Technologies	As directed on label.	Removes toxins from the body, boosts the immune system, improves overall physical and mental processes.
Free-form amino acid complex (Amino Balance from Anabol Naturals)	As directed on label, on an empty stomach.	To supply protein, important for construction and repair of all tissues. Use a formula containing both essential and nonessential amino acids.
Herpanacine from Diamond-Herpanacine Associates	As directed on label.	Contains antioxidants, amino acids, and herbs that promote overall skin health.

Kyo-Dophilus from Wakunaga	As directed on label.	A nondairy probiotic formula. Prevents the overgrowth of yeasts in the body.
Kyolic-EPA from Wakunaga	As directed on label.	Restores fatty acid balance. Repairs tissue and aids in healing.
Shark cartilage (BeneFin)	1 gram per 15 lbs of body weight daily, divided into 3 doses.	Reduces inflammation in eczema.
Vitamin A emulsion or capsules	100,000 IU daily for 1 month, then 50,000 IU daily for 2 weeks, then reduce to 25,000 IU daily. If you are pregnant, do not exceed 10,000 IU daily. 5,000 IU daily.	Needed for smooth skin. Aids in preventing dryness. Use emulsion form for easier assimilation and greater safety at high doses.
plus carotenoid complex	25,000 IU daily.	Antioxidants and precursors of vitamin A.
Vitamin D$_3$	400–1,000 IU daily.	Aids in healing of tissues.

HERBS

❑ Blackthorn, blueberry leaf, hawthorn berry, and rue contain flavonoids that are excellent for reducing inflammation.

❑ Chamomile can be taken internally or used to soothe the skin. It reduces inflammation.

❑ Poultices combining chaparral, dandelion, and yellow dock root can be helpful. *See* USING A POULTICE in Part Three.
   Note: Chaparral is recommended for external use only.

❑ The following herbs can be used in tea or capsule form: dandelion, goldenseal, myrrh, pau d'arco, and red clover. Alternate among them for best results.
   Caution: Do not take goldenseal on a daily basis for more than one week at a time, and do not use it during pregnancy. If you have a history of cardiovascular disease, diabetes, or glaucoma, use it only under a doctor's supervision.

❑ To relieve itching and promote healing, mix goldenseal root powder with vitamin E oil, then add a little honey until it is the consistency of a loose paste. Apply this mixture to the affected area.

❑ Gotu kola contains powerful antioxidants and promotes the formation of lipids and proteins that are essential for healthy skin.

❑ Grapeseed extract contains oligomeric proanthocyanadins (OPCs), which reduce inflammation and rid the body of toxins.

❑ Oregon grape root detoxifies the body and reduces inflammation.

RECOMMENDATIONS

❑ Add brown rice and millet to your diet.

❑ Avoid eggs, peanuts, soy foods, wheat, and dairy products.

❏ Also avoid sugar, strawberries, chocolate, white flour, fats, fried foods, and processed foods.

❏ Try a gluten-free diet for six weeks, then add gluten-containing foods back to the diet one at a time, and see if the condition changes. A gluten-free diet is often of therapeutic benefit in controlling dermatitis. (*See* CELIAC DISEASE in Part Two for the recommended diet.)

❏ Do not eat foods containing raw eggs, which contain avidin, a protein that binds to biotin and prevents it from being absorbed. Biotin is needed for skin and scalp disorders.

❏ Try keeping your house humidified and take fewer showers and baths. Showers and baths deplete the skin of its natural oils.

❏ Use a perfume-free moisturing lotion daily.

❏ For dermatitis of the scalp, make a strong, concentrated tea of rosemary, comfrey, tea tree oil (add the tea tree oil after the tea is made), dried nettles, and witch hazel, and apply it to the scalp after shampooing with a fragrance-free shampoo. Leave it on the scalp for ten or fifteen minutes.

❏ Massage tea tree oil antiseptic cream into the skin after contact with water or irritants.

❏ Keep the colon clean. Use a fiber supplement such as flaxseed, psyllium husk, or Aerobic Bulk Cleanse (ABC) from Aerobic Life Industries daily. Use occasional cleansing enemas for removing toxins for quicker healing. (*See* COLON CLEANSING and/or ENEMAS in Part Three.)

Note: Always take supplemental fiber separately from other supplements and medications.

CONSIDERATIONS

❏ Chemicals used in bubble bath products may cause dermatitis and may even irritate the tissues of the lower urinary tract sufficiently to cause bloody urine. This is most likely to occur if you soak in treated bathwater for too long.

❏ Primrose oil and vitamin B_6 (pyridoxine) have helped infants with dermatitis.

❏ Sensitivity to gluten is widespread, although it is often unrecognized. Research has shown that people suffering from virtually all skin disorders do better if they eliminate foods containing gluten and all dairy products from the diet.

❏ Food allergies can cause dermatitis. (*See* ALLERGIES in Part Two.)

❏ *See also* FUNGAL INFECTION; HIVES; POISON IVY/ POISON OAK/POISON SUMAC; PSORIASIS; ROSACEA; SCABIES; and/or SEBORRHEA, all in Part Two.

Detached Retina

See Dimness or Loss of Vision *under* EYE PROBLEMS.

Diabetes

Diabetes is a result of problems with the pancreatic hormone insulin. Insulin controls the amount of glucose (sugar) in the blood and the rate at which glucose is absorbed into the cells. The cells need glucose to produce energy. In people with diabetes, glucose builds up in the bloodstream instead of being taken into and used by the cells, leading to *hyperglycemia* (abnormally high levels of glucose in the blood). Eventually, hyperglycemia leads to damaged blood vessels, which in turn, may cause eye disease, heart disease, peripheral and autonomic neuropathy (nerve damage in the limbs and internal organs), and diabetic nephropathy (kidney disease).

There are two major types of diabetes. Type 1 (or insulin-dependent-diabetes mellitus [IDDM]) and type 2 (non-insulin-dependent diabetes mellitus [NIDDM]). *Type 1 diabetes* affects 5 to 10 percent of people with diabetes and usually starts at an early age. It is an autoimmune disease in which the body's immune system attacks and destroys the insulin-producing cells in the pancreas. Experts believe this may result from an immune response after a viral infection.

Type 2 diabetes, by far the most common form of diabetes, affects 90 to 95 percent of diabetes suffers. In type 2 diabetes, the pancreas does produce insulin in small quantities, but not enough to fuel the cells. The cells may also become resistant to the effects of what little insulin there is in the bloodstream. Many people have type 2 diabetes and are completely unaware of it. This type of diabetes usually begins in later years, although, unfortunately, it is now becoming more common in young people. Risk factors for developing type 2 diabetes include diet, weight, race, age, lack of exercise, and heredity. It is much more common among Latinos, American Indians, African-Americans, and American-Asians than Caucasians. In fact, over the last thirty years, the number of African-Americans diagnosed with diabetes has tripled.

Gestational diabetes is a form of the condition that develops during pregnancy, affecting about 4 percent of pregnant women. Hormonal changes during pregnancy can affect the body's resistance to insulin. Most often, this condition disappears after delivery, but it seems to be a sign that the woman is more likely to develop type 2 diabetes in later life. *Impaired glucose tolerance* (IGT) is a condition that affects about 11 percent of American adults. In people with IGT, blood glucose levels are above normal, but are not at diabetic levels. However, about 7 percent of people with IGT go on to develop type 2 diabetes.

According to figures published by the American Diabetes Association (ADA), 15.7 million people in America have diabetes. This disease is the sixth leading cause of death in the United States and the primary cause of blindness in people between the ages of twenty and seventy. The death rate for African-Americans with diabetes is 27 percent higher than the death rate for Caucasians who have the disease. If it is not properly controlled, diabetes can lead to heart disease, kidney disease, edema, nerve damage, and infections of the mouth, gums, lungs, skin, feet, bladder, and genital areas. Skin sores may develop and fail to heal properly.

People with diabetes are subject to episodes of both high and low blood sugar. The symptoms of *hyper*glycemia (too much glucose in the blood) often include fatigue, a constant need to urinate, extreme thirst, constantly feeling hungry, loss of weight, and problems with eyesight. Episodes of *hypo*glycemia (less than normal amounts of glucose in the blood), which strike suddenly, can be caused by a missed meal, too much exercise, or a reaction to too much insulin. The initial signs of hypoglycemia are hunger, dizziness, sweating, confusion, palpitations, and numbness or tingling of the lips. If not treated, the individual may go on to experience double vision, trembling, and disorientation, may act strangely, and may eventually lapse into a coma.

The major danger with diabetes, however, is not the disease itself, but the complications that can arise if insulin levels are not maintained at a constant level. Untreated, diabetes can lead to diabetic ketoacidosis (DKA) or hyperosmolar syndrome. DKA occurs when the body is so low in insulin that it starts using stored fat as fuel. When the fat breaks down, substances known as ketones are produced as a byproduct. In large quantities, ketones can cause body to become excessively acidic. Ketoacidosis is most often seen in people with type 1 diabetes. Symptoms include nausea, difficulty breathing, sweet breath, and confusion that can progress to coma. Hyperosmolar syndrome is a result of a combination of very high blood sugar levels (but without the presence of ketones) and dehydration. It is more common in older people with type 2 diabetes who are taking steroid medications. The condition may also be prompted by stress from a major illness. With hyperosmolar syndrome, blood sugar levels are so high that the blood thickens. Symptoms include confusion, tiredness, and coma. Hyperosmolar syndrome can sometimes be the first indication of diabetes in older adults. Both of these conditions require the immediate attention of a physician. Urinalysis can often detect unsuspected diabetes.

Unless otherwise specified, the dosages recommended here are for adults. For a child between the ages of twelve and seventeen, reduce the dose to three-quarters the recommended amount. For a child between six and twelve, use one-half the recommended dose, and for a child under the age of six, use one-quarter the recommended amount.

DIABETES SELF-TESTS

There are several ways to test yourself for diabetes. The tests for type 1 diabetes are also used for self-monitoring by persons diagnosed with the condition. Home testing tends to be less accurate than tests done in a doctor's office, however.

Type 1 Diabetes

To test for type 1 diabetes:

1. Purchase chemically treated plastic glucose testing strips at a drugstore.
2. Prick your finger and apply a drop of blood to the tip of the strip.
3. Wait one minute and compare the color on the strip to a color chart, which lists various glucose levels.

There are also electronic devices available that can analyze the test strip for you and give you a numerical readout of the glucose level. The Bayer Corporation of Elkhart, Indiana, manufactures two glucometer kits—Glucometer Elite and Glucometer Encore—for testing blood sugar in the convenience of your own home. You simply prick your finger with the spring-loaded needle, apply a drop of your blood to the test strip, and place it in the machine for analysis. This test gives you an immediate blood sugar result. It is a device that all people with diabetes should own.

The following is an approximate guideline for blood sugar levels (the measurement is milligrams of glucose to one-tenth liter of blood):

- 110 and under: normal.
- 110–126: impaired glucose tolerance/borderline.
- 126 and over for a two- or three-day period: diabetes

Type 2 Diabetes

People with type 2 diabetes often cannot perceive sweet tastes. This abnormality may play an important role in how individuals with diabetes perceive the taste of their food, and also in how well they comply with the dietary aspects of treatment. Because our society as a whole is addicted to sugar, this distorted taste perception is very common among the population in general.

The following test can detect an impaired ability to taste sweets:

1. Do not consume stimulants (coffee, tea, soda) or sweets for one hour before the test.
2. Fill seven identical glasses with 8 ounces of water each and label the glasses as having no sugar, 1/4 teaspoon sugar, 1/2 teaspoon sugar, 1 teaspoon sugar 1 1/2 teaspoons sugar, 2 teaspoons sugar, and 3 teaspoons sugar. Add the appropriate amount of sugar to each glass, then ask someone else to rearrange the order of the glasses and hide the labels.
3. Take a straw and sip from each glass, then write down the amount of sugar you think it contains. Between sips, rinse your mouth with pure water.

Healthy people generally notice a sweet taste when a teaspoon or less of sugar is added to 8 ounces of water. By contrast, people with adult-onset diabetes usually do not notice sweetness until 1 1/2 to 2 teaspoons of sugar have been added to the water.

NUTRIENTS

SUPPLEMENT	SUGGESTED DOSAGE	COMMENTS
Essential		
Alpha-lipoic acid	As directed on label.	For treatment of peripheral nerve damage in diabetic patients. Helps control blood sugar levels.
Chromium picolinate or	400–600 mcg daily.	Improves insulin's efficiency, which lowers blood sugar levels. A combination of chromium picolinate, vanadyl sulfate, and other vitamins and minerals that work synergistically to regulate blood sugar levels and correct deficiencies. *Caution:* If you have diabetes, consult with your physician before taking any supplement containing chromium.
Diabetic Nutrition Rx from Progressive Research Labs or	As directed on label.	
brewer's yeast with added chromium	As directed on label.	
Garlic (Kyolic from Wakunaga)	As directed on label.	Decreases and stabilizes blood sugar levels. Enhances immunity and improves circulation.
L-Carnitine	500 mg twice daily, on an empty stomach. Take with water. Do not take with milk. Take with 50 mg vitamin B_6 and 100 mg vitamin C for better absorption.	Mobilizes fat.
plus L-glutamine	500 mg twice daily, on an empty stomach.	Reduces the craving for sugars.
plus taurine	500 mg twice daily, on an empty stomach.	Aids in the release of insulin.
Quercetin (Activated Quercetin from Source Naturals, Quercitin-C from Ecological Formulas)	100 mg 3 times daily.	Helps protect the membranes of the lens of the eye from accumulations of polyols as a result of high glucose levels.
Raw adrenal glandular and	As directed on label.	Aids in rebuilding and nourishing these organs. (*See* GLANDULAR THERAPY in Part Three.)
raw pancreas glandular and	As directed on label.	
thyroid glandular	As directed on label.	
Vanadium	As directed on label.	Aids insulin's ability to move glucose into the cells. Use vanadyl sulfate form.
Vitamin B complex	50 mg of each major B vitamin 3 times daily (amounts of individual vitamins in a complex will vary). Do not exceed 300 mg daily from all supplements.	The B vitamins work best when taken together.
plus extra biotin and	50 mg daily.	Improves the metabolism of glucose.
inositol	50 mg daily.	Important for circulation and for prevention of atherosclerosis.
Vitamin B_{12} plus folic acid	As prescribed by physician or directed on label.	Needed to prevent diabetic neuropathy. Injections (under a doctor's supervision) are best. If injections are not available, use a lozenge or sublingual form.
Zinc	50–80 mg daily. Do not exceed a total of 100 mg daily from all supplements.	Deficiency has been associated with diabetes. Use zinc gluconate lozenges or OptiZinc for best absorption.

Very Important		
Coenzyme Q_{10} plus	80 mg daily.	Improves circulation and stabilizes blood sugar.
Coenzyme A from Coenzyme-A Technologies	As directed on label.	Works well with coenzyme Q_{10} in protecting the cells and removing toxic substances from the body.
Magnesium	750 mg daily.	Important for enzyme systems and pH balance. Protects against coronary artery spasm in arteriosclerosis. Increases energy levels. Low readings of magnesium are often found in people with diabetes, and are associated with the complications of eye disease.
Manganese	5–10 mg daily. Take separately from calcium.	Needed for repair of the pancreas. Also a cofactor in key enzymes of glucose metabolism. Deficiency is common in people with diabetes.
Psyllium husks or Aerobic Bulk Cleanse (ABC) from Aerobic Life Industries	As directed on label. Take with a large glass of water. Take separately from other supplements and medications.	Good fiber source and fat mobilizer.
Important		
Vitamin A with carotenoids	15,000 IU daily. If you are pregnant, do not exceed 10,000 IU daily.	An important antioxidant needed to maintain the health of the eyes. Use emulsion form for best absorption.
Vitamin C with bioflavonoids	3,000–6,000 mg daily.	Deficiency may lead to vascular problems in people with diabetes. Vitamin C may slow or prevent complications that occur in diabetes.
Vitamin E	400 IU and up daily.	Improves circulation and prevents complications through its antioxidant properties. Use d-alpha-tocopherol form.
Helpful		
Calcium	1,500 mg daily.	Important for pH balance.
Copper complex	As directed on label.	Aids in protein metabolism and in many enzyme systems.
Maitake extract	1–4 gm daily.	May help to normalize blood sugar levels.
Multienzyme complex plus	As directed on label. Take with meals.	To aid digestion. Proper digestion is essential in management of diabetes.
proteolytic enzymes	As directed on label. Take between meals.	
Pantethine	As directed on label.	A form of pantothenic acid that reduces LDL cholesterol and helps prevent buildup in the arteries.
Pycnogenol or	As directed on label.	A powerful antioxidant that also enhances the activity of vitamin C and strengthens connective tissue, including that of the cardiovascular system.
grape seed extract	As directed on label.	

HERBS

❏ Beanpod tea, made up of kidney, white, navy, lima, and northern beans, detoxifies the pancreas.

323

❑ Bitter melon (*Momordica charantia*), gudmar (*Gymnema sylvestre*), and gulvel (*Tinospora cordifo*) are herbal remedies used in Ayurvedic medicine to regulate blood sugar levels.

❑ Cedar berries are excellent nourishment for the pancreas.

❑ Dandelion root protects the liver, which converts nutrients into glucose.

Note: If you suffer from gallbladder problems, avoid large quantities of dandelion.

❑ Fenugreek seeds have been shown to reduce cholesterol and blood sugar levels.

❑ Ginseng tea is believed to lower the blood sugar level.
Caution: Do not use this herb if you have high blood pressure.

❑ Huckleberry helps to promote insulin production.

❑ Juniper berries have been found to lower blood glucose levels.

❑ Other herbs that may be beneficial for diabetes include bilberry, buchu, dandelion root, goldenseal, and uva ursi.

Caution: Do not take goldenseal on a daily basis for more than one week at a time, and do not use it during pregnancy. If you have a history of cardiovascular disease, diabetes, or glaucoma, use it only under a doctor's supervision.

RECOMMENDATIONS

❑ Eat a low-fat, high-fiber diet including plenty of raw fruits and vegetables as well as fresh vegetable juices. This reduces the need for insulin and also lowers the level of fats in the blood. Fiber helps to reduce blood sugar surges. For snacks, eat oat or rice bran crackers with nut butter or cheese. Legumes, root vegetables, and whole grains are also good. Remember to regulate your complex carbohydrate intake.

❑ Supplement your diet with spirulina. Spirulina helps to stabilize blood sugar levels. Other foods that help normalize blood sugar include berries, brewer's yeast, dairy products (especially cheese), egg yolks, fish, garlic, kelp, sauerkraut, soybeans, and vegetables.

❑ Get your protein from vegetable sources, such as grains and legumes. Fish and low-fat dairy products are also acceptable sources of protein.

❑ Avoid saturated fats and simple sugars (except when necessary to balance an insulin reaction).

❑ Eat more carbohydrates or reduce your insulin dosage before exercise. Exercise produces an insulinlike effect in the body. Talk to your doctor about the right approach for you.

❑ Do not take fish oil capsules or supplements containing large amounts of para-aminobenzoic acid (PABA), and avoid salt and white flour products. Consumption of these products results in an elevation of blood sugar.

❑ Do not take supplements containing the amino acid cysteine. It has the ability to break down the bonds of the hormone insulin and interferes with absorption of insulin by the cells.

❑ Do not take extremely large doses of vitamins B_1 (thiamine) and C. Excessive amounts may inactivate insulin. These vitamins may, however, be taken in normal amounts. Consult the Nutrients table, above, for recommendations.

❑ If symptoms of hyperglycemia develop, go to the emergency room of the nearest hospital. This is a potentially dangerous situation. Intravenous administration of proper fluids, electrolytes, and insulin may be required.

❑ Avoid taking large amounts of vitamin B_3 (niacin). However, small amounts (50 to 100 milligrams daily), taken by mouth, may be beneficial.

❑ If you have a child with diabetes, be sure his or her teacher knows how to respond to the warning signs of hypoglycemia and hyperglycemia.

❑ If symptoms of hypoglycemia develop, *immediately* consume fruit juice, soda pop, or anything else that contains sugar. If that fails to help within twenty minutes, repeat this regimen. If the second treatment fails, or if you cannot ingest food, seek immediate medical attention and/or administer a glucagon injection. Anyone who has insulin-dependent diabetes should always carry a glucagon kit and know how to use it.

❑ Avoid tobacco in any form; it constricts the blood vessels and inhibits circulation. Keep your feet clean, dry, and warm, and wear only white cotton socks and well-fitting shoes. Lack of oxygen (because of poor circulation) and peripheral nerve damage (with loss of pain sensation) are major factors in the development of diabetic foot ulcers. Try to avoid injury, and take measures to improve the circulation in the feet and legs.

❑ *See* CIRCULATORY PROBLEMS in Part Two.

CONSIDERATIONS

❑ To compensate for the lack of insulin production, a person with type 1 diabetes must inject insulin on a daily basis. Injections are necessary because insulin cannot be absorbed from the gastrointestinal tract into the bloodstream if taken orally. Insulin pumps and pens (individual, disposable prefilled insulin syringes in the form of a pen) are also available for the delivery of insulin. Because the management of type 1 diabetes is such a complex challenge, it is imperative that a person with this condition have a good relationship with the physician prescribing the insulin. There are many insulin formulations on the U.S. market, but all are variations of several basic types. The most commonly used are purified porcine (pork), purified bovine (beef), and recombinant DNA-origin (human) insulin. Purified porcine insulin is insulin derived from the pancreases of pigs that has undergone further purification; purified bovine insulin is cattle-pancreas-derived insulin that has undergone further purification. Recombinant DNA-origin insulin is genetically engineered by inserting the human gene for insulin production into a non-disease-producing laboratory strain of *Escherichia coli* bacteria or yeast.

❑ People with type 2 diabetes are less able than most people to perceive sweet tastes, and this may make it more difficult for them to lose weight. Because they do not recognize the sweet taste of substances, they often consume sugary products that they do not appreciate as sweet. If a person with type 2 diabetes attains a better understanding of food, exercises greater care in choosing foods, and reads food product labels carefully, he or she should be able to control the problem and avoid the need for treatment with drugs or insulin.

❑ Often, type 2 diabetes can be controlled by diet and exercise alone, but oral medications or injections of insulin can be added if regulating the diet does not work. Obesity is a major factor in type 2 diabetes, and a weight reduction program is often all that is required to control it.

❑ It was once thought that people with diabetes should avoid sweetened foods. For weight control, this is still the case. However, research has shown that sugar—a simple carbohydrate—does not cause the greatest increase in blood glucose. Eating baked potatoes or some breakfast cereals causes a greater rise in blood sugar. Indeed, carrots raise blood-sugar more than ice-cream does. Carbohydrates are converted quickly into glucose in the body. It is on this principle that many high-protein, low-carbohydrate diets are based. It is essential, therefore, that people with diabetes measure their intake of both simple and complex carbohydrates—not simply those coming from sugar.

❑ Insulin inhalers are now in development. The dose is inhaled through the mouth into the lungs, and from there, the dry or dissolved insulin can easily be absorbed into the bloodstream. The benefits to this method of ingestion, as compared with injection, are obvious. The drawbacks, however, are in accurately administering the correct dose in the correct form. The inhalers deliver only up to 10 percent of the drug into the lungs, making it more expensive because more insulin is needed. The size of the drug particles is also critical—if they are too small, the drug will bind together; if too large, the insulin will not be able to reach the lungs.

❑ Research indicates that supplementation with the hormone dehydroepiandrosterone in the form of 7-keto DHEA may help prevent diabetes. (*See* DHEA THERAPY in Part Three.)

❑ Hypothyroidism may be a leading cause of diabetes. Well-known researcher and author Stephen Langer, M.D., has noticed that neuropathies, together with other diabetic complications, disappear when thyroid hormone is administered. Many complications of diabetes and hypothyroidism are a result of clogged arteries, which prevent the blood from delivering nutrients and oxygen and carrying off waste and debris.

❑ Glycosylation—the binding of glucose and other sugars onto proteins in the blood, nerve cells, and lenses of the eyes—may be responsible for many of the long-term effects of diabetes. Researchers at the University of Surrey's School of Biological Sciences and the Academic Unit of Diabetes and Endocrinology of London's Whittington Hospital have shown that vitamin C may inhibit this destructive process. They say that if glycosylation is part of the normal aging process, taking vitamin C supplements may slow it.

❑ Magnet therapy helps some people with diabetes in coping with foot pain associated with the disorder. (*See* Magnet Therapy *under* PAIN CONTROL in Part Three.)

❑ A woman with diabetes who wants to become pregnant should watch her blood sugar levels long before she plans to conceive. The fetus has the greatest chance of developing birth defects during the first five to eight weeks of pregnancy, before most women know they are pregnant. It usually takes a few months to get the blood sugar under proper control; if a woman begins to monitor her blood sugar level the day she conceives, damage may already be done by the time it is under control.

❑ Retinopathy (damage to the retina) from diabetes is the leading cause of blindness in the United States. However, the incidence of blindness from diabetic retinopathy has dropped with the use of laser surgery. If people in the later stages of retinopathy are left untreated, almost 50 percent lose their sight within five years. Of those who receive laser treatment, only 5 percent lose their sight. Persons with diabetes should get annual retinal examinations to check on their condition.

❑ Diabetic nephropathy (damage to the kidneys caused by diabetes) is quite common, but is becoming less so, as people recognize the necessity of maintaining a stable blood sugar level. It is important to monitor kidney function periodically. Treating high blood pressure is important, as is eating a low-protein diet containing less than 40 grams of protein each day.

❑ Diabetic neuropathy (damage to the nerves caused by diabetes) usually affects the peripheral nerves, such as those in the feet, hands, and legs. Symptoms include numbness, tingling, and pain. Amitriptyline and desipramine, common antidepressant drugs, have proved to be successful in the treatment of this condition. They work by increasing levels of the neurochemical that carries messages between cells, thus increasing sensation. Autonomic neuropathy may lead, among other complaints, to a buildup of gastric juices in the stomach. Too much stomach acid can cause nausea and diarrhea, but the condition can be relieved by either antibiotic treatment or by eating smaller, low-fat meals. For men, neuropathy or circulatory problems can lead to erectile disfunction (ED). Sildenafil (Viagra) may be able to alleviate this problem. Your physician will probably want to do a stress test before prescribing this drug.

❑ In one study, large amounts of niacin raised blood

sugar levels in people with non-insulin-dependent diabetes by as much as 16 percent. Over time, this could cause dependence on insulin or medication. Niacin can also cause the level of uric acid in the blood to rise, indicating probable kidney dysfunction and an increased risk of gout. However, niacinamide, a form of niacin, slows down the destruction and enhances the regeneration of the insulin-producing beta cells in the pancreas, and therefore may be helpful for those with type 1 diabetes.

❏ Elevated glucose levels in the lens of the eye can result in the accumulation of substances called polyols, whose presence can ultimately cause damage to the lens. High polyol concentrations resulting from high glucose levels can persist even if glucose levels subsequently return to normal. Flavonoids, such as quercetin, help to inhibit the accumulation of polyols.

❏ Diabetes and high blood pressure often go hand in hand, and both can lead to kidney disease. In one recent study, hypertensive diabetics who took drugs called angiotensin converting enzyme (ACE) inhibitors cut their risk of developing serious kidney disease in half.

❏ Coronary heart disease is common in people with diabetes. Women with diabetes are particularly at risk. Elevated blood glucose in long-term diabetes is the primary factor that adversely affects the heart in people with diabetes. (See CARDIOVASCULAR DISEASE in Part Two.)

❏ Researchers at the University of Colorado Health Sciences Center found that smokers who have diabetes are two to three times more likely than their nonsmoking counterparts to develop kidney damage, often leading to the need for dialysis or a transplant. Smoking constricts blood vessels. In people with diabetes, this helps to push large protein molecules out of the vessels and into the kidneys. That can eventually lead to kidney failure.

❏ Rosiglitazone (Avandia) is a drug sometimes prescribed for type 2 diabetes. This drug controls blood sugar by adjusting the sensitivity of fat and muscle tissue to the insulin in the body.

❏ Many nutrients recommended for people with diabetes are available in combination supplements. One company that produces a line of specialty supplements for people with diabetes is Progressive Research Labs of Houston.

❏ It is vital for people who have diabetes to take care of their feet. Nerve damage can lead to lack of sensation in the feet, and once the skin is broken, sores there may not heal. Treatments for diabetic foot problems include becaplermin (Regranex), a topical gel that encourages tissue growth in the wound, and Dermagraft. Dermagraft is based on the collection of tissue-building cells from healthy sources and implanting them into the wound, stimulating one's own cells to heal the affected area.

❏ People with diabetes should be vigilant about blood fat and cholesterol levels. Optimum cholesterol levels for people with diabetes are LDL ("bad cholesterol"), about 100; HDL ("good cholesterol"), 45 or above; triglycerides, 200 or under.

❏ For more information on diabetes and its potential complications, contact any of the organizations listed under HEALTH AND MEDICAL ORGANIZATIONS in the Appendix.

Diabetic Retinopathy

See under EYE PROBLEMS.

Diarrhea

Diarrhea is characterized by frequent and loose, watery stools. Symptoms that may accompany diarrhea include vomiting, cramping, thirst, and abdominal pain. Some people run a fever as well. It is rarely a serious condition, except in young children and older adults. Diarrhea causes the loss of both fluids and electrolytes (minerals), which can lead to troublesome problems.

Diarrhea can exist alone or as a symptom of other problems. Among the many possible causes of diarrhea are incomplete digestion of food; food poisoning; food allergies; excess alcohol consumption; bacterial, viral, or other infection; and consumption of contaminated water. Caffeine, magnesium, laxatives, and sorbitol (for young children) are all known to cause diarrhea in some people. The use of certain drugs, including antibiotics such as tetracycline, clindamycin (Cleocin), or ampicillin can also contribute to diarrhea. Inflammatory bowel disease, such as ulcerative colitis, diverticulitis, or Crohn's disease; pancreatic disease; and cancer may all lead to severe intestinal upsets. Emotional stress also can cause diarrhea. Acute diarrhea accompanied by fever and mucus or blood in the stool can be a sign of infection or the presence of parasites.

Unless otherwise noted, the dosages recommended here are for adults. For a child between the ages of twelve and seventeen, reduce the dose to three-quarters of the recommended amount. For a child between the ages of six and twelve, use one-half the recommended dose, and for a child under six, use one-quarter of the recommended amount.

NUTRIENTS

SUPPLEMENT	SUGGESTED DOSAGE	COMMENTS
Very Important		
Aerobic Bulk Cleanse (ABC) from Aerobic Life Industries or	As directed on label.	To provide bulk that aids in forming stools.
psyllium seeds	4 capsules daily, at bedtime. Take with a large glass of water.	

Charcoal tablets	4 tablets every hour with water until the diarrhea subsides. Take separately from other supplements and medications.	Absorbs toxins from the colon and bloodstream and aids in firming stools. *Note:* Do not take for more than 3 days at a time.
Essential fatty acid complex	As directed on label.	Aids in forming stools.
Kelp	1,000 mg daily.	To replace minerals lost through diarrhea.
L-Glutamine	As directed on label.	Helps the gut to produce healthy new cells and boosts the immune system.
Potassium	99 mg daily.	To replace potassium lost in watery stools.
ProFlora whey from Wakunaga	As directed on label.	Essential for maintaining the proper pH of the colon flora. Alleviates diarrhea quickly.
Important		
Acidophilus (Kyo-Dophilus or Probiata from Wakunaga)	1 tsp in distilled water, twice daily, on an empty stomach.	Replaces lost "friendly" bacteria. Use a nondairy powder form.
Colloidal silver	As directed on label.	Acts as a natural alternative to antibiotics.
Garlic (Kyolic from Wakunaga)	2 capsules 3 times daily.	Kills bacteria and parasites. Enhances immunity.
Helpful		
Calcium	1,500 mg daily.	To replace calcium depleted from the body. Also aids in forming stools.
and magnesium	1,000 mg daily.	Needed for calcium uptake. Promotes pH balance.
and vitamin D$_3$	400 IU daily.	Needed for calcium uptake.
Multienzyme complex with pancreatin	As directed on label. Take with meals.	Needed for normal digestion.
Vitamin B complex	100 mg of each major B vitamin 3 times daily (amounts of individual vitamins in a complex will vary).	All B vitamins are necessary for digestion and absorption of nutrients. Sublingual forms are recommended for better absorption. Injections (under a doctor's supervision) may be necessary.
plus extra vitamin B$_1$ (thiamine) and	200 mg daily for 2 weeks.	
vitamin B$_3$ (niacin) and	50 mg daily.	
folic acid	50 mg daily.	
Vitamin C with bioflavonoids	500 mg 3 times daily.	Needed for healing and immunity. Use a buffered form.
Vitamin E	400–1,000 IU daily.	Protects the cell membranes that line the colon wall. Use d-alpha-tocopherol form.
Zinc	50 mg daily. Do not exceed a total of 100 mg daily from all supplements.	Aids in repair of damaged tissue of the digestive tract and enhances immune response. Use zinc gluconate lozenges or OptiZinc for best absorption.

HERBS

❏ If you suffer from occasional bouts of diarrhea, use blackberry root bark, chamomile, pau d'arco, and/or raspberry leaves. Herbs can be taken in tea form or added to applesauce, bananas, pineapple, or papaya juice.

Caution: Do not use chamomile on an ongoing basis, and avoid it completely if you are allergic to ragweed.

❏ Cayenne (capsicum) capsules, taken two to three times daily, may be beneficial.

❏ Fenugreek, taken as a tea, lubricates the intestines and reduces fever.

❏ Ginger tea is good for cramps and abdominal pain.

❏ Grapefruit seed extract has anti-parasitic properties.

❏ Marshmallow root tea (also known as malva tea) helps calm the stomach and soothe intestinal problems.

❏ Slippery elm bark, taken in tea or extract form, is soothing to the digestive tract.

❏ Wild oregano oil contains antibacterial, antifungal, antiparasitic, and antiviral agents.

RECOMMENDATIONS

❏ Drink plenty of liquids, such as hot carob drink, "green drinks," and plenty of quality water. Do not drink very hot or cold liquids. The prolonged loss of fluids as a result of diarrhea can lead to dehydration and loss of necessary minerals, such as sodium, potassium, and magnesium. Liquid gelatin, clear broth, sodas such as ginger ale or flat cola, and weak tea with honey can be substituted for water if necessary. Carrot juice is also good, and makes the stools less watery. Do not drink apple juice, as this can make diarrhea worse.

❏ Avoid high-fiber foods, which may stress the digestive system. Instead, stick to foods that are easy to digest, such as cooked potatoes, rice, bananas, applesauce, or toast.

❏ Drink 3 cups of rice water daily. To make rice water, boil ½ cup of brown rice in 3 cups of water for forty-five minutes. Strain out the rice and drink the water. Eat the rice as well. Rice helps to form stools and supplies needed B vitamins.

❏ Do not consume any dairy products (except for low-fat soured products). They are highly allergenic. Moreover, diarrhea causes a temporary loss of the enzyme needed to digest lactose (milk sugar). Limit your intake of fats and foods containing gluten, including barley, oats, rye, and wheat. Avoid alcohol, caffeine, and spicy foods.

❏ Let a mild case of diarrhea run its course. It is the body's way of cleaning out toxins, bacteria, and other foreign invaders. Do not take any medication to stop diarrhea for at least two days. Stick to a liquid diet for twenty-four hours to give the bowel a rest.

❏ Consider using homeopathic remedies. *Arsenicum album* is a homeopathic remedy for burning diarrhea that is troublesome at night. *Podophyllum* can be used for watery stools. *Sulfur* is excellent for diarrhea that comes on suddenly.

❑ Consult your health care provider if any of the following conditions occur: the diarrhea lasts for more than two days, there is blood in the stool, the stool looks like black tar, you have a fever above 101°F, you have severe abdominal or rectal pain, you suffer from dehydration as evidenced by dry mouth or wrinkled skin, or urination is reduced or stops in any eight-hour period. If an infant has a dry diaper for more than four hours accompanied by a fever, it is wise to seek the advice of your physician.

CONSIDERATIONS

❑ Carob powder is high in protein and helps halt diarrhea.

❑ When travelling abroad, do not drink the water unless you know it is safe. Avoid ice cubes, raw vegetables, dairy products, and unpeeled fruit. Use bottled water when you brush your teeth. Diarrhea is common when travelling in other countries, so it may be advisable to take certain preparations with you. Lactobacillus GG, a type of probiotic, is a natural alternative to both antibiotics or bismuth subsalicylate (Pepto-Bismol).

❑ Chronic diarrhea in very young children is evident if the child has five or more watery stools a day. A baby with diarrhea can become dehydrated very quickly and should be evaluated by a health care provider.

❑ Use of the vaccine against rotavirus, a type of virus that commonly causes diarrhea, especially in infants and small children, was halted after the National Centers for Disease Control and Prevention and the U.S. Food and Drug Administration (FDA) linked the vaccine to a rare type of bowel obstruction called *intussusception*. Further investigation is ongoing.

❑ If diarrhea is chronic or recurrent, an underlying problem such as a food allergy, infection, or intestinal parasites may be the cause. Allergy testing can determine if you have any food allergies. A stool culture can be done to check for infection or the presence of parasites.

Diverticulitis

Diverticulitis is a condition in which diverticula are perforated and become infected and inflamed. Diverticula are saclike pea- or grape-sized protrusions in the intestinal wall. They typically form if an individual suffers from frequent constipation. Eating a low-fiber diet, as is typical in industrialized countries such as the United States, may contribute to the development of diverticulitis. Without sufficient fiber to soften and add bulk, stools are harder to pass. Greatly increased pressure is required to force small portions of hard, dry stool through the bowel. This rise in pressure can cause pouches to form at weak points in the

wall of the colon. Once diverticula develop, they do not go away. The diverticula themselves cause no symptoms. Many people have diverticu*losis* (the pouchlike protrusions) and never develop diverticu*litis* (the inflamed pouches). However, if tiny cuts in the pouches become infected or inflamed, the result can be severe, causing fever, chills, nausea, and pain.

Diverticulitis can be either acute or chronic. Symptoms include cramping, bloating, tenderness on the left side of the abdomen that is relieved by passing gas or a bowel movement, constipation or diarrhea, nausea, and an almost continual need to eliminate. There may be blood in the stool. Peritonitis, an inflammation of the lining of the abdominal cavity, can develop if a diverticulum ruptures and intestinal contents flow into the abdomen.

Because the walls of the large intestine often weaken as a person ages, this is a condition affecting older rather than younger people. It usually strikes people between the ages of fifty and ninety. It affects millions of Americans, but many people do not even know they have the condition because they either experience no symptoms or accept their symptoms as simple indigestion.

Exactly why is not known, but it is known that smoking and stress make symptoms worse. In fact, this is a classic example of a stress-related disorder. Poor eating habits compound the problem. A poor diet, a family history of the disease, gallbladder disease, obesity, and coronary artery disease all increase the chances of developing diverticulitis.

There are several diagnostic tests available to help diagnose diverticulitis. A barium enema is a procedure in which the colon is filled with liquid barium and x-rays are taken to reveal pouches in the colon wall, narrowing of the colon, or other abnormalities. With sigmoidoscopy, a thin, flexible lighted tube is inserted into the rectum to give the physician a closer look at the lower colon. If necessary, tissue samples can be removed for examination. To see into other parts of the colon, a colonoscopy must be performed. This is similar to a sigmoidoscopy, but allows a view of the entire colon.

NUTRIENTS

SUPPLEMENT	SUGGESTED DOSAGE	COMMENTS
Essential		
Bio-Bifidus from American Biologics and	As directed on label.	To replace flora in the small intestine, primarily to improve assimilation.
Kyo-Dophilus from Wakunaga	As directed on label. Take on an empty stomach.	For bowel flora replacement to improve elimination and assimilation.
Fiber (oat bran, psyllium, ground flaxseeds, and Aerobic Bulk Cleanse (ABC) from Aerobic Life Industries are good sources)	As directed on label. Take 1 hour before meals with a large glass of liquid. Take separately from other supplements and medications.	Helps prevent constipation. Prevents infection by preventing accumulation of wastes in pouches in the colon walls.

Vitamin B complex	100 mg of each major B vitamin 3 times daily (amounts of individual vitamins in a complex will vary).	Needed for all enzyme systems in the body and for proper digestion. Use a hypoallergenic formula.
Very Important		
Multienzyme complex with pancreatin	As directed on label. Take with meals.	Needed to break down proteins. Use a formula high in pancreatin.
ProFlora whey from Wakunaga	2–3 tablespoons daily.	Helps prevent constipation and prevents infection by maintaining a proper colon pH balance.
Proteolytic enzymes	As directed on label. Take between meals.	Aids in digestion and reduces inflammation of the colon.
Important		
Dioxychlor from American Biologics	As directed on label.	An important antibacterial, antifungal, and antiviral agent.
Essential fatty acids (flaxseed oil, primrose oil, salmon oil, and Kyolic-EPA from Wakunaga are good sources)	As directed on label 3 times daily, before meals.	Improves lymphatic function and aids in protecting the cells lining the wall of the colon.
Garlic (Kyolic from Wakunaga)	2 capsules 3 times daily, with meals.	Aids in digestion and destroys unwanted bacteria and parasites. Use a yeast-free formula.
Kyo-Green from Wakunaga	As directed on label.	Aids in normal bowel function.
L-Glutamine	500 mg twice daily, on an empty stomach. Take with water or juice. Do not take with milk. Take with 50 mg vitamin B$_6$ and 100 mg vitamin C for better absorption.	A major metabolic fuel for the intestinal cells; maintains the villi, the absorption surfaces of the gut. (*See* AMINO ACIDS in Part One.)
Vitamin K or alfalfa	100 mcg daily.	Deficiency has been linked to intestinal disorders. *See under* Herbs, below.
Helpful		
Free-form amino acid complex (Amino Balance from Anabol Naturals)	As directed on label, on an empty stomach, 1/2 hour before meals.	To supply protein, needed for healing and repair of tissue.
Raw thymus glandular	As directed on label.	*See* GLANDULAR THERAPY in Part Three for its benefits. *Caution:* Do not give this supplement to a child.
Vitamin A with mixed carotenoids	25,000 IU daily. If you are pregnant, do not exceed 10,000 IU daily.	Protects and heals the lining of the colon.
Vitamin C with bioflavonoids	3,000–8,000 mg daily, in divided doses.	Reduces inflammation and boosts immune response. Use a buffered form.
Vitamin E	Up to 800 IU daily.	A powerful antioxidant that protects the mucous membranes. Use d-alpha-tocopherol form.

HERBS

❑ Alfalfa is a good natural source of vitamin K and valuable minerals, which are often deficient in people with intestinal disorders. It also contains chlorophyll, which aids healing. Take 2,000 milligrams daily in capsule or extract form.

❑ Aloe vera promotes the healing of inflamed areas. It also helps to prevent constipation. Drink 1/2 cup of aloe vera juice three times daily. It can be mixed with a cup of herbal tea if you wish.

❑ Bio-Rizin from American Biologics is a licorice extract that improves glandular function and helps relieve allergy symptoms. Take 10 to 20 drops twice daily.

❑ Pau d'arco has an antibacterial, cleansing, and healing effect. Drink two cups of pau d'arco tea daily.

❑ Other herbs beneficial for diverticulitis include cayenne (capsicum), chamomile, goldenseal, papaya, red clover, and yarrow extract or tea.

Caution: Do not use chamomile on an ongoing basis, as ragweed allergy may result. Avoid it completely if you are allergic to ragweed. Do not take goldenseal for more than one week at a time, and do not use it during pregnancy. If you have a history of cardiovascular disease, diabetes, or glaucoma, use it only under a doctor's supervision.

RECOMMENDATIONS

❑ The key to controlling this disorder is to consume an adequate amount of fiber and lots of quality water. You need at least 30 grams of fiber each day. You may prefer to supplement your diet with a bulk product and/or a stool softener that contains methylcellulose or psyllium, since these do not promote as much gas formation in the colon as other sources of fiber, especially wheat bran. Drink at least eight 8-ounce glasses of water daily. Herbal teas, broth, and live juices can account for some of the liquid needed. Liquid aids in keeping the pouchlike areas clean of toxic wastes, preventing inflammation.

❑ Eat a low-carbohydrate diet with high levels of protein from vegetable sources and fish. Do not eat grains, seeds, or nuts, except for well-cooked brown rice. These foods are hard to digest, resulting in bloating and gas. Also eliminate dairy products, red meat, sugar products, fried foods, spices, and processed foods.

❑ Eat plenty of green leafy vegetables. These are good sources of vitamin K. Obtaining this vitamin through diet is especially important for people with intestinal disorders.

❑ Eat garlic for its healing and detoxifying properties.

❑ During an acute attack of diverticulitis, your health care provider may recommend a low-fiber diet temporarily. Once the inflammation clears, you may slowly switch back to a high-fiber diet.

❏ When an attack or pain begins, give yourself a cleansing enema using 2 quarts of lukewarm water and the juice of a fresh lemon. (*See* ENEMAS in Part Three.) This helps to rid the colon of undigested and entrapped foods and to relieve pain.

❏ On the day of an acute attack, take 4 charcoal tablets or capsules with a large glass of water to absorb trapped gas. Charcoal tablets are available at health food stores. Always take charcoal separately from medications and other supplements, and do not take it for prolonged periods, as it absorbs beneficial nutrients as well as gas.

❏ During severe attacks, use liquid vitamin supplements for better assimilation and put all vegetables and fruits through a blender. Eat steamed vegetables only. Baby foods are good until healing is complete. Earth's Best produces organically grown baby foods that are available in health food stores and some supermarkets. Add supplemental fiber to the baby food. As healing progresses, gradually add raw fruits and vegetables to the diet. Drink carrot juice, cabbage juice, and "green drinks." Or take chlorophyll liquid or liquid alfalfa in juice.

❏ To relieve pain, massage the left side of the abdomen. Stand up and do stretching exercises.

❏ Clay tablets are beneficial. Take them as directed on the product label on an empty stomach upon arising.

❏ Check stools daily for blood. If the stool is black, take a portion of it to your physician for an analysis.

❏ Try to have a bowel movement at the same time each day. Take fiber first thing in the morning, before breakfast, to help the bowels move at this time.

Note: Always take supplemental fiber separately from other supplements and medications.

❏ Do not overuse laxatives; they can irritate the colon wall.

CONSIDERATIONS

❏ Food allergies are often a cause of intestinal disorders. Allergy testing is advised. (*See* ALLERGIES in Part Two.)

❏ If the diverticula are infected, your doctor may prescribe antibiotics. Be sure to consume plenty of soured products and some form of nondairy acidophilus if you are taking antibiotics.

❏ Fasting is beneficial. (*See* FASTING in Part Three.)

❏ *See also* CROHN'S DISEASE, IRRITABLE BOWEL SYNDROME, and ULCERATIVE COLITIS, all in Part Two.

Dizziness

See MÉNIÈRE'S DISEASE; VERTIGO. *See also under* PREGNANCY-RELATED PROBLEMS.

Dog Bite

A bite or scratch from a dog (or cat) that breaks the skin poses the danger of infection, especially if the wound is deep. Bites also carry the risk of rabies. Most household pets are immunized against rabies, but the possibility of infection still exists. It is also possible to contract a tetanus infection from an animal bite. *Clostridium tetani*, the microbe that causes tetanus, lives in the top layers of soil, and in the intestinal tracts of cows and horses, and easily infects wounds that result in reduced oxygen flow in the tissue, particularly crushing and puncture wounds.

A dog bite can be nothing more than a minor graze, or it can be so severe as to be life-threatening. Children are at most risk from dog bites, and children under five years of age are victims of the most severe attacks—many of them requiring hospitalization.

Unless otherwise stated, the dosages recommended here are for adults. For a child between the ages of twelve and seventeen, reduce the dose to three-quarters of the recommended amount. For a child between the ages of six and twelve, use one-half the recommended dose, and for a child under six, use one-quarter of the recommended amount.

NUTRIENTS

SUPPLEMENT	SUGGESTED DOSAGE	COMMENTS
Very Important		
Vitamin C with bioflavonoids	4,000–10,000 mg daily for 1 week, then reduce to 3,000 mg daily.	Fights infection. Important for repair of collagen and connective tissue.
Important		
Proteolytic enzymes or Inflazyme Forte from American Biologics	As directed on label. Take between meals. As directed on label.	Acts as an anti-inflammatory.
Helpful		
Colloidal silver	As directed on label.	To reduce the danger of infection. Can be taken internally or placed on a sterile bandage covering the wound.
Garlic (Kyolic from Wakunaga)	2 capsules 3 times daily.	Acts as a natural antibiotic.
L-Cysteine and L-methionine	500 mg each daily for 2 weeks. Take with water or juice on an empty stomach. Do not take with milk. Take with 50 mg vitamin B_6 and 100 mg vitamin C for better absorption.	Powerful detoxifying agents. (*See* AMINO ACIDS in Part One.)
Vira-Plex 135 from Enzymatic Therapy	As directed on label.	Aids in healing and fights infection.

Vitamin A plus mixed carotenoids plus vitamin E form.	25,000 IU daily. If you are pregnant, do not exceed 10,000 IU daily. 25,000 IU daily. 400 IU daily.	Powerful antioxidants that aid the immune system and assist healing of the skin. Use d-alpha-tocopherol
Vitamin B complex	50 mg of each major B vitamin 3 times daily (amounts of individual vitamins in a complex will vary).	Aids in tissue oxidation and antibody production.

HERBS

❑ Echinacea, goldenseal, pau d'arco, and red clover, taken in tea form, are good for dog bites. Goldenseal extract can also be applied directly on the affected area. This is a natural antibiotic that helps to fight infection.

Caution: Do not take goldenseal internally on a daily basis for more than one week at a time, and do not use it during pregnancy. If you have a history of cardiovascular disease, diabetes, or glaucoma, use it only under supervision.

RECOMMENDATIONS

❑ If you are bitten by a dog, the first thing you should do is remove the animal's saliva from the wound. Wash the area thoroughly with warm water, then add soap and wash for at least five minutes more. Rinse the wound for a few more minutes with plain water and cover it with a gauze dressing for twenty-four hours.

❑ See your health care provider to make sure that you do not need stitches or other professional treatment.

❑ If you know who the dog's owner is, inquire as to the animal's vaccination status. If the dog is unfamiliar, try to have someone confine it if possible so that its health can be checked and it can be placed under observation.

❑ Teach children how to behave around animals, and teach them not to approach strange animals. Never leave a young child alone with an animal—even the family pet.

CONSIDERATIONS

❑ Your physician may prescribe an oral antibiotic to prevent infection. If so, make sure that you take acidophilus to replace the "friendly" bacteria that antibiotics destroy. Your doctor will also likely recommend that you have a tetanus booster shot if you haven't had one in six years or more.

❑ In most states, dog bite incidents must be reported to the local health department, and the dog must then be kept under observation for any signs of rabies—viciousness, paralysis, growling, foaming at the mouth, or agitation. If the animal cannot be located and rabies ruled out, a series of rabies injections will be necessary.

Down Syndrome

Down syndrome is a condition caused by the presence of extra genetic material in the cells of a developing embryo. The disorder—named for English physician John Langdon Down—occurs in approximately 1 in every 800 to 1,000 live births, and usually results in mental retardation and distinctive physical abnormalities.

The incidence of Down syndrome increases with the age of the parents, especially if the mothers are thirty-four or older. The risk is also higher for children of parents who have already given birth to a Down syndrome child.

Down syndrome is usually caused by a phenomenon geneticists call nondisjunction, in which an error in cell division produces three copies of a chromosome—in this case, chromosome 21—instead of the normal two. In trisomy 21, which accounts for 95 percent of Down syndrome cases, the extra chromosome is due to an error in chromosome separation in the ovum before conception, although nondisjunction can also take place in the sperm. A small percentage of Down syndrome cases are linked to other kinds of chromosomal abnormalities, but all result in extra genetic material in some or all of the cells.

An infant born with Down syndrome typically—but not always—has characteristic physical traits such as a small head, poor muscle tone, a flat facial profile, slanted eyes, a depressed nose bridge, low-set ears, furrowed tongue, and a single deep crease across the center of the palm (known as a simian crease). People with Down syndrome are especially prone to having congenital heart disease and are more susceptible than most people to developing acute leukemia, thyroid disorders, and respiratory and digestive problems. While females with Down syndrome may menstruate and be fertile, males are almost always infertile.

Although the degree of mental retardation varies greatly among different individuals with Down syndrome, the average IQ falls within the range of 50 to 60. Generally, children with Down syndrome are able to learn everyday life skills and can be raised at home. Special education and training allow many individuals with Down syndrome to lead happy, useful, and love-filled lives. People with Down syndrome can live to middle or old age; however, as adults, they may be prone to developing Alzheimer's disease plus pneumonia and other lung diseases.

Unless otherwise specified, the dosages recommended here are for adults. For a child between the ages of twelve and seventeen, reduce the dose to three-quarters the recommended amount. For a child between six and twelve, use one-half the recommended dose, and for a child under the age of six, use one-quarter the recommended amount. Persons with malabsorption problems should consult a health care provider before starting any nutritional program.

Alternative Approaches for Down Syndrome

There are a number of revolutionary treatments to maximize the learning potential and physical capabilities of those with Down syndrome that have shown significant success and have been gaining increasing scientific attention in recent years.

NUTRITIONAL APPROACH

The use of nutritional supplementation to help boost the metabolism of those with Down syndrome began with North American physician Dr. Henry Turkel in the 1950s. To address the unique biochemistry of those with Down syndrome, he began treating affected children with a combination of vitamins, minerals, and hormones. Although his program achieved some success, his work was generally rejected or ignored by mainstream scientists.

However, a growing population of parents of children with Down syndrome continued to use Dr. Turkel's nutritional program. Eventually, Kent MacLeod, a pharmaceutical biochemist and owner of Nutri-Chem Labs in Ottawa, Canada, learned of Dr. Turkel's formula after a number of parents asked him to evaluate the protocol. MacLeod and the biochemical team at Nutri-Chem joined with Dr. Turkel and other researchers in further developing and refining the original supplement. A nutritional formula known as MSBPlus was the eventual result.

MSBPlus is a formula of vitamins, minerals, amino acids, antioxidants, and enzymes that targets essential nutrients missing from the biochemical makeup of the person with Down syndrome. This supplement, which can be custom-formulated to meet individual age and metabolic needs, has met with marked success. Research is ongoing. The University of Miami School of Medicine is now collaborating with Nutri-Chem on clinical trials and studies on Down syndrome. One long-term, double-blind study will examine the cognitive development and language skills of children with Down syndrome who are taking MSBPlus.

Nutri-Chem is also working with Dr. Marie Peeters, a pediatrician and former member of the Institute de Progenese in Paris. Dr. Peeters was an associate of Dr. Jerome LeJeune, the scientist who discovered the cause of Down syndrome. In an effort to further study the effects of nutritional supplements (particularly amino acids) on those with this disorder, Dr. Peeters is involved in clinical trials.

For additional information on MSBPlus formula, or to receive information on the connection between nutrition and Down syndrome, you can write to Nutri-Chem Labs, 1303 Richmond Road, Ottawa, Ontario K2B 7Y4, Canada; or call them at 613–820–9065 or 613–829–2226.

The work of Dr. Turkel also influenced Jack Warner, M.D., F.A.A.P., founder of Warner House, Inc., a not-for-profit center for the clinical study and treatment of Down syndrome. Together with medical colleagues, biochemists, and other medical professionals, Dr. Warner developed a metabolic treatment called HAP CAPS for children with Down syndrome. This formula is a supplemental yet integral part of a multidisciplinary treatment approach that includes examination and evaluation by a physical therapist, a developmental optometrist, a clinical psychologist, a speech advisor, and a nutritionist, under the recommendation of a primary care pediatrician, plus a system of periodic reports, tests, and doctors' observations. In addition to seeing patients regularly at the clinic in Fullerton, California, the Warner House staff also travels across the United States to meet with patients in many cities.

Dr. Warner reports that data from over twelve years of research and treatment show the Warner House treatment protocol has resulted in changes in the physical features of children with Down syndrome, a reduction in the frequency of infections that typically affect these children, and an improvement in their cognitive ability.

More information about Warner House can be obtained by writing to The Warner House, 1023 East Chapman Avenue, Fullerton, CA 92631; or by calling 714–441–2600.

DEVELOPMENTAL STIMULATION APPROACH

The Institutes for the Achievement of Human Potential in Philadelphia, Pennsylvania, offers parents of children with Down syndrome a specialized program for helping their children develop and maximize their potential. In this program, parents are the key players in a home therapeutic approach that involves providing simple yet intensive neurological stimulation for their children. A carefully designed nutritional regimen is also an integral part of the program.

Before beginning the program, parents attend a five-day course of lectures and demonstrations at The Institutes. They learn about the Developmental Profile, a measuring instrument that clearly shows visual, auditory, tactile, mobility, language, and manual abilities a child should attain by certain ages, and they learn specific techniques to use in working on different skill areas with their children. Once home, the parents carry out an individualized brain-development program tailored to the needs of their child. Carried out properly, these techniques have produced most encouraging results, often leading children with Down syndrome to perform even above levels exhibited by most average children.

More information on this program can be obtained by writing to The Registrar, The Institutes for the Achievement of Human Potential, 8801 Stenton Avenue, Philadelphia, PA 19118; or by calling 800–736–4663.

NUTRIENTS

SUPPLEMENT	SUGGESTED DOSAGE	COMMENTS
Aangamik DMG from FoodScience of Vermont	50 mg 4 times daily.	Promotes the utilization of oxygen.
Acetyl-L-carnitine (ALC)	100–500 mg daily.	A carnitine derivative produced naturally in the body, it is involved in carbohydrate and protein metabolism and in the transport of fats into the mitochondria. It increases levels of carnitine in tissues and even surpasses the metabolic potency of carnitine.
Coenzyme Q$_{10}$	10 mg daily.	Prevents heart damage by improving oxygenation of cells.
Essential fatty acids (Kyolic-EPA from Wakunaga, salmon oil, flaxseed oil, and primrose oil are good sources)	As directed on label. Take with meals.	Needed for proper brain and cardiovascular function.
Free-form amino acid complex	As directed on label.	To provide needed protein and bolster the immune system.
Garlic (Kyolic from Wakunaga)	As directed on label.	Natural antibiotic that helps the body to eliminate toxins and strengthens the cardiovascular system.
Kelp	As directed on label.	To supply minerals helpful in establishing thyroid balance.
Lecithin granules or	1 tsp 3 times daily.	Aids brain function.
capsules	2,400 mg 3 times daily.	
Multivitamin and mineral complex with	As directed on label.	All nutrients are needed for proper immune function.
vitamin A and	10,000 IU daily.	
mixed carotenoids and	15,000 IU daily.	
selenium	200 mcg daily.	
Potassium	200 mg daily.	Helps transmit nerve impulses.
Taurine Plus from American Biologics	500 mg daily, on an empty stomach. Take with water or juice. Do not take with milk. Take with 50 mg vitamin B$_6$ and 100 mg vitamin C for better absorption.	Reduces stress and regulates nervous system.
Vitamin B complex with	As directed on label.	Prevents and/or treats memory loss and increases learning capacity. Also protects against cardiovascular disease.
choline	100 mg daily.	
Vitamin C with bioflavonoids	3,000 mg daily.	Enhances immune function and reduces cholesterol levels.
Vitamin E	400 IU daily.	Boosts immune system and facilitates body's absorption of lecithin. Use d-alpha-tocopherol form.
Zinc plus	50 mg daily.	Needed for proper brain function and a healthy immune system.
copper	2–3 mg daily.	Needed to balance with zinc.

RECOMMENDATIONS

❏ Be patient when feeding a child with Down syndrome, and be sure to provide a balanced diet. Include fresh and whole foods that are rich in vegetable proteins, as well as foods that are high in magnesium, such as fresh green vegetables, figs, meat, fish and seafood, nuts and seeds, tofu, blackstrap molasses, apples, kelp, soybeans, cornmeal, rice, apricots, and brewer's yeast. Reduce consumption of foods high in gluten, such as wheat, rye, barley, and oats. Avoid refined foods, sugars, dairy products, and alcohol.

❏ Hold and nurture your child as much as possible.

❏ Provide plenty of exercise, including deep-breathing exercises, daily. This helps to oxygenate the brain.

❏ Provide environmental stimulation. Play music in your home, for example (studies suggest that classical music is best). Provide objects and toys that are safe to handle and that invite exploration. Talk to and interact with your child, and involve him or her as much as possible in whatever you happen to be doing (if you have other children, encourage them to do the same).

❏ Set realistic goals for your child, and remember the emotional needs of your other children.

❏ Use liquid or spray forms of supplements for a child with Down syndrome.

CONSIDERATIONS

❏ Some studies suggest that vitamin/mineral supplements and extra nutrients can be beneficial for people with Down syndrome. However, any kind of nutritional program should be designed with the help of a qualified physician or health care provider, who should take into account the individual makeup of any person with Down syndrome.

❏ Care for the child with Down syndrome depends on the degree of mental and physical impairment. Carefully planned programs to promote development of motor and mental skills are important. Since learning potential is greatest during infancy, an *early* stimulation program of exercises based on the child's ability is necessary for teaching gross motor skills.

❏ The risk of giving birth to a Down syndrome child increases markedly after the age of thirty-four. Amniocentesis may be recommended if you become pregnant past this age. (For additional information on amniocentesis and other types of prenatal testing, *see under* PREGNANCY-RELATED PROBLEMS in Part Two.)

❏ Additional information on Down syndrome, parent support groups, and early intervention programs for children with Down syndrome is available from The National Down Syndrome Society (*see* HEALTH AND MEDICAL ORGANIZATIONS in the Appendix).

Drug Addiction (Substance Abuse)

Addiction is said to exist when the body becomes so accustomed to the presence of a foreign substance that it can no longer function properly if the substance is withdrawn. Not everyone who uses drugs, legal or illegal, becomes addicted to them. The three most commonly used drugs—alcohol, tobacco, and caffeine—are legal and freely available, but they do not pose an addiction problem for all those who take them. Not everyone who drinks becomes an alcoholic; some people smoke only on weekends or special occasions; many people who drink coffee don't crave it all the time. Much research is focusing on the question of why some people become addicted while others do not, and scientists and nutritionists are providing some answers to the complex question of chemical dependency.

The reasons for addiction, according to most research, lie in the brain. A group of chemicals called neurotransmitters carry the signals between neurons in the brain. One of these neurotransmitters, dopamine, plays a pivotal role in transmitting feelings of satisfaction, arousal, and reward, so that every time we experience these feelings, we have the desire to replicate them by doing whatever it was that caused them before. This may account for the repetition inherent in addictive behavior.

Alcohol, nicotine, marijuana, cocaine, and amphetamines are a few of the substances that increase dopamine levels in the brain, and the more they are used, the more deeply these substances are associated with pleasure and reward, and the more profound the dependency. It is also thought that people who become addicted to a substance come to take less pleasure in things they used to enjoy. Through positron-emission tomography (PET) brain scans of addicted people, research has shown that their brains show less response to other pleasurable pursuits, such as listening to their favorite music, than do the brain scans of people not involved in substance abuse.

The pleasure elicited by whatever substance the individual is addicted to is so strong that it is difficult to eradicate, and even after years of abstinence, there are triggers that may cause the person to relapse. Research has shown that long-term drug abuse results in significant changes in brain function that persist long after an individual stops using drugs.

Signs of drug addiction can include a decreased desire to work and/or socialize, extreme drowsiness, inattentiveness, frequent mood swings, restlessness, personality changes, and a loss of appetite. Persons addicted to drugs may want to be alone, and lose their tempers easily. Drug withdrawal symptoms may include headache, insomnia, sensitivity to light and noise, diarrhea, hot and cold flashes, sweating, deep depression, irritability, irrational thinking, and disorientation. Not surprisingly, individuals who are addicted to drugs can end up centering their lives on avoiding the excruciating pain of withdrawal—that is, on assuring a continuing supply of the drug. This need to obtain the drug at all costs leads ultimately to a disintegration of normal life, including broken personal relationships, loss of employment, and even criminal behavior.

People who become chemically dependent do so at different rates, and research is showing that susceptibility to addiction may be, in part, hereditary. Complicating the phenomenon of addiction is the problem of drug tolerance. With prolonged drug use, the body often ends up needing more and more of the substance to produce the desired effect and to prevent withdrawal symptoms. Some users end up increasing the dosage to the point that they die, or come close to dying, from overdose. In addition, addiction almost always has a powerful psychological as well as a physical component.

The nutrient program outlined below is designed to help those recovering from drug addiction. Unless otherwise specified, the dosages recommended here are for adults. For a child under the age of seventeen, use one-half to three-quarters of the recommended amount.

NUTRIENTS

SUPPLEMENT	SUGGESTED DOSAGE	COMMENTS
Very Important		
Essential fatty acids complex	As directed on label.	Good for reversing the effects of malnourishment common in those with substance abuse problems.
Liquid Kyolic with B$_1$ and B$_{12}$ from Wakunaga	As directed on label.	Fights stress and protects the liver.
Neuro Logic from Wakunaga	As directed on label.	Nourishes the central nervous system. Detoxifies the system. Encourages normal brain function.
Vitamin B complex injections	2 cc daily or as prescribed by physician.	Needed when under stress to rebuild the liver. Injections (under a doctor's supervision) are most effective. If injections are not available, use a sublingual form.
plus extra vitamin B$_{12}$ or vitamin B complex	1 cc daily or as prescribed by physician. 100 mg of each major B vitamin daily (amounts of individual vitamins in a complex will vary).	Can give the same energy boost as a cup of coffee.
plus extra pantothenic acid (vitamin B$_5$) and	500 mg 3 times daily.	Essential for the adrenal glands and for reducing stress.
vitamin B$_3$ (niacinamide)	500 mg 3 times daily.	Important for brain function. *Caution:* Do not substitute niacin for niacinamide. Niacin should not be taken in such high doses.
Important		
Calcium and	1,500 mg at bedtime.	Nourishes the central nervous system and helps control tremors by calming the body. Use chelate forms.
magnesium	1,000 mg at bedtime.	

Free-form amino acid complex plus extra	As directed on label, on an empty stomach.	To supply needed protein in a readily assimilable form.
L-glutamine	500 mg 3 times daily, on an empty stomach.	Passes the blood-brain barrier to promote healthy mental functioning. Increases levels of gamma-aminobutyric acid (GABA), which has a calming effect.
and L-tyrosine	500 mg twice daily, on an empty stomach. Take these supplements with water or juice, not milk. Take with 50 mg vitamin B₆ and 100 mg vitamin C for better absorption.	Tyrosine and valerian root taken every 4 hours have given good results for cocaine withdrawal. (*See* AMINO ACIDS in Part One.) *Caution:* Do not take this supplement if you are taking an MAO inhibitor drug.
Gamma-amino-butyric acid (GABA)	As directed on label, on an empty stomach.	Acts as a relaxant and lessens cravings. (*See* AMINO ACIDS in Part One.)
Glutathione	As directed on label.	Aids in detoxifying drugs to reduce their harmful effects. Also reduces the desire for drugs or alcohol.
Lithium	As prescribed by physician.	A trace mineral that aids in relieving depression. Available by prescription only.
L-Phenylalanine	1,500 mg daily, taken upon arising.	Necessary as a brain fuel. Use for withdrawal symptoms. *Caution:* Do not take this supplement if you are pregnant or nursing, or suffer from panic attacks, diabetes, high blood pressure, or PKU.
S-Adenosylmethio-nine (SAMe)	As directed on label.	Aids in stress-relief, depression, eases pain, and produces antioxidant effects that can improve the health of the liver. *Caution:* Do not use if you have manic-depressive disorder or take prescription antidepressants.
Vitamin C with bioflavonoids	2,000 mg every 3 hours.	Detoxifies the system and lessens the craving for drugs. Use a buffered form such as sodium ascorbate. Intravenous administration (under a doctor's supervision) may be necessary.
Zinc	As directed on label.	Promotes a healthy immune system and protects the liver from damage.
Helpful		
5-Hydroxytryptophan (5-HTP)	As directed on label.	Aids with both stress and withdrawal symptoms.
Multivitamin and mineral complex	As directed on label.	All nutrients are needed in high amounts. Use a high-potency formula.

HERBS

❏ Burdock root and red clover aid in cleansing toxins from the bloodstream.

❏ Siberian ginseng helps those experiencing cocaine withdrawal.

Caution: Do not use this herb if you have hypoglycemia, high blood pressure, or a heart disorder.

❏ Milk thistle helps to detoxify the liver.

❏ Pueraria, a Chinese herb, has been used for centuries as a cure for alcoholism.

❏ St. John's wort is a good antidepressant and can help with withdrawal symptoms.

❏ Valerian root has a calming effect. Used with the amino acid tyrosine, it has been found to be helpful for those undergoing withdrawal from cocaine.

RECOMMENDATIONS

❏ Eat a well-balanced, nutrient-dense diet that emphasizes fresh, raw foods.

❏ Add high-protein drinks to the diet.

❏ Avoid heavily processed foods, all forms of sugar, and junk food. These foods are a quick source of energy, but are followed by a low feeling that may increase cravings for drugs.

❏ *See* FASTING in Part Three, and follow the instructions.

❏ Consider consulting a qualified acupuncturist. Acupuncture has been known to help addicts by decreasing stress, anxiety, and the craving for drugs.

CONSIDERATIONS

❏ There is no single treatment that will help all addicted people. Treatment needs to be tailored to fit the different needs and problems facing the individual.

❏ To minimize withdrawal symptoms, withdrawal from any drug should be done slowly. The dosage should be decreased gradually over a period of four weeks or longer. This task cannot be accomplished alone; most often hospitalization and/or professional help is required.

❏ Most people are aware that a drug overdose can kill, but many do not realize that these poisons kill in other ways as well. Angina, heart attack, coronary artery spasms, and life-threatening damage to the heart muscle may occur with the use of cocaine and heroin. All drugs weaken the immune system in one way or another. Chronic marijuana use can reduce the immune response by as much as 40 percent by damaging and destroying white blood cells. Without a strong immune system, the body is vulnerable to all kinds of infectious and degenerative diseases.

❏ Buprenorphine (Buprenex), a synthetic narcotic, taken either by itself or in combination with naloxone, a drug that prevents the "high" induced by narcotics, is sometimes prescribed for people who are dependent on opiates, and this treatment has shown some success. Methadone may also be prescribed as a substitute for illegal opiates.

❏ Many drug users suffer from malnutrition. Because drugs rob the body of necessary nutrients, those addicted to drugs need to take high doses of supplemental nutrients.

❏ Research has found that children of alcoholics are more

Substances That Rob the Body of Nutrients

Different substances deplete the body of different nutrients. Use the list below to determine which supplements you may need as a result of the use of prescription or over-the-counter drugs, including alcohol and caffeine.

Substance	Depleted Nutrients
Allopurinol (Zyloprim)	Iron.
Antacids	B-complex vitamins; calcium; phosphate; vitamins A and D.
Antibiotics, general (*See also* isoniazid, penicillin, sulfa drugs, and trimethoprim)	B-complex vitamins; vitamin K; "friendly" bacteria.
Antihistamines	Vitamin C.
Aspirin	B-complex vitamins; calcium; folic acid; iron; potassium, vitamins A and C.
Barbiturates	Vitamin C.
Beta-blockers (Corgard, Inderal, Lopressor, and others)	Choline; chromium; pantothenic acid (vitamin B_5).
Caffeine	Biotin; inositol; potassium; vitamin B_1 (thiamine); zinc.
Carbamazepine (Atretol, Tegretol)	Dilutes blood sodium.
Chlorthiazide (Aldoclor, Diuril, and others)	Magnesium; potassium.
Cimetidine (Tagamet)	Iron.
Clonidine (Catapres, Combipres)	B-complex vitamins; calcium.
Corticosteroids, general (*See also* prednisone)	Calcium; potassium; vitamins A, B_6, C, and D; zinc.
Digitalis preparations (Crystodigin, Digoxin, and others)	Vitamins B_1 (thiamine) and B_6 (pyridoxine); zinc.
Diuretics, general (*See also* chlorthiazide, spironolactone, thiazide diuretics, and triamterene)	Calcium; iodine; magnesium; potassium; vitamins B_2 (riboflavin) and C; zinc.
Estrogen preparations	Folic acid; vitamin B_6 (pyridoxine).
Ethanol (alcohol)	B-complex vitamins; magnesium; vitamins C, D, E, and K.
Fluoride	Vitamin C.
Glutethimide (Doriden)	Folic acid; vitamin B_6 (pyridoxine).
Guanethidine (Esimil, Ismelin)	Magnesium; potassium; vitamins B_2 (riboflavin) and B_6 (pyridoxine).
Hydralazine (Apresazide, Apresoline, and others)	Vitamin B_6 (pyridoxine).
Indomethacin (INH and others)	Vitamins B_3 (niacin) and B_6 (pyridoxine).
Laxatives (excluding herbs)	Potassium; vitamins A and K.
Lidocaine (Xylocaine)	Calcium; potassium.
Nitrate/nitrite coronary vasodilators	Niacin; pangamic acid; selenium; vitamins C and E.
Oral contraceptives	B-complex vitamins; vitamins C, D, and E.
Penicillin preparations	Vitamin B_3 (niacin); niacinamide; vitamin B_6 (pyridoxine).
Phenobarbital preparations	Folic acid; vitamin B_6 (pyridoxine); vitamin B_{12}; vitamins D and K.
Phenylbutazone (Cotylbutazone)	Folic acid; iodine.
Phenytoin (Dilantin)	Calcium; folic acid; vitamins B_{12}, C, D, and K.
Prednisone (Deltasone and others)	Potassium; vitamins B_6 (pyridoxine) and C; zinc.
Quinidine preparations	Choline; pantothenic acid (vitamin B_5); potassium; vitamin K.
Reserpine preparations	Phenylalanine; potassium; vitamins B_2 (riboflavin) and B_6 (pyridoxine).
Spironolactone (Aldactone and others)	Calcium; folic acid.
Sulfa drugs	Para-aminobenzoic acid (PABA); "friendly" bacteria.
Synthetic neurotransmitters	Magnesium; potassium; vitamins B_2 (riboflavin) and B_6 (pyridoxine).
Thiazide diuretics	Magnesium; potassium; vitamin B_2 (riboflavin); zinc.
Tobacco	Vitamins A, C, and E.
Triamterene (Dyrenium)	Calcium; folic acid.
Trimethoprim (Bactrim, Septra, and others)	Folic acid.

inclined than others to use drugs, including cocaine. These individuals are 400 times more likely to use drugs than those who do not have a family history of alcohol addiction.

❑ An individual can be addicted to substances other than illegal drugs. Many are addicted to nicotine, caffeine, colas, alcohol, sugar, and even certain foods. Although these addictions may not pose as great a health risk, withdrawal still may be painful and difficult. Those who use these substances may also be more susceptible to illness and disease because these addictive substances deplete the body of needed nutrients. (*See* Substances that Rob the Body of Nutrients on page 336.)

❑ A growing problem for substance abusers in these times, especially for those who use drugs intravenously and share needles, is the threat of AIDS (*see* AIDS in Part Two). Unfortunately, for long-term drug users, even this is not enough to deter them from continuing the habitual use of drugs.

❑ *See also* ALCOHOLISM and SMOKING DEPENDENCY in Part Two.

Dry Skin

A balance of oil and moisture is crucial for healthy, attractive skin. Oil is secreted by the sebaceous glands and lubricates the surface of the skin. Moisture is the water present inside the skin cells, and comes to the cells through the bloodstream. It is the water in the skin cells that keeps them plumped-up, healthy, and youthful-looking. Oil and moisture work together; there must be enough moisture in the skin cells, but there must also be enough oil to act as a shield, preventing excessive evaporation of moisture from the skin's top layers. Ichthyosis is one of several inherited skin conditions that cause the skin to lose moisture.

There are actually two types of dry skin: simple dry skin and complex dry skin. Simple dry skin results from a lack of natural oils. This condition most often affects women under the age of thirty-five. Complex dry skin lacks both oil and moisture, and is characterized by fine lines, brown spots, discolorations, enlarged pores, and sagging skin. It is usually associated with aging. The proteins that make up the skin—elastin, collagen, and keratin—may also be damaged by prolonged exposure to sunlight.

Dry skin tends to be dull-looking, even scaly and flaky, and readily develops wrinkles and fine lines. It usually feels "tight" and uncomfortable after washing unless some type of moisturizer or skin cream is applied. Chapping and cracking are signs of extremely dry, dehydrated skin.

Dry skin is most common on areas of the body that are exposed to the elements, such as the face and hands, but it can be a whole-body problem as well, especially in winter. It is probably primarily a genetic condition, but it may be caused (or aggravated) by a poor diet and by environmental factors such as exposure to sun, wind, cold, chemicals, or cosmetics, or excessive bathing with harsh soaps. Nutritional deficiencies, especially deficiencies of vitamin A and the B vitamins, can also contribute to dry skin. Fair-skinned people seem to be more likely than others to have dry skin, especially as they age; most people's skin tends to become thinner and drier as they get older. If all other causes for dry skin such as dermatitis, eczema, psoriasis, or seborrhea have been excluded, then it is most likely that the reason for dry skin lies in a combination of heredity, vitamin deficiencies, and poor nutrition. Many people have skin that is dry in some areas and oily in others. In the classic case of "combination skin," the skin on the forehead, nose, and chin tends to be oily, while the skin on the rest of the face is dry.

NUTRIENTS

SUPPLEMENT	SUGGESTED DOSAGE	COMMENTS
Very Important		
Liquid Kyolic with B$_1$ and B$_{12}$	As directed on label.	An anti-stress, anti-aging formula.
Primrose oil or Kyolic-EPA from Wakunaga	Up to 500 mg daily. As directed on label.	Contains linoleic acid, an essential fatty acid needed by the skin.
Vitamin A with mixed carotenoids or ACES + Zn from Carlson Labs	25,000 IU daily for 3 months, then reduce to 15,000 IU daily. If you are pregnant, do not exceed 10,000 IU daily. As directed on label.	Strengthens and protects the skin tissue. Contains antioxidants that protect the skin by neutralizing free radicals.
Vitamin B complex plus extra vitamin B$_{12}$	As directed on label. 1,000–2,000 mcg daily.	Anti-stress and anti-aging vitamins. Use a sublingual form.
Important		
Kelp	1,000–1,500 mg daily.	Supplies balanced minerals. Needed for good skin tone.
Vitamin E	Start with 400 IU daily and increase slowly to 800 IU daily.	Protects against free radicals. Used topically, it can minimize wrinkling. Use d-alpha-tocopherol form.
Zinc	50 mg daily. Do not exceed a total of 100 mg daily from all supplements.	Necessary for proper functioning of the oil-producing glands of the skin. Use zinc gluconate lozenges or OptiZinc for best absorption.
Helpful		
Ageless Beauty from Biotec Foods	As directed on label.	Protects the skin from free radical damage.
Collagen cream	Apply topically as directed on label.	Good for very dry skin. A nourishing cream that can restore a healthy tone to damaged skin.
Elastin	Apply topically as directed on label.	Helps prevent and smooth wrinkles.

Glucosamine sulfate or N-Acetylglucosamine (N-A-G from Source Naturals)	As directed on label. As directed on label.	Important for healthy skin and connective tissue.
Herpanacine from Diamond-Herpanacine Associates	As directed on label.	Contains antioxidants, amino acids, and herbs that promote skin health.
L-Cysteine	500 mg daily, on an empty stomach. Take with water or juice. Do not take with milk. Take with 50 mg vitamin B_6 and 100 mg vitamin C for better absorption.	Contains sulfur, needed for healthy skin. (See AMINO ACIDS in Part One.)
Lecithin granules or capsules	1 tbsp 3 times daily, before meals. 1,200 mg 3 times daily, before meals.	Needed for better absorption of the essential fatty acids.
Pycnogenol or grape seed extract	As directed on label. As directed on label.	A free radical scavenger that also strengthens collagen.
Selenium	200 mcg daily. If you are pregnant, do not exceed 40 mcg daily.	Encourages tissue elasticity and is a powerful antioxidant. Protects against ultraviolet-induced damage.
Superoxide dismutase (SOD)	As directed on label.	A free radical destroyer. Also good for brown age spots.
Vitamin C with bioflavonoids	3,000–5,000 mg daily, in divided doses.	Necessary for collagen production; strengthens the capillaries that feed the skin.

HERBS

❏ Used topically, aloe vera has excellent soothing, healing, and moisturizing properties. It also helps to slough off dead skin cells. Apply aloe vera gel topically on affected areas as directed on the product label.

❏ Calendula and comfrey have skin-softening properties. They can be used in a facial sauna or to make herbal or floral waters (see below). Comfrey also reduces redness and soothes irritated skin. Allantoin, an ingredient in many skin care products, is derived from comfrey.

Note: Comfrey is recommended for external use only.

❏ Spray an herbal or floral water mist on your skin throughout the day to replenish lost moisture. Almost all skin types, but particularly dry skin, benefit from lavender. You can purchase lavender water already made, or you can make your own by adding a few drops of essential oil to 4 ounces of distilled water, or by making an infusion of fresh lavender leaves and flowers.

❏ A weekly facial sauna using the herbs chamomile, lavender, and peppermint is good for dry skin. Using a glass or enameled pot, simmer a total of 2 to 4 tablespoons of dried or fresh herbs in 2 quarts of water. When the pot is steaming, place it on top of a trivet or thick potholder on a table, and sit with your face at a comfortable distance over the steam for fifteen minutes. You can use a towel to trap

the steam if you wish. After fifteen minutes, splash your face with cold water and allow your skin to air dry or pat it dry with a towel. Then either apply a good natural moisturizer or facial oil, or apply a clay mask (*see under* Recommendations, below). After the sauna, you can allow the herbal water to cool and save it for use as a toning lotion to be dabbed on your face with a cotton ball after cleansing.

RECOMMENDATIONS

❏ Eat a balanced diet that includes vegetables, fruits, grains, seeds, and nuts. Eat quality protein from vegetable sources. Increase your intake of raw foods.

❏ Eat foods high in sulfur, which helps to keep the skin smooth and youthful. Good sources include garlic, onions, eggs, and asparagus. Sulfur is also present in the amino acid L-cysteine, which can be purchased in pill form.

❏ Consume plenty of yellow and orange vegetables. These are high in beta-carotene, a precursor of vitamin A.

❏ Drink at least 2 quarts of quality water every day to keep the skin well hydrated.

❏ Avoid fried foods, animal fats, and heat-processed vegetable oils such as those sold in supermarkets. Use cold-pressed oils only. Beware of any oils that have been subjected to heat, whether in processing or cooking. Heating oils leads to the production of free radicals, which have a destructive effect on the skin. *Do* take supplemental essential fatty acids (*see under* Nutrients, above). This may be the best supplement available for dry skin, but be patient; it may take a month or more to see results.

❏ Do not drink soft drinks or eat sugar, chocolate, potato chips, or other junk foods.

❏ Avoid alcohol and caffeine. These substances have a diuretic effect, causing the body—including the skin cells—to lose fluids and essential minerals.

❏ Twice weekly, use a loofah sponge for the face and warm water to boost circulation and remove dead skin cells. Avoid using the loofah around your eyes, however.

❏ Always moisturize your skin after cleansing, and at other times throughout the day, if necessary, to keep it from drying out. Use a liquid moisturizer or facial oil that contains nutrients and other natural ingredients. Do not use solid, waxy moisturizing creams. Wrinkle Treatment Oil and Vitamin A Moisturizing Gel from Derma-E Products are both good for dry age lines caused by the sun and the skin's natural aging. The Wrinkle Treatment Oil is also good for cleansing the skin. The moisturizing gel is non-oily and fast-absorbing.

❏ Look for skin care products that contain humectants. Humectants are substances that attract water to the skin to hold in moisture. Natural humectants include vegetable glycerine, vitamin E, and panthenol, a form of pantothenic acid (vitamin B_5).

❏ Use a humidifier (or even a pan of water placed near a radiator) to humidify your environment, especially in winter. This helps to reduce the amount of moisture lost from the skin through evaporation.

❏ Once a week, use a facial mask to clarify the skin and remove dull, dry surface skin cells. (This can be done immediately after the facial sauna described under Herbs in this section.) Blend together well 1 teaspoon green clay powder (available in health food stores) and 1 teaspoon raw honey. Apply the mixture to your face, avoiding the eye area. Leave it on for fifteen minutes, then rinse well with lukewarm water. While your skin is still slightly damp, apply a natural skin oil or liquid moisturizer.

❏ If your skin is chapped or cracked, increase your consumption of water and essential fatty acids. Keep any chapped areas well lubricated and protected from the elements.

❏ For cracked, dry skin on the fingers, use calendula cream or oil with comfrey, vitamin E oil, and aloe vera. Apply the mixture to hands at bedtime, then wear plastic gloves overnight. Pure vitamin E oil can be found in health food stores.

❏ Do not smoke, and avoid secondhand smoke. Smoking has a harmful effect on the skin for several reasons. First, nicotine constricts the blood vessels, including the tiny capillaries that serve the skin. This deprives the skin of the oxygen and nutrients it needs for good health. Second, smoking involves the frequent repetition of certain facial postures, which eventually become etched in the skin in the form of wrinkles. The characteristic "smoker's face" has wrinkles radiating in a circle outward from the mouth. Smoking also can make the skin dry and leathery.

❏ Do not use harsh soaps, cold cream, or cleansing creams on your skin. Cleansing creams are made from hydrogenated oils, which can cause free radical damage to the skin, resulting in dryness and wrinkles. Instead, use pure olive, avocado, or almond oil to cleanse the skin. Pat the oil on, then wash it off with warm water and a soft cloth.

❏ Do not use very hot water when bathing or showering.

❏ As much as possible, stay out of the sun. The sun is responsible for most of the damage done to the skin. It causes dryness, wrinkles, and even rashes and blisters. Always apply a good sunscreen to all exposed areas of skin if you must be in the sun.

❏ To care for combination skin, simply treat the dry areas as dry skin and the oily areas as oily skin. *See* OILY SKIN in Part Two.

CONSIDERATIONS

❏ Dry skin can be a sign of an underactive thyroid. (*See* HYPOTHYROIDISM in Part Two.)

❏ Serious skin complications can arise for people with diabetes. (*See* DIABETES in Part Two.)

❏ Certain drugs, including diuretics, antispasmodics, and antihistamines, can contribute to dry skin.

❏ Balanced skin depends upon the production of natural moisturizing factors that help the skin attract and retain moisture. A group of acids known as alpha-hydroxy acids, applied topically, help to stimulate production of these naturally occurring substances. Alpha-hydroxy acids also encourage the formation of new skin cells. These acids occur naturally in apples, milk, sugar cane, citrus fruits, tomatoes, grapes, and blackberries. Of the alpha-hydroxy acids, lactic acid appears to be the best for improving moisturization, while glycolic acid is more effective at sloughing off dead skin cells and promoting cell renewal.

❏ Cocoa butter is a good skin cream and is not expensive. It also helps reduce skin wrinkling. Keep it in the refrigerator after opening.

❏ A deficiency of vitamin A can result in scaly skin, particularly on the hands and feet. Cod liver oil is a good source of vitamins A and D.

❏ GH3 cream from Gero Vita International, applied topically, is good for the prevention of wrinkles and can help with discoloration of the skin.

❏ Kinetin, a manufactured version of a plant hormone that prevents plants from withering, is proving effective in the treatment of fine facial lines.

❏ Hyper-C Serum from Jason Natural Cosmetics boosts collagen production and moisturizes and protects the skin.

❏ Pycnogenol Crème (or Gel) with Vitamins E, C, & A from Derma-E Products is good for moisturizing, softening, and protecting the skin. Derma-E makes Vitamin E Moisturizing Gel, a refreshing skin treatment, and Vitamin A Wrinkle Treatment for dry and aging skin.

❏ Tretinoin (Retin-A), applied topically, removes fine wrinkles and is also excellent for age spots, precancerous lesions, and sun-damaged skin. It is available by prescription only, and takes around six months to show results.

Dyspepsia

See INDIGESTION.

Dysthymia

See under DEPRESSION.

Ear Infection

It has been estimated that 75 percent of all children suffer from some type of ear infection by the age of three. *External otitis*, also known as swimmer's ear, affects the outer ear. It may be preceded by an upper respiratory infection or an allergic reaction to some foods, most commonly dairy products. The ear canal, extending from the eardrum to the outside, becomes inflamed and swollen. Symptoms can include slight fever, discharge from the ear, and pain, often severe and throbbing, that worsens when the earlobe is touched or pulled.

Middle ear infections (*otitis media*) are very common in infants and children. The site of this infection is behind the eardrum, where the small bones of the ear are located. Air pressure is regulated in this area by the eustachian or auditory tube, which runs from the ear to the back of the nasal cavity. If bacteria or viruses get into this space, the area becomes inflamed and fluid starts to build up, causing the sensation of pressure. Other symptoms include earache; sharp, dull, or throbbing pain; a feeling of fullness in the ear; and a fever as high as 103°F or higher. Children often pull at their ears in an attempt to relieve the pressure. High altitudes and cold temperatures increase discomfort and can worsen an infection.

A severe middle ear infection can cause perforation of the eardrum. If this happens, it can actually cause a sudden *reduction* in pain. This is because the pain of an ear infection results when pressure builds up in restricted spaces; this pressure on sensitive nerve endings causes pain. A perforated eardrum results in hearing loss and a discharge of bloody fluid from the ear.

Recurring ear infections are generally an indication that an original infection has been resistant to the prescribed treatment. In babies, earache is often associated with teething. Living in a household where someone smokes can be a contributing factor to ear problems in children.

Unless otherwise specified, the dosages recommended here are for adults. For a child between the ages of twelve and seventeen, reduce the dose to three-quarters the recommended amount. For a child between six and twelve, use one-half the recommended dose, and for a child under the age of six, use one-quarter the recommended amount.

NUTRIENTS

SUPPLEMENT	SUGGESTED DOSAGE	COMMENTS
Very Important		
AE Mulsion Forte from American Biologics	As directed on label.	For adults. Aids in controlling the infection.
or		
carotenoid complex	20,000 IU daily.	
or		
cod liver oil	1 tsp daily.	For children. A good source of vitamin A.
Colloidal silver	As directed on label.	A natural antibiotic. Can be taken orally or used as an earwash.
Manganese	10 mg daily. Take separately from calcium.	Deficiency has been linked to ear disorders.
Vitamin C with bioflavonoids	3,000–7,000 mg daily, in divided doses.	Boosts immunity and fights infection. Use an esterified or buffered form such as Ester-C or calcium or zinc ascorbate.
Zinc	10 mg in lozenge form 3 times daily for 5 days, then 50 mg daily in pill form. Do not exceed this amount.	Quickens immune response. Aids in reducing infection.
Important		
Dioxychlor from American Biologics	Add 3 drops to 10 drops distilled water to use as an earwash.	Important as an antibacterial, antifungal, and antiviral agent.
Primrose oil	1,000 mg daily for adults and children over 6; 500 mg daily for children under 6.	To reduce infection and inflammation.
or		
Kyolic-EPA from Wakunaga	As directed on label.	
Vitamin B complex	50 mg of each major B vitamin 3 times daily (amounts of individual vitamins in a complex will vary).	Essential for healing and immune function. A sublingual form is recommended.
plus extra vitamin B₆ (pyridoxine)	50 mg daily.	Important for immune function.
Vitamin E	Start with 200 IU daily and increase weekly until you reach 800 IU daily.	Enhances immune function. Use d-alpha-tocopherol form.
Helpful		
ThymuPlex #398 from Enzymatic Therapy	As directed on label.	Use if problem persists. Helps the immune system.

HERBS

❑ Take alcohol-free echinacea extract by mouth; this will generally end an ear infection if you catch it early.

❑ To alleviate pain, place a few drops of warm garlic oil or olive oil in the ear, then a drop or two of lobelia or mullein oil. You can plug the ear loosely with a cotton ball. You can also make a paste using onion powder or clay (from a health food store) and warm water, and apply the paste to the outside of the ear to relieve pain.

❑ Eardrops containing garlic, mullein, and St. John's wort are available at drug and health food stores

❑ Olive leaf extract helps the body fight infection.

❑ Place ½ dropperful of alcohol-free goldenseal extract in your mouth and swish it around for a few minutes before swallowing. Do this every three hours for three days. Alternating echinacea with goldenseal works wonders. For an infant, put the extract in formula or expressed breast milk, or in fruit-flavored sugar-free yogurt.

Caution: Do not take goldenseal on a daily basis for more

than one week at a time, and do not use it during pregnancy. If you have a history of cardiovascular disease, diabetes, or glaucoma, use it only under a doctor's supervision.

❑ Onion poultices are good for ear infections. (*See* USING A POULTICE in Part Three.)

RECOMMENDATIONS

❑ Avoid the most common allergenic foods: wheat, dairy products, corn, oranges, peanut butter, and all simple carbohydrates, including sugar, fruits, and fruit juices.

❑ To help reduce and prevent the development of food allergies, do not repeat foods frequently. A four-day rotation diet may be beneficial (*see* ALLERGIES in Part Two). With a young child, introduce new foods one at a time and watch carefully for any reaction.

❑ If a bottlefed baby has an ear infection, try eliminating milk and dairy products from the child's diet for thirty days to see if any benefits result. Try giving your baby soymilk, Rice Dream, or nut milk instead of cow's milk.

❑ Take garlic enemas if toxins accumulate to dangerous levels and cause the body to react. Signs of dangerous toxin levels include fever, chills, and general aches and pains. *See* ENEMAS in Part Three.

❑ Apply hot and cold compresses to the scalp just behind the ear.

❑ For ringing in the ears, mix 1 teaspoonful of salt and 1 teaspoonful of glycerine (sold in drugstores) in 1 pint of warm water. Use a nasal spray bottle to spray each nostril with the solution until it begins to drain into the back of the throat. Spray the throat with the mixture as well. Do this several times a day.

❑ If you suffer from a chronic cough that lasts more than three weeks, see your health care provider. A chronic cough can be caused by impacted earwax that exerts pressure on a nerve in the ear canal, stimulating the coughing reflex. A physician can easily see if you have excessive earwax buildup and can remove it using careful suction or warm water with a slender blunt curette, plus a special microscope to aid in guiding the removal.

❑ Otoscopes (for examining the inside of the ear) are available for home use. Your physician can show you how to use it. If you have a child who suffers from repeated ear infections, you may wish to look into a device called the EarCheck otitis media detector, manufactured by Safe Home Products (*see* MANUFACTURER AND DISTRIBUTER INFORMATION in the Appendix). This instrument detects the presence of a collection of fluid in the middle ear, a sign of middle ear infection, within five seconds.

❑ Earache Tablets from Hyland's is a homeopathic combination remedy containing *Belladonna, Calcarea carbonica, Chamomilla, Lycopodium, Pulsatilla,* and *Sulfur* that appears to work well in reducing pain and fever.

❑ Do not blow your nose if you have an ear infection. Keep the ear canal dry. Retained soap and water in the canal can be dangerous. Put cotton in the ear canal when showering or bathing. Do not go swimming until healing is complete.

❑ Avoid unsanitary conditions. An ear infection may result from lowered resistance due to a recent illness. Nonprescription ear drops may relieve the pain. A nasal spray may help open up the eustachian tube and relieve the pressure.

❑ If there are symptoms of dizziness, ringing in the ears, bleeding or a bloody discharge, sudden pain (or a sudden lessening of pain), and hearing loss in one or both ears, contact your health care provider immediately. These symptoms could indicate a ruptured eardrum.

CONSIDERATIONS

❑ Antibiotic therapy and/or surgical draining of the affected area may be necessary to heal an ear infection. However, some studies have shown that there is no significant overall difference in healing time or recurrence of ear infections between children treated with antibiotics and those not given antibiotics. In addition, many infants may also have reactions to the antibiotics used to treat ear infections, especially if they are used too frequently.

❑ In most cases, with proper treatment, a perforated eardrum heals naturally, with no permanent loss of hearing. An eardrum may rupture as a result of infection or due to sudden inward pressure to the ear from swimming, diving, a slap, a nearby explosion, or even a kiss over the ear.

❑ Breastfed babies are much less likely than bottlefed babies to suffer from ear infections.

❑ Ear problems are more common in the homes of smokers.

❑ *Branhamella catarrahalis* (B-cat), a common cause of ear infections, has developed strains that resist standard antibiotics. Fortunately, the antibiotic Augmentin (a combination of amoxicillin and clavulanate) can still destroy the B-cat bacterium.

❑ Ear infection is not the only cause of ear pain. Rapid changes in air pressure, such as occur during air travel, often cause ear pain and can even result in damage to the eardrum. This is called *aerotitis* or *barotitis media*. If an infection is present, the effects of pressure changes are magnified.

❑ Children who have frequent ear infections should be tested for food allergies. The role of allergies as a major cause of chronic otitis media has been firmly established. (*See* ALLERGIES in Part Two.)

Eating Disorders

See ANOREXIA NERVOSA; APPETITE, POOR; BULIMIA; OBESITY; UNDERWEIGHT.

Eczema

See DERMATITIS.

Edema

Edema is the accumulation of fluid in spaces between the cells in the soft tissue of the body. Any part of the body may develop edema. The swelling can be localized in the face, arms, and neck, or may involve the legs and ankles—a condition known as *dependent edema*. *Periorbital edema* is swelling around the eyes. *Corneal stroma* is edema of the cornea. Generalized edema is known as *anasarca*. *Preeclampsia* is a condition that occurs in approximately 5 percent of pregnant women, causing high blood pressure, fluid accumulation in the tissues, and albuminuria (protein in the urine).

The underlying causes of edema may be serious. Edema can indicate a much more profound illness, such as AIDS, cirrhosis of the liver, congestive heart failure, diabetes, or vena cava syndrome (narrowing of the vein that supplies blood from the upper body to the heart). More simply, edema can occur as the result of infection or prolonged bed rest. Fluid retention can also be caused by allergies.

NUTRIENTS

SUPPLEMENT	SUGGESTED DOSAGE	COMMENTS
Very Important		
Free-form amino acid complex (Amino Balance from Anabol Naturals)	As directed on label.	Sometimes edema is caused by inadequate protein assimilation. Protein deficiency has been linked to water retention.
Vitamin B complex	50–100 mg of each major B vitamin twice daily, with meals (amounts of individual vitamins in a complex will vary).	B vitamins work best when taken together.
plus extra vitamin B$_6$ (pyridoxine)	50 mg 3 times daily.	Reduces water retention.
Important		
Alfalfa		*See under* Herbs, below.
Calcium and magnesium	1,500 mg daily. 1,000 mg daily.	To replace minerals lost with correction of edema.
Silica	As directed on label.	A natural diuretic.

Helpful		
Bromelain	As directed on label, 3 times daily.	An enzyme derived from pineapples that helps digestion and allergies.
Garlic (Kyolic from Wakunaga)	2 capsules 3 times daily, with meals.	A detoxifier.
Kelp	1,000–1,500 mg daily.	Supplies needed minerals.
Kidney-Liver Complex #406 from Enzymatic Therapy	As directed on label.	Improves kidney function.
Potassium	99 mg daily.	Very important if taking diuretics. Helps to keep fluids on the inside of the cells.
Pycnogenol	As directed on label.	A powerful antioxidant that also strengthens the tissues of the circulatory system.
Superoxide dismutase (SOD)	As directed on label.	Helpful in heart and liver disorders.
Taurine	As directed on label.	Aids heart function.
Vitamin C with bioflavonoids	3,000–5,000 mg daily, in divided doses.	Essential for adrenal function and production of adrenal hormones, which are vital for proper fluid balance and control of edema.
Vitamin E	400 IU and up daily.	Aids circulation. Use d-alpha-tocopherol form.

HERBS

❑ Alfalfa is a good source of important minerals. It also contains chlorophyll, a potent detoxifier. Take 2,000 to 3,000 milligrams daily, in divided doses.

❑ Hawthorn berries, horsetail, juniper, and uva ursi are diuretics. By increasing the output of urine, they help to counteract edema.

❑ Horse chestnut has been shown to reduce post-surgical edema.

❑ Rose hips contain bioflavonoids helpful in the treatment of edema.

❑ SP-6 Cornsilk Blend from Solaray contains corn silk and other herbs that aid the body in expelling excess fluids. Take 2 capsules three times daily.

❑ Other herbs that can be beneficial if you are suffering from edema include butcher's broom, dandelion root, horsetail, juniper berries, lobelia, marshmallow, parsley, and pau d'arco tea.

Caution: Do not take lobelia internally on an ongoing basis.

RECOMMENDATIONS

❑ Eat a diet that is high in fiber.

❑ For protein, eat eggs, broiled white fish, and broiled skinless chicken or turkey. Consume small amounts of buttermilk, cottage cheese, kefir, and low-fat yogurt.

❑ Use kelp to supply needed minerals.

❏ Avoid alcohol, animal protein, beef, caffeine, chocolate, dairy products (except for those listed above), dried shellfish, fried foods, gravies, olives, pickles, salt, soy sauce, tobacco, white flour, and white sugar.

❏ If you have swelling of the legs and feet, sit with your feet up as often as you can. Wear support hose for swelling in the legs.

❏ Exercise daily and take hot baths or saunas twice a week.

❏ Avoid stress.

❏ *See* FASTING in Part Three and follow the program. Fasting flushes excess water from the tissues.

❏ If pressing with the fingers on your feet and ankles results in the formation of small "pits," consult your physician. This can be a sign of a serious health problem.

CONSIDERATIONS

❏ According to traditional Chinese medicine, avoiding raw foods, cold drinks, and fatty foods will help with water retention.

❏ Food allergy testing is recommended. (*See* ALLERGIES in Part Two.)

❏ *See also under* PREGNANCY-RELATED PROBLEMS in Part Two.

Emphysema

Emphysema is a degenerative lung disease that usually develops after many years of exposure to cigarette smoke or other toxins that pollute the air. It is one of a group of lung diseases referred to as *chronic obstructive pulmonary disease* (COPD). COPDs, which also include asthma and chronic bronchitis, can interfere with normal breathing. The predominant symptom of emphysema is shortness of breath and the feeling of not being able to get enough air during any kind of physical exertion.

In people with emphysema, damage to the alveoli (small air sacs in the lungs) causes the lungs to lose their elasticity. As a result, exhaling becomes difficult, and stale air remains trapped in the lungs, preventing the needed exchange of oxygen and carbon dioxide. A person with advanced emphysema may experience a near-constant state of breathlessness, chronic coughing and wheezing, and frequent discharge of sputum from the respiratory passages. Emphysema can also contribute to other health problems, such as lung infections and a condition called erythrocytosis, in which the blood contains abnormally high levels of red blood cells. Erythrocytosis can cause such symptoms as weakness, dizziness, fatigue, lightheadedness, headache, and vision problems.

Most people who are diagnosed with emphysema are long-term smokers. Symptoms may not occur until middle age, when the individual's ability to exercise or do heavy work begins to decline, and a productive cough begins. The symptoms may be subtle at first, but worsen with time.

In rare cases, emphysema is caused by a genetic condition that leads to a deficiency of a blood protein called alpha-1-antitrypsin. The overwhelming majority of cases, however, are related to smoking. Regular smoking, whether of tobacco or marijuana, causes chronic low-level inflammation of the lungs, which increases the chance of developing this progressive disease.

The American Lung Association estimates that 16 million Americans suffer from some form of COPD. COPD is the fourth leading cause of death in the United States, behind heart ailments, cancers, and stroke.

NUTRIENTS

SUPPLEMENT	SUGGESTED DOSAGE	COMMENTS
Essential		
Chlorophyll (Kyo-Green from Wakunaga is a good source)	As directed on label 3 times daily.	Aids in clear breathing.
Dimethylglycine (DMG) (Aangamik DMG from FoodScience of Vermont)	250 mg 3 times daily.	Increases endurance and provides oxygen to cells. Use a sublingual form.
Essential fatty acids (Kyolic-EPA from Wakunaga, salmon oil, flaxseed oil, and primrose oil are good sources)	As directed on label. Take with meals.	Essential for rebuilding and producing new cells.
Zinc plus copper	80 mg daily. Do not exceed a total of 100 mg daily from all supplements. 3 mg daily.	Works as an antioxidant with specific protective effects on lung proteins. Needed to balance with zinc.
Very Important		
Coenzyme Q10 plus Coenzyme A from Coenzyme-A Technologies	60 mg daily. As directed on label.	A powerful antioxidant; enhances oxygen in the lungs. Aids in removing toxins from the body.
Free-form amino acid complex	As directed on label.	Important for repair of lung tissue.
Garlic (Kyolic from Wakunaga)	2 capsules 3 times daily, with meals.	An immunity enhancer for protection against pneumonia.
L-Cysteine and L-glutathione and L-methionine	500 mg each twice daily, on an empty stomach. Take with water or juice. Do not take with milk. Take with 50 mg vitamin B6 and 100 mg vitamin C for better absorption.	To aid in repairing damaged lung tissue and act as antioxidants protecting lung tissue. (*See* AMINO ACIDS in Part One.)
Lung Complex #407 from Enzymatic Therapy	As directed on label.	*See* GLANDULAR THERAPY in Part Three for its benefits.
Lung Support Formula from Gero Vita	As directed on label.	Promotes healing and improved breathing.

Pycnogenol or grape seed extract	30 mg 3 times daily. As directed on label.	Powerful antioxidants that help protect the lungs.
Vitamin A plus carotenoid complex	25,000 IU daily. If you are pregnant, do not exceed 10,000 IU daily. As directed on label.	Needed for repair of lung tissues and for the immune system. Emulsion form is recommended for easier assimilation and greater safety at higher doses. Powerful antioxidants that protect against excess levels of free radicals.
Vitamin C with bioflavonoids	5,000–10,000 mg daily, in divided doses.	Strengthens immune response and aids healing of inflamed tissue.
Vitamin E emulsion or capsules	1,000 IU daily. Start with 400 IU daily and increase slowly to 1,600 IU daily. If you have heart problems, start with 200 IU daily and increase slowly to 800 IU daily.	An oxygen carrier and potent antioxidant. A deficiency can lead to destruction of cell membranes. Emulsion form is recommended for easier assimilation and greater safety at higher doses.
Helpful		
Aerobic 07 from Aerobic Life Industries	9 drops in water once daily.	Supplies oxygen and kills bacteria.
Beta-1,3-D-glucan	As directed on label.	Promotes healing and works as a highly effective free radical scavenger.
Calcium and magnesium	2,000 mg daily, at bedtime. 500–1,000 mg daily, at bedtime.	Act as a nerve tonic, protect nerve endings, and promote sound sleep. Use chelate forms.
Kelp	1,000–1,5000 mg daily.	Contains minerals needed for improved breathing and healing.
Multienzyme complex with pancreatin plus proteolytic enzymes or Inflazyme Forte from American Biologics or Oxy-5000 Forte from American Biologics	As directed on label. Take with meals. As directed on label. Take with meals. As directed on label. As directed on label.	To keep infection in check by cleansing the lungs. A balance of potent enzymes and cofactors as a powerful inflammatory inhibitor. A potent nutritional antioxidant for health and stress that destroys free radicals.

HERBS

❏ Astragalus, a Chinese herb also known as huang qi, accelerates healing in the bronchial tubes and promotes better breathing.

❏ ClearLungs from RidgeCrest Herbals is an herbal combination that helps provide relief from shortness of breath, tightness in the chest, and wheezing due to bronchial congestion. It is available in two formulas, with ephedra and without. Both have been found to be equally effective.

❏ Cordyceps may slow the progress of lung degeneration. Chinese medicine teaches that there is a synergistic connection between the kidneys and the lungs. Cordyceps

reinforces this connection, opens up the bronchioles, and produces greater oxygenization for the kidneys. Cordyceps from R-Garden Internationale is a good source of this herb.

❏ Ephedra (ma huang) is beneficial for respiratory disorders. Thyme is also very helpful.

Caution: Do not use ephedra if you suffer from anxiety, glaucoma, heart disease, high blood pressure, or insomnia, or if you are taking a monoamine oxidase (MAO) inhibitor drug for depression.

❏ Licorice extract increases energy levels and helps to improve organ function. Use an alcohol-free extract or Bio-Rizin from American Biologics.

Caution: If overused, licorice can elevate blood pressure. Do not use this herb on a daily basis for more than seven days in a row. Avoid it completely if you have high blood pressure.

❏ Other beneficial herbs for emphysema include alfalfa, fenugreek, fresh horseradish, mullein tea, and rosemary.

RECOMMENDATIONS

❏ Avoid any and all contact with tobacco. Tobacco smoke is the single most dangerous thing anyone suffering from emphysema can encounter. If you have emphysema and smoke, you must quit. Avoid areas where people smoke. Do not allow smoking in your home, your car, or anywhere near you.

❏ Eat a diet consisting of 50 percent raw foods. The other 50 percent should consist of soups, skinless chicken or turkey, fish, brown rice, millet, and whole grain cereals.

❏ Consume onions and garlic daily.

❏ Do not eat a typical American breakfast. Instead, sip hot, clear liquids (such as herbal teas) in the morning to help clear the mucus from the airways. Drink at least eight glasses of quality water daily. Using a psyllium-based fiber product or Aerobic Bulk Cleanse (ABC) from Aerobic Life Industries (a colon cleanser available in health food stores) is helpful after consuming the liquids. Mix ABC with a glass of juice and drink it quickly. This will help rid the colon of excess mucus and reduce gas and distention.

❏ Avoid fried and greasy foods, salt, and all foods that cause excess mucus to be formed in the gastrointestinal tract, lungs, sinuses, and nasal cavity. Foods that lead to the formation of mucus include meats, eggs, all dairy products and cheese, processed foods, tobacco, junk foods, and white flour products. Read labels carefully; these are sometimes "hidden" ingredients in food products.

❏ Avoid gas-forming foods such as legumes and cabbage. These foods cause abdominal distention that can interfere with breathing. Try using a product called Beano when you do eat foods that can cause gas. Place a few drops of the liquid on the first bite of food for best results.

❏ Avoid foods that require a great deal of chewing, such as meats and nuts. Chronic lung disease can make it difficult to breathe while chewing. If necessary, vegetables can be steamed to make them easier to eat.

❑ Get regular exercise. Daily exercise, especially walking, can be extremely beneficial for people with emphysema. It increases endurance, improves circulation, and generally leads to a reduced level of breathlessness. Start out with what you are able to do, even if it is only a minute or two of exercise every hour, then gradually increase the amount as you are able. Any exercise program should be started at a very low intensity and be gradually increased over time. Yoga or martial arts exercise, such as tai chi, may also be helpful.

❑ Humidify your home, especially if you experience a lot of congestion or have heavy discharges of sputum.

❑ Go on a cleansing fast periodically, using carrot, celery, spinach, kale, and all dark green fresh juices. *See* FASTING in Part Three.

❑ Use warm castor oil packs on the chest and back to help reduce mucus and enhance breathing. To make a castor oil pack, place a cup or so of castor oil in a pan and warm but do not boil it. Dip a piece of cheesecloth or other white cotton material into the oil until the cloth is saturated. Apply the cloth to the affected area and cover it with a piece of plastic that is larger in size than the cotton cloth, then place a warm cloth or a hot water bottle on top. Keep the pack in place for one-half to two hours, as needed.

❑ Rest and avoid stress. Get plenty of fresh air.

❑ Leave the house during major housecleaning and other major household projects, and remain away for at least two hours afterward. Housecleaning stirs up dust and mold.

❑ Do daily breathing exercises, which can improve lung function. A technique known as deep breathing involves inhaling through the nose while pulling the abdominal muscles inward in order to allow more air to be inhaled. Exhaling takes place steadily and slowly through the mouth while the tongue is pressed between the roof of the mouth and top of the teeth, so that slight pressure is felt through the windpipe and chest. A hissing sound is produced as the air is expelled through the lips. Exhaling should take at least twice as long as inhaling, so that all air is forced out. Do this for about ten minutes, two to three times daily. This will aid in an exchange of air in the lungs and improve breathing capacity.

❑ Because every extra chemical adds potential risk to the lungs, use only essential (and unscented) laundry products. Avoid perfume and anything containing fragrance. Avoid gas stoves as well; electric stoves are better for people with respiratory disorders. Choose flooring made from hardwood, ceramic tile, or stone rather than carpeting, which holds dust, mold, and many chemicals that get into the air and that can irritate the lungs. Avoid using window curtains and draperies, which also can harbor dust. Decorate with paint (new "odorless" formulas are now available) rather than wallpaper; the glues used to make the paper ad-

here to the wall can have volatile chemicals that may bother some people. Avoid plastic chairs, plastic dishes, and other plastic items in furnishing your home. Do not use aerosol products.

❑ Avoid air pollution. If your current working environment is dirty, dusty, or toxic to inhale, change jobs.

❑ Avoid hot, humid climates. If you must live in such a climate, continuous central air conditioning is essential. An air-conditioned car is also essential. Do not allow anyone to smoke or wear perfume in your car.

❑ Avoid letting furry or feathered animals into your home or car, as their hair and dander can irritate the lungs.

CONSIDERATIONS

❑ There is no known cure for emphysema, but the measures outlined in this section should slow the progression of the disease, ease discomfort, and make breathing a bit easier.

❑ Lung reduction surgery can be very effective in enhancing breathing function. This procedure involves making cuts in the damaged portions of the lungs and using a special stapling device that gives the healthy lung tissue more room to expand. In a similar procedure, surgeons section off the damaged lung tissue and buttress the folds using bovine pericardium (cow muscle) to enhance the viability of the tissue. Candidates for either type of surgery are carefully screened before being considered for treatment.

❑ In some cases, a lung transplant may be considered. This is a highly invasive, complex procedure that carries substantial risk. It is a viable option for only a small proportion of people with emphysema.

❑ Supplemental oxygen can benefit anyone with impaired lung function. Long-term oxygen therapy combats erythrocytosis and lowers the risk of heart failure.

❑ Older adults are at risk for magnesium deficiency, which can further compromise the ability to breathe. Taking magnesium supplements (500 to 1,000 milligrams daily) can significantly strengthen the muscles that power breathing and promote better oxygenation of the body's cells.

❑ The Air Supply personal air purifier from Wein Products is a miniature unit that is worn around the neck. It sets up an invisible pure air shield against microorganisms (such as viruses, bacteria, and mold) and micro-particles (including dust, pollen, and pollutants). It also eliminates vapors, smells, and harmful volatile compounds in the air. The Living Air XL-15 unit from Alpine Industries is an ionizing unit that purifies the air in the home or workplace.

❑ The University of Pennsylvania Hospital Department of Allergy reports that having an air conditioner and an electrostatic air cleaning machine in the bedroom of persons with respiratory disease is a major factor in the health of individuals with breathing trouble.

❑ A routine lung function test can determine lung capacity and other characteristics that can help identify various stages of emphysema. Several kinds of test are available:

- Arterial blood gas (ABG). An ABG is a blood test that measures amounts of carbon dioxide and oxygen in the blood. This test is used to assess more advanced stages of emphysema.

- Pulse oximetry. This test measures the amount of oxygen in the blood using a special light that is clipped onto a finger or earlobe.

- Spirometry. In this test, you take a deep breath and blow it out as quickly as possible through a tube that is connected to a machine that records airflow and capacity.

- X-ray. A plain chest x-ray and computerized axial tomography (CAT scan) can help diagnose moderate to severe cases of emphysema.

☐ *See also* ASCORBIC ACID FLUSH in Part Three and ENVIRONMENTAL TOXICITY in Part Two.

Endometriosis

Endometriosis is the abnormal growth of cells that form in the lining of the uterus. Some of these cells may, instead of being expelled from the body during the menstrual process, actually end up continuing their cycle elsewhere in the body. They then have no way of leaving the body, so the material builds up and may attach itself to other organs in the lower abdomen, such as the ovaries or bowel. This can produce a host of different symptoms, including in capacitating pain in the uterus, lower back, and organs in the pelvic cavity prior to and during the menses; intermittent pain throughout the menstrual cycle; painful intercourse; excessive bleeding, including the passing of large clots and shreds of tissue during the menses; nausea, vomiting, and constipation during the menses; dyschezia (difficulty in passing stools due to weak pelvic muscles and anal sphincter); dysuria (pain while urinating); and, sometimes, infertility. Because menstruation is typically heavy, iron-deficiency anemia is common. Women whose cycles are shorter than twenty-seven days and/or whose periods last longer than one week are at increased risk of anemia.

Growths of endometrial tissue outside of the uterine cavity occur most often in or on the ovaries, the fallopian tubes, the urinary bladder, the bowel, the pelvic floor, and/or the peritoneum (the membrane that lines the walls of the abdominal cavity), and within the uterine musculature. The most common site of endometriosis is believed to be the deep pelvic peritoneal cavity, or the cul-de-sac. The presence of endometrial implants outside the pelvic area is uncommon.

During the normal menstrual cycle, a continually changing hormonal environment stimulates the endometrium to grow in preparation for a possible pregnancy. This same cycle causes a follicle within one of the ovaries to ripen, and an egg is released. Fingerlike tissues on the fallopian tube grasp the egg, and the tiny, hairlike cilia inside the tube transport it toward the uterus, the lining of which is now spongy and well supplied with blood. If the egg is not fertilized within twenty-four hours or so of being released, the uterine lining proceeds to "die," to be sloughed off, and to pass through the vagina during the menses.

Though not inside the uterus, the abnormal implants of endometriosis also respond to the hormonal changes controlling menstruation. Like the uterine lining, these fragments build tissue each month, then break down and bleed. Unlike blood from the uterine lining, however, blood from the implants has no way to leave the body. Instead, it must be absorbed by surrounding tissue, which is a comparatively slow process. In the meantime, the blood accumulates in body cavities. The entire sequence, from bleeding through absorption, can be painful.

As the menstrual cycle recurs month after month, the implants may get bigger. They may seed new implants and form localized scar tissue and adhesions-scar tissue that attaches to pelvic organs and binds them together. This contributes to the pain of endometriosis, and it can cause extreme pain in a subsequent pregnancy, as the uterus enlarges and the organs within the abdomen are pushed into different positions. Sometimes a collection of blood called a sac or cyst forms. Endometrial or "chocolate" cysts are common on the ovaries. These are usually found to contain moderate amounts of oxidized blood, which looks something like chocolate syrup. If a cyst ruptures, it can cause excruciating pain.

No one knows what causes endometriosis, but several theories have been proposed. The *reflux menstruation theory* was developed by John Sampson, M.D., in 1920. According to this theory, menstrual fluid backs up into the fallopian tubes and drops into the peritoneal cavity, where endometrial cells implant themselves and grow. While this theory offers a possible answer to the question of what causes endometriosis, it has never been proved. Another popular theory states that endometriosis is caused when endometrial cells spread to other parts of the body through blood and lymphatic channels. Still another theory postulates that endometriosis is in effect a congenital condition (*see* An Alternative Theory and Treatment for Endometriosis on page 348).

Despite disagreement over the cause, more is known today about this condition than ever before. For example, research has shown that exposure to environmental polychlorinated biphenyls (PCBs) and dioxin, two types of hazardous waste materials, can cause spontaneous endometriosis. This may account for the rising incidence in the condition over the last few decades. Most women who suffer from endometriosis have never been pregnant, and as many as 30 to 40 percent of women who report infertility problems actually have endometriosis. According to the

Endometriosis Association, women who develop this condition have a history of more vaginal yeast infections, hay fever, eczema, and food sensitivities than most women. In addition, vulnerability to endometriosis appears to run in families. According to the *Journal of the American Medical Association,* an estimated 5 to 7 million American women, many of them young, suffer from endometriosis. Unfortunately, many women fail to seek medical help because they mistake the symptoms of this disease for normal menstrual discomfort.

Laparoscopy is the procedure most commonly used to diagnose endometriosis. This involves the insertion of a tiny lighted optical tube (a laparoscope or a smaller version, the microlaparoscope) through a small incision in the navel. The surgeon can then see inside the abdominal cavity. Laparoscopic procedures are usually done on an outpatient basis.

The nutrient program and other recommendations outlined below may help to keep endometriosis under control if it is diagnosed in the early stages.

NUTRIENTS

SUPPLEMENT	SUGGESTED DOSAGE	COMMENTS
Very Important		
Vitamin E	Start with 400 IU daily and increase slowly to 1,000 IU daily.	Aids hormonal balance. Use d-alpha-tocopherol form.
Vitamin K or alfalfa	200 mcg daily.	Needed for normal blood clotting. *See under* Herbs, below.
Important		
Essential fatty acids (primrose oil and Kyolic-EPA from Wakunaga are good sources)	1,500 mg daily.	Provides essential fatty acids such as gamma-linolenic acid (GLA) that aid in regulating hormonal and prostaglandin balance.
Iron	As directed by physician.	Iron-deficiency anemia is common in those with this disorder. Use ferrous fumarate form. *Caution:* Do not take iron unless anemia is diagnosed.
or Floradix Iron + Herbs from Salus Haus	As directed on label.	An easily assimilated and nontoxic source of iron.
Vitamin B complex plus extra pantothenic acid (vitamin B_5) and vitamin B_6 (pyridoxine)	As directed on label. 50 mg 3 times daily. 25 mg 3 times daily.	Promotes blood cell productivity and proper hormone balance. Relieves stress. Needed for proper adrenal function. Aids the body in removing excess fluids.
Vitamin C with bioflavonoids	2,000 mg 3 times daily.	Important in the healing process. Use a buffered form.
Zinc	50 mg daily. Do not exceed a total of 100 mg daily from all supplements.	For tissue repair and immune function. Use zinc gluconate lozenges or OptiZinc for best absorption.

Helpful		
Beta-1,3-D-glucan	As directed on label.	Stimulates the activity of macrophages, which can remove foreign cellular debris.
Calcium and magnesium	1,500 mg daily. 1,000 mg daily, at bedtime.	To supply needed minerals. Use chelate forms.
Kelp	1,000–1,500 mg daily.	To supply needed iron and other minerals.
Multivitamin and mineral complex	As directed on label.	All nutrients are required for repair and healing.

HERBS

❏ Alfalfa is a good source of vitamin K (necessary for blood clotting and healing) and needed minerals, including iron. Many women with endometriosis are iron-deficient.

❏ Astragalus, garlic, goldenseal, myrrh gum, pau d'arco, and red clover have antibiotic and antitumor properties.

❏ Burdock root, dong quai, and red raspberry leaf help to balance hormones.

❏ Nettle is rich in iron.

RECOMMENDATIONS

❏ Eat a diet consisting of 50 percent raw vegetables and fruits and including soy foods. In addition, eat only whole-grain products (no refined flour products) and raw nuts and seeds. A diet rich in soy and fiber is very important in managing endometriosis.

❏ Include "green drinks" made from dark green leafy vegetables in your diet.

❏ Avoid alcohol, caffeine, animal fats, butter, dairy products, fried foods, foods that contain additives, all hardened fats, junk foods or fast foods, red meats, poultry (except organically raised and skinless), refined and processed foods, salt, shellfish, and sugar.

❏ Fast for three days each month before the anticipated beginning of the menstrual period. Use steam-distilled water and fresh live juices. (*See* PREMENSTRUAL SYNDROME in Part Two and FASTING in Part Three.)

❏ Use a heating pad, hot water bottle, or a hot bath to help relieve pain. The warmth relaxes the muscles that cramp and cause pain.

❏ If you are taking medication for endometriosis, report any new or worsened symptoms to your doctor immediately, especially problems such as difficulty breathing or chest or leg pain. These symptoms may indicate the presence of a blood clot. Frequent checkups are needed to monitor possible side effects such as thinning of the bones. Be aware, however, that it is normal for endometriosis symptoms to worsen temporarily when a woman begins taking medicine.

347

An Alternative Theory and Treatment for Endometriosis

An alternative theory of the origin of endometriosis has been developed by David Redwine, M.D., of St. Charles Medical Center in Bend, Oregon. Dr. Redwine disagrees with those obstetrician/gynecologists who accept reflux menstruation as the cause of endometriosis. Instead, he proposes that endometriosis is actually a type of birth defect. During fetal development, cells that are destined to become part of the female reproductive organs differentiate and migrate toward the appropriate locations. But if the mechanisms that control this process do not function properly, some endometrial cells may be "left behind" in places they do not belong, where they become embedded and grow.

Initially, these bits of misplaced tissue are colorless, but over time the tissue begins to change into the lesions known as endometriosis, probably at least in part in response to stimulation from sex hormones. The lesions begin to change color and gradually become darker until they appear as the classic dark-colored implants found primarily in women in their thirties. Before they reach that stage, however, they may appear white, yellow, red, or brown, and many colors in between. Thus, according to Dr. Redwine, endometrial growths only *appear* to spread progressively throughout the pelvis—that is, they are there all the time, even before birth, but they are not usually recognized for what they are until they take on a sufficiently dark color, a process that occurs over time.

Based on his understanding of the disease, Dr. Redwine developed a treatment for endometriosis in which the implants are physically removed through surgery. Using a laparoscope, the surgeon examines the entire pelvic cavity and the entire peritoneal surface at very close range to identify any possible endometrial lesions. Then all suspected endometrial growths are removed. Each lesion is biopsied and a tissue sample analyzed in a laboratory to determine whether or not it is endometrial in origin. With this identification method, Dr. Redwine says that he has been able to demonstrate that lesions other than the black "powder-burn" lesions normally considered characteristic of the condition have been endometrial in origin.

Many women who undergo surgery for endometriosis are diagnosed with recurrences later. This would seem to support the idea that this is a progressive disease that tends to come back despite treatment. However, Dr. Redwine maintains that the reason so many women have recurring problems with endometriosis is that only a portion of their endometrial implants are removed in surgery. Most surgeons remove only the "typical" black powder-burn lesions and chocolate cysts. Dr. Redwine estimates that a surgeon who excises only the black lesions may leave from 50 to 60 percent of the actual disease behind. He has found that only 40 percent of his patients have the typical lesions, while 60 percent have the multicolored, "atypical" type. He believes that endometriosis is indeed curable, as long as *all* the lesions—both typical and atypical, and not only within the pelvic cavity, but on the peritoneum as well—are removed. His follow-up studies indicate that after surgery, approximately 75 percent of his patients experience complete relief of symptoms, and approximately 20 percent experience an improvement in symptoms so that what was disabling pain becomes only minimal pain. Only about 5 percent report no relief. Dr. Redwine's treatment is now used also by several other gynecological surgeons in the United States.

The following table outlines some of the key differences between Dr. Redwine's theory and conventional medical theory.

ENDOMETRIOSIS THEORIES CONTRASTED

Conventional Theory	Dr. Redwine's Theory
Caused by retrograde menstruation.	Caused by a defect in embryonic cell differentiation.
A progressive disease primarily of women over 30.	A static disease affecting women of all ages.
Associated with menstruation.	Independent of menstruation.
Causes infertility.	May be associated with infertility, but is not the actual cause of it.
Lesions bleed monthly.	Lesions do not bleed.
Most lesions are black.	Lesions may be clear, white, pink, red, brown, black, or multicolored. Most are not black.
Peritoneal implants are not considered to be endometrial in origin.	Peritoneal implants have been proved to be endometrial in origin.
Recurrence following removal of lesions is common.	Recurrence following removal of lesions is rare if both typical and atypical lesions are removed.
Hysterectomy is recommended for severe cases. Surgery provides undependable levels of relief.	Surgical removal of all typical and atypical lesions is the treatment of choice for this disorder, and can provide complete relief in up to 75 percent of cases.

Further information on Dr. Redwine and his approach to endometriosis treatment can be obtained by writing to the Endometriosis Treatment Program (*see* Endometriosis Association in HEALTH AND MEDICAL ORGANIZATIONS in the Appendix).

CONSIDERATIONS

❏ Daily moderate exercise such as walking or stretching is beneficial.

❏ If you suspect you may have endometriosis, you should see a gynecologist promptly so that the condition can be controlled at the earliest possible stage of development.

❏ Medical treatment recommended for endometriosis depends on how far the condition has progressed. Doctors may prescribe a drug called danazol (Danocrine), which stops the normal hormonal cycles, in an attempt to control the blood flow and pain, and in hopes of keeping the abnormal tissue from spreading and inducing the growths to heal and shrink. Some doctors prescribe oral contraceptives (birth control pills) for essentially the same reason. Danazol has been shown to improve symptoms for 89 percent of women who take it and to reduce the size and number of implants. Weight gain and a deepened voice are possible side effects, but are usually reversible when the medication is stopped. However, symptoms may also reappear after medication is stopped.

❏ Raloxifene (Evista), a drug approved initially to prevent bone loss in women, may block the manufacture of estrogen in the uterus lining, thus preventing the growth of endometriosis.

❏ Synthetic versions of a reproductive hormone, gonadatrophin-releasing hormone (GnRH), such as leuprolide (Lupron), nafarelin (Synarel), and goserelin (Zoladex) can be used. Taken for six months, these drugs may help to lessen the symptoms of endometriosis for a year or more. They work by stopping the production of estrogen. The side effects of GnRH are the same as the effects of menopause.

❏ If endometriosis is severe and disabling, or if drug therapy fails, and you do not wish to have any more children, hysterectomy may be recommended. However, hysterectomy does not always relieve all the symptoms, especially if there are implants of endometrial tissue throughout the pelvic region.

❏ An excision option less traumatic than hysterectomy that is used to treat milder cases is laparoscopy with laser surgery to identify and vaporize adhesions, cysts, and endometrial implants. The procedure has yet to be perfected; repeated laparoscopy may be necessary. Advances in this technique are being made at a rapid rate, however, and the need for repeat procedures may soon be a thing of the past.

❏ According to a report in the *Journal of the American Medical Association*, strenuous exercise lowers the level of estrogen in the body, and this may help suppress the symptoms of endometriosis. The more aerobic exercise a woman engages in and the earlier she starts, the lower her risk of developing the disease in the first place, according to a study of endometriosis led by Daniel W. Cramer of Brigham and Women's Hospital and Harvard Medical School. This study found that women who exercised more than seven hours a week had one-fifth the average risk of developing endometriosis. Unfortunately, this beneficial effect was limited to those who began exercising before the age of twenty-six.

❏ Because endometriosis depends on hormonal cycles, and pregnancy temporarily interrupts those cycles, many women find that their symptoms improve during pregnancy. In some cases, the improvement may be permanent, presumably because the break from cycles of growth, bleeding, and scarring finally allows the implants to heal and be shed. In other cases, however, the relief is only temporary, and once the hormonal cycles return to normal, the symptoms of endometriosis recur.

❏ Some nutrition researchers have theorized that endometriosis is related to an inability to absorb calcium properly. Another theory cites food allergies as part of the cause of endometriosis, and recommends removing all allergenic foods from the diet plus administering treatment for candida, using nystatin.

❏ Dioxins may be linked to endometriosis. Dioxins are chlorinated hydrocarbons and can be found in feminine hygiene products as a byproduct of the bleaching process. Dioxin can be absorbed into the body where it collects in fatty tissue. Pesticides are another source of dioxins, as are some types of waste incinerators.

❏ Endometriosis is a benign (noncancerous) condition, but research shows that women who have endometriosis are at greater risk of developing breast cancer, melanoma, lymphoma, and ovarian cancer than women who do not.

❏ *Adenomyosis* is a condition similar to endometriosis in some respects, but it is confined to the uterus. This condition is common in women who have had several children. The uterine wall does not contract as it should, and blood flow continues after menstruation. Endometrial ablation is a thirty-minute outpatient treatment for adenomyosis. In this procedure, a balloon is inserted into the uterus and filled with water. The water is heated, causing the blood vessels to seal, thus stopping the bleeding.

❏ For more information about endometriosis, you can contact the Endometriosis Association (*see* HEALTH AND MEDICAL ORGANIZATIONS in the Appendix).

Enlarged Prostate

See PROSTATITIS/ENLARGED PROSTATE.

Enuresis

See BED-WETTING.

Environmental Toxicity

Environmental issues such as global warming, ozone-layer depletion, and the overuse of pesticides and other chemicals are cause for concern—particularly as they affect the quality of our water and food supply and our level of exposure to radiation and toxic metals. The body's immune system can be the last line of defense against these environmental assaults. It is a complex network that protects us from infectious agents (viruses, bacteria, and other microorganisms), allergens (substances that induce allergic reactions), and other pathogens (substances that cause disease). When something foreign threatens the body, the body responds by forming antibodies and producing increased numbers of white blood cells to combat the intruder. The kidneys and liver work to rid the body of toxins. Thus, a properly functioning immune system is vital for good health, and proper nutrition is becoming increasingly important to help the body detoxify itself.

Certain minerals, such as calcium and zinc, are necessary to sustain life. Other minerals, like copper, are essential in small amounts but are toxic in greater amounts. Some minerals not only have no nutritional value but also are toxic in any amount. These toxic metals—lead, aluminum, cadmium, and mercury—pervade our environment and threaten our health, impairing the function of our organs. Pesticides, herbicides, insecticides, fungicides, fumigants, and fertilizers containing these metals and other toxic substances seep into our soil and food. Food additives, preservatives, and artificial coloring pervade the products in our supermarkets. Fruits and vegetables are sprayed, treated with ripening agents, and waxed to make them appear more appetizing. Toxic chemicals and hazardous waste have contaminated our air and water.

Indoor pollution is an especially serious issue. Studies conducted by the U.S. Environmental Protection Agency (EPA) have shown that indoor air pollution levels—in homes, schools, and workplaces—are often two to five times greater than outdoor levels, and sometimes as much as 100 times greater. People spend up to 90 percent of their time indoors, which increases their exposure to toxic elements. Such exposure is believed to have increased in recent years due to the construction of tightly closed, energy-efficient buildings and an increase in the use of synthetic building materials and chemical products. Indoor pollutants are as varied as the health problems they can cause. These substances include animal hair, asbestos, bedding, carbon monoxide, disinfectants, dust, electromagnetic fields, formaldehyde, hair sprays, household cleaning products, lead, low-level radiation from television screens and computer monitors., mold, paint, pesticides, pollen, radon, solvents, and tobacco smoke. Some products used in the home emit volatile components into the air, among them certain plastics (which emit styrene, solvents (ben-zene), carpets (4-phenylcyclohexene [4-PC]), and manufactured wood products such as pressed wood furniture and kitchen cabinets (formaldehyde). Permanent-press clothes and plastics emit traces of toxic vapors. Smoke from cigarettes, cigars, or pipes raises the level of toxic substances not only in the smoker, but also in those exposed to secondhand smoke. Exposure to any such substances can aggravate allergies and compromise the immune system, paving the way for the development of serious illness.

When pollutants in our environment invade our bodies, they can cause such reactions as watery eyes, diarrhea, nausea, upset stomach, and ringing in the ears. The symptoms of environmental toxicity are so varied that they also include asthma, bronchitis, stuffy nose, arthritis, fatigue, headache, eczema, and depression. If you suffer from chronic flulike symptoms, the culprit may not be a virus; you may be reacting to some material or item in your home or workplace. Exposure to environmental toxins has been linked to immune deficiency and cancer. In children, poor academic performance, and some behavioral, emotional, and learning disabilities have also been linked to indoor environmental pollution.

The symptoms of environmental toxicity and environmental allergies can be very similar, but the mechanisms that cause them are different. Allergies result from an overreaction by the immune system to some substance encountered in the environment. Environmental toxicity, on the other hand, is not a result of an immune system reaction, but a direct poisoning of tissues or cells, so that they can no longer function as they should. Allergic reactions usually begin to subside when contact with the offending allergen ceases, whereas toxicity-based problems can persist long afterwards, depending on the type and extent of the damage the toxins have caused.

NUTRIENTS

SUPPLEMENT	SUGGESTED DOSAGE	COMMENTS
Essential		
Coenzyme Q$_{10}$ plus Coenzyme A from Coenzyme-A Technologies	As directed on label. As directed on label.	Help the immune system detoxify many dangerous substances.
S-Adenosylmethionine (SAMe)	As directed on label.	Has antioxidant effects that can improve the health of the liver. *Caution:* Do not use if you have manic-depressive disorder or take prescription antidepressants.
Vitamin C with bioflavonoids and quercetin	3,000–10,000 mg daily, in divided doses.	Aids in removing toxins and heavy metals from the body.
Very Important		
Garlic (Kyolic from Wakunaga)	2 capsules 3 times daily.	A potent immunostimulant.

L-Cysteine and L-methionine plus L-carnitine and glutathione	500 mg each 3 times daily, on an empty stomach. Take with water or juice. Do not take with milk. Take with 50 mg vitamin B$_6$ and 100 mg vitamin C for better absorption.	To protect the lungs, heart, and liver by destroying free radicals and harmful substances.
Proteolytic enzymes plus pancreatic enzymes	As directed on label. Take between meals. As directed on label. Take with meals.	Important for proper digestion and detoxification.
Superoxide dismutase (SOD) (Cell Guard from Biotec Foods)	As directed on label.	A powerful antioxidant that protects against free radical formation and radiation.
Taurine Plus from American Biologics	As directed on label.	An important antioxidant and immune regulator, necessary for white blood cell activation and neurological function. Use the sublingual form.
Important		
Apple pectin	As directed on label.	Binds with toxins and heavy metals to remove them from the body.
Grape seed extract	As directed on label.	A powerful antioxidant.
Vitamin A plus carotenoid complex with beta-carotene plus vitamin E	25,000 IU daily for 1 month, then reduce to 15,000 IU daily. If you are pregnant, do not exceed 10,000 IU daily. As directed on label. 400–800 IU daily.	Vitamins A and E both act as powerful antioxidants and detoxifiers. Use emulsion forms for easier assimilation and greater safety at high doses. Antioxidants and precursors of vitamin A. Use d-alpha-tocopherol form.
Vitamin B complex plus extra pantothenic acid (vitamin B$_5$) and vitamin B$_6$ (pyridoxine) and niacinamide	100 mg of each major B vitamin 3 times daily, with meals (amounts of individual vitamins in a complex will vary). 100 mg 3 times daily. 50 mg 3 times daily. Up to 500 mg daily.	All B vitamins are vital for cellular function and repair; needed for proper digestion and to protect the lining of the digestive tract. Use a high-stress formula. Sublingual forms are recommended for best absorption.
Helpful		
Calcium plus copper and zinc	50 mg daily. 3 mg daily. 80 mg daily. Do not exceed a total of 100 mg daily from all supplements.	Minerals that aid the immune system. Use calcium pantothenate form. Use zinc gluconate lozenges or OptiZinc for best absorption.
Manganese	50 mg daily. Take separately from calcium.	Works with other trace minerals to aid the immune system. Use a chelate form.
Raw thymus glandular	500 mg daily.	Improves T cell production. (*See* GLANDULAR THERAPY in Part Three for its benefits.)

HERBS

❑ Burdock root and red clover assist in cleansing the bloodstream and lymphatic system.

❑ Milk thistle helps to protect the cells of the liver and also promotes the regeneration of damaged liver cells.

❑ Turmeric contains curcumin, which inhibits tumor growth and boosts the liver's ability to eliminate environmental toxins from the body.

RECOMMENDATIONS

❑ Include in your diet good sources of fiber, such as Aerobic Bulk Cleanse (ABC) from Aerobic Life Industries, oat bran, and wheat bran. Apple pectin also can be beneficial.

Note: Always take supplemental fiber separately from other supplements and medications.

❑ Drink only steam-distilled water.

❑ Try using an air cleaner or ionizer for symptomatic relief. These devices remove animal odors, bacteria, dust, pollen, smog, and smoke from the air. The Living Air XL-15 unit from Alpine Industries is an ionizing unit that is good for purifying the air in the home or workplace.

❑ Use nontoxic cleaning products whenever possible. Many disinfectants, drain cleaners, and other household chemicals have toxic properties. Fortunately there are environmentally friendly alternatives. For example, an effective, nontoxic disinfectant can be made at home by mixing ½ cup borax with 1 gallon hot water. Try clearing your drains by pouring ¼ cup baking soda down your drain and follow it with ½ cup vinegar. Close the drain until the fizzling stops and then flush with hot water.

❑ To reduce your exposure to natural gas, pesticides, radon, smoke, and other chemicals in the household, ventilate your home well. Replace particleboard subflooring with exterior-grade plywood that does not contain formaldehyde. The wood should then be sealed with a nontoxic sealant.

❑ Have your home and workplace tested for radon. Radon is a naturally occurring pollutant believed to be the second leading cause of lung cancer. Simple test kits are available at most hardware stores. If radon is found, measures such as sealing cracks and increasing ventilation in basement areas can often correct the problem.

❑ If you have any fuel-burning appliances, such as furnaces, hot water heaters, kerosene heaters or gas space heaters, be on the alert for carbon monoxide exposure. Be sure that all appliances are properly vented and that your house is well ventilated. Never run your car engine in the garage. Carbon monoxide is a colorless, odorless gas. When inhaled in sufficient quantities, it enters the bloodstream and combines with the hemoglobin in red blood cells, crowding out needed oxygen. Early symptoms of carbon monoxide poisoning include headaches, dizziness, nausea, vomiting, fatigue, and confusion. Continued exposure can lead to coma and, ultimately, death. About 500 Americans die each year from carbon monoxide poisoning, many due to motor vehicle exhaust. Portable carbon monoxide detectors can be purchased at hardware stores.

❏ Scrape any peeling paint inside and outside your home, using appropriate protective devices. Older paints contain toxic lead residue. (*See* LEAD POISONING in Part Two.)

❏ Change vacuum cleaner bags frequently. Most vacuum cleaner bags do a poor job of filtering out dust, pollen, dust mites, and other potentially harmful particles. When shopping for a new vacuum, look for models that encase the bag in a hard, impermeable shell.

❏ Do not smoke, and do not let anyone else smoke in your home or car.

❏ Do not use insect sprays or bug bombs. If you need the services of an exterminator, make sure that anyone you hire is licensed.

CONSIDERATIONS

❏ Most metal pots and pans used for cooking leave residues of metal in your food. Some of these metals—like iron from cast-iron skillets—can actually be beneficial. But other metals can be harmful. Some aluminum and coated cookware can leach off small amounts of metals that can be harmful over time.

❏ It is advisable to see an allergy specialist to have a radioallergosorbent test (RAST) if you experience any of the symptoms described above to rule out allergies as a cause of the problem. You may also want to have a hair analysis to determine the level of toxic substances in your system.

❏ Liver extract injections have produced good results for some people.

❏ Asbestos, once widely used in a variety of products and building materials, may still be present in buildings and homes that were built or renovated between 1900 and 1970. Asbestos is not dangerous if it is still intact and in solid form. It becomes dangerous when it breaks down and fibers are released into the air. The asbestos fibers—which are so small that they can pass through vacuum cleaner bags—can enter the lungs and get lodged in the delicate lung tissue. Asbestos exposure can cause a variety of illnesses, including lung cancer, asbestosis, and mesothelioma, a type of tumor. Cancers of the larynx, oral cavity, kidney, and colon are sometimes attributed to asbestos as well. Asbestos removal should be done only by qualified contractors.

❏ One household item that can cause a lot of problems is carpeting. Some of the chemicals commonly used in carpeting have been shown to have an adverse effect on health. One suspect chemical is 4-phenylcyclohexene (4-PC), a byproduct of the production of styrene-butadiene. This substance is used for the backing of many carpets. Breakdown products from styrene-butadiene are also potentially toxic. Shampooing carpeting can be particularly bad for your health. When you shampoo a carpet, the bottom stays damp well after the surface you walk on is dry. This dampness becomes a breeding ground for thousands of microorganisms that can wreak havoc on your system. The moisture can also seep into the floor beneath, which in many buildings consists of particleboard made from formaldehyde-based glue and processed wood. When the particleboard gets wet, the formaldehyde can be released into the air in the home.

❏ *See also* ALUMINUM TOXICITY; ARSENIC POISONING; CADMIUM TOXICITY; CHEMICAL POISONING; COPPER TOXICITY; FOODBORNE/WATERBORNE DISEASE; LEAD POISONING; MERCURY TOXICITY; and NICKEL TOXICITY, all in Part Two.

Epilepsy

Over 2 million people in America have epilepsy, a disorder characterized by recurring seizures. Seizures are a *symptom* of epilepsy, but not all people who have seizures have epilepsy, and even those who do may also have seizures that are not epileptic in nature. An epileptic seizure is a temporary malfunction of the brain caused by uncontrolled electrical activity from the nerve cells in the cerebral cortex. The seizures rarely damage the brain, but they can make life difficult.

The underlying cause, or causes, of epilepsy are relatively unknown. Seizures may occur for no apparent reason or may be triggered by a wide range of things, including exposure to an allergen; drug or alcohol withdrawal; fever; flashing lights; hunger; hypoglycemia; infection; lack of sleep; metabolic or nutritional imbalances; or trauma, especially head injury. There are several different types of seizures, including the following:

• *Absence (previously known as petit mal)*. This type of seizure is most common in children and teenagers. It is characterized by a blank stare lasting about half a minute; the person appears to be daydreaming. During this type of seizure, the individual is unaware of his or her surroundings. Staring or daydreaming in children should not be confused with absence seizures. If a child is daydreaming, he or she can be aroused by a simple touch or someone talking to him or her. A child having an absence seizure cannot.

• *Atonic (drop attack)*. A childhood seizure in which the child loses consciousness for about ten seconds and usually falls to the ground because of a complete loss of muscle tone.

• *Complex partial (temporal lobe)*. A blank stare, random activity, and a chewing motion are characteristic of this type of seizure. The person may be dazed and unaware of his or her surroundings, and may act oddly. There is no memory of this seizure. A person may experience a distinctive warning sign called an aura before this type of seizure. The aura is itself a form of partial seizure, but one in which the person retains awareness. The aura may be experienced as a peculiar odor, "butterflies" in the stomach, or a distorted sound. One man with epilepsy, an ardent racetrack gambler, said he always heard the roar of a crowd, followed by the name of a favorite racehorse, just before he lost consciousness.

- *Generalized tonic-clonic (previously known as grand mal).* This type of seizure is characterized by sudden cries, a fall, rigidity and jerking of the muscles, shallow breathing, and bluish skin. Loss of bladder control is possible. The seizure usually lasts two to five minutes, and is followed by confusion, fatigue, and/or memory loss. It can be frightening to witness, especially for the first-time observer.

- *Myoclonic.* Brief, massive muscle jerks occur.

- *Simple partial (Jacksonian).* Jerking begins in the fingers and toes and progresses up through the body. The person remains conscious.

- *Simple partial (sensory).* The person may see, hear, or sense things that do not exist. This may occur as a preliminary symptom of a generalized seizure.

Seizures in children can be particularly disturbing. They are the most common neurological problem affecting children—indeed, one-third of people with seizure disorders are children. Iodiopathic epilepsy (seizures of unknown cause) or febrile seizures (nonepileptic seizures induced by fever) affect about 3 percent of children. Angelman syndrome (a rare congenital disorder seen in children) is associated with seizures or tremors. Lennox-Gastaut syndrome is a severe seizure disorder that usually develops in children between the ages of one and eight. Seizures in very young children often stem from brain injury before birth, damage to the central nervous system, or metabolic inconsistencies. In older children, epilepsy is more likely to result from genetic factors, infections of the central nervous system, or head injury.

Nutritional supplementation is important for people with epilepsy. Unless otherwise specified, the dosages recommended here are for adults. For a child between twelve and seventeen, reduce the dose to three-quarters the recommended amount. For a child between six and twelve, use one-half the recommended dose, and for a child under the age of six, use one-quarter the recommended amount.

NUTRIENTS

SUPPLEMENT	SUGGESTED DOSAGE	COMMENTS
Essential		
Dimethylglycine (DMG)	As directed on label.	A powerful antioxidant. Increases oxygenation of tissues.
L-Carnitine	As directed on label.	An amino acid required to make protein and deliver essential fatty acids to the cells. Carnitine is depleted by anticonvulsant drugs.
L-Tyrosine	500 mg each 3 times daily, on an empty stomach. Take with water or juice. Do not take with milk. Take with 50 mg vitamin B$_6$ and 100 mg vitamin C for better absorption.	Important for proper brain function. *Caution:* Do not take tyrosine if you are taking an MAO inhibitor drug.
Magnesium	700 mg daily, in divided doses. Take between meals, on an empty stomach, with apple cider vinegar or betaine HCl.	Needed to calm the nervous system and muscle spasms. Use magnesium chloride form.
Selenium	As directed on label. If you are pregnant, do not exceed 40 mcg daily.	Low selenium levels result in a deficiency of glutathione peroxidase, an enzyme that detoxifies peroxides in the cells.
Taurine Plus from American Biologics	10–20 drops daily, in divided doses.	Taurine is an important antioxidant and immune regulator, necessary for white blood cell activation and neurological function. Use the sublingual form.
or taurine	As directed on label.	Levels of taurine are often low in people with seizure disorders. Taurine is an essential building block of all other amino acids.
Vitamin B complex	100 mg of each major B vitamin 3 times daily, with meals (amounts of individual vitamins in a complex will vary).	Extremely important in the functioning of the central nervous system. Injections (under a doctor's supervision) may be necessary.
plus extra vitamin B$_3$ (niacin)	50 mg daily.	Improves circulation and is helpful for many brain-related disorders.
and vitamin B$_6$ (pyridoxine)	100–600 mg 3 times daily, under the supervision of a health care professional.	Needed for normal brain function.
and vitamin B$_{12}$	1,000–2,000 mcg daily, on an empty stomach.	Involved in maintenance of the myelin sheaths that cover and protect nerve endings.
and folic acid	400 mcg daily. If you are taking anticonvulsants, do not exceed 400 mg daily from all sources.	A brain food vital for the health of the nervous system.
and pantothenic acid	500 mg daily.	The anti-stress vitamin.
Very Important		
Calcium	1,500 mg daily.	Important in normal nerve impulse transmission.
Liquid Kyolic with B$_1$ and B$_{12}$ from Wakunaga	As directed on label.	Increases energy and acts as an antioxidant.
Zinc	50–80 mg daily. Do not exceed a total of 100 mg daily from all supplements.	Protects the brain cells. Use zinc gluconate lozenges or OptiZinc for best absorption.
Important		
Coenzyme Q$_{10}$ plus	30 mg daily.	Improves brain oxygenation.
Coenzyme A from Coenzyme-A Technologies	As directed on label.	Works with coenzyme Q$_{10}$ for best results.
Oxy-5000 Forte from American Biologics	As directed on label.	A potent nutritional antioxidant for health and stress. Destroys free radicals.
Quercetin	As directed on label.	A flavonoid with anti-inflammatory and antioxidant properties. More powerful than vitamin C.

Helpful		
Chromium picolinate	200 mcg daily.	Important in maintaining stable cerebral glucose metabolism.
Kelp or alfalfa	1,000–1,500 mg daily.	For necessary mineral balance. See under Herbs, below.
Melatonin	Start with 2–3 mg daily, taken 2 hours or less before bedtime. If necessary, gradually increase the dosage until an effective level is reached.	Helpful if symptoms include insomnia.
Proteolytic enzymes plus multienzyme complex	As directed on label. Take between meals. As directed on label. Take with meals.	Aids in healing if inflammation is the cause of seizures. Aids digestion, helping to make needed nutrients available.
Raw thymus glandular and thyroid glandular	As directed on label. As directed on label.	Both the thymus and thyroid are important in proper brain function. (See GLANDULAR THERAPY in Part Three.)
Vitamin A with mixed carotenoids	25,000 IU daily. If you are pregnant, do not exceed 10,000 IU daily.	An important antioxidant that aids in protecting brain function.
Vitamin C with bioflavonoids	2,000–7,000 mg daily, in divided doses.	Vital to functioning of the adrenal glands, which are the anti-stress glands. A potent antioxidant.
Vitamin E	Start with 400 IU daily and gradually increase to 1,600 IU daily.	Aids circulation. Compensates for anticonvulsant-induced vitamin depletion. Emulsion form is recommended for easier assimilation and greater safety at high doses. Use d-alpha-tocopherol form.

HERBS

❑ Alfalfa is a good source of needed minerals. Take 2,000 milligrams daily in capsule or extract form.

❑ Black cohosh, hyssop, and lobelia are beneficial for people with epilepsy because they aid in controlling the central nervous system and have a calming effect. For best results, they should be used on an alternating basis.

Caution: Do not use black cohosh during pregnancy.

❑ *Avoid* the herb sage. This herb should not be used by anyone with a seizure disorder.

RECOMMENDATIONS

❑ Eat soured milk products like yogurt and kefir.

❑ Include beet greens, chard, eggs, green leafy vegetables, raw cheese, raw milk, raw nuts, seeds, and soybeans in the diet.

❑ Drink fresh "live" juices made from beets, carrots, green beans, green leafy vegetables, peas, red grapes, and seaweed for concentrated nutrients. (See JUICING in Part Three.)

❑ Eat small meals, do not drink large quantities of liquids at once, and take 2 tablespoons of olive oil daily.

❑ Avoid alcoholic beverages, animal protein, fried foods, artificial sweeteners such as aspartame (NutraSweet), caffeine, and nicotine. Avoid refined foods and sugar.

❑ If the bowels do not move each day, before going to bed, take a lemon enema using the juice of two lemons and 2 quarts of water. (See ENEMAS in Part Three.)

❑ Take an Epsom salts bath twice a week.

❑ Work toward self-care. Keep drug dosages as low as possible, and work toward becoming as free from drugs and seizures as possible. The correct diet and nutritional supplements are very important in the control of epilepsy.

❑ Get regular moderate exercise to improve circulation to the brain.

As much as possible, avoid stress and tension. Learn stress management techniques. (See STRESS in Part Two.)

❑ If you are present when someone is having a seizure:

• Do not restrain the person.

• Do not try to put anything in the person's mouth. A person having a seizure may bite his or her tongue, but this is not life threatening.

• Try to restrain a fall so that the person does not hit something as he or she collapses. Often, the person knows he or she is about to have a seizure, and you can ask him or her to sit on the floor, or help him or her to sit down, before a fall.

• Leave the person lying flat on a safe surface. Do not put anything under the person's head. If possible, turn the person onto his or her side, propping him or her in that position with cushions at the back during the seizure. This way, any saliva or blood from a bitten tongue will be able to flow freely out of the mouth.

• In case of loss of bladder or bowel control, if possible, loosely cover the person with a blanket to protect his or her privacy.

• Do not panic. Loosen any tight clothing to make the person more comfortable. Stay with the person until the seizure has stopped. He or she may be confused and tired immediately after the seizure.

• If the person has repeated seizures, one after the other, seek medical assistance. With a baby or young child, medical help should be sought immediately.

CONSIDERATIONS

❑ Most people who have epilepsy are aware of their condition and take medication to control the seizures. Possible side effects of antiseizure medications include blood disorders, fatigue, liver problems, and mental fatigue and/or fogginess.

❑ Other types of drugs can interact with antiseizure medications, lessening or intensifying the effects of one drug or the other. Alcohol, birth control pills, the antibiotic erythromycin, and some types of asthma, ulcer, and heart medicines are known to interact with certain epilepsy drugs.

Anyone who takes medication for epilepsy should always check with his or her doctor or pharmacist before taking other drugs, whether prescription or over-the-counter.

❏ Epilepsy is not the only cause of seizures. They can also be brought on by other factors, including alkalosis; excessive consumption of alcohol; arteriosclerosis; brain disorders such as a brain tumor, encephalitis, meningitis, or stroke; high fever (especially in children); the use of drugs; the formation of scar tissue as a result of an eye injury or a stroke; a lack of oxygen; and spasms of the blood vessels.

❏ High levels of aluminum have been found in the brains of some people with epilepsy. Studies in animals have shown that trace amounts of aluminum in the brain may initiate the type of disordered electrical activity that causes seizures. (See ALUMINUM TOXICITY in Part Two.)

❏ According to research done by Arizona State University's Biochemical Department, the artificial sweetener aspartame (NutraSweet) has been associated with seizures in some people. Toxic agents such as aluminum and lead may contribute to the problem.

❏ Doses of folic acid in excess of 400 micrograms per day may increase seizure activity in people with epilepsy, especially if they are taking the commonly prescribed anticonvulsant phenytoin (Dilantin).

❏ At least 90 percent of women who take epilepsy drugs during pregnancy give birth to normal, healthy infants. Because a seizure during pregnancy carries its own risks, most doctors advise pregnant women with epilepsy to continue taking their medication unless it is likely they will be seizure-free without it.

❏ Some good results have been reported using hyperbaric (high-pressure) oxygen therapy in treating people with epilepsy. (See HYPERBARIC OXYGEN THERAPY in Part Three.)

❏ If epilepsy is due to tiny tumors in the brain, a type of surgery known as lesionectomy may be recommended. Using a computer, a surgeon can view and vaporize the tiny tumors that cause some cases of epilepsy. This procedure can be performed with minimal damage to healthy tissue in the brain.

❏ Diastat, a gel form of diazepam (better known as Valium) designed for rectal administration, may be prescribed for people who suffer from multiple seizures on a regular basis. The gel takes only minutes to work and should be administered two to three minutes into a seizure.

❏ A specialized dietary program called the *ketogenic diet* has been used with considerable success to control seizures in children. This is a rigidly controlled diet that is high in fats and extremely low in carbohydrates and proteins, which forces the body to use fats rather than the usual carbohydrates to generate cellular energy. When fats are burned, byproducts called *ketones* are formed. Normally, ketosis—the presence of high levels of ketones in the body—occurs only in cases of starvation or uncontrolled di-

abetes mellitus. Eating a diet containing virtually no carbohydrates, however, can produce essentially the same effect, and also causes biochemical changes that enable the body's tissues to burn these ketones for needed energy. Although it is not known exactly how, this process appears to control seizure activity. The majority of children who have been put on this diet benefit from it, and many have been able to stop taking, or reduce their dosage of, antiseizure medication. Using this dietary program can be challenging for parents, however; the child's foods, liquids, medications, and even personal hygiene products such as toothpaste must be strictly controlled, and the program must be followed to the letter (even slight deviations can negate its effects). It should be undertaken only under the direct supervision of a physician who is experienced in its use. Information about the ketogenic diet is available from the Pediatric Epilepsy Center at Johns Hopkins Hospital (see HEALTH AND MEDICAL ORGANIZATIONS in the Appendix).

❏ Pseudoseizures, also known as psychogenic or nonepileptic attack disorder, are nonepileptic seizures and may be a symptom of a number of different psychological factors.

❏ Huntingon's disease (HD), also sometimes called Huntington's chorea, is a disorder that can cause tremors, jerking movements that may resemble myoclonic seizures. This is not a seizure disorder, however. HD is a result of a genetically transmitted chromosome irregularity that usually manifests itself during the third decade of life. There is no known cure for Huntington's disease, but following the diet designed for epilepsy may help slow the progression and ease symptoms of the condition.

Epstein-Barr Virus

See under CHRONIC FATIGUE SYNDROME; FIBROMYALGIA SYNDROME; MONONUCLEOSIS.

Eye Problems

Two of the most complex organs of the body, the eyes provide us with instantaneous visual feedback of the world around us. We have all experienced eye trouble at one time or another—eyes that are tired, bloodshot, dry, irritated, itchy, sensitive to light, or watery, to name just a few. While some eye disorders—nearsightedness or cataracts, for example—are localized problems, eye disturbances can be a symptom of disease elsewhere in the body. Watery eyes, for example, can be a symptom of the common cold; a thyroid problem may be indicated by protruding or bulging eyes and reading difficulties; dark circles under the eyes and eyes that are red, swollen, and/or watery may indicate al-

Maintaining Healthy Eyes

Like all other parts of the body, the eyes need to be nourished properly. In addition to making sure that the eyes are not strained by too much intense close work or inadequate light, proper eye care includes a healthy diet containing sufficient amounts of vitamins and minerals.

In order to promote good eyesight, you must make sure your diet contains the proper amounts of the B vitamins; vitamins A, C, and E; and the minerals selenium and zinc. Fresh fruits and vegetables are good sources of these vitamins and minerals; include plenty of these in your diet, especially yellow and yellow-orange foods such as carrots, yams, and cantaloupes. A well-balanced diet with plenty of fresh fruits and vegetables can help keep your eyes healthy.

NUTRIENTS

SUPPLEMENT	SUGGESTED DOSAGE	COMMENTS
Desiccated liver	As directed on label.	A good source of many important vitamins and minerals. Use only liver derived from organically raised beef.
Free-form amino acid complex plus	As directed on label.	For necessary protein. Free-form amino acids are assimilated best.
glutathione or	500 mg daily, on an empty stomach.	Powerful antioxidants that protect the lenses of the eyes.
N-acetylcysteine	500 mg daily, on an empty stomach. Take with water or juice. Do not take with milk. Take with 50 mg vitamin B$_6$ and 100 mg vitamin C for better absorption.	
Multivitamin and mineral complex with		All nutrients are needed in balance.
selenium	200 mcg daily. If you are pregnant, do not exceed 40 mcg daily.	Destroys free radicals that can damage the eyes.
Ocu-Care from Nature's Plus or	As directed on label.	These formulas provide many eye-strengthening nutrients, as well as protective and antioxidant substances, to support and nourish the eyes.
OcuGuard from Twinlab or	As directed on label.	
Visual Eyes from Source Naturals	As directed on label.	
Taurine Plus from American Biologics	As directed on label.	Taurine is associated with zinc in maintaining eye function. It is present in the retina of the eye in high concentrations. Use the sublingual form.
Vitamin A emulsion or	25,000 IU daily. If you are pregnant, do not exceed 10,000 IU daily.	Absolutely necessary for proper eye function. Protects the eye from free radicals. Emulsion form is recommended for easier assimilation and greater safety at higher doses.
capsules plus	15,000 IU daily.	
carotenoid complex with lutein and zeaxanthin	As directed on label.	Precursors of vitamin A.
Vitamin B complex	100 mg twice daily (amounts of individual vitamins in a complex will vary).	Needed for intracellular eye metabolism.
Vitamin C with bioflavonoids	2,000 mg 3 times daily.	An antioxidant that reduces intraocular pressure.
Vitamin E	400 IU daily.	Important in healing and immunity. Use d-alpha-tocopherol form.
Zinc	50 mg daily. Do not exceed a total of 100 mg daily from all supplements.	Deficiency has been linked to retinal detachment. Use zinc gluconate lozenges or OptiZinc for best absorption.

HERBS

❑ Bayberry bark, cayenne (capsicum), and red raspberry leaves, taken by mouth, are beneficial.

❑ Bilberry extract has been shown to improve both normal and night vision.

RECOMMENDATIONS

❑ Include the following in your diet: broccoli, raw cabbage, carrots, cauliflower, green vegetables, squash, sunflower seeds, and watercress.

❑ Drink fresh carrot juice. This can help to prevent or alleviate some eye problems.

❑ Eliminate sugar and white flour from your diet.

❑ If you wear glasses, wear clear spectacles that have been treated to keep out ultraviolet rays. This will help protect against damage from ultraviolet exposure. Avoid wearing tinted eyeglasses for this purpose, especially on a regular basis; dark glasses prevent needed light from entering the eyes. The functioning of the pineal gland, which plays an important role in the regulation of metabolism, behavior, and physiological functions, is largely governed by sunlight.

❑ Never use hair dyes containing coal tar on the eyelashes or eyebrows; doing so can cause injury or blindness. Although coal-tar dyes are legal, marketing them for the eyebrows and eyelashes is not.

❑ Be careful when using drugs, whether prescription or over-the-counter. Some may cause eye problems. Drugs that can cause damage to the optic nerve, retina, or other vital parts of the eye include the following:

• Adrenocorticotropic hormone, or ACTH (Acthar, Cortrosyn).

- Allopurinol (also sold under the brand name Zyloprim), which is used for gout.

- Anticoagulants such as heparin and warfarin (Coumadin).

- Aspirin.

- Corticosteroids, such as dexamethasone (Decadron), hydrocortisone (Cortenema, Hydrocortone, Solu-Cortef, VoSol HC), prednisolone (Blephamide, Hydeltra-T.B.A.), and prednisone (Deltasone).

- Chlorpropamide (Diabinese), which is used for non-insulin-dependent diabetes.

- Diuretics, antihistamines, and digitalis preparations. All of these can cause disturbances in color distinction.

- Indomethacin (Indocin), an arthritis medication.

- Marijuana.

- Nicotinic acid (niacin), if used for long periods.

- Streptomycin.

- Sulfa drugs.

- Tetracycline.

❑ Consult your health care provider if you develop any of the following conditions: change in pupil size; eye pain or pain on eye movement; impaired vision; intolerance to light; known exposure to gonorrhea or chlamydia; or swelling, tenderness, or redness around the eyes.

❑ If you have a baby or young child who exhibits any signs of eye infection, have the child evaluated by a professional.

CONSIDERATIONS

❑ There are three types of specialists who deal with the eyes:

1. Ophthalmologists are medical doctors who are eye specialists. They diagnose and treat eye disease, perform eye surgery, give eye tests, and prescribe corrective lenses.

2. Optometrists are not medical doctors, but they are licensed by the states to give eye tests and treat non-surgical eye problems. They can prescribe corrective lenses. In some states, they can prescribe medication as well.

3. Opticians fill prescriptions for glasses and contact lenses. Only twenty-six states require opticians to be licensed.

❑ Because the light-absorbing retinal pigment is composed of vitamin A and protein, which are continually being used up as images are formed, adequate supplies of these nutrients are vital for proper eye function.

❑ The combination of nicotine, sugar, and caffeine may temporarily affect vision.

❑ Ophthalmologist and author Gary Price Todd, M.D., says that the use of margarine and vegetable shortening is dangerous for those with certain eye disorders. Butter and vegetable oils can be used as substitutes. For those who must undergo eye surgery, he suggests taking a multivitamin and mineral supplement the evening before the operation, preferably a formula including 10,000 international units of vitamin A, 1,000 milligrams of vitamin C, and 1,200 international units of vitamin E. He recommends continued use of these nutrients, plus 2 milligrams of copper and 20 milligrams of zinc daily, after surgery. If there is bleeding involved or you are prone to bleeding, you should not take vitamin E two days or less before surgery. You can resume taking vitamin E after surgery.

❑ Sea mussel is a source of protein that aids in the functioning of eye tissues and the secretion of eye fluids.

❑ Zinc may help reduce vision loss because it is a factor in the metabolic functioning of several enzymes in the chorioretinal complex (the vascular coating of the eye). Never take more than 100 milligrams daily, however.

❑ According to a report in *Ocular Diagnosis and Therapy*, ocular abnormalities can be hastened by anti-infective agents, diazepam (Valium), haloperidol (Haldol), some antidepressants, quinine, and sulfa drugs.

❑ People who work at computers every day are at risk for eyestrain, headaches, blurred vision, dry or irritated eyes, sensitivity to light, double vision, and after-images.

❑ People who wear contact lenses need to take precautions against eye damage because of the increased risk of injury and infection associated with them.

❑ Two recent studies have shown that leaving contact lenses in place for more than twenty-four consecutive hours can result in ulcerative keratitis, a condition in which the cells of the cornea are rubbed away by the contact lens, leading to infection and scarring. If not properly treated, this condition can cause blindness. Users of extended-wear lenses are ten to fifteen times more likely than other people to develop ulcerative keratitis, according to *The New England Journal of Medicine*. If ordinary daily-wear lenses are left in place overnight, the risk rises to the same level.

❑ Abnormalities in one or more of the six muscles that move the eyes, or a lack of coordination among these muscles, can result in a cross-eyed or walleyed condition. These muscles can be exercised and relaxed to improve their function. The internal muscles likewise can be exercised to improve the focusing ability of the eyes, both near and far.

lergies; yellowing of the eyes from jaundice can be a sign of hepatitis, gallbladder disease, or gallstone blockage; droopy eyes are often an early sign of *myasthenia gravis,* a disorder in which the eye muscles weaken. A drastic difference in the sizes of the pupils can indicate a tumor somewhere in the body, whereas high blood pressure and diabetes may manifest themselves in periodic blurring of vision.

The eyeball is a sphere about an inch in diameter that is covered by a tough outer layer called the *sclera,* the "white of the eye." Underneath the sclera is the middle layer of the eye, the *choroid*, which contains the blood vessels that serve the eye. The front of the eye is covered by a transparent membrane called the *cornea*. Behind the cornea is a fluid-filled chamber called the *anterior chamber*; behind that—in the center of the sclera, on the front of the eyeball—is the highly pigmented *iris*, and in the center of the iris is the *pupil*. Behind the iris is the transparent *lens*. Inside, at the back of the eye, is the *retina*, a delicate light-sensitive membrane that is connected to the brain by the *optic nerve.*

The eye also contains two important fluids. The *ciliary body*, whose muscles are responsible for focusing the lens of the eye, also produces a waterlike substance called the *aqueous humor*, which fills the space between the cornea and the lens. The aqueous humor contains all of the constituents of blood except for red blood cells. The other fluid is the *vitreous humor*, a jellylike substance that fills the back of the eyeball, the space between the lens and the retina.

On the outside of the eyeball are six muscles that move the eyes. Under the upper eyelids are the lacrimal glands, which secrete tears. At the inner corners of the eyelids are the tear ducts, small openings through which the tears drain into the nose and the back of the throat. At the edges of the eyelids, where the eyelashes are, are glands that produce oils, sweat, and other secretions.

What we think of as the simple act of seeing is actually a complex, multistep process that goes on continuously and at breathtaking speed. Light enters the eye through the pupil, which changes size depending on the amount of light entering it. When there is very little light, the pupil dilates; in bright light, the pupil constricts. As light enters the eye, it is focused by the lens, which adjusts its shape by means of the action of the muscles and ligaments of the ciliary body. The lens becomes fatter or flatter depending upon the distance to the object being focused on. The lens projects light onto the retina, where special pigment absorbs the light and forms a corresponding image. Finally, this image is transmitted by means of the optic nerve to the brain, which interprets the image. Anything that interferes with any link in this chain of events can result in impaired vision.

Many cases of eye damage and vision loss are linked to underlying diseases of one type or another. Diabetes often leads to hemorrhages in the retina and the vitreous humor, eventually producing blindness. Early cataracts also may be related to diabetes. High blood pressure produces a gradual thickening of the blood vessels inside the eyes that can result in visual impairment and even blindness. Other factors linked to declining eyesight include too much sun exposure, poor nutrition, exposure to tobacco smoke or other pollutants, and dehydration.

One major contributor to eye trouble is poor diet, specifically the denatured, chemical- and preservative-laden foods that most Americans consume daily. A deficiency of just one vitamin can lead to various eye problems. Supplementation with the correct vitamins and minerals can help prevent or correct eye trouble. Some of these supplements also protect against the formation of free radicals, which

can damage the eyes. Specific eye problems that can be helped by supplementing the diet with vitamins and other nutrients are discussed in this section.

Unless otherwise specified, the nutrient dosages recommended are for adults. For a child between the ages of twelve and seventeen, reduce the dose to three-quarters of the recommended amount. For a child between six and twelve, use one-half of the recommended dose, and for a child under the age of six, use one-quarter of the recommended amount.

ASTIGMATISM

See under BLURRED VISION in this section.

BAGS UNDER THE EYES

Skin loses some of its elasticity with age, and muscles within the eyelids lose tone, causing what is known as bags under the eyes. In addition, fat can gather in the eyelid, and fluids can accumulate and cause swelling. Puffiness around the eyes can also be caused by allergies or excessive consumption of salt. Smoking can aggravate the problem.

Recommendations

❑ Avoid drinking fluids before bed.

❑ Avoid monosodium glutamate (MSG) and limit your salt intake.

❑ Do not smoke, and avoid secondhand smoke.

❑ Get plenty of sleep.

❑ Place a washcloth moistened in ice water, or a chilled gel-filled compress, over your eyes for fifteen minutes once or twice daily. You can also try using a lukewarm wet tea bag or cold cucumber slices. The cold shrinks the swollen blood vessels.

❑ *See* ALLERGIES in Part Two and take the self-test to determine allergens that may be causing the problem.

BITOT'S SPOTS

Bitot's spots are distinct elevated white patches on the conjunctiva, the membrane that covers most of the visible part of the eye. They may signify a severe deficiency of vitamin A.

NUTRIENTS

SUPPLEMENT	SUGGESTED DOSAGE	COMMENTS
Vitamin A	25,000 IU daily for two weeks, then 15,000 IU daily for 1 month, then reduce to 10,000 IU daily. If you are pregnant, do not exceed 10,000 IU daily.	Aids in dissolution of Bitot's spots, which may be caused by vitamin A deficiency. Use emulsion form for easier assimilation and greater safety at higher doses.
plus carotenoid complex with lutein and zeaxanthin	As directed on label.	

Recommendations

❏ Avoid eyestrain and smoke-filled rooms.

BLEPHARITIS

Blepharitis is an inflammation of the outer edges of the eyelids that causes redness, itching, burning, and, often, a sensation of having something in one's eye. Other possible symptoms include swelling of the eyelids, loss of eyelashes, excessive tearing, and sensitivity to light. Secretions may form crusts that "glue" the eyes together during sleep.

This condition may be caused by an infection of the eyelash follicles or glands at the outer edges of the eyelids. Eyestrain, poor hygiene, poor living and sleeping habits, poor nutrition, and systemic disease with resulting immunodepression commonly contribute to the problem. Blepharitis may also be associated with seborrhea of the face or scalp. (*See* SEBORRHEA in Part Two.)

NUTRIENTS

SUPPLEMENT	SUGGESTED DOSAGE	COMMENTS
Inflazyme Forte from American Biologics	As directed on label.	Aids in reducing inflammation.
Vitamin A	25,000 IU daily. If you are pregnant, do not exceed 10,000 IU daily.	Important in all eye disorders.
plus carotenoid complex with lutein and zeaxanthin	As directed on label.	Important antioxidants and precursors of vitamin A.
Vitamin C with bioflavonoids	6,000 mg daily, in divided doses.	A powerful antioxidant that protects the eyes and reduces inflammation.
Zinc	50 mg daily. Do not exceed a total of 100 mg daily from all supplements.	Needed for proper immune function. Use zinc gluconate lozenges or OptiZinc for best absorption.

Herbs

❏ Warm eyebright, goldenseal, or mullein compresses are soothing and help reduce inflammation. Prepare a tea using one of these herbs, cool it to a comfortably warm temperature, and soak a clean cloth or a piece of sterile cotton in it to make the compress. Apply the compress and relax for ten to fifteen minutes. Then make a fresh compress and gently wipe the edge of the eyelid and the area around and between the eyelashes to remove any scaly matter or dandruff-like debris. Do this twice a day or as needed. Use each compress only once before laundering or discarding it.

Recommendations

❏ Eat a well-balanced diet that emphasizes fresh, raw vegetables, plus grains, legumes, and fresh fruits.

❏ Keep the eyelids clean, especially along the edges (see the procedure described under Herbs, above), but do not touch or rub your eyes except when necessary. Always wash your hands before touching your eyes.

❏ Get sufficient sleep, and avoid eyestrain. Anything that increases eye fatigue makes the discomfort worse.

Considerations

❏ *See also* SEBORRHEA in Part Two.

BLOODSHOT EYES

Bloodshot eyes occur when the small blood vessels on the surface of the eye become inflamed and congested with blood, usually in response to an insufficient supply of oxygen in the cornea or tissues covering the eyes. They are usually a consequence of eyestrain, fatigue, and improper diet, especially the consumption of alcohol. But they can also indicate bodywide capillary fragility, the presence of a blood clot, or high blood pressure.

A bloodshot appearance can also result from deficiencies in vitamins B_2 (riboflavin) and B_6 (pyridoxine), and the amino acids histidine, lysine, or phenylalanine. Once the body receives the nutrients it needs, the congestion in the blood vessels should disappear.

NUTRIENTS

SUPPLEMENT	SUGGESTED DOSAGE	COMMENTS
Vitamin A	25,000 IU daily. If you are pregnant, do not exceed 10,000 IU daily.	Needed for all eye disorders.
plus carotenoid complex with lutein and zeaxanthin	As directed on label.	
Vitamin B complex	100 mg of each major B vitamin 3 times daily (amounts of individual vitamins in a complex will vary).	Deficiencies have been linked to bloodshot eyes.
plus free-form amino acid complex	As directed on label.	Use a formula containing both essential and nonessential amino acids.
Vitamin C with bioflavonoids	1,000–2,500 mg 4 times daily.	Important antioxidants and necessary free radical destroyers. Required for tissue growth and repair.

Herbs

❏ Use raspberry leaf to alleviate redness and irritation. Prepare a raspberry leaf tea, allow it to cool, and soak a clean cloth or piece of sterile cotton in the tea to make a compress. Apply the compress to the eyes with the lids closed for ten minutes or as needed.

BLURRED VISION

Vision may become blurred for any of a number of reasons.

Refractive error (nearsightedness, farsightedness, and/or astigmatism) results in chronically blurry vision that can usually be overcome with corrective lenses. Eyestrain, fatigue, and excessive tearing can result in a temporary blurring of vision. A disturbance in the fluid balance in the body can also result in blurry vision.

A recurring tendency to periodic blurring can result from an inadequate supply of the light-sensitive pigment in the eye called rhodopsin, or visual purple, which is composed of vitamin A and protein. Any light that enters the eyes breaks down part of the visual purple, and the products of this purposeful breakdown set up nerve impulses that tell the brain what the eyes are seeing. If there is not enough pigment present, a time delay occurs between the time the eyes focus on an object and the time the brain forms an image of it. This is experienced as a blurring of vision.

NUTRIENTS

SUPPLEMENT	SUGGESTED DOSAGE	COMMENTS
Potassium	99 mg daily.	Needed to maintain proper fluid balance.
Vitamin A plus carotenoid complex with lutein and zeaxanthin	25,000 IU daily. If you are pregnant, do not exceed 10,000 IU daily. As directed on label.	Necessary for pigment formation and proper balance of intraocular fluid. Needed for all eye disorders.

Considerations

❑ Laser surgery is an increasingly popular method for correcting refractive errors that cause myopia (nearsightedness), hyperopia (farsightedness), and astigmatism (distorted vision). Two laser surgery procedures—*photorefractive keratectomy* (PRK) and *laser in situ keratomileusis* (LASIK)—may be used to correct mild to moderate nearsightedness. Both are outpatient procedures with relatively short recovery times. Both also have very high rates of success, but neither procedure is foolproof. Some people have improved vision as a result of the laser surgery, but still have to wear corrective lenses afterward. Others have to have follow-up surgery to improve results. In rare cases, people who have laser surgery end up with worse vision. People who tend to heal slowly or who have ongoing medical problems such as glaucoma or diabetes are not good candidates for laser surgery. The same is true of those with uncontrolled high blood pressure, autoimmune diseases, or certain eye diseases involving the cornea or retina. Pregnant women should not have refractive surgery of any kind because the refraction of the eye may change during pregnancy.

CATARACTS

A cataract is a clouding of the eye's lens that can lead to vision problems. If the lens of the eye thickens and becomes clouded or opaque, it becomes unable to focus or admit light properly. Some causes of cataracts include aging, diabetes, heavy metal poisoning, exposure to radiation, injury to the eye, and the use of certain drugs, such as steroids.

The main symptom of a developing cataract is a gradual, painless loss of vision. Cataracts are the number one cause of blindness in the world, although the vast majority of cataract conditions can be successfully treated with surgery. Occasionally, a cataract may swell and cause secondary glaucoma.

The most common form of cataract is the senile cataract, which typically affects people over sixty-five. This type of cataract is often caused by free radical damage. Exposure to ultraviolet rays and low-level radiation from x-rays leads to the formation of reactive chemical fragments in the eye's lens. The resistance of the lens begins to decline in older people. Free radicals attack the structural proteins, enzymes, and cell membranes of the lens. The free radicals in our food, water, and environment are probably a major factor in the increasing number of cataracts in our population.

NUTRIENTS

SUPPLEMENT	SUGGESTED DOSAGE	COMMENTS
Copper and manganese	3 mg daily. 10 mg daily. Take separately from calcium.	These minerals are important for proper healing and for retarding the growth of cataracts.
Glutathione	As directed on label.	An amino acid that is a potent antioxidant and aids in maintaining a healthy lens and protects against toxins. Has been shown to slow the progression of cataracts.
Grape seed extract	As directed on label.	A powerful antioxidant.
L-Lysine	As directed on label, on an empty stomach. Take with water or juice. Do not take with milk. Take with 50 mg vitamin B_6 and 100 mg vitamin C for better absorption.	Important in collagen formation, which is necessary for lens repair. Also neutralizes viruses implicated in lens damage. *Caution:* Do not take lysine for longer than 6 months at a time.
Pantothenic acid (vitamin B_5)	500 mg daily.	An anti-stress vitamin.
Selenium	200 mcg daily. If you are pregnant, do not exceed 40 mcg daily.	An important free radical destroyer that works synergistically with vitamin E.
Vitamin A plus carotenoid complex with lutein and zeaxanthin	25,000 IU daily. If you are pregnant, do not exceed 10,000 IU daily. As directed on label.	Vital for normal visual function. Precursors of vitamin A. Needed for all eye disorders.
Vitamin B complex plus extra vitamin B_1 (thiamine) and vitamin B_2 (riboflavin)	As directed on label. 50 mg daily. 50 mg daily.	B vitamins work best when taken together. Important for intracellular eye metabolism. Deficiency has been linked to cataracts.

Vitamin C with bioflavonoids	3,000 mg 4 times daily.	A necessary free radical destroyer that also lowers intraocular pressure.
Vitamin E	400 IU daily.	An important free radical destroyer. Has been shown to arrest and reverse cataract formation in some cases. Use d-alpha-tocopherol form.
Zinc	50 mg daily. Do not exceed a total of 100 mg daily from all supplements.	Protects against light-induced damage. Use zinc gluconate lozenges or OptiZinc for best absorption.

Herbs

❑ Bilberry extract, taken orally, supplies bioflavonoids that aid in removing toxic chemicals from the retina of the eye.

❑ Ginkgo biloba improves microcapillary circulation.

Recommendations

❑ Increase your consumption of green leafy vegetables, especially collard greens, kale, mustard greens, spinach, and turnip greens; legumes; yellow vegetables; flavonoid-rich berries such as blueberries, blackberries, and cherries; and foods rich in vitamins E and C, such as raw fruits and vegetables.

❑ Avoid dairy products, saturated fats, and any fats or oils that have been subjected to heat, whether by cooking or processing. These foods promote formation of free radicals, which can damage the lens. Use cold-pressed vegetable oils only.

❑ Drink quality water, preferably steam-distilled water. This is absolutely necessary in cataract prevention. Avoid fluoridated and chlorinated water. Even water from deeply driven wells may not be safe, since many aquifers (underground water sources), especially those located near or under farmland, are contaminated with toxic residue from farm runoff.

❑ Avoid direct sunlight. Wear a a wide-brimmed hat when outdoors, and protect your eyes by wearing sunglasses (polarized) that block ultraviolet rays. Make sure the sunglasses are large enough to adequately protect your eyes.

❑ If you have cataracts, avoid antihistamines.

Considerations

❑ Several studies have found that people who eat foods rich in lutein and zeaxanthin—broccoli, collard greens, kale, mustard greens, spinach, and turnip greens—are much less likely to develop age-related cataracts than those who do not include these foods in their diets. These foods also are effective in reducing risk of macular degeneration. Researchers believe lutein and zeaxanthin act as anti-oxidants, protecting the cells in the eyes from free radical damage.

❑ Taking vitamin C supplements for at least a decade and eating a diet rich in antioxidants can lower the risk of cataracts, according to researchers at the Harvard Medical School.

❑ A study published by the *Journal of Pineal Research* showed that melatonin was very effective in preventing laboratory-induced cataracts in rats. A control group of rats not given melatonin developed cataracts in 89 percent of the cases, whereas only 7 percent of the rats that had received melatonin developed cataracts. It is known that melatonin production slows with age, and most cataract cases develop in people who are sixty or older. Melatonin is known to be a powerful antioxidant, with the ability to permeate every level of the cell. Its effectiveness against cataract formation in humans needs to be studied further, however.

❑ A number of heavy metals increase in concentration in the lenses of both aging people and people with cataracts. Cadmium, for instance, is found at levels two or three times higher than normal in lenses with cataracts. Concentrations of other metals, such as cobalt, nickel, iridium, and bromine, also are elevated.

❑ An article in *Science* magazine reported that the single greatest cause of cataracts is the body's inability to cope with food sugars. Lactose (milk sugar) was the worst offender, followed by refined white sugar. Many eye specialists note that most people with cataracts eat diets that include substantial amounts of dairy products and refined white sugar. Cataracts can also develop if the diet is inadequate and prolonged stress is endured.

❑ People who are deficient in the enzyme that converts galactose into glucose (ordinary blood sugar) develop cataracts much sooner than the rest of the population.

❑ Smoking is a risk factor for cataracts, probably because the free radicals it generates increase the oxidant stress on the body. A study of cigarette smoking and the risk of cataracts reported in the *Journal of the American Medical Association* found a significant association between smoking and the incidence of cataracts.

❑ The conventional treatment for cataracts is surgery. In cataract surgery, the eye's own dysfunctional lens is removed, and usually is replaced with a prosthetic intraocular lens implant made of plastic or silicone. The lens may be removed whole, or a surgical procedure called phacoemulsification (often called the "phaco" technique) may be used. In this operation, the surgeon makes one minuscule incision, inserts the tip of a vibrating instrument into the cataract, and beats it until it turns liquid. The liquid is then sucked out and a new lens is implanted. With this type of surgery, the incision is only one-tenth of an inch long, compared to conventional one-third inch or one-half inch incisions. Another method used is extracapsular surgery, in which a slightly longer incision is made on the side of the cornea. The surgeon then removes the hard center of the lens, and the remainder of the lens is removed by suction.

COLORBLINDNESS

Colorblindness is a general term for the inability to see colors as most people see them. Specialized cells in the retina known as cones, which are vital for translating light waves into a perception of color, may be completely or partially lacking, or may not function properly, resulting in colorblindness. There are different types and varying severities of this condition. Most colorblind people confuse certain colors (they may not be able to tell red from green, for example); in rare cases, an individual may see no color at all. Some can distinguish colors only in certain lights.

There are also certain diseases, including pernicious anemia and sickle cell disease, as well as a number of different medications, that can cause disturbances in color vision.

Because few people are tested for color vision, colorblindness is probably an underdiagnosed condition, especially among women. In most cases, colorblindness is present from birth, although the dimming of vision caused by cataracts can diminish a person's ability to distinguish colors later in life.

NUTRIENTS

SUPPLEMENT	SUGGESTED DOSAGE	COMMENTS
Vitamin A plus carotenoid complex with lutein	25,000 IU daily. If you are pregnant, do not exceed 10,000 IU daily. As directed on label.	May be helpful because it is essential for proper functioning of the cones in the retina. Also improves night blindness. Use emulsion form, which is safe at higher doses than capsules.
Vitamin B$_{12}$	1,000–2,000 mcg daily.	Deficiency can lead to yellow-blue colorblindness.

CONJUNCTIVITIS (PINKEYE)

Conjunctivitis is an inflammation of the conjunctiva—the membrane that lines the eyelid and wraps around to cover most of the white of the eye. The eyes may appear swollen and bloodshot; they are often itchy and irritated. Because the infected membrane is often filled with pus, the eyelids are apt to stick together after being closed for an extended period.

Factors that can contribute to conjunctivitis include bacterial infection, virus, injury to the eye, allergies, and exposure to substances that are irritating to the eye, such as fumes, smoke, contact lens solutions, chlorine from swimming pools, chemicals, makeup, or any other foreign substance that enters the eye. Conjunctivitis is highly contagious if it is caused by a viral infection.

NUTRIENTS

SUPPLEMENT	SUGGESTED DOSAGE	COMMENTS
Vitamin A plus carotenoid complex with lutein and zeaxanthin	25,000 IU daily for 1 month; then reduce to 15,000 IU daily. If you are pregnant, do not exceed 10,000 IU daily. As directed on label.	Vitamin A, vitamin C, and zinc all help to promote immunity, which is especially important in common viral conjunctivitis. Use an emulsion form for easier assimilation and greater safety at high doses.
Vitamin C with bioflavonoids	2,000–6,000 mg daily, in divided doses.	Protects the eye from further inflammation. Enhances healing.
Zinc	50 mg daily. Do not exceed a total of 100 mg daily from all supplements.	Enhances immune response. Use zinc gluconate lozenges or OptiZinc for best absorption.

Herbs

❑ Calendula, chamomile, fennel, and/or eyebright herbal teas can be used to make hot compresses. Eyebright can also be taken orally in capsule or tea form. It is good for any eye irritation or inflammation. The tea can also be used to rinse the eyes.

❑ Goldenseal, used as an alternative or in addition to eyebright, is very useful if conjunctivitis is caused by infection.

Caution: Do not take goldenseal internally on a daily basis for more than one week at a time. Do not use it during pregnancy.

Recommendations

❑ Increase your consumption of green leafy vegetables—especially collard greens, kale, mustard greens, spinach, and turnip greens; legumes; yellow vegetables; flavonoid-rich berries such as blueberries, blackberries, and cherries; and foods rich in vitamins E and C, such as raw fruits and vegetables.

❑ Apply hot compresses several times a day. Many of the microorganisms that cause conjunctivitis cannot tolerate heat. For greater benefit, use one of the herbal teas recommended above to make the compresses.

❑ If pain or blurred vision occurs, seek medical attention immediately. These can be signs of a more serious problem.

❑ If your eyelids are swollen, try peeling and grating a fresh potato, wrapping it with gauze, and placing it over your eyes. This acts as an astringent and has a healing effect.

Considerations

❑ Pinkeye associated with hay fever can be treated with prescription drops containing steroids.

❏ A bacterial infection is typically treated with antibiotics if the eye does not improve within four days of using compresses and taking supplements.

CORNEAL ULCER

If the cornea—the membrane covering the front of the eye—is damaged, the eye becomes inflamed and vulnerable to infection that can result in ulceration. Damage may occur as a result of injury, a foreign body in the eye, or excessive or inappropriate wearing of contact lenses. The infections that can result in ulceration of the cornea may be caused by viruses, bacteria, or fungi.

NUTRIENTS

SUPPLEMENT	SUGGESTED DOSAGE	COMMENTS
Vitamin A plus carotenoid complex with lutein and zeaxanthin	25,000 IU daily. If you are pregnant, do not exceed 10,000 IU daily. As directed on label.	Needed for all eye disorders.
Vitamin C with bioflavonoids	6,000 mg daily, in divided doses.	A healing and antiviral substance.

Recommendations

❏ If you suspect that a corneal ulcer may be developing, consult a physician immediately.

DIABETIC RETINOPATHY

Diabetes can cause retinopathy, a disorder in which some of the tiny capillaries that nourish the retina leak fluid or blood that can damage the rod and cone cells. New capillaries then begin to form in the injured area, and these also interfere with vision. Problems with the blood vessels can cause retinal hemorrhage (leakage from the vessels that transmit the fluids of the eye), microaneurysms (abnormally enlarged blood vessels in the eye), retinal edema (the accumulation of fluid in the eye), and perhaps, loss of vision. Diabetic retinopathy affects about 7 million Americans and causes blindness among about 7,000 each year. Unfortunately, there are few warning signs; the condition usually causes no symptoms until it is relatively advanced.

NUTRIENTS

SUPPLEMENT	SUGGESTED DOSAGE	COMMENTS
Vitamin A plus carotenoid complex with lutein and zeaxanthin	25,000 IU daily. If you are pregnant, do not exceed 10,000 IU daily. As directed on label.	Needed for all eye disorders.
Shark cartilage (BeneFin)	1 gm per 15 lbs of body weight daily, divided into 3 doses. If you cannot tolerate taking it orally, it can be administered rectally in a retention enema.	To prevent or possibly halt the progression of the condition by inhibiting the growth of tiny blood vessels in the eye that contribute to vision loss.

Recommendations

❏ *See* DIABETES in Part Two and follow the dietary recommendations.

❏ If you have diabetes, make sure to have an annual eye examination to detect the onset of retinopathy. If the disorder is detected in time, laser surgery to seal leaking blood vessels can help stem vision loss.

Considerations

❏ One study reported that people with insulin-dependent (type 1) diabetes who controlled their blood sugar levels tightly were able to slow the pace of retinopathy by about 60 percent.

❏ Researchers at the National Eye Institute induced a condition resembling diabetic retinopathy in dogs and then treated the animals with an experimental drug called sorbinil, which suppresses the action of an enzyme that converts excess sugar in the blood into an alcohol that seems to damage the retinal blood vessels. In this study, the sorbinil treatment totally blocked the progression of retinopathy.

DIMNESS OR LOSS OF VISION

Many different conditions can lead to a dimming or loss of vision. Among the most common are cataracts, glaucoma, and diabetic retinopathy. Macular degeneration and retinitis pigmentosa are less common, but do occur with some frequency. There are others as well. *Retinal detachment* causes a loss of vision often compared to having a curtain drawn across one's field of vision. Loss of vision may be preceded by a shower of "sparks" or lightning-like flashes of light, or by a dramatic increase in the number of black floaters in the field of vision. (*See* FLOATERS in this section.) *Uveitis* is an inflammation in the middle layer of the eye, which consists of the iris, the ciliary body, and the choroid. In many cases it is caused by an underlying systemic disease such as rheumatoid arthritis or infection. Pain and redness may be present, but often symptoms consist primarily of diminished or hazy vision. Another condition that can lead to loss of vision is *blockage of a blood vessel serving the retina,* usually by a blood clot. Visual loss is generally sudden if the affected blood vessel is an artery, but it may be less rapid if the blocked vessel is a vein. Usually only one eye is affected.

Inflammation of the optic nerve is another possible cause of vision loss. Such inflammation may occur as a result of a systemic illness or infection, but in many cases the cause cannot be determined. This condition usually affects only one eye but it may affect both, causing varying degrees of vision loss over the course of a few days. *Toxic amblyopia* is a condition in which a toxic reaction damages the optic nerve, creating a small "hole" in the field of vision that enlarges over a period of time and may even lead to blindness. In most cases, both eyes are affected. This disorder is most common in people who smoke—in fact, it is sometimes referred to as *tobacco amblyopia*—and is seen most often in pipe smokers. It may also occur in those who consume excessive amounts of alcohol or who come into contact with lead, methanol, chloramphenicol, digitalis, ethambutol, and other chemicals.

Recommendations

❏ If any of the above symptoms develop, consult a physician. For most of these conditions, prompt treatment may help to preserve sight or at least slow vision loss.

❏ Do not smoke, and avoid those who do. Even people who have already developed toxic amblyopia as a result of smoking can have their vision improve if they quit.

Considerations

❏ The syndromes discussed here are usually painless. Physical discomfort is not a reliable indicator of visual health. Regular ophthalmic examinations are recommended for everyone over thirty-five.

❏ *See also* CATARACTS; DIABETIC RETINOPATHY; GLAUCOMA; MACULAR DEGENERATION; and RETINITIS PIGMENTOSA in this section.

DRY EYES

Dry eyes occur when the tear ducts do not produce enough fluid (tears) to keep the eyes moist, resulting in burning and irritation. This problem is more common in women than in men, and women's susceptibility increases after menopause. Contact lens wearers are particularly prone to developing dry eye problems. Dry eyes generally stem from a lack of vitamin A, and are more likely to affect people over the age of sixty-five. Some drugs are known to inhibit tear production or change the composition of tears, including antihistamines, decongestants, and various drugs used to control Parkinson's disease and high blood pressure.

NUTRIENTS

SUPPLEMENT	SUGGESTED DOSAGE	COMMENTS
Primrose oil	1,000 mg 2–3 times daily.	A source of essential fatty acids.
Vitamin A ointment and/or	As directed on label.	Beneficial for eyes that seem dry and scratchy. Tears contain vitamin A.
vitamin A	25,000 IU daily. If you are pregnant, do not exceed 10,000 IU daily.	
plus carotenoid complex with lutein and zeaxanthin	As directed on label.	Needed for all eye disorders.

Recommendations

❏ Drink at least eight glasses (sixty-four ounces) of water every day. Steam-distilled water is best.

❏ See your health care provider if you have dry eyes. It may be a symptom of a more serious condition, such as rheumatoid arthritis or lupus. Also, constant irritation to the eye as a result of dryness can result in injury and damage.

❏ If your tear ducts are swollen, add more calcium to your diet and avoid processed foods.

❏ Artificial tears are safe and effective for keeping the eyes moist. Choose a product that is preservative-free, such as Cellufresh from Allergan, Dry Eye Therapy from Bausch & Lomb, or Tears Naturale from Alcon.

❏ Similasan Eye Drops #1 and #2 are soothing homeopathic eyedrops containing *Belladonna, Euphrasia,* and *Mercurius sublamitus;* and *Apis mellifica, Euphrasia,* and *Sabadilla,* respectively.

❏ Use a humidifier to add moisture to the dry air.

❏ Wear wraparound glasses on windy days.

❏ Avoid cigarette smoke and other types of smoke.

❏ Avoid products that claim they can "get the red out." Some over-the-counter drops used to relieve red and sore eyes contain vasoconstrictors that can further dry your eyes, especially if used for an extended period of time.

❏ Limit your use of hair dryers. Allow your hair to dry naturally. Shield your eyes from direct heat blasts from hair dryers and other heat sources.

Considerations

❏ In some cases, an ophthalmologist may perform a procedure to close the internal tear ducts, through which some tears drain from the eyes into the nose, to conserve tears and keep the eyes moist.

❏ Contact lenses made of a material called sulfoxide hydrogel may hold promise for people who currently cannot wear contact lenses because they are prone to dry eyes or frequent eye infections. The new material holds more water than current lens materials. It is currently being tested in clinical trials.

❏ Sjögren's syndrome is a disorder that can cause dryness in the eyes.

EYESTRAIN

Eyestrain causes a dull, aching sensation around and behind the eyes that can expand into a generalized headache. It may feel painful or fatiguing to focus the eyes. Eyestrain is commonly a result of overuse of the eyes for activities requiring close, precise focus, such as reading or computer work. People in certain occupations, such as jewelers, are particularly prone to eyestrain. Wearing improper lenses (whether the wrong prescription or an incorrectly made pair of glasses) can also cause eyestrain.

Acute closed-angle glaucoma can cause pain around the eyes as well, but the sensation is usually sharp and throbbing and accompanied by other symptoms. Most other eye disorders, even serious ones, cause little or no discomfort.

NUTRIENTS

SUPPLEMENT	SUGGESTED DOSAGE	COMMENTS
Vitamin A	25,000 IU daily. If you are pregnant, do not exceed 10,000 IU daily.	Needed for all eye disorders.
plus carotenoid complex with lutein and zeaxanthin	As directed on label.	
Vitamin B complex	50–100 mg of each major B vitamin daily (amounts of individual vitamins in a complex will vary).	Improves intraocular cellular metabolism.
plus extra vitamin B₂ (riboflavin)	25 mg 3 times daily.	Helps to alleviate eye fatigue.

Herbs

❑ Taking eyebright in capsule or tea form can be helpful. Eyebright tea can also be used to rinse the eyes.

❑ Goldenseal can be used as an alternative or in addition to eyebright.

Caution: Do not take goldenseal internally on a daily basis for more than one week at a time, do not use it during pregnancy, and use it with caution if you are allergic to ragweed.

Recommendations

❑ Lie down, close your eyes, and place a cold compress over your eyes. Relax for ten minutes or longer, replacing the compress with a fresh one as necessary. This often helps to alleviate discomfort. You can also try using a wet tea bag or cold cucumber slices. The cold shrinks the swollen blood vessels.

❑ Take measures to avoid eyestrain. Try to vary your tasks so that your eyes change focusing distance every so often. When doing close work for prolonged periods, take periodic "focus breaks." Every twenty minutes or so, look away from your work and focus your eyes on something in the distance for a minute or two.

❑ If you work with computers for long periods of time, take a five- or ten-minute break every hour. Focus on distant objects as often as possible. Position the computer monitor to reduce glare from all light sources. Try a glare-reduction filter that carries a seal of approval by the American Optometric Association. If possible, use an active-matrix LCD flat display, which is sharper and brighter than a typical CRT-based display.

❑ Get sufficient sleep. Fatigue promotes eyestrain.

❑ If pain is severe and comes on suddenly, and especially if vision is disturbed or the pain is accompanied by nausea and vomiting, seek professional help at once. This may be a sign of an acute glaucoma attack. (*See* GLAUCOMA in Part Two.)

FLOATERS

Bits of cellular debris floating within the eye are commonly referred to as floaters. Because these floaters cast shadows over the retina, the individual sees small specks that move slowly before the eyes, especially in certain lights and against certain backgrounds. Older adults and nearsighted people are most likely to complain of floaters. Most floaters eventually become less noticeable and are considered benign. Floaters that coalesce into long, stringy strands may be caused by a disorder called *fibrillar degeneration of the vitreous.* This condition is usually caused by excessive exposure to sunlight.

NUTRIENTS

SUPPLEMENT	SUGGESTED DOSAGE	COMMENTS
Apple pectin	As directed on label.	Chelates heavy metals that can circulate through the eyes.
L-Methionine	As directed on label, on an empty stomach. Take with water or juice. Do not take with milk. Take with 50 mg vitamin B₆ and 100 mg vitamin C for better absorption.	Chelates heavy metals. (*See* AMINO ACIDS in Part One.)
Oxy-5000 Forte from American Biologics	As directed on label.	A potent nutritional antioxidant for health and stress that destroys free radicals.
Vitamin A	25,000 IU daily. If you are pregnant, do not exceed 10,000 IU daily.	Needed for all eye disorders.
plus carotenoid complex with lutein and zeaxanthin	As directed on label.	

Recommendations

❑ It is normal to see a few floaters at times, but if you suddenly see a large number of them, consult an ophthalmologist. This may be a sign of developing retinal detachment. Delaying treatment can result in a detached retina requiring lengthy surgery.

GLAUCOMA

Glaucoma is a serious eye disease marked by an increase in the pressure that the fluids within the eyeball exert on other parts of the eye. If this pressure is unrelieved, it may harm the retina and ultimately damage the optic nerve, resulting in vision loss, even blindness. It is most common in people over thirty-five, in nearsighted people, and in people with high blood pressure. *See* GLAUCOMA in Part Two for a more complete discussion of this condition.

HYPEROPIA

See under BLURRED VISION in this section.

ITCHY OR TIRED EYES

Itchy or tired eyes can be the result of many different factors, including allergies, eyestrain, fatigue, infection (conjunctivitis), and an inadequate supply of oxygen to the cornea and outer eye tissues.

NUTRIENTS

SUPPLEMENT	SUGGESTED DOSAGE	COMMENTS
Vitamin A	25,000 IU daily. If you are pregnant, do not exceed 10,000 IU daily.	Needed for all eye disorders.
plus carotenoid complex with lutein and zeaxanthin	As directed on label.	
Vitamin B complex plus extra	50–100 mg daily.	Improves intraocular cellular metabolism.
vitamin B$_2$ (riboflavin)	50 mg daily.	Helps improve oxygenation of eye tissues.

Recommendations

❏ For quick relief of occasional itchy or tired eyes, close your eyes and apply a cold compress. Leave the compress in place for ten minutes. Compresses can be used as often as necessary.

Considerations

❏ If the problem is a recurrent one, allergies are a likely culprit. (*See* ALLERGIES in Part Two.)

❏ If itching and aching are accompanied by a bright pink or red color and thick secretions, you may have conjunctivitis. (*See* CONJUNCTIVITIS in this section.)

❏ If itchy and tired eyes persist over a long period of time, there may be an underlying nutritional cause. Supplement your diet with the B vitamins as described under Nutrients, above.

MACULAR DEGENERATION

This disorder causes a progressive visual loss due to degeneration of the macula, the portion of the retina responsible for fine vision. Macular degeneration is the leading cause of severe visual loss in the United States and Europe in people over fifty-five years old. This loss of vision may appear suddenly or it may progress slowly. Usually peripheral and color vision are unaffected.

There are two types of macular degeneration: atrophic (or "dry") and exudative ("wet"). In the latter type, the degeneration of the macula is accompanied by hemorrhaging or leaking of fluid from a network of tiny blood vessels that develop under the center of the retina. This results in scarring and loss of vision.

Macular degeneration is probably the result of free radical damage similar to the type of damage that induces cataracts. Factors that predispose a person to developing macular degeneration include aging, atherosclerosis, hypertension, and environmental toxins. Heredity may play a role as well.

NUTRIENTS

SUPPLEMENT	SUGGESTED DOSAGE	COMMENTS
Coenzyme Q$_{10}$ plus	60 mg daily.	Powerful antioxidants protect against macular degeneration.
Coenzyme A from Coenzyme-A Technologies	As directed on label.	
Grape seed extract	As directed on label.	A powerful antioxidant that protects against free radical damage.
Orbitol from Neways	As directed on label.	Contains bilberry, eyebright, beta-carotene and many other nutrients for the eyes.
Selenium	400 mcg daily.	An important antioxidant.
Shark cartilage (BeneFin)	1 gm per 15 lbs of body weight daily, divided into 3 doses. If you cannot tolerate taking it orally, it can be administered rectally in a retention enema.	To prevent and possibly halt the progression of exudative macular degeneration by inhibiting the growth of tiny blood vessels in the eye that contribute to vision loss.
Vitamin A plus	25,000 IU daily.	Potent antioxidant and important in eye function.
carotenoid complex with lutein and zeaxanthin	As directed on label.	Use emulsion form for easier assimilation and greater safety at high doses.
Vitamin C plus bioflavonoids	1,000–2,500 mg 4 times daily.	An important antioxidant and a necessary free radical destroyer. Prevents eye damage; also relieves pressure from cataracts.
Vitamin E	600–800 IU daily.	An important antioxidant and free radical destroyer. Use d-alpha-tocopherol form.
Zinc plus	45–80 mg daily. Do not exceed a total of 100 mg daily from all supplements.	Deficiency has been linked to eye disorders. Use zinc picolinate form.
copper	3 mg daily.	Needed to balance with zinc.

Herbs

❏ Clinical studies have shown that taking bilberry extract (160 milligrams and up daily) and eating fresh blueberries (8 to 10 ounces per day), plus taking ginkgo biloba extract and zinc, can help halt the loss of vision. Blueberries are rich in valuable bioflavonoids. Treatment at an early stage is most effective.

Recommendations

❑ Increase your consumption of green, leafy vegetables, especially collard greens, kale, mustard greens, spinach, and turnip greens; legumes; yellow vegetables; flavonoid-rich berries such as blueberries, blackberries, and cherries; and foods rich in vitamins E and C, such as raw fruits and vegetables.

❑ Avoid alcohol, cigarette smoke, all sugars, saturated fats, and foods containing fats and oils that have been subjected to heat and/or exposed to the air, such as fried foods, hamburgers, luncheon meats, and roasted nuts.

Considerations

❑ In a study reported in the *Archives of Ophthalmology*, ophthalmologists at Louisiana State University Medical School tested the effects of supplemental zinc on people suffering from macular degeneration. Half the group received a 100-milligram tablet of zinc twice a day; the other half received a placebo. After twelve to twenty-four months, the zinc group showed significantly less deterioration than the placebo group.

❑ Antioxidant nutrients are known to protect against macular degeneration, but two in particular—lutein and zeaxanthin—are believed to play a critical role in the prevention of the disease. A study by Johanna M. Seddon, M.D., of the Massachusetts Eye and Ear Infirmary in Boston, compared the diets of 356 patients with macular degeneration with 520 patients with other eye diseases. The data revealed that beta-carotene was not especially effective, but that lutein and zeaxanthin were. Some foods that contain lutein and zeaxanthin are collard greens, kale, mustard greens, and turnip greens.

MUCUS IN THE EYES

A number of different conditions can cause mucus to accumulate in the eyes, such as allergies, head colds, and infection (conjunctivitis).

Herbs

❑ Gently and carefully wash each eye with diluted alcohol-free goldenseal extract or cool goldenseal tea.

Caution: Do not use goldenseal during pregnancy, and use it with caution if you are allergic to ragweed.

MYOPIA

See under BLURRED VISION in this section.

PHOTOPHOBIA

Photophobia is an abnormal inability of the eyes to tolerate light; exposure to light hurts the eyes. It is more common in people with light-colored eyes, and usually is not a serious problem. In some cases, however, it may be associated with

irritation or damage to the cornea, acute glaucoma, or uveitis. It can also be a symptom of developing measles.

NUTRIENTS

SUPPLEMENT	SUGGESTED DOSAGE	COMMENTS
Vitamin A plus carotenoid complex with lutein and zeaxanthin	25,000 IU daily. If you are pregnant, do not exceed 10,000 IU daily. As directed on label.	Needed for all eye disorders.

Considerations

❑ *See also* GLAUCOMA and/or MEASLES, both in Part Two.

❑ *See also* the discussion of uveitis *under* Dimness or Loss of Vision in this section.

PINKEYE

See CONJUNCTIVITIS in this section.

RETINAL EDEMA

See DIABETIC RETINOPATHY in this section.

RETINAL HEMORRHAGE

See DIABETIC RETINOPATHY in this section.

RETINITIS PIGMENTOSA

Retinitis pigmentosa is a group of inherited diseases that affects approximately one of every 3,700 people. The retina is the innermost layer that lines the eyeball. It contains photoreceptor cells that are directly connected to the brain by the optic nerve. Retinitis pigmentosa causes these photoreceptor cells to degenerate over time. The first symptom usually is loss of night vision, beginning in adolescence or young adulthood. This is followed by loss of peripheral vision and, ultimately, blindness, which sets in anywhere between the ages of thirty and eighty. *Usher syndrome* is a variation of retinitis pigmentosa that also impairs hearing. (*See* HEARING LOSS in Part Two).

NUTRIENTS

SUPPLEMENT	SUGGESTED DOSAGE	COMMENTS
Coenzyme Q_{10}	60 mg daily.	A powerful antioxidant that can improve retinitis pigmentosa symptoms.
Vitamin A plus carotenoid complex with lutein and zeaxanthin	15,000 IU daily. If you are pregnant, do not exceed 10,000 IU daily. As directed on label.	Helpful for all eye disorders. Use emulsion form for easier assimilation and greater safety at higher doses.

Recommendations

❏ Get a thorough eye evaluation by an eye care professional who specializes in retinitis pigmentosa. An accurate diagnosis can sometimes be difficult to obtain, but it is getting more reliable through better awareness and more sophisticated technology.

Considerations

❏ High doses of vitamin A may be able to slow the loss of remaining eyesight by about 20 percent per year in some cases, according to a 1993 study led by Eliot Berson, M.D., professor of ophthalmology at Harvard Medical School. At the same time, the study found that high doses of supplemental vitamin E (400 international units or more daily) can be detrimental to people with retinitis pigmentosa.

❏ Retinal cell transplantation and gene therapy are still in the preliminary stages of research, but both may prove to be effective in treating retinitis pigmentosa. Photoreceptor cells have been successfully transplanted into the retinas of animals. The Foundation Fighting Blindness reports that it remains to be seen whether or not this procedure would be effective with retinitis pigmentosa-type disorders. Meanwhile, researchers have identified many of the mutated genes that contribute to retinitis pigmentosa. It may become possible in the future to use gene therapy—replace defective genes with normal ones—to treat the disorder.

❏ More information on this disorder can be obtained by calling the Foundation Fighting Blindness (see HEALTH AND MEDICAL ORGANIZATIONS in the Appendix.)

SCOTOMA

A scotoma is a blind spot in the visual field. Unless a scotoma is large or is located in the center of the field of vision, it may not be noticed. However, a professional can detect scotomas with a type of examination called a visual field test.

Scotomas are considered a symptom of disease, not a disease in themselves. They may be a sign of a problem with the retina or damage to the optic nerve, such as that caused by glaucoma.

NUTRIENTS

SUPPLEMENT	SUGGESTED DOSAGE	COMMENTS
Vitamin A plus carotenoid complex with lutein and zeaxanthin	25,000 IU daily for 2 months. If you are pregnant, do not exceed 10,000 IU daily. As directed on label.	Essential for eye health. Use emulsion form for easier assimilation and greater safety at higher doses.

SHINGLES (HERPES ZOSTER)

Shingles is an infection caused by the varicella-zoster virus, a member of the herpes family and the same virus that causes chickenpox. The characteristic symptom is a rash of painful blisters. Shingles can appear anywhere on the body. If it occurs on the forehead near the eyes or on the tip of the nose, the eyes are likely to become involved, and damage to the cornea can occur. Taking the proper supplements when blisters first appear can make the blisters dry up quickly, and the discomfort may be alleviated.

NUTRIENTS

SUPPLEMENT	SUGGESTED DOSAGE	COMMENTS
L-Lysine	1,000 mg daily, on an empty stomach. Take with water or juice. Do not take with milk. Take with 50 mg vitamin B6 and 100 mg vitamin C for better absorption.	Fights herpesviruses. (See AMINO ACIDS in Part One.) Caution: Do not take lysine longer than 6 months at a time.
Vitamin A plus carotenoid complex with lutein and zeaxanthin	25,000 IU daily. If you are pregnant, do not exceed 10,000 IU daily. As directed on label.	Needed for all eye disorders.
Vitamin B12	1,000–2,000 mcg daily, on an empty stomach.	Prevents damage to the nerves in the eyes. Use a lozenge or sublingual form.
Vitamin C with bioflavonoids	2,000–6,000 mg daily and up.	An antiviral and immune system enhancer.
Vitamin E	1,000 IU daily. If you have high blood pressure and have not taken vitamin E previously, start with 400 IU daily and slowly increase to 800 IU daily.	Helps to prevent scarring and tissue damage. Use d-alpha-tocopherol form.

Recommendations

❏ If shingles appear on the forehead near the eyes or on the tip of the nose, seek treatment from an ophthalmologist.

❏ Apply zinc oxide cream to the blisters and the affected area. After the blisters have healed over, apply aloe vera gel and vitamin E to the area.

Considerations

❏ If zinc oxide, aloe vera gel, and/or vitamin E do not work to heal the blisters within three days, intravenous injections of 25 grams of vitamin C should provide relief almost immediately.

❏ See also SHINGLES in Part Two.

STYE

A stye is a bacterial infection within an oil gland on the edge of the eyelid. Because the tissues of the eye become inflamed from the infection, the stye takes on the appearance of a small pimple. This pimple gradually comes to a head, opens, and drains. Early treatment speeds the healing process and helps to avoid further complications.

Herbs

❑ Prepare raspberry leaf tea and use it as an eyewash to alleviate styes.

Recommendations

❑ Apply a hot compress to the affected area for ten minutes four to six times daily to help relieve discomfort and bring the stye to a head so that it can drain and healing can begin.

❑ If you suffer from styes frequently, supplement your diet with vitamin A. Recurring styes are often a sign of vitamin A deficiency.

Considerations

❑ If a stye does not heal promptly, it may need to be drained. This is a procedure that must be done by a health care professional. *Do not* squeeze the lump or attempt to drain it at home. This can cause the infection to spread into the bloodstream, leading to systemic illness.

❑ In severe and/or stubborn cases, treatment with antibiotics may be necessary.

THINNING EYELASHES

Many problems can lead to a thinning or even the total loss of the eyelashes. Among these are allergies, especially contact allergies to eye makeup; the use of certain drugs; exposure to environmental toxins; hypothyroidism; eye surgery; a poor diet and/or nutritional deficiencies; and trauma.

NUTRIENTS

SUPPLEMENT	SUGGESTED DOSAGE	COMMENTS
Vitamin A	25,000 IU daily. If you are pregnant, do not exceed 10,000 IU daily.	Promotes healthy skin and hair.
plus carotenoid complex with lutein and zeaxanthin	As directed on label.	Needed for all eye disorders.
Vitamin B complex plus extra	50–100 mg daily.	The B vitamins help prevent loss of eyelashes.
vitamin B₂ (riboflavin) and	As directed on label.	
vitamin B₃ (niacin) plus	As directed on label.	
brewer's yeast	2 tbsp daily.	A good source of B vitamins.

Recommendations

❑ Gently rub vitamin E oil on your eyelashes and into your eyelids at bedtime. This helps to thicken the lashes and promote normal growth.

ULCERATED EYE

See CORNEAL ULCER in this section.

ULCERATED EYELID

If an eyelid is scratched and the scratch becomes infected, an ulcerated area may develop. Ulcerated eyelids also can occur as a result of chronic blepharitis.

XEROPHTHALMIA

Xerophthalmia is an inflammation of the cornea that is associated with nutritional deficiency, especially a deficiency of vitamin A. The cornea becomes dry, and infection and/or ulceration may set in. Bitot's spots may appear, and night blindness may occur.

NUTRIENTS

SUPPLEMENT	SUGGESTED DOSAGE	COMMENTS
Vitamin A	25,000 daily. If you are pregnant, do not exceed 10,000 IU daily.	Specifically for dry eyes.
plus carotenoid complex with lutein and zeaxanthin	As directed on label.	Needed for all eye disorders.
Vitamin B₆ (pyridoxine) and	50 mg daily.	Nutrients that work well together to heal dry eyes.
vitamin C with bioflavonoids and	2,000–14,000 mg daily, in divided doses.	
zinc	50 mg daily. Do not exceed a total of 100 mg daily from all supplements.	Use zinc gluconate lozenges or OptiZinc for best absorption.

Considerations

❑ *See also* Bitot's Spots in this section.

Fatigue

See CHRONIC FATIGUE SYNDROME.

Fever

A fever is an elevation in body temperature. Fever is not a disease, but a symptom that may indicate the presence of disease.

Normal body temperature ranges from 97°F to 99°F. It varies from individual to individual. Rectal temperature is usually about 1°F higher than oral temperature, and body temperature varies in the course of the day—it usually increases in the afternoon. Women have a higher temperature after ovulation than before ovulation.

One should not have undue concern unless body temperature rises above 102°F (103°F in children). Often, running a temperature is helpful to the body. This defense mechanism of the body acts to destroy harmful microbes. A part of the brain called the hypothalamus regulates body temperature by regulating heat loss, mainly from the skin. When destructive microbes or tumor cells invade the body, the immune cells rushing to fight them release proteins that tell the hypothalamus to raise the temperature. Moderate temperatures (under 103°F for adults) encourage the body to manufacture more immune cells.

There are some situations, however, in which fever can cause problems. A high fever (104°F or higher) may pose a risk for people with cardiac problems, since it makes the heart beat faster and work harder, and can cause irregular heart rhythms, chest pain, or heart attack. Fever over 106°F, especially for prolonged periods, can cause dehydration and brain injury.

Unless otherwise specified, the dosages recommended here are for adults. For a child between the ages of twelve and seventeen, reduce the dose to three-quarters the recommended amount. For a child between six and twelve, use one-half the recommended dose, and for a child under the age of six, use one-quarter the recommended amount.

NUTRIENTS

SUPPLEMENT	SUGGESTED DOSAGE	COMMENTS
Very Important		
Dioxychlor from American Biologics	Take sublingually, as directed on label.	An important antibacterial, antifungal, and antiviral agent.
Inflazyme Forte from American Biologics	As directed on label.	A balanced, potent enzyme complex that moderates the inflammatory response.
Vitamin A emulsion or	As directed on label.	Essential in immune system function. Needed to fight infection and to strengthen the immune system. Emulsion form is recommended because it enters the system more quickly.
capsules with carotenoids	For adults: 25,000 IU daily. If you are pregnant or nursing, do not exceed 10,000 IU daily. For children over 2 years: 1,000–10,000 IU daily	
Important		
Bio-Bifidus from American Biologics	As directed on label.	For bowel flora replacement to improve elimination and assimilation.
Free-form amino acid complex (Amino Balance from Anabol Naturals or Amino Blend from Carlson Labs)	As directed on label 3 times daily, on an empty stomach. Take with 50 mg each of vitamins B₆ and C for better absorption.	A readily absorbed form of protein that helps repair tissue damaged by fever.
Taurine Plus from American Biologics	As directed on label.	An important antioxidant and immune regulator, necessary for white blood cell activation and neurological function. Use the sublingual form.

Vitamin C with bioflavonoids	5,000–20,000 daily, in divided doses. *See* ASCORBIC ACID FLUSH in Part Three.	To flush out toxins and reduce fever. For a child, use calcium ascorbate form—it does not produce heavy diarrhea.
Helpful		
Garlic (Kyolic from Wakunaga)	2 capsules 3 times daily.	A natural antibiotic and powerful immunostimulant.
Royal jelly	As directed on label 3 times daily.	Has antifungal properties and improves adrenal function.
Spiru-tein from Nature's Plus	As directed on label, between meals.	A protein drink that contains all the amino acids, vitamins, and minerals needed for nourishment.

HERBS

❏ To bring a high fever down, use catnip tea enemas twice daily. These also relieve constipation and congestion, which keep fever up. (*See* ENEMAS in Part Three.)

❏ Catnip tea with dandelion and lobelia, taken in tea or extract form, is good for lowering fever. Lobelia can also be used on its own. Taking ½ teaspoon of lobelia extract or tincture every four hours helps to lower fever. If an upset stomach occurs, cut the dosage back to ¼ teaspoon.

Caution: Do not take lobelia internally on an ongoing basis.

❏ Elderberry tea and hot steam baths may help.

❏ You can make a poultice from echinacea root to lower fever. (*See* USING A POULTICE in Part Three.)

❏ A combination of hyssop, licorice root, thyme, and yarrow tea can help a fever.

Caution: Do not use licorice on a daily basis for more than seven days in a row. Avoid it completely if you have high blood pressure.

❏ Other beneficial herbs include blackthorn, echinacea, fenugreek seed, feverfew, ginger, and poke root.

Caution: Do not use feverfew during pregnancy.

RECOMMENDATIONS

❏ Replace fluid loss by drinking as much quality water as you can. This will also help to bring down body temperature.

❏ Get plenty of rest.

❏ Avoid radical changes in atmospheric temperature.

❏ Drink plenty of distilled water and juices, but avoid solid food until the fever breaks.

❏ While feverish, avoid taking any supplements that contain iron or zinc. When an infection is present, the body attempts to "hide" iron in the tissues in an attempt to keep the infecting organism from using it for nourishment. Taking a supplement containing iron therefore causes undue strain on a body that is fighting an infection. Zinc is not properly absorbed while a fever is present.

❑ Take cool sponge baths. Do not use rubbing alcohol to cool off, however; it gives off noxious fumes.

❑ To induce sweating, which may shorten the length of the fever, wrap up in a warm blanket or robe for twenty minutes. Replace lost fluids as soon as you can. However, lowering a fever is not always the best thing to do in an otherwise healthy adult.

❑ *Belladonna* and *Aconite napellus* are homeopathic remedies used to reduce fever. Use a 12x strength and dilute 5 drops of one or both of these remedies in a glass of water. Take this every half-hour or as needed.

❑ As long as a fever does not get too high (above 102°F), let it run its course. It helps to fight infection and eliminate toxins.

❑ If body temperature rises above 102°F (103°F in a child), take measures to reduce the fever, and consult your health care provider. This can be a sign of a serious condition.

❑ If baby of three months or under has a temperature of 103°F or higher, take the child to a doctor immediately. In a child of any age, fever accompanied by a stiff neck, swelling of the throat, or disorientation needs immediate attention from a physician as these symptoms may indicate meningitis.

❑ See a health care professional immediately if you develop a fever associated with any of the following:

• Frequent urination, a burning sensation while urinating, or blood in the urine.

• Pain concentrated in one area of the abdomen.

• Shaking chills or alternating chills and sweats.

• Severe headache and vomiting.

• Profuse watery diarrhea lasting more than twenty-four hours.

• Swollen glands or rashes.

❑ Never give aspirin to a child with a fever. (*See* REYE'S SYNDROME in Part Two.)

CONSIDERATIONS

❑ Lingering or recurring flulike symptoms can be associated with diabetes (especially in children), hepatitis, Lyme disease, or mononucleosis (especially in adolescents). (*See* CHRONIC FATIGUE SYNDROME; DIABETES; HEPATITIS; LYME DISEASE; and/or MONONUCLEOSIS in Part Two.)

❑ Vigorous exercise, in which the muscles generate heat faster than the body can dissipate it, can cause a temporary rise in temperature.

Fibrocystic Breasts

Fibrocystic breasts is a noncancerous condition characterized by the presence of cysts, or lumps, in the breasts. This condition is also known as *fibrocystic changes, chronic cystic mastitis, mammary dysphasia,* and—although it is not actually a disease—*fibrocystic disease.* It is caused by monthly changes in levels of estrogen and progesterone. It affects more than half of all women of childbearing age, most often between the ages of thirty and fifty.

Fibrocystic breasts are characterized by the presence of round lumps or cysts that move freely and are either firm or soft. Symptoms include tenderness and lumpiness in the breasts. The discomfort is usually most pronounced before menstruation.

Normally, fluids from breast tissues are collected and transported out of the breasts by means of the lymphatic system. However, if there is more fluid than the system can cope with, small spaces in the breast may fill with fluid. Fibrous tissue surrounds them and thickens like a scar, forming cysts. Many breast cysts swell before and during menstruation, and the resulting pressure can cause a feeling of fullness, a dull ache, increased sensitivity, or a burning sensation. Some women also experience significant pain.

Breast cysts may change in size, but they are benign. A cyst is tender and moves freely—it feels like an eyeball behind the lid. In contrast, a cancerous growth usually does not move freely, is most often not tender, and does not go away.

Most cysts are harmless. In fact, the normal structure of the breasts has a lumpy texture. However, this does not mean that any lumps should be disregarded. Each woman should be familiar with the normal feel of and cyclical changes in her breasts so that she can easily detect any new lumps. Ideally, she should check her breasts weekly, and if any new lumps become apparent between menstrual cycles, she should consult her health care practitioner promptly.

A physician can diagnose fibrocystic breasts with a simple office procedure. Using a fine needle, he or she attempts to remove fluid from the lump. If fluid is present, the lump is a cyst. A biopsy may be recommended to determine the risk, if any, of developing cancer. Routine mammograms are usually recommended as well.

NUTRIENTS

SUPPLEMENT	SUGGESTED DOSAGE	COMMENTS
Essential		
Coenzyme Q10 plus	As directed on label.	Powerful antioxidants that help to remove toxins from the body, boost the immune system, and improve overall physical and mental processes.
Coenzyme A from Coenzyme-A Technologies	As directed on label.	
Kelp	1,500–2,000 mg daily, in divided doses.	A rich source of iodine. Iodine deficiency has been linked to fibrocystic breasts.
Primrose oil	1,500 mg daily.	May reduce the size of the lumps.

Vitamin E	400–600 IU daily.	Protects the breast tissue because of its antioxidant ability. Use d-alpha-tocopherol form.
Very Important		
Vitamin A	15,000 IU daily, with meals. If you are pregnant, do not exceed 10,000 IU daily.	Needed for the ductal system of the breast.
plus carotenoid complex with beta-carotene	As directed on label.	Antioxidants and precursors of vitamin A.
Vitamin B complex	50 mg of each major B vitamin 3 times daily, with meals (amounts of individual vitamins in a complex will vary).	B-complex vitamins are important for all enzyme systems in the body.
plus extra vitamin B$_6$ (pyridoxine)	50 mg 3 times daily.	Needed for proper fluid balance and hormone regulation.
Important		
Vitamin C with bioflavonoids	2,000–4,000 mg daily, in divided doses.	Needed for proper immune function, tissue repair, and adrenal hormone balance.
Zinc	50 mg daily. Do not exceed a total of 100 mg daily from all supplements.	For repair of tissues and immune function. Use zinc gluconate lozenges or OptiZinc for best absorption.
Helpful		
Multimineral complex	As directed on label.	Balanced body minerals are important.
Proteolytic enzymes plus bromelain	As directed on label. Take with meals and between meals. As directed on label.	To reduce inflammation and soreness due to swelling.

HERBS

❏ The following herbs are good for fibrocystic breasts: echinacea, goldenseal, mullein, pau d'arco, red clover, squaw vine, and turmeric (curcumin).

Caution: Do not take goldenseal internally on a daily basis for more than one week at a time, as it may disturb normal intestinal flora. Do not use it during pregnancy, and use it with caution if you are allergic to ragweed.

❏ Use poke root or sage poultices to relieve breast inflammation and soreness. (*See* USING A POULTICE in Part Three.)

Note: Poke root is recommended for external use only.

RECOMMENDATIONS

❏ Eat a low-fat, high-fiber diet. Eat more raw foods, including seeds, nuts, and grains. Be sure nuts have not been subjected to heat. Include in your diet three or more servings daily of apples, bananas, grapes, grapefruit, raw nuts, seeds, fresh vegetables, and yogurt. Whole grains and beans should also be an important part of the diet.

❏ Include in your diet foods that are high in germanium, such as garlic, shiitake mushrooms, and onions. Germa-nium helps to improve tissue oxygenation at the cellular level.

❏ Do not consume any coffee, tea (except herbal teas), cola drinks, or chocolate. These foods contain caffeine, which has been implicated in fibrocystic breasts. Also avoid alcohol, animal products (especially meats and animal fats), cooking oils from supermarket shelves, fried foods, salt, sugar, tobacco, and all white flour products.

CONSIDERATIONS

❏ Good results have been achieved using primrose oil to reduce the size of cysts.

❏ According to research done by Dr. John Peter Minton of the Department of Surgery at Ohio State University College of Medicine, Columbus, women who eliminate caffeine-containing substances from their diets have a high rate of success in eliminating cysts.

❏ The drug danazol (Danocrine), a hormone, acts through the pituitary gland, reducing the function of the ovaries. This in turn decreases the amount of estrogen in the breast, shrinking the lumps. Danocrine is not effective for all women, but about 60 percent notice results within a few weeks. Many report less pain or tenderness. The drug may have some unpleasant effects, however. It should be used only if the suggestions above fail to give the desired results.

❏ Thyroid function is important in fibrocystic breasts; iodine deficiency can cause an underactive thyroid and has also been linked to fibrocystic changes. (*See* HYPOTHY-ROIDISM in Part Two.) Other factors include hormonal imbalance and abnormal production of breast milk brought about by high levels of the hormone estrogen.

❏ The National Cancer Institute recommends that all women examine their own breasts once a month. Self-examination should be done five to ten days after menstruation, after all swelling has subsided. Postmenopausal women should conduct a self-examination on the same date every month.

Fibroids, Uterine

Uterine fibroids (also called *leiomyomas* or *myomas*) are benign growths that can form on the interior muscular wall as well as the exterior of the uterus. This disorder involves not only the uterus but sometimes the cervix as well. The term *fibroid* may be somewhat misleading because the tumor cells are not fibrous. They are abnormal muscle cells. Their position within the uterus determines what they are called—submucosal, intramural, or subserosal. Fibroids attached to the uterus by a stalk are referred to as *pedunculated*.

It is estimated that 20 to 30 percent of all women develop fibroid tumors. For reasons not yet understood, they tend to form during the late thirties and early forties, and then to shrink after menopause. This would seem to suggest that estrogen is involved in the process. However, all women produce estrogen, but only some develop fibroid tumors. The presence of fibroid tumors does seem to have something to do with genetics, since they are known to run in families. African-American women are over three times more likely to develop fibroids than women of other ethnic backgrounds.

Most women who have fibroid tumors never even know it, unless they are discovered during the course of a routine pelvic examination. In roughly half of all cases, fibroid tumors cause no symptoms at all. In other cases, however, these growths can cause abnormally heavy and frequent menstrual periods. Other possible signs and symptoms include anemia, bleeding between periods, fatigue and weakness as a result of blood loss, increased vaginal discharge, and painful sexual intercourse or bleeding after intercourse. Depending upon their precise location, fibroids can cause pain in the legs, back, and/or pelvis, and exert pressure upon the bowels or the bladder, or even block the urethra, producing kidney obstruction.

NUTRIENTS

SUPPLEMENT	SUGGESTED DOSAGE	COMMENTS
Coenzyme Q$_{10}$	30 mg daily.	Promotes immune function and tissue oxygenation.
Floradix Iron + Herbs from Salus Haus	As directed on label. Do not take at the same time as vitamin E; iron depletes vitamin E in the body.	To supply iron in easily assimilable natural formula. Women with heavy menstrual flow as a result of fibroids are often anemic.
Garlic (Kyolic from Wakunaga)	As directed on label.	Powerful immune stimulant and antioxidant. Inhibits tumor growth.
L-Arginine

and
L-lysine | 500 mg daily, on an empty stomach. Take with water or juice. Do not take with milk. Take with 50 mg vitamin B$_6$ and 100 mg vitamin C for better absorption.

500 mg daily, on an empty stomach. | Enhances immune function and may retard tumor growth. See AMINO ACIDS in Part One.

Needed to balance with arginine. |
| Maitake extract and/or shiitake extract | As directed on label.

As directed on label. | To strengthen the body and improve overall health; have potent immunostimulant properties that inhibit tumor growth. |
| Multivitamin and mineral complex | As directed on label. | All nutrients are necessary in balance. |
| Vitamin A

with mixed carotenoids | 25,000 IU daily. If you are pregnant, do not exceed 10,000 IU daily. | Important in immune function and to promote tissue repair. Use emulsion form for easier assimilation and greater safety at higher doses. |
| Vitamin C with bioflavonoids | 3,000–10,000 mg daily, in divided doses. | Promotes immune function and acts as an antioxidant. |
| Zinc

plus
copper | 30–80 mg daily. Do not exceed a total of 100 mg daily from all supplements.

3 mg daily. | Needed for a healthy immune system.

Needed to balance with zinc. |

HERBS

❑ Dandelion root, milk thistle, scutellaria (also known as Chinese skullcap) root, and turmeric rhizome are all powerful antioxidants that support the liver while promoting the elimination of toxins.

❑ Green tea is a powerful antioxidant with anticancer properties.

❑ Red clover and burdock root both aid in cleansing the bloodstream.

RECOMMENDATIONS

❑ If you have unpleasant symptoms such as those outlined in this section, or if menstrual bleeding is so heavy that you saturate a sanitary pad or tampon more often than once an hour, consult your health care practitioner.

❑ If a fibroid is found, do not take oral contraceptives with a high estrogen content. High-estrogen birth control pills may stimulate the growth of fibroid tumors. Consider other forms of contraception, such as condoms and foam, a diaphragm, or a cervical cap.

CONSIDERATIONS

❑ Fibroids are almost never malignant, so treatment is not usually required as long as they remain relatively small and do not produce unpleasant symptoms.

❑ Women with fibroids may have higher levels of human growth hormone than other women.

❑ A woman's chance of developing fibroids may be decreased if she avoids the use of oral contraceptives.

❑ In the past, it was a matter of general practice to perform surgery to remove fibroids if they grew to a point that the uterus was enlarged to the same extent it would be in a twelfth-week pregnancy. Increasingly, however, physicians are becoming more reluctant to remove these tumors based solely upon the "twelve-week rule" unless they are causing medical problems for the patient. Since these tumors usually shrink with the onset of menopause, the problem may well take care of itself over time.

❑ Over 30 percent of the hysterectomies performed in the U.S. are done to remove fibroid tumors. An alternative to hysterectomy is a procedure known as myomectomy. This operation removes the fibroids, but leaves the uterus intact. This is an attractive alternative for a woman who wishes to bear children in the future, although it can be performed on any woman, regardless of age or childbearing desires. Myomectomy is more exacting surgery and places greater demands on the woman during recovery. There is also a slightly higher chance of complications with myomectomy than with hysterectomy, and the results are not always permanent. There is an estimated 50-percent chance that new tumors will form later, although they probably will not grow as large as the original fibroid tumors. If fibroids recur and cause symptoms, a repeat myomectomy can be performed.

❑ *Laparoscopic myolysis* is a procedure that may be recommended for the treatment of larger fibroids. In this technique, the surgeon uses a laser or electric current, delivered by means of special needles, to burn the fibroid and shrink it. This can be done on an outpatient basis.

❑ *Uterine fibroid embolization* (UFE) is a technique that involves making a tiny incision in the groin and placing a catheter into the femoral artery. The catheter is then guided up into the blood vessels that supply the fibroid. The idea is to cut off the blood supply to the fibroid, thus making it shrink. This technique is relatively new and the results so far have been inconclusive.

❑ *Hysteroscopic resection* can be used to remove uterine fibroids. In this procedure, a surgical instrument is inserted though the vagina into the uterus, the fibroids are removed vaginally, and the remaining area is cauterized. This can be performed on an outpatient basis.

❑ Any woman pondering a hysterectomy should give the matter close and careful consideration, and should ask her physician about less radical ways to treat fibroids. There are alternative procedures that may be suitable for some women. Some 650,000 hysterectomies are performed each year in the United States, many of them unnecessary. (*See* HYSTERECTOMY-RELATED PROBLEMS in Part Two.)

Fibromyalgia Syndrome

Fibromyalgia syndrome (FMS) is a rheumatic disorder characterized by chronic achy muscular pain that has no obvious physical cause. It most commonly affects the lower back, the neck, the shoulders, the back of the head, the upper chest, and/or the thighs, although any area or areas of the body may be involved. The pain is usually described as burning, throbbing, shooting, and stabbing. The pain and stiffness is often greater in the morning than at other times of day, and it may be accompanied by chronic headaches, strange sensations in the skin, insomnia, irritable bowel syndrome, and temporomandibular joint syndrome (TMJ). Other symptoms often experienced by people with fibromyalgia include premenstrual syndrome, painful periods, anxiety, palpitations, memory impairment, irritable bladder, skin sensitivities, dry eyes and mouth, a need for frequent changes in eyeglass prescription, dizziness, and impaired coordination. Such activities as lifting

and climbing stairs are often very difficult and painful. Depression often accompanies this disorder, and stress may trigger the development of problems similar to those associated with cardiovascular disease and adrenal gland disorders. Because the immune system is typically compromised in this disorder, opportunistic viral and bacterial infections are common as well.

The most distinctive feature of fibromyalgia, one that differentiates it from similar conditions, is the existence of certain "tender points"—eighteen specific spots where the muscles are abnormally tender to the touch. The eighteen points tend to cluster around the neck, shoulders, chest, knees, elbows region, and hips, and include the following:

- Around the lower vertebra of the neck.

- At the insertion of the second rib.

- Around the upper part of the thigh bone.

- In the middle of the knee joint.

- In muscles connected to the base of the skull.

- In muscles of the neck and upper back.

- In muscles of the mid-back.

- On the side of the elbow.

- In the upper and outer muscles of the buttocks.

There are 5 to 6 million people known to be suffering from FMS in the United States. However, the real number of cases is probably much higher, as this condition is often misdiagnosed. Fibromyalgia manifests itself in similar ways to chronic fatigue syndrome (CFS), chemical sensitivities, rheumatoid arthritis, and chronic myofascial pain (shortened muscle fiber syndrome). As a result, it often takes a long time for a proper diagnosis to be made. In the past, FMS was known as *fibrositis* or *fibromyositis*, but both of these terms are now considered inappropriate because they imply inflammation of some sort (the suffix *-itis* is medical terminology for "inflamation") and inflammation does not exist in fibromyalgia.

Most people with fibromyalgia also have an associated sleep disorder known as alpha-EEG anomaly. In this disorder, the individual's deep sleep periods are interrupted by bouts of waking-type brain activity, resulting in poor sleep. Some people with fibromyalgia are plagued by other sleep disorders as well, such as sleep apnea, restless leg syndrome, bruxism, and sleep myoclonus (a sudden rapid contraction of a muscle or a group of muscles during sleep or as one is falling asleep). Not surprisingly, given all these sleep difficulties, people with fibromyalgia often suffer from chronic fatigue that can range from mild to incapacitating. Other disorders common in people with fibromyalgia include the following:

- Chemical and/or food allergies.

- Dizziness and loss of balance.

- Extreme fatigue.

- Headaches.

- Irritable bowel syndrome (diarrhea and/or constipation, often alternating).

- Jaw pain.

- Memory loss and difficulty in concentrating.

- Menstrual pain.

- Sensitivity to bright lights or loud noises.

- Sensitivity to dairy products.

- Skin sensitivities.

- Stiffness in the morning and, often, when walking.

Fibromyalgia is much more common in females than in males, and most often begins in young adulthood. In most cases, symptoms come on gradually and slowly increase in intensity. They can be triggered (or made worse) by a number of different factors, including overexertion, stress, lack of exercise, anxiety, depression, lack of sleep, grief, trauma, extremes of temperature and/or humidity, and infectious illness. In the majority of cases, symptoms are severe enough to interfere with normal daily activities; a significant number of people with fibromyalgia are actually disabled by the condition. The course of the disorder is unpredictable. Some cases clear up on their own, some become chronic, and some go through cycles of flare-ups alternating with periods of apparent remission.

The cause or causes of fibromyalgia are not known, and there are no tests that can diagnose FMS with complete certainty. Some evidence points to a problem with the immune system; certain immunologic abnormalities are common among people with fibromyalgia. Their significance and relationship to the syndrome are not understood, however. A disturbance in brain chemistry may also be involved; many people who develop fibromyalgia have a history of clinical depression. Some research has found FMS is more likely to occur in people who have a history of sexual abuse, domestic violence, and even alcoholism. Other possible causes that have been proposed include infection with the Epstein-Barr virus (EBV), the virus that causes infectious mononucleosis, or with the fungus *Candida albicans*; chronic mercury poisoning from amalgam dental fillings; anemia; parasites; hypoglycemia; and hypothyroidism. Some experts believe that fibromyalgia may be related to chronic fatigue syndrome (CFS), which causes similar symptoms, except that in fibromyalgia, muscle pain predominates over fatigue, whereas in CFS, fatigue predominates over pain. FMS has even been misdiagnosed as multiple sclerosis or Parkinson's disease.

Because malabsorption problems are common in people with this disorder, higher than normal doses of all supplemental nutrients are needed. Wherever possible, it is best to use sublingual vitamins and other supplements because they are more easily absorbed than tablets or capsules.

NUTRIENTS

SUPPLEMENT	SUGGESTED DOSAGE	COMMENTS
Essential		
Acidophilus (Kyo-Dophilus from Wakunaga is a good source) or Bifido Factor from Natren	As directed on label.	Candida infection is common in people with fibromyalgia. Acidophilus Probiotics replace "friendly" bacteria destroyed by candida. Use a nondairy formula.
Coenzyme Q10	75 mg daily.	Improves oxygenation of tissues, enhances the effectiveness of the immune system, and protects the heart. Works with coenzyme Q10 to increase energy supply to the cells.
plus Coenzyme A from Coenzyme-A Technologies	As directed on label.	
Lecithin	As directed on label, with meals.	Promotes energy, enhances immunity, aids in brain function, and improves circulation.
Malic acid and magnesium	As directed on label.	Involved in energy production in many cells of the body, including the muscle cells. Needed for sugar metabolism.
Manganese	5 mg daily. Take separately from calcium.	Influences the metabolic rate by its involvement in the pituitary-hypothalamic-thyroid axis.
Nicotinamide adenine dinucleotide (NADH) (Enada)	10–15 mg first thing in the morning on an empty stomach.	Increases level of energy.
Proteolytic enzymes or Inflazyme Forte from American Biologics or Wobenzym N from Marlyn Nutraceuticals	As directed on label, 6 times daily, with meals, between meals, and at bedtime.	Reduces inflammation and improves absorption of foods, especially protein, which is needed for tissue repair.
Vitamin A with mixed carotenoids plus vitamin E or ACES + Zn from Carlson Labs	25,000 IU daily for 1 month, then slowly reduce to 10,000 IU daily. If you are pregnant, do not exceed 10,000 IU daily. 800 IU daily for 1 month, then slowly reduce to 400 IU daily. As directed on label.	Powerful free radical scavengers that protect the body's cells and enhance immune function. Use emulsion forms for easier assimilation. Use d-alpha-tocopherol form. Contains vitamins A, C, and E plus the minerals selenium and zinc, to protect immune function.
Vitamin C with bioflavonoids	5,000–10,000 mg daily.	Has a powerful antiviral effect and increases the body's energy level. Use a buffered form.
Very Important		
Dimethylglycine (DMG) (Aangamik DMG from FoodScience of Vermont)	50 mg 3 times daily.	Enhances oxygen utilization by the muscles and destroys free radicals that can damage cells.
5-Hydroxy L-tryptophan (5-HTP)	50 mg daily for 1 week, then increase to 100 mg daily.	Enhances synthesis of serotonin in the brain. Excellent for pain relief. *Caution:* Do not use if you take an MAO inhibitor, commonly prescribed for depression.

Free-form amino acid complex (Amino Balance from Anabol Naturals or Amino Blend from Carlson Labs)	As directed on label.	To supply protein essential for repair and rebuilding of muscle tissue and for proper brain function. Use a formula containing all the essential amino acids.
Garlic (Kyolic from Wakunaga) plus Kyo-Green from Wakunaga	2 capsules 3 times daily, with meals. As directed on label.	Promotes immune function and increases energy. Also destroys common parasites. To improve digestion and cleanse the bloodstream.
Grape seed extract or Pycnogenol	As directed on label. As directed on label.	Powerful antioxidants that protect the muscles from free radical damage and enhance immunity.
Methylsulfonyl-methane (MSM)	As directed on label.	Provides support for tendons, ligaments, and muscles. *Note:* Because this supplement contains sulfur, you may notice an odor to your urine.
Methylsulfonyl-methane (MSM) cream	As directed on label.	Relieves pain.
S-Adenosylmethio-nine (SAMe)	As directed on label.	Aids in stress-relief, depression, eases pain, and produces antioxidant effects that can improve the health of your liver. *Caution:* Do not use if you have manic-depressive disorder or take prescription antidepressants.
Vitamin B complex injections	2 cc twice weekly for 1 month or as prescribed by physician.	Essential for increased energy and normal brain function. Injections (under doctor's supervision) are best. All injectables can be combined in a single syringe.
plus extra vitamin B$_6$ (pyridoxine) and vitamin B$_{12}$	1/4 cc twice weekly for 1 month or as prescribed by physician. 1 cc twice weekly for 1 month or as prescribed by physician.	
plus raw liver extract	2 cc twice weekly for 1 month or as prescribed by physician.	A source of B vitamins and iron. *Caution:* Do not take a supplement containing iron unless prescribed by your physician.
or vitamin B complex	100 mg of each major B vitamin 3 times daily, with meals (amounts of individual vitamins in a complex will vary).	If injections are not available, or once the course of injections has been completed, use a sublingual form of all the B vitamins listed.

Important

Calcium and magnesium and vitamin D$_3$ or Bone Support from Synergy Plus plus potassium and selenium	2,000 mg daily. 1,000 mg daily. 400 IU daily. As directed on label. 99 mg daily. 200 mcg daily. If you are pregnant, do not exceed 40 mcg daily.	Needed for proper functioning of all muscles, including the heart; relieves muscle spasms and pain. Deficiencies are common in people with this disorder. Contains calcium and magnesium plus other minerals to aid absorption. Involved in proper muscle function. An important antioxidant.
and zinc plus copper	50 mg daily. Do not exceed a total of 100 mg daily from all supplements. 3 mg daily.	Needed for proper functioning of the immune system. Needed to balance with zinc.

Capricin from Probiologic or Probiata from Wakunaga	As directed on label.	To combat candida, which is associated with fibromyalgia.
Chromium	200–400 mcg daily.	To help balance blood sugar levels and aid in preventing night sweats.
Creatine	As directed on label. Do not take with fruit juices, as this combination produces creatinine, which is difficult for the kidneys to process.	To combat muscle depletion. Should be used in conjunction with a balanced, nutrititious diet.
DL-phenylalanine (DLPA)	500 mg daily every other week.	Can be very effective for controlling pain. Also increases mental alertness. *Caution:* Do not take this supplement if you are pregnant or nursing, or suffer from panic attacks, diabetes, high blood pressure, or PKU.
Essential fatty acids (black currant seed oil, flaxseed oil, Kyolic-EPA from Wakunaga, and primrose oil are good sources)	As directed on label 3 times daily, with meals.	Protects against cell damage. Helps to reduce pain and fatigue.
Fibroplex from Metagenics	As directed on label.	A formula containing vitamins B$_1$ and B$_6$ plus magnesium, manganese, and malic acid.
Fibro-X from Olympian Labs	As directed on label.	To relieve pain. Contains many nutrients listed in this table, plus shark cartilage.
Gamma-amino-butyric acid (GABA) or GABA Plus from Twinlab	As directed on label. As directed on label.	For proper control of brain function and to control anxiety. Contains a combination of GABA, inositol, and niacinamide.
Kelp	As directed on label.	Contains minerals that support the thyroid.
L-Leucine plus L-isoleucine and L-valine plus L-carnitine	500 mg each daily, on an empty stomach. Take with water or juice. Do not take with milk. Take with 50 mg vitamin B$_6$ and 100 mg vitamin C for better absorption. As directed on label	These amino acids are found primarily in muscle tissue. They are available in combination formulas. (*See* AMINO ACIDS in Part One.) Increases energy.
L-Tyrosine	500–1,000 mg daily, at bedtime.	Helps to relieve depression and aids in relaxing the muscles. *Caution:* Do not take this supplement if you are taking an MAO inhibitor drug.
Melatonin	As directed on label, 1–2 hours or less before bedtime.	Promotes sound sleep. A sustained release formula is best. Take a sublingual form during the night if you wake up and cannot go back to sleep.
Multivitamin and mineral complex plus carotenoid complex (Advanced Carotenoid Complex from Solgar)	As directed on label. 15,000 IU daily.	All nutrients are necessary in balance. Use a high-potency hypoallergenic formula.
Ocu-Care from Nature's Plus	As directed on label.	Contains essential nutrients to protect and nourish the eyes.

Raw thymus glandular and	As directed on label.	To boost the immune system. (*See* GLANDULAR THERAPY in Part Three.)
raw spleen glandular plus	As directed on label.	
multiglandular complex	As directed on label.	
Reishi extract	As directed on label.	A mushroom extract that helps the body deal with stress and increases energy levels.
Taurine	500 mg daily, on an empty stomach.	An important antioxidant and immune system regulator necessary for white blood cell activation and neurological function.
Vanadyl sulfate	As directed on label.	Protects the muscles and reduces overall body fatigue.

HERBS

❑ Astragalus and echinacea enhance immune function.

❑ Black walnut and garlic aid in removing parasites.

❑ Boswellia is excellent for morning stiffness and joint pain.

❑ Teas brewed from burdock root, dandelion, and red clover promote healing by cleansing the bloodstream and enhancing immune function. Combine or alternate these herbal teas, and drink 4 to 6 cups daily.

❑ Calendula or rosemary oil (or a combination of the two), diluted with an equal amount of water or vegetable oil and massaged into the skin, helps to relieve pain.

❑ Topical applications of cayenne (capsicum) powder mixed with wintergreen oil can help relieve muscle pain. Cayenne contains capsaicin, a substance that appears to inhibit the release of neurotransmitters responsible for communicating pain sensations. Use 1 part cayenne powder to 3 parts wintergreen oil. Cayenne can also be taken orally, in capsule form.

❑ Put 4 to 6 ounces of ginger powder into a moderately hot bath. This will induce sweating and help remove toxins from the body. Drinking hot ginger tea will have the same effect.

❑ Ginkgo biloba improves circulation and brain function.

❑ Kava kava decreases anxiety and elevates the mood.

❑ Licorice root supports the glandular system, especially the adrenal glands.
    Caution: If overused, licorice can elevate blood pressure. Do not use this herb on a daily basis for more than seven days in a row. Avoid it if you have high blood pressure.

❑ Milk thistle protects the liver.

❑ Pau d'arco, taken in tea or tablet form, is good for treating candida infection.

❑ Skullcap and valerian root improve sleep.

❑ White willow bark is good for relieving pain.

RECOMMENDATIONS

❑ Eat a well-balanced diet of 50 percent raw foods and fresh "live" juices. The diet should consist mostly of vegetables, fruits, whole grains (primarily millet and brown rice), raw nuts and seeds, soy products, skinless turkey or chicken, and deep-water fish. These quality foods supply nutrients that renew energy and build immunity.

❑ Include pomegranates and pomegranate juice in your diet. They have anti-inflammatory and antioxidant properties.

❑ Eat four to five small meals daily to keep a steady supply of protein and carbohydrates available for proper muscle function. If the body does not have enough fuel for energy, it will rob the muscles of essential nutrients, causing muscle wasting and pain.

❑ Drink plenty of liquids to help flush out toxins. The best choices are steam-distilled water and herbal teas. Fresh vegetable juices supply necessary vitamins and minerals.

❑ Limit your consumption of green peppers, eggplant, tomatoes, and white potatoes. These foods contain solanine, which interferes with enzymes in the muscles, and may cause pain and discomfort.

❑ Do not eat meat, dairy products, or any other foods that are high in saturated fats. Saturated fats raise cholesterol levels and interfere with circulation. They also promote the inflammatory response and increase pain. Also avoid fried foods, processed foods, shellfish, dairy foods, and white flour products such as bread and pasta.

❑ Do not consume any caffeine, alcohol, or sugar. Eating sugar in any form—including fructose and honey—promotes fatigue, increases pain, and disturbs sleep. If these substances have been a regular part of your diet, your symptoms may actually get worse for a short period as a result of the "withdrawal" effect, but after that, you should experience a noticeable improvement in your condition.

❑ Avoid wheat and brewer's yeast until your symptoms improve.

❑ Use wheatgrass retention enemas to detoxify the system. To make the enema, add 1 ounce of wheatgrass juice to 1 cup of warm water. If fresh wheatgrass is not available, powdered Sweet Wheat from Sweet Wheat, Inc. is a good substitute. Use this treatment every other day for two weeks. (*See* ENEMAS in part Three.)

❑ Maintain a regular program of moderate exercise. A daily walk followed by some gentle stretching exercises is good. If you have been sedentary before, start slowly and be careful not to overexert yourself; this can aggravate symptoms. Keep in mind that what you need is some amount of daily exercise, *not* a strenuous workout two or three times a week. Once your body is accustomed to regular exercise, symptoms are likely to improve. Moderate exercise and stretching help to keep muscles flexible and prevent joints from stiffening up.

❑ Be sure to give your body sufficient rest. Set aside at least eight hours for sleep each night.

❑ Take a hot shower or a bath upon arising to stimulate circulation and help relieve morning stiffness. Or alternate between hot water and cold water while showering. Recent studies have shown cold showers to be beneficial for relieving the pain of fibromyalgia. Hot baths help to relax the muscles.

❑ Consider trying massage therapy, which can help to relax muscles and reduce stiffness of the joints.

❑ Take chlorophyll in tablet form or in "green drinks" such as Kyo-Green from Wakunaga of America. Spiru-tein from Nature's Plus is a good protein drink to use between meals to aid in maintaining energy levels and to reduce muscle pain.

❑ Have your doctor check your thyroid function. Symptoms of hypothyroidism can mimic those of FMS.

CONSIDERATIONS

❑ Chronic pain sufferers, especially those with fibromyalgia and chronic fatigue syndrome, tend to be deficient in magnesium.

❑ Common painkillers such as aspirin, acetaminophen, and ibuprofen are not usually effective at relieving the pain of fibromyalgia. Other approaches, including attention to diet, exercise, and nutritional supplementation, are more likely to be of benefit.

❑ Many different disorders can cause symptoms similar to those of fibromyalgia, including anemia, depression, hepatitis, and Lyme disease, among others. Anyone who experiences muscular pain and/or fatigue that persists for longer than a week or two should consult a health care professional. There may be an underlying medical disorder that requires treatment.

❑ Recent research points to the possible involvement of chemical and/or food sensitivities in fibromyalgia, chronic fatigue syndrome, and the pain associated with these disorders. This would hardly be surprising, as humans have been exposed to more chemicals in the last fifty years than in all the rest of our history combined.

❑ Studies are being conducted on the possible role of a genetic defect that interferes with the formation of adenosine triphosphate (ATP, the source of cellular energy) in this disorder.

❑ Some experts suggest that people with fibromyalgia should *avoid* salt-free diets.

❑ Plant sterols and sterolins (plant fats that are present in fruits, vegetables, seeds, and nuts) stimulate the immune system, thus helping the body fight off infection.

❑ Because malabsorption problems are common in this disorder, all nutrients are needed in greater than normal amounts, and a proper diet is essential. Colon cleansing is recommended to rid the gastrointestinal tract of mucus and debris, and so improve nutrient absorption. (*See* COLON CLEANSING in Part Three.)

❑ Many doctors prescribe low-dose antidepressants for fibromyalgia. These drugs can be beneficial in some cases, but can also cause a number of side effects, such as drowsiness. Other medical treatments that may or may not be of help to any given individual include muscle relaxants and/or local anesthetic sprays or injections for relief of pain. Antianxiety drugs are sometimes prescribed as well. These drugs can cause a loss of equilibrium.

❑ Physical therapy, relaxation techniques, exercise therapy, massage therapy, deep heat therapy, and biofeedback are all helpful in some cases. Massage therapy is particularly beneficial for improved muscle function and pain relief. If you are diagnosed with fibromyalgia, it is wise to seek out a health care practitioner who has specific experience in the management and treatment of this condition.

❑ Food allergies can exacerbate the discomfort of many disorders. (*See* ALLERGIES in Part Two.)

❑ *See also* CHRONIC FATIGUE SYNDROME and DEPRESSION in Part Two. *See also* PAIN CONTROL in Part Three.

❑ For names and addresses of organizations that can provide further information about fibromyalgia, *see* HEALTH AND MEDICAL INFORMATION in the Appendix.

Flu

See INFLUENZA.

Foodborne/ Waterborne Disease

Food- or waterborne disease occurs when a person consumes substances containing harmful toxins, chemicals, parasites, or microorganisms (usually bacteria). Foodborne illness, commonly referred to as *food poisoning*, causes some 6.5 million known cases of illness and 9,000 deaths every year in the United States. The actual number of cases is almost certainly well above any reported number, because people often mistake the symptoms of food poisoning for a simple upset stomach.

Symptoms of food poisoning may include nausea, vomiting, abdominal cramps and diarrhea, even chills, fever, severe headache, and worse, lasting from a few hours to a few days. Some types of food poisoning, such as botulism, are more serious, especially for elderly people and children. In addition, many cases of food poisoning lead to chronic health disorders, such as reactive arthritis and chronic immune deficiency. Pathogenic and toxigenic organisms—those that can cause disease and those that can produce harmful toxins—are silent threats because nothing about the taste, odor, or appearance of the food indicates their presence. All types of bacteria can potentially become toxigenic.

There are different types of food poisoning, depending on the agent that causes it (for a quick summary of some of these, *see* Types of Food Poisoning, page 381).

The most common type is salmonellosis, or *Salmonella* infection. Between 2 and 4 million cases are treated every year in the United States. *Salmonella* bacteria are part of the natural intestinal flora of many animals. They are easily transmitted through the food supply, the hands of food preparers, and the surfaces of objects such as knives and tabletops. Salmonellosis is typically associated with eggs. External contamination from fecal matter, once a common source of salmonellosis, has almost been eliminated as a cause due to more stringent testing and inspection regimens implemented in the 1970s. The principal danger now comes from eggs because *Salmonella enteritidis,* the organism responsible for the majority of Salmonella infections, is now present in the ovaries of a significant percentage of egg-producing hens in the United States, and it contaminates the eggs before the shells form. Thus, eggs do not need to be cracked or unclean on the outside to be contaminated. Foods made from raw eggs, including Caesar salad dressing, eggnog, hollandaise sauce, and ice cream have also been found to contain these bacteria. Of thirty-five outbreaks of illness that were reported over a two-year period and determined to be food poisoning, twenty-four were traced to contaminated eggs or foods containing these infected eggs. Salmonellosis as a result of the consumption of raw clams, oysters, and sushi made from raw fish has also been reported. Although this does not occur as often as *Salmonella* infection from eggs, meat, and poultry, it does happen.

Symptoms of *Salmonella* infection can range from mild abdominal pain to severe diarrhea and dehydration to typhoid-like fever. Symptoms usually develop within eight to thirty-six hours of eating contaminated foods. Diarrhea is often the first sign. *Salmonella* can also weaken the immune system and cause kidney and cardiovascular damage as well as arthritis.

Outbreaks of salmonellosis occur primarily in the warmer months. Most cases are the result of the consumption of contaminated foods, primarily chicken, eggs, beef, and pork products. People who eat raw or incompletely cooked meats are at greater risk of developing the disorder. Cooks who first handle raw meat or poultry and then handle other foods, without washing their hands in between, endanger others; cooks who lick their hands or fingers after handling raw meat or poultry put themselves at risk of *Salmonella* infection. People taking antibiotics are also at greater risk. Antibiotics can effectively treat bacterial infections, but, paradoxically, they can also promote infection by destroying good, competing bacteria and permitting the growth of bacteria that are antibiotic resistant. People with AIDS are twenty times more likely to suffer from salmonellosis than other population groups.

After *Salmonella, Staphylococcus aureus* is the second most frequent cause of foodborne illness. Staphylococci are responsible for approximately 25 percent of all cases of food poisoning. *Staphylococcus* (staph) infection can manifest itself in a variety of ways, from food poisoning to skin infections to septicemia (blood infection). In severe cases, it can be life threatening. This microorganism is commonly found in the nose and throat, but if a food product becomes contaminated with the bacteria (by being sneezed or coughed on, for example), the bacteria can grow and produce an enterotoxin, a toxin that specifically targets the cells of the intestines. It is this toxin, rather than the bacteria itself, that causes the food poisoning. Symptoms include diarrhea, nausea, vomiting, abdominal cramps, and prostration, usually beginning from two to eight hours after consumption of the contaminated food. Staphylococcal toxin is found most often in meat, poultry, egg products, tuna, potato and macaroni salads, and cream-filled pastries.

The bacterium *Clostridium botulinum*, which commonly inhabits the soil in the form of harmless spores, can cause a particularly dangerous type of food poisoning. Of the various types of food poisoning, botulism is the among the most severe. It affects the central nervous system. As with *Staphylococcus*, it is not the bacteria but rather toxins produced by the bacteria that cause the poisoning—and like staph, the bacteria can infect surface wounds. Woundborne botulism is not common, but it can occur if an open sore becomes infected with the botulism bacteria. People who use intravenous drugs can also be infected by using dirty or shared needles. Infant botulism is a type of the disorder that usually affects children under twelve months of age. It can occur if a young child ingests anything contaminated by botulism spores. This can include soil, cistern water, dust, and even some foods, such as honey.

The toxins produced by *C. botulinum* block the transmission of impulses from nerves to muscles, thus paralyzing the muscles. The paralysis often begins with the muscles that are responsible for eye movement, swallowing, and speech, and progresses to those in the torso and the extremities. Early symptoms of botulism include extreme weakness, double vision, droopy eyelids, and trouble swallowing. These symptoms typically appear twelve to forty-eight hours after ingestion of the contaminated food. Eventually, muscle weakness affecting the entire body, including the muscles required for breathing, can result. Paralysis and death may occur in severe cases.

There are seven recognized types of botulin bacteria, designated A, B, C, D, E, F, and G. The A, B, E, and F varieties cause human botulism. Types C and D are isolated to animals. Type G has been found in soil samples in Argentina, but no cases of illness involving type G have yet been reported. A total of about 110 cases of botulism are reported each year. Of these, 72 percent are infant botulism,

25 percent are foodborne botulism, and the remainder are woundborne botulism.

Botulin toxin has been found in home-canned foods with a low acidity level, such as asparagus, beets, corn, and green beans. Less common sources include chopped garlic in oil, tomatoes, handled and then baked potatoes kept in aluminium foil, and home-canned or fermented fish. A bulging lid or cracked jar can be a sign that the food within is contaminated, but botulism can occur even if a food container shows no signs of damage. Keeping certain foods at room temperature for prolonged periods can also be a problem. In one reported case, a restaurant allowed a large batch of sautéed onions to be kept out throughout the day, instead of keeping them refrigerated, and small amounts were used as needed. Several people became very ill from botulin toxin in the onions.

Freezing, drying, and treatment with chemicals such as sodium nitrite prevent *C. botulinum* spores from growing and producing toxins. Although it does not kill the spores themselves, heating food to a temperature of at least 176°F for thirty minutes prevents food poisoning by destroying the lethal toxins.

Another microorganism that can cause food poisoning is *Campylobacter jejuni*. With this type of food poisoning, people tend not to associate the illness with food because it takes three to five days for the bacteria to produce symptoms, which include abdominal cramps, diarrhea, fever, and possibly blood in the stool. *C. jejuni* can be present in the intestinal tracts of apparently healthy cattle, sheep, chickens, turkeys, dogs, and cats, and can be contracted by eating or drinking food or water that has somehow become contaminated by the feces of an infected person or animal. Chickens, turkeys, and waterfowl are the most common carriers. Fortunately, heat destroys these bacteria, so it is possible to avoid this type of food poisoning by eating meat only if has been cooked thoroughly.

Another type of bacteria that can cause food poisoning is *Clostridium perfringens,* sometimes called the "food-service germ." It is one of the most common causes of foodborne illness. This microorganism thrives in previously cooked food that is kept for a long time at room temperature. Meat products and gravy are the most likely sources of the toxin. As foods cool, the bacteria multiply, forming spores and generating toxins. The toxins are often heat resistant. The symptoms of *C. perfringens* poisoning usually are limited to mild nausea and vomiting that last a day or less, but that can be a very serious problem for older adults or people with Crohn's disease or HIV.

Not all foodborne illness is the result of bacterial contamination. *Giardia lamblia* is a protozoan (single-celled parasitic microorganism) that infects the small intestine. Giardiasis is associated with the consumption of contaminated water. It can also be transmitted to raw foods that have grown in contaminated water. Cool, moist environments are conducive to the growth of this microorganism. Symptoms generally occur within one to three weeks of infection and include diarrhea, constipation, abdominal pain, flatulence, loss of appetite, nausea, and vomiting. Norwalk virus is a very common virus that can be transmitted in food and water, and that causes many cases of diarrhea in both children and adults. The hepatitis A and E viruses can be transmitted by direct contact with fecal matter or with foods contaminated by fecal matter. They can also be transmitted by contaminated water. *Trichinella spiralis* is a parasitic roundworm that causes the infection known as trichinosis. It is most often the result of eating raw or improperly cooked or processed pork or pork products (ham and sausage) and wild game.

Escherichia coli (E. coli) is a type of bacteria naturally found in the intestines of human and some animals, where it actually serves a useful function—it helps to suppress harmful bacteria and aid in the absorption of vitamins. But sometimes, under the right circumstances, *E. coli* can cause serious illness. The reason for the change from benign or friendly to pathogenic is not known. But this can be a very serious illness, particularly for the very young, the elderly, and those with compromised immune systems. This bacteria has been found in meat, vegetables, and some unpasteurized juices or fruits.

Scombroid poisoning (also called histamine poisoning) is a relatively rare type of food poisoning that can occur after the consumption of fish such as tuna, mackerel, mahi mahi, sardines, bluefish, and abalone. After a fish is caught, decomposition carried on by bacteria in the fish can trigger the production of high levels of a chemical called histamine. When the fish is eaten, in a matter of minutes the histamine can cause symptoms including facial flushing, nausea, vomiting, abdominal pain, and/or hives. Fortunately, symptoms usually subside in twenty-four hours. Vibriobacteria, which comprise a group of different species of bacteria that can cause food poisoning, are mostly found in raw or improperly cooked fish and shellfish.

Thanks to our food safety, labeling, and inspection laws, our supermarket shelves are stocked with a nearly endless variety of foods that must meet strict government standards. Yet the truth is that food poisoning remains a major problem in this country, and it strikes with a frequency that is both surprising and alarming. The CDC offers several reasons for this. First, food animals are now raised in very close, confined quarters, a situation that is conducive to the spread of bacteria such as *Salmonella*. At the same time, food processing is becoming more and more centralized, so a single ingredient that is tainted with a contaminant can eventually show up in a multitude of different products. The United States now also imports record amounts of food from overseas, often from developing countries where proper hygiene in food production may not be as reliable as it is in this country.

Then there is the matter of food preparation. An increasing number of Americans are simply unaware of the prevalence of potentially dangerous microorganisms in the food supply, and lack knowledge of basic techniques for han-

Types of Food Poisoning

There are many different types of food poisoning, some more common than others. The following is a summary of some of these, together with the relative incidence and typical symptoms of each.

Type	Relative Incidence	Symptoms	Time Between Exposure and Onset of Symptoms
Bacterial Origin			
Botulism	Rare.	Double vision; difficulty speaking, breathing, and swallowing; nausea, vomiting, and abdominal pain; diarrhea; muscular weakness.	12–48 hours, but may be as long as 8 days.
Campylobacter infection	Common.	Muscular pain, nausea, vomiting, fever, abdominal cramps.	2–10 days.
Clostridium perfringens poisoning	Common.	Diarrhea, abdominal cramps.	9–15 hours.
Escherichia coli (*E. coli*) poisoning	Common.	Diarrhea, abdominal cramps, vomiting.	1–7 days
Listeriosis	Rare.	Flulike symptoms, including fever, chills; can cause spontaneous abortion or stillbirth; can cause severe illness in newborns and immune-depressed people.	2–4 weeks.
Salmonellosis	Common.	Nausea, vomiting, diarrhea, abdominal cramps, fever, headache.	6–48 hours.
Staphylococcal food poisoning	Common.	Vomiting, diarrhea; occasionally weakness, dizziness.	30 minutes–8 hours.
Vibriobacteria	Not common, but occurs in occasional outbreaks during warmer months.	Diarrhea, fever, chills, cramps, headache, vomiting.	4–96 hours.
Parasitic Origin			
Giardiasis	Common.	Nausea, gas, abdominal pain and/or cramping, diarrhea; in severe cases, malabsorption problems and weight loss.	1–3 weeks.
Trichinosis	Rare.	Fever, edema of eyelids, muscle pain.	1–2 days.
Viral Origin			
Hepatitis A/ hepatitis E	Sporadic outbreaks.	Fever, nausea, lethargy, and pain in abdominal area. Hepatitis A infection may cause jaundice.	For hepatitis A, 10–50 days. For hepatitis E, 2–9 weeks.
Norwalk virus infection	Common.	Nausea, vomiting, diarrhea, headache.	1–2 days.
Rotavirus	Common.	Vomiting, diarrhea, possible temporary lactose intolerance.	1–3 days.
Toxin-Caused Scombroid poisoning	Uncommon.	Headache, dizziness, burning throat, hives, nausea, vomiting, abdominal pain.	5 minutes–1 hour.

Tips for Preventing Food Poisoning

Here are some fast, easy rules to help prevent food poisoning at home and while eating out:

• Keep food either hot or cold. Leaving food at room temperature encourages the growth of bacteria.

• Keep perishable products refrigerated. Oils containing herbs or garlic should also be refrigerated.

• Refrigerate leftovers as soon as possible. Do not refrigerate foods in the same containers they were cooked or served in; transfer leftovers into clean containers so that they will cool more quickly.

• Organize your refrigerator so that raw meats are kept away from, or do not drip blood onto, other foods.

• Cook meat, poultry, and seafood thoroughly. Meats should be cooked to an internal temperature of at least 165°F.

• If you bake potatoes in aluminum, keep them either hot or refrigerated.

• Never use raw eggs that are cracked.

• Wash your hands before handling food, and after handling raw meat or poultry. Harmful bacteria can be transmitted if you handle food after diapering a baby or blowing your nose.

• Keep two cutting boards, one for meat and the other for vegetables. This will prevent the transfer of bacteria from meat to vegetables. At least three times a week, wash your cutting boards with a solution of 1/4 cup of 3 percent hydrogen peroxide and 2 gallons of water. As an alternative, you can use a mixture of 1/2 cup of chlorine bleach and 1 quart of water, then rinse the board thoroughly with clean water.

• Go home directly after grocery shopping, especially in warm weather. Store foods immediately according to the instructions on the labels.

• Clean any utensil that has come in contact with raw hamburger, poultry, eggs, or seafood. Such utensils should not be allowed to come into contact with other foods until they have been disinfected.

• Wash out lunch boxes and Thermos bottles after every use.

• Beware of bulging cans, cracked jars, or loose lids on products. These can indicate botulism. Throw away cans that are bulging, rusted, bent, or sticky. Beware of cracks in jars and leaks in paper packaging, and exercise caution when consuming home-canned foods.

• When reheating food, bring it to a rapid boil, if possible, and cook it at that temperature for at least four minutes.

• Set your refrigerator temperature at 40°F or below. Freezers should be set at 0°F or below.

• Wash kitchen towels and sponges with a bleach-and-water solution (1 part bleach to 20 parts water) daily.

• Do not leave foods such as mayonnaise, salad dressing, and milk products at room temperature or, worse, out in the sun. Be especially careful at picnics and cookouts.

• Do not give honey to a young baby. This can lead to infant botulism, in which botulinal spores colonize the digestive tract and produce botulin toxin there. Honey is safe for babies after age one.

• Mold commonly grows on spoiled food products. The following foods should be avoided if mold is growing on them: bacon, bread, cured luncheon meats, soft dairy products, flour, canned ham, hot dogs, dried nuts, peanut butter, roast poultry, soft vegetables, and whole grains. Throw away any cooked or raw foods that are covered with mold.

• Thaw all frozen foods, especially meats and poultry, in the refrigerator, not at room temperature.

• Eat hamburger and other meats only if they have been cooked at least until they turn brown. Meat or poultry that is even a little pink in color may still harbor bacteria. To ensure that all bacteria have been destroyed, it is best to cook meat until it is well done.

• When preparing a chicken or turkey with dressing, do not stuff the bird until you are ready to put it in the oven. Either cook the stuffing separately or place it in the poultry *immediately* before putting it in the oven and then remove it as soon as the bird is done.

• Exercise caution when eating at restaurants and salad bars. Do not eat at salad bars that do not look fresh and clean or that do not have protective glass over them. Avoid the following foods when eating at salad bars: chicken, fish, creamed foods, foods containing mayonnaise, undercooked foods, and soups that are not kept at near-boiling temperatures.

• Before eating out, take 2 garlic tablets to help prevent food poisoning, as well as a product called ACES + Zn from Carlson Labs to destroy any free radicals created by unknown toxins and oxidized fats in the food.

dling, preparing, and storing food safely. Most cases of food poisoning are easily preventable, provided you know how (*see* Tips for Preventing Food Poisoning above). Also, more and more Americans, rather than eating meals prepared at home, purchase ready-made food at restaurants and from takeout establishments.

If you contract food- or waterborne illness, the following supplements should be helpful. Unless otherwise specified, the dosages recommended here are for adults. For a child between the ages of twelve and seventeen, reduce the dose to three-quarters the recommended amount. For a child between six and twelve, use one-half the recommended dose, and for a child under the age of six, use one-quarter the recommended amount.

NUTRIENTS

SUPPLEMENT	SUGGESTED DOSAGE	COMMENTS
Very Important		
Charcoal tablets	5 tablets at first signs of illness and again 6 hours later. Take separately from other medications and supplements.	Removes toxic substances from the colon and bloodstream.
Garlic (Kyolic from Wakunaga)	2 capsules 3 times daily, with meals.	A powerful detoxifier that also destroys bacteria in the colon.
Potassium	99 mg daily.	To restore proper electrolyte balance.
Vitamin C with bioflavonoids plus	8,000 mg daily, in divided doses.	Detoxifies the body and aids in removing bacteria and toxins.
vitamin E	600 IU daily.	Reduces symptoms by enhancing immune function. Use d-alpha-tocopherol form.
Important		
Acidophilus (Kyo-Dophilus from Wakunaga is a good source)	As directed on label, twice daily, on an empty stomach.	Replaces essential intestinal bacteria. Use a nondairy source.
Aerobic 07 from Aerobic Life Industries	20 drops in a glass of water every 3 hours.	Destroys harmful bacteria such as Salmonella.
Fiber (Aerobic Bulk Cleanse [ABC] from Aerobic Life Industries and oat bran are good sources)	As directed on label 6 hours after second dose of charcoal tablets and twice daily thereafter. Take separately from other supplements and medications.	Removes bacteria that have attached themselves to the colon walls, preventing them from entering the bloodstream; this reduces symptoms and speeds recovery.
Kelp	1,000–1,500 mg daily.	Contains needed minerals to restore electrolytes.
L-cysteine and L-methionine and selenium and superoxide dismutase (SOD) plus	500 mg each daily, on an empty stomach. Take with 50 mg each of vitamins B$_6$ and C for better absorption. 200 mcg daily. If you are pregnant, do not exceed 40 mcg daily. 5,000 mg daily.	All of these nutrients are essential in immune function.
glutathione	500 mg daily.	A powerful antioxidant.

HERBS

❏ At the first sign of food poisoning, take a dropperful of alcohol-free goldenseal extract. Repeat this every four hours for one day. Goldenseal is a natural antibiotic that aids in destroying bacteria in the colon.

Caution: Do not take goldenseal internally on a daily basis for more than one week at a time, do not use it during pregnancy, and use it with caution if you are allergic to ragweed.

❏ Milk thistle and red clover aid in liver and blood cleansing.

❏ Use lobelia tea enemas to rid the body of the poison. (*See* ENEMAS in Part Three.) Adding a dropperful of alcohol-free goldenseal extract to the enema is beneficial as well.

RECOMMENDATIONS

❏ If you suspect food poisoning, call your regional poison control center immediately. Poison control centers can be reached twenty-four hours a day, and can provide you with up-to-date information regarding treatment. It is a good idea to keep the number of your local center posted by your telephone and/or entered into your telephone's automatic dialing program.

❏ At the first suspicion of food poisoning, protect your immune system by taking 6 charcoal tablets. These are available at most health food stores and should be kept on hand for emergencies. The agents in these tablets circulate through the bloodstream and help to neutralize and eliminate poisons. After six hours, take 6 more tablets. Consume a lot of quality water to aid in flushing toxins from the system.

❏ Use cleansing enemas to remove toxins from the colon and bloodstream. (*See* ENEMAS in Part Three.)

❏ If vomiting occurs, make sure that the individual does not choke. If vomiting does not subside in twenty-four hours, collect a sample of the vomit for analysis to aid in pinpointing the cause of the illness.

❏ If you have been vomiting and have diarrhea, you may become seriously dehydrated. Replace lost fluids and electrolytes with clean water or other liquids designed specifically for rehydration.

❏ If you suspect that you have been poisoned by food from a public restaurant or other eating place, contact your local health department right away. It may be possible to save others from food poisoning.

❏ For some cases of poisoning, it may be desirable to induce vomiting to help expel the toxin that is the cause of the problem. Keep syrup of ipecac (available in drugstores) on hand for this purpose.

Caution: Syrup of ipecac should be used only at the direction of a physician or poison control center.

❏ If symptoms of food poisoning are severe or prolonged, consult your health care provider.

CONSIDERATIONS

❏ David Hill, a microbiologist at England's University of Wolverhampton, monitored all the bacteria present in the intestines and found that in the presence of garlic, disease-causing microbes were eliminated. According to Hill, the sulfur compounds in garlic are the secret weapon that knocks out dangerous bacteria.

❑ It was once believed that nylon or plastic cutting boards were preferable to the wooden variety. Since then, research has indicated that wood is probably better after all. Researchers have discovered that when cutting boards are contaminated with organisms that can cause food poisoning, almost all the bacteria on the wooden boards die off within three minutes, while almost none die on the plastic ones. For added security, you can wash your wooden cutting board periodically with hydrogen peroxide and water or a bleach-and-water solution. The ideal solution is to use one cutting board exclusively for vegetables and one for meat (*see* Tips for Preventing Food Poisoning on page 382). Glass cutting boards are probably safest of all.

❑ Certain strains of bacteria found in eggs are not destroyed if the eggs are poached, prepared over-easy, or sunny-side up.

❑ The overwhelming majority (an estimated 90 percent) of cases of botulism in the United States are attributable to improper home-canning techniques. The best safeguard against this illness is to avoid all home-canned meats, fruits, and vegetables unless they have been prepared in a pressure cooker in scrupulous accordance with the manufacturer's directions. The old "stovetop" method of home canning is *not* a reliable way to seal the jar lids properly.

❑ Food allergies are a common cause of illness and stomach upsets. For instance, a person who experiences severe headache and vomiting soon after eating may be suffering from food allergies. If this is the case, you should be able to develop a pattern associated with certain foods. (*See* ALLERGIES in Part Two.) In the meantime, charcoal tablets and a coffee retention enema can help rid the body of substances that cause allergic reactions.

❑ Interestingly, botulin toxin, one of the most potent toxins known to man, has been attracting attention from the medical community as a potential therapeutic tool. The U.S. Food and Drug Administration recently approved the use of a purified form of botulin toxin as a drug to treat two muscle disorders that affect the eyes, *blepharospasm* (uncontrollable muscle spasms of the eyelids) and *strabismus* (a tendency of one eye to deviate from parallelism with the other). A tiny amount of the toxin is injected directly into the muscles to paralyze them, reducing symptoms.

Fracture

A fracture is a break or a crack in a bone. If the skin over the bone remains intact, a fracture is referred to as a *closed* or *simple fracture;* if the bone breaks the skin, it is termed an *open* or *compound fracture.* A fracture may cause extreme pain and tenderness in the injured area; swelling; a protruding bone or blood under the skin; and numbness, tingling, or

paralysis below the fracture. A major fracture, such as of an arm or leg, may also cause a loss of the pulse below the fracture, as well as weakness and an inability to bear weight. Broken arms, fingers, or legs may be bent out of alignment.

Fractures occur most often in the very young and in older adults. Indeed, fractures pose an increasing problem as we grow older and our bones become more brittle. Falls account for 87 percent of all fractures in people aged sixty-five or older. An estimated 300,000 hip fractures occur in people over fifty years of age each year. People aged eighty-five or older are fifteen times more likely to suffer from a fracture if they fall than people between sixty and sixty-five. Osteoporosis is a factor in many of these cases.

Hip fractures are by far the most troublesome fractures for older adults, and, unfortunately, many cannot live an independent life after a hip fracture.

A broken bone calls for prompt professional help. After a bone has been set, the following supplements and other recommendations will aid in healing. Unless otherwise specified, the dosages recommended here are for adults. For a child between the ages of twelve and seventeen, reduce the dose to three-quarters the recommended amount. For a child between six and twelve, use one-half the recommended dose, and for a child under the age of six, use one-quarter the recommended amount.

NUTRIENTS

SUPPLEMENT	SUGGESTED DOSAGE	COMMENTS
Very Important		
Bone Builder With Boron from Ethical Nutrients	As directed on label.	A microcrystalline hydroxyapatite concentrate (MCHC) that contains the organic protein-calcium matrix of raw bone. Available only through health care professionals.
Bone Support from Synergy Plus or Bone Defense from KAL	As directed on label. Take with calcium and magnesium below. As directed on label.	To supply essential nutrients for bone health.
Boron	3 mg daily. Do not exceed this amount.	Important in bone health and healing. Studies show boron can increase calcium uptake by as much as 30 percent.
Calcium and	1,000–2,000 mg daily, in divided doses, after meals and at bedtime.	Vital for proper bone repair.
magnesium and	1,000 mg daily.	Needed to balance with calcium.
potassium	99 mg daily	Useful for maintaining good muscle and heart function.
Glucosamine and chondroitin plus	As directed on label.	Helps the body maintain joint flexibility by building cartilage.
methylsulfonyl-methane (MSM)	As directed on label.	Makes cell walls permeable, allowing water and nutrients to freely flow into cells and allowing wastes and toxins to properly flow out.

Kelp	1,000–1,500 mg daily.	Rich in calcium and minerals in a natural balance.
Neonatal Multi-Gland from Biotics Research	As directed on label.	Promotes healing. *See* GLANDULAR THERAPY in Part Three for its benefits.
Proteolytic enzymes	As directed on label. Take between meals and with meals.	Taken between meals, reduces inflammation. Taken with meals, aids digestion of proteins. *Caution:* Do not give this supplement to a child under 16 years of age.
S-Adenosylmethio- nine (SAMe)	As directed on label.	A natural alternative to prescribed antidepressants. Can also be used in a lower dose as an anti-inflammatory agent for joint stiffness. *Caution:* Do not use if you have manic-depressive disorder or take prescription antidepressants.
Silica or horsetail	As directed on label.	Supplies silicon, needed for calcium uptake and connective tissue repair. *See under* Herbs, below.
Vitamin C with bioflavonoids	3,000–6,000 mg daily, in divided doses.	Important in repair of bones, connective tissue, and muscles.
Vitamin D$_3$	400–1,000 IU daily.	Needed for calcium absorption and bone repair. May help to prevent fractures.
Zinc	80 mg daily. Do not exceed a total of 100 mg daily from all supplements.	Important in tissue repair. Use zinc gluconate lozenges or zinc methionate (OptiZinc) for best absorption.
Helpful		
Free-form amino acid complex (Amino Balance from Anabol Naturals or Amino Blend from Carlson Labs)	As directed on label.	Speeds healing.
Octacosanol	3,000 mg daily.	Improves tissue oxygenation.
Raw liver extract	As directed on label.	Supplies balanced B vitamins and other needed vitamins and minerals. (*See* GLANDULAR THERAPY in Part Three.)
Vitamin A with mixed carotenoids	25,000 IU daily until healed. If you are pregnant, do not exceed 10,000 IU daily.	Protein is not utilized without vitamin A. Use emulsion form for easier assimilation and greater safety at higher doses.
Vitamin B complex plus extra pantothenic acid (vitamin B$_5$)	As directed on label. 100 mg 3 times daily.	Helps maintain healthy muscle tone and proper brain function. Important for older adults because these nutrients are less well absorbed as we age. Anti-stress vitamin. Aids in vitamin utilization.

HERBS

❏ Boswellia, an herb used commonly in Ayurvedic medicine, aids in the process of recovery from a fracture, easing pain and acting as an excellent anti-inflammatory.

❏ Horsetail extract is a good source of silica, which enhances the utilization of calcium and promotes healing and repair.

❏ Turmeric paste makes a good poultice. Combine turmeric with a little hot water and apply it to the site of the injury on a gauze dressing. This is also good for bruises and helps to reduce swelling. A poultice of fresh mullein leaves is also good. (*See* USING A POULTICE in Part Three.)

RECOMMENDATIONS

❏ Eat half of a fresh pineapple every day until the fracture is healed. Pineapple contains bromelain, an enzyme that acts to reduce swelling and inflammation. Use only fresh pineapple, not canned or processed. If you don't like pineapple, the food supplement bromelain will provide the same benefits. Bromelain should be taken on an empty stomach.

❏ Avoid red meat, as well as colas and any other products containing caffeine. Foods with preservatives should also be avoided due to their phosphorus content. Phosphorus can lead to bone loss.

❏ Use clay poultices for bruises and swelling.

❏ Make your home safer by taking measures such as the following:

• Use non-slippery floor coverings. If you have carpets that are not fitted, make sure the edges are taped down.

• Make sure you have enough light so that you can see properly.

• Keep your path clear. If you have pets, they should be trained to keep out of your way. Do not leave things on the floor.

• Wipe up any spilled liquids immediately.

• Wear shoes or slippers with rubber soles.

• Take extra precautions when using the stairs. Install handrails if necessary.

• Keep the telephone in a readily accessible place. Do not rush to answer it. Portable phones are available with a simple large red button that will connect you directly with the 911 emergency number.

• Medical alert devices that are worn around the neck are also available for people living alone.

• Talk to your physician about the medications you are taking and discuss whether they might impair your balance or orientation.

❏ If you are in any discomfort after a fall, have an x-ray taken of the painful area. If there is a fracture, you need to have it attended to immediately.

❏ If you suffer a hip fracture, ask your physician about nerve blocks before you have an operation to fix it. A nerve block can lessen the amount of oral analgesic administered during surgery.

CONSIDERATIONS

❑ Ultrasound therapy after a fracture may speed healing by as much as 45 percent. The device has been approved by the FDA but only, at present, for wrist and shinbone fractures. This treatment is applied at home through a window in the cast. This treatment is expensive, however, and may not be covered by some insurance policies.

❑ *See also* OSTEOPOROSIS and SPRAINS, STRAINS, AND OTHER INJURIES OF THE MUSCLES AND JOINTS in Part Two.

Frigidity

Frigidity is the inability to experience pleasure from sexual intercourse, characterized by a general lack of sexual desire and responsiveness. The term *frigidity* is most often used to describe sexual dysfunction in women. It is usually of psychological origin, stemming from fear, anxiety, guilt, depression, conflict with one's mate, and/or feelings of inferiority. Early traumatic sexual experience or other unpleasant childhood and adolescent episodes are often factors. Frigidity may also be a result of physiological factors. Some women find intercourse painful due to insufficient lubrication, inadequate stimulation, underlying illness or infection, or some other physical cause. The pain causes them to fear and shrink from sexual contact. Vitamin deficiency can cause a deficiency in estrogen levels and result in improper lubrication. A chronic illness, some medications, low testosterone levels, and certain medical conditions can also greatly diminish sexual desire. The supplement program outlined below should help.

NUTRIENTS

SUPPLEMENT	SUGGESTED DOSAGE	COMMENTS
Very Important		
Kelp	2,000–2,500 mg daily.	A good source of iodine and other important minerals.
Vitamin B complex	100 mg of each major B vitamin twice daily (amounts of individual vitamins in a complex will vary).	Calms the nervous system and aids in reducing anxiety.
Vitamin E	Start with 200–400 IU daily and increase slowly to 1,600 IU daily.	Necessary for the functioning of the reproductive system and glands. Use d-alpha-tocopherol form.
Helpful		
Fish liver oil	As directed on label. Take with meals.	Supplies vitamins A and D.
Lecithin granules or capsules	1 tbsp 3 times daily, with meals. 2,400 mg 3 times daily, with meals.	Contains essential fatty acids and aids in proper nerve function.
L-Phenylalanine and L-tyrosine	500 mg each daily, on an empty stomach. Take with water or juice. Do not take with milk. Take with 50 mg vitamin B$_6$ and 100 mg vitamin C for better absorption. Do not exceed the recommended dosage.	Amino acids needed for synthesis of crucial neurotransmitters involved in mood and nervous system function. *Caution:* Do not take phenylalanine if you are pregnant or nursing a baby, or if you suffer from panic attacks, diabetes, high blood pressure, or PKU. Do not take tyrosine if you are taking an MAO inhibitor drug.
Para-aminobenzoic acid (PABA)	100 mg daily.	A B vitamin that stimulates vital life functions.
Vitamin C with bioflavonoids	3,000–6,000 mg daily, in divided doses.	Important in glandular function and stress response.
Zinc plus copper	50–80 mg daily. Do not exceed a total of 100 mg daily from all supplements. 3 mg daily.	Zinc deficiency can result in impaired sexual function. Use zinc gluconate lozenges or OptiZinc for best absorption. Needed to balance with zinc.

HERBS

❑ Chives contain minerals required for the manufacture of sex hormones.

❑ Damiana is the "woman's sexuality herb"—one of the most popular of plant aphrodisiacs. It contains alkaloids that directly stimulate the nerves and organs and have a testosterone-like effect. Damiana is excellent for supporting the sexual organs and enhancing sexual pleasure. For best results, place a dropperful of damiana extract under your tongue an hour or two before sexual activity. It may take several days for the difference to become apparent.

❑ Kava kava, traditionally valued for its mellowing effects, may help with issues of anxiety and nervousness.
Caution: This herb can cause drowsiness. It is not recommended for pregnant women or nursing mothers, and it should not be taken together with other substances that act on the central nervous system, such as alcohol, barbiturates, antidepressants, and antipsychotic drugs.

❑ Wild yam contains a natural steroid called dehydroepiandrosterone (DHEA) that rejuvenates and gives vigor to lovemaking. Take it for two weeks, then stop for two weeks, and so on.

❑ Other herbs that are good for promoting energy and sexuality include fo-ti, gotu kola, sarsaparilla, saw palmetto, and Siberian ginseng.
Caution: Do not use Siberian ginseng if you have hypoglycemia, high blood pressure, or a heart disorder.

RECOMMENDATIONS

❑ Make sure to include the following in your diet: alfalfa sprouts; avocados; eggs that come fresh from hens (not those stored cold in the supermarket); olive oil; pumpkin seeds and other seeds and nuts; soy and sesame oil; and wheat.

❑ Try taking supplemental bee pollen to increase energy.
Caution: Bee pollen may cause an allergic reaction in

some people. Start with a small amount at first, and discontinue use if a rash, wheezing, discomfort, or other symptom occurs.

❏ Avoid poultry, red meat, and sugar products.

❏ Avoid smoggy conditions. Smog is highly toxic and dangerous; it adversely affects immune function and hormonal activity, as well as a host of other body functions.

CONSIDERATIONS

❏ There are medical alternatives that can help some women by alleviating painful intercourse. Painful intercourse may also be a sign of certain gynecological diseases.

❏ If frigidity is due to interpersonal conflict or psychological causes, help from a couples counselor or other mental health professional is advised.

❏ Sexual dysfunction in men can be caused by psychological issues, but is usually described as a form of impotence instead of "frigidity." Psychological impotence in men can be based on early sexual trauma, anxiety, fear, guilt, and other psychologicial conflicts. (*See* IMPOTENCE in Part Two.)

❏ Depression or hypothyroidism may be the underlying problem. (*See* DEPRESSION and HYPOTHYROIDISM in Part Two.)

Fungal Infection

Certain types of fungi (most commonly candida and tinea) can infect the skin and/or mucous membranes; they can also grow under the nails, between the toes, or on internal surfaces of the colon and other organs.

Fungal infection of the skin is most common in places where skin tends to be moist and one skin surface is in contact with another, such as the groin area (*"jock itch"*) and between the toes (*"athlete's foot"*). A type of scalp infection known as *tinea capitis* is found mainly in schoolchildren, although adults also may be affected. Moist, possibly itchy, red patches anywhere on the body can indicate fungal infection. In babies, a fungal infection can manifest itself as diaper rash that makes the skin bright red in light-skinned babies and darker brown in dark-skinned babies.

Fungal infection of the mouth is referred to as *oral thrush*, a condition in which creamy-looking white patches form on the tongue and the mucous membranes of the mouth. If the patches are scraped off, bleeding may result. This condition is most common in infants and in those with compromised immune systems.

Nursing mothers sometimes develop a *candida infection of the nipples* that causes severe pain while feeding. This can be further complicated if the baby develops oral thrush; it can lead to a "ping-pong" effect in which mother and baby continually reinfect each other.

Fungal infection under the nails (*paronychia*) or between the toes may cause discoloration and swelling, and the nails may become raised above the surface of the nail bed. In fungal infection of the vagina (*yeast infection*), a cheesy discharge is present, usually accompanied by intense itching.

Ringworm, also known as tinea infection, is a fungal infection of the skin or scalp. Caused by various species of fungi—mainly microspora, trichophyta, and epidermophyta, it is characterized by the development of small red spots that grow to a size of about one-quarter inch in diameter. As the spots expand, the centers tend to heal and clear while the borders are raised, red, and scaly, giving them a ringlike appearance. Like other fungal infections, ringworm can be very itchy.

Recurrent fungal infections are a common sign of depressed immune function. The people most likely to be affected are those who have diseases such as diabetes or cancer, or who are infected with human immunodeficiency virus (HIV). Women who use oral contraceptives and people taking antibiotics are at higher risk as well, as are people who are obese and/or who perspire heavily.

Unless otherwise specified, the dosages recommended here are for adults. For a child between the ages of twelve and seventeen, reduce the dose to three-quarters the recommended amount. For a child between six and twelve, use one-half the recommended dose, and for a child under the age of six, use one-quarter the recommended amount.

NUTRIENTS

SUPPLEMENT	SUGGESTED DOSAGE	COMMENTS
Essential		
Acidophilus (Kyo-Dophilus and Probiata by from Wakunaga are good sources)	As directed on label.	Supplies the "friendly" bacteria that are usually deficient in people with fungal infections.
Garlic (Kyolic from Wakunaga)	2 capsules 3 times daily, with meals.	Neutralizes most fungi.
Kyolic-EPA from Wakunga	As directed on label.	For relief of pain and inflammation.
Important		
Colostrum (New Life Colostrum from Symbiotics [original and high-Ig formulas], and Colostrum Specific from Jarrow Formulas are good sources)	As directed on label.	Possesses healing properties, boosts the immune system, and fights fungal infection.
Vitamin B complex plus extra pantothenic acid (vitamin B₅)	50 mg 3 times daily, with meals. 50 mg 3 times daily.	Needed for correctly balanced "friendly" bacteria in the body. Plays a role in the formation of antibodies and aids in the utilization of nutrients.
Vitamin C with bioflavonoids	5,000–20,000 mg daily, in divided doses. (*See* ASCORBIC ACID FLUSH in Part Three.)	Needed for proper immune function.

Vitamin E	400–800 IU daily.	Needed for proper immune function. Use emulsion for easier assimilation. Use d-alpha-tocopherol form.
Zinc	50 mg daily. Do not exceed a total of 100 mg daily from all supplements.	Needed for proper immune function. Use zinc gluconate lozenges or OptiZinc for best absorption.
Helpful		
Essential fatty acids (black currant seed oil, primrose oil, and salmon oil are good sources)	As directed on label.	For relief of pain and inflammation.
Vitamin A with mixed carotenoids	25,000 IU daily. If you are pregnant, do not exceed 10,000 IU daily.	Aids healing of skin and mucous membranes. Needed for proper immune function.

HERBS

❏ Berberine is a phytochemical that has antifungal action. Goldenseal, a berberine-containing herb, works against a variety of fungi, including candida. Bloodroot, another herb that contains berberine, has shown action against skin fungi and is also an anti-inflammatory. Other herbs that contain berberine and are recommended for fungal infections include barberry, Oregon grape, and yellowroot.

❏ Horopito, or pepper tree (*Pseudowintera colorata*), a shrub native to New Zealand, contains polygodial, an antifungal agent that has been shown to act against bacteria as well. The leaves can be bruised, steamed, and applied topically to treat skin diseases such as ringworm. *Licaria puchuri-major,* a medicinal plant found in the Brazilian rainforest, has been found to augment the antifungal activity of polygodial and increase its effectiveness against fungal infection.

❏ Kolorex from Nature's Sources is an herbal product that has been shown to be effective in treating ringworm and tinea fungi infections. It is available in both capsule and cream form.

❏ Pau d'arco has strong antifungal properties. Drink 3 cups of pau d'arco tea daily.

❏ For toenail or fingernail fungus, soak nails in a mixture of pau d'arco and goldenseal. In a wide pan, make pau d'arco tea using 6 tea bags and a gallon of water. Bring to boil, then allow to cool to a very warm but tolerable temperature. Add the contents of 4 capsules of goldenseal. Soak your feet or hands in this mixture for fifteen minutes twice a day.

❏ Tea tree oil is a natural antifungal for external use. It can be applied to the affected area several times a day, either full strength or diluted with distilled water or cold-pressed vegetable oil. For trichomonal vaginitis or vaginal candidiasis, apply a few drops of the oil on a tampon, or mix it with water and use it as a douche. You can also use black walnut extract.

❏ Wild oregano oil is a powerful antifungal agent that has the ability to destroy even resistant forms of fungi.

RECOMMENDATIONS

❏ Eat a diet of 60 to 70 percent raw foods. Eat plenty of fresh vegetables and moderate amounts of broiled fish and broiled skinless chicken.

❏ Do not eat any foods containing sugar or refined carbohydrates. Fungi thrive on sugar.

❏ Eliminate those foods from the diet that tend to promote secretion of mucus, especially meat and dairy products.

❏ Avoid cola drinks, grains, processed foods, and fried, greasy foods.

❏ See FASTING in Part Three and follow the program.

❏ Keep the skin clean and dry. Expose the affected area to the air as much as possible.

❏ Wear clean cotton clothing and underwear. Do not wear clothing or use towels more than once without washing them, preferably in hot water with chlorine bleach added.

❏ To replace necessary "friendly" bacteria in the colon, use an *L. bifidus* retention enema. See ENEMAS in Part Three.

❏ Try not to allow an infected area of the body to come in contact with healthy skin. People who have fungal infections in one area often also have infections in other areas.

❏ If you are nursing a baby and your baby has thrush, *or* you develop sharp, shooting pains during feedings, *or* both, consult both your child's and your own health care provider. You may have a fungal infection. Both you and your baby should be treated to ensure a cure.

❏ To treat ringworm, use a sterile pad and apply colloidal silver to the affected area. Hands and feet can also be soaked in this solution, a natural antibiotic that destroys some 650 different microorganisms.

❏ For ringworm, mix 1/2 clove crushed garlic with 1/4 cup vegetable oil. Coat the affected area with honey, then apply the garlic mixture (avoid healthy skin). Cover loosely with sterile gauze that allows air to penetrate. Leave in place for four hours.

❏ If you have been treating a fungal infection on your own and you develop symptoms of a worsening infection, such as increased redness and swelling or fever, consult your physician. You may have developed a bacterial infection on top of the fungal infection.

❏ For fungal infections underneath the fingernails, soak your nails in a mixture of 50 percent white distilled vinegar and 50 percent pure water for ten to twenty minutes daily.

CONSIDERATIONS

❏ There are numerous topical antifungal preparations

available in drug stores. However, we believe that garlic is safer and works just as well, if not better, than these drugs.

❑ See also ATHLETE'S FOOT; CANDIDIASIS; and/or YEAST INFECTION in Part Two.

Gallbladder Disorders

The gallbladder is a three- to four-inch-long pear-shaped organ located on the right side of the body, directly under the liver. One of the functions of the liver is to remove poisonous substances from the blood so that they can be expelled from the body. The liver excretes all these gathered toxins in a digestive agent called bile. Bile also contains cholesterol, bile salts, lecithin, and other substances. The bile—about one pint of it every day—goes first to the gallbladder, which holds it until food arrives in the small intestine. The gallbladder then releases the bile, which passes through the cystic and bile ducts into the small intestine. Ultimately, the toxins are passed out of the body through the feces.

Abnormal concentration of bile acids, cholesterol, and phospholipids in the bile can cause the formation of gallstones. The presence of gallstones is known to doctors as *cholelithiasis*. It has been estimated that 20 million Americans have gallstones. In fact, one in ten people have gallstones without knowing it. However, if a stone is pushed out of the gallbladder and lodges in the bile duct, this can cause nausea, vomiting, and pain in the upper right abdominal region. These symptoms often arise after the individual has eaten fried or fatty foods.

Gallstones can range from the size of a tiny grain of sand to larger than a pea-sized mass. Seventy-five percent of gallstones are cholesterol stones, with the remaining 25 percent being pigment stones. Pigment stones are composed of calcium salts. Although the cause of pigment stones is unknown, factors such as intestinal surgery, cirrhosis of the liver, and blood disorders can increase the rate risk.

The presence of gallstones creates a possibility that *cholecystitis*, inflammation of the gallbladder, may develop. This can cause severe pain in the upper right abdomen and/or across the chest, possibly accompanied by fever, nausea, and vomiting. Other symptoms of gallbladder disease include constant pain below the breastbone that shoots into the right or left shoulder area and radiates into the back. The pain can last from thirty minutes to several hours. The urine may be tea- or coffee-colored, and there may be shaking, chills, and jaundice (a yellowish discoloration of the skin and eyes). Gallbladder attacks occur often in the evening and can take place sporadically. Abdominal pain that occurs on a daily basis may be a problem unrelated to the gallbladder. A gallbladder attack may mimic a heart attack, with severe pain in the chest area. *Biliary dyskinesia* is a condition in which all the symptoms of gallbladder disease are present, but there are no stones.

Inflammation of the gallbladder requires immediate treatment. If left untreated, it can be life threatening. If you experience pain in your upper abdomen that lasts for more than an hour, your doctor may recommend an ultrasound to confirm signs of gallbladder disease.

NUTRIENTS

SUPPLEMENT	SUGGESTED DOSAGE	COMMENTS
Alfalfa		*See under* Herbs, below.
Essential fatty acid complex or Kyolic-EPA from Wakunaga	As directed on label.	Important constituents of every living cell. Needed for repair and prevention of gallstones.
Lecithin granules or capsules	1 tbsp 3 times daily, before meals. 1,200 mg 3 times daily, before meals.	A fat emulsifier; aids digestion of fats.
L-Glycine	500 mg daily, on an empty stomach. Take with water or juice. Do not take with milk. Take with 50 mg vitamin B$_6$ and 100 mg vitamin C for better absorption.	Essential for the biosynthesis of nucleic and bile acids. (*See* AMINO ACIDS in Part One.)
Multienzyme complex with ox bile (D.A. #34 from Carlson Labs)	As directed on label. Take before meals.	Aids in digestion if too little bile is secreted from the gallbladder. Ox bile is needed especially if you have had gallbladder removal surgery. *Caution:* Do not give this supplement to a child. If you have a history of ulcers, do not use a formula containing HCl.
Taurine Plus from American Biologics	As directed on label.	Necessary for the formation of an important bile acid and may prevent the formation of gallstones. Use the liquid form.
Vitamin A with carotenoids	25,000 IU daily. If you are pregnant, do not exceed 10,000 IU daily.	Needed for repair of tissues. Use emulsion form for easier assimilation.
Vitamin B complex plus extra vitamin B$_{12}$ and choline and inositol	50 mg 3 times daily, with meals. 2,000 mcg daily. 500 mg daily. 500 mg daily.	All B vitamins are necessary for proper digestion. Use a high-potency formula. Important in cholesterol metabolism and liver and gallbladder function.
Vitamin C with bioflavonoids	3,000 mg daily.	Deficiency can lead to gallstones.
Vitamin D$_3$	400 IU daily.	Gallbladder malfunction interferes with vitamin D absorption.
Vitamin E	600 IU daily.	Prevents fats from becoming rancid. Use d-alpha-tocopherol form.

HERBS

❑ Alfalfa cleanses the liver and supplies necessary vitamins and minerals. Twice a day for two days, take 1,000 milligrams in tablet or capsule form with a glass of warm water.

❑ Peppermint oil capsules are used in Europe to cleanse the gallbladder.

❑ If you have gallstones, or are prone to developing them, turmeric can reduce your risk of further problems.

❑ Other beneficial herbs include barberry root bark, catnip, cramp bark, dandelion, fennel, ginger root, horsetail, parsley, and wild yam.

Caution: Do not use barberry during pregnancy.

RECOMMENDATIONS

❑ If you have an attack, drink 1 tablespoon of apple cider in a glass of apple juice. This should relieve the pain quickly. If the pain does not subside, go to the emergency room to rule out other disorders such as gastroesophogeal reflux disease (GERD) or heart problems.

❑ For inflammation of the gallbladder, eat no solid food for a few days. Consume only distilled or spring water. Then drink juices such as pear, beet, and apple for three days. Then add solid foods: shredded raw beets with 2 tablespoons of olive oil, fresh lemon juice, and freshly made uncooked applesauce made in a blender or food processor. Apple juice aids in softening gallstones.

❑ For gallstones, take 3 tablespoons of olive oil with the juice of a lemon before bed and upon awakening. Stones are often passed and eliminated in the stool with this technique—look for them. You can use grapefruit juice instead. To relieve acute pain, try using hot castor oil packs on the gallbladder area. Place castor oil in a pan and heat but do not boil it. Dip a piece of cheesecloth or other white cotton material into the oil until the cloth is saturated. Apply the cloth to the affected area and cover it with a piece of plastic that is larger in size than the cotton cloth. Place a heating pad over the plastic and use it to keep the pack warm. Keep the pack in place for one-half to two hours, as needed.

❑ Eat a diet consisting of 75 percent raw foods. Include in the diet applesauce, eggs, yogurt, cottage cheese, broiled fish, fresh apples, and beets.

❑ To cleanse the system, consume as much pure apple juice as possible for five days. Add pear juice occasionally. Beet juice also cleanses the liver.

❑ Avoid sugar and products containing sugar. People who consume an excessive amount of sugar are much more likely to form gallstones. Avoid all animal fat and meat, saturated fats (found primarily in meat), full-fat dairy products, fried foods, spicy foods, margarine, soft drinks, commercial oils, chocolate, and refined carbohydrates.

❑ While you have pain, nausea and/or vomiting, and fever, follow a fasting program and use coffee enemas for a few days. The coffee enema is important. You can also use garlic in the enema. (*See* ENEMAS and FASTING in Part Three.)

❑ A detoxification program for the liver and colon is important for improved gallbladder function. Use cleansing enemas if you have chronic problems.

❑ Do not overeat. Obesity and gallbladder disease are related. Females age forty and over who are overweight and who have had children are more likely than most people to suffer from disorders of the gallbladder.

CONSIDERATIONS

❑ Rapid weight changes can cause gallbladder problems. A study published in the *Annals of Internal Medicine* revealed that yo-yo dieting—that is, repeatedly losing and gaining weight due to dieting—increases the risk of gallstones and the necessity for surgery by as much as 70 percent.

❑ The recommended treatment for gallstones used to be surgical removal of the gallbladder. However, if gallstones show up on an x-ray but do not cause symptoms, there is no need for surgery.

❑ A gallstone may slip into a bile duct, one of the structures that drain the gallbladder and the liver. If this occurs, extraction or surgical removal by a technique called *laparoscopic cholecystectomy* may be necessary. Also known as keyhole surgery, this is the now most common method of removing the gallbladder. The surgeon uses a trocar (a hollow tube) and enters the abdomen through the navel. Three more of these tubes are inserted into the abdomen so that instruments can be inserted through them. The surgeon inserts a laparoscope (a small camera) through one of these tubes, so that he or she can see inside the patient without the large incision normally required to remove a gallbladder. The procedure requires four small incisions in total, instead of a single six- to nine-inch incision, and recovery time is said to be greatly reduced. However, research from Washington University suggests that people with a history of gallbladder inflammation or ten or more gallbladder attacks, or who are over sixty-five years of age, may be more likely to have complications with this type of surgery. If complications do arise after surgery, this may be because the gallbladder was not in fact the source of the initial problem, or because of a bile leak.

❑ Sometimes stones in the gallbladder can be fragmented or dissolved without surgery, using the drug deoxycholic acid or lithotripsy (the use of sound waves to break up stones). Bile acid preparations used to dissolve stones work very slowly and can be used only on small stones.

❑ Eighty percent of gallstones produce no symptoms and require no treatment. Discuss any recommended treatment with your doctor and surgeon and make sure an operation is absolutely necessary before proceeding.

❑ Physical activity can reduce the risk of gallstones by 20 to 40 percent.

❑ A study reported in the *Journal of the American Medical Association* found that drinking three cups of coffee a day may lower men's (and possibly women's) risk of developing gallstones. However, it is not recommended that you start drinking more coffee due to the results of one study.

□ People with pigment stones, which consist of calcium salts, should probably avoid using calcium supplements, although some researchers believe it is all right for them to continue taking calcium supplements.

□ Gallstones run in families. Women are twice as likely to form gallstones as men.

Gangrene

Gangrene is a condition in which body tissues die, and ultimately decay, as a result of an inadequate oxygen supply. It can affect any body part, but most frequently affects extremities—the toes, feet, fingers, hands, and arms. Gangrene of the internal organs is especially dangerous.

There are two types of gangrene: wet gangrene and dry gangrene. Wet gangrene is the result of a wound or injury that becomes infected with bacteria. The infection prevents adequate venous drainage, depriving the area of needed blood supply and oxygen. The disruption in oxygen supply in turn promotes the infection. Symptoms of wet gangrene include severe and rapidly worsening pain, swelling, and tenderness in the area. As the infection progresses, the affected tissue changes color, usually from pink to deep red to gray-green or purple. Left untreated, wet gangrene can lead to shock and death in a matter of days. Fortunately, careful hygiene can usually prevent this type of gangrene.

Dry gangrene does not involve bacterial infection. It is caused by stopped or reduced blood flow, which results in oxygen-deprived tissue. Reduced blood flow may be caused by injury, hardening of the arteries, poor circulation, diabetes, or blockage in a blood vessel. The condition most often occurs in the feet and toes. Symptoms of the most common type of dry gangrene are a dull, aching pain and coldness in the area. Pain and pallor of the affected area are early signs.

Sometimes gangrene is caused by frostbite. In frostbite, the oxygen-deprived area dies, but the gangrene does not spread to any other area. As the flesh dies, it may be painful, but once the skin is dead, it becomes numb and slowly darkens.

The risk of developing gangrene is higher than normal for people with diabetes, who smoke or drink excessively, or who have poor circulation in general. Proper nutrition and a healthy lifestyle decrease the likelihood of developing gangrene and also aid in recovery should you require surgery for this condition.

Unless otherwise specified, the dosages recommended here are for adults. For a child between the ages of twelve and seventeen, reduce the dose to three-quarters of the recommended amount. For a child between six and twelve, use one-half of the recommended dose, and for a child under the age of six, use one-quarter of the recommended amount.

NUTRIENTS

SUPPLEMENT	SUGGESTED DOSAGE	COMMENTS
Essential		
Dimethylglycine (DMG) (Aangamik DMG from FoodScience of Vermont)	100 mg 3 times daily.	Enhances oxygen utilization by affected tissue.
Dioxychlor from American Biologics	As directed on label.	Antiviral, antifungal, and anti-bacterial. Assists the immune system in defending against invading microorganisms, with little or no toxicity to normal tissues.
Garlic (Kyolic from Wakunaga)	As directed on label.	Speeds healing and increases circulation. Cleanses the blood. Use the liquid form.
Methylsulfonyl-methane (MSM)	As directed on label.	Aids in the healing of injuries and can help to detoxify the body on a cellular level. It has also been found to be an aid to the organs, connective tissue, and immune functions.
plus vitamin C with bioflavonoids	5,000–20,000 mg daily. See ASCORBIC ACID FLUSH in Part Three.	For tissue repair and improved circulation. Improves the benefits of MSM.
Silicon (BioSil from Jarrow Technologies)	As directed on label.	Needed for skin and tissue repair.
Very Important		
Chlorophyll (Liquid Chlorophyll from American Biologics)	As directed on label.	A source of minerals, enzymes, and vitamins. Also used as a blood detoxifier and nutrient.
Coenzyme Q$_{10}$ plus Coenzyme A from Coenzyme-A Technologies	As directed on label.	Powerful antioxidants that help to improve circulation and boost the immune system.
Essential fatty acids (flaxseed, primrose, and salmon oils are good sources)	As directed on label.	Protects and aids in the repair of new tissues and cells.
Free-form essential amino acid complex plus extra	As directed on label.	For repair of tissues.
L-arginine	As directed on label.	Facilitates natural synthesis of nitric oxide, which promotes healthy blood vessels. Note: Do not use if you are pregnant or have cataracts, colitis, or a viral infection such as herpes.
Kyo-Green from Wakunaga	As directed on label.	Acts as a blood cleanser and builds up the blood supply.
Micellized Vitamin A emulsion from American Biologics	As directed on label.	Vitamin A is essential for tissue repair; vitamin E improves circulation. Both enhance immune function. Use this emulsion form for easier assimilation and safety at higher doses.
Proteolytic enzymes	As directed on label. Take with meals and between meals.	Aids in damaged tissue "cleanup" and repair. Caution: Do not give this supplement to a child under 16 years of age.

Vitamin E	400–600 IU daily.	Improves circulation. Use d-alpha-tocopherol form.
Important		
Kelp	1,000–1,500 mg daily.	A rich source of chlorophyll and minerals good for circulation. A blood cleanser.
Helpful		
Aerobic 07 from Aerobic Life Industries	As directed on label. Also apply a few drops directly on the affected area.	A stabilized oxygen product. Kills infecting bacteria.
Beta-1,3-D-glucan	As directed on label.	Helps to recruit immune T cells to the site of infection and aids in the growth of new blood vessels.
Calcium and magnesium	2,000 mg daily. 1,000 mg daily.	For connective tissue repair. Dilates blood vessels, improving blood flow. Needed to balance with calcium.
Multivitamin and mineral complex with potassium	As directed on label.	All nutrients are necessary for healing. Helps reduce tissue swelling.
Zinc	50–80 mg daily. Do not exceed a total of 100 mg daily from all supplements.	Speeds healing. Necessary for tissue repair and immune function. Use zinc gluconate lozenges or zinc methionate (OptiZinc) for best absorption.

HERBS

❑ Butcher's broom is important for circulation.

❑ Bromelain and tumeric (curcumin) are good for reducing swelling and inflammation.

❑ Olive leaf is good for fighting infections.

❑ Other beneficial herbs include bayberry, cayenne (capsicum), echinacea, ginkgo biloba, goldenseal, and red seal.

Caution: Do not take goldenseal internally on a daily basis for more than one week at a time, as it may disturb normal intestinal flora. Do not use it during pregnancy, and use it with caution if you are allergic to ragweed.

RECOMMENDATIONS

❑ Eat a high-protein, high-calorie diet to promote fast tissue repair.

❑ Include in the diet foods that are high in germanium, such as garlic, shiitake mushrooms, and onions. Germanium helps to improve tissue oxygenation.

❑ Drink six to eight glasses of quality water (preferably steam-distilled) every day.

❑ Add "green drinks" made from vegetables to your diet. (*See* JUICING in Part Three.)

❑ If you smoke, stop. Avoid all contact with tobacco.

❑ If you have diabetes, be vigilant in your treatment.

❑ If an injured area becomes red, swollen, and painful, or develops an odor, see your health care practitioner without delay.

CONSIDERATIONS

❑ The only treatment for established gangrene is surgical removal of the affected area.

❑ For wet gangrene, treatment with antibiotics and surgical removal of the dead tissue are usually necessary. Hyperbaric oxygen therapy may be employed as well. (*See* HYPERBARIC OXYGEN THERAPY in Part Three.)

❑ Slowly developing dry gangrene may be reversed by arterial surgery. Chelation is an alternative. (*See* CHELATION THERAPY in Part Three.) If an acute arterial obstruction is involved, emergency surgery must be performed.

❑ *See also* ARTERIOSCLEROSIS and CIRCULATORY PROBLEMS in Part Two.

❑ Raynaud's syndrome, a condition that affects the small arteries of the fingers and toes, can lead to gangrene if not treated. *See* RAYNAUD'S DISEASE/RAYNAUD'S PHENOMENON in Part Two for a more complete discussion of this condition.

Gas

See HEARTBURN/GASTROESOPHAGEAL REFLUX DISEASE (GERD); INDIGESTION (DYSPEPSIA). *See also under* PREGNANCY-RELATED PROBLEMS.

Gastroenteritis

See FOODBORNE/WATERBORNE DISEASE. *See also under* INFLUENZA.

Gastroesophageal Reflux Disease (GERD)

See HEARTBURN/GASTROESOPHAGEAL REFLUX DISEASE (GERD).

German Measles (Rubella)

German measles, or rubella, is a contagious viral disease that generally produces mild symptoms but is potentially dangerous to a fetus if a pregnant woman contracts the disease during the first trimester. Before a rubella vaccine was developed in the late 1960s, thousands of babies in the United States were born with severe birth defects because their mothers were exposed to the virus. Today, most children receive a vaccine that protects against measles, mumps, and rubella, but the virus exists worldwide and outbreaks still occur sporadically, usually in large population areas.

German measles mostly affects children, adolescents, and young adults. It initially causes swelling of the lymph glands in the neck and behind the ears. Other symptoms include coughing, fatigue, headache, mild fever, muscle aches, and stiffness, mainly in the neck. A pink rash often develops, usually starting on the face and neck and then spreading to the rest of the body. The rash typically lasts for about three days. The virus usually runs its course in five to seven days, and is generally not treated. A person who has had German measles has a lifetime immunity against the virus.

The communicable period probably begins two to four days before the rash appears, and the virus most often disappears from the nose and throat by the time the rash on the body disappears, one to three days after the onset of symptoms. However, because of the danger it poses to pregnant women, German measles should be considered contagious from one week before the rash appears until one week after the rash fades.

Unless otherwise specified, the dosages recommended here are for adults. For a child between the ages of twelve and seventeen, reduce the dose to three-quarters the recommended amount. For a child between six and twelve, use one-half the recommended dose, and for a child under the age of six, use one-quarter the recommended amount.

NUTRIENTS

SUPPLEMENT	SUGGESTED DOSAGE	COMMENTS
Helpful		
Bio-Strath from Nature's Answer	As directed on label.	Acts as a tonic. Contains the vitamin B complex. Use the liquid form.
Calcium and magnesium	As directed on label. As directed on label.	Needed for tissue repair.
Essential fatty acids (flaxseed oil, Kyolic-EPA from Wakunaga, primrose oil, and salmon oil are good sources)	As directed on label.	Helps prevent scarring and healing tissue cells.
Garlic (Kyolic from Wakunaga)	2 capsules 3 times daily, with meals.	Improves immune function.
Kyo-Dophilus or Probiata from Wakunaga	As directed on label.	Aids in normal bowel function. Allows survival and rapid passage of "friendly" bacteria through the stomach into the small intestine. Use a dairy-free, yeast-free formula.
Micellized Vitamin A emulsion from American Biologics	As directed on label.	Supplies vitamins A and E, needed to reduce infection and repair tissues. For a child under 10, substitute cod liver oil.
Proteolytic enzymes	As directed on label. Take on an empty stomach. Also take between meals.	Reduces infection and aids digestion. *Caution:* Do not give this supplement to a child.
Raw thymus glandular plus adrenal glandular	500 mg twice daily. As directed on label.	To stimulate the immune system. *Caution:* Do not give these supplements to a child.
Vitamin C with bioflavonoids	5,000–20,000 mg daily, in divided doses. *See* ASCORBIC ACID FLUSH in Part Three.	Very important for immune function. Controls fever and infection. Has antiviral properties. Use ascorbate or esterified form.
Zinc lozenges	1 15-mg lozenge 3 times daily for 4 days. Then reduce to 1 lozenge daily. Use this dosage for adults and for children over 5.	For immune response and tissue repair.

HERBS

❏ If necessary, catnip tea or garlic enemas can be used to lower fever. (*See* ENEMAS in Part Three.)

❏ Clove and peppermint tea aid in relieving symptoms.

❏ Alcohol-free goldenseal extract, placed directly under the tongue, aids in destroying bacteria and viruses and also relieves coughing. Use 3 drops for a child from three to ten years of age; for an adult or a child over ten, use one dropperful. Hold the extract under the tongue for a few minutes, then swallow. Repeat this three times daily for three days. As an alternative, use an echinacea and goldenseal combination extract, available in health food stores. Echinacea is good for the immune response.

Caution: Do not take goldenseal internally on a daily basis for more than one week at a time. Do not use it during pregnancy.

❏ Take $\frac{1}{2}$ teaspoon of lobelia extract every four to five hours for pain.

Caution: Do not take lobelia internally on an ongoing basis.

❏ Maitake, reishi, and shiitake mushrooms are all effective in boosting the body's immune system.

❏ Olive leaf extract is good for reducing symptoms and controlling the virus.

RECOMMENDATIONS

❏ Drink plenty of fluids such as water, juices, and vegetable broths.

❏ Avoid processed foods.

❏ Rest until the rash and fever have disappeared.

❏ Avoid contact with healthy individuals, especially women of childbearing age and their children, until one week after the rash disappears.

❏ *Do not* give aspirin to a child with German measles. *See* REYE'S SYNDROME in Part Two.

CONSIDERATIONS

❑ Antibiotics are useless against viruses, so they are not called for in the treatment of German measles.

❑ A person infected with German measles should be kept isolated in a dimly lit room. Extra care should be taken if a rash breaks out close to the eyes.

❑ A woman who has had German measles will pass immunity to any child she has for the first year of his or her life.

❑ Immunity to German measles can be determined by a blood test. Any woman who wishes to become pregnant and who is not sure whether she has achieved immunity to German measles should be tested and vaccinated, if necessary. Pregnancy must then be avoided for at least three months following immunization.

❑ It is a good idea for any woman who is (or who may be) pregnant to take precautions to avoid exposure to anyone who has, or has recently been exposed to, German measles. A pregnant woman who suspects she may have been exposed to German measles and who knows she has not achieved immunity (either through vaccination or from having the disease) should consult her doctor immediately concerning a gamma-globulin injection. If given soon after exposure, gamma-globulin may reduce the severity of the illness or even prevent it from developing.

❑ Many doctors believe that children should be immunized against German measles at about 15 months of age and again a few years later. Nonpregnant women of childbearing age are advised to be immunized also. People who should *not* be immunized include women who may be pregnant and individuals with impaired immune function, such as those with AIDS or cancer, or those currently taking cortisone or anticancer drugs or undergoing radiation therapy. Those with an illness that causes a fever should defer vaccination until healthy.

Gingivitis

See under PERIODONTAL DISEASE.

Glaucoma

Glaucoma is a group of diseases that affect the optic nerve and can lead to irreversible vision loss. It is usually, but not always, associated with elevated fluid pressure within the eye. All forms of glaucoma can cause damage to the optic nerve and lead to vision loss, even blindness, if left untreated.

Over 2 million Americans are affected by glaucoma. It is one of the leading causes of blindness, and is expected to become more prevalent in years to come due to the growing population of older adults. Those at greatest risk are people over the age of sixty; people of African ancestry; and people with diabetes, high blood pressure, severe myopia (nearsightedness), or a family history of glaucoma. Smokers also have an elevated risk, as do those who have sustained eye injuries or who have used steroids for an extended period of time.

As many as 3 percent of Americans are believed to have open-angle glaucoma, the most common form of the disease. Yet because this disorder causes no symptoms until it is quite advanced, only about half of those who have it are aware of it. In open-angle glaucoma, there is no physical blockage and the structures of the eye appear normal, but the drainage of fluid nevertheless is inadequate to keep the intraocular pressure at a normal level. The most pronounced symptoms of open-angle glaucoma are the gradual loss or "darkening" of peripheral vision and a marked decrease in night vision or the ability of the eye to adjust to darkness. Peripheral vision is the ability to see "out of the corner of the eye." The loss of this ability leaves a person with "tunnel vision." Other possible symptoms include chronic low-grade headaches (often mistaken for tension headaches), the need for frequent changes in eyeglass prescription, and/or seeing halos around electric lights.

A far less common, yet more serious, form of glaucoma is *closed-angle glaucoma*. Closed-angle glaucoma is much more insidious than open-angle forms because it almost never manifests any symptoms until very late in the condition. By that time, vision may be irreversibly damaged. Closed-angle glaucoma accounts for about 15 percent of all cases. Attacks of this type of glaucoma occur when the channels through which the eye's fluids drain suddenly become constricted or obstructed. This is usually due to narrowing or hardening of the exit channels from the eyes, and it results in extreme pain, poor vision, and even blindness. It is considered a medical emergency. Early warning signs that a problem may be developing include eye pain or discomfort mainly in the morning, blurred vision, seeing halos around lights, and inability of the pupils to adjust to a dark room. Symptoms of the acute attack itself include throbbing eye pain and loss of sight, especially peripheral vision; pupils that are fixed in a mildly dilated condition and do not respond to light properly; and a sharp increase in the pressure in the inner eye, especially on one side. These symptoms come on very rapidly and may be accompanied by nausea and even vomiting. Permanent vision damage can occur in as little as three to five days, making treatment within the first twenty-four to forty-eight hours imperative.

In some cases, glaucoma manifests itself even though there is normal fluid pressure within the eye. This form of glaucoma is called *normotensive* (normal-tension), and accounts for about 15 percent of all cases. With this condition, the optic nerve is damaged and vision is impaired much the same way as open-angle glaucoma, but without the increased fluid pressure. This has led many researchers to shift their focus in recent years to the optic nerve itself. Mechanisms other than pressure may cause changes in the eye that can cause damage to the optic nerve.

Glaucoma probably has many causes. Many scientists believe it may be closely linked to stress and nutritional problems, or disorders such as diabetes and high blood pressure. Some suspect that excessive amounts of glutamic acid, a nonessential amino acid also known as glutamate, may be involved. Glaucoma has also been linked with a deficiency in nitric oxide, a molecule that is critical for healthy blood vessels. Problems with collagen, the most abundant protein in the human body, have been linked to glaucoma. Collagen acts to increase the strength and elasticity of tissues in the body, especially those of the eye. Collagen and tissue abnormalities at the back of the eye contribute to the "clogging" of the tissues through which intraocular fluid normally drains. The result is elevated inner eye pressure that leads to glaucoma and related vision loss. Conditions characterized by errors of collagen metabolism are frequently associated with eye disorders.

Experts now believe that a simple pressure test is inadequate for diagnosis of glaucoma. An eye exam should also include a close examination of the optic nerve itself while the pupil is dilated, plus a test of the peripheral vision to see if any vision loss has occurred. People who are at risk for glaucoma should be tested frequently so that any loss of peripheral vision can be documented early.

NUTRIENTS

SUPPLEMENT	SUGGESTED DOSAGE	COMMENTS
Very Important		
Choline and inositol or	1,000–2,000 mg daily.	Important B vitamins for the eyes and brain.
lecithin	As directed on label.	A good source of choline and inositol.
Essential fatty acids (flaxseed oil, Kyolic-EPA from Wakunaga, primrose oil, and salmon oil are good sources)	As directed on label. Take with meals.	Protects and aids repair of new tissues and cells.
Glutathione	500 mg twice daily, on an empty stomach. Take with 50 mg vitamin B_6 and 100 mg vitamin C for better absorption.	A powerful antioxidant that protects the lens and maintains the molecular integrity of the lens fiber membranes.
Rutin	50 mg 3 times daily.	An important bioflavonoid that works with vitamin C and aids in reducing pain and intraocular pressure.
Vitamin A plus carotenoid complex with lutein and zeaxanthin	50,000 IU daily. If you are pregnant, do not exceed 10,000 IU daily. As directed on label.	Needed for good eyesight. Essential in formation of visual purple, the substance necessary for night vision.
Vitamin B complex plus extra pantothenic acid (vitamin B_5)	100 mg of each major B vitamin 3 times daily (amounts of individual vitamins a complex will vary). 100 mg 3 times daily.	B vitamins work best when taken together. Use a sublingual form or injections (under a doctor's supervision). Whenever stress is a factor, B-complex injections are a good idea. Anti-stress vitamin needed for the adrenal glands, and an essential constituent of coenzyme A, needed for many vital metabolic processes.
Vitamin C with bioflavonoids	10,000–15,000 mg daily, in divided doses. Under a doctor's supervision, you can increase the dose to 30,000 mg daily.	Reduces intraocular pressure.
Vitamin E plus L-Arginine	400 IU daily. As directed on label.	Helpful in removing particles from the lens of the eye. Has antioxidant properties to protect the lens and other eye tissues. Use d-alpha-tocopherol form. Facilitates natural synthesis of nitric oxide, which promotes healthy blood vessels. *Note:* Avoid arginine if you are pregnant or have cataracts, colitis, or a viral infection such as herpes.
Helpful		
Alpha-lipoic acid	150 mg daily.	An important antioxidant. Improves visual functions.
Magnesium	500–1,000 mg daily.	Dilates blood vessels, enhancing flow to the eyes.
Multivitamin and mineral complex with selenium	As directed on label. 200 mcg daily.	All nutrients are needed to aid in healing and to reduce intraocular pressure. A potent antioxidant that works with vitamin E.
Taurine Plus from American Biologics	As directed on label.	An antioxidant that protects the lens of the eye.
Zinc	50 mg daily. Do not exceed a total of 100 mg daily from all supplements.	Essential in activating vitamin A from the liver. Very beneficial in glaucoma therapy. Use zinc sulfate form.

HERBS

❏ Bilberry contains flavonoids and nutrients needed to protect the eyes from further damage. Fresh blueberries and red raspberry leaf can be used also.

❏ Chickweed and eyebright are good for all eye disorders.

❏ *Coleus forskohli*, an Ayurvedic herb, has been shown to reduce eye pressure.

Caution: Do not take this herb if you have prostate cancer.

❏ Eye baths using warm fennel tea, alternating with chamomile and eyebright, are helpful. Or use an eye dropper and apply three drops to each eye three times a day. Always dilute any herbal preparations used in the eyes with high-quality water.

Caution: Do not use chamomile on an ongoing basis, as ragweed allergy may result. Avoid it completely if you are allergic to ragweed.

❑ A combination of ginkgo biloba extract and zinc sulfate may slow progressive vision loss.

❑ Jaborandi is a rainforest herb that contains pilocarpine, used for over 120 years to relieve intraocular pressure in glaucoma.

Caution: Do not use this herb if you have pleurisy, are nursing, or have excess fatty tissue around the heart.

❑ Rose hips supply valuable flavonoids and vitamin C.

❑ *Avoid* the herbs ephedra (ma huang) and licorice.

RECOMMENDATIONS

❑ Follow the supplementation program outlined above.

❑ Exercise regularly. Research has shown that people with open-angle glaucoma patients who exercise at least three times a week can reduce intraocular pressure by 20 percent or more. If they stop exercising, the pressure begins to build up again. Exercise does not appear to have the same benefits for people with closed-angle glaucoma.

❑ If your ophthalmologist recommends medication to control glaucoma and it is working to your satisfaction, continue to use it faithfully. Also take vitamin C in high doses, but only under supervision.

❑ If you are using eyedrops to reduce intraocular pressure, make sure you know how to administer the eye drops properly to ensure that your eyes receive a sufficient amount of the medication. If improperly administered, eye drops can roll off the eye, spill down your cheek, or even get absorbed into your own tear duct. It can be difficult to gauge how effective you are at administering your own eyedrops. Ask your ophthalmologist for help in finding the best method. It also helps to occasionally have someone watch you administer the drops to make sure they are getting into the eye. It is also a good idea to close your eye gently for a minute or two after administering eye drops to give time for the medication to be absorbed.

❑ Avoid prolonged eye stress such as watching television, reading, and using a computer for long periods. If you must engage in close work for any length of time, take periodic "focus breaks." Every twenty minutes or so, raise your eyes and focus on something in the distance for a minute or so.

❑ Avoid tobacco smoke, coffee, alcohol, nicotine, and all caffeine.

❑ Drink only small amounts of liquid at any given time.

❑ Avoid taking high doses of niacin (over a total of 200 milligrams daily).

CONSIDERATIONS

❑ There is no cure for glaucoma, and any damage to vision is irreversible. Chronic open-angle glaucoma can often be controlled through the use of medication, usually in the form of eye drops. Several types of these medications are available. Often an ophthalmologist has to experiment a lit-tle to find the specific one that works most effectively for a particular individual. However, many people with glaucoma find that the eye drops cause severe headaches and other side effects. This problem can often be alleviated by changing the prescription. If headaches persist, it may help to adjust the schedule for taking the medication so that it interferes with normal activities as little as possible.

❑ Several studies have shown that smoking marijuana can help reduce intraocular pressure. However, marijuana is not recommended in the treatment of glaucoma for a variety of reasons, not least of which is its illegal status. Marijuana tends to increase the heart rate and lower blood pressure, which could compromise blood flow to the optic nerve. Also, the mechanisms by which marijuana lowers intraocular pressure are not fully understood, nor has it been shown that marijuana can work as safely and effectively as many FDA-approved drugs currently on the market.

❑ If eyedrops fail to control intraocular pressure, a doctor may use a procedure called laser trabeculoplasty. With this technique, a laser beam makes tiny holes in the meshwork through which the aqueous fluid normally drains, opening up blocked drainage channels.

❑ Surgery has certain advantages over medication, such as reduced out-of-pocket costs. However, it has disadvantages as well. An estimated 40 percent of people who undergo surgery for glaucoma experience no improvement, and the procedure may have to be repeated; approximately 15 percent report a decline in their quality of life after surgery.

❑ For acute closed-angle glaucoma attacks, surgery is usually necessary. Even though only one eye may be affected initially, the ophthalmologist performing the surgery will likely recommend that you have the surgical procedure on both eyes to prevent a second attack.

❑ The conventional treatment for acute closed-angle glaucoma is to immediately reduce eye pressure by employing an osmotic diuretic agent, followed by surgery. These osmotic agents (applied as eyedrops) almost always act immediately to alleviate symptoms. However, surgery is still recommended because without it, the attacks are likely to recur, and each attack can cause additional irreversible vision damage. Using only osmotic agents can lull a person into thinking that his or her condition is improving while in fact it is worsening rapidly.

❑ Agents that act to dilate the pupils, such as ephedra and belladonna, should be avoided at all costs.

❑ Vitamin C supplementation has been demonstrated to lower intraocular pressure in several clinical studies. Nearly normal tension levels have been achieved in some people who were unresponsive to conventional therapies. Intravenous administration of vitamin C has yielded even greater initial pressure reduction, but close monitoring by a physician is necessary to determine the required dosage. The role vitamin C plays in collagen formation may be the key to its action.

❏ Bioflavonoid supplementation prevents the breakdown of vitamin C in the body before it is metabolized. It also improves capillary integrity and stabilizes the collagen matrix by preventing free radical damage. The bioflavonoid rutin is known to help in lowering ocular pressure when used in conjunction with conventional drugs. Bilberry extract is particularly rich in this beneficial flavonoid compound. Is also good for diabetic retinopathy.

❏ Corticosteroids can induce glaucoma by destroying collagen structures in the eye. If you must take corticosteroids, you should take the smallest amount possible and for the shortest possible time. If you have glaucoma, you should avoid these medications entirely.

❏ There are many types of glaucoma medications available. Most are in eyedrop form and are administered several times a day. Types of medications your doctor may prescribe include:

• Miotics, which increase the outflow of aqueous (liquid) from the eye. Examples include pilocarpine (Adsorbocarpine, Ocu-Carpine, Piloptic, and others), carbachol (Carbastat, Carboptic, and others), and echothiophate (Phospholine Iodine).

• Epinephrine compounds, which lower intraocular pressure by increasing the outflow of aqueous from the eye.

• Beta-blockers, which can reduce the amount of aqueous humor produced in the eye. Examples include betaxolol (Betoptic) and timolol (Timoptic).

• Carbonic anhydrase inhibitors and alpha-adrenergic agonists, which also work to reduce the amount of aqueous humor. Examples include acetazolamide (Dazamide, Diamox, and others) and methazolamide (Neptazane).

• Prostaglandin analogs, which work near the drainage area of the eye to increase the secondary route of aqueous outflow to lower pressure. Latanoprost (Xalatan) is one such drug.

Many of the same medications used to treat open-angle glaucoma are also used to treat angle-closure glaucoma. Several medications that help to reduce intraocular pressure can have potentially serious side effects, such as headaches or respiratory problems.

❏ Beta-blocking eyedrops, which are often prescribed for people with glaucoma, have a number of undesirable side effects. They tend to cause unfavorable changes in blood fats, lowering the proportion of high-density lipoproteins—the so-called "good" cholesterol—to low-density lipoproteins, or "bad" cholesterol. In addition, the incidence of hip fracture among beta-blocker users is roughly three times greater than that seen in the general population. This is attributed to the dizziness and fainting experienced by some people who take these medications. Vision loss compounds the risk of falls and other accidents. Hip fracture is a major health threat among postmenopausal women.

❏ Some laser surgery treatments are being used to improve fluid drainage in the eyes, frequently in conjunction with other medications. Other surgical procedures have a fairly high success rate, but are usually used only when traditional medications fail.

❏ The best way to prevent vision loss due to glaucoma is to receive regular eye exams from a qualified ophthalmologist—especially if you fall into one of the risk categories mentioned earlier in this section.

❏ For names and addresses of organizations that can provide additional information about glaucoma, *see* HEALTH AND MEDICAL ORGANIZATIONS in the Appendix.

Glomerulonephritis

See under KIDNEY DISEASE (RENAL FAILURE).

Gout

Gout is a common type of arthritis that occurs when there is too much uric acid (sodium urate) in the blood, tissues, and urine. Uric acid is the end product of the metabolism of a class of chemicals known as purines. In people with gout, the body does not produce enough of the digestive enzyme uricase, which oxidizes relatively insoluble uric acid into a highly soluble compound. As a result, uric acid accumulates in the blood and tissues and, ultimately, crystallizes.

When it crystallizes, uric acid takes on a shape like that of a needle and, like a needle, it jabs its way into the joints. It seems to prefer the joint of the big toe, but other joints can be vulnerable as well, including the mid-foot, ankle, knee, wrist, and even the fingers. Uric acid is more likely to crystallize at lower temperatures, which may explain why roughly 90 percent of gout attacks affect cooler extremities like the big toe. Acute pain is usually the first symptom. Then the affected joints become inflamed, almost infected-looking—red, swollen, hot, and extremely sensitive to the touch. Repeated attacks of gout over a long period of time can lead to joint damage.

It should be noted that uric acid is *not* a fundamentally harmful substance, but a powerful antioxidant, almost as effective as vitamin C, that helps to protect cells from oxidative damage. It is only when levels become abnormally elevated that it becomes problematic. Approximately 70 percent of people who suffer from gout produce too much uric acid, and 30 percent cannot properly eliminate it from their bodies. About 25 percent have a family history of gout. Elevated levels of uric acid in the blood can also be an indicator of poor kidney function.

Uric acid is a byproduct of certain foods, so gout is

closely related to diet. Obesity and an improper diet increase the risk of developing gout. Gout has been called the rich man's disease, since it is associated with too much rich food and alcohol. But in fact it affects people from all walks of life, most commonly men between the ages of forty and fifty. It may be inherited or brought on by crash dieting, drinking, certain medications, overeating, stress, surgery, or injury to a joint. Approximately 90 percent of the people who suffer from gout are male. Uric acid kidney stones may be a related problem.

Diagnosing gout can be difficult when the symptoms appear in the joints—several other diseases can mimic gout, including rheumatoid arthritis and infections. Pseudogout (false gout), another form of arthritis, produces joint inflammation, redness, and swelling in the larger joints (usually the knees, wrists, or ankles) caused by the development of calcium pyrophosphate dihydrate crystals in one or more joints. The best way to get a definitive diagnosis of gout is for a physician to insert a needle into the affected joint, remove some fluid, and examine the fluid under a microscope for the characteristic uric acid crystals.

NUTRIENTS

SUPPLEMENT	SUGGESTED DOSAGE	COMMENTS
Very Important		
Essential fatty acids (Kyolic-EPA from Wakunaga is a good source)	As directed on label. Take with meals.	Needed to repair tissues, aid in healing, and restore proper fatty acid balance. An excess of saturated fats is often behind this disorder.
Liquid Kyolic with B_1 and B_{12} from Wakunaga	As directed on label.	Stress reducer. Antioxidant free radical quencher. Excellent for joint problems.
Proteolylic enzymes (Wobenzym N from Marlyn Nutraceuticals or Inflazyme Forte from American Biologics)	2 capsules with meals and 2 capsules between meals.	Taking with meals improves digestion of protein; taking between meals reduces inflammation.
Vitamin B complex	100 mg of each major B vitamin twice daily. (amounts of individual vitamins in a complex will vary).	Needed for proper digestion and all bodily enzyme systems.
plus extra pantothenic acid (vitamin B_5) and	500 mg daily, in divided doses.	The anti-stress vitamin.
folic acid	400–800 mcg daily.	An important aid in nucleo-protein metabolism.
Vitamin C with bioflavonoids	3,000–5,000 mg daily, in divided doses.	Lowers serum uric acid levels.
Vitamin E	400 mg daily.	Improves circulation. Use d-alpha-tocopherol form.
Important		
Free-form amino acid complex	As directed on label.	Uric acid production increases if essential amino acids are lacking. Use a supplement containing all the essential amino acids.

Kelp or alfalfa	1,000–1,500 mg daily.	Contains complete protein and vital minerals to reduce serum uric acid. *See under* Herbs, below.
Micellized Vitamin A emulsion from American Biologics	As directed on label.	Aids in reducing uric acid in the blood and is a potent antioxidant.
Potassium	99 mg daily.	Needed for proper mineral balance.
Pycnogenol or grape seed extract	As directed on label. As directed on label.	Powerful antioxidants.
Superoxide dismutase (SOD)	As directed on label, on an empty stomach (first thing in the morning is best). Take with a full glass of water.	An antioxidant and potent free radical destroyer.
Zinc	50–80 mg daily. Do not exceed a total of 100 mg daily from all supplements.	Important in protein metabolism and tissue repair. Use zinc gluconate lozenges or OptiZinc for best absorption.
Helpful		
Calcium and magnesium	1,500 mg daily. 750 mg daily.	To reduce stress caused by this disorder. Works well during sleep. Use chelate forms.
Glucosamine and chondroitin plus methylsulfonyl-methane (MSM)	As directed on label.	Important for joint tissue. Has anti-inflammatory and pain-relieving properties.
Sea cucumber (bêche-de-mer)	As directed on label.	Marine animals that have been used as an arthritis treatment in China for thousands of years.

HERBS

❏ Alfalfa is a good source of minerals and other nutrients that help to reduce serum uric acid. Take 2,000 to 3,000 milligrams daily in tablet or capsule form.

❏ Bilberry extract is a good source of anthocyanidins and proanthocyanidins—powerful antioxidant compounds.

❏ Boswellia and turmeric (curcumin) have powerful anti-inflammatory properties.

❏ Apply cayenne (capsicum) powder, mixed with enough wintergreen oil to make a paste, to affected areas to relieve inflammation and pain. This may cause a stinging sensation at first, but with repeated use, pain should diminish markedly. Cayenne can also be taken in capsule or liquid form.

❏ Celery seed extract contains numerous anti-inflammatory compounds.

❏ Try using chamomile, lady's mantle (yarrow), peppermint, or skullcap, in either capsule or tea form.

❏ Devil's claw and yucca can aid in relieving pain.

❏ Other beneficial herbs include birch, burdock, colchicum tincture, hyssop, and juniper.

RECOMMENDATIONS

❏ When an attack of gout strikes, eat only raw fruits and vegetables for two weeks. Juices are best. Frozen or fresh cherry juice is excellent. Also drink celery juice diluted with distilled water—use distilled water only, not tap water. Blueberries, cherries, and strawberries neutralize uric acid and have antioxidant properties, so eat lots of them. Also include grains, seeds, and nuts in your diet.

❏ Maintain a diet low in purines at all times. Purines are organic compounds that contribute to uric acid formation. Purine-rich foods to avoid include anchovies, mackerel, shellfish, asparagus, consommé, herring, meat gravies and broths, mushrooms, mussels, sardines, peanuts, baker's and brewer's yeast, mincemeat, and sweetbreads. Thyme and thyroid extracts can also pose a problem if taken for long periods of time.

❏ Enjoy foods like rice, millet, starchy vegetables, green vegetables, corn, cornbread, fruit, cheese, eggs, nuts, and milk.

❏ Consume plenty of quality water. Fluid intake promotes the excretion of uric acid.

❏ Eat no meat of any kind, including organ meats. Meat contains extremely high amounts of uric acid.

❏ Consume no alcohol. Alcohol both increases the production of uric acid and reduces uric acid elimination. Beer and wine also contain yeast.

❏ Do not eat any fried foods, roasted nuts, or any other foods containing (or cooked with) oil that has been subjected to heat. When heated, oils become rancid. Rancid fats quickly destroy vitamin E, resulting in the release of increased amounts of uric acid.

❏ Avoid rich foods such as cakes and pies. Leave white flour and sugar products out of your diet.

❏ Avoid the amino acid glycine. Glycine can be converted into uric acid more rapidly in people who suffer from gout.

❏ Limit your intake of caffeine, cauliflower, dried beans, lentils, fish, eggs, oatmeal, peas, poultry, spinach, and yeast products.

❏ If you are overweight, lose the excess pounds. Losing weight lowers serum uric acid levels. Avoid very restricted weight loss diets (crash diets), however. Abruptly cutting back on foods or fasting for longer than three days may result in increased uric acid levels.

❏ Consider using homeopathic remedies. One helpful homeopathic regimen for gout involves using a combination of *Belladonna* for severe pain, *Arnica* for less intense pain, and *Rhus toxicodendron* for joint pain and itching. Use 3x to 12x strength and take one dose of each three times each day.

❏ Avoid taking high doses of niacin (over 50 milligrams daily).

CONSIDERATIONS

❏ Very few women develop gout. Most of those who do are in their seventies, when estrogen levels are low.

❏ Some people can have high levels of uric acid with no gout symptoms.

❏ Dimethylsulfoxide (DMSO) is helpful for flare-ups of gout. This oily liquid is applied topically and is reportedly very effective at relieving pain and reducing swelling.

Note: Only DMSO from a health food store should be used. Commercial-grade DMSO found in hardware stores is not suitable for healing purposes. The use of DMSO may result in a garlicky body odor. This is temporary, and is not a cause for concern.

❏ Treatment with honeybee venom has provided relief for some gout sufferers. In this practice, called *apitherapy*, honeybee venom is administered by injection, either with a hypodermic needle or by the bees themselves. The venom appears to act as both an anti-inflammatory and immune system stimulant. Further information is available from the American Apitherapy Society (*see* HEALTH AND MEDICAL ORGANIZATIONS in the Appendix). Bee venom is also available in cream form as Bee Venom Balm from Aerobic Life Industries. You should not use this product if you are allergic to bee stings.

❏ Deficiencies of certain nutrients can provoke an attack. A deficiency of pantothenic acid (vitamin B_5) produces excessive amounts of uric acid. A study in animals found that a diet deficient in vitamin A can produce gout. Vitamin E deficiency causes damage to the nuclei of cells that produce uric acid, causing more uric acid to form.

❏ People who have candida infections, or who have taken antibiotics on and off for long periods, often have increased levels of uric acid in their blood.

❏ Because of the cellular destruction associated with chemotherapy in cancer treatment, uric acid is often released in extreme amounts, resulting in gouty arthritis.

❏ In rare cases, a secondary type of gout called saturnine gout can result from a toxic overload in the body.

❏ Allopurinol (Zyloprim), which inhibits uric acid synthesis, is often prescribed for gout. This drug has been linked directly to skin eruptions, inflammation of the blood vessels, and liver toxicity. If you have kidney problems, treatment with this drug should be carefully monitored.

❏ Colchicine, a drug derived from the autumn crocus (*Colchicum autumnale*), is used to both alleviate acute attacks and prevent further attacks from occurring. While often dramatically effective, this drug can cause serious side effects and toxicity, especially when taken in high doses and/or for prolonged periods. Another medication sometimes prescribed for gout is indomethacin (Indocin), a nonsteroidal anti-inflammatory drug (NSAID). Possible side effects include confusion and headache.

❏ Cortisone is commonly prescribed for relief of acute attacks. However, this may put added strain on the adrenal glands, which are already under stress as a result of this painful disorder.

❏ For pseudogout, injections of nonsteroidal anti-inflammatory drugs and steroids directly into the joint may provide relief. Unfortunately, there is no thorough procedure to extract the calcium crystals that cause this condition.

❏ *See also* ARTHRITIS in Part Two and PAIN CONTROL in Part Three.

Graves' Disease

See under HYPERTHYROIDISM.

Growth Problems

Growth problems usually occur when the pituitary gland fails to function as it should. The pituitary gland distributes hormones, including the growth hormone *somatotropin*, to various parts of the body. Somatotropin stimulates the growth of muscle and bone in growing children.

Either overproduction or underproduction of this hormone can cause growth abnormalities. The secretion of too little growth hormone by the pituitary causes dwarfism; too much causes the body to grow in an exaggerated fashion, resulting in abnormally large hands, feet, and jaw. Some cases of malfunction of the pituitary are caused by the growth of a tumor on the gland.

In some cases, growth problems are caused by the failure of the thyroid gland to function properly. The thymus gland may also be involved. If the thymus gland of an infant is damaged, development is retarded and the child has a greater than normal susceptibility to infection. Nutrition can also play a significant role in the growth and development of a child.

Dwarfism is a condition characterized by abnormally short stature. In some cases, individuals are very small, but normally proportioned; in others, the limbs are short as compared to the size of the rest of the body. Causes of dwarfism include unrecognized or untreated congenital hypothyroidism (once known as cretinism), Down syndrome, achondroplasia, hypochondroplasia, and spinal tuberculosis.

Achondroplasia is a primary bone disorder caused by chemical changes within a single gene. People with achondroplasia have large heads and arms and legs that are short in comparison with the length of the trunk. They usually also have a large forehead, a flat area between the eyes, and a protruding jaw. Often, the teeth are crowded together. In most cases, intelligence is normal, although motor development may occur a bit more slowly than normal. Both children and adults with achondroplasia must be particularly attentive to diet and nutrition, as obesity can often be a problem. People with achondroplasia are at greater than normal risk for a number of other health problems as well, including certain neurolgic and respiratory problems, orthopedic problems, fatigue, and numbness or pain in the lower back and thighs.

Congenital hypothyroidism is a condition characterized by the absence of sufficient quantities of thyroxine, a hormone secreted by the thyroid gland. In most cases, this is a result of the absence of a thyroid gland, an inborn defect. If congenital hypothyroidism is not detected and treated within a very short time, a number of developmental abnormalities may result, including short stature, disproportionately short arms and legs, coarse hair, and mental retardation.

Gigantism is a growth disorder characterized by an abnormally great height, usually due to excessive cartilage and bone formation at the ends of the long bones. Pituitary gigantism is the most common form of this condition. It is a result of the pituitary gland secreting excessive amounts of growth hormone.

Nutritional imbalances, delayed puberty, obesity, and certain diseases (including congenital heart disorders and chronic kidney failure) can be other factors involved in growth problems. If you are concerned about your child's growth rate, you should have him or her examined to determine if there is a problem and, if so, what the exact nature of the problem is. It is important to remember that some people are just naturally shorter or taller than average.

Unless otherwise specified, the dosages recommended here are for adults and teenagers over age seventeen. For a child between ages twelve and seventeen, use three-quarters of the recommended amount. For a child between six and twelve, use half the recommended dose. For a child under six, use a quarter of the recommended dose.

NUTRIENTS

SUPPLEMENT	SUGGESTED DOSAGE	COMMENTS
Very Important		
Alfalfa		*See under* Herbs, below.
Cod liver oil	As directed on label.	Contains vitamins A and D, needed for proper growth and for strong tissues and bones.
Essential fatty acid complex *or*	As directed on label.	For normal growth.
primrose oil	As directed on label.	
Kelp	As directed on label.	Contains natural iodine. An iodine deficiency can cause growth problems.
L-Lysine	As directed on label, on an empty stomach. Take with water or juice. Do not take with milk. Take with 50 mg vitamin B$_6$ and 100 mg vitamin C for better absorption.	Needed for normal growth and bone development. (*See* AMINO ACIDS in Part One.) *Caution:* Do not take this supplement for longer than 6 months at a time.

Zinc	As directed on label. Do not exceed a total of 100 mg daily from all supplements.	Deficiency has been linked to growth problems. Use zinc gluconate lozenges or OptiZinc for best absorption.
Important		
Calcium and magnesium	As directed on label. As directed on label.	Needed for normal bone growth.
Free-form amino acid complex	As directed on label.	Deficiency has been linked to growth disorders.
Raw pituitary glandular	As directed on label.	For children. Stimulates growth.
Helpful		
Bio-Bifidus from American Biologics	As directed on label.	For bowel flora replacement to improve assimilation and elimination.
L-Ornithine	As directed by physician.	Helps promote release of growth hormone. Use only under a physician's supervision.
Multiglandular complex	As directed on label.	For the endocrine, hormonal, and enzyme systems.
Vitamin B complex	50 mg of each major B vitamin daily (amounts of individual vitamins in a complex will vary).	B vitamins work best when taken together.
plus extra vitamin B$_6$ (pyridoxine)	50 mg 3 times daily, with meals.	Needed for uptake of the amino acids and for proper growth.

HERBS

❏ Alfalfa is a valuable source of vitamins, minerals, and other nutrients that promote the proper functioning of the pituitary gland. It can be taken in tablet or capsule form, as well as eaten in a natural form such as alfalfa sprouts.

RECOMMENDATIONS

❏ Eat a well-balanced diet high in healthful sources of protein. Protein is necessary for growth.

❏ Include in the diet foods high in the amino acid arginine. Arginine is used by the body to synthesize another amino acid, ornithine, which promotes the release of growth hormone. Good food sources of arginine include carob, coconut, dairy products, gelatin, oats, peanuts, soybeans, walnuts, wheat, and wheat germ.

CONSIDERATIONS

❏ When evaluating a child's growth, it is the overall growth pattern, rather than size, that is important. If a child seems to "fall off" a previously steady growth curve, he or she should be evaluated for possible nutritional deficiencies and other underlying health problems.

❏ There is currently no treatment to promote growth in people with achondroplasia. Therapy is directed toward prevention and treatment of complications.

❏ Surgery is now being performed on an experimental

basis to lengthen the arms and legs of those with androchdroplasia. It is an arduous procedure, often involving many complications.

❏ The addition of iodine to public drinking water supplies has shown a decrease in the occurrence of neonatal and congenital hypothyroidism in some areas of the United States.

❏ If growth is slowed because of insufficient growth hormone production, a doctor may prescribe growth hormone therapy.

❏ If growth problems are the result of a tumor of the pituitary gland, surgical removal or treatment of the tumor with drugs or by other means, may be recommended.

❏ *Kwashiorkor* is a protein/calorie deficiency disorder that causes children to grow slowly and have very little resistance to disease. It is most common among very poor people in developing countries. However, it can occur anywhere if a child's protein and/or calorie requirements are not met over a period of time. If detected early, it can be treated. Malabsorption syndromes, such as that associated with celiac disease, can cause similar problems even though nutritional intake appears to be adequate.

❏ High levels of lead, a toxic metal, may cause growth problems. A hair analysis can be done to rule out this metal toxicity. (*See* LEAD POISONING in Part Two and HAIR ANALYSIS in Part Three.)

❏ A large amount of research is being done on growth problems. Interestingly, some studies have indicated that shorter people may live longer than people of average height.

❏ *See also* HYPERTHYROIDISM and HYPOTHYROIDISM in Part Two.

Gum Disease

See under PERIODONTAL DISEASE. *See also* Bleeding Gums *under* PREGNANCY-RELATED PROBLEMS.

Hair Loss

Baldness or loss of hair is referred to as *alopecia. Alopecia totalis* means loss of all the scalp hair. *Alopecia universalis* means loss of all body hair, including eyebrows and eyelashes. If hair falls out in patches, it is termed *alopecia areata.* This condition is usually temporary and rarely leads to baldness. Factors that are involved in hair loss include heredity, hormones, and aging. Researchers have yet to determine the exact cause of hair loss, but some scientists believe the body's immune system mistakes hair follicles for foreign tissue and attacks them. Many suspect a genetic component.

A less dramatic, but more prevalent, type of hair loss is *androgenetic alopecia* (AGA), or male pattern baldness. AGA is common in men. As the name implies, a genetic or hereditary predisposition to the disorder and the presence of androgens—male sex hormones—are involved in this condition. Research indicates that the hair follicles of individuals susceptible to AGA may have receptors programmed to slow down or shut off hair production under the influence of androgens.

Women sometimes have the same type of hair loss, but it is not usually as extensive and most often does not occur until after menopause. All women experience some hair thinning as they grow older, especially after menopause, but in some it begins as early as puberty. In addition, most women lose some hair two or three months after having a baby because hormonal changes prevent normal hair loss during pregnancy.

A species of tiny mite, *Demodex follicularum*, may be the cause of, or a contributing factor to, balding. These mites are present in virtually all hair follicles by the time a person reaches middle age, and in most cases cause no harm. Researchers believe that the difference between people who lose their hair and those who do not may lie in how the scalp reacts to the presence of these mites. If the body initiates the inflammatory response as it tries to reject the mites, this may close down the hair follicles, thus killing the mites but also killing the hair.

In addition to heredity, factors that promote hair loss include poor circulation, acute illness, surgery, radiation exposure, skin disease, sudden weight loss, high fever, iron deficiency, diabetes, thyroid disease, drugs such as those used in chemotherapy, stress, poor diet, ringworm and other fungal infections, stress, chemicals such as hair dyes, and vitamin deficiencies.

NUTRIENTS

SUPPLEMENT	SUGGESTED DOSAGE	COMMENTS
Very Important		
Essential fatty acids (flaxseed oil, Kyolic-EPA from Wakunaga, primrose oil, and salmon oil are good sources)	As directed on label.	Improves hair texture. Prevents dry, brittle hair.
Raw thymus glandular	500 mg daily.	Stimulates immune function and improves functioning capacity of glands. *Caution:* Do not give this supplement to a child.
Ultra Hair from Nature's Plus	As directed on label.	Contains nutrients necessary to stimulate hair growth. If the condition is not severe, you can use this complex alone.
Vitamin B complex with vitamin B$_3$ (niacin)	50 mg 3 times daily.	B vitamins are important for the health and growth of the hair.
and pantothenic acid (vitamin B$_5$)	50 mg 3 times daily.	
and vitamin B$_6$ (pyridoxine) plus extra	50 mg 3 times daily.	
biotin	300 mcg daily. Also use hair care products containing biotin.	Deficiencies have been linked to skin disorders and hair loss.
and inositol	100 mg twice daily.	Vital for hair growth.
and methylsulfonyl-methane (MSM)	As directed on label.	Aids with the manufacture of keratin, a protein that is the major component of hair.
Vitamin C with bioflavonoids	3,000–10,000 mg daily.	Aids in improving scalp circulation. Helps with the antioxidant action in hair follicles.
Vitamin E	Start with 400 IU daily and slowly increase to 800–1,000 IU daily.	Increases oxygen uptake, which improves circulation to the scalp. Improves health and growth of hair. Use d-alpha-tocopherol form.
Zinc	50–100 mg daily. Do not exceed this amount.	Stimulates hair growth by enhancing immune function. Use zinc gluconate lozenges or OptiZinc for best absorption.
Important		
Coenzyme Q$_{10}$ plus Coenzyme A from Coenzyme-A Technologies	60 mg daily.	Improves scalp circulation. Increases tissue oxygenation.
Dimethylglycine (DMG) (Aangamik DMG from FoodScience of Vermont)	100 mg daily.	Good for circulation to the scalp.
Kelp	500 mg daily.	Supplies needed minerals for proper hair growth.
Helpful		
Copper	3 mg daily.	Works with zinc to aid in hair growth. Use a chelate form.
Dioxychlor from American Biologics	5 drops in water twice daily.	Destroys harmful bacteria and supplies oxygen to the tissues.
Grape seed extract	As directed on label.	A powerful antioxidant to protect hair follicles from free radical damage.
L-Cysteine and L-methionine plus glutathione	500 mg each twice daily, on an empty stomach. Take with water or juice. Do not take with milk. Take with 50 mg vitamin B$_6$ and 100 mg vitamin C for better absorption.	Improves quality, texture, and growth of hair. Helps prevent hair from falling out, and also promotes blood supply to the scalp. (*See* AMINO ACIDS in Part One.)
Methylsulfonyl-methane (MSM)	As directed on label.	Required for the building blocks of protein, which provides stronger hair.
Silica (Body Essential Silica gel from NatureWorks or BioSil from Jarrow Formulas)	As directed on label.	Aids in hair growth and also makes the hair stronger.

HERBS

❑ Use apple cider vinegar and sage tea as a rinse to help hair grow.

❑ Ginkgo biloba improves circulation to the scalp.

❑ Horsetail is a good source of silica, necessary for strong, shiny hair.

❑ Green tea, pygeum, and saw palmetto may aid in reducing hair loss.

❑ Tea tree oil combats bacteria and mites that may cause hair loss. Massage 10 drops into the scalp, then shampoo your hair in the usual fashion.

RECOMMENDATIONS

❑ Eat a diet high in fruits and vegetables and low in starch. This may help to slow down the process of hair loss. Fruits and vegetables contain flavonoids, many of which are antioxidants that may provide protection for the hair follicles and encourage hair growth.

❑ Eat plenty of foods high in biotin and/or take supplemental biotin as recommended under Nutrients in this entry. Biotin is needed for healthy hair and skin, and may even prevent hair loss in some men. Good food sources of biotin include brewer's yeast, brown rice, bulgur, green peas, lentils, oats, soybeans, sunflower seeds, and walnuts.

❑ Include soy foods such as soybeans, tempeh, and tofu in your diet. Soy foods appear to inhibit the formation of dihydrotestosterone, a hormone implicated in the process of hair loss.

❑ Do not eat foods containing raw eggs. Raw eggs not only pose a risk of *Salmonella* infection (*see* FOODBORNE/WATERBORNE DISEASE in Part Two), but are high in avidin, a protein that binds biotin and prevents it from being absorbed. Cooked eggs are acceptable.

❑ Lie head down on a slant board fifteen minutes a day to allow the blood to reach your scalp. Massage your scalp daily.

❑ Use shampoos and conditioners that contain biotin and silica. Aloe vera gel, vitamins C and E, and jojoba oils also are very good for the hair. Conditioners containing chamomile, marigold, ginseng, and/or passionflower help to keep hair healthy as well.

❑ Be careful of using products that are not natural on the hair. Allergic reactions to chemicals in these products occur frequently. Alternate among several different hair care products, using only all-natural and pH-balanced formulas. Most health food stores carry a variety of natural hair care products.

❑ Hair is fragile when it is wet. Gently pat your hair dry and squeeze out remaining moisture with a towel.

❑ Cover your hair when it is exposed to sunlight. Long exposure to sunlight and seawater can damage the hair.

❑ Avoid rough treatment. Do not use a brush or fine-toothed comb, or towel-dry your hair. Also, do not use a blow dryer or other heated appliances on your hair; let it dry naturally. Do not comb your hair until it is dry, as wet hair tends to break off. Use a pick to put wet hair in place. Do not wear tight ponytails, cornrows, or other styles that pull on the hair.

❑ Avoid crash diets and diets that neglect any of the food groups. These can cause deficiencies in nutrients that are detrimental to the hair.

❑ If you are losing large amounts of hair, see a physician.

CONSIDERATIONS

❑ It is normal to lose 50 to 100 hairs a day.

❑ Taking large doses of vitamin A (100,000 IU or more daily) for a long period can trigger hair loss, but stopping the vitamin A will reverse the problem. Often the hair grows back when the cause is corrected.

❑ Pregnancy, a high concentration of metals in the body, and autoimmune diseases can sometimes cause hair loss.

❑ Hypothyroidism can cause hair loss. (*See* HYPOTHYROIDISM in Part Two.)

❑ Hair transplantation can be a very successful treatment for hair loss if you have enough of your own hair to graft onto the bald area. Make sure to find a physician skilled in the technique if you decide to pursue a hair transplant.

❑ Rogaine, a topical solution developed by the Upjohn Company and containing 2 percent minoxidil, has been approved by the FDA for the treatment of male pattern baldness. This product is now available over the counter in drugstores. However, this drug may cause heart changes if used for long periods of time, researchers at the University of Toronto report. Also, although using minoxidil does result in hair growth, the quality of the hair is usually poor and hair growth ceases when use is discontinued.

❑ Finasteride (Propecia), a prescription medication, is said to be effective for younger men with male pattern baldness who have at least half of their hair remaining. It usually takes at least three months to be effective, and results last only as long as the medication is continued.

❑ In some people with alopecia areata, cortisone injections into the hairless patches of the head can trigger hair growth. Anthralin (Dritho-Scalp) cream, applied to the scalp and washed off after an hour, can sometimes stimulate hair growth after a few months of use. For extensive alopecia areata, a treatment called psoralen plus ultraviolet A radiation therapy, abbreviated PUVA, may be recommended. It involves the administration of light-sensitizing medication followed by exposure to ultraviolet-A light rays.

❑ Researchers at Cornell University say that gene therapy may someday be used to stimulate hair growth. They have discovered that hair follicles that have genetically been "turned off" can, in effect, be "turned on" again.

❏ For names and addresses of organizations that can provide more information on treatments for alopecia areata, *see* HEALTH AND MEDICAL ORGANIZATIONS in the Appendix.

Halitosis (Bad Breath)

Halitosis is typically caused by poor dental hygiene. However, other factors may be involved, including gum disease, tooth decay, heavy metal buildup, infection of the respiratory tract (throat, lungs, nose, and windpipe), improper diet, constipation, smoking, fever, diabetes, foreign bacteria in the mouth, indigestion, inadequate protein digestion, liver or kidney malfunction, postnasal drip, stress, and too much unfriendly bacteria in the colon. Halitosis can also be caused by a buildup of toxins in the gastrointestinal tract, salivary gland disorders, chronic bronchitis, sinusitis, or diabetes. Dieting, alcohol abuse, or fasting can cause bad breath as well. "Morning breath" results from dehydration and a reduction in the amount of saliva, which is needed to wash away bacteria in the mouth. Dieters and people who are fasting may experience bad breath because the lack of food causes the body to break down stored fat and protein for fuel; metabolic wastes resulting from that process have an unpleasant odor as they are exhaled from the lungs.

NUTRIENTS

SUPPLEMENT	SUGGESTED DOSAGE	COMMENTS
Very Important		
Aerobic Bulk Cleanse from Aerobic Life Industries or oat bran or psyllium husks or rice bran	1 tbsp in juice or water twice daily, on an empty stomach. Take separately from other supplements and medications.	For needed fiber. Fiber removes toxins from the colon that can result in bad breath.
Chlorophyll (alfalfa liquid, wheatgrass, and barley juice are good sources) or	1 tbsp in juice twice daily. Chlorophyll can also be used as a mouth rinse—add 1 tbsp to ½ glass of water.	"Green drinks" are one of the best ways to combat bad breath.
Kyo-Green from Wakunaga	As directed on label.	Contains chlorophyll to cleanse the body of toxins.
Vitamin C with bioflavonoids	2,000–6,000 mg daily.	Important in healing mouth and gum disease and in preventing bleeding gums. Also rids the body of excess mucus and toxins that can cause bad breath.
Important		
Acidophilus (Kyo-Dophilus and Probiata from Wakunaga are good sources)	As directed on label. Take on an empty stomach.	Needed to replenish "friendly" bacteria in the colon. Insufficient "friendly" bacteria and an overabundance of harmful bacteria can cause bad breath.
Garlic (Kyolic from Wakunaga)	2 capsules 4 times daily, with meals and at bedtime.	Acts as a natural antibiotic, destroying foreign bacteria in both the mouth and colon. Use an odorless form.
Zinc	30 mg 3 times daily. Do not exceed 100 mg daily.	Has an antibacterial effect and neutralizes sulfur compounds, a common cause of mouth odor.
Helpful		
Bee propolis	As directed on label.	Aids in healing the gums, aids control of infection in the body, and has an antibacterial effect.
Vitamin A plus carotenoid complex	15,000 IU daily. If you are pregnant, do not exceed 10,000 IU daily. As directed on label.	Needed for control of infection and in healing of the mouth.
Vitamin B complex plus extra vitamin B₃ (niacin)	100 mg of each major B vitamin daily (amounts of individual vitamins in a complex will vary). 50 mg 3 times daily. Do not exceed this amount.	Needed for proper digestion. Dilates tiny capillaries to help blood flow to infection sites. *Caution:* Do not take niacin if you have a liver disorder, gout, or high blood pressure.
and vitamin B₆ (pyridoxine)	50 mg daily.	Needed for all enzyme systems in the body.

HERBS

❏ Alfalfa supplies chlorophyll, which cleanses the bloodstream and colon, where bad breath often begins. Take 500 to 1,000 mg in tablet form or 1 tablespoon of liquid in juice or water three times daily.

❏ Gum disease is a major factor in bad breath. If infection is present, place alcohol-free goldenseal extract on a small piece of cotton and place the cotton over infected gums or mouth sores. Do this for two hours per day for three days. It should quickly heal the infected parts.

❏ Use myrrh (to brush your teeth and rinse your mouth), peppermint, rosemary, and sage.

Caution: Do not use sage if you suffer from epilepsy or other seizure disorder.

❏ Chewing a sprig of parsley after meals is an excellent treatment for bad breath. Parsley is rich in chlorophyll, the active ingredient in many popular breath mints.

❏ Other herbs that may be helpful for bad breath include anise, cloves, fennel, and parsley.

RECOMMENDATIONS

❏ Go on a five-day raw foods diet. After the fast, eat at least 50 percent of your food raw every day. This is a good routine diet to adhere to on an ongoing basis.

❏ Drink generous amounts of quality water.

❏ Avoid spicy foods, whose odors can linger for hours. Foods like anchovies, blue cheese, Camembert, garlic, onions, pastrami, pepperoni, Roquefort cheese, salami, and tuna leave oils in the mouth that can release odor for up to twenty-four hours, no matter how much you brush or gargle. Beer, coffee, whiskey, and wine leave residues that stick to the soft, sticky plaque on teeth and get into the digestive system. Each exhalation releases their odor back into the air.

❑ Avoid foods that get stuck between the teeth easily or that cause tooth decay, such as meat, stringy vegetables, and sweets, especially sticky sweets.

❑ Go on a cleansing fast with fresh lemon juice and water to detoxify the system. (*See* FASTING in Part Three.)

❑ Brush your teeth *and tongue* after every meal.

❑ Use a tongue scraper to help remove bacterial plaque and shed dead cells and food debris from the surface of the tongue.

❑ Replace your toothbrush every month, as well as after any infectious illness, to prevent bacteria buildup.

❑ Use dental floss and a chlorophyll mouthwash daily.

❑ Use Stim-U-Dent wooden toothpicks, available in most drugstores, after every meal to massage between the teeth. This is important for the prevention of gum disease.

❑ Keep your toothbrush clean. Between uses, store it in hydrogen peroxide or grapefruit seed extract to kill germs (if using hydrogen peroxide, rinse it well before brushing). There are bacteria-destroying toothbrush sanitizers available that turn on automatically at intervals throughout the day.

❑ Do not use commercial mouthwashes. Most contain nothing more than flavoring, dye, and alcohol. While they may kill the bacteria that cause bad breath, the bacteria soon return in greater force. Mouthwashes can also irritate the gums, tongue, and mucous membranes in the mouth.

❑ Bad breath may be a sign of an underlying health problem. Consult your health care provider for a thorough checkup if the suggestions in this section do not improve the condition.

CONSIDERATIONS

❑ *See also* PERIODONTAL DISEASE; SINUSITIS; and/or SORE THROAT in Part Two.

Hay Fever

Hay fever (allergic rhinitis) is an allergic response to pollen or mold that affects the mucous membranes of the nose, eyes, and air passages. Symptoms include itchy, red eyes; watery discharge from the nose and eyes; sneezing; fatigue; and nervous irritability. Many of the symptoms of hay fever are similar to those of the common cold. However, allergies cause a distinctive clear, thin nasal discharge, whereas secretions caused by colds usually become thick and yellow-green as the illness progresses. Also, colds are often associated with mild fever and are usually gone within a

week, while allergy sufferers often have a feeling of being "wiped out" for weeks on end.

At least 32 million Americans suffer from the seasonal sneezes, runny nose, and itchy eyes that come with hay fever. There are actually three hay fever seasons, distinguished by the different types of pollen present at different times. Tree pollens appear first, usually between February and May, depending on the local climate. The biggest problems come later in spring and in summer, when trees, weeds, and grass pollens—and people—are out at the same time. The fall is ragweed pollen season. Depending on which pollen or pollens an individual is allergic to, hay fever may be present at any or all of these times.

People who suffer from hay fever often also suffer from other so-called atopic disorders, such as asthma and dermatitis. Those who suffer from hay fever symptoms throughout the year are said to have *perennial rhinitis*. Animal hair, dust, feathers, fungus spores, molds, and/or some other environmental agent may trigger the symptoms. A susceptibility to hay fever tends to be inherited.

People prone to allergies are most often aware of the time of year and conditions under which they are most sensitive. For a definitive diagnosis, the radioallergosorbent (RAST) test is easily done and gives reliable results.

The nutrient program outlined below is beneficial for hay fever. Hay fever sufferers should always choose hypoallergenic supplements. Unless otherwise specified, the dosages recommended here are for adults. For a child between the ages of twelve and seventeen, reduce the dose to three-quarters the recommended amount. For a child between six and twelve, use one-half the recommended dose, and for a child under the age of six, use one-quarter the recommended amount.

NUTRIENTS

SUPPLEMENT	SUGGESTED DOSAGE	COMMENTS
Very Important		
Bromelain (Ultra Bromelain from Nature's Plus or Mega Bromelain from Twinlab)	1,000 mg 3 times daily, between meals.	Reduces inflammation associated with hay fever symptoms.
Coenzyme Q10	30 mg twice daily.	Improves oxygenation and immunity.
Quercetin	400 mg twice daily, before meals.	A bioflavonoid that stabilizes the membranes of the cells that release histamine, which triggers allergic symptoms.
or		
Activated Quercetin from Source Naturals	As directed on label.	Contains quercetin plus bromelain and vitamin C for better absorption.
or		
AntiAllergy formula from Freeda Vitamins	As directed on label.	A combination of quercetin, calcium pantothenate, and calcium ascorbate.
Raw thymus glandular plus adrenal glandular	500 mg twice daily. As directed on label.	To promote immune function. *Caution:* Do not give these supplements to a child under 16 years of age.

Vitamin A with mixed carotenoids	25,000 IU daily. If you are pregnant, do not exceed 10,000 IU daily.	Powerful immunostimulants. An emulsion form is recommended for easier assimilation and greater safety at high doses.
Vitamin B complex plus extra pantothenic acid (vitamin B$_5$) and vitamin B$_6$ (pyridoxine)	As directed on label. 100 mg 3 times daily. 50 mg twice daily.	All B vitamins are necessary for proper functioning of the immune system. Use hypoallergenic formulas.
Vitamin C with bioflavonoids	3,000–10,000 mg 3 times daily.	A potent immunostimulant and anti-inflammatory. Use an esterified or buffered form.

Important

Proteolytic enzymes	As directed on label. Take with meals and between meals.	Necessary for digestion of essential nutrients that boost immune function. *Caution:* Do not give this supplement to a child.
Zinc	50–80 mg daily. Do not exceed a total of 100 mg daily from all supplements.	Boosts immune function. Use zinc gluconate lozenges or OptiZinc for best absorption.

Helpful

Aller Bee-Gone from CC Pollen	As directed on label.	A combination of herbs, enzymes, and nutrients to fight acute symptoms.
Calcium and magnesium	1,500 mg daily. 1,000 mg daily.	Minerals that have a calming effect on the system.
Dioxychlor DC-3 from American Biologics or Aerobic 07 from Aerobic Life Industries	5 drops in water twice daily. Also use topically: mix 30 drops in 2 oz water and instill 1 dropperful in each nostril. As directed on label.	To supply stabilized oxygen and fight bacteria, fungi, and viruses.
Garlic (Kyolic from Wakunaga)	As directed on label.	Helpful for sinus inflammation. Use a liquid formula.
Kelp	As directed on label twice daily.	A rich source of minerals.
Manganese	10–30 mg daily. Take separately from calcium.	Aids in metabolism of vitamins, minerals, enzymes, and carbohydrates.
Pycnogenol or grape seed extract	As directed on label.	Powerful free radical scavengers that also act as anti-inflammatories and enhance the activity of vitamin C.
Superoxide dismutase (SOD) (Cell Guard from Biotec Foods)	As directed on label.	A powerful antioxidant.
Vitamin E	400–800 IU daily.	Boosts the immune system Use d-alpha-tocopherol form.

HERBS

❏ Alfalfa supplies chlorophyll and vitamin K. Use a liquid form. Take 1 tablespoon in juice or water twice daily.

❏ Bio-Rizin from American Biologics contains licorice extract, which improves energy levels and helps relieve allergy symptoms. Take 10 to 20 drops twice daily or as needed.

Caution: Do not use licorice for more than seven days at a time. Avoid it completely if you have high blood pressure.

❏ For red, itchy eyes, place slices of cool cucumbers over the eyes. Rotate this treatment with steeped, cooled black tea bags placed directly on the eyelids.

❏ Ephedra helps to relieve bronchial spasms, congestion, and coughing. However, it is not a cure for allergies, and long-term use may weaken the adrenal glands.

Caution: Do not use this herb if you suffer from anxiety, glaucoma, heart disease, high blood pressure, or insomnia, or if you are taking a monoamine oxidase (MAO) inhibitor drug for depression.

❏ Eucalyptus oil can relieve congestion if used in a steam inhalation (*see* STEAM INHALATION in Part Three) or added to bath water.

❏ Alcohol-free eyebright and lady's mantle (yarrow) liquid extracts are good for relieving hay fever symptoms. Use 20 to 30 drops two times daily to make a tea or place the extract under your tongue and hold it there for a few minutes before swallowing. Drink a glass of water after you take the extract.

❏ If your throat is itchy or you feel a need to cough, use alcohol-free goldenseal extract. Hold a dropperful in your mouth for a few minutes, then swallow. This will halt a sore throat.

Caution: Do not take goldenseal internally on a daily basis for more than one week at a time, as it may disturb normal intestinal flora. Do not use it during pregnancy, and use it with caution if you are allergic to ragweed.

❏ Horehound, mullein leaf, stinging nettle, and/or wild cherry bark help to ward off severe allergic reactions.

❏ Use turmeric to reduce inflammation.

❏ Nettle leaf is very good for all types of allergies.

❏ Noni juice aids in relieving symptoms of hay fever.

RECOMMENDATIONS

❏ The best defense against hay fever is to try to avoid the substance that is causing your allergies.

❏ Eat more fruits (especially bananas), vegetables, grains, and raw nuts and seeds. Stay on a high-fiber diet.

❏ If you enjoy the flavor of horseradish, use it liberally. Horseradish is good for a runny nose and congestion.

❏ Eat yogurt or any soured products three times a week. Homemade yogurt is best. However, beware of the possibility that you may be allergic to casein, the principal protein found in milk.

❏ Consume no cakes, chocolate, coffee, dairy products (except yogurt), packaged or canned foods, pies, soft drinks, sugar, tobacco, white flour products, or any junk food.

❏ Avoid tobacco smoke, which irritates the lungs and eyes, and alcohol, which increases the production of mucus.

❏ When allergy season arrives, spend as little time as possible outdoors. Keep windows and doors closed during the day, with air conditioning on if possible.

❏ Use your car air conditioner when you drive. Especially avoid going outside in the afternoon. If you exercise or play sports outside, do it in the morning rather than in the afternoon; grasses pollinate in midday and the wind keeps the pollen floating until it drops to the ground at night.

❏ Try to avoid working in the yard—wear a mask and goggles if you do to keep the pollen from getting into your eyes. Avoid placing laundry outdoors to dry, as the pollen collects on the surface of fabrics.

❏ Shower and change your clothes when you come indoors after spending time outside. Pollen can stick to your hair, especially on a windy day. Washing your hair also helps.

❏ Consider using homeopathic remedies. *Sabadilla* is good for watery eyes, runny nose, and a dry throat. Another good choice for these symptoms is *Wyethia*.

❏ Perform a cleansing fast. *See* FASTING in Part Three.

❏ Keep pets either inside or outside. Dogs and cats can pick up pollen on their fur and bring it indoors with them.

❏ Try using a good-quality air purifier and filter in your home. The Air Supply personal air purifier from Wein Products is a miniature unit that is worn around the neck. It sets up an invisible pure air shield against microorganisms (such as viruses, bacteria, and mold) and microparticles (including dust, pollen, and pollutants) in the air. It also eliminates vapors, smells, and harmful volatile compounds in the air. The Living Air XL-15 unit from Alpine Industries is an ionizing unit that is good for purifying the air in the home or workplace.

CONSIDERATIONS

❏ The best and safest way to control allergies is the natural way—by avoiding allergens and taking steps to normalize immune function and prevent or lessen the symptoms. Allergies can usually be controlled if you are willing to make changes in your lifestyle, diet, and mental state.

❏ A study at the University of California–Davis found that eating yogurt every day significantly reduced the incidence of hay fever attacks, especially those triggered by grass pollens.

❏ If you are a man with facial hair, cleaning your mustache and/or beard with soap and water or shampoo twice a day will cut down on the symptoms associated with hay fever.

❏ Researchers at Giessen University in Germany found that three bananas contain enough magnesium—180 milligrams—to quell a hay fever attack. Other foods rich in magnesium are kidney beans, soybeans, almonds, lima beans, whole-wheat flour, brown rice, molasses, and peas. Magnesium can also be taken in supplement form.

❏ Antihistamines are the most commonly recommended conventional treatment for hay fever. They can reduce itching in the eyes, ears, and throat; dry up a runny nose; and reduce sneezing attacks. However, they can also cause drowsiness, depression, and other side effects. Newer antihistamines, such as terfenadine (Seldane), astemizole (Hismanal), and loratidine (Claritin) do not cause drowsiness and depression. But they are expensive and available only by prescription, and they might not work for everyone. Do not take these with grapefruit juice.

❏ Steroid drugs are even more powerful suppressors of allergic reactions than antihistamines. Doctors often prescribe the steroid beclomethasone in nasal inhalers sold under the brand names Beconase and Vancenase. These can be very effective in relieving symptoms, but some of the steroids are bound to get into the rest of the body. Steroids suppress immune function.

❏ Some physicians recommend desensitization shots for people with hay fever. These are expensive, painful, and not risk-free. And a disappointingly low percentage of people experience satisfactory relief, even after years of injections. The typical person requires weekly shots for up to a year and monthly shots for up to five years, at a total cost that can run into the thousands of dollars.

❏ The following types of treatments are available for hay fever sufferers: antihistamines, decongestants, topical corticosteroids, leukotriene antagonists, immunotherapy, and surgery (for those with structural problems in which airways are open, making medications ineffective). Unfortunately, most of these treatments have drawbacks. You should consider them only if your symptoms substantially interfere with the quality of your daily life.

❏ The U.S. Food and Drug Administration (FDA) released a warning about the prescription antihistamine astemizole (Hismanal). When taken with certain other medications or at higher than recommended doses, astemizole can increase the risk of death from irregular heartbeat, drug interactions, or anaphylactic shock. Astemizole should *not* be taken together with indinavir (Crixivan, a drug used to treat HIV and AIDS), mibefradil (Posicor, used for hypertension), the antibiotics clarithromycin (Biaxin) and troleandomycin (TAO), some antidepressants, and a number of other drugs. Astemizole also should not be used by people with liver disorders, and it should not be taken with grapefruit juice. The manufacturer has since changed its product labeling to inform users about the drug's potential adverse effects.

❏ *See also* ALLERGIES in Part Two and ASCORBIC ACID FLUSH in Part Three.

Headache

Virtually everyone gets a headache at one time or another. An estimated 17.6 percent of women and 6 percent of men in the United States experience headaches on more than an occasional basis, and some 20 million regularly experience cluster and migraine headaches. Headaches are as common—and as difficult to cure—as the common cold and flu. Common causes of headache include stress; tension; anxiety; allergies; constipation; coffee consumption; eyestrain; hunger; sinus pressure; muscle tension; hormonal imbalances; temporomandibular joint (TMJ) syndrome; trauma to the head; nutritional deficiencies; the use of alcohol, drugs, or tobacco; fever; and exposure to irritants such as pollution, perfume, or after-shave lotions. Migraines result from a disturbance in the blood circulation in the head. (*See* MIGRAINE in Part Two.)

Headache experts estimate that about 90 percent of all headaches are tension headaches and 6 percent are migraines. Tension headaches, as the name implies, are caused by muscular tension. Another type of headache is the cluster headache. These are severe, recurring headaches that strike about 1 million Americans, and are widely considered to be the most painful type of headache.

Headaches can also be a sign of an underlying health problem. People who suffer from frequent headaches may be reacting to certain foods and food additives, such as wheat, chocolate, monosodium glutamate (MSG), sulfites (used in restaurants on salad bars), sugar, hot dogs, luncheon meats, dairy products, nuts, citric acid, fermented foods (cheeses, sour cream, yogurt), alcohol, vinegar, and/or marinated foods. Other possibilities to consider are anemia, bowel problems, brain disorders such as tumors, bruxism (tooth-grinding), hypertension (high blood pressure), hypoglycemia (low blood sugar), sinusitis, spinal misalignment, toxic overdoses of vitamin A, vitamin B deficiency, and diseases of the eye, nose, and throat. Dehydration also can cause headaches—often accompanied by a feeling of being flushed, a warm face, and a sense of heaviness in the head.

Unless otherwise specified, the dosages recommended here are for adults. For a child between the ages of twelve and seventeen, reduce the dose to three-quarters the recommended amount. For a child between six and twelve, use one-half the recommended dose, and for a child under the age of six, use one-quarter the recommended amount.

NUTRIENTS

SUPPLEMENT	SUGGESTED DOSAGE	COMMENTS
Helpful		
Bromelain	500 mg as needed.	An enzyme that helps to regulate the inflammatory response.
Calcium and magnesium	1,500 mg daily. 1,000 mg daily.	Minerals that help to alleviate muscular tension. Use chelated forms. Deficiency may be a cause of migraines. Relaxes muscles and blood vessels.
Coenzyme Q$_{10}$ plus Coenzyme A from Coenzyme-A Technologies	30 mg twice daily. As directed on label.	Improves tissue oxygenation. Supports the immune system's detoxification of many dangerous substances, increases energy, and facilitates the manufacture of connective tissue.
Dimethylglycine (DMG) (Aangamik DMG from FoodScience of Vermont)	125 mg twice daily.	Improves tissue oxygenation. Use a sublingual form.
DL-Phenylalanine (DLPA)	750 mg daily.	For pain relief. *Caution:* Do not take this supplement if you are pregnant or nursing a baby, or if you suffer from panic attacks, diabetes, high blood pressure, or PKU.
5-Hydroxy L-tryptophan (5-HTP)	As directed on label.	Many clinical studies have shown excellent results with both tension headaches and migraines.
Glucosamine sulfate	As directed on label.	A natural alternative to aspirin and other nonsteroidal anti-inflammatory drugs (NSAIDs).
L-Tyrosine plus L-glutamine plus quercetin	As directed on label. 500 mg twice daily. 500 mg twice daily.	For relief of cluster headaches. *Caution:* Do not take tyrosine if you are taking an MAO inhibitor drug, commonly prescribed for depression.
Methylsulfonyl-methane (MSM)	As directed on label.	Relieves pain.
Potassium	99 mg daily.	For the proper sodium and potassium balance, which is needed to avoid water retention. Water retention may put undue pressure on the brain.
Primrose oil	500 mg 3–4 times daily.	Supplies essential fatty acids, which promote healthy circulation, help regulate the inflammatory response, and relieve pain.
Vitamin B$_3$ (niacin) and niacinamide	Up to 300 mg combined daily. Do not exceed this amount. Stop and maintain the dosage that provides relief.	Improves circulation and aids in the functioning of the nervous system. Professional supervision is advised. *Caution:* Do not take niacin if you have a liver disorder, gout, or high blood pressure.
Vitamin B complex plus extra vitamin B$_6$ (pyridoxine)	50 mg of each major B vitamin 3 times daily (amounts of individual vitamins in a complex will vary). 50 mg 3 times daily.	B vitamins work best when taken together. Use a yeast-free formula. In severe cases, injections (under a doctor's supervision) may be advisable. Removes excess water from tissues.
Vitamin C with bioflavonoids	2,000–8,000 mg daily, in divided doses.	Protects against harmful effects of pollution and aids production of anti-stress hormones. Use an esterified or buffered form.

Vitamin E	Start with 400 IU daily and increase slowly to 1,200 IU daily.	Improves circulation. Use d-alpha-tocopherol form.

HERBS

❑ Cayenne thins the blood, which reduces pain and allows beneficial blood flow.

❑ Chamomile relaxes muscles and soothes tension.

❑ A salve made from ginger, peppermint oil, and wintergreen oil rubbed on the nape of the neck and temples can help relieve tension headaches. For sinus headaches, rub the salve across the sinus area.

❑ Ginkgo biloba extract improves circulation to the brain, and may be helpful for certain types of headache.

❑ Guarana can alleviate cluster headaches.

❑ Several clinical studies have shown ginger to be helpful for pain relief.

❑ Jamaica dogweed is good for sinus headaches.

❑ Kava kava is helpful for tension headaches.

❑ Meadowsweet is an anti-inflammatory agent.

❑ Periwinkle flower has been found to increase the cerebral flow of oxygen, which helps to alleviate headache pain.

❑ Skullcap acts as an antispasmodic agent and has a sedative effect. It is good for headaches related to muscular tension and spasms.

❑ Valerian root is a good sedative to take during a headache.

❑ Other herbs that may help relieve headache pain include brigham, burdock root, fenugreek, feverfew, goldenseal, lavender, lobelia, marshmallow, mint, rosemary, skullcap, and thyme.

Caution: Do not use feverfew during pregnancy. Do not take goldenseal internally on a daily basis for more than one week at a time, do not use it during pregnancy, and use it with caution if you are allergic to ragweed. Do not take lobelia internally on an ongoing basis.

RECOMMENDATIONS

❑ Eat a well-balanced diet, including protein with every meal. Avoid chewing gum; consuming ice cream, iced beverages, or salt; and guard against excessive sun exposure.

❑ Try eliminating foods containing tyramine and the amino acid phenylalanine. Then reintroduce one food at a time and see which ones produce headaches. Phenylalanine is found in aspartame (Equal, NutraSweet), monosodium glutamate (MSG), and nitrites (preservatives found in hot dogs and luncheon meats). Foods that contain tyramine include alcoholic beverages, bananas, cheese, chicken, chocolate, citrus fruits, cold cuts, herring, onions, peanut butter, pork, smoked fish, sour cream, vinegar, wine, and fresh-baked yeast products. Tyramine causes the blood pressure to rise, resulting in a dull headache.

❑ Practice deep-breathing exercises. A lack of oxygen can cause headaches. (*See* BREATHING EXERCISES *under* PAIN CONTROL in Part Three.)

❑ Maintain good posture habits.

❑ Use fiber daily and a cleansing enema weekly. (*See* COLON CLEANSING and ENEMAS in Part Three.)

Note: Always take supplemental fiber separately from other supplements and medications.

❑ If you feel a headache coming on, drink a large glass of water every three hours until symptoms subside.

❑ When a headache strikes, take a cleansing enema. This removes the toxins that cause many headaches. If not eliminated, toxins can be absorbed into the bloodstream and circulated throughout the body. For a headache brought on by fasting, use a coffee retention enema. *See* ENEMAS in Part Three.

❑ Apply cold compresses to the spot from which the pain is radiating. This helps relieve headaches by constricting blood vessels and easing muscle spasms. Leave a damp washcloth in the freezer for ten minutes or use a cold gel-pack.

❑ Use a heating pad, hot water bottle, or hot towel to relax neck and shoulder muscles, which can cause tension when they are too tight.

❑ Use a homeopathic remedy suitable for the particular headache symptoms you are experiencing. *Belladonna* helps with sudden, severe pain that is worse on the right side of the body. *Natrum muriaticum* is recommended for tension headaches and periodic headaches. *Sanguinaria* is good for pain that is sharp and splitting. *Arsenicum album, kali bichromium, Mecurius solubilis,* and *Pulsatilla* all encourage drainage of the sinuses.

❑ Acupressure is helpful for tension headaches and pain. Take your thumb and press up firmly underneath your skull, at the back of your neck, for one to two minutes.

❑ For headaches caused by sinus congestion, try self-massage. By applying pressure to specific areas of the head, you can open up the sinuses and ease tension. Rub the area surrounding the bones just above and below the eyes, and massage the cheeks directly in line with these points. Lean your head forward slightly to facilitate sinus drainage. Applying heat to the sinuses, either with compresses or with steam inhalation, can also be beneficial.

❑ Always seek and treat the cause of the headache, not the symptom. Long-term overreliance on aspirin, acetaminophen, and other nonprescription painkillers can make chronic headaches worse by interfering with the brain's natural ability to fight headaches. If you are using nonprescription painkillers more than four times a week, talk to your health care provider about other ways to control the pain.

❑ If you experience a headache that does not subside, but instead progressively worsens over the course of a week,

Types of Headaches

Headaches come in a number of forms, differentiated by their causes and specific symptoms. The appropriate treatment depends on the type of headache. The table below lists some of the more common types of headaches and possible treatments for them.

Type of Headache	Symptoms	Causes	Treatment
Aneurysm-associated headache	Early symptoms mimic those of cluster headaches and migraines. If an aneurysm ruptures, it can cause sudden extreme pain, double vision, rigid neck, and stroke leading to unconsciousness.	A balloonlike bulge or weak spot on a blood vessel wall; high blood pressure.	Keep blood pressure low. If found early, surgery may be necessary.
Arthritis headache	Pain at the back of the head or neck, made worse by movement; inflammation of joints and shoulder and/or neck muscles.	Unknown.	Take feverfew supplements. *Caution:* Do not use feverfew during pregnancy
Bilious headache	Dull pain in forehead and throbbing temples.	Indigestion; overeating; lack of exercise.	Colon cleansing may be helpful. (*See* COLON CLEANSING in Part Three.)
Caffeine headache	Throbbing pain caused by blood vessels that have dilated.	Caffeine withdrawal.	Ingest a small amount of caffeine, then taper off.
Cluster headache	Severe, throbbing pain on one side of the head around the eye area, flushing of the face, tearing of eyes, nasal congestion, occurring 1–3 times a day over a period of weeks or months and lasting from a few minutes to several hours each time. One of the most painful headaches.	Stress, alcohol, smoking.	Take supplemental L-tyrosine, DL-phenylalanine, ginkgo biloba extract, L-glutamine, quercetin.*Caution:* Do not take L-tyrosine if you are taking an MAO inhibitor drug. Do not take phenylalanine if you are pregnant or suffer from panic attacks, diabetes, high blood pressure, or phenylketonuria (PKU).
Exertion headache	Generalized headache during or after physical exertion such as running or sexual intercourse, or passive exertion such as sneezing or coughing.	Usually related to migraine or cluster headaches. About 10 percent are related to organic diseases such as tumors or blood vessel malformation.	Take nutritional supplements; apply ice packs at the site of pain. If the pain goes away after exercising and exertion, see your physician.
Eyestrain headache	Usually frontal pain on both sides.	Overuse of the eyes; eye muscle imbalance; uncorrected vision; astigmatism.	Correct vision.
Fever headache	Headache develops with fever due to inflammation of blood vessels of the head.	Infection.	Reduce fever, apply ice packs.
Hangover headache	Migrainelike, with throbbing pain and nausea.	Alcohol causes dehydration and dilation of blood vessels in the brain.	Drink plenty of quality water. Take a B-complex supplement. Apply ice to neck.

Type of Headache	Symptoms	Causes	Treatment
Hunger headache	Strikes just before mealtime due to low blood sugar, muscle tension, and rebound dilation of blood vessels.	Skipping meals; too-stringent dieting.	Eat regular meals with adequate amounts of complex carbohydrates and protein.
Hypertension headache	Dull, generalized pain affecting a large area of the head and aggravated by movement or exertion.	Severe high blood pressure.	Get blood pressure under control.
Menstrual headache	Migraine-type pain shortly before, during, or after menstruation, or at midcycle, at time of ovulation.	Variation in estrogen levels.	Take supplements of vitamin B_6, potassium, and extra magnesium.
Migraine, classic	Similar to common migraine, but preceded by auras such as visual disturbances, numbness in arms or legs, smelling of strange odors, hallucinations.	Excessive dilation or contraction of blood vessels of the brain.	*See* MIGRAINE in Part Two.
Migraine, common	Severe throbbing pain, often on one side of the head; nausea; vomiting; cold hands; dizziness; sensitivity to light and sounds.	Excessive dilation or contraction of blood vessels of the brain.	*See* MIGRAINE in Part Two.
Sinus headache	Gnawing, nagging pain over nasal/sinus area, often increasing in severity as the day goes by. Fever and discolored mucus may be present.	Allergies, infection, nasal polyps, food allergies. Often caused by blocked sinus ducts or acute sinus infection.	Increase intake of vitamins A and C; use moist heat to help get sinuses to drain.
Temporal headache	Jabbing, burning, boring pain; pain in temple or around ear on chewing; weight loss; flulike symptoms; problems with eyesight. Usually seen in people over 55. Untreated, can lead to blindness, stroke, heart attack, or a tear in the aorta.	Inflammation of temporal arteries.	Consult physician for steroid therapy.
Temporo-mandibular joint (TMJ) headache	Temporal, above-ear, or facial pain; muscle temple pain upon awakening.	Stress, contraction of one side of face; clicking or malocclusion (poor popping of jaw; neck or upper back pain; bite), jaw clenching, gum chewing.	Reduce stress; use relaxation techniques, biofeedback, nutritional supplements, ice packs.
Tension headache	Constant pain, in one area or all over the head; sore muscles with trigger points in neck and upper back; lightheadedness; dizziness. The most common type of headache.	Emotional stress, anxiety, worry, depression, anger, food allergies, poor posture, too-shallow breathing.	Apply ice packs on neck and upper back; take supplements of vitamin C with bioflavonoids, DLPA, bromelain, magnesium, primrose oil, and ginger for relief of muscle spasms.
Tic douloureux	Short, jabbing pains around the mouth, jaw, or forehead. More common in women over 55 years old.	Unknown.	Take nutritional supplements. In some cases, surgery may be necessary.
Tumor headaches	Progressively worsening pain; projectile problems with vision, speech, and equilibrium; personality changes.	Usually unknown.	Surgery and/or radiation.
Vascular headaches	Throbbing on one side of the head, sensitivity to light and often nausea. Related to cluster headaches and migraines.	Disturbances in the blood vessels.	Lie down and keep your blood pressure under control.

consult your physician. This can be a sign of an underlying organic problem such as a tumor.

❑ To help prevent headaches, eat small meals and eat between meals to help stabilize wide swings in blood sugar. Include almonds, almond milk, watercress, parsley, fennel, garlic, cherries, and pineapple in your diet.

❑ Be sure to get sufficient sleep. Inositol and/or calcium, if taken before bedtime, aid sleeping. A grapefruit half also helps. Do not eat sweet fruit or anything else sweet after 5:00 P.M.

❑ If you suffer from headaches while taking birth control pills, talk to your doctor about switching to a low-estrogen formulation or going off the pills for a while. Oral contraceptives can cause a vitamin B_6 deficiency that results in headaches and migraines.

❑ If you must eat a food to which you suspect you may be sensitive, use charcoal tablets (from a health food store). Take five tablets within an hour before eating and three tablets after eating. As soon as possible, take a cleansing enema and a coffee retention enema. If you have severe headaches after consuming a food, this will relieve it quickly by eliminating the allergenic substances. Do not take charcoal tablets daily, however, as they also absorb the good nutrients.

❑ If any of the following symptoms accompany the headache, consult your health care provider: blurred vision, confusion or loss of speech, fever and stiffness in the neck, sensitivity to light, pressure behind the eyes that is relieved by vomiting, pressure in the facial sinus area, throbbing of the head and temples, a pounding heartbeat, visual color changes, and feeling as though your head will explode. Seek immediate medical attention if you experience a sudden, severe headache like a "thunderclap," or if you experience a headache after a head injury, even a minor fall or bump. Chronic headache pain that worsens after coughing, exertion, straining, or sudden movement is also reason to seek professional attention.

❑ If you suffer from more than the occasional tension headache, keep a headache log to help your health care provider diagnose your condition. Keep the log for at least two months, noting the time of each headache and describing the pain (throbbing or dull), its severity, location, and duration.

❑ If you get a headache every time you exercise, see your health care provider to rule out heart problems. A headache that begins with exercise and then subsides after rest can be a cardiac headache.

CONSIDERATIONS

❑ Headaches are often caused by allergies. A food allergy diary can help identify offending foods. (*See* ALLERGIES in Part Two.)

❑ Poor vertebral alignment may cause reduced blood flow to the brain. This is often caused by flat feet or by wearing high heels. Chiropractic adjustment can help.

❑ Routine chiropractic spinal manipulation and deep neck muscle massage can reduce the frequency of headaches and the need for pain-relieving medications.

❑ Regular exercise can help prevent headaches caused by tension and may also reduce the frequency and severity of migraines. But headaches with organic causes can be made worse by exercise. Talk to your health care provider about your headaches before using exercise to control the pain.

❑ Researchers are studying the possibility that the trigeminal nerve pathway (the site of the nerve responsible for sensation in the face, mouth, and nasal cavity) and the brain chemical serotonin are factors in severe headaches. Disturbances in serotonin levels are associated with most headaches. In migraines, serotonin levels increase before onset and then decrease during the headache phase. In chronic tension headaches, serotonin levels remain low all the time. As a result of lower serotonin levels, an impulse moves along the trigeminal nerve to blood vessels in the meninges, the brain's outer covering. This causes blood vessels in the meninges to dilate and become inflamed and swollen. The result is a headache.

❑ The drug sumatriptan (Imitrex) is sometimes prescribed for relief of migraines. This drug works by increasing the amount of serotonin in the brain. It is relatively expensive, however, and must be administered by injection (it is sold in the form of a home injection kit). Possible side effects include increased heart rate, elevated blood pressure, and a feeling of tightness in the chest, jaw, or neck.

❑ Some doctors prescribe the drug lidocaine (Anestacon, Xylocaine) for cluster headaches. Used in nose drop form, it gives relief in minutes.

❑ In one study, twenty adults suffering from long-term cluster headaches squirted a capsaicin solution in their noses daily for five days. Within ten days of the last dose, there was a 67 percent drop in the number of attacks.

❑ Research shows that sleeping in a bedroom kept at a cooler temperature can help prevent cluster headaches. Headaches are more frequent when environmental heat increases body temperature, which causes blood vessels to dilate.

❑ One study showed taking 10 milligrams of melatonin near bedtime to be effective in reducing the frequency of episodic cluster headaches. Chronic cluster headaches did not show improvement with this treatment, however.

❑ Women who suffer from migraines may benefit from using progesterone cream topically.

❑ There are a number of common misdiagnoses of headache, including sinus pain, allergies, and temporomandibular joint syndrome (TMJ). What many people think are sinus headaches are really migraines. Sinus infections can cause brief, intense bouts of head pain, but recurring headaches are more likely to be tension headaches, migraines, or cluster headaches. Facial pain, pain in the temples, or pain above the ear is sometimes diagnosed as temporomandibular joint (TMJ) headache, caused by the joint of the jawbone being out of alignment. But this too may actually be one of the common types of headache, which may be triggered or aggravated by the joint.

❑ Carbon monoxide poisoning can cause headache, in addition to nausea, vomiting, and neurological problems. Some 200 Americans die each year, and another 10,000 are treated in emergency rooms, for carbon monoxide exposure from leaking furnaces, gas ranges, and water heaters. Early signs of carbon monoxide poisoning are sometimes misdiagnosed. One way to protect yourself is to invest in a carbon monoxide detector. These can be purchased at hardware stores.

❑ *See also* HYPOGLYCEMIA; MIGRAINE; PAIN CONTROL; and TMJ SYNDROME, all in Part Two.

❑ For the names and addresses of organizations that can provide additional information and other services for people with headaches, see HEALTH AND MEDICAL ORGANIZATIONS in the Appendix.

Hearing Loss

Loss of hearing occurs when the passage of sound waves to the brain is impaired. Hearing loss may be partial or complete, temporary or permanent, depending on the cause. Hearing loss is not technically the same thing as deafness, or hearing deficit. While hearing loss can lead to hearing deficit, deafness is an inability to hear that most often occurs at, or before, birth or as a result of a major illness or infection.

Hearing loss is divided into three categories: conductive hearing loss, sensorineural hearing loss, and central hearing loss. Conductive hearing loss occurs when the passage of sound waves is impeded in the external or middle ear. It may result from factors such as earwax buildup, middle ear infection and inflammation, Paget's disease, arthritis, or trauma to the eardrum. Sensorineural hearing loss is a consequence of damage to the structures or pathways of the inner ear. It may result from damage to the acoustic nerve (the eighth cranial nerve, also known as the auditory nerve), which carries information from the inner ear to the brain, or from damage to tiny cells called hair cells in the inner ear. The hair cells are responsible for translating sound waves into nerve impulses for transmission to the brain. If the hair cells die, they are unable to repair themselves and the resulting hearing loss is permanent. Sensorineural hearing loss can be present from birth, or it can be caused by certain prescription medications including certain antibiotics, nonsterodial anti-inflammatory drugs (NSAIDs), aspirin taken over along period of time in

high doses, quinine, viral infection of the inner ear, and Ménierè's disease. This type of hearing loss affects both the acuity and clarity of hearing. Initially, it is noticed at higher pitches, and then, as it progresses, it is noticed at lower pitches, where speech is heard. It is also possible to have mixed hearing loss, in which both conductive and sensorineural loss are present. Neural hearing loss usually occurs as a result of a brain tumor or stroke. Central hearing loss is very rare and is usually due to severe brain damage.

Hearing loss can be sudden or gradual, occurring over a period of days, weeks, or years. Infection, trauma, changes in atmospheric pressure, and earwax buildup or impaction can cause a sudden loss of hearing. Infection and inflammation often follow an upper respiratory infection or trauma to the ear, such as from the overuse or improper use of cotton swabs. Bathing or swimming in water that is overly chlorinated or contains high levels of bacteria and/or fungi can also lead to ear infections. Persistent and recurrent ear infections are often linked to fungal infection (candidiasis) and are frequently seen in people with allergies, cancer, diabetes, or other chronic diseases.

If hearing loss develops gradually, the individual experiencing it may be unaware of it until it reaches a fairly advanced stage. In fact, it is not uncommon for friends and family members to notice signs of hearing loss before the person experiencing it does. Some signs that may point to a hearing problem include seeming inattentiveness, unusually loud speech, irrelevant comments, inappropriate responses to questions or environmental sounds, requests for statements to be repeated, a tendency to turn one ear toward sound, and unusual voice quality.

One-third of people over the age of sixty-five have problems with their hearing. Aging is the major factor in loss of the ability to hear the full range of frequencies in everyday communication. Loss of the ability to hear high-frequency noises usually comes first. This type of age-related hearing impairment is called *presbycusis*. Presbycusis can be caused by a change in the blood supply to the ear due to heart disease, some diabetic conditions, or circulatory problems.

Suspected hearing deficits in infants deserve close and immediate attention, as an undiagnosed hearing impairment can lead to delayed and/or diminished acquisition of language skills and, possibly, learning disabilities. Risk factors for hearing loss in infancy include a family history of hearing loss; known hereditary disorders; congenital abnormalities of the ears, nose, or throat; maternal exposure to rubella or syphilis, or to ototoxic drugs such as tobramycin (Nebcin), streptomycin, gentamicin (Garamycin), quinine (Quinamm), furosemide (Lasix), or ethacrynic acid (Edecrin); and birth-related problems such as prematurity, trauma and/or lack of oxygen during delivery, low birth weight, Usher syndrome, or jaundice. *Otitis media* (middle ear infection) is the most common cause of hearing loss in children. For the most part, this is temporary, but chronic or recurrent ear infections can cause permanent hearing loss due to inflammation and infection of the middle ear. (*See*

EAR INFECTION in Part Two.) Sensorineural hearing loss in children can also be caused by childhood diseases such as meningitis, mumps, and rubella. Signs of hearing problems in infancy include failure to blink or startle at loud noises; failure to turn the head toward familiar sounds; a consistent ability to sleep through loud noises; greater responsiveness to loud noises than to voices; a failure to babble, coo, or squeal; and monotonal babbling. In toddlers, warning signs include failure to speak clearly by age two, showing no interest in being read to or in playing word games, habitual yelling or shrieking when communicating or playing, greater responsiveness to facial expressions than to speech, shyness or withdrawal (often misinterpreted as inattentiveness, dreaminess, and/or stubbornness), and frequent confusion and puzzlement. In older children, signs of hearing loss are similar to those in adulthood—a failure to respond to verbal requests, inappropriate responses to questions or other sound stimuli, and a seeming inattentiveness.

Hearing loss caused by exposure to loud noises (noise pollution) is an increasing problem in our society today. When the delicate mechanisms of the inner ear are assaulted by loud noises, a phenomenon called *temporary threshold shift* (TTS) occurs. If you have ever walked away from a concert or a construction site with a buzzing or hissing in your ears, or with everything sounding as if you are underwater, you have experienced temporary threshold shift. When this condition occurs, you hear only noises above a certain level. While overnight rest usually restores normal hearing, this is a sign that damage has occurred to the hair cells in your inner ear. If this type of damage is lengthy and/or repeated, *permanent threshold shift* (PTS), with permanent damage and hearing loss, is the result. There are a number of terms—some clinical, some informal—used to distinguish among the sources of noise-related hearing loss. *Boilermaker's ear* is a condition caused by heavy exposure to broad-band noise. The affected individual loses the ability to hear high-frequency sounds and has difficulty in understanding spoken words. *Diplacusis* is a form of hearing loss experienced as sound distortion—the pitch of a given tone is heard differently by each ear. *Hyperacusis* is an extreme sensitivity to loud noises that can be caused by damage to the eardrum. *Sociocusis* is a term used to denote hearing loss from non-work-related exposure to noise. Most people who develop noise-related hearing loss say they were unaware that anything was wrong until they developed tinnitus or speech became inaudible, but in fact, the damage begins long before that and temporary threshold shift is a clear sign of it.

Noise-related hearing loss is common in train engineers, military personnel, and workers subjected to constant industrial noise, as well as in hunters and musicians, especially rock musicians. Recent National Institutes of Health (NIH) statistics indicate that as much as one-third of all hearing loss is associated with loud noises, and while conclusive data are as yet lacking, many researchers believe that more young people are losing their hearing today than in previous years. The National Center for Health Statistics reports that young people account for one-third of today's hearing loss statistics. They also report that in most cases, this type of hearing loss could have been prevented.

Tinnitus is a condition that occurs in about 85 percent of people with hearing loss. It is experienced as constant or recurring ringing, buzzing, or hissing noises not caused by anything in the external environment. It is now thought that the noise originates in the brain and not in the ear, as was previously believed. If the ear is damaged by exposure to loud noises or certain medications (including aspirin), the brain may try to compensate and end up producing electrical signals that a person hears as a ringing noise in the ears.

Unless otherwise specified, the dosages recommended here are for adults. For a child between the ages of twelve and seventeen, reduce the dose to three-quarters the recommended amount. For a child between six and twelve, use one-half the recommended dose, and for a child under the age of six, use one-quarter the recommended amount.

HEARING LOSS SELF-TEST

The following is a quick test for hearing loss that you can do easily on your own: Rub your thumb and index finger together a few inches from your ear. If you can hear a scratching sound, your hearing is probably intact. If not, you may be experiencing hearing loss. Consult a doctor or audiologist for further evaluation.

NUTRIENTS

SUPPLEMENT	SUGGESTED DOSAGE	COMMENTS
Important		
Coenzyme Q₁₀	30 mg daily.	Powerful antioxidant. Crucial in the effectiveness of the immune system and circulation to the ears.
plus Coenzyme A from Coenzyme-A Technologies	As directed on label.	Works well with coenzyme Q₁₀ in supporting the immune system.
Colloidal silver	As directed on label.	Excellent antiviral agent. Can also be used as ear drops for infection or inflammation.
Magnesium	1,500 mg daily	Prevents damage to the hair cells in the inner ear.
Manganese	10 mg daily.	Deficiency has been linked to ear disorders.
Multivitamin and mineral complex	As directed on label.	To provide a balance of all nutrients.
Potassium	99 mg daily.	Important for a healthy nervous system and transmission of nerve impulses.
Ultimate Oil from Nature's Secret	As directed on label.	Blend of essential fatty acids. Helps reduce tendency to produce excessive amounts of earwax.

Vitamin A	15,000 IU daily. If you are pregnant, do not exceed 10,000 IU daily.	To boost immunity, increase resistance to infection, and strengthen mucous membranes. Studies have shown benefits to hearing-impaired people from taking vitamin A. Antioxidants and precursors of vitamin A.
plus carotenoid complex	15,000 IU daily.	
Vitamin B complex injections or	As prescribed by physician.	Essential for healing; reduces ear pressure. Injections (under a doctor's supervision) are best. If injections are not available, use a sublingual form.
vitamin B complex	50 mg of each major B vitamin 3 times daily (amounts of individual vitamins in a complex will vary).	
plus extra folic acid and	400 mcg daily.	Often depleted in people with hearing loss.
vitamin B₁₂	1,000–2,000 mcg daily.	
Vitamin C with bioflavonoids plus	3,000–6,000 mg daily.	Needed for proper immune function and to aid in preventing ear infections.
N-acetylcysteine	As directed on label.	To remove excess fluids from the ear canal.
Vitamin E	600 IU daily.	Powerful antioxidant that increases circulation. Use d-alpha-tocopherol form.
Zinc lozenges	50 mg daily. Do not exceed a total of 100 mg daily from all supplements.	Quickens immune response; aids in reducing infection.

HERBS

❑ Bayberry bark, burdock root, goldenseal, hawthorn leaf and flower, and myrrh gum purify the blood and counteract infection.

Caution: Do not take goldenseal internally on a daily basis for more than one week at a time, as it may disturb normal intestinal flora. Do not use it during pregnancy, and use it with caution if you are allergic to ragweed.

❑ Echinacea aids poor equilibrium and reduces dizziness. It also fights infection and helps reduce congestion. It can be taken in tea or capsule form.

❑ Ephedra, eucalyptus, hyssop, mullein, and thyme have decongestant properties, which may alleviate ringing in ears.

❑ Ginkgo biloba helps to reduce dizziness and improve hearing loss related to reduced blood flow. Other herbs that may help to improve circulation and blood flow to the ear area include butcher's broom, cayenne, chamomile, ginger root, turmeric, and yarrow.

❑ To soothe inflammation and fight infection, mullein oil can be used as ear drops. If mullein is not available, garlic oil or liquid extract (Kyolic) may be substituted.

RECOMMENDATIONS

❑ Eat fresh pineapple frequently to reduce inflammation. Also include plenty of garlic, kelp, and sea vegetables in your diet.

❑ Limit your consumption of alcohol and sugars, which encourage the growth of yeast. This is particularly important if you have recurrent ear infections and have been treated with antibiotics. Also eliminate or keep to a minimum your intake of caffeine, chocolate, and sodium.

❑ For earwax buildup, clean or irrigate your ears using either a solution of 1 part vinegar to 1 part warm water, or a few drops of hydrogen peroxide. Using an eyedropper, place a few drops in your ear, allow them to settle for a minute, then drain. Repeat the process with the other ear. Do this two or three times a day. Do not use cotton swabs to clean inside the ear canal, as this can push wax further into the ear canal and exacerbate the problem. If the wax is hard and dry, apply garlic oil for a day or two to soften it. Then wash out the ear with a steady stream of warm water. Be patient, continue to irrigate the ear canal, and flush with warm water. Most cases of ear wax buildup can be treated by this method. Another method of removing excess ear wax, called ear candling, uses special candles available at health food stores. Instructions for the procedure are included with the candles. The candling procedure requires assistance, so do not attempt this by yourself.

❑ For an ear infection, put 2 to 4 drops of warm (not hot) liquid garlic extract in the affected ear. (If both ears are infected, do not use the same dropper for both ears, as it may spread infection.) This treatment is very helpful for children.

❑ If you are experiencing ear pain, tug on your earlobe. If this tug makes the ear hurt, you probably have an ear infection and should seek medical treatment. If the tug on the lobe does not hurt, the pain may be due to a dental problem.

❑ When flying, chew gum during the plane's descent to prevent the discomfort and hearing loss associated with changes in atmospheric pressure. Or pop your ears by holding your nose and *gently* blowing air through your closed mouth. This clears the eustachian tubes. A decongestant such as pseudoephedrine (found in Sudafed and other products) may also be helpful, but remember, these medications are dehydrating (and so is the lack of humidity in an airplane cabin). If you use them, be sure to drink plenty of water and juice during the flight, and skip the cocktail and coffee, as alcohol and caffeine also are dehydrating.

❑ Always wear ear protection (disposable plugs or earphone-style headset) when using loud appliances such as power tools or lawn mowers; and when you know you will be exposed to sudden loud noises, such as when shooting a gun.

❑ Protect your hearing when listening to music. A general guideline is to keep the volume low enough that you can easily hear the telephone and other sounds over the music. If you are using a personal stereo unit with headphones, you should be the only one able to hear your music. If someone standing next to you can hear it, it's too loud.

❑ Take measures to reduce your cholesterol level. Studies

suggest that people with high cholesterol levels have greater hearing loss as they age than people with normal cholesterol levels. (*See* HIGH CHOLESTEROL in Part Two.)

❑ If you are prone to ear infections, wear ear plugs while swimming.

❑ If you are planning to become pregnant, make sure you have achieved immunity to German measles, either through having had the disease or through vaccination. A doctor can perform a blood test to determine immunity. If vaccination is necessary, you must guard against becoming pregnant for at least three months to avoid the risk of serious birth defects, such as hearing loss.

❑ If you become ill during pregnancy and medication is required, question your doctor or pharmacist thoroughly about possible effects on the developing fetus and do some research on your own. This will reduce the risk of giving birth to a child with impaired hearing.

❑ If you have an infant, pay very close attention to his or her reactions to noises. If you have any doubt about your child's hearing, consult your physician. Be aware, however, that many physicians are not expert at picking up on hearing loss. If your doctor seems too quick to dismiss your concerns, talk to another doctor. Keep in mind that early detection is vitally important; detection of hearing loss before a child's first birthday greatly reduces the chances that he or she will be disadvantaged by hearing problems in the years to come.

❑ If you have experienced permanent hearing loss, advise family members, friends, and coworkers to speak slowly and distinctly, and avoid shouting. Depending on the nature of the hearing loss, a hearing aid may be helpful. Although 28 million Americans are known to be hearing impaired, only 6 million use a hearing aid. There are now several different types of hearing aids on the market, including the following:

• Behind-the-ear (BTE) devices. These hook behind the ear and a tube carries the sound to an microphone fitted in the ear. The earpiece can also be attached to a pair of glasses. BTE devices work well, but some people find them aesthetically unappealing.

• In-the-ear (ITE) devices. These are placed partly in the outer portion of the ear and partly in the ear canal. They are less obvious than BTE hearing aids. They can cause problems with feedback, however, because the microphone part is so close to the receiver and the controls are rather small.

• In-the-canal (ITC) devices. As the name suggests, these are placed in the ear canal so they are difficult to see. This makes them very popular, but they too have problems with feedback due to the close proximity of the microphone and the receiver.

• Digital devices. These represent the most exciting potential advance in hearing aid technology. They are able to suppress background noise, which is something other hear-

ing aids cannot do. Unfortunately, the price of these devices, at least at present, is prohibitively high, and more work is needed before they exceed the efficacy of the older analogue hearing aids.

❑ Hearing loss due to infection that has destroyed or damaged the sound-conducting mechanism of the inner ear can now be corrected with surgery. Surgeons can rebuild the damaged section with artificial bone and restore the eardrum to its original state.

❑ Researchers at the Massachusetts Institute of Technology (MIT) are working on cochlear implants to send messages to a tiny computer worn on the body. The messages are intended to stimulate the auditory nerve fibers, allowing hearing-impaired individuals to hear normal everyday sounds.

CONSIDERATIONS

❑ Appropriate treatment for hearing loss depends on the underlying cause.

❑ Food allergies, especially allergies to wheat and dairy products, can be the culprit in recurrent middle ear infections. (*See* ALLERGIES in Part Two.)

❑ You can minimize the level of hearing loss you will experience as you grow older if you reduce your exposure to loud noises in the earlier years of your life. Hearing can also be improved with proper diet and supplements.

❑ If you have to raise your voice to be heard over your surroundings, your environment is too noisy. You should try to limit your exposure to such places. If such exposure cannot be avoided, you should wear ear protection.

❑ Most cases of early childhood hearing deficit are first detected by the parents, not health care providers.

❑ The Occupational Safety and Health Administration (OSHA) has established guidelines for workplace noise levels. For any eight-hour day, the noise level should not be above 90 decibels (dBA). Protective headphones should be provided if noise levels exceed 85 dBA for any period of time.

❑ The average rock concert or stereo headset set at full blast (about 100 decibels) can damage your hearing in as little as half an hour. Similar damage can occur after about two hours spent in a video game arcade.

❑ Some researchers say that in addition to causing hearing loss, constant exposure to noise may lead to (or exacerbate) impaired vision, impotence, heart disease, psychological disorders, and other health problems.

❑ Any hearing loss that does not resolve on its own within two weeks should be evaluated by a professional. Some of the symptoms associated with hearing loss can be a sign of a serious health problem that requires treatment.

❑ If you are concerned about your hearing, you can arrange to take a free hearing test over the telephone. The

Dial a Hearing Screening Test is provided as public service by Occupational Hearing Services (*see* HEALTH AND MEDICAL ORGANIZATIONS in the Appendix). It is not a definitive test, but can give some indication as to whether you have a hearing problem you may need to talk to a hearing specialist about.

❑   *See also* EAR INFECTION and MÉNIÈRE'S DISEASE in Part Two.

Heart Attack

Every year, a staggering 1.6 million Americans have heart attacks and over 30 percent of them die. The heart is a muscle that pumps blood around the body. It is made up of four separate chambers, two *atria* and two *ventricles*. Between the four chambers are valves that allow the blood to flow in one direction only—forward. With each beat of the heart, the right ventricle pumps deoxygenated blood to the lungs while the left ventricle pumps oxygenated blood into the arteries for circulation around the body. The heart in turn depends on oxygenated blood coming to it through the coronary arteries (the arteries around the heart) for necessary oxygen and nutrients. If the coronary arteries are constricted due to atherosclerosis (the deposit of fatty plaques in the arteries), an embolus (a piece of tissue or air lodged in the artery), or a thrombus (a blood clot in the artery), the heart may be deprived of sufficient oxygen, causing a heart attack. The medical term for a heart attack is *myocardial infarction* (death of cardiac tissue). When the supply of blood to the heart is sharply reduced or cut off, the heart is deprived of needed oxygen. If blood flow is not restored within minutes, portions of the heart muscle begin to die, permanently damaging the heart muscle. Because this happens when the coronary arteries cannot provide the heart with sufficient oxygen, physicians also commonly refer to a heart attack as a "coronary."

With the onset of a heart attack, the primary symptom is a consistent deep, often severe, pain in the chest that can spread to the left arm, neck, jaw, or the area between the shoulder blades. The pain may be present for up to twelve hours. Many people who have had heart attacks describe it as a heavy, substernal pressure that makes it feel as if the chest is being squeezed. Other possible symptoms include shortness of breath, sweating, nausea, and vomiting. In addition, a heart attack can cause abnormal heartbeat rhythms called arrhythmias. But the symptoms often are not at all as clear as this. They may also vary from person to person, and from heart attack to heart attack. This cannot be emphasized enough—especially for women, who are more likely to have "atypical" symptoms such as pain between the shoulder blades rather than crushing chest pain, and who therefore tend to delay seeking treatment or help.

There are three basic scenarios that can produce a heart attack. The first, and by far the most common, is partial or complete blockage of one of the arteries that supply the heart with oxygen, most often by a blood clot. Usually the arteries have been narrowed by years of coronary artery disease in which plaque, which is composed of cholesterol-rich fatty deposits, proteins, calcium, and excess smooth muscle cells, builds up on the arterial walls. The arterial walls thicken, inhibiting the flow of blood to the heart muscle. The roughening of arterial walls by deposits of plaque not only narrows the arteries, but also makes it easier for blood clots to form along their inner surfaces. When a clot grows, or detaches from its place of origin and travels through the blood vessels, it may block a coronary artery completely, resulting in a heart attack.

In the second heart attack scenario, an arrhythmia may set in, so that the heart is no longer pumping enough blood to ensure its own supply.

In the third, a weak spot in a blood vessel, called an aneurysm, may rupture, causing internal bleeding and disrupting normal blood flow.

No one knows exactly why some people develop heart disease and others do not, but a number of significant clues and risk factors have been identified. One risk factor that has been receiving a great deal of attention is homocysteine, an amino acid formed as a result of the metabolism of another amino acid, methionine, which is essential for normal growth and normal metabolism. Homocysteine in turn is converted back into methionine in a constant recycling process. The proper balance between homocysteine and methionine is essential. Too much homocysteine is toxic to the vascular system, and is very strongly associated with atherosclerosis. High homocysteine levels can be detected in over 20 percent of people with heart disease.

High levels of blood fats—specifically, certain lipoproteins and triglycerides—are also associated with an increased risk of heart disease. Lipoproteins are molecules that transport cholesterol in the bloodstream. There are two principal types: low-density lipoprotein (LDL) and high-density lipoprotein (HDL). High levels of LDL can lead to the formation of fatty plaques that can narrow the arteries and cause reduced blood flow. Lipoprotein(a) is a cholesterol-carrying protein closely related to LDL. It appears to be an important contributing factor in atherosclerosis, although the reason for this is not clear. High levels of HDL, on the other hand, appear to carry cholesterol away from the arteries and back to the liver for processing. Triglycerides are lipids (fats) that bind to proteins to form the high- and low-density lipoproteins. As with LDL, high triglyceride levels are associated with atherosclerosis and heart attack. Eating too many fatty foods, drinking too much alcohol, or having high insulin levels can result in elevated triglyceride levels.

Another possible factor in heart disease is an insufficient supply of antioxidants. Antioxidants render free radicals harmless and help the body dispose of toxic substances that may cause cellular damage. High levels of fibrinogen, a blood-clotting protein, may also be involved. If fibrinogen levels are high, the blood is more likely to form clots that obstruct blood flow, resulting in heart attack or stroke.

Still other research into the origins of heart disease focuses on the possible role of infectious bacteria. The presence of the bacteria *Helicobacter pylori (H. pylori)*, normally associated with ulcers, has been found to be present in a significant number of people who have suffered heart attack. *Chlamydia pneumoniae*, a type of bacteria responsible for nearly 10 percent of cases of pneumonia, may also be associated with an increased likelihood of developing heart disease. Researchers believe that the chronic presence of low levels of these bacteria may result in chronic low-level inflammation in the blood vessels, which in turn makes them more vulnerable to developing deposits of fatty plaques. In support of this hypothesis, high levels of a substance called C-reactive protein (CRP) have been found helpful in predicting an individual's potential for developing heart disease. CRP is released into the bloodstream when the blood vessels serving the heart have been damaged due to inflammation. Another sign of inflammation is a substance known as intracellular adhesion molecule (ICAM-1) or CD54. A type of molecule found on the surface of certain cells, ICAM-1 interacts with other body chemicals to trigger the inflammatory process. The more prevalent ICAM-1 is, the more likely you are to develop atherosclerosis, although CRP levels are still considered a better indicator of inflammation than ICAM-1 levels.

In general, persons considered to be at greater than normal risk of heart attack are those with a family history of heart disease; those who smoke and/or abuse drugs; people with diabetes, high blood pressure, high blood cholesterol and/or triglyceride levels, or high homocysteine levels; sedentary people; and those who are under stress and/or who have "type A" personalities.

One third of all heart attacks occur without warning. The remainder are preceded by months or even years of symptoms, most commonly angina pectoris—chest pain that is typically aggravated by stress or physical exertion and relieved by rest. Like a heart attack, angina is caused by a lack of oxygen in the heart muscle, but the extent of oxygen deprivation is not sufficient to actually damage heart tissue. Many people complain of intermittent angina, shortness of breath, and/or unusual fatigue in the days or weeks leading up to a heart attack. A constant sensation of heartburn that persists for days and from which antacids provide no relief can be a sign of an impending heart attack.

The dietary, nutritional, and lifestyle recommendations in this section are designed to help prevent, or to support recovery from, a heart attack. They are not meant as a substitute for proper emergency treatment. If you think you may be having a heart attack, do not waste any time in seeking medical assistance. Any delay in obtaining help can result in greater damage to the heart.

NUTRIENTS

SUPPLEMENT	SUGGESTED DOSAGE	COMMENTS
Essential		
Aerobic Heart from Aerobic Life Industries	As directed on label.	Lowers homocysteine levels—vital for maintaining a healthy heart.
Alpha-linolenic acid (ALA)	As directed on label.	An omega-3 fatty found in a long-term French study to lower the risk of a fatal heart attack by over one-third.
Alpha-lipoic acid	As directed on label.	An antioxidant that lowers LDL levels.
Chinese red yeast rice extract	As directed on label.	Promotes blood circulation and regulates cholesterol levels.
Coenzyme Q$_{10}$	100 mg daily.	Improves heart muscle oxygenation and may help prevent second heart attacks.
or Q-Gel	As directed on label.	A patented form of coenzyme Q$_{10}$ that is more easily absorbed than standard forms, so you can take less with the same effect.
plus Coenzyme A from Coenzyme-A Technologies	As directed on label.	Works well with coenzyme Q$_{10}$ to streamline metabolism, ease depression and fatigue, increase energy, support adrenal glands, process fats, remove toxins from the body, and boost the immune system.
Grape seed extract or Pycnogenol	150–300 mg daily.	Powerful antioxidants. Reduces the clotting tendency of the blood. Best used in combination with phosphatidyl choline, a natural component of lecithin.
Inositol hexaphosphate (IP$_6$)	As directed on label.	Protects the heart by preventing blood clots and reducing cholesterol and triglyceride levels.
L-Arginine	As directed on label.	An amino acid that boosts production of nitric oxide, which dilates the arteries to allow better blood flow. *Note:* If you are prone to herpes outbreaks, do not take L-arginine without L-lysine.
Lecithin	As directed on label.	Contains choline and inositol, important parts of the vitamin B complex. Aids in lowering cholesterol levels.
Potassium	99 mg twice a day.	Needed to maintain regular heart rhythm. Lowers cholesterol.
S-Adenosylmethionine (SAMe)	As directed on label.	A natural antidepressant (depression has been linked to heart disease). Lowers homocysteine levels. *Note:* If you take SAMe, be careful to maintain a correct balance of vitamins B$_6$ and B$_{12}$ and folic acid.
or trimethylglycine (TMG)	As directed on label.	Is converted into SAMe in the body. Lowers homocysteine levels.
Selenium	300 mcg daily. If you are pregnant, do not exceed 40 mcg daily.	Deficiency has been implicated in heart disease.

Vitamin B complex	50 mg of each major B vitamin 3 times daily. (amounts of individual vitamins in a complex will vary).	B vitamins work best when taken together.
plus extra vitamin B$_3$ (niacin) and	50 mg daily.	B vitamins that lower homocysteine levels. Sublingual forms are best.
vitamin B$_6$ (pyridoxine) and	50 mg daily.	
vitamin B$_{12}$ and	1,000–2,000 mcg daily.	
folic acid	400 mcg daily. If you take anticonvulsant medication for epilepsy, do not exceed 400 mcg of folic acid per day from all sources, as it may induce seizures.	Deficiency of folic acid in the heart muscle leads to heart disease. Low folate levels may be more dangerous than high cholesterol for people with heart disease.
or No Shot B-6/B-12/ Folic from Superior Source	As directed on label.	A combination of these three important B vitamins.
Vitamin E capsules or liquid vitiman E with tocotrienols	Start with 200 IU daily, and increase slowly to 800 IU daily. As directed on label.	A powerful antioxidant that improves circulation and thins the blood, reducing the risk of clots. Use d-alpha-tocopherol form. *Note:* If you take prescription blood-thinners, consult your doctor before taking supplemental vitamin E.

Very Important		
Acetyl-L-carnitine or L-carnitine plus L-cysteine and L-methionine	500 mg each daily, on an empty stomach. Take with water or juice. Do not take with milk. Take with 50 mg vitamin B$_6$ and 100 mg vitamin C for better absorption.	To reduce blood lipid levels, increase cellular glutathione and coenzyme Q$_{10}$, protect against lipid peroxidation, and assist in the breakdown of fats, preventing fatty buildup in the arteries, which helps restore blood flow to the heart.
Calcium and magnesium	1,500 mg daily. 1,000 mg daily, in divided doses, between meals and at bedtime.	Important for maintaining proper heart rhythm and blood pressure. Use chelate or citrate forms.
Cardio Logic from Wakunaga	As directed on label.	Increases oxygenation of heart tissue.
Chromium	100 mcg daily.	Helps raise levels of HDL ("good cholesterol").
Essential fatty acids (Kyolic-EPA from Wakanuga, primrose oil, and salmon oil are good sources)	As directed on label.	Protects heart muscle cells. Reduces triglyceride levels in the blood.
Garlic (Kyolic from Wakunaga)	2 capsules 3 times daily.	Beneficial for the heart, promotes circulation, and aids in reducing high blood pressure.
Glucosamine Plus from FoodScience of Vermont	As directed on label.	Plays an important role in the formation of heart valves.
Heart Science from Source Naturals	As directed on label.	Contains antioxidants, cholesterol-fighters, herbs, and vitamins that work together to promote cardio-vascular function.
Multienzyme complex	As directed on label. Take with meals.	For proper digestion and to prevent heartburn.

Proteolytic enzymes	As directed on label 3 times daily. Take between meals for better protein absorption.	Anti-inflammatory agents that prevent free radical damage to the arteries.
Sea mussel	As directed on label.	Aids in the functioning of the cardiovascular system, the lymphatic system, and the endocrine system.
7-Keto DHEA	As directed on label.	Has been found to reduce depression.
Vitamin A with mixed carotenoids	As directed on label. If you are pregnant, do not exceed 10,000 IU daily.	Helps prevent free radical damage to the arteries. Use emulsion form for easier assimilation.
Zinc plus copper	50 mg daily. Do not exceed a total of 100 mg daily from all supplements. 3 mg daily.	Necessary for proper balance with copper and for thiamine utilization. Use a chelate form. Deficiency has been linked to heart disease.

Important		
Dimethylglycine (DMG) (Aangamik DMG from FoodScience of Vermont)	As directed on label.	Improves oxygenation of heart tissue.
Vitamin C with bioflavonoids	3,000–6,000 mg daily.	Aids in thinning the blood. Prevents blood clots and free radical damage.

HERBS

❑ Alfalfa, borage seed, horsetail, nettle, and pau d'arco are rich in minerals necessary for proper regulation of heart rhythm.

❑ Black cohosh, oat straw, passionflower, valerian root, skullcap, and wood betony are calming herbs that may help to regulate arrhythmias.

❑ Butcher's broom, hawthorn berries and leaf, mother-wort, and red sage strengthen the heart muscle.

❑ Cayenne (capsicum), ginger root, and ginkgo biloba strengthen the heart and are helpful for chest pain.

Note: If you take prescription blood-thinning medica-tion, consult your health care provider before using ginkgo.

❑ Cordyceps is a Chinese herb that lowers both blood pressure and LDL ("bad cholesterol") levels.

❑ Gotu kola, primrose, and rosemary are helpful in man-aging angina.

❑ Green tea has superb antioxidant properties. Drinking 10 to 20 cups a day can provide protection against heart dis-ease and many other illnesses.

Note: If you take prescription blood-thinners, consult your doctor before taking green tea in capsule form. Green tea capsules—not the tea itself—contain fairly large quan-tities of vitamin K, which promotes blood clotting.

❑ Turmeric contains curcumin, an anti-inflammatory that also lowers blood cholesterol.

RECOMMENDATIONS

❏ If you think you may be having a heart attack follow the steps outlined below:

• Stop what you are doing and sit down.

• Assess the situation. Try to remain calm. If there is someone else around you, let him or her know what is happening. If there is no one else there and you are still feeling pain or discomfort after a few minutes, or if you are sweating and weak without any other obvious symptoms, call for emergency help and tell the person on the other end of the line that you may be having a heart attack. *Do not* drive yourself to hospital. *Do not* delay getting treatment.

• After calling for medical help, if you are unable to leave your telephone number and address, you may want to leave the telephone off the hook so that your number and address can be traced. If you have given your address and telephone number successfully, hang up and call a friend or relative who may be of assistance.

• If you have nitroglycerin tablets, take one every five minutes, up to three tablets in total. If you have aspirin in the house, take one and chew it. This may prevent a blood clot.

• If a friend or relative is with you, have him or her check your pulse and respiration (breathing) at regular intervals. If your pulse or breathing stops, this person should start cardiopulmonary resuscitation (CPR) immediately. He or she should then call the emergency number again, so that when the ambulance arrives, emergency personnel know that this is indeed a heart attack.

• If it is later established that the episode was *not* a heart attack, consider having your potential for a heart attack assessed by a doctor to relieve any doubts and concerns you may have.

❏ If you have suffered a heart attack, or if you are considered at risk for a heart attack, modify your diet. Important dietary measures include the following:

• Make sure your diet is high in fiber. Not all types of fiber decrease the risk of heart attack, however. The most beneficial fiber appears to come from whole-grain breakfast cereals.

• Eat lots of foods that are rich in vitamins B_6 and B_{12} and folic acid, which are needed to keep homocysteine levels in check. Vitamins B_6 and B_{12} come naturally from leafy green vegetables and fruits. Folic acid can be found in some breakfast cereals, asparagus, spinach, chickpeas, and beans.

• Include almonds, brewer's yeast, grains, and sesame seeds in your diet.

• Enjoy onions frequently. Onions—especially red onions—contain valuable antioxidants. Chop them and allow them to stand for ten minutes before cooking for optimal benefit.

• Add kelp and sea vegetables to your diet for necessary minerals. Drink fresh vegetable juices.

• Drink steam-distilled water only.

• Do not eat red meat, salt, sugars, or white flour. A diet high in red meat can elevate homocysteine levels. Eat soy-based protein foods instead. Soy protein can effectively lower high LDL cholesterol levels.

• Avoid salt, sugars, and white flour. Refined sugars produce adverse reactions in all cells by causing wide variations in blood sugar. The high surges are followed by hypoglycemic drops, causing dangerous instability in vital intracellular sugar levels.

• Eliminate fried foods, coffee, black tea, colas, and other stimulants from the diet.

• Refrain from excessive alcohol use, as it has an adverse effect on the heart. Drinking alcohol in moderation may actually be heart-healthy, but do not start to drink if you have not done so before—the potential benefit simply does not justify it.

• Sip barley water throughout the day for its healing and fortifying properties. (*See* THERAPEUTIC LIQUIDS in Part Three.)

❏ Fast three days a month to cleanse and detoxify the body. (*See* FASTING in Part Three, and follow the program.)

❏ To relieve stress and promote relaxation, add a few drops of lavender, sandalwood, or ylang ylang essential oil to a bath, or simply place a few drops on a tissue and inhale the aroma from time to time throughout the day.

❏ *Arnica* is a homeopathic remedy used to support recovery from a heart attack

❏ Do not smoke. Avoid secondhand smoke.

❏ If you think you may be at risk for cardiovascular disease, you should discuss the following tests with your doctor:

• Antibodies for *H. pylori* and *C. pneumoniae*.

• Antioxidant level.

• C-reactive protein (CRP). Normal levels of CRP are 0.8 mg/dL or less.

• Fibrinogen level.

• High-density lipoprotein (HDL) and low-density lipoprotein (LDL) levels. Desirable HDL levels are 60 milligrams per deciliter of blood (mg/dL) or *higher*. Desirable LDL levels are 130 mg/dL or *lower*.

• Homocysteine level. Homocysteine levels should be around 7 micromoles per liter (μmol/L).

• Lipoprotein(a) (Lp[a]). Normal levels of Lp(a) are 30 mg/dL and under.

• Thyroid hormone level. The thyroid gland secretes the hormones thyroxine (T_4) and triiodothyronine (T_3). These two hormones, along with many other functions, maintain cardiac output, rate, and force.

• Triglyceride level. Desirable triglyceride levels are 150 mg/dL or less. Levels up to 200 may be considered acceptable.

CONSIDERATIONS

❑ Heart attacks are directly related to a number of other conditions, such as arteriosclerosis, circulatory problems, hypertension (high blood pressure), high cholesterol, and cardiovascular disorders (including aneurysms, angina pectoris, and arryhythmias). These conditions are discussed separately in Part Two. It is advisable to refer to all of the sections on these interrelated diseases to learn about all aspects of, and contributing causes to, heart attacks.

❑ A guide to some of the language doctors use in talking about cardiovascular disease and heart attacks appears on page 272. This is not a definitive list, but it may provide a handy reference guide for major terms and tests for heart attacks.

❑ It is highly recommended that at least one person in every household receive thorough training in CPR.

❑ A technique known as thermography can be used to test for the presence of atherosclerosis by detecting fluctuations in the temperature of the arteries. In healthy arteries, the temperature remains constant, while in arteries that contain plaque, the temperature is different in diseased areas and the healthy areas. Another test for detecting harmful levels of calcium or plaque buildup in the arteries is gated helical computerized tomography (GHCT) scanning. Ask your doctor if he or she thinks either of these is a test you should have.

❑ Tirofiban (Aggrastat) is an injectable drug that may help people recover from acute cardiac episodes, including severe angina or severe chest pain. It is a type of agent called a glycoprotein blocker that stops blood from clotting. Trials conducted in New Zealand found that tirofiban was more effective at preventing a second fatal heart attack than aspirin or heparin.

❑ Some compounds known as plant sterols and stanols have been shown to lower LDL cholesterol levels and can be found in some types of margarine and salad dressing. They are also available in tablet form.

❑ Very large doses of vitamin D—over 1,000 international units daily—can be dangerous for people with heart disease. In large quantities, vitamin D is toxic and can cause hypercalcemia (excessively high levels of calcium in the blood), which in turn may lead to deposits of calcium in the arteries.

❑ There is ongoing debate about whether or not taking synthetic estrogen protects the heart after menopause. Some studies have suggested that it may, but there have also been studies showing it may actually increase the risk of a heart attack.

❑ There are many different medications that may be prescribed for people with heart disease. These include the following:

• Angiotensin-converting enzyme (ACE) inhibitors inhibit the formation of the hormone angiotensin, which narrows the blood vessels. Angiotensin II receptor blockers interfere with the action, rather than the formation, of the same hormone.

• Anticoagulants (blood thinners) are commonly prescribed for people in particular danger of developing blood clots, such as people who are bedridden, cancer patients, people with certain types of arrhythmias, and those who have had heart valve replacement surgery. There are also newer drugs known as platelet-aggregation inhibitors that may be prescribed for the same purposes.

• Beta-blockers induce the heart to beat more slowly and with less force.

• Calcium channel blockers relax blood-vessel muscle.

• Central adrenergic inhibitors (central-acting agents) prevent the nervous system from increasing heart rate and narrowing blood vessels.

• Diuretics (water pills) help the kidneys get rid of sodium and water, reducing the volume of blood in the body and, therefore, the strain on the heart.

❑ Helidac is a treatment for *H. pylori,* which is now seen as a culprit in heart disease. It is a prescription medication that contains three different drugs: bismuth subsalicylate, the active ingredient in Pepto-Bismol); metronidazole, an antibacterial and antiparasitic drug; and the antibiotic tetracycline.

❑ Most people who have heart attacks experience the characteristic chest pain. However, not all do. Some people have a sensation that feels like indigestion; others have no noticeable symptoms at all. This phenomenon is often referred to as a "silent" heart attack. Elderly people and people with diabetes are probably more likely than others to have this type of heart attack.

❑ Many illnesses can mimic heart attacks, such as a gallbladder attack, fibromyalgia that causes pain in the chest wall, or gastroesophageal reflux disease (GERD), but if you have chest pain, you must see a physician. Chest pain or even ill-defined symptoms that you cannot explain just may be a heart attack—these are not conditions you can afford to ignore.

❑ In some cases, heart attacks are caused by spasms of the arteries that suddenly shut off the flow of blood to the heart.

❑ Sensible, moderate exercise and a proper diet with nutritional supplements can prevent arteriosclerosis of the coronary arteries and myocardial infarction.

Caution: If you are over thirty-five and/or have been sedentary for some time, consult with your health care provider before beginning an exercise program.

❑ Studies have shown that people who take supplemental coenzyme Q_{10} following a heart attack are less likely than those who did not to have a second attack within five years.

❑ Researchers have found that eating just an ounce of

walnuts a day (about seven nuts) may reduce the risk of a heart attack by 8 to 10 percent.

❑ A heart attack is not the same thing as heart failure. In heart failure, the heart does not supply enough blood to the body; in a heart attack, the heart does not receive enough blood to meet its needs. However, the damage produced by a heart attack can lead to heart failure.

❑ Heart attacks are not, as many think, a "male" disorder. In fact, of all Americans who suffer heart attacks, 44 percent of women die within a year, whereas only 27 percent of men do. Heart attacks, not cancer, are the leading cause of death for American women. Twice as many women die of heart attacks each year as die from all forms of cancer combined.

❑ An underactive thyroid may increase the risk of heart attacks. An article in the February 2000 issue of the *Annals of Internal Medicine* reported that women who had a condition termed *subclinical hypothyroidism* were about two times more likely to suffer from blockage in the aorta that could lead to a heart attack than women who had normally functioning thyroids.

❑ Depression and heart attacks often go hand-in-hand. It is therefore wise to actively treat depression.

❑ *See* ARTERIOSCLEROSIS/ATHEROSCLEROSIS; CARDIOVASCULAR DISEASE; CIRCULATORY PROBLEMS; HIGH BLOOD PRESSURE (HYPERTENSION); HIGH CHOLESTEROL; and RHEUMATIC FEVER, all in Part Two.

❑ *See also* CHELATION THERAPY in Part Three.

Heart Disease

See CARDIOVASCULAR DISEASE; HEART ATTACK.

Heartburn/Gastroesophageal Reflux Disease (GERD)

Heartburn is a burning sensation and pain in the stomach and/or chest, behind the breastbone. It may be accompanied by bloating, gas, nausea, shortness of breath, and/or an acidic or sour taste in the throat. Approximately 60 million Americans suffer from heartburn. It often occurs when hydrochloric acid, which is used by the stomach to digest food, backs up into the esophagus (the tube between the throat and stomach), causing sensitive tissues to become irritated. Normally, the esophageal sphincter muscle pinches itself shut and prevents stomach acid from surging upward. However, if the sphincter is not functioning properly, the acid can slip past it and into the esophagus. This is gas-

troesophageal reflux. Conditions that affect the esophagus and cause a reflux of stomach acids into the esophagus are now referred to as *gastroesophageal reflux disease* (GERD) rather than dyspepsia, chronic heartburn, or acid indigestion. GERD can strike anyone, at any age. GERD can scar the esophagus, and if stomach acids make their way into the lungs, it can cause asthma-like symptoms. GERD can also lead to a condition called *Barrett's esophagus*, which is characterized by changes in the cells lining the esophagus that can induce cancer.

People with hiatal hernia often experience heartburn. It can also be triggered by excessive consumption of spicy foods, fatty or fried foods, alcohol, coffee, citrus fruits, chocolate, or tomato-based foods. Ulcers, gallbladder problems, stress, allergies, and enzyme deficiencies are other possible contributing factors.

NUTRIENTS

SUPPLEMENT	SUGGESTED DOSAGE	COMMENTS
Very Important		
Pancreatin plus bromelain	As directed on label. Take with meals. As directed on label.	Enzymes necessary for proper digestion.
Papaya tablets	As directed on label.	To relieve symptoms. Use chewable tablets from a health food store.
Vitamin B complex plus extra vitamin B₁₂	50 mg of each major B vitamin 3 times daily, with meals (amounts of individual vitamins in a complex will vary). 1,000–2,000 mcg daily.	Needed for proper digestion. Use lozenge or sublingual forms.
Helpful		
Acid-Ease from Prevail	As directed on label.	A soothing plant enzyme and herb formula that aids in the breakdown and assimilation of foods.
Acidophilus (Probiata from Wakunaga)	As directed on label.	Replaces friendly bacteria in the stomach.
Calcium and magnesium and potassium	300 mg twice daily. 150–200 mg twice daily. 100 mg twice daily.	These minerals have an alkalizing effect that binds up stomach acid. Take these together between meals. Use calcium carbonate or calcium chelate form.
Methylsulfonyl-methane (MSM)	As directed on label.	Relieves hyperacidity without disturbing the normal acid-alkaline balance.

HERBS

❑ Aloe vera juice aids healing of the intestinal tract.

❑ Catnip, fennel, ginger, marshmallow root, and papaya tea all aid in proper digestion and act as a buffer to stop heartburn.

❑ Drinking chamomile tea can relieve esophageal irritation.

❏ Deglycyrrhizinated licorice (DGL) has effectively treated both heartburn and ulcers of the stomach and esophagus.

Caution: Do not use licorice if you have high blood pressure.

RECOMMENDATIONS

❏ At the first sign of heartburn, drink a large glass of water. This often helps.

❏ Try raw potato juice. Do not peel the potato—just wash it and put it in the juicer. (*See* JUICING in Part Three.) Mix the juice with an equal amount of water. Drink it immediately after preparation, three times a day.

❏ Try drinking a glass of fresh cabbage or celery juice every day.

❏ Change your eating habits. Eat more raw vegetables. Eat smaller, more frequent meals. Chew your food well. Eat slowly and enjoy your food. Following a disciplined diet is an important aspect of managing GERD.

❏ Sip 1 tablespoon of raw apple cider vinegar, mixed with a glass of water, while eating a meal. Do not drink any other liquids with meals.

❏ Eat fresh papaya and/or pineapple to aid digestion. Chew a few of the papaya seeds as well.

❏ Do not eat for three hours before bedtime. Wait at least three hours after eating before lying down.

❏ Avoid acidic foods such as citrus fruits and juices (*see* ACID/ALKALI IMBALANCE in Part Two).

❏ Do not consume carbonated beverages, fats, fried foods, processed foods, peppermint, spearmint, tobacco, tomatoes, onions, caffeine products, sugar, or spicy or highly seasoned foods. These seem to be the main cause of heartburn.

❏ *See* FASTING in Part Three and follow the instructions. *Also see* the self-tests *under* ACID/ALKALI IMBALANCE and CARDIOVASCULAR DISEASE in Part Two.

❏ Do not take a multienzyme complex containing hydrochloric acid (HCl).

❏ Maintain an exercise program that includes walking, biking, or low-impact aerobics. Avoid running and weight lifting as these activities put pressure on the stomach. Do not exercise after eating, however.

❏ Elevate the head of your bed.

❏ As much as possible, avoid stress and anger.

❏ If you are taking any medications, ask your doctor if heartburn may be a side effect.

❏ Do not wear clothes that fit tightly around the waist. Do not wear tight clothing to bed.

❏ Do not ignore symptoms of GERD. This condition can cause serious health problems. If heartburn lasts longer than two weeks, you should seek medical attention.

❏ The early symptoms of angina and heart attack sometimes mimic those of "acid stomach." If symptoms persist, if the pain begins to travel down into your left arm, or if the sensation is accompanied by a feeling of weakness, dizziness, or shortness of breath, seek emergency medical help at once. (*See* HEART ATTACK in Part Two.)

CONSIDERATIONS

❏ Estrogens can weaken the esophageal hiatus muscle, which keeps stomach acids in the stomach. Women who are pregnant and women who take birth control pills that contain estrogen and progesterone are therefore more likely to suffer from heartburn.

❏ People with certain illnesses, such as cancer, often have excessive amounts of acid in their systems. The consumption of too much processed and cooked food can also create an acidic environment in the body.

❏ Aspirin and ibuprofen can cause heartburn.

❏ Lying on your left side can help relieve heartburn. This keeps the stomach below the esophagus, helping to keep it acid-free.

❏ Antacids often provide relief of symptoms. However, in so doing, they may mask an underlying problem. In addition, many over-the-counter antacids contain excessive amounts of sodium, aluminum, calcium, and magnesium. With prolonged use of these products, dangerous mineral imbalances can occur. Excess sodium can aggravate hypertension, and excess aluminum has been implicated in Alzheimer's disease. Reading the label of the antacids you intend to use will provide you with information concerning possible harmful ingredients contained in the product. Some types of antacids and the products they are found in are:

• Aluminum salts or gels: AlternaGEL, Amphojel.

• Aluminum-magnesium mixtures: Aludrox, Di-Gel, Gaviscon, Gelusil, Maalox, Mylanta, Riopan.

• Calcium carbonate: Alka-Mints, Chooz, Titralac, Tums.

• Calcium-magnesium mixtures: Rolaids.

• Magnesium salts or gels: Phillips' Milk of Magnesia.

• Sodium bicarbonate: Alka-Seltzer, Bromo Seltzer, Citrocarbonate.

❏ Calcium carbonate works as an antacid and contains no aluminum.

❏ A product called Acid-Ease, from Prevail Corporation, has shown promising results. It can be purchased at health food stores. Acid-Ease is aluminum-free.

❏ Drugs that suppress the production of stomach acid are sometimes recommended for people who suffer from frequent heartburn. These include cimetidine (Tagamet), famotidine (Pepcid), nizatidine (Axid), omeprazole (Prilosec), and ranitidine (Zantac). It has been suggested that long-term use of these medications may lead to damage to the stomach lining, thus increasing the risk of benign or malignant tumors. According to an item in the *Johns Hopkins Medical Letter,* excessive (more than 3 grams a day) and prolonged use of the heartburn medication cimetidine may cause impotence or breast enlargement. These conditions usually go away when the medication is discontinued.

❑ One study showed that 57 percent of heartburn sufferers had hiatal hernias, almost half had damage to the esophageal lining, and 6 percent had developed *Barrett's esophagus.*

❑ If you are taking antacids more than three times a week, you should consult your physician.

❑ Free information about GERD is available from the American College of Gastroenterology (*see* HEALTH AND MEDICAL ORGANIZATIONS in the Appendix).

❑ *See also* PEPTIC ULCER in Part Two. *Also see under* PREGNANCY-RELATED PROBLEMS in Part Two.

Heel or Bone Spur

A bone spur is a pointed growth on a bone, most commonly in the heel. Extreme stress and strain on the heel bone and soft tissues are the main causes of heel spurs. The stress results in inflammation of the plantar fascia, a ligament on the bottom of the foot that attaches the ball of the foot to the heel bone. This condition is known as plantar fasciitis. If it is not relieved, the repeated pulling of the ligament aggravates the heel bone and eventually the body, in an attempt to protect itself, forms a bone spur. The most common sign of a bone spur is severe pain with the first step in the morning and after periods of inactivity.

Bone spurs can be caused by, or be associated with, physical injury, obesity, gout, lupus, muscle inflammation, nerve problems (such as tarsal tunnel syndrome), strain of the plantar arch, or excessive exercise, standing, or walking. Heel spurs are also common in people who have alkalosis, arthritis, neuritis, or tendinitis. A bone spur may be caused by calcium deposits in unwanted areas of the body. Most people who have heel disorders are middle-aged or overweight. Shoes that are uncomfortable, fit poorly, or lack cushioning for the heel may contribute to the pain.

X-rays may reveal a bony spur within the heel. The presence of this may lead to the formation of tiny tumors at the end of several nerves, and these may be very painful.

NUTRIENTS

SUPPLEMENT	SUGGESTED DOSAGE	COMMENTS
Very Important		
Betaine hydro-chloride (HCl)	As directed on label.	Needed for proper calcium uptake. A deficiency of HCl is more common in elderly people. *Caution:* Do not use HCl if you have a history of ulcers.
Calcium and magnesium	1,500 mg daily. 750 mg daily.	A proper balance of calcium and magnesium helps prevent abnormal calcium deposition. Use chelate or aspartate forms.
Important		
Proteolytic enzymes or Inflazyme Forte from American Biologics or Intenzyme Forte from Biotics Research	As directed on label. As directed on label. As directed on label.	To aid in absorption of nutrients and in control of inflammation and irritation. *Caution:* Do not give these supplements to a child.
Vitamin C with bioflavonoids	2,000–4,000 mg daily.	Acts as an anti-inflammatory; important for collagen and connective tissue.
Helpful		
Bioflavonoids	100 mg daily.	Vitamin C activators that also help relieve pain.
Methylsulfonyl-methane (MSM)	As directed on label. It can be applied as a cream or taken by mouth in the pill form.	Very effective for pain relief.
Vitamin B complex plus extra vitamin B6 (pyridoxine)	50–100 mg of each major B vitamin daily (amounts of individual vitamins in a complex will vary). 50 mg daily.	B vitamins work best when taken together. Necessary for production of hydrochloric acid, which helps prevent bone spurs by aiding proper calcium absorption.

HERBS

❑ Use arnica and chamomile to bathe the foot. You can also wrap the herbs in a cloth and apply it to the affected area as a poultice. (*See* USING A POULTICE in Part Three.)

❑ Bromelain, derived from pineapple, and curcumin, from turmeric, reduce pain and inflammation.

RECOMMENDATIONS

❑ Drink steam-distilled water only.

❑ Do not eat any citrus fruits, especially oranges. Eliminate alcohol, coffee, and sugar from your diet. These inhibit the healing process and upset the body's mineral balance.

❑ To alleviate pain, try stretching exercises; deep, localized massage; physical therapy; and anti-inflammatory herbs. You can also use hot linseed oil packs. Place linseed oil in a pan and heat but do not boil it. Dip a piece of cheesecloth or other white cotton material into the oil until the cloth is saturated. Apply the cloth to the affected area and cover it with a piece of plastic that is larger in size than the cotton cloth. Place a heating pad over the plastic and use it to keep the pack warm. Keep the pack in place for one-half to two hours, as needed.

❑ Ice massages on the bottoms of the feet can be helpful. Alternate between hot and cold foot baths.

❑ Select well-made, rubber-heeled shoes; these are better for the feet than leather. Choose footwear for comfort—not for looks. Some jogging shoes can be very comfortable. Adding heel cushions to footwear helps to relieve pain.

❑ Use night splints to provide a mild, constant stretching function across the sole of the foot at night while sleeping.

❑ If you normally walk or jog for exercise, try bicycling or swimming instead.

❑ Avoid walking on hard surfaces such as concrete, wood, or hard floors without carpeting.

CONSIDERATIONS

❑ A two-week raw food fast or a cleansing fast can be beneficial. (*See* FASTING in Part Three.)

❑ It is best not to have a heel spur surgically removed unless it is extremely irritating or painful.

❑ Steroid injections have been the used to treat this condition. They are not without potential complications, however. They may cause loss of the fatty tissue pad at the bottom of the heel and bring about a condition that is painful and irreversible.

❑ Foot surgery is a last-resort option that is usually reserved for extremely rare, severe cases. An incision is made over the heel to release the attached fascia from the heel bone. Recovery time is approximately six to ten weeks before walking can be resumed comfortably.

❑ *See also* ARTHRITIS in Part Two.

Hemophilia

In a healthy individual, a minor bump can damage a blood vessel, causing blood to leak into the surrounding tissue, producing a bruise. A process called hemostasis (coagulation) plugs the hole in the damaged vessel and forms a clot that stops the blood loss and limits the size of the bruise.

In people with hemophilia and related problems, bleeding can take a very different course. The blood does not clot normally because one or another of the blood proteins that collaborate to repair damaged vessels and form clots is defective, deficient, or totally absent. Approximately 20,000 people in the United States suffer from hemophilia.

There are two main types of hemophilia. They are classified according to the particular protein, or clotting factor, that is deficient. Hemophilia A, caused by a deficiency of factor VIII, accounts for almost 80 percent of people with this disorder. It is usually inherited by male children of mothers who are carriers. Hemophilia B, sometimes called *Christmas disease,* is caused by a problem with clotting factor IX. It too is passed on by carrier mothers to male children. It is also possible to have a bleeding disorder due to

factor XI deficiency. Unlike hemophilia A and B, this problem can be carried by either the male or female parent, and can be passed on to both male and female offspring.

The idea that people with hemophilia can bleed to death from a minor cut or injury is a misconception. In fact, external bleeding is seldom a serious problem. People with hemophilia may bleed somewhat longer than other people, but minor bleeding episodes can generally be controlled by ordinary first aid measures.

Injuries also commonly cause bleeding inside the body—bleeding we may neither see nor feel. Unchecked internal bleeding can be serious—even life threatening—for a person with hemophilia. Blood that leaks into the knee joint, a common site of internal bleeding, can cause painful swelling. Repeated bleeding eventually destroys the cartilage that enables the knee to work smoothly and easily. The joint becomes permanently stiff and painful, the result of hemophilic arthritis. Other joints—the ankle, wrist, or elbow—can be similarly affected by internal bleeding. People with hemophilia can also bleed into muscle and other soft tissue. Internal bleeding can ultimately obstruct air passages or damage the brain or other vital organs.

Hemophilia can be mild, moderate, or severe, depending on how impaired an individual's production of clotting factors is. In severe hemophilia, clotting factor activity is less than 1 percent of normal. Injury, surgery, or dental care can present significant problems for such people. Spontaneous bleeding can require infusion of clotting factor concentrate as often as several times a week. People with moderate hemophilia (factor levels between 1 and 5 percent of normal) do not usually experience spontaneous bleeding, but even a minor injury, if untreated, can cause prolonged bleeding. In mild hemophilia, factor activity ranges between 5 and 50 percent of normal. Bleeding can be expected from surgery, major dental care, or trauma. These individuals rarely bleed into joints, and their disease usually does not interfere with normal living.

The National Hemophilia Foundation estimates that nearly 450 American boys with hemophilia are born each year. The number of females with hemophilia is not known. Hemophilia primarily affects males and is passed down through females because the two primary genes involved in the production of clotting factors are located on the X chromosome. And while females have two X chromosomes, males have only one. For a female to develop the disease, both of her X chromosomes would have to carry the defective gene (which is unlikely), whereas a male has only a single X chromosome, so if one of its clotting factor genes is defective, he will be affected.

A woman who has one defective gene will not develop hemophilia herself, but is a carrier of the condition. All children of (female) carriers have a 50-percent chance of inheriting the defective gene. For sons, this means a 50-percent chance of developing the disease; for daughters, it means a 50-percent chance of being carriers, like their mothers. For the children of (male) hemophiliacs, the story is somewhat different. Sons are not affected (unless the mother is a carrier), but daughters always become carriers. For hemophilia to occur in a female, she would have to have both a father with the condition and a mother who either has hemophilia or is a carrier.

People with hemophilia are commonly treated with plasma concentrates prepared from pooled blood plasma. As a result, as many as two-thirds of all Americans with hemophilia became infected with HIV before the virus was identified and a screening test developed. Blood donors are now screened for HIV and clotting factor products are routinely subjected to heat to minimize, if not eliminate, the risk of transmission of the virus, but the chance of contracting HIV understandably remains a source of concern for people with hemophilia. Hepatitis viruses have also been a problem for people using blood products.

Unless otherwise specified, the dosages recommended here are for adults. For a child between the ages of twelve and seventeen, reduce the dose to three-quarters the recommended amount. For a child between six and twelve, use one-half the recommended dose, and for a child under the age of six, use one-quarter the recommended amount.

NUTRIENTS

SUPPLEMENT	SUGGESTED DOSAGE	COMMENTS
Helpful		
Calcium and	1,500 mg daily.	Essential for blood clotting.
magnesium	1,000 mg daily.	Needed to balance with calcium.
Liver extract injections or	1 cc once weekly or as prescribed by physician.	Contains vital nutrients for blood clotting.
raw liver extract	As directed on label.	
Multivitamin and mineral complex	As directed on label.	Provides necessary vitamins and minerals.
Vitamin B complex plus extra	As directed on label.	All B vitamins are essential in blood formation and clotting.
vitamin B$_3$ (niacin) and	As directed on label.	*Caution:* Do not take niacin if you have a liver disorder,
niacinamide	As directed on label.	gout, or high blood pressure.
Vitamin C with bioflavonoids	3,000 mg daily.	Important in normal blood coagulation.
Vitamin K or	300 mcg daily.	Essential in blood clotting mechanism.
alfalfa		*See under* Herbs, below.

HERBS

❑ Alfalfa is a good source of vitamin K, which is vital in the process of blood clotting. It can be taken in tablet form or eaten in a natural form, such as alfalfa sprouts.

RECOMMENDATIONS

❑ Eat a diet high in vitamin K. Foods that contain a measurable amount of this vitamin are alfalfa, broccoli, cauli-

flower, egg yolks, kale, liver, spinach, and all green leafy vegetables.

❑ "Green drinks" made from the vegetables listed above are very healthful. Drink one of these each day for vitamin K and other essential clotting factors.

❑ Be alert for early warning signs of internal bleeding, including a bubbling or tingling sensation or a feeling of warmth, tightness, or stiffness in the affected area. A blow to the head, headache, confusion, drowsiness, or other evidence of neurological impairment may signal intracranial bleeding.

❑ Wear an identity bracelet so that, in an emergency, people will know that you have hemophilia.

❑ *Do not* take aspirin. Aspirin is an anticlotting agent.

❑ If you care for an infant or toddler with hemophilia, be alert for signs of joint or muscle pain caused by internal bleeding. The child may cry for no apparent reason, refuse to use an arm or leg, refuse to walk, or have swelling or excessive bruising. If you suspect internal bleeding, seek treatment immediately.

CONSIDERATIONS

❑ Treatment of hemophilia consists of intravenous infusions of the missing clotting factor. This is now usually done at home. How much antihemophilic factor an individual needs and when depends on the severity of his disease.

❑ Gene therapy may hold the key to curing hemophilia, although the factor VIII gene is extremely complex, and it may be some time before scientists are able to replace these defective genes in people with hemophilia.

❑ For names and addresses of organizations that may be of assistance in obtaining information and/or treatment options, *see* HEALTH AND MEDICAL ORGANIZATIONS in the Appendix.

Hemorrhoids

Hemorrhoids are swollen veins around the anus and in the rectum (the very lowest portion of the colon) that may protrude from the anus. The word *hemorrhoid* comes from *hemo* (Greek for "blood") and *rrhoos* ("discharging"). They are also known as piles, from the Latin word *pila*, meaning "ball." Hemorrhoids are very much like varicose veins; they enlarge and lose their elasticity, resulting in saclike protrusions into the anal canal. They are not tumors or growths. They can be caused, and aggravated, by sitting or standing for prolonged periods, violent coughing, lifting heavy objects (or lifting even relatively light objects improperly), and straining at bowel movements (especially when constipated, although bouts of diarrhea accompanied by involuntary spasms can exacerbate the problem). Other factors that can cause or contribute to the formation of hemorrhoids include obesity, lack of exercise, liver damage, food allergies, and insufficient consumption of dietary fiber. Hemorrhoids are common during pregnancy and after childbirth. Hormonal changes and pressure exerted by the growing fetus may be the reason. Approximately half of all Americans have had hemorrhoids by the age of fifty. The incidence increases with age until age seventy, then begins to decrease again.

The most common symptoms of hemorrhoids include itching, burning, pain, inflammation, swelling, irritation, seepage, and bleeding. The bleeding, which is usually bright red during bowel movements, can be startling, even frightening. Although it does signal that something is amiss in the digestive system, rectal bleeding is not necessarily an indication of serious disease.

There are different types of hemorrhoids, depending on their location, severity, and the amount of pain, discomfort, or aggravation they cause. These are:

• *External.* These develop under the skin at the opening of the anal cavity. They may form a hard lump and cause painful swelling if a blood clot forms. When an external hemorrhoid swells, the tissue in the area becomes firm but sensitive and turns blue or purple in color. This type of hemorrhoid most often affects younger people and can be extremely painful.

• *Internal.* Internal hemorrhoids are located inside the rectum. They are usually painless, especially if located above the anorectal line, because rectal tissues lack nerve fibers. Internal hemorrhoids do, however, tend to bleed. When they do, the blood appears bright red.

• *Prolapsed.* A prolapsed hemorrhoid is an internal hemorrhoid that collapses and protrudes outside the anus, often accompanied by a mucous discharge and heavy bleeding. Prolapsed hemorrhoids can become *thrombosed*— that is, they can form clots within that prevent their receding. Thrombosed hemorrhoids can also be excruciatingly painful.

As far as we know, hemorrhoids are unique to human beings. No other creature develops this problem. This can be taken as an indication that our dietary and nutritional habits probably play a greater role in this disorder than anything else. Between 50 and 75 percent of this country's population develop hemorrhoids at one time or another, although many may be unaware of them. Hemorrhoids can occur at any age, but they tend to become more common as people age. Among younger people, pregnant women and women who have had children seem to be the most susceptible. The tendency to develop hemorrhoids also appears to be hereditary. Although hemorrhoids can be quite painful, they do not usually pose a serious threat to health.

NUTRIENTS

SUPPLEMENT	SUGGESTED DOSAGE	COMMENTS
Very Important		
Aerobic Bulk Cleanse from Aerobic Life Industries	As directed on label. Mix with ½ fruit juice and ½ aloe vera juice, and drink it down quickly before the fiber thickens. Take separately from other supplements and medications.	Keeps the colon clean, relieving pressure on the rectum.
Calcium	1,500 mg daily.	Essential for blood clotting. Helps prevent cancer of the colon. Use calcium chelate or asporotate form.
and magnesium	750 mg daily.	Needed to balance with calcium.
Vitamin C plus	3,000–5,000 mg daily.	Aids in healing and normal blood clotting.
mixed bioflavonoids with hesperidin and rutin	100 mg 3 times daily.	
Vitamin E	600 IU daily.	Promotes normal blood clotting and healing. Use d-alpha-tocopherol form.
Important		
Vitamin B complex	50–100 mg of each major B vitamin 3 times daily, with meals (amounts of individual vitamins in a complex will vary).	All B vitamins are vital for digestion. Improved digestion results in reduced stress on the rectum. Use lozenge or sublingual forms.
plus extra vitamin B6 (pyridoxine)	50 mg 3 times daily, with meals.	
and vitamin B12 plus	1,000 mcg twice daily.	
choline and inositol	50 mg each twice daily.	
Helpful		
Coenzyme Q10	100 mg daily.	Increases cellular oxygenation and assists in healing.
Dimethylglycine (DMG) (Aangamik DMG from FoodScience of Vermont)	125 mg twice daily.	Improves cellular oxygenation.
Garlic (Kyolic from Wakunaga)	As directed on label.	A natural antibiotic and immune system stimulant. Use the liquid form.
Key-E Suppositories from Carlson Labs	As directed on label.	Shrinks inflamed hemorrhoidal tissue.
Potassium	99 mg daily.	Constipation, which can cause hemorrhoids, is common in those with potassium deficiencies.
Shark cartilage (BeneFin)	1 gram per 15 lbs of body weight daily, divided into 3 doses. Can be taken either orally or rectally, in a retention enema.	Treats pain and inflammation.
Vitamin A with mixed carotenoids	15,000 IU daily. If you are pregnant, do not exceed 10,000 IU daily.	Aids in healing of mucous membranes and tissues.

Vitamin D$_3$	600 IU daily.	Aids in healing of mucous membranes and tissues. Also needed for calcium absorption.

HERBS

❑ Aloe vera gel, applied directly on the anus, has properties similar to aspirin. It can relieve pain and soothe the burning sensation. The fresh pulp is best.

❑ Bayberry, goldenseal root, myrrh, and white oak, used in a salve form, work like conventional hemorrhoid preparations—possibly better.

❑ A paste made from powdered comfrey root can be used in a poultice to heal bleeding hemorrhoids.

Note: Comfrey is recommended for external use only.

❑ An elderberry poultice can relieve the pain associated with hemorrhoids. A mullein poultice can be used as well. (*See* USING A POULTICE in Part Three.)

❑ Brew a strong, warm tea using the herb lady's mantle (yarrow), and apply with a cotton ball several times a day.

❑ Witch hazel is helpful because of its astringent properties. Apply it three times daily with a sterile cotton pad to shrink the swollen vein.

❑ Other beneficial herbs include buckthorn bark, collinsonia root, parsley, red grape vine leaves, and stone root. These can be taken in capsule or tea form.

RECOMMENDATIONS

❑ Eat foods that are high in dietary fiber, such as wheat bran, fresh fruits, and nearly all vegetables. Apples, beets, Brazil nuts, broccoli, foods in the cabbage family, carrots, green beans, guar gum, oat bran, lima beans, pears, peas, psyllium seed, and whole grains are recommended. A high-fiber diet is probably the most important consideration in the treatment and prevention of hemorrhoids.

❑ To help bleeding hemorrhoids, eat foods such as alfalfa, blackstrap molasses, and dark green leafy vegetables, which are high in vitamin K.

❑ Drink plenty of liquids, especially water (preferably steam-distilled). Water is the best, most natural stool softener in existence. It also helps prevent constipation.

❑ Avoid fats, animal products, coffee, alcohol, and hot spices. Red meat and high-protein diets are especially hard on the lower digestive tract.

❑ Take 1 or 2 tablespoons of flaxseed oil daily. Flaxseed oil helps to soften stools.

❑ If you decide to use a fiber supplement, start with a moderate amount and increase your intake gradually. If you take too much at first, this will cause painful bloating, gas, and possibly diarrhea.

Note: Always take supplemental fiber separately from other supplements and medications.

❑ Use cayenne (capsicum) and garlic enemas to keep the bowels clean. A plain warm water enema is fast acting and relieves discomfort in most cases. (*See* ENEMAS in Part Three.)

❑ Use a peeled clove of garlic as a suppository three times a week. You can also use raw potato suppositories to help heal hemorrhoids and relieve pain. Peel a potato and cut it into small cone-shaped pieces.

❑ If you are bothered by persistent bleeding, take vitamin and mineral supplements to prevent anemia. An iron supplement together with a powerful vitamin B complex and vitamin C will keep the blood healthy. A sublingual B complex, such as Perfect B from Pharmaceutical Purveyors of Oklahoma or Coenzymate B Complex from Source Naturals, is among the most efficiently absorbed forms of the B vitamins.

❑ Learn not to strain when moving the bowels. Keep the bowels clean and avoid constipation. Don't sit on the commode for longer than ten minutes at a time, as this causes blood to pool in the hemorrhoidal veins.

❑ Cleanse the problem area frequently with warm water. A hot bath for fifteen minutes a day is quite helpful. Do not add bath beads, oils, or bubbles to the water, as this can irritate sensitive tissues. Many people add Epsom salts, but this has no proven clinical value. It is the warm water that reduces swelling and eases the pain. Avoid using soap products to cleanse the anus.

❑ Warm sitz baths are especially beneficial. Take a mineral sitz bath daily. (*See* SITZ BATH in Part Three.) We recommend Batherapy from Para Laboratories/Queen Helene, a powder that contains many valuable minerals and is added to bath water. This can be found in many health food stores.

❑ Sit on a soft cushion, not on hard surfaces. Use an ordinary cushion, not a donut-shaped one. The old-fashioned inflated doughnut cushion actually increases pressure upon the hemorrhoidal blood vessels, aggravating the swelling and bleeding.

❑ Learn proper lifting techniques. Bend your knees, not your back. Do not hold your breath as you lift; this puts enormous strain and pressure upon the hemorrhoidal vessels. Instead, take a deep breath and exhale at the moment of lifting. Make your thighs do the work, not your back. Avoid heavy lifting as much as possible.

❑ Get regular moderate exercise.

❑ Avoid strong or harsh laxatives. Most of these products induce unnecessary straining at bowel movements and often "overdo" their jobs by creating a condition similar to diarrhea. Also, using chemical laxatives does not provide the healthful benefits that natural substances provide. Laxative products can also cause the bowels to become dependent upon them for normal functioning, much like an addiction. Instead of chemical preparations, use a stool softener such as aloe vera or prune juice if constipation or straining at defecation are a problem.

❑ Avoid using rough toilet paper. Use moistened toilet paper or baby wipes instead.

❑ Avoid sitting or standing for prolonged periods of time. If sitting for extended periods of time cannot be avoided, take frequent breaks to stretch and move around (this is also good for circulation, the back, and the legs).

❑ Do not use products containing ibuprofen or aspirin for hemorrhoid pain—they can encourage bleeding. Instead, choose pain medications such as acetaminophen (in Tylenol, Datril, Valadol, and other products).

❑ If home treatments bring no relief, consult your health care provider, especially if the problem is recurrent and bleeding persists for more than three days. Although the amount of blood loss might seem insignificant, even a slow loss of blood will eventually result in anemia and its associated problems. (See ANEMIA in Part Two.) In addition, persistent rectal bleeding can lead to infections and even a compromised immune system. If the blood is dark red, it can indicate a more serious problem such as an abscess, an anal fissure, a fistula, or cancer. Anal fissures are common in people with Crohn's disease.

CONSIDERATIONS

❑ Depending upon the location and severity of the problem, physicians today use the following treatment approaches in dealing with hemorrhoids:

• *Bipolar electrocoagulation.* Also called BiCap coagulation, this procedure uses spurts of electrical current to shrink hemorrhoids. It is comparable to infrared photocoagulation in that it has the equivalent advantages and disadvantages.

• *Conservative measures.* A dietary regimen with fiber supplements and self-help treatments is helpful in most cases, except in instances where a hemorrhoid has thrombosed.

• *Infrared photocoagulation.* This involves the employment of infrared heat to treat minor internal hemorrhoids. It is less painful than ligation but is not always as effective.

• *Injection sclerotherapy.* In this procedure, used to shrink internal hemorrhoids and stop bleeding, a solution containing either quinine and urea or phenol is injected directly into the hemorrhoids.

• *Laser treatment.* This approach has gained popularity over the last several years as the easiest and least painful method of dealing with internal hemorrhoids. There is controversy about its efficacy, however. Repeated treatments are frequently required. Most researchers believe that more study should be done to improve effectiveness before laser treatment is routinely recommended.

• *Ligation.* This is now the most common treatment approach for internal hemorrhoids. A small rubber band is used to tie off the base of the blood vessel. Once blood circulation is eliminated from the offending vessel, it soon detaches and the rubber band is eliminated with body waste. This approach often requires repeat treatments and is painful.

• *Surgery.* Some hemorrhoids are not helped very much by any of the above approaches and respond to nothing short of aggressive surgery. If you have very painful hemorrhoids or are losing significant amounts of blood, you should receive a thorough examination from a physician, preferably a proctologist, as soon as possible. Improved surgical techniques have resulted in less painful operations and quicker recovery periods than in the past. Surgery is completely effective in about 95 percent of cases. However, additional surgery may be required if the hemorrhoids recur.

❑ Anurex is a chemical-free product that helps give prompt, soothing, and lasting relief from the burning, itching, and bleeding caused by hemorrhoids. It is a small plastic device that contains a permanently sealed cold-retaining gel. It works best if kept in the freezer. When placed at the site of pain, it imparts a controlled degree of cooling to the inflamed tissue. Each Anurex device is reusable for up to six months. This product can be found in many pharmacies and health food stores, or can be ordered directly from Anurex Labs (see MANUFACTURER AND DISTRIBUTOR INFORMATION in the Appendix).

❑ Nitroglycerin, a blood-vessel dilator used for heart pain (angina pectoris) seems to relieve pain following hemorrhoidectomy (surgical removal of hermorrhoids). Some doctors prescribe it for hemorrhoid sufferers. However, its approval for this use is still under study. Another experimental treatment for hemorrhoids involves the use of local injections of botulinum toxin (Botox), but this has drawbacks such as the loss of control of the anal sphincter.

❑ Key-E suppositories from Carlson Labs are good for relief of itching and pain.

❑ Eating certain foods, especially beets, can cause the stool to become reddish and can be mistaken for blood.

❑ The most common cause of anal itching is tissue trauma resulting from the use of harsh toilet paper. *Candida albicans,* allergies, and parasitic infections can also cause anal itching.

❑ See also under PREGNANCY-RELATED PROBLEMS in Part Two.

Hepatitis

Hepatitis is an inflammation of the liver, usually caused by a viral infection. The liver is responsible for filtering out from the bloodstream harmful substances such as dead cells, toxins, fats, an overabundance of hormones, and a yellowish substance called bilirubin that is a byproduct of the breakdown of old red blood cells. If the liver is inflamed, tender, and enlarged, it becomes unable to function normally. As a result, toxins that would normally be filtered out by the liver build up in the body, and certain nutrients are not processed and stored as they should be. The symptoms of hepatitis include fever, weakness, nausea, vomiting, headache, appetite loss, muscle aches, joint pains, drowsiness, dark urine, light-colored stools, abdominal discomfort, and often, jaundice (yellowing of the skin due to an accumulation of bilirubin) and elevated liver enzymes in the blood. Flulike symptoms may be mild or severe.

There are different types of hepatitis, classified according to the virus that causes the condition. Scientists have identified the viruses responsible for three leading types of the disease, called hepatitis A, hepatitis B, and hepatitis C. There are also other, less common types known as hepatitis D, hepatitis E, and hepatitis G. All are contagious to some extent.

Hepatitis A, also known as infectious hepatitis, is easily spread through person-to-person contact, fecal contamination of food or water, and raw shellfish taken from polluted water. It is contagious between two to three weeks before, and one week after, jaundice appears.

Hepatitis B, also referred to as serum hepatitis, is spread through contact with infected blood (for example, from mother to child at birth or through the use of contaminated syringes, needles, and transfused blood) from adults to children living together in close contact, through sexual activity, and through blood transfusions. Most people—75 percent—recover from hepatitis B, although 25 percent go on to develop cirrhosis or cancer of the liver.

Hepatitis C, the most serious form of hepatitis, accounts for 8,000 to 10,000 deaths a year in America. It is estimated that 4 million Americans are infected with the hepatitis C virus (HCV) and this disease is the primary reason for liver transplants in this country. Hepatitis C is four times more prevalent than AIDS and twenty times easier to catch. About 85 percent of infections lead to chronic liver disease. The virus causes slowly progressing but ultimately devastating damage to the liver. In addition, people with HCV often have elevated levels of iron in the liver. This also can cause liver damage. Tests can detect HCV antibodies in donated blood, but an infected individual may take up to six months to develop the antibodies, so it is still impossible to identify all infected blood. The U.S. Food and Drug Administration (FDA) maintains that only 7 percent of current hepatitis C cases were acquired as a result of blood transfusions, and that the risk of contacting the virus from a unit of blood is about 1 in 100,000. The incidence of hepatitis C infection from blood transfusions or the use of blood products has decreased since 1992, when screening was introduced, but there is always a risk—and the lack of testing before 1992 has left a huge legacy of HVC-infected people. The most common means of HCV transmission after blood transfusions before 1992 are sharing needles, intravenous drug use, and sexual contact. HCV can also be transmitted from mother to child during childbirth.

Hepatitis D, or delta hepatitis, occurs in some people already infected with hepatitis B. It is the least common of all the hepatitis viruses, but the most serious because there are two types of hepatitis working together. It can be transmitted through sexual contact or from mother to child at birth.

Hepatitis E is rare in the United States, but more common in other parts of the world, notably Mexico, India, and Asian and African countries. It is usually spread through fecal contamination and appears to be dangerous for pregnant women, but generally does not lead to chronic hepatitis in others.

It is also possible to develop hepatitis as a result of exposure to certain toxins or alcohol or drug use, including the overuse of over-the-counter medications such as acetaminophen or ibuprofen. This is called *toxic hepatitis*. Environmental toxins absorbed through the skin can also damage the liver. Chlorinated hydrocarbons and arsenic are examples of severe hepatotoxic agents. In toxic hepatitis, the amount of exposure to the toxin determines the extent of liver damage.

NUTRIENTS

SUPPLEMENT	SUGGESTED DOSAGE	COMMENTS
Essential		
Alpha-lipoic acid (ALA)	As directed on label.	Has antioxidant properties that protect the liver.
Beta-1,3-D-glucan	As directed on label.	An excellent antioxidant. Stimulates the activity of macrophages, which surround and digest cellular debris.
Free-form amino acid complex (Amino Balance from Anabol Naturals)	As directed on label.	To supply necessary protein. The liver breaks down protein; taking free-form amino acids takes strain off the liver.
Glutathione plus	500 mg twice daily, on an empty stomach.	Protects the liver.
L-arginine and	As directed on label.	Detoxifies the liver.
L-cysteine and L-methionine	500 mg each twice daily, on an empty stomach. Take with water or juice. Do not take with milk. Take with 50 mg vitamin B_6 and 100 mg vitamin C for better absorption.	Detoxifies harmful hepatotoxins and protects glutathione. (*See* AMINO ACIDS in Part One.)
Inositol hexaphosphate (IP_6)	As directed on label.	A powerful antioxidant that has many positive effects on the body, including protecting the liver. Also known as phytic acid.
Liquid Kyolic with B_1 and B_{12} from Wakunaga	As directed on label.	Powerful liver protectors and potent antioxidants.
Raw liver extract or desiccated liver	As directed on label. As directed on label.	Promotes liver function. (*See* GLANDULAR THERAPY in Part Three.) Consider injections (under a doctor's supervision).
S-Adenosylmethionine (SAMe) or trimethylglycine (TMG)	As directed on label. As directed on label.	Promotes the health of the liver. Needed for conversion of harmful homocysteine into methionine, the basis for production of SAMe.

Selenium Forte from American Biologics	As directed on label.	Studies have shown selenium to protect against liver cancer.
Very Important		
Coenzyme Q$_{10}$ plus Coenzyme A from Coenzyme-A Technologies	60 mg daily.	Counteracts immunosuppression and enhances tissue oxygenation.
Dimethylglycine (DMG) (Aangamik DMG from FoodScience of Vermont)	As directed on label.	Improves cellular oxygen concentration.
Lecithin granules or capsules	1 tbsp 3 times daily, before meals. 1,200 mg 3 times daily, before meals.	Protects cells of the liver and is a fat mobilizer. Aids in preventing fatty liver.
Multivitamin complex with vitamin B complex plus extra vitamin B$_{12}$ plus chloline and inositol	50–100 mg of each major B vitamin 3 times daily, with meals (amounts of individual vitamins in a complex will vary). Do not exceed a total of 100 mg vitamin B$_3$ (niacin) in any one day until healing is complete. 1,000 mcg twice daily. As directed on label.	All nutrients are necessary in balance. All B vitamins are absolutely essential for normal liver function. Sublingual forms are recommended. Injections (under a doctor's supervision) may be necessary, especially of vitamin B$_{12}$ and folic acid.
Superoxide dismutase (SOD) or Cell Guard from Biotec Foods or Oxy-5000 Forte from American Biologics	As directed on label. As directed on label. As directed on label.	Powerful antioxidants that neutralize damaging superoxide free radicals, improving liver function.
Vitamin C with bioflavonoids	5,000–10,000 mg daily and up.	A powerful antiviral agent. Studies show improvement quickly with high doses.
Vitamin E	Start with 400 IU daily and increase to 1,200 IU daily over the course of 1 month.	A potent antioxidant. Use d-alpha-tocopherol form.
Important		
Calcium and magnesium	1,500 mg daily. 1,000 mg daily.	Essential for blood clotting, which is a problem for people with liver disease. Use chelated forms. Do not use bone meal.
Essential fatty acids (primrose oil and salmon oil are good sources) or shark liver oil or squalene or Kyolic-EPA from Wakunaga	As directed on label. As directed on label. As directed on label. As directed on label.	Important sources of essential lipids. To combat inflammation of the liver and lowers serum fats.
Multienzyme complex with betaine hydrochloride (HCl)	As directed on label.	Important for proper digestion.

Helpful		
Maitake extract or reishi extract or shiitake extract	As directed on label. As directed on label. As directed on label.	To boost the immune system and fight viral infection.
Raw pancreas glandular	As directed on label.	Aids in digestion and pancreatic function.
7-Keto DHEA	50–75 mg daily.	Increases antibody and interleukin-2 formation.
Vitamin A (Micellized Vitamin A emulsion from American Biologics)	25,000 IU daily. If you are pregnant, do not exceed 10,000 IU daily.	Needed for healing. Use an emulsion form for easier assimilation and greater safety. Avoid using beta-carotene or capsule forms of vitamin A until healing is complete.

HERBS

❑ Artichoke increases the effectiveness of liver function.

❑ Ayurvedic medicine has used beets to promote the regeneration of liver cells.

❑ Burdock and dandelion are important for cleansing the liver and the bloodstream.

❑ Studies have shown licorice to be effective in treating viral hepatitis, particularly chronic active hepatitis, due to its well-documented antiviral activity.

Caution: Do not use this herb on a daily basis for more than seven days in a row. Avoid if you have high blood pressure.

❑ Ligustrum is an immune restorative and anti-inflammatory agent.

❑ Milk thistle extract contains silymarin, a flavonoid that has been shown to aid in healing and rebuilding the liver. It can be taken in capsule or alcohol-free extract form. Take 200 to 400 milligrams three times daily.

❑ Olive leaf extract is a potent antifungal agent.

❑ Phyllanthus, an Ayurvedic herb, is useful for hepatitis B. After an initial bout with the virus, you can become symptom-free but still remain a carrier of the disease. This herb is said to eradicate carrier-status hepatitis B in some cases.

❑ Schizandra is a Chinese herb used to protect the liver.

❑ Scutellaria, also known as Baikal skullcap or Chinese skullcap, is a Chinese herb that is a powerful antioxidant.

❑ Turmeric is a potent anti-inflammatory.

❑ Other herbs beneficial for hepatitis include black radish, green tea, red clover, and yellow dock.

RECOMMENDATIONS

❑ Eat a raw vegetable and fruit diet for two to four weeks. Start this diet with a cleansing fast. (*See* FASTING in Part Three.)

❏ Include artichokes in the diet. Artichokes protect the liver. Globe artichoke extract also is available.

❏ Drink "green drinks," carrot juice, and beet juice. (*See* JUICING in Part Three.)

❏ Drink only steam-distilled water.

❏ Consume no alcohol in any form. Propylene glycol is a compound related to alcohol that is commonly used in medicines that are supposed to be alcohol-free. It too should be avoided.

❏ Avoid all fats, sugar, and highly processed foods.

❏ Avoid all raw fish and shellfish, and eat no animal protein. Also avoid chemicals and food additives.

❏ Get plenty of bed rest.

❏ Use chlorophyll-containing enemas such as fresh wheatgrass juice or Kyo-Green from Wakunaga, three times a week. Use one pint and retain it for fifteen minutes. (*See* ENEMAS in Part Three.)

❏ Keep a person with hepatitis A in isolation to avoid spreading the infection. Wash hands and all clothing often. The clothing and bed linens of a person with hepatitis A require special handling. Wash them separately from other laundry in hot water with chlorine bleach or a disinfectant added. Because the feces are infectious, bathrooms should be decontaminated frequently. Clean toilets and floors with a disinfectant.

❏ Especially when traveling, beware of contaminated water or foods from polluted waters.

❏ Do not take any drugs that have not been prescribed by your doctor. Read package inserts carefully for information regarding liver toxicity.

CONSIDERATIONS

❏ Taking excessive amounts of vitamin A over long periods may cause liver enzyme levels to become elevated. Anyone who has been taking over 50,000 international units of vitamin A daily for over a year should reduce his or her intake or switch to an emulsion form, which is less harmful to the liver.

❏ If you have hepatitis C, it is best to reduce the iron levels in the body before starting any treatment. High iron levels inhibit therapy for the liver.

❏ Catechin, a flavonoid found in green and black Indian teas, has been shown to decrease serum bilirubin levels in people with all types of acute viral hepatitis.

❏ Liver extract supplements contain nutritional substances that aid liver regeneration. Only products derived from organically raised beef should be used.

❏ In laboratory experiments, injections of whole liver cells have rapidly repaired liver tissue in experimental animals with lethal, acute liver failure.

❏ Silymarin, the active ingredient in milk thistle, has been known to lower liver enzymes and reverse the kind of liver damage common in people with hepatitis C. Some studies have found that milk thistle can cure liver cancer in rats.

❏ Ribavirin (Virazole) and interferon may be prescribed for hepatitis C and are proving to be effective in the treatment of this disease.

❏ Hepatitis is diagnosed by means of a blood test. In some cases, it may be necessary to double-check a test for the hepatitis C virus by means of a test called the RIBA HCV 3.0 Strip Immunoblot Assay (SIA).

❏ A home test called the Home Access Hepatitis C Check is available. It can be purchased in drugstores or ordered directly from the manufacturer, Ab Diagnostics (*see* MANUFACTURER AND DISTRIBUTOR INFORMATION in the Appendix).

❏ Ultraviolet blood irradiation therapy (UBIT) is said to improve the oxygenation of tissue, help with inflammation, stimulate the immune system, and fight viral infection. This treatment, which has been approved by the FDA, consists of bombarding the blood with ultraviolet light. It appears to render the virus inactive. This treatment is offered by Bradford Research Institute in Chula Vista, California (*see* HEALTH AND MEDICAL ORGANIZATIONS in the Appendix).

❏ If you require surgery and may need a blood transfusion, discuss this with your doctor or surgeon. You may be able to bank your own blood or the blood of a relative or friend before the procedure.

❏ There is a vaccine available to protect against hepatitis A. It is recommended for members of high-risk groups such as those suffering from liver disease, those in contact with hepatitis A–infected people, those who engage in anal sex with multiple partners, and those travelling to areas where hepatitis A is common, including Africa, the Middle East, the Caribbean, and South and Central America. The U.S. Centers for Disease Control (CDC) now recommends that children living in high-risk states in this country be vaccinated against this disease as well. The high-risk states include Arizona, Alaska, California, Idaho, New Mexico, Oregon, South Dakota, and Washington. Some other states have *areas* where hepatitis A is common. Ask your health care provider about possible side effects from the vaccine.

❏ There is a vaccine available that gives protection against hepatitis B for approximately five years. Ask your health care provider about both the benefits and side effects.

❏ Because the hepatitis C virus has many genotypes, or forms, and can mutate rapidly, no vaccine has yet been developed to successfully protect against this virus. Likewise, there are no vaccines against hepatitis D or E.

Herpes Zoster

See SHINGLES. *See also under* EYE PROBLEMS.

Herpesvirus Infection

There are at least seven types of herpesviruses. Herpes simplex type 1 (HSV-1) and type 2 (HSV-2) cause cold sores and genital herpes. Many experts suspect HSV-1 may be involved in Bell's palsy and some other neurological disorders. Herpes zoster is responsible for chickenpox and shingles. Cytomegalovirus, another member of the herpes family, can cause some cardiovascular diseases and eye disorders, and is particularly dangerous to developing fetuses, newborns, and people with depressed immune systems. The Epstein-Barr virus (EBV) is the virus that causes infectious mononucleosis. Human herpesvirus type 6 (HHV-6) and 7 (HHV-7) are suspected of being capable of triggering autoimmune disorders, including multiple sclerosis, and roseola, a common illness of early childhood. Human herpesvirus type 8 (HHV-8) is very closely related to the Epstein-Barr virus, and may lead to cancer of the bone, chronic fatigue syndrome, Kaposi's sarcoma, and infection of the lymphatic system. This section primarily addresses genital herpes.

Genital herpes is the most prevalent sexually transmitted disease in the United States. More than 45 million Americans—one out of every five persons over the age of twelve—have it, though more than half never develop serious symptoms. This viral infection can range in severity from a silent infection to a serious inflammation of the liver with fever. It is especially dangerous to infants. A baby whose mother is infected can pick up the virus in the birth canal, creating a risk of brain damage, blindness, and death.

For those whose symptoms do not remain dormant, genital herpes causes outbreaks of red, sensitive skin; itching; burning; and painful, fluid-filled blisters that are highly infectious until they are completely healed, which can take up to three weeks. It is, however, fairly common to have virtually no symptoms of the infection.

A mild tingling and burning in the vaginal area may be the first sign of genital herpes in women. Within a matter of a few hours, blisters develop around the rectum, clitoris, and cervix, and in the vagina. There is often a watery discharge from the urethra and pain when urinating. In men, blisters break out on the penis, groin, and scrotum, often with a urethral discharge and painful urination. Sometimes the penis and foreskin swell. A man may also have tender, swollen lymph nodes in the groin.

The first attack of genital herpes usually comes within twenty days after exposure to the virus. It may be so mild that it isn't noticed, or it may cause itching and burning at the site of viral entry as well as painful sores that can last a week or more, plus fever, headache, and other flulike symptoms. After a few days, pus erupts from the blisters and painful ulcers form. These sores crust over and dry while healing. Usually, they leave no scars.

It has traditionally been believed that HSV-1 causes cold sores and skin eruptions and HSV-2 is responsible for genital herpes. The difference between HSV-1 and HSV-2 is often debated, however. The current theory is that the two viruses are more alike than once was thought—the two viruses share about 50 percent of their DNA—but that they do have different characteristics. For example, when HSV-1 is in a dormant state, the virus usually establishes its home in the nerve cells near the ear, so it is more inclined to cause an outbreak around the mouth. HSV-2, on the other hand, prefers to live near the base of the spine, so when an outbreak occurs, it is more likely to occur in the genital area. The two viral agents can, however, live in either place, and it has been suggested that social pressures are the real reason we like to think of the two as being very different. Many people have a tendency to associate genital herpes with a promiscuous lifestyle (which in fact is not justified) but the same stigma is not attached to cold sores.

If HSV-1 exchanges its usual site with HSV-2, or vice versa, outbreaks are normally less severe. If you have a sexual partner who has a genital HSV-1 infection and you have genital HSV-2, you can contract HSV-1, but it is extremely rare that HSV-1 is transmitted to a person who already has HSV-2. Oral sex with a person who has genital HSV-2 is unlikely to result in an HSV-2 infection affecting the mouth. HSV-2 is almost wholly transmitted through genital sex.

Experts now believe that HSV-2 can be transmitted even when an infected individual is experiencing no symptoms. In the first year after infection, people shed the virus between 6 and 10 percent of the time when there are no visible signs of the infection, a phenomenon called *asymptomatic viral shedding.*

Although it is a serious illness, herpes is not normally life threatening. Having the virus means that you have to adjust your lifestyle to protect yourself and others, but there are few cases of herpes infecting other organs of the body. Because the incidence of genital herpes is increasing so profoundly—some 20 percent of the U.S. population is now said to be infected—it is extremely important to be aware of the disease and to protect yourself against it. If you already have the infection, it is equally important to protect yourself as much as you can from repeated outbreaks and to avoid passing the infection on to others.

NUTRIENTS

SUPPLEMENT	SUGGESTED DOSAGE	COMMENTS
Very Important		
Beta 1,3-D-glucan	As directed on label.	Useful for treating any bacterial, viral, or fungal disease. Stimulates the activity of macrophages, immune cells that surround and digest invading microorganisms and cellular debris.
Coenzyme A from Coenzyme-A Technologies	As directed on label.	Supports the immune system's detoxification of many dangerous substances.

Herp-Eeze from Olympian Labs	As directed on label.	Possesses antiviral, anti-inflammatory, and antioxidant properties for the treatment of herpes.
L-Lysine	1,500 mg daily, on an empty stomach. Take with water or juice. Do not take with milk. Take with 50 mg vitamin B₆ and 100 mg vitamin C for better absorption.	When the amount of lysine present exceeds the amount of arginine, the growth of the herpes virus is inhibited. (*See* AMINO ACIDS in Part One.) *Caution:* Do not take this supplement for longer than 6 months at a time without a break. Resume the therapy again if you have further outbreaks.
Dioxychlor Oxy C-2 Gel from American Biologics	Apply to affected areas as directed on label.	A useful antiviral, antifungal, and bactericide.
VIR-L-Lysine from Global Health Services	As directed on label.	Contains L-lysine, bee pollen, and pituitary and adrenal tissue, and has been found to help keep herpes in remission.
Vitamin A with mixed carotenoids	25,000 IU daily. If you are pregnant, do not exceed 10,000 IU daily.	Important for healing. Prevents spreading of infection. Use emulsion form for easier assimilation and greater safety at higher doses.
Vitamin B complex	50 mg of each major B vitamin and up, 3 times daily (amounts of individual vitamins in a complex will vary).	Combats the virus and helps to keep it from spreading. Also works with lysine to prevent outbreaks. Use hypoallergenic form.
Vitamin C plus bioflavonoids	5,000–10,000 mg daily. 30–60 mg daily, in divided doses.	Needed to prevent sores and inhibit the growth of the virus. Use an esterified or buffered form. Works with vitamin C.
Zinc	50–100 mg daily, in divided doses. Do not exceed 100 mg daily.	Boosts immune function. For genital herpes, use a chelate form. For oral herpes, use zinc gluconate lozenges.

Important

Acidophilus (Kyo-Dophilus from Wakunaga is a good source)	As directed on label, 3 times daily, on an empty stomach.	Needed for the production of the B vitamins. Prevents overgrowth of harmful micro-organisms in the intestines. Use a nondairy formula.
Dioxychlor from American Biologics	As directed on label.	An important antiviral, anti-bacterial, and antifungal agent.
Egg lecithin	As directed on label.	Helps control the virus.
Essential fatty acids (primrose oil, salmon oil, and Kyolic-EPA from Wakunaga are good sources)	As directed on label.	Needed for cell protection.
Garlic (Kyolic from Wakunaga)	3 tablets 3 times daily, with meals.	An immune system stimulant and a natural antibiotic.
Superoxide dismutase (SOD) or Cell Guard from Biotec Foods	As directed on label. As directed on label.	Reduces infection and speeds healing. A powerful free radical destroyer. An antioxidant complex that contains SOD.
Vitamin E	600 IU daily.	Important in healing. Prevents spread of the infection. Use emulsion form for easier assimilation. Use d-alpha-tocopherol form.

Helpful

Calcium and magnesium	1,500 mg daily. 750 mg daily.	To relieve stress and anxiety. Use chelated forms.
Dimethylglycine (DMG) (Aangamik DMG from FoodScience of Vermont)	2 tablets dissolved in the mouth twice daily.	Enhances utilization of oxygen by tissue.
Maitake extract or shiitake extract or reishi extract	As directed on label. As directed on label. As directed on label.	Mushroom extracts that have immune-boosting and antiviral properties.
Multivitamin and mineral supplement	As directed on label.	Needed to enhance healing. Take a hypoallergenic form.
Proteolytic enzymes	As directed on label 2–3 times daily. Take between meals.	Helps protect against infection; works on undigested food remaining in the colon. *Caution:* Do not give this supplement to a child.
Raw thymus glandular	500 mg twice daily.	Enhances immune function. *Caution:* Do not give this supplement to a child.

HERBS

❑ Astragalus, or huang qi, enhances the immune system and acts as an antibiotic.

❑ Applying black walnut or goldenseal extract to the affected area may help.

❑ Cat's claw has immune-enhancing properties and acts against viral infection.

❑ Goldenseal is a natural antibiotic. It can be taken in capsule or tea form.

Caution: Do not take goldenseal internally on a daily basis for more than one week at a time, do not use it during pregnancy, and use with caution if you are allergic to ragweed.

❑ Larreastat is a trademarked herbal remedy derived from chaparral that is said to have antioxidant, antiviral, and anti-inflammatory properties.

❑ Licorice root inhibits both the growth and cell-damaging effects of herpes simplex. If you are using licorice, increase your potassium intake.

Caution: Do not use this herb on a daily basis for more than seven days in a row. Avoid it completely if you have high blood pressure.

❑ Olive leaf extract appears to help curb the growth of viral diseases such as herpes.

❑ Red marine algae contains antiviral carbohydrates that are effective, both topically and orally, for the treatment of herpes.

❑ Spirulina contains phytonutrients that appear to boost the immune system.

❑ Tea tree oil is a powerful natural antiseptic. During a

herpes outbreak, dab it lightly on the affected area several times a day, either full strength or, if that is too strong, diluted with distilled water or cold-pressed vegetable oil. Do not get tea tree oil close to the eye area.

❑ Other herbs useful for herpes treatment include cayenne (capsicum), echinacea, myrrh, red clover, and St. John's wort.

RECOMMENDATIONS

❑ Avoid alcohol, processed foods, colas, white flour products, sugar, refined carbohydrates, coffee, and drugs to lessen the chance of an outbreak. Herbal teas are beneficial (see Herbs, above), but all other teas should be avoided.

❑ Drink steam-distilled water.

❑ Eat the following in moderation during outbreaks: almonds, barley, cashews, cereals (grains), chicken, chocolate, corn, dairy products, meat, nuts and seeds, oats, and peanuts. These contain L-arginine, an amino acid that suppresses L-lysine, the amino acid that retards virus growth.

❑ Do not consume citrus fruits and juices while the virus is active.

❑ Get plenty of rest. Stress reduction is important.

❑ To ease swelling and pain in the genital area, use ice packs. Warm Epsom salts or baking soda baths help itching and pain. After the bath, pat dry gently and keep the lesions dry.

❑ Apply vitamin E and vitamin A, alternately, directly on the sores. Or try using L-lysine cream from a health food store.

❑ Wear cotton underwear. Practice good genital hygiene—keep clean and dry.

❑ If you have active lesions, refrain from sex until the sores have completely healed. Do not have intercourse with a person with visible genital lesions of any kind.

❑ If you are pregnant and know you have genital herpes, tell your health care provider. If an attack occurs late in the pregnancy, your baby may have to be delivered by cesarean section to protect against exposure during birth. If there are no lesions present, the risk to the baby is probably low.

CONSIDERATIONS

❑ Genital herpes infections in women increase the risk of cervical cancer. Women with herpes should be conscientious about having Pap smears done periodically, as recommended by a qualified health care provider.

❑ A virus identified by the National Cancer Institute as the human B cell lymphotropic virus (HBLV) is believed to be a member of the herpesvirus family and may also be a factor in fatigue.

❑ Research suggests that capsaicin may be able to prevent outbreaks of genital lesions.

❑ High levels of the amino acid arginine may cause outbreaks of herpes. Foods containing arginine include chocolate, peanuts, and soybeans.

❑ Dimethylsulfoxide (DMSO), a byproduct of wood processing, is a liquid that can be applied topically to relieve pain and promote the healing of herpes outbreaks.

Note: Only DMSO from a health food store should be used. Commercial-grade DMSO found in hardware stores is not suitable for healing purposes. The use of DMSO may result in a garlicky body odor. This is temporary and is not a cause for concern.

❑ The antiviral drug acyclovir (Zovirax) has been shown to relieve symptoms and reduce the severity and frequency of outbreaks. This drug is available by prescription only and comes in capsule and lotion forms. It can be used for both oral and genital herpes. The capsules are usually taken every four hours for ten days. Applying the lotion when an imminent outbreak is first sensed usually weakens the attack. In studies conducted by the National Institutes of Health, taking 400 milligrams of acyclovir twice daily for four months reduced cold sore episodes by 52 percent, and when outbreaks did occur, the blisters healed approximately twice as fast as normal. Caution should be practiced if the drug is taken on a regular basis, however. When the drug is stopped, a "rebound" effect may result in a more serious outbreak than usual. Two other antiviral agents, valacyclovir (Valtrex) and famciclovir (Famvir) also may be prescribed for herpes.

❑ A vaccine for genital herpes is currently undergoing testing. It is called disabled infectious single cycle (DISC) HSV.

❑ Isotretinoin, a derivative of vitamin A, has given dramatic results with herpes simplex infections.

❑ Some physicians have used butylated hydroxytoluene (BHT) to treat herpes. This can have dangerous consequences, however, especially if taken on an empty stomach. Irritation and even perforation of the stomach can result. We do not recommend this treatment for herpes.

❑ Choraphor is a trademarked topical antiseptic formula containing ammoniated acid sulfate and trace minerals that is said to promote an immune response to herpes and clear up outbreaks. It has not yet undergone clinical testing, however.

❑ See also COLD SORES; SEXUALLY TRANSMITTED DISEASE; and SHINGLES in Part Two.

Hiatal Hernia

See under HEARTBURN/GASTROESOPHAGEAL REFLUX DISEASE (GERD).

High Blood Pressure (Hypertension)

When the heart pumps blood through the arteries, the blood presses against the walls of the blood vessels. In people who suffer from hypertension, this pressure is abnormally high.

Whether blood pressure is high, low, or normal depends on several factors: the output from the heart, the resistance to blood flow of the blood vessels, the volume of blood, and blood distribution to the various organs. All of these factors in turn can be affected by the activities of the nervous system and certain hormones.

If blood pressure is elevated, the heart must work harder to pump an adequate amount of blood to all the tissues of the body. Ultimately, the condition often leads to kidney failure, heart failure, and stroke. In addition, high blood pressure is often associated with coronary heart disease, arteriosclerosis, kidney disorders, obesity, diabetes, hyperthyroidism, and adrenal tumors.

About 35 million Americans have high blood pressure. An estimated 15 million are not aware that they are hypertensive, and of the people who do know that they have a problem, only two out of every five receive adequate treatment for this potentially dangerous condition. According to the U.S. Public Health Service, hypertension affects more than half of all Americans over the age of sixty-five. The percentage of the African-American population with high blood pressure is approximately one-third higher than that for whites. African-Americans between the ages of twenty-four and forty-four are *eighteen times* more likely than whites to develop kidney failure due to hypertension. One-third of all African-American women, and a slightly higher percentage of African-American men, have hypertension, as compared with under one-fifth and roughly one-fourth of white men. While high blood pressure was once thought of as a "man's disease," in fact women are very nearly as likely to suffer from this condition as men are, and more women than men die from complications of high blood pressure because women and, to some extent, their medical practioners, often ignore or fail to detect their high blood pressure until it is too late.

Because high blood pressure usually causes no symptoms until complications develop, it is known as the "silent killer." Warning signs associated with advanced hypertension may include headaches, sweating, rapid pulse, shortness of breath, dizziness, and visual disturbances.

Blood pressure is usually divided into two categories, designated *primary* and *secondary*. Primary hypertension is high blood pressure that is not due to another underlying disease. The precise cause is unknown, but a number of definite risk factors have been identified. These include cigarette smoking, stress, obesity, excessive use of stimulants such as coffee or tea, drug abuse, and high sodium intake. The use of oral contraceptives used to be considered a contributing factor, but with the low-dose pills now available, this is not as much a problem as it once was. Because too much water retention can exert pressure on the blood vessels, those who consume foods high in sodium may be at a greater risk for high blood pressure. Elevated blood pressure is also common in people who are overweight. Blood pressure can rise due to stress as well, because stress causes the walls of the arteries to constrict. Also, those with a family history of hypertension are more likely to suffer from high blood pressure.

When persistently elevated blood pressure arises as a result of another underlying health problem, such as a hormonal abnormality or an inherited narrowing of the aorta, it is called secondary hypertension. A person may also have secondary hypertension because the blood vessels are chronically constricted or have lost elasticity from a buildup of fatty plaque on the inside walls of the vessel, a condition known as atherosclerosis. Arteriosclerosis and atherosclerosis are common precursors of hypertension. The narrowing and/or hardening of the arteries makes circulation of blood through the vessels difficult. As a result, blood pressure becomes elevated. Secondary hypertension can also be caused by poor kidney function, which results in the retention of excess sodium and fluid in the body. This increase in blood volume within the vessels causes elevated blood pressure levels. The kidneys may also elevate blood pressure by secreting substances that cause blood vessels to constrict.

To diagnose high blood pressure, a physician uses a device called a *sphygmomanometer*. Blood pressure is represented as a pair of numbers. The first is the *systolic* pressure, which is the pressure exerted by the blood when the heart beats, forcing blood into the blood vessels. This reading indicates blood pressure at its highest. The second reading is the *diastolic* pressure, which is recorded when the heart is at rest in between beats, when the blood pressure is at its lowest. Both figures represent the height (in millimeters, or mm) that a column of mercury (Hg) reaches under the pressure exerted by the blood. The combined blood pressure reading is then expressed as a ratio of systolic blood pressure to diastolic blood pressure.

It is impossible for a health care provider to make a correct diagnosis of high blood pressure with a single reading. The test must be repeated throughout the day to be accurate. Home testing is best because it enables you to monitor your condition periodically. Measuring blood pressure at home on a regular schedule may:

• Help determine whether your blood pressure is high only when taken during a medical visit.

• Enable you to collaborate with your health care provider in controlling your high blood pressure.

• Reduce the frequency with which you need to visit your health care provider for blood pressure evaluation.

Blood pressure monitoring devices fall into two basic categories: mechanical gauges and automated electronic gauges. The mechanical gauge is the type most often used in physicians' offices. It consists of an instrument to measure the pressure, an air bladder (inflatable cuff), and a pressure bulb with a release valve to pump up the cuff. The standard-size arm cuff on blood pressure monitors fits arms up to thirteen inches around (if your arm is larger than this, you will need to obtain a larger cuff). With most of these devices, the pressure is read on a gauge dial.

Mechanical gauges are much less expensive than electronic ones and many physicians feel they give more accurate readings, at least in the hands of an experienced user. However, if you use this type of device to take your own blood pressure, you must pump up the cuff with one hand, read a dial, and listen with a stethoscope more or less simultaneously (see How to Measure Your Blood Pressure on page 439). In other words, using these devices correctly requires dexterity, good eyesight, acute hearing, and some training and practice.

An alternative to the mechanical gauge is the digital sphygmomanometer. With this device, the machine automatically gauges your blood pressure when the cuff is inflated and presents the result in a digital format. These are more expensive than the mechanical types, but because they are much easier to use accurately, they are generally preferred for home use.

There are also other electronic devices available, including wrist and finger cuff monitors. Although they are easy to operate, most doctors do not recommend them because they tend to be less accurate and also more sensitive to the effects of temperature and poor blood circulation.

NUTRIENTS

SUPPLEMENT	SUGGESTED DOSAGE	COMMENTS
Essential		
Calcium and	1,500–3,000 mg daily.	Deficiencies have been linked to high blood pressure.
magnesium and	750–1,000 mg daily.	
potassium	As directed on label.	If you are taking cortisone or high blood pressure medication, take extra potassium to counteract depletion of this mineral.
Coenzyme Q10 plus	As directed on label.	Improves heart function.
Coenzyme A from Coenzyme-A Technologies	As directed on label.	Works effectively with coenzyme Q10 to support the immune system's detoxification of many dangerous substances.
Essential fatty acids (black currant seed oil, flaxseed oil, olive oil, primrose oil, and Kyolic-EPA from Wakunaga are good sources)	As directed on label.	Important for circulation and for lowering blood pressure.
Garlic (Kyolic from Wakunaga)	2 capsules 3 times daily.	Effective in lowering blood pressure.
L-Arginine	As directed on label.	Shown to play an increasingly important role in heart health by lowering blood pressure and cholesterol levels.
L-Carnitine plus	500 mg twice daily, on an empty stomach.	Transports long fatty acid chains. Together with L-glutamic acid and L-glutamine, aids in preventing heart disease. To detoxify ammonia and aid in preventing heart disease. (See AMINO ACIDS in Part One.)
L-glutamic acid and L-glutamine	500 mg each daily, on an empty stomach. Take with water or juice. Do not take with milk. Take with 50 mg vitamin B6 and 100 mg vitamin C for better absorption.	
Selenium	200 mcg daily.	Deficiency has been linked to heart disease.
Vitamin E	Start with 100 IU daily and add 100 IU daily each month, until you reach 400 IU daily.	Improves heart function. Vitamin E also acts as a blood thinning agent; use with caution if you are taking prescription blood-thinners. Use d-alpha-tocopherol form.
and/or octacosonol	As directed on label.	Use emulsion form for easier assimilation and greater safety at high doses.
Very Important		
Vitamin C with bioflavonoids	3,000–6,000 mg daily, in divided doses.	Improves adrenal function; reduces blood-clotting tendencies.
Important		
Lecithin granules or	1 tbsp 3 times daily, before meals.	To emulsify fat, improve liver function, and lower blood pressure.
capsules or	1,200 mg 3 times daily, before meals.	
lipotropic factors	As directed on label.	
Helpful		
Bromelain	As directed on label.	An enzyme that aids in the digestion of fats.
Chinese red yeast rice extract	As directed on label.	Has cholesterol-lowering properties.
Kelp	1,000–1,500 mg daily.	A good source of minerals and natural iodine.
Kyo-Green from Wakunaga	As directed on label twice daily.	This concentrated barley and wheatgrass juice contains important nutrients.
Maitake extract or	As directed on label.	To help reduce high blood pressure and prevent heart disease.
shiitake extract or	As directed on label.	
reishi extract	As directed on label.	
Multivitamin and mineral complex with		All nutrients are needed in balance.
vitamin A and	15,000 IU daily. If you are pregnant, do not exceed 10,000 IU daily.	
zinc	50 mg daily.	
Proteolytic enzymes	As directed on label. Take with meals and between meals.	Aids in cleansing the circulatory system. Completes protein digestion.

Raw heart glandular plus	As directed on label.	Strengthens the heart.
Bio-Cardiozyme Forte from Biotics Research or	As directed on label.	A complex that strengthens the heart muscle.
Heart Science from Source Naturals	As directed on label.	Contains antioxidants, cholesterol-fighters, herbs, and vitamins that work together to promote cardiovascular function.
Vitamin B complex	100 mg of each major B vitamin twice daily, with meals (amounts of individual vitamins in a complex will vary).	Important for circulatory function and for lowering blood pressure. Take niacin only under the supervision of a physician.
plus extra vitamin B₃ (niacin) and	50 mg twice daily.	
choline and	50 mg twice daily.	
inositol	50 mg twice daily.	
Vitamin B₆	50 mg 3 times daily.	Reduces water content in tissues to relieve pressure on the cardiovascular system.

HERBS

❏ Use cayenne (capsicum), chamomile, fennel, hawthorn berries, parsley, and rosemary for high blood pressure.

Caution: Do not use chamomile on an ongoing basis, as ragweed allergy may result. Avoid it completely if you are allergic to ragweed.

❏ Hops and valerian root are good for calming the nerves.

❏ Drink 3 cups of suma tea daily.

❏ *Avoid* the herbs ephedra (ma huang) and licorice, as these herbs can elevate blood pressure.

RECOMMENDATIONS

❏ Follow a strict salt-free diet. This is essential for lowering blood pressure. Lowering your salt intake is not enough; eliminate all salt from your diet. Read labels carefully and avoid those food products that have "salt," "soda," "sodium," or the symbol "Na" on the label. Some foods and food additives that should be avoided on this diet include monosodium glutamate (Accent, MSG); baking soda; canned vegetables (unless marked sodium- or salt-free); commercially prepared foods; over-the-counter medications that contain ibuprofen (such as Advil or Nuprin); diet soft drinks; foods with mold inhibitors, preservatives, and/or sugar substitutes; meat tenderizers; softened water; and soy sauce.

❏ Eat a high-fiber diet and take supplemental fiber. Oat bran is a good source of fiber.

Note: Always take supplemental fiber separately from other supplements and medications.

❏ Eat plenty of fruits and vegetables, such as apples, asparagus, bananas, broccoli, cabbage, cantaloupe, eggplant, garlic, grapefruit, green leafy vegetables, melons, peas, prunes, raisins, squash, and sweet potatoes.

❏ Include fresh "live" juices in the diet. The following juices are healthful: beet, carrot, celery, currant, cranberry, citrus fruit, parsley, spinach, and watermelon.

❏ Eat grains like brown rice, buckwheat, millet, and oats.

❏ Drink steam-distilled water only.

❏ Take 2 tablespoons of flaxseed oil daily.

❏ Avoid all animal fats. Bacon, beef, bouillons, chicken liver, corned beef, dairy products, gravies, pork, sausage, and smoked or processed meats are prohibited. The only acceptable animal foods are broiled white fish and skinless turkey or chicken, and these should be consumed in moderation only. Get protein from vegetable sources, grains, and legumes instead.

❏ Avoid foods such as aged cheeses, aged meats, anchovies, avocados, chocolate, fava beans, pickled herring, sherry, sour cream, wine, and yogurt.

❏ Avoid all alcohol, caffeine, and tobacco.

❏ If you are taking an MAO inhibitor (one of a class of drugs prescribed to counter depression, lower blood pressure, and treat infections and cancer), avoid the chemical tyramine and its precursor, tyrosine. Combining MAO inhibitors with tyramine causes the blood pressure to soar and could cause a stroke. Tyramine-containing foods include almonds, avocados, bananas, beef or chicken liver, beer, cheese (including cottage cheese), chocolate, coffee, fava beans, herring, meat tenderizer, peanuts, pickles, pineapples, pumpkin seeds, raisins, sausage, sesame seeds, sour cream, soy sauce, wine, yeast extracts (including brewer's yeast), yogurt, and other foods. In general, any high-protein food that has undergone aging, pickling, fermentation, or similar processes should be avoided. Over-the-counter cold and allergy remedies should also be avoided.

❏ Keep your weight down. If you are overweight, take steps to lose the excess pounds. (*See* OBESITY in Part Two.)

❏ Fast for three to five days each month. Periodic cleansing fasts help to detoxify the body. (*See* FASTING in Part Three.)

❏ Get regular light to moderate exercise. Take care not to overexert yourself, especially in hot or humid weather.

Caution: Consult with your health care provider before beginning a new exercise regimen, particularly if you have been sedentary for some time.

❏ Be sure to get sufficient sleep.

❏ Have your blood pressure checked at least every four to six months. Because hypertension often shows no signs, regular blood pressure checks by a professional are important, especially if you are in a high-risk category.

❏ If you are pregnant, have your blood pressure monitored frequently by your health care provider. Untreated hypertension in pregnancy can progress suddenly and pose a serious threat to both mother and child.

❑ Do not take antihistamines except under a physician's direction.

❑ Do not take supplements containing the amino acids phenylalanine or tyrosine. Also avoid the artificial sweetener aspartame (Equal, NutraSweet), which contains phenylalanine.

❑ As much as possible, avoid stress.

CONSIDERATIONS

❑ Hypertension is directly related to a number of other conditions, such as arteriosclerosis, cardiovascular disease, heart attack, and high cholesterol. These conditions are dis-

How to Measure Your Blood Pressure

Your blood pressure measurement actually tells you how much pressure it takes to stop the flow of blood through your arteries. This is assumed to be equivalent to the pressure at the pump end, the heart.

Blood pressure is measured at two points in the heart's pumping rhythm: *systolic pressure* is taken at the moment the heart beats; *diastolic pressure* is taken when the heart is at rest between beats. To measure blood pressure, the soft, inflatable cuff of the sphygmomanometer is wrapped around the upper arm and inflated. Systolic pressure is measured when there is no longer a pulse in the arm beyond the cuff. Then the cuff is deflated and the diastolic pressure is taken when the blood flows freely once more. The combined pressure is usually expressed as a fraction—120/80, for example.

Ideally, blood pressure should be taken with the arm bare. A tight sleeve may constrict the arm or make it impossible to apply the blood pressure cuff properly. The cuff should be placed around the arm about one inch above the bend in the elbow. Before beginning to work with the sphygmomanometer, check the following four items:

1. Be sure that the sphygmomanometer reads 0 when there is no pressure in the system.

2. Check to be sure that the needle stays in place when the valve is closed.

3. Check the valve screw to make sure that it operates smoothly.

4. Inspect your stethoscope for cracks or leaks in the tubing, earpieces, bell, or diaphragm.

You should first feel for the blood pressure. Find the radial pulse, on the thumb side of the wrist. Then inflate the cuff 30 mm Hg beyond the point where the pulse is obliterated. Open the valve and release 2–3 mm Hg per second. When the pulsations of the radial pulse again become palpable, this is the systolic pressure. The diastolic blood pressure occurs when vibrations in the artery cease. Diastolic pressure is much more difficult to obtain.

Next, use the stethoscope to take the blood pressure. Follow this procedure:

1. Position the disc of the stethoscope snugly against the skin where the elbow bends—a little to the left of center on the right arm, and a little to the right of center on the left arm. There should be no gaps between the stethoscope and the skin, but you should not apply any undue pressure. Make sure that the stethoscope is not touching the cuff at any point.

2. Position the earpieces of the stethoscope in your ears (with the earpieces directed forward).

3. Hold the stethoscope disc snugly in position with one hand while you pump the cuff with the other hand.

4. Pump the cuff until the gauge registers about 30 mm Hg above the point where you felt the pulse disappear earlier, or about 200 mm Hg.

5. Loosen the valve slightly and permit the pressure to drop slowly. Listen carefully for the first sound of a beat—the number on the scale when you hear the first beat is the systolic pressure. (If you think that you missed the first beat or are unsure, tighten the valve again and pump the cuff up; repeat the process, listening carefully.)

6. Continue to deflate the cuff slowly until the last sound of blood pumping through the blood vessels is heard. When you hear no more blood flowing, the number on the scale is the diastolic pressure.

When taking your blood pressure, follow these general guidelines for best results:

• Avoid eating, smoking, or exercising for at least one-half hour before measuring your blood pressure.

• Test yourself at about the same times each day. Plan ahead to give yourself time to get over any feelings of anger or anxiety.

• Sit quietly and eliminate extraneous noise.

• Follow the manufacturer's instructions carefully.

• Position your arm at heart level, palm up. If you are using a cuff device, wrap the cuff just above the elbow—with your sleeve rolled up above the cuff—and be sure it is not too tight.

• Make sure the hoses from the cuff are not tangled or pinched.

• Take care not to move the hoses during the reading.

• Wait at least five minutes in between readings, with the cuff fully deflated.

• Take the device along on medical visits once a year or more to check its accuracy against your physician's measurements.

cussed separately in Part Two. It is advisable to refer to all of the sections on these interrelated conditions mentioned, even if you are concerned with only one of these illnesses.

❑ Because the use of diuretic drugs causes increased urinary excretion of magnesium, it can cause hypomagnesemia in elderly people. Magnesium is needed in conjunction with calcium to prevent bone deterioration, as well as to maintain a normal heart rhythm and muscular contraction. Losses of potassium due to diuretics may be dangerous, causing heart malfunction. Herbal diuretics are far safer. Consult your physician before using diuretics.

❑ People with hypertension often suffer from sleep apnea, in which they stop breathing for ten seconds or more throughout the night. Apnea is associated with loud snoring and restless sleep, and can cause the individual to feel excessively sleepy during the day. Evaluation and treatment of apnea may help reduce high blood pressure.

❑ Some risks for hypertension cannot be changed—a family history of the disease, for instance. However, many risk factors can be avoided by making changes in diet and lifestyle.

❑ According to the National Stroke Association, hypertension is the most important controllable risk factor for stroke, increasing the risk of stroke by seven times.

❑ Approximately 80 million Americans have increased sensitivity to dietary sodium. African-Americans in particular are prone to salt-sensitive hypertension.

❑ Research has revealed that people with variations in two specific genes are twice as likely to develop high blood pressure from salt consumption. This discovery may make it possible to identify children prone to high blood pressure; if such people can be identified in early childhood, it may be possible to modify their diets so that they can avoid developing high blood pressure later in life.

❑ Heavy snorers are more likely to have high blood pressure or angina than silent sleepers. Research suggests that snorers may suffer from a malfunctioning of the part of the brain responsible for fluent breathing; this can put an unnatural strain on the heart and lungs due to oxygen shortage.

❑ Researchers at the State University of New York found that the lower the level of magnesium in the body, the higher the blood pressure. This double-blind, placebo-controlled trial showed that taking supplemental magnesium can result in a significant, dose-dependent reduction in both systolic and diastolic blood pressure.

❑ Apple pectin aids in reducing blood pressure.

❑ A synthetic heart hormone that appears to be very effective in lowering blood pressure is currently undergoing testing at some twenty-five medical centers.

❑ Certain colors have a beneficial effect on blood pressure. (See COLOR THERAPY in Part Three.) Music also can be used to reduce stress and thereby lower blood pressure. (See MUSIC AND SOUND THERAPY in Part Three.)

❑ Taking medication for high blood pressure may lead to low blood pressure (hypotension). Hypotension can cause fainting, fatigue, and weakness, possibly with nausea, sweating, and restlessness preceding a loss of consciousness. *Postural hypotension*, which is a very temporary lowering of blood pressure, is usually caused by standing up too suddenly. This leads to dizziness and wears off quickly. For older adults, low blood pressure can simply result from eating. This is called *postprandial hypotension*, and it happens because blood is diverted to the gastrointestinal tract to help with digesting the food. In older people, the heart is not as efficient at increasing blood flow by pumping more quickly, so, with too much blood going to help with digesting a meal, there is too little traveling to the brain. Drinking lots of fluids increases blood volume, which may alleviate this condition. In some cases, low blood pressure can be a sign of heart disease or blood loss, especially a sudden loss of blood such as in an accident. In very many cases though, low blood pressure is a sign of good health, especially in younger people.

❑ *See also* ARTERIOSCLEROSIS/ATHEROSCLEROSIS; CARDIOVASCULAR DISEASE; CIRCULATORY PROBLEMS; and HEART ATTACK in Part Two.

High Cholesterol

A high blood cholesterol level, especially elevated low-density lipoproteins (LDL), is considered to be a contributor to plaque building up in the arteries and impeded blood flow to the brain, kidneys, genitals, extremities, and heart. It is among the primary causes of heart disease, because cholesterol produces deposits in arteries. High cholesterol levels may also be implicated in gallstones, impotence (although it is often the drugs prescribed to deal with high cholesterol that causes this), mental impairment, and high blood pressure.

Cholesterol is an essential part of every cell structure and is needed for proper brain and nerve function. It is also the basis for the manufacture of sex hormones. Cholesterol is manufactured in the liver and transported through the bloodstream to the sites where it is needed. It is a fatty substance and, because blood is mainly water, it has to latch on to molecules called lipoproteins to travel around successfully. Low-density lipoproteins (LDLs) are the major transporters of cholesterol in the bloodstream and, because LDLs seem to encourage the deposit of cholesterol in the arteries, it is known as "bad cholesterol." High-density lipoproteins (HDLs), on the other hand, are considered to be "good cholesterol" because they carry unneeded cholesterol away from the cells and back to the liver, where it is broken down for removal from the body. If everything is functioning as it should, this system remains in balance.

However, if there is too much cholesterol for the HDLs to pick up promptly, or if there are not enough HDLs to do the job, cholesterol can form plaque that sticks to artery walls and may eventually cause heart disease.

It is important to distinguish between serum cholesterol and dietary cholesterol. Serum cholesterol is the cholesterol in the bloodstream. Dietary cholesterol is cholesterol that is present in food. While eating foods high in dietary cholesterol can raise serum cholesterol, it is not the only source of serum cholesterol. Indeed, you would have some amount of serum cholesterol even if you never ate any food containing dietary cholesterol because the body produces its own cholesterol.

Cholesterol levels are greatly influenced by diet, but they are also affected by your genetic makeup. The consumption of foods high in cholesterol and/or saturated fat increases cholesterol levels, while a vegetarian diet, regular exercise, and the nutrients niacin and vitamin C may lower cholesterol.

The National Cholesterol Education Program has set the "safe" level of total serum cholesterol (including both LDL and HDL) at 200 milligrams per deciliter of blood (mg/dl). A reading above 200 indicates an increased potential for developing heart disease. A level of 200 to 239 is borderline, and levels over 240 are considered to indicate high risk. The normal HDL level for adult men in the United States is 45 to 50 mg/dl, and that for women is 50 to 60 mg/dl. It is suggested that higher HDL levels, such as 70 or 80 mg/dl, may protect against heart disease. An HDL level under 35 mg/dl is considered risky. So if you have a cholesterol reading of 200, with HDL at 80 and LDL at 120, you are considered at low risk for heart disease. On the other hand, even if you have a total cholesterol level well under 200, if your HDL level is under 35, you would still be considered at increased risk of developing cardiovascular disease. In other words, as your HDL decreases, your potential for heart problems intensifies, even if your total is on the low side.

CHOLESTEROL LEVEL SELF-TEST

A test called the Advanced Care Cholesterol Kit, produced by Johnson & Johnson, can be used to check your cholesterol level at home. It is available in drugstores without a prescription, and it gives a cholesterol reading in fifteen minutes. Be aware that the results can be skewed if you wait longer than five minutes after blood is drawn to perform the test or if you have taken the test four hours after taking a 500-milligram dose of vitamin C or after taking acetaminophen. This test shows total cholesteral level only. It is 97 percent accurate.

The test contains pads that are the size of a credit card and have a chemical reagent zone. When a drop of blood is placed on the surface of the pad, the reagents react with enzymes in the blood and the treated zone changes color. The color of the zone is then matched against a color-coded chart to find the serum cholesterol level.

If you have high cholesterol, follow the nutritional guidelines and recommendations in this section, and consult your health care provider.

NUTRIENTS

SUPPLEMENT	SUGGESTED DOSAGE	COMMENTS
Very Important		
Apple pectin	As directed on label.	Lowers cholesterol levels by binding fats and heavy metals.
Calcium	As directed on label.	To prevent hypocalcemia, or low calcium levels. Use calcium aspartate form.
Chinese red yeast rice extract	As directed on label.	Has cholesterol-lowering properties.
Chromium picolinate	400–600 mcg daily.	Lowers total cholesterol levels and improves HDL-to-LDL ratio.
Coenzyme Q$_{10}$ plus	60 mg daily.	Improves circulation.
Coenzyme A from Coenzyme-A Technologies	As directed on label.	Works well with coenzyme Q$_{10}$ to streamline metabolism, process fats, remove toxins from the body, and boost the immune system.
Fiber (oat bran and guar gum are good sources)	As directed on label, ½ hour before the first meal of the day. Take separately from other supplements and medications.	Helps to lower cholesterol.
Garlic (Kyolic from Wakunaga)	2 capsules 3 times daily.	Lowers cholesterol levels and blood pressure.
L-Carnitine	As directed on label.	Studies conducted using 4 grams of carnitine daily for 12 months showed lowered death rates and lowered cholesterol levels in heart attack patients.
Lecithin granules or capsules	1 tbsp 3 times daily, before meals. 1,200 mg 3 times daily, before meals.	Lowers cholesterol. A fat emulsifier.
Lipotropic factors	As directed on label.	Substances that prevent fat deposits (as in atherosclerosis).
Vitamin A with mixed carotenoids	As directed on label.	If you are taking cholesterol-lowering drugs, your lycopene levels will be reduced. Lycopene is one of the carotenoids that boosts the immune system.
Vitamin B complex plus extra vitamin B$_1$ (thiamine) and vitamin B$_3$ (niacin)	As directed on label. 300 mg daily. Do not exceed this amount.	B vitamins work best when taken together. Important in controlling cholesterol levels. Lowers cholesterol. Do not use a sustained-release formula, and do not substitute niacinamide for niacin. *Caution:* Do not take niacin if you have a liver disorder, gout, or high blood pressure.
Vitamin C with bioflavonoids	3,000–8,000 mg daily, in divided doses.	Lowers cholesterol.
Vitamin E	Begin with 200 IU daily and slowly increase dosage to 1,000 IU daily.	Improves circulation. Use an emulsion form for rapid assimilation. Use d-alpha-tocopherol form.

Helpful		
Essential fatty acids (black currant seed oil, borage oil, primrose oil, and Kyolic-EPA from Wakunaga are good sources)	As directed on label. Take with vitamin E as recommended above.	Reduces LDL level and thins the blood.
Heart Science from Source Naturals	As directed on label.	Contains antioxidants to lower cholesterol, plus herbs, vitamins, and other nutrients that protect the heart and promote healthy cardiovascular function.
Proteolytic enzymes	As directed on label. Take with meals and between meals.	Aids digestion. *Caution:* Do not give this supplement to a child.
Selenium	200 mcg daily. If you are pregnant, do not exceed 40 mcg daily.	Deficiency has been linked to heart disease.
Shiitake extract or reishi extract	As directed on label. As directed on label.	Helps to control and lower cholesterol levels.

HERBS

❏ Cayenne (capsicum), goldenseal, and hawthorn berries help to lower cholesterol.

Caution: Do not take goldenseal internally on a daily basis for more than one week at a time, do not use it during pregnancy, and use with caution if you are allergic to ragweed.

❏ Spirulina, taken on a daily basis, has been shown to lower cholesterol.

RECOMMENDATIONS

❏ Include the following cholesterol-lowering foods in your diet: apples, bananas, carrots, cold-water fish, dried beans, garlic, grapefruit, and olive oil.

❏ Make sure to take in plenty of fiber in the form of fruits, vegetables, and whole grains. Water-soluble dietary fiber is very important in reducing serum cholesterol. It is found in barley, beans, brown rice, fruits, glucomannan, guar gum, and oats. Oat bran and brown rice bran are the best foods for lowering cholesterol. Whole-grain cereals (in moderation) and brown rice are good as well. Since fiber absorbs the minerals from the food it is in, take extra minerals separately from the fiber.

❏ Drink fresh juices, especially carrot, celery, and beet juices. Carrot juice helps to flush out fat from the bile in the liver and this helps lower cholesterol.

❏ Go on a monthly spirulina fast, with carrot and celery juice or lemon and steam-distilled water. (*See* FASTING in Part Three.)

❏ Use only unrefined cold- or expeller-pressed oils. Cold-pressed oils are those that have never been heated above 110°F during processing—at this temperature, enzyme destruction begins. Use vegetable oils that are liquid at room temperature, such as olive, soybean, flaxseed, primrose, and black currant seed oil. Olive oil is recommended.

❏ Do not eat any nuts except raw, unsalted walnuts and almonds. Almonds are rich in the amino acid arginine, and were found in one study to cut cholesterol levels by sixteen points over a four-week period.

❏ Reduce the amount of saturated fat and cholesterol in your diet. Saturated fats include all fats of animal origin as well as coconut and palm kernel oils. Eliminate from the diet all hydrogenated fats and hardened fats and oils such as margarine, lard, and butter. Margarine that contains plant sterols, however, is a healthy option. Consume no heated fats or processed oils, and avoid animal products (especially pork and pork products) and fried or fatty foods. Always read food product labels carefully. You may consume nonfat milk, low-fat cottage cheese, and skinless white poultry meat (preferably turkey), but only in moderation.

❏ Do not consume alcohol, cakes, candy, carbonated drinks, coffee, gravies, nondairy creamers, pies, processed or refined foods, refined carbohydrates, tea, tobacco, or white bread.

❏ Get regular moderate exercise. Always consult with your health care provider before beginning any new exercise program.

❏ Try to avoid stress and sustained tension. Learn stress-management techniques. (*See* STRESS in Part Two.)

CONSIDERATIONS

❏ High cholesterol is directly related to conditions such as arteriosclerosis, cardiovascular disease, circulatory problems, heart attack, and hypertension. These conditions are discussed separately in Part Two. It is advisable to refer to all of the sections on these interrelated diseases to learn about all aspects of, and contributing causes to, high cholesterol.

❏ Meat and dairy products are primary sources of dietary cholesterol. Vegetables and fruits are free of cholesterol.

❏ Many people use margarine or vegetable shortening as substitutes for butter because they contain no cholesterol. However, these products contain compounds called cis- and trans-fatty acids that become oxidized when exposed to heat and can clog the arteries. They have been linked to the formation of damaging free radicals.

❏ In large amounts, coffee can elevate blood cholesterol levels, more than doubling the risk of heart disease. According to a report published in *The New England Journal of Medicine*, observation of 15,000 coffee drinkers revealed that as the intake of coffee rises, the amount of cholesterol in the blood goes up.

❏ Cream substitutes (nondairy coffee creamers) are actually poor alternatives to cholesterol-heavy dairy products.

Many contain coconut oil, which is a highly saturated fat. Soymilk or almond milk is preferable.

❑ The body does need some fats, but they must be the right kind. Good fats supply essential fatty acids, which are a very important link in our health chain. Fats supply energy, and they stay in the digestive tract for longer periods than proteins or carbohydrates, giving a feeling of fullness. They act as an intestinal lubricant, generate body heat, and carry the fat-soluble vitamins A, D, E, and K in the body. The protective myelin sheaths that protect nerve fibers are composed of fats. All cell membranes are composed of fats as well. Unfortunately, most Americans consume much too much of the wrong fats—that is, saturated, hydrogenated, and heated fats—which are linked to obesity, cardiovascular disease, and certain types of cancer.

❑ Human growth hormone therapy has been found to decrease cholesterol levels. (*See* GROWTH HORMONE THERAPY in Part Three.)

❑ Many fast-food restaurants use beef tallow (fat) to make their hamburgers, fish, chicken, and French-fried potatoes. Not only do these fried foods contain high amounts of cholesterol, but this fat is subjected to high temperatures in the deep-frying process, resulting in oxidation and the formation of free radicals. Heating fat, especially frying food in fat, also produces toxic trans-fatty acids, which seem to behave much like saturated fats in clogging the arteries and raising blood cholesterol levels.

❑ Certain drugs can elevate cholesterol levels. These include steroids, high-dose oral contraceptives, furosemide (Lasix) and other diuretics, and levodopa (L-dopa, sold under the brand names Dopar, Larodopa, and Sinemet), which is used to treat Parkinson's disease. Beta-blockers, often prescribed to control high blood pressure, can cause unfavorable changes in the ratio of LDL to HDL in the blood. Check with your physician if you are taking any of these medications, or any other medications, that might affect high cholesterol levels.

❑ Some people claim that taking charcoal tablets lowers blood cholesterol. However, charcoal also absorbs good nutrients along with the cholesterol. Activated charcoal should not be consumed daily, and it should not be taken at the same time as other supplements or medications. Other "experts" recommend taking fish oil capsules to lower cholesterol, but fish oil is 100-percent fat, and the evidence is lacking that the ingestion of fish oil reduces serum fats.

❑ Pure virgin olive oil appears to help reduce serum cholesterol. A monounsaturated-fatty-acid-rich diet that includes olive oil may be the reason for the low serum cholesterol levels found in people living in Italy and Greece.

❑ Studies have shown that diets consisting of grains, fruits, and vegetables result in lower blood cholesterol levels. In the United States and northern Europe, where people consume large amounts of meat and dairy products,

extremely high rates of heart and circulatory disease are present. Even children in these nations show signs of progressive vascular disease due to hypercholesterolemia (an excess of cholesterol in the blood).

❑ There are a number of cholesterol-lowering drugs on the market. Available by prescription only, these tend to be costly, and they can have serious side effects. We believe that these drugs should be used only as a last resort. The sensible way to keep the serum fats within a safe range is to follow a diet that excludes animal fats (including meat, milk, and all dairy products) and includes ample amounts of fiber and bulk (whole grains, fruits, and vegetables).

❑ Sunlight, or rather the lack of it, has been shown to have adverse effects on cholesterol levels.

❑ Some people have hereditary disorders that prevent even the healthiest diet from lowering LDL levels. For these people, researchers are working on a device that uses an enzyme to break down LDL and accelerate its removal before it can fasten onto artery walls to form plaque. The device would be implanted under the skin to control the LDL levels in the blood.

❑ There are opposing theories about high cholesterol levels. Some medical practitioners believe that it has little to do with heart disease and that a direct correlation has never been fully established. Studies in India, Guatemala, Poland, and the United States claim to have proved that there is no relationship between atherosclerosis and cholesterol levels. However, it is probably best to take cholesterol levels seriously, and also to consider other tests that may help to assess your likelihood of developing heart disease as outlined in HEART ATTACKS in Part Two.

❑ *See also* ARTERIOSCLEROSIS/ATHEROSCLEROSIS; CARDIO-VASCULAR DISEASE; CIRCULATORY PROBLEMS; HEART ATTACK; and HYPERTENSION, all in Part Two. Also see CHELATION THERAPY in Part Three.

Human Immunodeficiency Virus

See AIDS.

Hives

Hives, called *urticaria* by the medical profession, is a skin condition that is characterized by sudden outbreaks of red, itchy welts on the skin. Any area of the body may be affected. The welts may vary in appearance, from tiny, goose-bump-like spots to rashes that cover significant areas of the body. Hives usually go away within a few hours to two days, but in rare cases they become chronic and may last for six weeks or more.

Many cases of hives are brought on as allergic reactions and coincide with the release of histamine in the body. The release of histamine into the skin produces an inflammatory reaction, with itching, swelling, and redness. Hives can cause significant discomfort, but it does not cause injury or damage to any vital organs.

The skin is the largest organ of the body. It is an important part of the excretory system. The skin acts in conjunction with other systems in the body to remove toxins and waste. Hives can be a natural reaction to the presence of a foreign substance in the body. However, an offending substance need not enter the body to trigger an outbreak of hives. Merely coming into contact with various substances, such as pesticides, soaps, shampoos, hair sprays, residues from laundry products or dry cleaning chemicals on clothing, or any other of a vast array of other seemingly innocuous household items can unleash a maddening attack of hives.

The severity of a hives outbreak can vary from case to case as well as from person to person. Some people can break out in hives if they merely touch a certain type of plant or bush; others may develop hives only with considerable exposure, such as overconsumption of a certain food. Chemicals are a major cause of hives for many people; anything from perfumes to household cleaners can trigger a reaction, as can nervous conditions, stress, certain foods, and alcohol.

Viruses also can cause hives. Hepatitis B and Epstein-Barr virus, the virus that causes infectious mononucleosis, are the two most common culprits. Some bacterial infections likewise can cause outbreaks of hives, both chronic and acute. An association between *Candida albicans* and chronic hives has been established in several clinical studies over the past twenty years.

Antibiotics such as penicillin and related compounds are the most common cause of drug-induced hives. At least 10 percent of the American population is thought to be allergic to penicillin. Nearly one-quarter of those people will develop hives, *angioedema* (a condition that is similar to hives but affects deeper layers of the skin and causes larger wheals), *laryngeal angiodema* (angioedema that affects the throat, and can have an adverse effect on breathing), or anaphylaxis (a systemic allergic reaction causing generalized itching and difficulty breathing) if they ingest penicillin.

The following are some of the drugs and other substances that most commonly cause outbreaks of hives in susceptible people. This list is not exhaustive, and we do not mean to imply that these items *will* cause a hives outbreak, only that they at least contribute to the condition in some people:

- *Animals,* especially animal dander and dog saliva.

- *Aspirin.*

- *Allopurinol* (Zyloprim), a gout medication.

- *Antimony,* a metallic element that is present in various metal alloys.

- *Antipyrine,* an agent used to relieve pain and inflammation.

- *Barbiturates.*

- *BHA and BHT,* preservatives used in many food products.

- *Bismuth,* another metallic element present in certain metal alloys.

- *Cancer,* especially leukemia.

- *Chloral hydrate,* a sedative used in the treatment of tetany.

- *Chlorpromazine* (Thorazine), a tranquilizer and antiemetic.

- *Cologne or perfume.*

- *Corticotropin* (also known as adrenocorticotropic hormone, or ACTH, and sold for medicinal purposes under the brand names Acthar and Cortrosyn).

- *Environmental factors,* especially heat, cold, water, and sunlight.

- *Eucalyptus,* a tree whose leaves yield an aromatic oil that is used in cough remedies and other medicines.

- *Exercise.*

- *Fluorides,* which are found in certain dental care products and in fluoridated drinking water.

- *Food allergies,* especially allergies to shellfish, eggs, fruits, and various nuts.

- *Food colorings and preservatives.*

- *Gold.*

- *Griseofulvin* (Fulvicin, Grisactin, and others), an antifungal medication.

- *Hyperthyroidism.*

- *Infections,* especially strep infections, hepatitis, and parasites.

- *Insect bites.*

- *Insulin.*

- *Iodines,* used in certain antiseptics and dyes.

- *Liver extract.*

- *Makeup.*

- *Menthol,* an extract of peppermint oil used in perfumes, as a mild anesthetic, and as a mint flavoring in candy and cigarettes.

- *Meprobamate* (Miltown, Equanil, Meprospan), a tranquilizer.

- *Mercury,* a toxic metallic element found in dental fillings, certain antacids, and some first-aid preparations, among other things.

- *Morphine.*

- *Opium.*

- *Para-aminosalicylic acid,* an anti-inflammatory drug.

- *Penicillin.*
- *Phenacetin,* an ingredient in some pain medications.
- *Phenobarbital,* a sedative and anticonvulsant.
- *Pilocarpine,* a glaucoma medication.
- *Plants.*
- *Poliomyelitis vaccine.*
- *Potassium sulfocyanate,* a preservative.
- *Preservatives.*
- *Procaine* (Novocain), an anesthetic.
- *Promethazine* (Phenergan), an antihistamine, sedative, and antiemetic.
- *Quinine,* used in quinine water and antimalaria medications.
- *Reserpine,* a heart medication.
- *Saccharin,* an artificial sweetener found in Sweet'n Low, many toothpastes, and many dietetic and "sugarless" products.
- *Salicylates,* chemicals used as food flavorings and preservatives.
- *Soaps,* including laundry soap.
- *Shampoo.*
- *Sulfites,* chemicals used as food preservatives and in the production of dried fruits such as raisins.
- *Tartrazine,* a food dye and an ingredient in Alka-Seltzer.
- *Thiamine hydrochloride,* an ingredient in some cough medicines.

Other hives-provoking substances are being identified with increasing frequency. Meat, dairy, and poultry products, especially in frozen or fast foods, are increasingly being associated with hives, probably because many farmers and ranchers routinely give their livestock antibiotics in an effort to prevent disease or infection. These antibiotics are not affected by subsequent freezing, processing, or cooking. Allergic reactions have been traced to antibiotics in milk, soft drinks, and even frozen dinners.

Unless otherwise specified, the dosages recommended here are for adults. For a child between the ages of twelve and seventeen, reduce the dose to three-quarters the recommended amount. For a child between six and twelve, use one-half the recommended dose, and for a child under the age of six, use one-quarter the recommended amount.

NUTRIENTS

SUPPLEMENT	SUGGESTED DOSAGE	COMMENTS
Helpful		
Acidophilus (Probiata from Wakunaga)	As directed on label.	Reduces allergic reactions and helps replenish "friendly" bacteria. Use a nondairy formula.
Flaxseed oil or primrose oil	1,000 mg twice daily. 1,000 mg twice daily.	Has anti-inflammatory effects.
Garlic (Kyolic from Wakunaga)	As directed on label.	Aids in destroying bacteria.
Herpanacine from Diamond-Herpanacine Associates	As directed on label.	A nutrient and herb combination that supports overall skin health.
Multivitamin and mineral complex	As directed on label.	To correct any nutrient or mineral deficiencies that may be contributing to outbreaks. Use a hypoallergenic formula.
Quercetin or AntiAllergy formula from Freeda Vitamins	As directed on label. As directed on label.	Reduces inflammation and reactions to substances that may cause hives. A combination of quercetin, calcium pantothenate, and calcium ascorbate.
Vitamin B complex plus extra pantothenic acid (vitamin B_5) and vitamin B_{12}	As directed on label, with meals. (Note: a complex will vary in amounts.) 250 mg 3–4 times daily at first outbreak. Reduce to 1–2 times daily when hives subside. 1,000–2,000 mcg daily.	Needed for the functioning of the nervous system and for healthy skin. Aids with the body's immune response. Prevents nerve damage and promotes normal growth of the skin. Use a lozenge or sublingual form.
Vitamin C with bioflavonoids	1,000 mg 3 times daily.	Enhances immune response; acts as an anti-inflammatory.
Vitamin D_3	400 IU daily.	To reduce outbreaks.
Vitamin E and zinc	600 IU daily. 50 mg daily. Do not exceed a total of 100 mg daily from all supplements.	A powerful antioxidant that improves circulation to the skin tissues. Use d-alpha-tocopherol form. Promotes a healthy immune system and healing of skin tissues. Needed for proper concentrations of vitamin E in the blood. Use zinc gluconate lozenges or OptiZinc for best absorption.

HERBS

❑ Alfalfa, bilberry extract, cat's claw, chamomile, echinacea, ginseng, licorice, nettle, sarsaparilla, and yellow dock are all beneficial to the hives sufferer. Alfalfa can also be used as a preventive blood tonic. It cleanses the blood and helps keep the body free of toxins.

Caution: Do not use chamomile on an ongoing basis, and avoid it completely if you are allergic to ragweed. Do not use ginseng or licorice if you have high blood pressure.

❑ Applying aloe vera gel to the affected area can be helpful.

❑ Black nightshade leaves may help. Wash and boil the leaves in water, put them on a cloth, and apply as a poultice to the affected area. (*See* USING A POULTICE in Part Three.)

Caution: Do not take this herb internally, and avoid getting it in your eyes.

❑ The leaves and the bark of the red alder tree, when brewed into a strong tea, can help hives. Apply it locally to the affected area, and take a couple of tablespoons internally as well. Reapply several times daily until the hives abate. Red alder contains the astringent tannin.

RECOMMENDATIONS

❏ Avoid alcohol and all processed foods, which put added stress on the body by depleting nutrients. Also avoid dairy products, eggs, chicken, and nuts. Especially avoid foods high in saturated fats, cholesterol, and sugar.

❏ Do not take any medications (including aspirin, pain killers, sedatives, laxatives, cough syrups, and antacids) that are not prescribed for you.

❏ Use only hypoallergenic skin care products.

❏ For the typical case of hives, avoid using prednisone or other steroids. Instead, use the nutrients and herbs listed above. Try nettle first.

❏ For topical treatment, use cornstarch or colloidal oatmeal added to bath water. A good oatmeal product for this purpose is Aveeno Bath Treatment, available at drugstores. Bathing in cool water with baking soda added also may relieve symptoms.

❏ Take a cool shower when you see the first signs of hives appearing. Make sure that it is cool, not hot. This may slow the spreading of hives.

❏ Wear loose-fitting clothing.

❏ Try using homeopathic remedies. *Bovista, Cantharis,* and *Rhus toxicodendron* are homeopathic remedies that may alleviate symptoms of hives.

❏ If you have had hives for longer than six weeks, or if you are developing an acute case of hives, consult your health care provider.

❏ If sun exposure is the cause of your hives, apply a strong sunscreen—this will usually alleviate the problem.

❏ If hives develop in your mouth or throat, and especially if it causes swelling around the throat or interferes with swallowing or breathing *to any extent at all,* seek medical help immediately. Go to the emergency room of the nearest hospital or call for emergency assistance. Hives can signal or accompany the onset of anaphylaxis, a dangerous allergic reaction that can block the breathing passages. The possibility of anaphylaxis is what makes allergies to insect stings, such as those from bees, a potentially serious concern. If you have ever had this type of reaction, you should be under a physician's care and have an epinephrine injection kit on hand. Make sure you know how to use it, and keep the kit with you at all times.

CONSIDERATIONS

❏ Many people who suffer acute attacks find at least temporary relief from the symptoms of hives by taking antihistamines such as hydroxyzine (Atarax, Vistaril), chlorpheniramine (Chlor-Trimeton, Teldrin, and others), or diphenhydramine (Benadryl and others). Chronic sufferers have less success with this approach, as antihistamines are suppressive agents and may actually contribute to the persistence of hives. Antihistamines in gel or spray form can be applied topically for immediate but temporary relief of itchiness or burning.

❏ Depending on the nature and severity of the symptoms, health care providers may prescribe antihistamines, cortisone, or a bronchodilator such as terbutaline or ephedrine for people with hives. They may also prescribe sedatives for anxiety in severe cases.

❏ If a hives outbreak is the result of a food or drug that you have ingested, you obviously do not want that substance in your body again. If you cannot isolate whatever food or drug it might be that causes hives, having a physician do some blood work to find the allergen may be your only solution, even though this approach can be relatively expensive.

❏ Occasionally, hives can persist for weeks or even months, resisting all attempts at treatment. For this reason alone, it is best to learn what the cause of the outbreak is in order to avoid it. If you suffer from chronic hives and cannot isolate the cause, eliminating all the possible allergens from your home may be your only resort. This can be a long, drawn-out, and painstaking process. (*See* ALLERGIES in Part Two.)

❏ Chronic hives may be linked to *Candida albicans*. If you suspect this may be the cause of hives, adopting a yeast-free diet can be of some benefit. (*See* CANDIDIASIS in Part Two.)

❏ An elimination diet is important. (*See* ALLERGIES in Part Two.)

Hot Flashes

See under MENOPAUSAL AND PERIMENOPAUSAL PROBLEMS.

Hypertension

See HIGH BLOOD PRESSURE.

Hyperthyroidism

This disorder occurs when the thyroid gland produces too much thyroid hormone, resulting in an overactive metabolic state. All of the body's processes speed up with this disorder. Symptoms of hyperthyroidism include nervousness, irritability, a constant feeling of being hot, increased perspiration, insomnia and fatigue, increased frequency of bowel movements, less frequent menstruation and decreased menstrual flow, weakness, hair and weight loss, change in skin thickness, separation of the nails from the nail bed, hand tremors, intolerance of heat, rapid heartbeat, goiter, and, sometimes, protruding eyeballs. Hyperthyroidism is sometimes also called *thyrotoxicosis*. The most common type of this disorder is *Graves' disease*

The thyroid gland is the body's internal thermostat. It regulates the temperature by secreting two hormones that control how quickly the body burns calories and uses energy. If the thyroid secretes too much hormone, hyperthyroidism results; too little hormone results in hypothyroidism. Many cases of hypothyroidism and hyperthyroidism are believed to result from an abnormal immune response. The exact cause is not understood, but the immune system can produce antibodies that invade and attack the thyroid, disrupting hormone production. Hyperthyroidism can also be caused by lumps or tumors that form on the thyroid and disrupt hormone production. Infection or inflammation of the thyroid can cause temporary hyperthyroidism, as can certain prescription drugs.

Hyperthyroidism is not as common as hypothyroidism. Both of these thyroid disorders affect women more often than men. A malfunctioning thyroid can be the underlying cause of many recurring illnesses.

Unless otherwise specified, the dosages recommended here are for adults. For a child between the ages of twelve and seventeen, reduce the dose to three-quarters of the recommended amount. For a child between six and twelve, use one-half of the recommended dose, and for a child under the age of six, use one-quarter of the recommended amount.

NUTRIENTS

SUPPLEMENT	SUGGESTED DOSAGE	COMMENTS
Very Important		
Multivitamin and mineral complex	As directed on label.	Increased amounts of vitamins and minerals are needed for this "hyper" metabolic condition. Use a super-high-potency formula.
Vitamin B complex	50 mg of each major B vitamin 3 times daily, with meals (amounts of individual vitamins in a complex will vary).	Needed for thyroid function. Injections (under a doctor's supervision) may be necessary.
plus extra vitamin B₁ (thiamine) and	50 mg twice daily.	Needed for blood formation and energy levels.
vitamin B₂ (riboflavin) and	50 mg twice daily.	Required for normal functioning of all cells, glands, and organs in the body.
vitamin B₆ (pyridoxine)	50 mg twice daily.	Activates many enzymes and is needed for immune function and antibody production.
Helpful		
Brewer's yeast	1–3 tbsp daily and up.	Rich in many basic nutrients, especially the B vitamins.
Essential fatty acids (Kyolic-EPA from Wakunaga is a good source)	As directed on label.	Needed for correct glandular function.
Lecithin granules or capsules	1 tbsp 3 times daily, before meals. 1,200 mg 3 times daily, before meals.	Aids in digestion of fats and protects the lining of all cells and organs.
Vitamin C with bioflavonoids	3,000–5,000 mg daily and up.	Especially important in this stressful condition.
Vitamin E	400 IU daily. Do not exceed this amount.	An antioxidant and necessary nutrient. However, excessive amounts may stimulate the thyroid gland. Use d-alpha-tocopherol form.

RECOMMENDATIONS

❑ Eat plenty of the following foods: broccoli, Brussels sprouts, cabbage, cauliflower, kale, mustard greens, peaches, pears, rutabagas, soybeans, spinach, and turnips. These help to suppress thyroid hormone production.

❑ Avoid dairy products for at least three months. Also avoid stimulants, coffee, tea, nicotine, and soft drinks.

❑ Be wary of treatment with radioactive sodium iodine (iodine 131, or I-131), which is often recommended for this condition. Severe side effects have been known to accompany the use of I-131. Also, do not rush into surgery. Try improving your diet first.

CONSIDERATIONS

❑ Along with other bodily processes, digestion speeds up with this disorder. Malabsorption occurs, so a proper diet is important.

❑ Researchers in England studied ten people who were being treated for Parkinson's disease and found that all of them also had hyperthyroidism. Once the thyroid condition was treated, the Parkinson's disease improved dramatically.

❑ If a goiter affects breathing or swallowing, surgery may be needed to remove part or all of the thyroid. It may be necessary to take thyroid hormone pills after surgery.

❑ The pituitary gland, parathyroid glands, and sex glands all work together and are influenced by thyroid function. If there is a problem in one place, they all may be affected.

❑ The parathyroid glands, small endocrine glands that are positioned near or within the rear surface of the thyroid, secrete parathyroid hormone (PTH), which aids in controlling calcium levels. Hyperparathyroidism is a rare disorder in which these apple-seed-sized organs become enlarged and overactive. When too much PTH is released, excess calcium leaches out of the bones and into the blood. Routine blood tests may reveal excess calcium in the blood. If left untreated, it can lead to other problems such as bone pain and kidney stones. The standard treatment for this disorder is surgery. Permanent hoarseness is a possible side effect, if the nerves supplying the voice box are injured.

❏ An undiagnosed thyroid condition can be mistaken for menopausal symptoms. Symptoms such as fatigue, mood swings, and depression are often present in both circumstances. If you are experiencing menopausal symptoms, you should have your thyroid function tested.

❏ For names and addresses of organizations that can provide additional information about thyroid disorders, see HEALTH AND MEDICAL ORGANIZATIONS in the Appendix.

Hypoglycemia (Low Blood Sugar)

Hypoglycemia, or low blood sugar, is a condition in which there is an abnormally low level of glucose (sugar) in the blood. *Reactive hypoglycemia* occurs when blood sugar drops to abnormally low levels two to five hours after eating a meal. Symptoms of reactive hypoglycemia include sweating, tremors, rapid heartbeat, anxiety, and hunger. Most often, this results from the oversecretion of insulin by the pancreas. Insulin facilitates the transport of glucose from the bloodstream into the cells, especially those of muscle and fatty tissue, and causes glucose to be synthesized in the liver. If the pancreas is not functioning properly, normal carbohydrate metabolism is impossible. As the blood sugar drops, stress hormones such as adrenaline and cortisol kick in at high levels to prevent the blood sugar level from dropping dramatically. Another type of hypoglycemia is known as *fasting hypoglycemia*. This occurs as a result of abstaining from food for eight or more hours. The symptoms are often more severe than those of reactive hypoglycemia and can include seizures, loss of consciousness, and a loss of mental acuity. Liver disease or a tumor of the pancreas is generally the underlying cause of this type of hypoglycemia.

A person suffering from hypoglycemia may display any or all of the following symptoms: fatigue, dizziness, heart palpitations, nausea, blurred vision, an inability to concentrate, lightheadedness, headache, irritability, fainting spells, depression, anxiety, cravings for sweets, confusion, night sweats, weakness in the legs, swollen feet, a feeling of tightness in chest, constant hunger, pain in various parts of the body (especially the eyes), nervous habits, mental disturbances, and insomnia. People with hypoglycemia can become very aggressive and lose their tempers easily. Any or all of these symptoms may occur a few hours after eating sweets or fats. The onset and severity of symptoms are directly related to the length of time since the last meal was eaten and the type of foods that meal contained.

More and more Americans today may have this condi-

tion, due to poor dietary habits that include eating large quantities of simple carbohydrates, sugars, alcohol, caffeine, and soft drinks, and insufficient amounts of complex carbohydrates. High stress levels are believed to be a contributing factor in the increasing incidence of hypoglycemia.

Hypoglycemia can be inherited, but most often it is precipitated by an inadequate diet. This is referred to as *functional hypoglycemia (FH)*. Many other bodily disorders can cause hypoglycemic problems as well, among them adrenal insufficiency, thyroid disorders, pituitary disorders, kidney disease, and pancreatitis. Immune deficiency and candidiasis are strongly linked to hypoglycemia. Glucose intolerance and hyperinsulinemia (high blood insulin levels), producing hypoglycemia, frequently occur in people with chronic liver failure. Other common causes are smoking and the consumption of large amounts of caffeine, found in colas, chocolate, and coffee. Though it may seem paradoxical, low blood sugar can also be an early sign of diabetes (high blood sugar).

Diagnosis of hypoglycemia can be difficult because the symptoms often mimic those of other disorders, including adrenal dysfunction, allergies, asthma, candidiasis, chronic fatigue syndrome, digestive or intestinal disorders, eating disorders, food allergies, hypothyroidism, kidney failure, malabsorption syndrome, menopause, mental disorders, neurological problems, nutritional deficiencies, sepsis (blood infection), stress, and weight problems.

To diagnose hypoglycemia, a health care provider may perform a glucose tolerance test (GTT). However, many people have symptoms of hypoglycemia even though the results of a five-hour GTT are within normal limits. A useful diagnostic test may be to follow the dietary and nutritional supplement regimen outlined in this section and see if symptoms improve.

NUTRIENTS

SUPPLEMENT	SUGGESTED DOSAGE	COMMENTS
Very Important		
Brewer's yeast	As directed on label.	Aids in stabilizing blood sugar levels.
Chromium picolinate	300–600 mcg daily.	Vital in glucose metabolism. Essential for optimal insulin activity.
Kyo-Dophilus from Wakunaga	As directed on label.	To replace the friendly bacteria lacking in this disorder. Use the liquid form.
Garlic (Kyolic from Wakunaga)	As directed on label.	Very good for relieving low blood sugar when an attack occurs.
Glutathione	As directed on label.	A compound consisting of three amino acids that is associated with the breakdown of glucose into energy.
Pancreatin	As directed on label. Take with meals.	For proper protein digestion. Use a high-potency formula.

Proteolytic enzymes	As directed on label. Take between meals.	People with this disorder often fail to digest protein properly, resulting in "leaky gut syndrome" and allergies. *Caution:* Do not give this supplement to a child.
Quercetin	As directed on label.	Aids in stopping allergic reactions. Helpful if food allergies are a factor.
Vitamin B complex	50–100 mg of each major B vitamin daily and up (amounts of individual vitamins in a complex will vary).	Important in carbohydrate and protein metabolism, and proper digestion and absorption of foods; helps the body tolerate foods that produce low blood sugar reactions. Also helps counteract the effects of malabsorption disorders, common in people with hypoglycemia.
plus extra vitamin B_1 (thiamine) and	100 mg daily.	Aids in the production of hydrochloric acid, needed for proper digestion.
vitamin B_3 (niacin)	100 mg daily. Do not exceed this amount.	Aids in the functioning of the nervous system and in proper digestion. *Caution:* Do not take niacin if you have a liver disorder, gout, or high blood pressure.
and pantothenic acid (vitamin B_5) and	1,000 mg daily, in divided doses.	Important in adrenal gland function and conversion of glucose to energy.
vitamin B_{12}	1,000–2,000 mcg daily, on an empty stomach.	Crucial for prevention of anemia, common because malabsorption disorders result in deficiency.
Zinc	50 mg daily. Do not exceed a total of 100 mg daily from all supplements.	Needed for proper release of insulin. People with hypoglycemia are often zinc deficient. Use zinc gluconate lozenges or OptiZinc for best absorption.

Important		
L-Carnitine plus	As directed on label.	Converts stored body fat into energy.
L-cysteine and	As directed on label.	Blocks the action of insulin, which lowers blood sugar.
L-glutamine	1,000 mg daily, on an empty stomach. Take with water or juice. Do not take with milk. Take with 50 mg vitamin B_6 and 100 mg vitamin C for better absorption.	Reduces cravings for sugar.
Magnesium plus	750 mg daily, in divided doses, after meals and at bedtime.	Important in carbohydrate (sugar) metabolism.
calcium	1,500 mg daily, in divided doses, after meals and at bedtime.	Works with magnesium and aids in preventing colon cancer.
Manganese	As directed on label. Take separately from calcium.	Important for the maintenance of blood glucose levels. Most people with hypoglycemia have low levels of this trace mineral in their blood.
Vitamin C with bioflavonoids	3,000–8,000 mg daily, in divided doses.	For adrenal insufficiency, common in people with hypoglycemia.
Vitamin E	400 IU and up.	Improves energy and circulation. Use d-alpha-tocopherol form.

Helpful		
Aerobic Bulk Cleanse from Aerobic Life Industries or psyllium husks	As directed on label. Take with aloe vera juice on an empty stomach in the morning. Take separately from other supplements and medications.	Aids in slowing down blood sugar reactions and keeping the colon clean.
Liver extract injections or desiccated liver	1 cc twice weekly for 3 months, then once weekly for 2 months or more, or as prescribed by physician. As directed on label.	Liver glandulars supply B vitamins and other valuable nutrients.
Multivitamin and mineral complex	As directed on label.	All nutrients are required for healing.
Cravex from Natrol	As directed on label.	Controls sugar cravings and helps balance metabolism.

HERBS

❑ The following herbs help to normalize blood sugar: angostura bitters (or any combination of bitters), artichoke leaf, and gentian root.

❑ To help your body respond to stress, try astragalus or licorice root.

Caution: If overused, licorice can elevate blood pressure. Do not use this herb on a daily basis for more than seven days in a row. Avoid it completely if you have high blood pressure or are pregnant or nursing.

❑ Bilberry and wild yam aid in controlling insulin levels.

❑ Dandelion root is an excellent source of calcium and supports the pancreas and liver.

❑ Gudmar (*Gymnema sylvestre*), an Ayurvedic herb, suppresses the intestinal absorption of saccharides, which prevents blood sugar fluctuations.

❑ Licorice nourishes the adrenal glands.

Caution: Do not use this herb on a daily basis for more than seven days in a row. Avoid if you have high blood pressure or are pregnant or nursing.

❑ Milk thistle rejuvenates the liver.

❑ Other beneficial herbs include echinacea, parsley, pau d'arco, raspberry leaves, and uva ursi.

RECOMMENDATIONS

❑ Remove from the diet all alcohol, canned and packaged foods, refined and processed foods, dried fruits, salt, sugar, saturated fats, soft drinks, and white flour. Also avoid foods that contain artificial colors or preservatives.

❑ Avoid sweet fruits and juices such as grape and prune. If you drink these, mix the juice with an equal amount of water.

❑ Sweeten food with natural sweeteners such as stevia, a South American herb available in liquid form that is 200 times sweeter than sugar. Other acceptable sweeteners include barley malt syrup, molasses, and brown rice syrup.

❏ Eat a diet high in fiber and include large amounts of vegetables, especially broccoli, carrots, Jerusalem artichokes, raw spinach, squash, and string beans. Vegetables should be eaten raw or steamed. Also eat beans, brown rice, oats, oat bran, lentils, potatoes, soy products (tofu), and fruits, especially apples, apricots, avocados, bananas, cantaloupes, grapefruits, lemons, and persimmons.

❏ For protein, eat low-fat cottage cheese, fish, grains, kefir, raw cheese, raw nuts, seeds, skinless white turkey or white chicken breast, and low-fat yogurt.

❏ Eat starchy foods such as corn, hominy, noodles, pasta, white rice, and yams in moderation only.

❏ Include maitake mushrooms in your diet. They are beneficial for helping the body adapt to stress.

❏ Do not eat fatty foods such as bacon, cold cuts, fried foods, gravies, ham, sausage, or dairy products (except for low-fat soured products).

❏ Do not go without food or consume large, heavy meals. Eat six to eight small meals throughout the day. Some people find that eating a small snack before bedtime helps.

❏ Use a rotation diet; food allergies are often linked to hypoglycemia and can make the symptoms more pronounced. (See ALLERGIES in Part Two.)

❏ Try taking 200 micrograms of chromium picolinate daily. This can alleviate many symptoms and raise blood glucose levels if symptoms occur after sugar or a heavy meal is consumed. Chromium, also known as glucose tolerance factor or GTF, has been known to alleviate sudden shock.

❏ During a low blood sugar reaction, eat something that combines fiber with a protein food, such as bran or rice crackers with raw cheese or almond butter.

❏ Instead of eating applesauce, have a whole apple, which has more fiber. The fiber in the apple will inhibit fluctuations in blood sugar. Fiber alone (found in popcorn, oat bran, rice bran, crackers, ground flaxseed, and psyllium husks) will slow down a hypoglycemic reaction. Take fiber half an hour before meals. Spirulina tablets taken between meals further help to stabilize blood sugar.

❏ Maintain a regular exercise regimen. This helps to maintain steady blood sugar levels. Eat one to three hours prior to exercise.

❏ Stress is a major factor in hypoglycemia, as it affects adrenal function and blood sugar levels. Practice stress reduction by meditating, listening to soothing music, getting a massage, or using deep breathing techniques.

❏ Fast once a month with fresh vegetable juices and a series of lemon juice enemas. (See FASTING and ENEMAS in Part Three.) To prevent a low blood sugar reaction while fasting, use spirulina or a protein powder supplement. Many people find this makes them start to feel better very quickly.

CONSIDERATIONS

❏ Avocados contain a seven-carbon sugar that depresses insulin production, which make them an excellent choice for people with hypoglycemia.

❏ The production of insulin is affected by the functioning of the adrenal glands. The adrenal glands produce epinephrine, which acts to "turn off" insulin production, among other things. If the adrenal glands are overstressed and exhausted, they cannot function properly and an overabundance of insulin may result. This causes the blood sugar level to sink below normal, creating a low energy syndrome in the body.

❏ Injections of vitamin B complex plus extra vitamin B_6 (pyridoxine) and liver extract have produced good results for those with hypoglycemia. Liver extract supplements contain a nutritional substance that aids liver regeneration. Only liver from organically raised beef should be used.

❏ Hypoglycemia can mimic menopausal symptoms, especially since it often escalates during midlife.

❏ In rare cases, hypoglycemia can be triggered by large doses of aspirin or by sulfonamides (sulfa drugs), a class of antibiotics often prescribed for urinary tract infections.

❏ People who are most prone to hypoglycemia are those taking medications for high blood sugar or diabetes.

❏ Hypoglycemia is often the underlying cause of misdiagnosed cases of attention deficit disorder (ADD). (See ATTENTION DEFICIT DISORDER [ADD]/ATTENTION DEFICIT HYPERACTIVITY DISORDER [ADHD] in Part Two.)

❏ It is estimated that half the people with hypoglycemia who are over fifty have reduced thyroid function and hypothyroidism. (See HYPOTHYROIDISM in Part Two.)

❏ Caffeine, alcohol, and tobacco cause profound swings in blood sugar levels. Insomnia can result if any type of sugar is consumed after dinner. Consuming sugar at any time tends to cause drowsiness and fatigue.

❏ Some studies have shown that reducing the amount of meat protein in the diet and adding some starches, such as potatoes, may be beneficial.

❏ Milk allergy is common as this disorder progresses. Allergy testing is recommended. (See ALLERGIES in Part Two.)

Hypothyroidism

Hypothyroidism is caused by an underproduction of thyroid hormone. Symptoms include fatigue, loss of appetite, inability to tolerate cold, a slow heart rate, weight gain, painful premenstrual periods, a milky discharge from the breasts, fertility problems, muscle weakness, muscle cramps, dry and scaly skin, a yellow-orange coloration in the skin (particularly on the palms of the hands), yellow bumps on the eyelids, hair loss (including the eyebrows), recurrent infections, migraines, hoarseness, respiratory infections, constipation, depression, difficulty concentrating, slow speech, goiter, and drooping, swollen eyes. The most common symptoms are fatigue and intolerance to cold. If you consistently feel cold while others around you are hot, you may be suffering from reduced thyroid function.

The thyroid gland is the body's internal thermostat, regulating the temperature by secreting two hormones that control how quickly the body burns calories and uses energy. If the thyroid secretes too much hormone, hyperthyroidism results; too little hormone results in hypothyroidism. Hypothyroidism affects about 13 million people in the United States, about 90 percent of whom are women. Women between the ages of thirty and fifty seem to be most prone to this condition. It is estimated that one in eight women will develop a thyroid condition at some point in her lifetime. Thyroid problems can cause many recurring illnesses and fatigue. The thyroid can be affected by poor diet, fluoride in the water, excessive consumption of unsaturated fats, endurance exercise, pesticide residues on fruits and vegetables, radiation from x-rays, alcohol, and drugs.

A condition called *Hashimoto's disease* is believed to be the most common cause of underactive thyroid. In this disorder, the body in effect becomes allergic to thyroid hormone. It then produces antibodies against its own thyroid tissue. Hashimoto's disease is a common cause of goiter, a swelling of the thyroid gland, among adults, and it can occur in association with other disorders, such as pernicious anemia, lupus, yeast infections, and rheumatoid arthritis. Congenital hypothyroidism in children, if left untreated, can lead to mental retardation and dwarfism. Generally, however, hypothyroidism is detected within a baby's first few months, when routine blood tests are performed.

A rare condition that can result from long-term undiagnosed hypothyroidism is called *myxedema coma*. The coma can occur during illness, after an accident, from exposure to cold, or as a result of the ingestion of narcotics and/or sedatives. This is a medical emergency that requires immediate treatment.

Measuring levels of different hormones in the blood can determine if the thyroid gland is working properly. A physician may order a blood test to measure levels of thyroid hormone or thyroid-stimulating hormone (TSH). This hormone is secreted by the pituitary gland and in turn helps regulate thyroid hormone production. Even a minuscule drop in thyroid function registers as a distinctly elevated TSH level. Most endocrinologists believe that TSH levels rise when a person is in the earliest stages of thyroid failure.

An iodine absorption test may also be performed. This test involves ingesting a small amount of radioactive iodine. An x-ray then shows how much of the iodine was absorbed by the thyroid. A low uptake of the iodine may indicate hypothyroidism.

Unless otherwise specified, the dosages recommended in this section are for adults. For a child between the ages of twelve and seventeen, reduce the dose to three-quarters of the recommended amount. For a child between six and twelve, use one-half of the recommended dose, and for a child under the age of six, use one-quarter of the recommended amount.

THYROID SELF-TEST

To test yourself for an underactive thyroid, keep a thermometer by your bed at night. When you awaken in the morning, place the thermometer under your arm and hold it there for fifteen minutes. Keep still and quiet. Any motion can upset your temperature reading. A temperature of 97.6°F or lower may indicate an underactive thyroid. Keep a temperature log for five days. If your readings are consistently low, consult your health care provider.

NUTRIENTS

SUPPLEMENT	SUGGESTED DOSAGE	COMMENTS
Essential		
Kelp	2,000–3,000 mg daily.	Contains iodine, the basic substance of thyroid hormone.
L-Tyrosine	500 mg twice daily, on an empty stomach. Take with water or juice. Do not take with milk. Take with 50 mg vitamin B$_6$ and 100 mg vitamin C for better absorption.	Low plasma levels have been associated with hypothyroidism. (*See* AMINO ACIDS in Part One.)
Very Important		
Multi-Glandular from American Biologics	As directed on label.	A nutritional supplement for the endocrine, hormonal, and enzyme systems.
Raw thyroid glandular	As prescribed by physician.	To replace deficient thyroid hormone (*see* GLANDULAR THERAPY in Part Three). Natural thyroid extract such as Armour Desiccated Thyroid Tablets is best. Available by prescription only.
ThyroStart from Silver Sage	As directed on label.	An herbal supplement that contains ingredients to support the thyroid, including iodine.
Important		
Vitamin B complex	100 mg of each major B vitamin 3 times daily, with meals (amounts of individual vitamins in a complex will vary).	B vitamins improve cellular oxygenation and energy and are needed for proper digestion, immune function, red blood cell formation, and thyroid function.
plus extra vitamin B$_2$ (riboflavin) and	50 mg twice daily.	
vitamin B$_{12}$	1,000–2,000 mcg 3 times daily, on an empty stomach.	Use a lozenge or sublingual form for best absorption.
Helpful		
Brewer's yeast	As directed on label.	Rich in basic nutrients, especially B vitamins.

Essential fatty acids (Kyolic-EPA from Wakunaga is a good source)	As directed on label.	Necessary for proper functioning of the thyroid gland.
Iron	As directed by physician. Take with 100 mg vitamin C for better absorption.	Essential for enzyme and hemoglobin production. Use ferrous chelate form. *Caution:* Do not take iron unless anemia has been diagnosed.
or Floradix Iron + Herbs from Salus Haus	As directed on label.	A natural, nontoxic form of iron from food sources.
Selenium	As directed on label. If you are pregnant, do not exceed 40 mcg daily.	A vital antioxidant that protects the immune system.
Vitamin A with mixed carotenoids plus	15,000 IU daily. If you are pregnant, do not exceed 10,000 IU daily.	Needed for proper immune function and for healthy eyes, skin, and hair. May be taken in a multivitamin complex.
natural beta-carotene or	15,000 IU daily.	Antioxidant and precursor of vitamin A.
carotenoid complex (Betatene)	As directed on label.	*Note:* If you have diabetes, omit the beta-carotene; people with diabetes cannot convert beta-carotene into vitamin A.
Vitamin C with bioflavonoids	500 mg 4 times daily. Do not exceed this amount.	Needed for immune function and stress hormone production. *Caution:* Do not take extremely high doses of vitamin C—this may affect the production of thyroid hormone.
Vitamin E	400 IU daily. Do not exceed this amount.	An important antioxidant that improves circulation and immune response. Use d-alpha-tocopherol form.
Zinc	50 mg daily. Do not exceed a total of 100 mg daily from all supplements.	An immune system stimulant. Use zinc gluconate lozenges or OptiZinc for best absorption.

HERBS

❑ Bayberry, black cohosh, and goldenseal can help this thyroid condition.

Caution: Do not take goldenseal internally on a daily basis for more than one week at a time, do not use it during pregnancy, and use it with caution if you are allergic to ragweed.

❑ Gentian and mugwort extracts are helpful for hypothyroidism.

❑ Herbal bitters such as Swedish bitters may help alleviate the symptoms associated with thyroid malfunctions.

RECOMMENDATIONS

❑ Include in your diet apricots, dates, egg yolks, molasses, parsley, potatoes, prunes, raw seeds, and whole grains. Eat fish or chicken and raw milk and cheeses.

❑ Eat these foods in moderation: broccoli, Brussels sprouts, cabbage, kale, mustard greens, peaches, pears, radishes, spinach, and turnips. If you have severe symptoms, omit these foods entirely. They may further suppress thyroid function.

❑ Avoid processed and refined foods, including white flour and sugar.

❑ Drink steam-distilled water only.

❑ Begin a moderate exercise program such as yoga or walking.

❑ Do not take sulfa drugs or antihistamines unless specifically directed to do so by a physician.

❑ Avoid fluoride (including that found in toothpaste and tap water) and chlorine (also found in tap water). Chlorine, fluoride, and iodine are chemically related. Chlorine and fluoride block iodine receptors in the thyroid gland, resulting in reduced iodine-containing hormone production and finally in hypothyroidism.

❑ Taking the homeopathic remedy *Calcarea carbonica* may help. It can sometimes increase thyroid function.

❑ Because thyroid medication can interact with other medications, take them several hours apart. Ask your physician if any other medications will interfere with the effectiveness of your thyroid prescription. Sucralfate (Carafate), an ulcer medication; aluminum hydroxide (an antacid found in Alu-Tab, Amphojel, and Nephrox), and two drugs used to lower cholesterol, cholestyramine (Questran) and colestipol (Colestid), are some of the drugs that affect thyroid medications. Do not take thyroid medication with carbonate supplements or calcium as they can block the absorption of thyroxine (T_4).

CONSIDERATIONS

❑ Because sugar intolerance, menopause, and depression can cause many of the same symptoms of thyroid disorders, a simple thyroid test should be considered to rule out any errors in diagnosis.

❑ Treatment for a regular morning temperature of 96°F is 3 to 4 grains of Armour Desiccated Thyroid Tablets (available by prescription) daily. A person with a regular morning temperature of 97°F should take 1 to 2 grains. If you have side effects, speak to your physician about reducing the dosage.

❑ Synthroid and Levothroid are synthetic versions of T_4 that are most frequently prescribed by physicians for people with hypothyroidism. Some side effects of these medications include headache, irritability, nervousness, loss of sleep, diarrhea, weight loss, and changes in appetite. If a person shows no response to this medication, the physician may prescribe liothyronine (Cytomel). It contains T_3, which is needed to regulate metabolism. A study done at the University of Massachusetts found that thyroxine can cause a loss of bone mass.

❑ The conventional treatment for Hashimoto's disease is usually a prescription of a thyroid hormone that must be taken for the duration of one's lifetime.

❑ The presence of too much thyroid hormone in the system can cause a condition known as *thyroid storm*. The heart rate increases rapidly and, in exceptionally severe cases, a heart attack can occur.

❑ Recent evidence indicates that an underactive thyroid may put you at an increased risk of heart attack—even if your thyroid is only slightly underactive.

❑ Applying a natural progesterone cream, which is available at most health food stores, may increase thyroid activity.

❑ Lithium, a trace mineral used as a drug to treat manic-depressive disorders, can sometimes cause thyroid malfunction.

❑ Wilson's syndrome is a condition that results from a problem in the conversion of one thyroid hormone, T_4, to another thyroid hormone, T_3. This causes symptoms of decreased thyroid function, especially triggered by significant physical or emotional stress. These symptoms can be debilitating, and may persist even after the stress has passed. People with Wilson's syndrome have many of the symptoms of hypothyroidism, including low body temperature, fatigue, headaches, menstrual dysfunction, memory loss, loss of concentration, loss of sex drive, anxiety and panic attacks, depression, unhealthy nails, dry skin, frequent infections, allergies, insomnia, intolerance to cold, and lack of energy and motivation. Their blood test results are often normal, however. (*See* WILSON'S DISEASE in Part Two).

❑ For names and addresses of organizations that can provide more information about thyroid disorders, *see* HEALTH AND MEDICAL ORGANIZATIONS in the Appendix.

Hysterectomy-Related Problems

Hysterectomy is the surgical removal of the uterus. This is done for many different reasons. A common reason is fibroid tumors, benign growths in the uterus that can cause problems. Over 30 percent of the hysterectomies performed in the United States are done to remove fibroids. (*See* FIBROIDS, UTERINE in Part Two.) Other conditions for which hysterectomy is performed include endometriosis (20 percent) and prolapse of the uterus (16 to 18 percent).

Many people question the fact that over 650,000 hysterectomies are performed in the United States each year. Very few of these operations are performed because of a life-threatening situation, and it is likely that many of them are actually unnecessary. Per capita, half as many hysterectomies are performed in Great Britain as in the United States, and, statistically, American women show no health benefits for their higher incidence of surgery. Outside the United States, very few hysterectomies are performed for what doctors often term "quality of life" reasons. Hysterec-

tomy effectively and permanently causes sterility, and this may be a motive (conscious or unconscious) for some women and/or their doctors to make this choice. Financial motives may be another possibility. U.S. Department of Health and Human Services statistics show that far fewer hysterectomies are performed under managed care plans, in which doctors receive a set fee for their services each year, than in situations in which surgeons are compensated directly for each operation performed.

The symptoms that lead women to consider hysterectomy are varied but include the following: a constant heavy, bloated feeling; urinary tract problems or incontinence; unusually long and heavy menstrual periods; unusual swelling in the abdominal region (due to fibroid tumors); infertility (due to fibroid tumors or endometriosis); complications of childbirth; cancer; and intolerance to the drug therapy usually prescribed for endometriosis.

The following are three different ways in which hysterectomy may be performed:

• *Total hysterectomy.* In this procedure, the cervix is removed along with the uterus.

• *Partial (also known as subtotal or supracervical) hysterectomy.* In partial hysterectomy, the uterus is removed but the cervix and other female reproductive organs remain intact.

• *Pan (or radical) hysterectomy.* In this, the most extensive form of hysterectomy, the ovaries, cervix, supporting ligaments, tissues, fallopian tubes, upper portion of the vagina, pelvic lymph nodes, and uterus are removed.

To remove the uterus surgically, doctors may choose one of the following three options:

• *Abdominal hysterectomy.* In some circumstances, the physician may choose to perform the hysterectomy by making an incision in the abdomen. This option is usually chosen if the woman undergoing the procedure has a large ovarian cyst or tumor. It is the most invasive type of hysterectomy, and the most traumatic due to the incision in the abdomen.

• *Total laparoscopic hysterectomy* (TLH). This involves performing the entire operation with a laparoscope (a tiny telescope), inserted through a very small incision in the navel and using small surgical instruments. This is used in situations in which the doctor needs an extensive picture of the pelvic region.

• *Vaginal hysterectomy.* In this type of procedure, the uterus is removed through the vagina. A doctor may choose to perform the procedure using a laparoscope. This method is called the *laparoscopically assisted vaginal hysterectomy* (LAH).

Many women who have hysterectomies experience significant problems as a result. The most obvious of these occurs when the ovaries are removed together with the uterus; menopause begins abruptly, with its attendant difficulties and discomforts, because the body is suddenly deprived of estrogen. This hormonal loss in turn can lead to a greatly increased risk of bone mass loss, which often precedes osteoporosis, and to an increased likelihood of heart disease, as well as depression, urinary tract problems, joint pain, headaches, dizziness, insomnia, and fatigue.

Even women who retain their ovaries often experience a drastic reduction in estrogen production, and menopause comes earlier—sometimes years earlier—than it would have naturally. This is believed to be because the supply of blood to the ovaries is disrupted and decreased by removal of the uterus. Over half of women who have ovary-sparing "partial" hysterectomies experience early menopause.

Another problem common among women who have undergone hysterectomy is diminished sexual interest and desire after surgery. Research indicates that one-third of all women who have hysterectomies find their sexual desire and enjoyment greatly diminished. Removal of the ovaries may result in loss of sexuality because they secrete about half of a woman's supply of androgens, hormones that are responsible for sex drive in both men and women. However, diminished sexuality may occur whether or not the ovaries are removed. In Finland, studies have shown that the removal of the cervix in hysterectomy also resulted in diminished capacity for orgasm. Hormone replacement therapy can alleviate this problem.

Not all of the problems that can follow hysterectomy are directly hormone related. Some women experience depression because of the knowledge that once the uterus is gone, it is too late to change one's mind about having children. Also, no surgical procedure is entirely 100-percent safe, foolproof, or guaranteed. There is a 50-percent chance of at least one minor postoperative complication (usually fever, bleeding, or wound trouble). It is estimated that 1 woman in 1,000 who has a hysterectomy will die as a result of complications, and 10 percent of the women who have this surgery will require a blood transfusion. If there is a possibility that you may require a transfusion as a result of this type of surgery, you should talk to your doctor about donating your own blood for use during the operation. (*See* HEPATITIS in Part Two for information about blood transfusions).

The following supplements can help to counteract the unpleasant side effects of hysterectomy.

NUTRIENTS

SUPPLEMENT	SUGGESTED DOSAGE	COMMENTS
Very Important		
Boron	3 mg daily. Do not exceed this amount.	Aids in calcium absorption and prevention of bone loss that can occur after hysterectomy.
Calcium and magnesium	2,000 mg daily, at bedtime. 1,000 mg daily, at bedtime.	Lack of estrogen hinders calcium uptake. Needed for the central nervous system. Enhances calcium absorption.
Essential fatty acids (primrose oil is a good source)	1,000 mg 3 times daily.	Helps the body manufacture estrogen.
Garlic (Kyolic from Wakunaga)	As directed on label.	May inhibit tumor growth.
Potassium	99 mg daily.	Needed if hot flashes occur to replace electrolytes lost through perspiration.
Raw thymus glandular	As directed on label.	Potentiates immune function.
Vitamin B complex	100 mg of each major B vitamin twice daily, with meals (amounts of individual vitamins in a complex will vary).	Needed for the nervous system and to reduce stress. Use a high-stress formula. Injections (under a doctor's supervision) may be necessary.
Vitamin C with bioflavonoids	3,000–6,000 mg and up daily, in divided doses.	An anti-stress vitamin also needed for tissue repair.
Vitamin E	Start with 400 IU daily and increase slowly to 1,200 IU daily. For hot flashes, find the dosage that eases symptoms and stay at that level.	Important in estrogen production. Use d-alpha-tocopherol form. *Caution:* Do not take this supplement for 2 weeks prior to surgery.
Important		
L-Arginine and L-lysine	500 mg each daily, on an empty stomach. Take with water or juice. Do not take with milk. Take with 50 mg vitamin B$_6$ and 100 mg vitamin C for better absorption.	Essential amino acids important in recovery after surgery. Both are needed to avoid an imbalance in amino acids. (*See* AMINO ACIDS in Part One.)
Micellized Vitamin A emulsion from American Biologics plus carotenoid complex plus zinc	50,000 IU daily. 50 mg daily. Do not exceed a total of 100 mg daily from all supplements.	Important in immune function and to promote tissue repair. Use emulsion form for easier assimilation and greater safety at higher doses. Boosts the immune system. Use zinc gluconate lozenges or zinc methionate (OptiZinc) for best absorption.
Helpful		
Melatonin	As directed on label.	This hormone stimulates the immune system and is important in the production of estrogen, testosterone, and, possibly, other hormones.
Multiglandular complex (Cytozyme-F from Biotics Research)	As directed on label.	Aids in glandular function.
Multivitamin and mineral complex	As directed on label.	Restores the essential vitamins and minerals to balance.

HERBS

❑ Herbs that act as natural estrogen promoters include anise, dong quai, fennel, fenugreek, ginseng, licorice, red clover, sage, suma, and wild yam.

Caution: Do not use sage if you have any kind of seizure disorder.

❑ Menocom is an herbal menopause complex containing helpful herbs, vitamins, and minerals.

❑ The following herbs may alleviate symptoms of ovarian cysts and uterine fibroids: black cohosh, black haw, blue cohosh, dandelion root, lady's mantle (yarrow), milk thistle, and pau d'arco.

❑ St. John's wort is helpful for depression.

RECOMMENDATIONS

❑ Adopt a hypoglycemic diet; eat plenty of foods that are high in fiber, such as vegetables, whole grains, and high-fiber fruits, plus fish, skinless white turkey or chicken breast, soy products, and low-fat yogurt, kefir, and cottage cheese for protein. Eat starchy foods in moderation only. Do not consume any refined sugar, white flour, alcohol, processed foods, saturated fats, or foods containing artificial colors, preservatives, or other additives. Eat six to eight small meals spaced regularly throughout the day, rather than two or three larger meals. *See* HYPOGLYCEMIA in Part Two for additional suggestions.

❑ Avoid caffeine, colas, dairy products (except for low-fat soured products), processed foods, red meat, and sugar.

❑ Use vitamin E to help prevent incisional scarring and relieve itching and discomfort in the area surrounding the stitches. Open a vitamin E capsule and apply the oil along the incision (but not on the stitches themselves).

❑ If you are considering a hysterectomy, give the matter close and careful consideration. Seek wise counsel and second opinions. Check into alternative treatments. Remember, once the operation has been performed, it is impossible to restore the uterus if you find the symptoms unacceptable or unbearable. The results of a hysterectomy are irreversible.

CONSIDERATIONS

❑ Women over forty who have hysterectomies performed often have their ovaries removed as well, supposedly as a precaution against the later development of ovarian cancer. However, many health care professionals question the logic of doing this; ovarian cancer is relatively rare.

❑ Estrogen replacement therapy is often recommended following a hysterectomy. For some women, it is, unfortunately, unavoidable, because of severe posthysterectomy symptoms. Not all women can tolerate estrogen replacement. In our opinion, synthetic estrogens are potentially dangerous because they are strongly linked to breast cancer and cardiovascular disease. Natural estrogens, on the other hand, are safe and effective. Natural estrogen promoters include anise, dong quai, fennel, fenugreek, ginseng, licorice, primrose oil, red clover, sage, suma, and wild yam. (*See* MENOPAUSAL AND PERIMENOPAUSAL PROBLEMS in Part Two.)

❑ A hysterectomy usually requires four or five days in the hospital followed by approximately six weeks of at-home recuperation. Recovery can be more painful if the surgeon makes a vertical incision as opposed to a horizontal one. In addition, the scar that results from a vertical incision acts as a lifelong reminder of the surgery (a horizontal incision can be hidden below the pubic hairline).

❑ Evidence is mounting that there is a higher incidence of cardiovascular disorders, osteoporosis, and Alzheimer's disease among women who have undergone hysterectomies.

❑ Some doctors advocate performing hysterectomies on women with fibroid tumors because they say that the fibroids block access to the ovaries during pelvic exams, which might delay a possible diagnosis of ovarian cancer. This position is no longer valid, however, because technology allows the use of ultrasound to examine the ovaries for any abnormality. If fibroid tumors need to be removed, a myomectomy should be considered and opted for if at all possible (*see* FIBROIDS, UTERINE in Part Two).

❑ There are instances in which hysterectomy proves advantageous. Some women manage to avoid the major hormonal changes that are so common after surgery, and in addition to no longer being bothered with monthly menses, they may feel liberated because they no longer need to fear becoming pregnant and have more fulfilling sex lives as a result. However, these women are probably in the minority.

❑ While over half of the women who have their ovaries left in place still experience drastic estrogen loss, this is not always permanent. A vitamin and mineral supplement regimen can reduce the risk of severe estrogen deprivation. Remember the natural estrogen promoters discussed in this section.

❑ If you do require hormone replacement to control symptoms after a hysterectomy, take the lowest dose possible. Ask your doctor for a combined hormone containing estrogen and progesterone to help reduce the risk of cancer.

❑ Dr. Betty Kamen, an expert in women's health problems, says that progesterone, not estrogen, should be the hormone of choice for replacement therapy.

❑ *See also* MENOPAUSE-RELATED PROBLEMS in Part Two.

❑ *See also* PREPARING FOR AND RECOVERING FROM SURGERY in Part Three.

Immune System, Weakened

See WEAKENED IMMUNE SYSTEM.

Impotence

Impotence, or chronic erectile disfunction (ED), is no longer a taboo subject. It is estimated that 30 million American men suffer from ED and, for a great majority of them, the problem is solvable. A man is considered impotent if he does not have the ability to achieve or maintain an erection adequate for normal sexual intercourse. Erections result from a complex combination of brain stimuli, blood vessel and nerve function, and hormonal actions. Anything that interferes with any of these factors can lead to impotence, and that can include arteriosclerosis, or peripheral vascular disease; the use of certain medications listed later in this section; alcohol, or cigarettes; a history of sexually transmitted disease; and chronic illness such as diabetes or high blood pressure.

Impotence is extremely common in men who have diabetes; the estimate is that 50 percent of men with diabetes are impotent and that the other 50 percent will become impotent over time. Hormonal imbalances such as low levels of thryoid hormone may also contribute to the problem. Low levels of the hormone testosterone are rarely the cause of ED. Testosterone is responsible for the process of desire, not for ED—but of course, lack of desire may be the problem. If desire is not there in the first place, it is difficult to either get or maintain an erection. Loss of libido (sexual desire) may be caused by depression, illness, or medications, and of course, a waning attraction to one's partner.

ED may be chronic or recurring, or it may occur as a single isolated incident. One or two occurrences, however, are rarely thought of as impotence, although they may be upsetting at the time. Most of the men who have this problem are age forty or over (one in three men over sixty is affected), but those under forty may also have the problem.

In the past, it was assumed that impotence was primarily a psychological problem, but many therapists and physicians today believe that as many as 85 percent of all cases of impotence have some physical basis. The Association for Male Sexual Dysfunction recognizes over 200 drugs that may cause impotence. Some of the most common are alcohol, antidepressants, antihistamines, antihypertensives, blood-pressure medication, cancer chemotherapy, diuretics, narcotics, nicotine, sedatives, steroids (if abused), stomach acid inhibitors, and ulcer medications. Atherosclerosis, or hardening of the arteries (one type of arteriosclerosis), poses a risk to the condition of both the heart and the penis (impotence can, in fact, be a symptom of this disorder). Most people today know smoking and eating fatty foods lead to the production of plaques that clog arteries and block the flow of blood to the heart. These plaques also can block the arteries leading to the genitals, interfering with the ability to attain an erection.

NUTRIENTS

SUPPLEMENT	SUGGESTED DOSAGE	COMMENTS
Essential		
Essential fatty acid complex	As directed on label.	Aids in the formation of sperm and seminal fluid in the prostate gland.
Iodine or kelp	As directed on label (usually 150 mg daily). 2,000–3,000 mg daily.	Iodine is a component of the thyroid hormones and necessary for development of the reproductive organs. Toxicity will result if taken in large quantities.
Selenium	As directed on label.	Found in high concentration in the testicles. *Caution:* Do not take this supplement if you have heart, liver, or kidney disease.
Vitamin C with bioflavonoids	500 mg 3 times daily.	Helps boost testosterone levels.
Vitamin E	Start with 200 IU daily and slowly increase to 400–1,000 IU daily.	Increases circulation. Use d-alpha-tocopherol form. *Caution:* Vitamin E is a blood-thinning agent. Do not use if you take prescription blood thinners.
Zinc	80 mg daily. Do not exceed this amount.	Important in prostate gland function and reproductive organ growth. Also helps boost testosterone levels. Use zinc gluconate lozenges or OptiZinc for best absorption.
Important		
Dimethylglycine (DMG) (Aangamik DMG from FoodScience of Vermont)	As directed on label.	Increases oxygen supply in the blood to all tissues. Blood vessels must be dilated for an erection to occur. Use a sublingual form.
GH3 from Gero Vita	As directed on label.	Stimulates the activity of sex hormones. *Caution:* Do not use GH3 if you are allergic to sulfites.
Multi-Glandular from American Biologics	As directed on label.	A supplement for the endrocine, hormonal, and enzyme systems.
Octacosanol	1,000–2,000 mcg 3 times weekly.	Natural source of vitamin E. Good for hormone production.
Helpful		
L-Tyrosine	500 mg twice daily, on an empty stomach. Take with water or juice. Do not take with milk. Take with 50 mg vitamin B_6 and 100 mg vitamin C for better absorption.	Helps stabilize moods and alleviate stress. (*See* AMINO ACIDS in Part One.) *Caution:* Do not take tyrosine if you are taking an MAO inhibitor drug.
Raw orchic glandular	As directed on label.	Glandular extracts from the male reproductive organs that promote their function. (*See* GLANDULAR THERAPY in Part Three.)
Vitamin A plus	15,000 IU daily.	Antioxidants that enhance immunity.
mixed carotenoids or	15,000 IU daily.	Antioxidants and vitamin A precursors.
carotenoid complex (Betatene)	As directed on label.	
Vitamin B complex	50 mg of each major B vitamin 3 times daily (amounts of individual vitamins in a complex will vary).	Needed for a healthy nervous system. B vitamins are important in all cell activities.
plus extra vitamin B_6 (pyridoxine)	50 mg 3 times daily.	Required for the synthesis of of RNA and DNA, which govern cellular reproduction.

HERBS

❏ Ashwagandha and schizandra, both Ayurvedic herbs, are said to ensure potency and increase fertility.

❏ Damiana is good for improving blood flow to the genital area and increasing desire.

❏ Sarsaparilla contains a testosterone-like substance for men.

❏ Wild yam contains natural steroids that rejuvenate and give vigor to lovemaking. Steroids are what help exercise to burn off more weight. This hormone is found in the human body as dehydroepiandrosterone (DHEA). Take twice the amount recommended on the label for two weeks, then stop for two weeks. Continue this on-and-off cycle, taking the recommended amount.

❏ Yohimbe bark is said to expand the blood vessels in the penis and increase blood flow. It also claims to increase nitrous oxide (NO), which is important for producing an erection.

Caution: Do not take yohimbe if you have high blood pressure.

❏ Other herbs that may be beneficial include dong quai, gotu kola, hydrangea root, pygeum, saw palmetto, and/or Siberian ginseng.

❏ There are a number of herbal products on the market that claim to help sexual potency:

• Prostata from Gero Vita International normalizes prostate function, increasing libido and erectile ability.

• Saw Palmetto Supreme from Gaia Herbs is an herbal tincture that helps to normalize prostate function.

• SensualiTea from UniTea Herbs contains damiana, sarsaparilla, and licorice root. It can be found in many health food stores that sell bulk herbs.

• Stamina from HerbaSway Therapeutic Formulas, an herbal formula containing yohimbe, yin-yang-huo (also known as horny goatweed), ginseng, and other herbs, is said to both enhance performance and increase stamina.

• Super Herbal V contains many of the herbs listed above, as does Super Libido Formula. Both are sold under a variety of brand names.

• Viagrin from Fountain of Youth Technologies is a blend of yin-yang-huo and other herbs that is said to increase erectile ability and promote endurance. It may also help restore sexual desire in women.

• Virility Two from KAL contains damiana, gotu kola, Jamaican ginger, oak grass powder, sarsaparilla, and yohimbe.

RECOMMENDATIONS

❏ Eat a healthy, well-balanced diet. Include in the diet pumpkin seeds, bee pollen, or royal jelly.

Caution: Bee pollen may cause an allergic reaction in some individuals. Start with a small amount, and discontinue use if a rash, wheezing, discomfort, or other symptom occurs.

❏ Avoid alcohol, particularly before sexual encounters.

❏ Do not consume animal fats, sugar, or fried or junk foods.

❏ Do not smoke. Avoid being around cigarette smoke.

❏ Avoid stress.

❏ Consult a urologist for testing to determine whether impotence is caused by an underlying illness that requires treatment.

❏ Consider possible psychological factors that may be contributing to impotence, especially repressed anger or a fear of intimacy. Exploring psychological issues with a qualified therapist can help.

❏ If you suspect impotence may be related to a drug you are taking, discuss this with your physician. There may be satisfactory alternatives that will not cause this problem. Certain blood pressure medications and tranquilizers often cause erectile difficulties. The drugs cimetidine (Tagamet) and ranitidine (Zantac), which are used to treat ulcers and heartburn, also have significant side effects in some men.

Caution: Do not stop taking a prescription drug or change the dosage without consulting your physician.

❏ Investigate the possibility of heavy metal intoxication. A hair analysis can reveal possible heavy metal poisoning. (*See* HAIR ANALYSIS in Part Three.)

❏ Keep in mind that sexual function changes with age. As you age, you may require more stimulation and a longer period of time to achieve an erection.

CONSIDERATIONS

❏ A study done at the Boston University School of Medicine linked overall health to impotence. Researchers studied the medical histories of 1,300 men aged forty to seventy years. They found some impotence in a total of 52 percent of those under study. Men who were being treated for heart disease, high blood pressure, or diabetes were one and a half to four times more likely than the overall group to be completely impotent later in life. The situation was even worse for men with heart disease or hypertension who also smoked.

❏ Alcohol intake decreases the body's ability to produce testosterone. Research at Chicago Medical School revealed that drinking alcohol may cause the hormonal equivalent of menopause in men. Alcohol not only affects sexual function, but also helps set the stage for a heart attack and other dangerous conditions.

❏ Arteriosclerosis, which restricts blood supply to the penis and to the nerves that govern sexual arousal, may result in a "failure to perform." If impotence is related to clogged blood vessels, a diet low in fats can actually help reverse the problem. (*See* ARTERIOSCLEROSIS/ATHEROSCLE-

ROSIS, CARDIOVASCULAR DISEASE, and/or CIRCULATORY PROBLEMS in Part Two.)

❑ A study done at Boston University showed that men who smoked one pack of cigarettes a day for five years were 15 percent more likely to develop clogging in the arteries that serve the penis, a situation that can cause impotence. In addition, heavy smoking decreases sexual capability by damaging the tiny blood vessels in the penis. The use of marijuana and cocaine can also result in impotence.

❑ Duplex ultrasonography, a noninvasive method of measuring penile blood flow, is a reliable method of determining whether arterial occlusion plays a role in impotence. If your doctor believes atherosclerosis to be the underlying problem, he or she may advise vascular surgery to improve blood flow to the penis.

❑ According to figures from impotence organizations, only about 5 percent of the estimated 30 million men affected are aware of therapy options.

❑ Urologists differ in the types of treatment they recommend for impotence, but many opt first for nonsurgical treatment.

❑ Sildenafil (Viagra) is probably the best known drug for dealing with ED. It is not, however, a drug that will make you feel like having sex, but rather a drug that will help you to have an erection. In other words, if desire is not there, it will not help. Partners of men who take Viagra may have difficulty adjusting to the higher level of potency shown by their partners, so taking an enhancement drug such as sildenafil should always be discussed with your partner. Sildenafil may not be suitable for men with certain cardiovascular or blood disorders, or for men with advanced kidney or liver disease. There are some concerns about sildenafil and high blood pressure.

❑ Apomorphine (Uprima) is a newer prescription drug for impotence that works through the brain to produce erections—unlike sildenafil, which works by increasing blood flow to the penis. This drug too can have side effects, most notably nausea, vomiting, dizziness, or sweating.

❑ Injections of the drugs papaverine (Pavabid) and phentolamine (Regitine) or prostaglandin E1 (PGE1) into the base of the penis before intercourse have proven roughly 80 percent effective in producing "satisfactory erection" in impotent men who have tried it. The drug alprostadil also is available in an injection kit (Caverject). These drugs work by relaxing smooth muscle, which causes the blood vessels in the penis to dilate, promoting an erection that can last an hour or more. Possible side effects include priapism (prolonged, painful erections). Also, although the injections are done with a tiny needle, and are supposed to be painless when done properly (proper technique is crucial), this prospect is unappealing to many men. A less invasive technique involves instilling alprostadil into the urethra with a suppository applied with a tiny plunger.

❑ Yohimbine (sold under the brand names Dayto, Yocon, and Yohimex) is a prescription drug that has been approved by the FDA for treatment of impotence. Its effectiveness is questionable, however. Many experts consider it to be, in essence, a placebo. Yohimbine has an effect on the body similar to that of adrenaline; it speeds up the heartbeat and elevates blood pressure. Beware of yohimbine if you have high blood pressure.

❑ If impotence is linked to high levels of the hormone prolactin, bromocriptine (Parlodel) may be prescribed to correct the problem.

❑ A number of vacuum devices are used to promote erection. With these devices, a cylinder is placed over the penis and a hand pump is used to create a vacuum in the cylinder. This in turn causes blood to flow into the penis, creating an erection. The user then puts a constriction band around the base of the penis, causing the erection to last up to thirty minutes. These devices are available by prescription only. Problems abound with this technique, however.

❑ Some men turn to inflatable penile implants to mechanically create erections. Penile implants are surgically installed devices that are made of silicone or polyurethane. One type is made of two semirigid but bendable rods; another type consists of a pump, a fluid-filled reservoir, and two cylinders into which the fluid is pumped to create an erection. There have been many reports of problems with inflatable devices. With the development of more effective agents, implants are now considered to be a last resort, to be tried only when all other methods have failed.

❑ Dr. Robert Frankt of Budapest University in Hungary found a great increase in sexual vitality and energy in men using a combination of two herbs, green oats (Avena sativa) and stinging nettle. "Feeling one's oats" is an expression that originated centuries ago, and probably with good reason; a study by the Institute for Advanced Study of Human Sexuality found that men who suffered from reduced sexual desire and diminished performance were helped by green oats. Nettle is full of vital minerals and is good also for allergies, depression, hypoglycemia, prostate and urinary tract disorders, and a host of other problems.

❑ Premature ejaculation (PE) is considered sexual dysfunction. It is not the same thing as impotence, but it too can diminish the quality of one's sex life. Premature ejaculation—reaching orgasm too quickly to satisfy one's partner—is thought to be a learned trait, acquired through the habit of masturbation and immediate gratification, that can be unlearned through counseling. However, if PE begins suddenly, when there was no history of it before, it is probably due to problems with the arteries and veins that run to the penis. Venous leaks may be one of these problems because the extra blood that should be going to the penis and making it erect is draining away, so it is difficult to maintain a good erection for any length of time. This problem is common with older men.

□ *Peyronie's disease* results in a twisting of the penis when it is erect. This is due to plaque or scars blocking the tunica albuginea, a membrane containing the corpora cavernosa, the two long, thin chambers in the penis that fill with blood and create the erection. This prevents the penis from retaining its overall elasticity. When erect, the penis may look deformed and contorted.

□ *See also* HYPERTHYROIDISM and HYPOTHYROIDISM in Part Two.

Incontinence

Incontinence (loss of bladder control) is a common complaint. There are many factors that can cause this annoying problem. Incontinence can be either acute or persistent. Acute incontinence is most often caused by an infection. Persistent incontinence develops over time and tends to last longer. There are several different types of persistent incontinence, among them stress incontinence, urge incontinence, functional incontinence, reflex incontinence, and total incontinence.

Stress incontinence is the most common bladder control problem. This is leakage that occurs when a person coughs, sneezes, laughs, lifts a heavy object, or otherwise increases pressure in the lower abdomen. The bladder is rarely completely emptied. Dribbling is more common than complete evacuation of the bladder. This problem is a result of weakened pelvic muscles, which can be due to aging, obesity, and/or pregnancy.

Urge incontinence is the result of an overactive bladder. The detrusor muscle, which surrounds the bladder, may involuntary contract and begin the flow of urine. Frequent urination is common with this type of incontinence, as is nocturnal urination, especially in men. Difficulty urinating may also be due to prostate inflammation. Possible underlying causes of urge incontinence include a history of pelvic inflammatory disease, abdominal surgery, stimulants such alcohol and coffee, and bladder infection. It may also be due to prostate problems.

Functional incontinence is characterized by an uncontrollable urge to empty the bladder before you can reach the bathroom. It can be caused by stress; changes in environment, such as having to stay in the hospital and not being able to get to the bathroom in time; and mobility restrictions. Some individuals are not aware when their bladders are full, and this loss of sensation can lead to urine leakage. This is reflex incontinence, and it is most often due to spinal cord injury or other neurological impairment. Total incontinence is the unpredictable loss of urine at all times. It can be caused by neurological dysfunction, abdominal surgery, spinal cord injury, or an anatomical defect.

Incontinence is most common in people over fifty, but loss of bladder control can occur at any age, especially in pregnant women. It is wrong to assume that loss of bladder control is an inevitable part of getting older. It is also wrong to assume that nothing can be done about this problem.

NUTRIENTS

SUPPLEMENT	SUGGESTED DOSAGE	COMMENTS
Very Important		
Free-form amino acid complex	As directed on label.	Helps to strengthen bladder muscle. Use a product made from a vegetable source.
Important		
Calcium and magnesium	1,500 mg daily. 350 mg daily.	To aid in controlling bladder spasms.
Helpful		
Multivitamin and mineral complex with vitamin B complex	As directed on label.	Aids in relieving stress and supplies all needed nutrients.
Potassium	99 mg daily.	Aids in balancing sodium and potassium in the body.
Vitamin A and vitamin E	As directed on label. If you are pregnant, do not exceed 10,000 IU daily. 600 IU daily.	To aid in normalizing bladder muscle function. Use d-alpha-tocopherol form.
Zinc	80 mg daily. Do not exceed a total of 100 mg daily from all supplements.	For improved bladder function. Also enhances the immune system.

HERBS

□ Kidney Bladder Formula from Nature's Way and SP-6 Cornsilk Blend from Solaray are herbal formulas that have a diuretic effect and reduce bladder spasms. Take 2 capsules twice daily.

RECOMMENDATIONS

□ Stay away from alcohol, caffeine, carbonated beverages, coffee, chocolate, refined or processed foods, and simple sugars. Chemicals in food, drugs, and impure water have an adverse effect on the bladder.

□ If you are overweight, adopt a healthy weight-loss diet and exercise program to help you lose the excess pounds. Obesity is a common factor in incontinence. (*See* OBESITY in Part Two.)

□ Do not delay emptying the bladder. Making sure that you urinate every two to three waking hours—"voiding by the clock"—can help.

□ Do not use "feminine hygiene sprays," packaged douches, bubble baths, or tampons, sanitary pads, or toilet paper containing fragrance. The chemicals these products contain are potentially irritating.

□ Do pelvic exercises such as Kegel's exercises (*see under* PROLAPSE OF THE UTERUS in Part Two). These are useful because weak pelvic muscles are often involved in bladder control problems. Daily exercises can strengthen pelvic muscles and improve bladder control. Exercising your muscles for just five minutes three times a day can make a big difference. The National Kidney and Urologic Diseases Information Clearinghouse (*see* HEALTH AND MEDICAL ORGANIZATIONS in the Appendix) can supply very useful information on all types of pelvic exercises.

CONSIDERATIONS

❏ Anyone who is experiencing bladder control problems should consult a physician to check for possible underlying causes and investigate the possibilities for treatment. The appropriate type of treatment depends on the type of bladder control problem.

❏ *Cantharis* is a homeopathic remedy for pain during urination and for frequent urination.

❏ Tolterodine (Detrol), an antispasmodic drug, may be prescribed for some types of incontinence. Muscle relaxers and calcium channel blockers may be tried as well.

❏ Local injections of Botilinum toxin (BoTox) are sometimes recommended for men who have bladder control difficulties related to prostate problems.

❏ For names and addresses of organizations that can provide additional information on incontinence and its treatments, *see* HEALTH AND MEDICAL ORGANIZATIONS in the Appendix.

Indigestion (Dyspepsia)

Indigestion may be a symptom of a disorder in the stomach or the intestines, or it may be a disorder in itself. Symptoms can include abdominal pain, allergic symptoms, belching, a bloated feeling, a burning sensation after eating, chronic bowel irritation, chronic fatigue, constipation, diarrhea, gas, insomnia, joint and muscle pain, nausea, rumbling noises, skin disorders, sugar cravings, and vomiting. Heartburn often accompanies indigestion.

Swallowing air—by chewing with the mouth open, talking while chewing, or gulping down food—can cause indigestion. Drinking liquids with meals contributes to indigestion because it dilutes the enzymes needed for digestion (a lack of digestive enzymes can cause intestinal problems). Certain foods and beverages can cause indigestion because they are irritating to the digestive tract. These include alcohol, caffeine, greasy, spicy, or refined foods, and vinegar. Other factors that can cause or contribute to indigestion include intestinal obstruction, lack of friendly bacteria, malabsorption, peptic ulcers, and disorders of the gallbladder, liver, or pancreas. Food allergies and intolerances (such as lactose intolerance) also can cause indigestion.

If food is not digested properly, it ferments in the stomach and upper intestines, producing hydrogen, carbon dioxide, and organic acids. These acids do not help digestion, but are factors in gas and bloating. Foods high in complex carbohydrates, such as grains and legumes, are the primary foods responsible for gas because they are difficult to digest, and therefore are more likely to yield undigested particles on which the intestinal bacteria act. Undigested food and bacteria present in the gut can produce toxins that can damage the mucosal lining, causing *leaky gut syndrome*. This condition occurs when particles of undigested food normally eliminated in the feces pass through tiny rips in the intestinal lining and get absorbed into the system, causing severe digestive distress. Contributing factors include abnormal intestinal flora (candida), food allergies, regular alcohol consumption, and parasites, chemicals or drugs that irritate the small intestines. Psychological factors such as anxiety, stress, worry, or disappointment can disturb the nervous mechanism that controls the contractions of stomach and intestinal muscles.

STOMACH ACID SELF-TEST

Hydrochloric acid (HCl), which is produced by glands in the stomach, is necessary for the breakdown and digestion of many foods. Insufficient amounts of HCl can lead to indigestion. HCl levels often decline with age.

You can determine if you need more hydrochloric acid with this simple test. Take a tablespoon of apple cider vinegar or lemon juice. If this makes your indigestion go away, then you need more stomach acid. If it makes your symptoms worse, then you have too much acid, and you should take care not to take any supplements that contain HCl.

NUTRIENTS

SUPPLEMENT	SUGGESTED DOSAGE	COMMENTS
Very Important		
Glucomannan or Aerobic Bulk Cleanse from Aerobic Life Industries	1 tbsp in a full glass of liquid upon arising. Take separately from other supplements and medications.	Colon cleansers that aid in normal stool formation.
Proteolytic enzymes or Inflazyme Forte from American Biologics or pancreatin	As directed on label, with each meal. Take $\frac{1}{2}$ the recommended dose with snacks.	To aid in the breakdown of protein for proper absorption. Important for combating gas and bloating. *Caution:* Do not give these supplements to a child.
Important		
Acidophilus (Kyo-Dophilus and Probiata from Wakunaga and All Flora from New Chapter are good sources)	As directed on label, $\frac{1}{2}$ hour before each meal.	Necessary for normal digestion. Use a nondairy formula.

Garlic (Kyolic from Wakunaga)	2 capsules 3 times daily, with meals.	Aids in digestion and destroys unwanted bacteria in the bowel.
Omega-3 fatty acids (Intestamend from Health From The Sun is a good source)	As directed on label.	Maintains proper digestive function.
Vitamin B complex	100 mg of each major B vitamin 3 times daily, with meals (amounts of individual vitamins in a complex will vary).	Essential for normal digestion.
plus extra vitamin B$_1$ (thiamine) and	50 mg 3 times daily.	Enhances production of hydrochloric acid.
vitamin B$_6$ and	150 mg twice daily.	Digesting protein increases need for this vitamin, which is required for HCl production.
vitamin B$_{12}$	1,000 mcg twice daily.	Important for proper digestion. Use a lozenge or sublingual form.

Helpful		
AbsorbAid from Nature's Sources	As directed on label.	To prevent acid reflux.
Activated charcoal	As directed on label.	To absorb intestinal gas.
Alfalfa		See under Herbs, below.
Copper	2–3 mg daily.	Required for protein metabolism.
Hydrochloric acid (HCl)	As directed on label.	Required for protein digestion.
L-Carnitine	As directed on label.	Carries fat into the cells for breakdown into energy.
Lecithin granules or	1 tbsp 3 times daily, before meals.	Fat emulsifiers that aid in the breakdown of fats.
capsules or	1,200 mg 3 times daily, before meals.	
phosphatidyl choline	As directed on label.	Restores gastrointestinal mucosa by strengthening the mucosal lining.
L-Methionine	As directed on label, on an empty stomach. Take with water or juice. Do not take with milk. Take with 50 mg vitamin B$_6$ and 100 mg vitamin C for better absorption.	A potent liver detoxifier. (See AMINO ACIDS in Part One.)
Manganese	3–10 mg daily.	Required for fat and carbohydrate metabolism.
Multienzyme complex	As directed on label. Take with meals.	To improve digestion. Do not use a formula containing HCl.
N-Acetylcysteine (NAC)	500–1,000 mg daily, on an empty stomach with a small amount of B$_6$ and vitamin C.	Essential for repair of the large, and especially the small, intestines. Also detoxifies harmful substances.
ProFlora whey from Wakunaga	As directed on label.	Feeds the beneficial bacteria in the colon and maintains a proper pH. Note: Do not use this supplement if you have diabetes.
Selenium	100–300 mcg daily. If you are pregnant, do not exceed 40 mcg daily.	Required for proper pancreatic function.
Zinc	20–50 mg daily.	Required for proper carbohydrate digestion and protein metabolism.

HERBS

❏ Acid-Ease from Prevail Corporation is an herbal formula that aids in the breakdown and assimilation of foods, and also contains natural plant enzymes to ease heartburn. It can be taken between meals if needed.

❏ Alfalfa supplies needed vitamin K and trace minerals. It can be taken in liquid or tablet form.

❏ Aloe vera is good for heartburn and other gastrointestinal symptoms. Take 1/4 cup of aloe vera juice on an empty stomach in the morning and again at bedtime.

❏ Anise seeds can help relieve a sour stomach. Chew the whole seeds or grind them and sprinkle on food.

❏ Catnip, chamomile, fennel, fenugreek, goldenseal, papaya, and peppermint are all good for indigestion.
   Caution: Do not use chamomile on an ongoing basis, and avoid it completely if you are allergic to ragweed. Do not take goldenseal internally on a daily basis for more than one week, do not use it during pregnancy, and use it with caution if you are allergic to ragweed.

❏ Ginger is a time-honored remedy for nausea.

❏ A few sprigs of fresh parsley, or 1/4 teaspoon of dried, taken with a glass of warm water, can help relieve indigestion.

❏ Slippery elm is good for inflammation of the colon; use it as an enema for fast relief. (*See* ENEMAS in Part Three.)

❏ Tum-Ease from New Chapter is an herbal formula that enhances digestion.

RECOMMENDATIONS

❏ If you are prone to indigestion, consume well-balanced meals with plenty of fiber-rich foods such as fresh fruits, vegetables, and whole grains.

❏ Include in your diet fresh papaya (which contains papain) and fresh pineapple (which contains bromelain). These are good sources of beneficial digestive enzymes.

❏ Add acidophilus to your diet. Acidophilus can be useful for indigestion because a shortage of the "friendly" bacteria is often the cause. Open 10 capsules or use 1 tablespoon of powdered formula. Neo-Flora from New Chapter and Kyo-Dophilus from Wakunaga are nondairy products that can be used if you have a reaction to dairy products. Acidophilus used as an enema hardly ever results in a problem. You may experience some rumbling and slight disturbance for an hour or so, but it will subside. (*See* ENEMAS in Part Three.)

❏ For disorders such as gas, bloating, and heartburn, try brown rice and/or barley broth. Use 5 parts water to 1 part grain, and boil the mixture, uncovered, for ten minutes. Then put the lid on and simmer for fifty-five minutes more. Strain and cool the liquid. Sip this throughout the day.

❏ Limit your intake of lentils, peanuts, and soybeans. They contain an enzyme inhibitor.

❑ Avoid bakery products, beans, caffeine, carbonated beverages, citrus juices, fried and fatty foods, pasta, peppers, potato chips and other snack foods, red meat, refined carbohydrates (sugar), tomatoes, and salty or spicy foods.

❑ Do not eat dairy products, junk foods, or processed foods. These cause excess mucus formation, which results in inadequate digestion of protein.

❑ For upper gastrointestinal gas, take pancreatin; for lower gastrointestinal gas, take supplemental trace minerals. If you have gas, use the juice of one fresh lemon in a quart of lukewarm water as an enema to balance the body's pH. If gas is constant for days, use an *L. bifidus* enema. This should relieve the problem within hours. (*See* ENEMAS in Part Three.)

❑ For relief of occasional digestive difficulties, use charcoal tablets, available in health food stores. These are good for absorbing gas and toxins. Because they can interfere with the absorption of other medications and nutrients, they should be taken separately, and they should not be taken for long periods of time. Occasional use is not harmful and has no side effects.

❑ If stools are foul-smelling and are accompanied by a burning sensation in the anus, follow a fasting program. This is often a sign that the colon contains toxic material. (*See* ENEMAS and FASTING in Part Three.)

❑ If you have had abdominal surgery (such as a bowel shortened), take pancreatin to help digest foods. If you have hypoglycemia (low blood sugar), you also need pancreatin. After meals, if you have a stuffed feeling and a rumbling or gurgling with bloating and gas, use pancreatin.

❑ If the results of the stomach acid self-test showed that you need more hydrochloric acid, sip 1 tablespoon of pure apple cider vinegar in a glass of water with each meal to aid digestion.

❑ Chew your food thoroughly. Digestion starts in the mouth, and chewing signals the rest of the digestive system to prepare to break down the food for absorption.

❑ Do not eat when you are upset or overtired.

❑ Do not drink liquids while eating. This dilutes the stomach juices and prevents proper digestion.

❑ Find out which foods your body has trouble digesting, and stay away from foods that cause a reaction. (*See* ALLERGIES in Part Two.)

❑ If you are experiencing an excess of acid backup with heartburn symptoms, see your doctor to rule out gastroesophageal reflux disease (GERD) or heartburn.

❑ If you develop heartburn and the symptoms persist, consult your health care provider. If the pain begins to travel down your left arm, or if the sensation is accompanied by a feeling of weakness, dizziness, or shortness of breath, seek emergency medical help. The early symptoms of a heart attack can be very much like those of indigestion, particularly heartburn, and as a result, many people mistakenly dismiss them. (*See* HEART ATTACK in Part Two.)

CONSIDERATIONS

❑ Fructooligosaccharides (FOS) have been clinically proven to promote the growth of friendly intestinal bacteria.

❑ Drinking the juice of a lemon in a cup of water first thing in the morning is good for healing and for purifying the blood.

❑ Exercise, such as brisk walking or stretching, aids the digestive process.

❑ Food combinations are important. Proteins and starches are a poor combination, as are vegetables and fruits. Milk should not be consumed with meals. Foods containing sugar, such as fruit, should not be consumed with proteins or starches.

❑ Older people often lack sufficient hydrochloric acid and pancreatin to digest foods properly.

❑ Many people take antacids to relieve the discomfort of indigestion and heartburn, but these medications may actually make matters worse. Antacids neutralize the acid in the stomach, preventing proper digestion and interfering with the absorption of nutrients. This only leads to continued indigestion. Antacids are useless for gas and bloating.

❑ Most antacids sold in the United States contain aluminum compounds, calcium carbonate, magnesium compounds, or sodium bicarbonate. Aluminum-based antacids can cause constipation. Calcium carbonate can cause a rebound effect in which the stomach produces more acid than before once the antacid's effects wear off. Magnesium compounds can cause diarrhea. Sodium bicarbonate can cause gas and bloating.

❑ Beano from AkPharma, Inc. and Be Sure from Wakunaga of America Company are good for preventing gas. These products must be taken with the first bite of food to be effective.

❑ The *Johns Hopkins Medical Letter* reported that reversible impotence or breast enlargement may result from prolonged, excessive (more than 3 grams a day) use of the heartburn medication cimetidine (Tagamet).

❑ *See also* ENZYMES in Part One.

❑ *See also* ALLERGIES in Part Two and take the self-test.

❑ *See also* DIVERTICULITIS; FOODBORNE/WATERBORNE DISEASE; GALLBLADDER DISORDERS; HEARTBURN/GASTROESOPHAGEAL REFLUX DISEASE (GERD); IRRITABLE BOWEL SYNDROME; LACTOSE INTOLERANCE; MOTION SICKNESS; PANCREATITIS; PEPTIC ULCER; and/or ULCERATIVE COLITIS, all in Part Two.

Infertility

Infertility is usually defined as the failure to conceive after a year or more of regular sexual activity during the time of ovulation. It may also refer to the inability to carry a pregnancy to term. Infertility affects some 6.1 million American couples, and pinpointing the exact cause of the problem can be difficult. Ovulation, fertilization, and the journey of the fertilized ovum through the fallopian tube and finally into the uterus are highly intricate processes. Many events must work together perfectly for pregnancy to occur.

In 40 percent of infertile couples, problems affecting the male partner are either partially or wholly the cause of infertility. For men, infertility is most often the result of a low sperm count or an anatomical abnormality. A variety of factors can result in a low sperm count, including alcohol consumption; endocrine disorders; exposure to toxins, radiation, or excessive heat; recent acute illness or prolonged fever; testicular injury; and, very rarely, mumps-induced wasting of the testicles. Varicoceles, abnormal enlargements of veins that drain the testicles, can cause infertility in men because the veins of the testes no longer moderate the temperature of the testicles correctly, and this can negatively affect sperm.

For women, the most common causes of infertility include ovulatory failure or defect, blocked fallopian tubes, endometriosis, and uterine fibroids. Some women develop antibodies to their partners' sperm, in effect becoming allergic to them. Chlamydia, a sexually transmitted disease that strikes 4 million Americans a year, causes many cases of infertility. Psychological issues, such as stress or fear of parenthood, may contribute to infertility as well, although stress is usually the result of infertility, not the cause of it.

The following are the most common reasons couples are unable to conceive:

- The woman has endometriosis.

- The man has abnormal sperm, a low sperm count, or erectile disfunction.

- The woman's fallopian tubes are blocked.

- Ovulation takes place rarely or irregularly.

- The couple is unable to have complete sexual intercourse.

- The cervical mucous attacks and kills the sperm.

- The woman does not manufacture enough progesterone to carry a baby to term.

- The woman is over thirty-four (fertility declines rapidly after that age).

Often, more than one cause for infertility is found, and in approximately 20 percent of cases, nothing that would seem to inhibit conception can be found.

OVULATION TIMING SELF-TEST

If you wish to become pregnant, there are a number of tests available over the counter that can help you determine the best time to attempt to conceive. These tests predict the time of ovulation by detecting the release of luteinizing hormone (LH), which in turn triggers the release of the egg.

A chemically treated dipstick detects the LH in urine samples. If the hormone has been released, the stick changes color. After a positive result, ovulation takes place within twelve to thirty-six hours. Remember, however, that no test is 100-percent accurate.

Unless otherwise specified, the following nutrients in this section are recommended for either or both partners.

NUTRIENTS

SUPPLEMENT	SUGGESTED DOSAGE	COMMENTS
Essential		
Selenium	200–400 mcg daily. If you become pregnant, cut back to no more than 40 mcg daily.	Deficiency leads to reduced sperm count and has been linked to sterility in men and infertility in women.
Vitamin C with bioflavonoids	2,000–6,000 daily, in divided doses.	Important in sperm production. Keeps the sperm from clumping and makes them more motile.
Vitamin E	Start with 200 IU daily and increase gradually to 400–1,000 IU daily.	Needed for balanced hormone production. Has been known as the "sex vitamin" that carries oxygen to the sex organs and increases sperm count. Use d-alpha-tocopherol form.
Zinc	80 mg daily. Do not exceed a total of 100 mg daily from all supplements.	Important for the functioning of the reproductive organs. Zinc is found in high concentrations in semen.
Important		
Dimethylglycine (DMG) (Aangamik DMG from FoodScience of Vermont)	As directed on label.	Increases oxygen supply in the blood to all tissues. Use a sublingual form.
Octacosanol	As directed on label.	The heart of wheat germ. Aids in hormone production.
Phosphatidyl choline	1,000 mg daily.	Improves the transmission of messages from the brain to the genitals, thus increasing sex drive.
Helpful		
Essential fatty acids (Kyolic-EPA from Wakunaga is a good source)	As directed on label.	Essential for normal glandular function and activity, especially for the reproductive system.
L-Arginine plus	As directed on label.	Increases sperm count and plays a role in sperm motility.
L-cysteine and	As directed on label.	Sulfur-containing amino acids that are effective free radical destroyers and chelating agents that protect glandular and hormonal function.
L-methionine plus	As directed on label.	

L-tyrosine	500 mg daily, on an empty stomach. Take with water or juice. Do not take with milk. Take with 50 mg vitamin B$_6$ and 100 mg vitamin C for better absorption.	Alleviates stress and aids in stabilizing moods. (*See* AMINO ACIDS in Part One.) *Caution:* Do not take tyrosine if you are taking an MAO inhibitor drug.
plus acetylcholine	As directed on label.	Increases sexual pleasure.
Manganese	As directed on label. Take separately from calcium.	Maintains sex hormone production.
Proteolytic enzymes	As directed on label. Take between meals.	Aids in the breakdown of foods. Facilitates absorption of nutrients.
Pycnogenol or grape seed extract	As directed on label. As directed on label.	Powerful antioxidant bioflavonoids that may increase sperm count.
Raw orchic glandular	As directed on label.	For men. Supports testicular function. (*See* GLANDULAR THERAPY in Part Three.)
Raw ovarian glandular	As directed on label.	For women. Supports ovarian function. (*See* GLANDULAR THERAPY in Part Three.)
7-Keto DHEA	As directed on label.	Improves libido.
Vitamin A plus carotenoid complex (Betatene)	15,000 IU daily. As directed on label.	Important in reproductive gland function. Antioxidants and vitamin A precursors.
Vitamin B complex plus extra pantothenic acid (vitamin B$_5$) and vitamin B$_6$ (pyridoxine) and para-aminobenzoic acid (PABA) and folic acid and vitamin B$_{12}$	50 mg of each major B vitamin daily (amounts of individual vitamins in a complex will vary). As directed on label. 50 mg 3 times daily. 50 mg daily. 400 mcg daily. 2,000 mcg daily.	Important in reproductive gland function. Maintains sex hormone production. Helpful for stress. Needed for the synthesis of RNA and DNA. Plays a role in restoring fertility in some women. Protects the egg, sperm, and genetic material. Maintains fertility. Use a sublingual form.

HERBS

❏ Astragalus extract has been reported to stimulate sperm motility.

Caution: Do not use this herb in the presence of a fever.

❏ Damiana, ginseng, sarsaparilla, saw palmetto, and yohimbe enhance sexual function in men. Damiana, dong quai, false unicorn root, ginseng, gotu kola, licorice root, and wild yam root are good for women.

Caution: Do not use ginseng or licorice if you have high blood pressure.

❏ Green oat (*Avena sativa*) extract is an excellent aid if the reason for infertility is the man's inability to maintain an erection.

❏ Yin-yang-huo (*Aceranthus sagittatum*), a Chinese herb also known as horny goat weed is a male aphrodisiac, and may increase sperm count and semen density.

❏ Heavy use of echinacea, ginkgo biloba, and St. John's wort may cause infertility in men, and should be avoided.

RECOMMENDATIONS

❏ Avoid all alcohol; it reduces sperm count in men and can prevent implantation of the fertilized egg in women.

❏ Avoid douching, as this appears to reduce fertility.

❏ Do not take any drugs except those prescribed by your physician. Inform your physician if you are attempting to have a baby. He/she will be able to advise you if your medications may inhibit conception or may be dangerous for the fetus.

❏ Do not smoke, and avoid being around cigarette smoke.

❏ A balanced diet is important. Do not consume animal fats, fried foods, sugar, or junk foods. Do eat pumpkin seeds, bee pollen, or royal jelly.

Caution: Bee pollen may cause an allergic reaction in some people. Start with a small amount, and discontinue use if a rash, wheezing, discomfort, or other symptom occurs.

❏ Some artificial lubricants can prevent the sperm from reaching the cervix. Saliva may also have a detrimental affect on spermatozoa.

❏ Investigate the possibility of heavy metal intoxication, which may affect ovulation. A hair analysis can reveal heavy metal poisoning. (*See* HAIR ANALYSIS in Part Three.)

❏ Infertility is stressful, but do all you can to reduce the stresses in your life. Learn stress management techniques to help you deal with stresses that cannot be avoided. (*See* STRESS in Part Two.)

CONSIDERATIONS

❏ Because there are so many causes of infertility, in most cases the opinion of a qualified health care professional is needed.

❏ Sperm factors account for approximately 40 percent of all cases of infertility. Some causes of sperm inadequacy (recent illness, endocrine disorders) may be temporary or reversible, but others are not. Except for artificial insemination, orthodox drug therapy is ineffective in such cases.

❏ Varicoceles are sometimes treatable with surgery, and fertility can sometimes be restored.

❏ The ulcer medications cimetidine (Tagamet) and ranitidine (Zantac) may decrease the sperm count and even produce impotence.

❏ Strict adherence to a gluten-free diet has enabled some previously sterile men to become fathers. A gluten-free diet has also enabled women who were previously unable to conceive to become pregnant. *See* CELIAC DISEASE in Part Two for more information about a gluten-free diet.

Fertility Tests

There are a number of tests—some for men, some for women—that may be performed if conception does not occur within a twelve-month period. It is both easier and more cost-effective to test the male partner first before going on to the more invasive techniques needed to test the female partner. The following table lists some of the most frequently performed fertility tests.

Tests Performed on Men

TEST	DESCRIPTION
Endrocrine test	Blood tests are done to determine levels of follicle-stimulating hormone (FSH), luteinizing hormone (LH), and thyroid hormones (T). LH levels are tested only if T levels are abnormal.
Postcoital test	The partners have sexual intercourse and the ejaculate is tested for surviving sperm.
Semen analysis	A sample of semen is examined no longer than one hour after ejaculation. It is tested for sperm motility (the percentage of sperm that are swimming) and morphology (the percentage that are normally shaped).
Sperm penetration test	Sperm is tested to see if it has the ability to penetrate hamster egg cells. This indicates the sperm's ability to penetrate the partner's egg.
Testicular biopsy	A sample of testicular tissue is examined under a microscope to determine the condition of the sperm, or to determine if sperm are being made.
X-ray	This test is done to check for damage to the ducts in the male responsible for transporting the sperm to the penis.

Tests Performed on Women

TEST	DESCRIPTION
Endometrial biopsy	A tiny sample of the endometrium (the lining of the uterus) is taken in the later part of the menstrual cycle and tested to see if there is enough progesterone in the lining as it matures. If not, the condition is called luteal phase defect. It can be treated with hormone therapy.
FSH test	A blood sample is taken on day three of the menstrual cycle and tested for FSH. FSH levels increase as a woman reaches menopause. If there is a high FSH level, pregnancy is unlikely.
Hysterosalpingo-gram (HSG)	Dye is inserted through the cervix into the fallopian tubes and uterus, and an x-ray is taken to determine whether the tubes are open and if the uterus is a normal shape.
Laparoscopy	A surgical procedure in which a physician examines the reproductive organs by means of a tiny scope. If scar tissue or endometrial buildup is found, it can be removed by means of the scope as well.
Postcoital test (PCT, Sims-Huhner Test)	The partners have intercourse 2–8 hours before this test. A sample of cervical mucus and tissue is removed and examined to determine whether the mucus or the cervix is prohibiting fertilization. Undergoing a PCT is much the same as having a Pap smear.
Transvaginal ultrasound	A probe is inserted into the vagina to look for fibroid tumors or ovarian cysts. This can also be done to track early pregnancies.

❏ Marijuana and cocaine lower sperm count.

❏ The transdermal use of natural progesterone cream may benefit infertile women.

❏ Researchers at Britain's Medical Research Council and Edinburgh University scientists have found a clue to male infertility: gene defects that interfere with proper sperm production. Located on the Y chromosome, these genes are involved in producing a protein that contributes to fertility. Infertility results when a mutation disrupts the gene's normal functioning. More research may lead to new infertility treatments, including gene therapy.

❏ If a woman has developed antibodies to her partner's sperm, it may help to have him use a condom for at least thirty days. The sperm antibodies should then decrease, and intercourse without the use of a condom during the time of ovulation may lead to conception.

❏ Conception is more likely if the woman is on the bottom during intercourse.

❑ Sperm count reaches its highest level after two or three days of abstinence from any sexual activity, but sperm that remains in a man's body for longer than a month is less effective at fertilizing an egg.

❑ A woman who suffers from such premenstrual symptoms as bloating and breast tenderness is probably ovulating, so if she is having difficulty becoming pregnant, the cause probably lies elsewhere.

❑ More women are waiting to bear children in later reproductive years. However, a woman's fertility begins to decrease when she reaches her thirties.

❑ Para-aminobenzoic acid (PABA) stimulates the pituitary gland and sometimes restores fertility to some women who cannot conceive.

❑ Caffeine consumption may prevent some women from becoming pregnant.

❑ Procedures known as transcervical balloon tuboplasty (TBT) and selective fallopian tube canalization have roughly 90-percent success rates in removing obstructions of the fallopian tubes. TBT is similar to the artery-clearing technique called angioplasty. A tiny balloon is inserted into the tube by means of a catheter; when the catheter reaches the blockage, the balloon is inflated to stretch and clear the blocked section of the tube. The procedure may be performed in about fifteen minutes under either local or general anesthesia. Because this procedure is relatively non-invasive (no incision is required), the risks involved are few. However, there is a chance that a tube may become blocked again. This happens in approximately 20 percent of the women who undergo the procedure. Fallopian tube canalization produces similar results to those of TBT.

❑ Assisted reproductive techniques (ART) may be tried if all other methods have been attempted. These techniques include the following:

• Gamete intrafallopian tube transfer (GIFT). In this technique, eggs and sperm are mixed and put into the fallopian tube immediately, without waiting to see if fertilization has taken place.

• Intracytoplasmic sperm injection (ICSI). In this procedure, which may be used if the man has a low sperm count or too many abnormal sperm, the woman is injected with healthy sperm extracted from the testes.

• In vitro fertilization (IVF). Here a woman's eggs are fertilized outside the womb and inserted into the uterus. This is usually done if the fallopian tubes are blocked.

• Zygote intrafallopian tube transfer (ZIFT). Eggs and sperm are combined, and if an egg is fertilized, it is inserted into the fallopian tube.

❑ A University of Michigan study indicated that intense exercise may result in a drop in the production of hormones involved in potency, fertility, and sex drive.

❑ The use of donor eggs to impregnate women who can-

not conceive on their own is controversial and is extremely expensive.

❑ Your health care provider must get your consent before performing diagnostic tests to determine the cause of infertility. There may be risks involved any time you penetrate the body using a tube, needle, or viewing instrument, or expose the body to the radiation, drugs, anesthetics, and dye materials used in certain imaging techniques. The risks of any given procedure vary depending on your age and health status, and the skill of the practitioner.

Inflammation

Inflammation is a natural reaction to injury or infection. The affected tissues swell, redden, become warm and tender, and may be painful. Things that can trigger inflammation include drug overuse, environmental toxins, free radical damage, infections, injury, trauma, and bacterial, fungal, or viral infection, to name a few. Unfortunately, it is often difficult to identify the sources of inflammation.

Any organ or tissue of the body, internal or external, can become inflamed. Internal inflammation is often caused by bacterial infection, but can also be caused by disorders such as allergies, arthritis, asthma, autoimmune diseases, Crohn's disease, inflammatory bowel disorders, osteoarthritis, peptic ulcer disease, or ulcerative colitis. External inflammation is most often the result of injury, but can also result from (or be aggravated by) allergies, infection, and other factors.

NUTRIENTS

SUPPLEMENT	SUGGESTED DOSAGE	COMMENTS
Essential		
Vitamin B complex	50 mg of each major B vitamin 3 times daily (amounts of individual vitamins in a complex will vary).	Needed for tissue repair.
plus extra vitamin B₁₂	2,000 mcg daily.	
Vitamin C with bioflavonoids	3,000–6,000 mg daily, in divided doses.	Essential to the healing process and in reducing inflammation. Use a buffered form.
Very Important		
Carotenoid complex	As directed on label.	Strengthens the immune response.
Essential fatty acids (evening primrose oil, flaxseed oil, and fish oils are good sources)	As directed on label.	Reduces inflammation.
Grape seed extract	As directed on label.	Powerful antioxidant.
Proteolytic enzymes or Inflazyme Forte from American Biologics	As directed on label, between meals and at bedtime, for 1 month. 2 tablets twice daily, between meals.	Aids in controlling inflammation.

Superoxide dismutase (SOD)	As directed on label.	A high-potency free radical scavenger that reduces infection and inflammation.
Zinc	50 mg daily. Do not exceed a total of 100 mg daily from all supplements.	Helps to control inflammation and promotes healing. Use zinc gluconate lozenges or OptiZinc for best absorption.
Important		
Bromelain	As directed on label. Take on an empty stomach with 100–500 mg magnesium and 500 mg L-cysteine to enhance results. Take separately from copper and iron.	Has anti-inflammatory activity and increases the breakdown of fibrin, which forms around the inflamed area, blocking the blood and lymphatic vessels and leading to swelling.
Garlic (Kyolic from Wakunaga)	2 capsules 3 times daily, with meals.	Has natural anti-inflammatory properties.
Micellized Vitamin A emulsion from American Biologics	As directed on label.	Supplies vitamins A and E in easily assimilable emulsion form to destroy free radicals, boost the immune system, and help the body to use oxygen efficiently.
Multimineral complex	As directed on label.	Supplies important minerals. Needed to reduce stress. Use a formula high in calcium.
Silica or horsetail	As directed on label, twice daily.	Supplies silicon, which aids in absorption of calcium and repair of connective tissues. See under Herbs, below.
Helpful		
Beta-1,3-D-glucan	As directed on label.	Boosts immune function and fights inflammation.
Kelp or alfalfa	1,000–1,500 mg daily.	Contains a balance of essential minerals plus chlorophyll, which cleanses the blood. See under Herbs, below.
Raw thymus glandular	As directed on label.	Improves thymus function— important for immune function.
Selenium	200 mcg daily. If you are pregnant, do not exceed 40 mcg daily.	A powerful antioxidant and aid in inflammation reduction.
VitaCarte from Phoenix BioLabs	As directed on label.	Contains bovine cartilage, which has been shown to be effective in reducing inflammation.
Vitamin E	400–600 IU daily.	Effective antioxidant and reducer of inflammation. Use d-alpha-tocopherol form.

HERBS

❑ Alfalfa is a good source of minerals and chlorophyll.

❑ Aloe vera juice is helpful for inflammation.

❑ Bilberry contains flavonoids that reduce inflammation.

❑ Boswellia and turmeric (curcumin) help to reduce inflammation.

❑ Cat's claw is good for inflammation and healing.

❑ Echinacea, ginger, goldenseal, pau d'arco, red clover, and yucca are all good for inflammation.

Caution: Do not take goldenseal internally on a daily basis for more than one week at a time, do not use during pregnancy, and use with caution if you are allergic to ragweed.

❑ A poultice that combines fenugreek, flaxseed, and slippery elm can be applied directly to the affected area to subdue inflammation. As an alternative, a goldenseal or mustard poultice can be used. *See* USING A POULTICE in Part Three.

❑ Horsetail extract is a good source of silica, beneficial for healing and repair of bones and connective tissue.

❑ Olive leaf extract eases inflammation and is good for any bacterial infection.

RECOMMENDATIONS

❑ Eat a diet composed of 75 percent raw foods, and drink plenty of herbal teas and juices.

❑ Eat foods high in flavonoids, which are powerful antioxidants and useful for inflammation reduction. Spinach and blueberries are excellent sources of flavonoids. Strawberries contain smaller amounts. Quercetin, found in onions, is good for inflammation as well.

❑ Consume half of a fresh pineapple or fresh papaya daily. Pineapple contains bromelain and papaya contains papain, both enzymes that reduce swelling and inflammation. It should reduce the pain and swelling in two to six days. Only fresh pineapple or papaya (not canned) is effective. Bromelain is also available in pill form.

❑ Eat coldwater fish such as herring, mackerel, salmon, and sardines, as they are rich sources of essential fatty acids.

❑ Limit saturated fats and salt.

❑ Avoid cola, sugar, white flour products, and junk foods.

❑ For quick results, *see* FASTING in Part Three and follow the program.

CONSIDERATIONS

❑ Bacterial arthritis, which causes painful inflammation of the joints, is usually associated with an infection elsewhere in the body, such as in the lungs, kidney, or gallbladder.

❑ The complex sugar beta-1,3-D-glucan (found in the cell walls of baker's yeast, and a variety of fungi, such as maitake and reishi mushrooms) has proven to be a powerful immune booster. When beta-1,3-D-glucan attaches to the receptor site on macrophage cells, these immune cells are activated to attack and destroy invading organisms and reduce infection and inflammation.

❑ The traditional methods for relieving inflammation are positioning the affected part properly (including splinting, if necessary), applying heat and/or ice (heat and cold therapies), taking painkillers along with nutritional supplements, and getting plenty of rest. Nonsteroidal anti-inflammatory drugs (NSAIDs) are prescribed to 70 to 80 million people a year for chronic inflammation.

☐ *See also* ABSCESS; ARTHRITIS; and SPRAINS, STRAINS, AND OTHER INJURIES OF THE MUSCLES AND JOINTS, all in Part Two.

☐ *See also* PAIN CONTROL in Part Three.

Influenza

Influenza, better known as "the flu," is a highly contagious viral infection of the upper respiratory tract. There are two types of influenza viruses, designated type A and type B, that cause this acute infection of the throat, nose, bronchial tubes, lungs, and middle ear. The virus enters the body's airways through mucous membranes in the nose, eyes, or mouth. Because this illness can be spread easily by coughing and sneezing, influenza epidemics are very common, especially in winter. During an epidemic, from 25 to more than 50 percent of the population can become infected. The flu is unpredictable and can strike anyone, at any age. More than 200 different individual strains of virus can cause colds and flu, and strains of these viruses are constantly changing, so vaccinations against influenza have been only partly successful in preventing outbreaks of the disease.

The symptoms of influenza begin much like those of the common cold—body aches, cough, fatigue, headache, and hot and cold sweats. In many cases, a fever develops, and you may feel unbearably hot one moment and chilled and shaking the next. Most influenza sufferers have a dry throat and cough. Nausea and vomiting may occur as well. Often, a person with the flu is so weak and so uncomfortable that he or she does not feel like eating or doing anything else. Colds last for about one week to ten days, on average, but the flu lasts longer—up to twelve days or more, followed by a week or more of residual coughing and fatigue.

Influenza is rarely dangerous in healthy adults sixty years of age or younger, but it does make a person more susceptible to pneumonia, ear infections, and sinus trouble. The disease is linked to 20,000 deaths in the United States every year. Among people sixty-five or older, serious respiratory infections such as influenza and pneumonia are the fifth leading cause of death, so the flu is clearly a serious infection for older people. High-risk flu groups also include those of any age with weakened immune systems or with chronic conditions such as heart or lung disease.

Unless otherwise specified, the dosages recommended here are for adults. For a child between the ages of twelve and seventeen, reduce the dose to three-quarters of the recommended amount. For a child between six and twelve, use one-half of the recommended dose, and for a child under the age of six, use one-quarter of the recommended amount.

NUTRIENTS

SUPPLEMENT	SUGGESTED DOSAGE	COMMENTS
Essential		
ACES + Zn from Carlson Labs	As directed on label.	Contains vitamins A, C, and E, plus selenium and zinc. Take this supplement in addition to zinc lozenges as directed below.
Vitamin A	15,000 IU daily. If you are pregnant, do not exceed 10,000 IU daily.	A powerful antioxidant and immunity booster.
plus natural beta-carotene	15,000 IU daily.	Antioxidants and precursors of vitamin A.
or carotenoid complex (Betatene)	As directed on label.	
Vitamin C with bioflavonoids	5,000–20,000 mg daily, in divided doses. (*See* ASCORBIC ACID FLUSH in Part Three.)	Strengthens the immune system by increasing the number and quality of white blood cells. For a child, use buffered vitamin C or calcium ascorbate.
Zinc lozenges	For adults and children over 6 years of age, one 15-mg lozenge every two hours for 2 days, starting at the first signs of the flu. Then reduce dosage to a total of 80 mg or less daily.	A potent immunostimulant that nourishes the cells. Keep these on hand and use them as soon as symptoms develop.
Important		
Colloidal silver	As directed on label.	Good for viral infections. Promotes healing.
Free-form amino acid complex	As directed on label.	Helps to repair tissue and control fever. Free-form amino acids are rapidly absorbed into the body.
Garlic (Kyolic from Wakunaga)	2 capsules 3 times daily.	Has antiviral and antibacterial properties.
L-Lysine	500 mg daily, on an empty stomach. Take with water or juice. Do not take with milk. Take with 50 mg vitamin B$_6$ and 100 mg vitamin C for better absorption.	Aids in combating viral infection and preventing outbreaks of cold sores in and around the mouth, common when the body is under stress from illness. (*See* AMINO ACIDS in Part One.) *Caution:* Do not take lysine longer than 6 months at a time.
N-acetylcysteine (NAC)	As directed on label.	Thins mucus and aids in preventing respiratory disease.
Helpful		
Dioxychlor from American Biologics	10–20 drops sublingually, 1–2 times daily. Also, add 20 drops to 1 oz water and instill a dropperful in each nostril daily.	An important antibacterial, antifungal, and antiviral agent. Especially good for older adults.
Maitake extract	As directed on label.	Helps to boost immunity and fight viral infection.
or shiitake extract	As directed on label.	
or reishi extract	As directed on label.	
Multivitamin and mineral complex with vitamin B complex	100 mg of each major B vitamin daily (amounts of individual vitamins in a complex will vary).	All vitamins are needed for healing. Necessary in all cellular and enzyme functions. Reduces stress caused by viral infection.
and selenium	200 mcg daily. If you are pregnant, do not exceed 40 mcg daily.	Boosts the immune response, enhancing the body's ability to fight infection.

HERBS

❏ Astragalus, black cherry, echinacea, ginger, goldenseal, pau d'arco, slippery elm, and yarrow tea are good for influenza. Combining peppermint tea with any of these herbal teas is effective for helping to open up the nasal passages. Echinacea is also good for children.

Caution: Do not take goldenseal internally on a daily basis for more than one week at a time, do not use it during pregnancy, and use it with caution if you are allergic to ragweed.

❏ The herb boneset works as an expectorant and eliminates mucus from the lungs.

❏ If it is necessary to lower fever, take catnip tea enemas and 1/4–1/2 teaspoon lobelia tincture every three to four hours until fever drops. This is good for children also.

Caution: Do not use this mixture if you are pregnant or breastfeeding, and do not give it to a child under one year old. Do not take lobelia internally on an ongoing basis.

❏ Cat's claw may cut the duration of the flu. Cold-X10 from Olympian Labs is a complex that contains cat's claw and many nutrients effective against flu and colds.

❏ Cayenne (capsicum) helps to keep mucus flowing, aiding in preventing congestion and headaches. Simply add a bit of cayenne powder to soups and other foods.

❏ ClearLungs from RidgeCrest Herbals is a Chinese herbal formula designed to provide nutrients to the lungs.

❏ The Chinese mushroom cordyceps is available in a tonic formula to support the lungs.

❏ At the first sign of a cough, place one dropperful of alcohol-free echinacea and goldenseal extract in your mouth and hold it there for five to ten minutes. Repeat this every hour for three to four hours. This stops the virus from multiplying.

❏ Alcohol-free echinacea and goldenseal combination extract is recommended for children. Give a child 4 to 6 drops of combination extract in water or juice every four hours for three days. Echinacea is very effective at enhancing the body's own natural defenses. Goldenseal is a natural antibiotic and helps to relieve congestion.

❏ Elderberry has antiviral properties and reduces flu symptoms.

❏ Ephedra (ma huang) is beneficial for relief of congestion and coughing.

Caution: Do not use this herb if you suffer from anxiety, glaucoma, heart disease, high blood pressure, or insomnia, or if you are taking a monoamine oxidase (MAO) inhibitor drug.

❏ Eucalyptus oil is beneficial for relieving congestion. Put 5 drops in a hot bath or 6 drops in a cup of boiling water, put a towel over your head, and inhale the vapors.

❏ Fenugreek breaks up phlegm and mucus, and slippery elm helps remove them from the body.

❏ Fenu-Thyme from Nature's Way helps to rid the nose and sinuses of mucus by loosening it so it can flow easily. It does not dry up the mucus, so healing is faster.

❏ Lung Tonic Extract by Herbs Etc. is a mixture of herbs designed to protect the lungs.

❏ Maitake, shiitake, and reishi mushrooms possess beta-1,3-D-glucan, a type of polysaccharide that stimulates the immune cells. Their immune-boosting power makes them essential for fighting the flu.

❏ Olive leaf extract enhances immune function and fights all types of infection, including the flu virus.

❏ For cough and sore throat, mix 1 tablespoon of slippery elm bark powder with 1 cup of boiling water and 1/2 cup honey. Take 1 teaspoon of this mixture every three to four hours. It can be taken either hot or cold, as you prefer.

RECOMMENDATIONS

❏ Consume plenty of fluids, especially fresh juices, herbal teas, soups, and quality water, to prevent dehydration and help flush out the body. To shorten the length of the flu, go on a liquid diet emphasizing hot herbal teas and hot broth for one or two days.

❏ Take hot chicken or turkey soup. This is grandmother's old remedy and it is still good today. Add a bit of cayenne pepper to help prevent and break up congestion. Avoid dairy products, mucus-forming foods, and sugar.

❏ Sleep and rest as much as possible.

❏ In treating a sore throat, avoid using aspirin chewing gum and aspirin gargles. Aspirin applied directly to mucous membranes does not reduce pain and can act as an irritant.

❏ Do not take zinc at the same time you eat or drink citrus fruits or juices. It will diminish the effectiveness of the zinc. Do consume a lot of other types of fruit.

❏ Do not take iron supplements while a fever exists.

❏ Do not give aspirin to a child who has the flu. The combination of aspirin and a viral illness has been linked to the development of Reye's syndrome, a potentially dangerous complication. (*See* REYE'S SYNDROME in Part Two.)

❏ Fever is one of the body's major defense mechanisms against the flu. Flu viruses do not survive well in a warmer environment. If you have a fever, do not try to suppress it, unless it is over 103°F.

❏ If you consume alcoholic beverages even occasionally, or if you have liver or kidney disease, be cautious about using the painkiller acetaminophen (Tylenol, Datril, and others). The combination of alcohol and acetaminophen has been associated with serious liver problems.

❏ If you are over sixty-five, see your health care provider. Influenza can cause serious complications for people in this age group.

❏ Since flu viruses are often transmitted by way of the hands, wash your hands frequently with an antibacterial soap. Rinse and dry your hands thoroughly and keep them away from your eyes, nose, and mouth. If you sneeze, use a disposable tissue.

❏ Buy a new toothbrush—toothbrushes can harbor viruses and prolong the illness.

❏ Try one or more of the following homeopathic remedies to ease flu symptoms:

• *Anas barbariae* (Oscillococcinum), a homeopathic treatment, works very well if taken at the first signs of the flu.

• *Aconitum napellus*, *Belladonna*, and *Eupatorium perfoliatum* help to ease flu symptoms.

• HP 2 from Metagenics is a homeopathic combination remedy containing *Aconite*, *Bryonia*, *Eucalyptus globulus*, *Eupatorium perfoliatum*, *Ipecacuanha*, *Gelsemium*, *Phosphorus*, and *Pulsatilla*, to relieve chills, fatigue, fever, headache, nasal congestion, sneezing, and overall aching and discomfort. You should not use this formula if you are pregnant.

CONSIDERATIONS

❏ Antibiotics are useless against viral illnesses like influenza. The best way to get rid of the flu or any other infectious illness is to attack it head-on by strengthening the immune system. The thymus and the adrenal glands are the power seat of the immune system. When the body is getting sick, or is already sick, it is under stress, and stress taxes the immune system. Researchers have linked vulnerability to colds and flu to psychological stress.

❏ Zanamivir (Relenza), an inhaled antiviral drug, battles flu symptoms and shortens the duration of the illness. It has also been shown to be effective in preventing the flu in both strains of influenza. Another medication, oseltamivir (Tamiflu) has shown comparable results. Both of these medications may be beneficial for people with immune system problems.

❏ We do not recommend flu shots in general. Their usefulness is questionable, and the side effects may be worse than the flu would be. Enhancement of immune function is preferable—and safer. If you are allergic to eggs or chicken, you should definitely avoid flu shots, as the vaccine is produced from chicken embryos.

❏ Children who have the flu frequently should be checked for thyroid malfunctions. (*See* HYPOTHYROIDISM in Part Two.)

❏ The term "stomach flu" is commonly used to refer to another condition, gastroenteritis. This is not influenza, but an acute inflammation of the lining of the stomach. Gastroenteritis is characterized by diarrhea, vomiting, and abdominal cramps that vary in severity, and may be accompanied by fever, chills, head and body aches, chest pain and cough, and extreme fatigue. It may be caused by a number of different factors, including food poisoning, viral infection, alcohol intoxication, sensitivity to drugs, and certain allergies. This type of illness usually runs its course in one or two days.

❏ *See also* COMMON COLD and PNEUMONIA, both in Part Two.

Insect Allergy

There are only a few stinging insects in the United States that can cause an allergic reaction: honeybees, hornets, yellow jackets, bumblebees, wasps, spiders, and ants. Insects of the group known as *hymenoptera*, which includes bees, wasps, hornets, and ants, cause an allergic reaction in 5 out of 1,000 people. This reaction is known as an insect venom allergy, and it can be dangerous, even life threatening. The yellow jacket and honeybee are the cause of most allergic reactions to insects.

Allergic reactions to stings can cause wheezing, tightness in the throat, nausea, diarrhea, hives, itching, pain and swelling in the joints, respiratory distress, and vascular swelling. In a person with a mild allergy to venom, the reaction can occur within a few minutes, but when a person experiences a severe allergic reaction, the symptoms can take longer to appear (ten to twenty minutes). If the reaction to the venom is delayed, symptoms such as fever, hives, inflamed lymph glands, and joint pain can occur. In some circumstances, a person who is highly allergic to insect venom can go into shock (circulatory collapse) and die within minutes. Signs that a dangerous reaction is developing include confusion, difficulty swallowing, extreme drop in blood pressure, hoarseness, labored breathing, severe anxiety, severe swelling, weakness, and a feeling of impending disaster. A more severe reaction can also result in closing of the airway, producing unconsciousness.

Some biting insects, such as mosquitoes, can cause allergic skin reactions that appear as scaly and itchy eczema.

NUTRIENTS

SUPPLEMENT	SUGGESTED DOSAGE	COMMENTS
Essential		
Quercetin (Activated Quercetin from Source Naturals)	As directed on label.	A unique bioflavonoid that reduces allergic reactions.
Vitamin C with bioflavonoids	5,000–20,000 mg daily, in divided doses. (*See* ASCORBIC ACID FLUSH in Part Three.)	Acts as an anti-inflammatory and helps fight the toxicity of insect venom. For a child, use buffered vitamin C or calcium ascorbate.
Helpful		
Aller Bee-Gone from CC Pollen	As directed on label.	A combination of herbs, enzymes, and nutrients designed to fight acute allergic symptoms.

| Inflazyme Forte from American Biologics | As directed on label. | A potent enzyme and powerful inflammatory inhibitor. |

HERBS

❑ Calendula is an excellent topical cream to apply to skin irritations.

❑ Herbal flea-repellent pet collars contain oils of cedar, citronella, eucalyptus, pennyroyal, rosemary, and rue. These herbs may be effective insect repellents for humans as well.

Caution: Do not use pennyroyal or rue during pregnancy. Avoid excessive and/or prolonged use.

❑ Lavender may help relieve itching.

❑ Tea tree oil can be rubbed on exposed areas of skin to deter insects. It can also be applied to bites. If pure tea tree oil is too strong, dilute it with canola oil or another low-fragrance vegetable oil until a tolerable strength is achieved.

RECOMMENDATIONS

❑ If you have ever had an allergic reaction to an insect sting, you should have access to an epinephrine (adrenaline) kit at all times. Have your physician prescribe an emergency treatment kit and instruct you in its proper use. Epinephrine raises the blood pressure and speeds the heart rate, counteracting the allergic response. It is best administered via a preloaded syringe found in injection kits. Your emergency kit should also include antihistamine tablets and an identification card listing your medical information.

❑ To avoid insect stings, wear plain, light-colored clothing when spending time outdoors—avoid wearing anything that is flowered or dark. Do not wear shiny jewelry, and do not use hair spray, perfume, scented soaps, or suntan lotion. Avoid wearing sandals or loose-fitting clothes.

❑ Avoid areas where bees are concentrated, such as orchards and flower gardens.

❑ If you are bothered by a yellow jacket, do not squash it; doing so releases a chemical that attracts other yellow jackets and wasps. It is best to leave these insects alone, or to find and destroy the nest after dark, when they are less active.

❑ If you do get stung, *immediately and carefully* remove any stinger left in the skin. It is best not to pull the stinger out. Instead, gently and carefully scrape or tease it out with a sterilized knife. If no knife is readily available, you can use a fingernail or even the edge of a credit card instead. After a sting, be alert for signs that a reaction is developing. Reactions can occur in minutes or hours, and they can progress very quickly. If you have any doubts about your condition, seek treatment at once.

❑ As soon as possible after a bite or sting, soften charcoal tablets or capsules (these can be obtained from health food stores) in warm water and make a paste. Apply this paste to the site and cover it with a clean wet piece of gauze or cotton. It is a good idea to take a few charcoal tablets with you whenever you will be spending time outdoors.

❑ Apply a cold ice pack on the sting to reduce swelling and inflammation.

❑ To neutralize the effects of the venom, apply a paste made of baking soda and lemon juice or vinegar to the affected area.

❑ *Apis mellifica,* a homeopathic remedy, is good for wasp or bee stings. When taken promptly after a bite, it helps to prevent severe swelling and anaphylactic shock. It works quickly and can be used when waiting for medical attention. Another homeopathic remedy, *Silica,* is useful if a stinger is embedded deep in the skin; it forces the object out of the body in a few hours.

CONSIDERATIONS

❑ Sometimes brewer's yeast or garlic rubbed on the skin deters insects. Eating garlic may help also.

❑ A venom extractor called the Lil Sucker is available from Terra Tech (*see* MANUFACTURER AND DISTRIBUTOR INFORMATION in the Appendix). It is small enough to fit inside a pocket or purse. If you get stung, it produces a vacuum that sucks the venom out within two minutes. The end of the extractor can also be used to remove a honeybee stinger.

❑ Antihistamines given by injection or by mouth following a sting can reduce later-appearing symptoms.

❑ When a person has had a severe allergic reaction, the treatment usually involves an injection of adrenaline (epinephrine) and/or cardiopulmonary resuscitation. Corticosteroids may be prescribed to diminish swelling and reduce the hives.

❑ If you are diagnosed with an insect allergy, your physician may suggest immunotherapy, which involves building up tolerance to the venom. Small doses of the venom are introduced into the body over a period of time until your system can tolerate the toxin.

❑ *See also* BEE STING; INSECT BITE; and/or SPIDER BITE in Part Two.

Insect Bite

Many different insects bite, including mosquitoes, fire ants, fleas, gnats, and ticks. Most insect bites are a nuisance, causing localized itching and redness, but are relatively harmless. Others can be serious. Tick bites can spread diseases such as babesiosis, Lyme disease, or Rocky Mountain spotted fever. In some places (principally in developing countries), mosquito bites may transmit malaria and yellow fever, as well as viruses that cause encephalitis, an inflammation of the brain. Spiders, while not technically insects, can cause similar bites. The black widow and brown recluse are two of the most poisonous spiders. Bees, hornets, and yellow jackets may sting in self-defense or to subdue their prey (see BEE STING in Part Two). There are also stings that can be obtained from aquatic life such as jellyfish, sea anemones, and some types of coral.

Unless otherwise specified, the dosages recommended here are for adults. For a child between the ages of twelve and seventeen, reduce the dose to three-quarters the recommended amount. For a child between six and twelve, use one-half the recommended dose, and for a child under the age of six, use one-quarter the recommended amount.

NUTRIENTS

SUPPLEMENT	SUGGESTED DOSAGE	COMMENTS
Essential		
Bromelain plus curcumin	400–500 mg 3 times daily. As directed on label.	Reduces inflammation, swelling, and pain. Has anti-inflammatory properties.
Grape seed extract	75 mg daily.	An effective anti-inflammatory and powerful antioxidant.
Quercetin (Activated Quercetin from Source Naturals)	300–400 mg every 4 hours.	A unique bioflavonoid that reduces allergic reactions.
Vitamin C with bioflavonoids	5,000–20,000 mg daily, in divided doses. (*See* ASCORBIC ACID FLUSH in Part Three.)	An anti-inflammatory that is helpful for relieving the toxicity of bites. For a child, use buffered vitamin C or calcium ascorbate.

HERBS

❑ Calendula ointment is an excellent insect repellent and counterirritant. You can also try cedar, eucalyptus, and/or tea tree oils. These are available in oil, spray, and lotion form.

❑ Citronella candles are good for repelling mosquitoes.

❑ Goldenseal and tea tree oil are natural insect repellants and are beneficial when applied to affected areas.

❑ Poultices made with lobelia and charcoal tablets (found in health food stores) are helpful for insect bites. (*See* USING A POULTICE in Part Three.)

❑ Pennyroyal oil helps to repel insects.

Caution: Do not use this herb during pregnancy. Avoid excessive and/or prolonged use.

RECOMMENDATIONS

❑ For ant, mosquito, or chigger (mite) bites, wash the area thoroughly with soap and water. For chigger bites, use a brush and scrub. Then apply a paste made of baking soda and water. Use ice packs if swelling occurs and, if bitten on an arm or leg, elevate the affected limb to decrease swelling.

❑ For tick bites, remove the tick as quickly as you can. The sooner the tick is removed, the less chance there is of contracting any disease the tick may be carrying. Using tweezers, grasp the head of the tick firmly, as close to the skin as possible, and pull straight back with the tweezers. Try not to leave the head or any other part of the tick embedded in the skin. Do not touch the tick with your hands. Once it has been removed, scrub the bite with soap and water. *Do not* try to burn the tick out, or use home remedies like kerosene, turpentine, or petroleum jelly.

❑ Make a paste using a charcoal capsule and a few drops of goldenseal extract and place it on a piece of gauze. Apply the gauze to the bite and cover it with a bandage. This will draw out the poisons and aid in fast relief. Do this immediately after being bitten, if possible.

❑ Apply calamine lotion to help relieve itching.

❑ Rub a cut onion on an insect bite to provide a powerful antioxidant treatment.

❑ Take a dose of homeopathic *Apis mellifica* promptly after a bite. It works quickly to help prevent severe swelling.

❑ If you have been bitten by a spider you suspect may be a black widow or a brown recluse, seek medical attention immediately. If possible, take the spider with you for identification.

❑ Treat jellyfish and sea-anemone stings by removing the tentacles with a cloth or gloves; rinse with seawater, then place vinegar or rubbing alcohol on the affected area. Meat tenderizer also takes the sting away. Remove sea-urchin barbs with tweezers or by rubbing with soap and water. Apply warm compresses to extract the toxins. Coral injuries are very dangerous and should get immediate medical attention. Remove coral fragments with tweezers, wash with soap and water, and keep the affected limb stationary.

❑ To avoid mosquito bites, eat fish, brown rice, brewer's yeast, blackstrap molasses, or wheat germ before spending time outside. These foods are rich in vitamin B_1 (thiamine). Carbon dioxide, estrogens, moisture, sweat, and warmth attract mosquitoes. They appear to be repelled by the B vitamins, which are excreted through the skin, and especially by thiamine, so as an alternative, take thiamine supplements.

❑ To avoid many insect bites, try taking a chlorine bleach bath before going out. Add 1 cup of bleach per tub of water. Insects dislike the smell. Swimming in a pool treated with chlorine also works. Rubbing brewer's yeast or garlic on the skin may deter insects as well.

❑ Avoid walking barefoot outside.

❑ Avoid all refined sugar, which causes the skin to give off a sweet smell that attracts mosquitoes.

❑ Avoid alcoholic drinks. Alcohol causes the skin to flush and the blood vessels to dilate, which attracts mosquitoes and horseflies.

❑ Avoid using perfume, hair spray, and other cosmetics. These attract insects.

❑ Avoid wearing bright colors.

❏ Wear clothing that covers your arms and legs (although mosquitoes can bite through cotton clothing).

❏ Apply citrus juice to exposed areas to repel mosquitoes.

CONSIDERATIONS

❏ Diethyl toluamide (DEET) works to repel chiggers, ticks, and mosquitoes. It is probably the most effective insect repellent known, but it is also potentially quite toxic and it can destroy substances such as plastics and synthetic fabrics, so it must be used with care and only in accordance with package directions. Never apply a product that has more than 35 percent DEET to the skin. Children are especially at risk for problems due to this potentially hazardous chemical, so their skin exposure to it should be strictly limited. To be safe, apply DEET to clothing and use it sparingly, if at all, on the skin.

❏ If you spend much time outdoors, you may want to purchase a vacuum pump called the Lil Sucker from Terra Tech to extract the poison from insect bites. This pump is painless to use, and in one study, 94 percent of participants who used it had either no reaction or a minor one to an insect bite.

❏ If you are in the wilderness, or anywhere without access to the above remedies, the old folk remedy of immediately applying mud to a sting can help to neutralize the pain and swelling.

❏ We do not recommend using electric insect-repelling devices ("bug zappers"). They kill biting bugs, but not black flies and mosquitoes. Many of the insects they kill are an important part of the daily diet of birds. If you feel you must use one of these devices, do not place it near children's play areas, barbecue grills, or picnic tables. When insects like houseflies get zapped, the parts can spray as far as seven feet, spreading bacteria and viruses.

❏ Information on poisonings from insect bites can be obtained from the Centers for Disease Control in Atlanta (*see* HEALTH AND MEDICAL ORGANIZATIONS in the Appendix).

❏ *See also* BEE STING; INSECT ALLERGY; LYME DISEASE; and/or SPIDER BITE, all in Part Two.

Insomnia

Habitual sleeplessness is classified as insomnia. Failure to get an entire night's sleep on most nights over a one-month period can be considered chronic insomnia. It affects one out of ten Americans (about 40 million) and approximately 30 percent of healthy seniors. Insomnia can take the form of being unable to fall asleep when you first go to bed or waking during the night and being unable to go back to sleep. While insomnia can be very frustrating, it is hardly dangerous and is usually only a temporary annoyance, although in some cases sleep-related problems can last for months or even years.

Chronic insomnia is often a symptom of a serious underlying medical disorder. Fifty percent of insomnia cases can be attributed to depression and psychological disorders, such as anxiety, stress, or grief. Insomnia can result from a wide variety of causes, including arthritis, asthma, breathing problems, hypoglycemia, hyperthyroidism, indigestion, kidney or heart disease, muscle aches, Parkinson's disease, or physical pain. Caffeine consumption, jet lag, and the use of certain drugs, including many antidepressants, the antiseizure medication phenytoin (Dilantin), most appetite suppressants, beta-blockers (medications used for high blood pressure and heart ailments), the decongestant pseudoephedrine (found in many cold and allergy remedies), and thyroid hormone replacement drugs can also lead to insomnia.

A lack of the nutrients calcium and magnesium can cause you to wake up after a few hours and not be able to return to sleep. Systemic disorders involving the brain, digestive system, endocrine system, heart, kidneys, liver, lungs, and pancreas all may affect sleep, as can poor nutritional habits and eating too close to bedtime. A sedentary lifestyle can be a major contributor to sleep disorders.

While one or two sleepless nights can cause irritability and daytime sleepiness, with decreased ability to perform creative or repetitive tasks, most people can adapt to short-term periods of sleep deprivation. After more than three days, however, sleep deprivation begins to cause a more serious deterioration in overall performance and can even result in mild personality changes. If chronic, inadequate sleep compromises productivity, creates problems in relationships, and can contribute to other health problems.

There are no hard and fast rules about how much sleep is enough, because every individual's requirements are different. Some people can function on as little as five hours of sleep a night, while others seem to perform better with nine, ten, or even more hours of sleep. Most adults need about eight hours of sleep nightly in order to feel refreshed and operate at peak efficiency during the day. Children, especially very young children and adolescents, generally require more sleep than adults to be at their best. It is not uncommon for people to sleep less as they get older, especially after the age of sixty.

Millions of people have trouble getting to sleep due to a condition commonly known as *restless leg syndrome* (RLS). For reasons unknown, when these people are in bed, their legs jerk, twitch, and kick involuntarily. Restless leg syndrome has also been linked to the painful nighttime leg muscle cramps that afflict so many people. A deficiency of magnesium may be involved in RLS, and some research strongly suggests that anemia may play a major role in this annoying disorder.

Sleep apnea affects about 20 million Americans and is a potentially serious sleep disorder. This problem is commonly associated with snoring and extremely irregular breathing throughout the night. In sleep apnea, breathing actually stops for as long as two minutes at a time while the individual is asleep. When breathing stops, the level of oxygen in the blood drops, resulting in oxygen deprivation. The individual then awakens, startled and gasping. A person with sleep apnea may awaken as many as 200 times throughout the night. The affected individual may not remember these awakenings, but anyone else who is awake at the time can naturally become alarmed when a person with sleep apnea stops breathing. In the less common form, central sleep apnea, breathing is stopped, not because the airway is closed, but because the diaphragm and chest muscles stop working.

Aside from disrupting normal sleep and causing extreme sleepiness during the day, sleep apnea is associated with other, more serious, health problems. People who have sleep apnea tend to have higher than normal blood pressure and are more likely to have strokes than the general population, and they also face an increased risk of heart disease, although the reason or reasons for these links are not known. People with sleep apnea also seem to have a higher-than-normal incidence of emotional and psychotic disorders. Experts attribute this to what they call a "dream deficit"—a lack of adequate rapid-eye-movement (REM) sleep, the stage of sleep in which dreaming occurs. A person with sleep apnea often cannot settle into REM sleep for even the eight to twelve seconds it takes to have a normal, healthy dream. While there is much about the phenomenon of dreaming that is not understood, it is known that prolonged periods of REM-sleep deprivation can induce various psychoses and other serious emotional disorders.

NUTRIENTS

SUPPLEMENT	SUGGESTED DOSAGE	COMMENTS
Important		
Calcium	1,500–2,000 mg daily, in divided doses, after meals and at bedtime.	Has a calming effect. Use calcium lactate or calcium chelate form (do not use lactate form if you are allergic to dairy products).
and magnesium	1,000 mg daily.	Needed to balance with calcium and relax the muscles.
Melatonin	Start with 1.5 mg daily, taken 2 hours or less before bedtime. If this is not effective, gradually increase the dosage until an effective level is reached (up to 5 mg daily).	A natural hormone that promotes sound sleep. Use it only occasionally and do not give it to children.
Helpful		
Vitamin B complex plus extra	As directed on label.	Helps to promote a restful state.
pantothenic acid (vitamin B$_5$) and	50 mg daily.	Good for relieving stress.
inositol and	100 mg daily, at bedtime.	Enhances REM sleep.
niacinamide	100 mg.	Promotes serotonin production.

Vitamin C with bioflavonoids	500 mg daily.	Very important for reducing stress.
Zinc	15 mg daily.	Aids in the recovery of body tissues while sleeping.

HERBS

❑ California poppy, hops, kava kava, lemon balm, passionflower, skullcap, and valerian root, taken in capsule or extract form, are all good for helping to overcome insomnia. Valerian root has become the favorite among many experts. It is best not to rely on one herb on a regular basis, but to rotate among several. Take these herbs before bedtime.

❑ The combination of California poppy, passionflower, and valerian promote sound sleep and beneficial REM sleep. California poppy and chamomile will strengthen the nervous system to calm you before bedtime.

❑ Catnip and chamomile have mild sedative properties. These herbs are safe even for children if taken in tea form. For adults, drinking chamomile tea several times throughout the day helps to calm and tone the nervous system, promoting restful sleep.

Caution: Do not use chamomile on an ongoing basis. Avoid it completely if you are allergic to ragweed.

❑ Kava kava is a good relaxant. If stress or anxiety is the reason for your insomnia, this herb can help you develop better sleep patterns.

❑ A combination herbal extract such as Slumber from Nature's Answer or Silent Night from Nature's Way can be helpful.

RECOMMENDATIONS

❑ In the evening, eat bananas, dates, figs, milk, nut butter, tuna, turkey, and whole grain crackers, or yogurt. These foods are high in tryptophan, which promotes sleep. Eating a grapefruit half at bedtime also helps.

❑ Avoid alcohol. A small amount can help induce sleep initially, but it invariably disrupts deeper sleep cycles later.

❑ Avoid tobacco. While smoking may seem to have a calming effect, nicotine is actually a neurostimulant and can cause sleep problems.

❑ Avoid stimulants, such as caffeine-containing beverages, after lunch.

❑ Avoid heavy meals three hours before bedtime.

❑ Avoid bacon, cheese, chocolate, eggplant, ham, potatoes, sauerkraut, sugar, sausage, spinach, tomatoes, and wine close to bedtime. These foods contain tyramine, which increases the release of norepinephrine, a brain stimulant.

❑ Avoid taking nasal decongestants and other cold medications late in the day. While many ingredients in these preparations are known to cause drowsiness, they can have the opposite effect on some people and act as a stimulant.

❑ Establish a set of habits and follow them consistently to establish a healthy sleep cycle. Among them:

• Go to bed only when you are sleepy.

• Do not stay in bed if you are not sleepy. Get up and move to another room and read, watch television, or do something quietly until you are really sleepy.

• Use the bedroom only for sleep and sex—not for reading, working, eating, or watching television.

• Set an alarm clock and get out of bed at the same time every morning, no matter how you slept the night before. Once normal sleep patterns are reestablished, most people find that they have no need for an alarm clock.

• Do not nap during the day if this isn't a normal thing for you to do.

• Exercise regularly in the late afternoon or early evening—but not right before bedtime. Physical exertion is an excellent way to make your body tired so that sleep comes about more easily.

• Take a hot bath (not a shower) an hour or two before bedtime. For further relaxation, put several drops of a soothing essential oil such as chamomile (if you are not allergic to ragweed) in the bath water. (*See* AROMATHERAPY AND ESSENTIAL OILS in Part Three.)

• Keep the bedroom comfortable and quiet. If *too much* quiet is the problem, try running a fan or playing a radio softly in the background. There are also devices available that generate "white noise" sounds like the ocean surf or a steady rain that help people who are "quiet-sensitive" to sleep.

• Learn to put worries out of your mind. If you have occasional trouble getting to sleep, concentrate on pleasant memories and thoughts. Recreate a pleasurable time or event in your life and relive it in your mind. Learning a relaxation technique such as meditation or the use of guided imagery is extremely helpful in getting sleep patterns back to normal for many people.

❑ For occasional sleeplessness, try using melatonin, Calcium Night from Source Naturals, or one of the herbs recommended above. These are effective and safe sleep-promoters.

❑ One of the best remedies for insomnia is taking 5 milligrams of melatonin one hour before bedtime. If you feel groggy in the morning, reduce the dosage the next time you use it. Certain drugs frequently prescribed for older adults, including beta-blockers (for high blood pressure) and even aspirin, can lower melatonin levels.

Caution: Do not overuse melatonin. According to some recent reports, more than occasional use of melatonin can permanently stop the body's own production of this vital hormone.

❑ If you snore, try sleeping on your side. Sleep on a couch for a few nights to become accustomed to sleeping on your side.

CONSIDERATIONS

❑ During sleep, the body's systems are still controlling basic functions. Nutrients are essential for the body and are used during the sleep cycle.

❑ A lack of sleep can encourage serious illness and cause premature aging. Experts recommend at least eight hours of sleep per night.

❑ *Women's Health Advisor* reports that an estimated 10 percent of all Americans suffer from restless legs syndrome (RLS), a disorder marked by uncomfortable urges to move the legs, especially just before falling asleep. Various treatments have been attempted for restless leg syndrome, but nothing seems to work consistently for everyone. The drug pramipexole (Mirapex) has shown positive benefits for some people with this condition. We believe that taking the proper vitamin and mineral supplements is the best approach to this problem. The supplements that help this condition more than anything are calcium, potassium, magnesium, and zinc. The following nutrients may prevent restless leg syndrome and leg cramps: 400 milligrams of B complex, 1,000 milligrams of magnesium, and 400 international units of vitamin E (d-alpha-tocopherol) per day.

❑ Regardless of how many hours of sleep you get each night, if you wake up easily in the morning, and especially if you rarely (or ever) need the services of your alarm clock, and if you can make it through the entire day without seeming to run out of steam or feeling drowsy after sitting quietly or reading for a while, you are probably getting enough sleep.

❑ Research psychologist Dr. James Penland believes that a large number of women are suffering from copper and iron deficiencies, and that these deficiencies can cause insomnia. A hair analysis can reveal whether you have a deficiency. (*See* HAIR ANALYSIS in Part Three.)

❑ The hormonal shifts that occur during premenstrual syndrome and menopause may trigger insomnia. Estrogen affects the production and balance of the brain chemicals responsible for wakefulness.

❑ 5-Hydroxy L-tryptophan (5-HTP) and the amino acid tryptophan are helpful for insomnia and depression. For more information, *see under* AMINO ACIDS and NATURAL FOOD SUPPLEMENTS in Part One.

❑ Dehydroepiandrosterone (DHEA) is a naturally occurring hormone that improves the quality of sleep. (*See* DHEA THERAPY in Part Three.)

❑ Anyone who snores excessively should be evaluated for sleep apnea. Many cases of sleep apnea respond to such measures as allergy treatment, weight reduction, or a simple laser surgery procedure to remove obstructions in the nasal passages.

❑ Mild cases of obstructional sleep apnea can sometimes be treated with lifestyle and diet changes. Oral devices are available for mild cases to prevent obstruction of the airway by holding the tongue or jaw forward.

❑ An effective treatment for snoring is the use of radio waves to reduce the soft palate tissue that obstructs the air passage in the mouth. In this technique, a health care practitioner inserts a probe into the back of the mouth and the radio waves are directed at the palate.

❑ Millions of Americans consciously choose to skimp on their sleep in the mistaken belief that sleeping fewer hours allows them to be more productive. Many people even look on the fact that they can "get by" on so few hours of sleep as a badge of honor. In fact, however, they are likely doing themselves a great deal of harm in the long run. Moreover, the night owls who sleep less to accomplish more are actually less creative and less productive than those who get adequate amounts of sleep. Dr. Richard Bootzin, professor of psychology and director of the insomnia clinic at the University of Arizona Sleep Disorders Center, conducted long-term research into normal sleep habits and patterns. He discovered that people who get seven to eight hours of sleep each night live longer, happier, healthier lives than those who skimp on their sleep.

❑ Sleep therapists and other experts are greatly divided about the virtues of napping. While some maintain that napping is not necessary for people who are well rested, others say it is a natural human tendency and should not be discouraged. There have been studies that seem to demonstrate that productivity is higher and the incidence of accidents lower in countries where napping is common. Consistency is probably the most important factor. While it is usually most advisable to consolidate all sleeping into one time period, if you regularly take an afternoon nap and you do not suffer from any sleeping disorders, then giving up naps might actually cause a disruption in your sleeping habits. If you nap, keep your naps short—less than an hour—and make sure that they are a *regular* part of the daily routine, not a now-and-then proposition.

❑ Sleep experts advise that people with insomnia avoid caffeine, but many people who are accustomed to drinking coffee late in the day and in the evening hours have been known to have their sleep cycles disrupted if they give up drinking coffee. This seems to bear out the idea that maintaining a steady routine is the most important factor in establishing a healthy sleep pattern. Of course, this applies only to those who are not experiencing any difficulties with their sleeping habits. Anyone who develops a bout of insomnia should consider eliminating all caffeine from his or her diet.

❑ Many people who suffer from insomnia resort to sleeping pills, whether over-the-counter or prescription medica-

tions. Sleeping pills do not cure insomnia, however, and they can interfere with REM sleep. The continued use of pharmacological sleeping aids can eventually lead to disruption of all the deeper stages of sleep. Researchers have found that up to 50 percent of people who take sleeping pills on a regular basis actually find that their insomnia becomes worse. The persistent use of sleeping pills also leads to dependency, either psychological or physical. The use of sleep medication should therefore be reserved for those whose insomnia has a physical basis, and then only as a temporary solution.

❑ Tranquilizers like the benzodiazepines and similar medications are being prescribed for insomnia because they pose a lower risk of overdose than sedatives. The most prescribed include quazepam (Doral), estazolam (ProSom), flurazepam (Dalmane), temazepam (Restoril), and triazolam (Halcion). Triazolam can cause mental confusion and even amnesia. There have also been reports that drugs such as temazepam, secobarbital (Seconal), flurazepam, and diazepam (Valium) may lead to confusion, sluggishness, restlessness, and heightened anxiety, as well as prolonged sedation and drug dependency.

❑ Zolpidem (Ambien) is a different type of sleep-aid drug. Its manufacturer claims that it does not inhibit or disrupt the deep-sleep cycles, like REM.

❑ People who take sleeping pills on a regular basis are 50 percent more likely than other people to die in accidents. Drowsiness accounts for 200,000 to 400,000 automobile accidents every year, and is responsible for two-thirds of all industrial mishaps, most common among shift workers in the early morning hours. Sleeping pills are also the third most commonly used means in suicide and are implicated in one-third of all drug-related suicide attempts and deaths.

❑ Over-the-counter sleep aids can cause a wide range of side effects, including agitation, confusion, depression, dry mouth, and worsening of symptoms of enlarged prostate.

❑ *See also under* PREGNANCY-RELATED PROBLEMS.

Irritable Bowel Syndrome

Irritable bowel syndrome (IBS) is the most common digestive disorder seen by physicians. It is estimated that about one in five adult Americans has symptoms of IBS, although fewer than half of them seek a physician's help for it. Twice as many women suffer from the condition as men. IBS, also sometimes called *intestinal neurosis, mucous colitis, spastic colitis,* or *spastic colon,* usually affects people between the ages of twenty-five and forty-five.

In IBS, the normally rhythmic muscular contractions of

the digestive tract become irregular and uncoordinated. This interferes with the normal movement of food and waste material, and leads to the accumulation of mucus and toxins in the intestine. This accumulated material sets up a partial obstruction of the digestive tract, trapping gas and stools, which in turn causes bloating, distention, and constipation. IBS may affect the entire gastrointestinal tract, from the mouth through the colon. There are no physical signs of disease in bowel tissue with this disorder, and its cause is unknown, but one theory is that irregularities in the intestinal hormones responsible for bowel motility, cholecystokinin (CCK), motilin, and vasoactive intestinal peptide (VIP), are behind this disorder. According to this theory, people with IBS have abnormal contractions of the smooth muscle of the digestive tract. Some scientists believe a virus or bacterium may play a role. Lifestyle factors such as stress and diet are probably common causes, as are food allergies. The overuse of antibiotics, antacids, or laxatives, which disturb the bacterial microflora of the bowel, may also be a factor.

Symptoms of IBS may include abdominal pain, anorexia, bloating, constipation and/or diarrhea (often alternating), flatulence, intolerances to certain foods, mucus in the stools, and nausea. Pain is often triggered by eating and may be relieved by a bowel movement. Because of the pain, diarrhea, nausea, and sometimes severe headaches and even vomiting, a person with IBS may dread eating. Whether or not an individual with IBS eats normally, malnutrition may result because nutrients often are not absorbed properly. As a result, people with IBS require as much as 30 percent more protein than normal, as well as an increased intake of minerals and trace elements, which can quickly be depleted by diarrhea.

Many other diseases can be related to IBS, including candidiasis, colon cancer, diabetes mellitus, gallbladder disease, malabsorption disorders, pancreatic insufficiency, ulcers, and the parasitic infections amebiasis and giardiasis. Over 100 different disorders may be linked to the systemic effects of IBS. One disorder that is linked in about 25 percent of adults with IBS is arthritis, usually peripheral arthritis, which affects the ankles, knees, and wrists. Less frequently, the spine is affected. IBS can also be related to skin disorders, but this is unusual. Some people with IBS have abnormalities in the levels of liver enzymes in their blood.

Diagnosis of irritable bowel syndrome requires ruling out disorders that can cause similar symptoms, such as celiac disease, colon cancer or benign tumors, Crohn's disease, depression, diverticulitis, endometriosis, fecal impaction, food poisoning, infectious diarrhea, ischemic or ulcerative colitis, and lactose intolerance. A physician may recommend one or more of a variety of procedures to do this, including barium enema, colonoscopy, rectal biopsy, sigmoidoscopy, and stool examination to check for the presence of bacteria, blood, and/or parasites.

Irritable bowel syndrome is painful, but not serious, and most people who have it can lead active, productive lives if they change their diets, get regular exercise, and replace needed nutrients.

NUTRIENTS

SUPPLEMENT	SUGGESTED DOSAGE	COMMENTS
Very Important		
Essential fatty acids (flaxseed oil and primrose oil are good sources)	As directed on label.	Needed to protect the intestinal lining.
L-Glutamine	500 mg twice daily, on an empty stomach. Take with water or juice. Do not take with milk. Take with 50 mg vitamin B$_6$ and 100 mg vitamin C for better absorption.	A major metabolic fuel for the intestinal cells; maintains the villi, the absorption surfaces of the gut. (See AMINO ACIDS in Part One.)
Vitamin B complex	50–100 mg of each major B vitamin 3 times daily, with meals (amounts of individual vitamins in a complex will vary).	Needed for proper muscle tone in the gastrointestinal tract.
plus extra vitamin B$_{12}$	1,000–2,000 mcg daily.	Needed for proper absorption of foods, protein synthesis, and metabolism of carbohydrates and fats, and to prevent anemia. Use a lozenge or sublingual form.
Important		
Acidophilus (Probiata from Wakunaga) or Bio-Bifidus from American Biologics	As directed on label. As directed on label.	To replenish the "friendly" bacteria. Needed for digestion and for the manufacture of the B vitamins. Use a nondairy formula.
Colostrum (New Life Colostrum from Symbiotics and Colostrum Specific from Jarrow Formulas are good sources)	As directed on label.	Heals intestinal lining and aids in nutrient absorption.
Fiber (oat bran, flaxseeds, psyllium seeds, and Aerobic Bulk Cleanse from Aerobic Life Industries are good sources)	As directed on label. Take separately from other supplements and medications.	Has both a healing and cleansing effect. Avoid wheat bran, as it may be too irritating.
Free-form amino acid complex	As directed on label.	Necessary for repair of mucous membranes of the intestines.
Garlic (Kyolic from Wakunaga)	As directed on label.	Aids in digestion and destruction of toxins in the colon. Liquid form is best.
Multivitamin and mineral complex	As directed on label.	Supplies those nutrients lost or not absorbed. Use a hypoallergenic formula.
N-Acetylglucosamine (N-A-G from Source Naturals)	As directed on label.	A major constituent of the intestinal lining and of the barrier layer that protects the intestinal lining from digestive enzymes and other potentially damaging intestinal contents.

Proteolytic enzymes with pancreatin	As directed on label.	To aid in protein digestion and prevention of "leaky gut syndrome." Also aids in reducing inflammation. Use a formula that is low in HCl and high in pancreatin.
Quercetin	As directed on label.	Helps control the allergic response to foods.
Ultra Clear Sustain from Metagenics	As directed on label.	A complex that provides nutritional support for gastrointestinal mucosa. Available only through health care professionals.
Helpful		
Calcium and magnesium	2,000 mg daily. 1,000 mg daily.	Helps the "nervous stomach" and the central nervous system. Aids in preventing colon cancer. Use chelate forms.
Dioxychlor from American Biologics	As directed on label.	Destroys foreign bacteria in the digestive tract and carries oxygen to the tissues.
Shark cartilage (BeneFin)	As directed on label. If you cannot tolerate taking it orally, it can be administered rectally in a retention enema.	Fights growth and metastasis of cancerous tumors. IBS is associated with an increased risk of colon cancer.

HERBS

❑ If you have IBS, it is wise to treat your liver as well as your digestive tract, preferably with silymarin (milk thistle extract). Licorice can also be used. Other beneficial herbs are burdock root and red clover, which are good for cleansing the bloodstream, and thereby the liver.

Caution: If overused, licorice can elevate blood pressure. Do not use this herb on a daily basis for more than seven days in a row. Avoid it completely if you have high blood pressure.

❑ Alfalfa contains vitamin K, needed to build intestinal flora for proper digestion, and chlorophyll for healing and cleansing of the bloodstream. It can be taken in liquid or tablet form.

❑ Aloe vera is healing to the digestive tract. Used in combination with Aerobic Bulk Cleanse (ABC) from Aerobic Life Industries, it helps to keep the colon walls clean of excess mucus and slow down food reactions. Take 1/2 cup of aloe vera juice three times daily, on an empty stomach.

❑ Peppermint aids in healing and digestion, and also relieves upset stomach and gas or that "too-full" feeling. It must be taken in enteric-coated capsule form to prevent the oil from being released before it reaches the colon. Do not take any other form, or heartburn may result.

❑ Skullcap and valerian root are helpful for the nerves that regulate intestinal muscle function. These are good taken at bedtime or when an upset occurs.

❑ Other herbs that can be beneficial for irritable bowel syndrome include balm, chamomile, fenugreek, ginger, goldenseal, lobelia, marshmallow, pau d'arco, rose hips, and slippery elm.

Caution: Do not use chamomile or lobelia on an ongoing basis. Avoid chamomile completely if you are allergic to ragweed. Do not take goldenseal internally on a daily basis for more than one week at a time, do not use it in large quantities during pregnancy, and use it with caution if you are allergic to ragweed.

RECOMMENDATIONS

❑ Eat a high-fiber diet including plenty of fruits and vegetables, plus whole grains (especially brown rice) and legumes.

❑ Use supplemental fiber. Psyllium powder regulates bowel movements and should be used daily. Also use oat bran and ground flaxseeds daily, on an alternating basis.

❑ Avoid animal fats, butter, all carbonated beverages, coffee and all other substances containing caffeine, candy, chocolate, all dairy products, fried foods, ice cream, all junk foods, the additives mannitol and sorbitol, margarine, nuts, orange and grapefruit juices, pastries, all processed foods, seeds, spicy foods, sugar, sugar-free chewing gum, and wheat bran and wheat products. These foods encourage the secretion of mucus by the membranes and prevent the uptake of nutrients.

❑ Limit your consumption of gas-producing foods such as beans, broccoli, and cabbage if they cause any problems.

❑ Avoid alcohol and tobacco; these irritate the linings of the stomach and colon.

❑ When an intestinal upset occurs, switch to a bland diet. Put vegetables and nonacidic fruits through a food processor or blender. Organic baby food is good. If you are on a soft diet, take some type of fiber and a protein supplement.

❑ To relieve occasional gas and bloating, use charcoal tablets (available in health food stores). Take 5 tablets as soon as this problem arises. Do not use charcoal daily, however, because it also absorbs needed nutrients, and do not take it at the same time as other supplements or medications.

❑ For excessive gas and bloating that lingers, read the section on ENEMAS in Part Three and follow the instructions for the retention enema. This will replace the "friendly" bacteria very quickly and resolve the problem. Exercise, such as stretching exercises, swimming, or walking, is also important.

❑ Check to see if you have food allergies; they are important factors in this disorder. Eliminating allergenic foods from the diet relieves symptoms in many cases. (*See* ALLERGIES in Part Two.)

❑ Chew your food well. Do not overeat or eat in a hurry.

❑ Practice deep-breathing exercises. Shallow breathing reduces the oxygen available for proper bowel function.

❑ Wear loose-fitting clothing. Do not wear anything that is tight around the waist.

❑ Do not eat right before going to bed. Wait one or two hours after eating before lying down.

❑ *See* ACID/ALKALI IMBALANCE in Part Two and take the self-test. Significant acidosis may occur with IBS.

CONSIDERATIONS

❑ Eating the correct diet, using supplemental fiber, and drinking plenty of quality water are very important in controlling IBS. Early recognition of the disease, good nutrition, and a positive outlook help minimize complications.

❑ It takes between twelve and fifteen hours for food to be completely processed. Food such as meat can take longer, whereas fresh foods, raw foods, or lightly steamed foods are processed much more quickly.

❑ Certain foods irritate the wall of the intestinal tract. Lactose (milk sugar) is a common culprit, as are all dairy products. Avoid grains, nuts, and seeds until symptoms subside. Always chew these types of foods until they are almost liquified in the mouth.

❑ IBS should not be confused with the more serious bowel disorders, such as Crohn's disease and ulcerative colitis. These are also inflammatory bowel diseases but, unlike IBS, they result in demonstrable lesions in the digestive tract. Crohn's disease affects the entire length and thickness of the wall of the large and/or small intestine; ulcerative colitis affects the lining of the large intestine, the last five to seven feet of the digestive tract. (*See* CROHN'S DISEASE and/or ULCERATIVE COLITIS, both in Part Two.)

❑ People with irritable bowel syndrome are also likely to have associated conditions such as dysphagia (difficulty swallowing), gastroesophageal reflux, globus sensation (a feeling of having a ball in the throat), gynecological problems, heartburn, noncardiac chest pain, and urologic dysfunction.

❑ An imbalance of gut flora is common for those with irritable bowel syndrome. Usually, the pathogenic flora outnumber the friendly bacteria.

❑ People with IBS should receive regular physical examinations. This disorder has been linked to a higher-than-normal incidence of colon cancer and diverticulitis.

❑ If IBS causes chronic diarrhea, electrolyte and trace mineral deficiencies are likely. (*See* DIARRHEA in Part Two for suggested mineral supplementation. *See also* MALABSORPTION SYNDROME in Part Two.)

❑ Certain drugs can aggravate the malabsorption problems often present with IBS. These include antibiotics, corticosteroids, cholestyramine (Questran), and sulfasalazine (Azulfidine), among others. These drugs increase the need for nutritional supplements.

❑ Antispasmodic drugs (Di-Spaz, Lomotil) and antidiarrheal drugs (Imodium) slow the function of the gastrointestinal tract and are regularly prescribed for irritable bowel syndrome. However, they have serious side effects and can induce dependency. Some health practitioners have also prescribed highly addictive tranquilizers and antidepressants.

❑ Many people with irritable bowel syndrome have experienced improvements in symptoms after using Chinese herbal medicine (CHM).

❑ Research and testing have found not only that breathing exercises can control IBS, but that people who practice stress management have fewer and less severe attacks. Stress management also relieves symptoms. (*See* STRESS in Part Two. *Also see* Breathing Exercises *under* PAIN CONTROL in Part Three.)

❑ The symptoms of IBS are similar to those of many other disorders, including cancer. If dietary modification and natural remedies yield no relief, it is wise to consult a physician to rule out some other underlying problem. We recommend this only after natural remedies have been tried, however.

❑ *See also* DIVERTICULITIS; HEARTBURN; and/or INDIGESTION in Part Two.

Jaundice

Jaundice is a yellowing of the skin and eyes that is caused by a buildup of bilirubin in the blood. Bilirubin is a yellow-brown substance that results from the breakdown of old red blood cells. If this waste product is not removed from the bloodstream by the liver, as it should be, a backup of bilirubin in the blood occurs, producing a yellowing of the skin and the whites of the eyes. The urine may be darker than normal, while the stools may appear lighter. Jaundice may be accompanied by edema (fluid retention) in the trunk of the body, fatigue, generalized itching, nausea, rashes on the skin, and vomiting.

Jaundice is not a disease in itself, but a sign of any one of several blood or liver disorders. Among the conditions that can cause jaundice are cirrhosis of the liver, pernicious anemia, hepatitis, and hemolysis (abnormal destruction of red blood cells). Jaundice can also be a sign of an obstruction in the path of the bile flow, from the liver through the bile ducts to the gallbladder and then to the intestinal tract. If the biliary tract is obstructed, the bile (which contains bilirubin) passes back into the bloodstream instead of into the digestive system, producing jaundice. Occasionally, jaundice is caused by some form of parasitic infestation such as tapeworm or hookworm, or a bite from a flea or mosquito that carries a viral, bacterial, or parasitic infection. It can also be caused by a tumor, a gallstone, or inflammation.

Some degree of jaundice is common in newborn babies, especially premature babies, and is not considered serious. It occurs because a new baby's liver is limited in its ability to process bilirubin, and in most cases soon resolves itself.

NUTRIENTS

SUPPLEMENT	SUGGESTED DOSAGE	COMMENTS
Very Important		
Coenzyme Q$_{10}$	As directed on label.	Promotes tissue oxygenation and removes toxic substances from the body.
plus Coenzyme A from Coenzyme-A Technologies	As directed on label.	Works with coenzyme Q$_{10}$ to support the immune system's detoxification of many dangerous substances.
Colostrum (New Life Colostrum from Symbiotics)	As directed on label.	Improves immune function and protects the liver.
Grape seed extract	As directed on label.	A powerful antioxidant that aids the liver in removing toxic substances from the body.
Kyo-Dophilus from Wakunaga	As directed on label.	Protects the liver and the intestinal tract.
Kyolic from Wakunaga	As directed on label.	Potent immune enhancer.
L-Glutathione and L-methionine	500 mg each daily, on an empty stomach. Take with water or juice. Do not take with milk. Take with 50 mg vitamin B$_6$ and 100 mg vitamin C for better absorption.	Substances that work together to protect the liver. (*See* AMINO ACIDS in Part One.)
Liquid Kyolic with B$_1$ and B$_{12}$ from Wakunaga	As directed on label.	An excellent liver detoxifier.
Raw liver extract	As directed on label.	Aids in building the liver. (*See* GLANDULAR THERAPY in Part Three.) Use liver from organically raised beef.
S-Adenosylmethionine (SAMe)	As directed on label.	Aids in stress-relief, depression, eases pain, and produces antioxidant effects that can improve the health of the liver. *Caution:* Do not use it you have manic-depressive disorder or take prescription antidepressants.
Vitamin B complex	50 mg of each major B vitamin three times daily (amounts of individual vitamins in a complex will vary).	The B vitamins are necessary for proper digestion, absorption of nutrients, and formation of red blood cells. They help to maintain the health of the eyes, and liver, and skin. Use a high-potency formula.
Vitamin C with bioflavonoids	3,000–6,000 mg daily.	Vitamin C combines with toxic substances, renders them harmless, and removes them from the body.

HERBS

❑ Burdock root and red clover aid in cleansing the blood.

❑ Celandine, chaparral, and dandelion aid in cleansing the liver.

❑ Oregano is good for relieving jaundice.

❑ Silymarin, an active flavonoid extracted from the herb milk thistle, is known to repair damaged tissues in the liver. Liv-R-Actin from Nature's Plus is a good source of silymarin.

RECOMMENDATIONS

❑ Eat only raw vegetables and fruits for one week. Then eat a diet consisting of 75 percent raw food for a month. Take fresh lemon enemas daily during this period. (*See* ENEMAS in Part Three.)

❑ Use the spices coriander and turmeric in your cooking. These are good liver cleansers.

❑ Drink the following juices: lemon juice and water, beet and beet greens, and dandelion or black radish extract. All are good for rebuilding and cleansing the liver.

❑ Never consume raw or undercooked fish, meat, or poultry. All raw fish pose a risk of infection from bacteria, parasites, and viruses.

❑ Do not consume *any* alcohol. Alcohol places a great strain on the liver, which can aggravate the condition further.

CONSIDERATIONS

❑ If jaundice is a result of a tumor or gallstone, surgery may be necessary to correct the problem.

❑ To diagnose the problem that is causing jaundice, your physician may perform a blood test, liver biopsy, or ultrasound scan of the liver.

❑ *See* CIRRHOSIS OF THE LIVER and HEPATITIS, both in Part Two, for additional nutritional and dietary suggestions.

Jock Itch

See under FUNGAL INFECTION.

Kaposi's Sarcoma

See under SKIN CANCER.

Kidney Disease (Renal Failure)

Kidneys remove waste products from the body, keep body

chemicals in balance, and help maintain the body's water balance. There are a number of different renal (kidney) problems that may occur. The kidneys may be damaged by exposure to certain drugs or toxins, including heavy metals, solvents, chemotherapy agents, snake or insect venom, poisonous mushrooms, and pesticides. Renal failure can also accompany or result from many other disorders, such as congestive heart failure, diabetes, chronic hypertension, liver disease, lupus, and sickle-cell anemia.

Bright's disease is a kidney disease marked by the presence of blood protein in the urine, along with hypertension and edema (retention of water in the tissues). *Glomerulonephritis* is an inflammation of tiny blood vessels within the kidney that filter out wastes from the blood. This may occur as a result of an immunological response to infection, such as a *Streptococcus* throat infection. *Pyelonephritis* is a kidney infection that may be caused by a birth defect. Both glomerulonephritis and pyelonephritis can be chronic or acute, and can be serious. *Hydronephrosis* is a condition in which the kidney and the renal pelvis (the structure into which urine is discharged from the kidney) become filled with urine due to an obstruction of urinary flow. *Polycystic kidney disease* (PKD) is an inherited disease in which cysts grow on the kidneys, rendering them incapable of functioning. *Kidney stones* are mineral accumulations (primarily calcium) in the kidneys. In *renal tubular acidosis,* the kidneys fail to reabsorb bicarbonate normally, causing impaired ammonia production and acid excretion. Severe acidosis, potassium depletion, and bone disorders may result. *Nephrotic syndrome* is not a disease in itself, but can be a sign of kidney disease. It is marked by edema and excess protein in the urine. It can be caused by lesions of glomeruli (small structures in the kidney made of capillaries) that become inflamed, or by chronic diseases such as diabetes or lupus.

One important symptom of kidney problems is edema. Edema results when the kidneys produce less urine because they are unable to properly excrete salt and other wastes, and fluid builds up in the body. Ankles and hands may swell, and the person becomes short of breath. Toxic wastes may accumulate in the bloodstream due to kidney malfunction, a condition known as *uremia.* Symptoms of kidney problems include abdominal pain, appetite loss, back pain, chills, fever, fluid retention (bloating), nausea, urinary urgency, and vomiting. The urine may be cloudy or bloody. Back pain may be sudden and intense, occurring just above the waist and running down the groin.

The following supplements aid in controlling urinary tract infection and help maintain proper kidney function. Unless otherwise specified, the dosages recommended here are for adults. For a child between the ages of twelve and seventeen, reduce the dose to three-quarters of the recommended amount. For a child between six and twelve, use one-half of the recommended dose, and for a child under the age of six, use one-quarter of the recommended amount.

NUTRIENTS

SUPPLEMENT	SUGGESTED DOSAGE	COMMENTS
Very Important		
Acidophilus (Kyo-Dophilus from Wakunaga is a good source)	As directed on label, 3 times daily. Take on an empty stomach.	Especially important if taking antibiotics.
Coenzyme A from Coenzyme-A Technologies	As directed on label.	Acts as an antioxidant and removes harmful substances from the body.
Vitamin B$_6$ (pyridoxine) plus choline and inositol (IP$_6$)	50 mg 3 times daily. 50 mg daily. 100 mg daily.	To reduce fluid retention.
Vitamin C with bioflavonoids	2,000–4,000 mg daily.	Acidifies the urine, boosts immune function, and aids healing.
Helpful		
Calcium and magnesium	1,500 mg daily. 750 mg daily.	For proper mineral balance; calcium and magnesium should be in a 2-to-1 ratio in the body. Do not use bone meal, oyster shells, or dolomite as a source. Important in water absorption.
L-Arginine and L-methionine	500 mg 4 times daily. As directed on label, on an empty stomach. Take with water or juice. Do not take with milk. Take with 50 mg vitamin B$_6$ and 100 mg vitamin C for better absorption.	For kidney disease. For improved kidney circulation. (*See* AMINO ACIDS in Part One.)
Lecithin granules or capsules	1 tbsp 3 times daily, before meals. 1,200 mg 3 times daily, before meals.	Needed for nephritis.
Multienzyme complex plus hydrochloric acid (HCl)	As directed on label. As directed on label.	Necessary for digestion. *Caution:* Do not give this supplement to a child under 16 years except as directed by physician. Particularly important for elderly people, who tend to be deficient. *Caution:* Do not take HCl if you have a history of ulcers.
Multimineral complex	As directed on label.	Corrects mineral depletion, common with kidney disease. Use high-potency formula.
Potassium	99 mg daily.	Acts as a kidney stimulant. Needed for nephritis. *Note:* Omit this supplement if serum potassium is elevated.
Vitamin A with mixed carotenoids	100,000 IU daily for 3 days, then 50,000 IU daily for 5 days, then reduce to 25,000 IU daily. If you are pregnant, do not exceed 10,000 IU daily.	Important in healing of urinary tract lining and in immune function. Use emulsion form for easier assimilation and greater safety at high doses. Do not take this amount in pill form.

Vitamin B complex	100 mg of each major B vitamin daily (amounts of individual vitamins in a complex will vary).	B vitamins work best when taken together. Use a high-potency formula.
plus extra vitamin B₂ (riboflavin)	25 mg 3 times daily.	Needed for nephritis.
Vitamin E emulsion or capsules	800 IU daily. Start with 200 IU daily and gradually increase to 1,000 IU daily.	Promotes immune function. An important free radical destroyer. Use d-alpha-tocopherol form.
Zinc	50–80 mg daily. Do not exceed 100 mg daily from all supplements.	An immunostimulant necessary for healing and an important inhibitor of crystallization and crystal growth. Use zinc gluconate lozenges or OptiZinc for best absorption.
plus copper	3 mg daily.	Needed to balance with zinc.

HERBS

❑ Buchu tea is good. Do not boil it, however.

❑ Celery and parsley seeds are natural diuretics. Taken in combination, they are especially helpful if high uric acid levels are present in the blood. Eating large amounts of animal proteins makes one susceptible to high levels of uric acid. These two herbs help keep them in check.

❑ Cranberries contain substances that acidify the urine, destroy bacteria buildup, and promote healing of the bladder. Drink at least 8 ounces of cranberry juice three times daily. Use only pure, unsweetened juice (available at health food stores). Do not substitute a commercial cranberry juice cocktail product; these contain large amounts of sugar. If natural cranberry juice is not available, cranberry capsules can be used as a substitute.

❑ Dandelion root extract aids in excretion of the kidney's waste products and is very beneficial for nephritis.

❑ The herbs hydrangea and uva ursi are excellent natural diuretics. One of the best first steps in cleaning out the urinary tract and keeping it healthy is to help it flush itself. Voiding the urinary tract keeps harmful deposits of calcium or other mineral salts from forming obstructions. Uva ursi is also slightly germicidal, so if there are any bacteria present, they will likely be destroyed by it.

❑ Marshmallow tea helps to cleanse the kidneys. Drink 1 quart daily.

❑ SP-6 Cornsilk Blend from Solaray helps reduce water retention. Kidney Bladder Formula from Nature's Way is also a good herbal diuretic.

❑ Other herbs that are beneficial for kidney problems include goldenrod tea, juniper berries, marshmallow root, nettle, parsley, red clover, and watermelon seed tea.

RECOMMENDATIONS

❑ Consume a diet composed of 75 percent raw foods. Eat asparagus, bananas, celery, cucumbers, garlic, papaya, parsley, potatoes, and watercress. Watermelon and pump-

kin seeds are also beneficial. Watermelon should be eaten by itself so that it passes through the system quickly; if it stays in the body too long, toxins begin to form. Also eat sprouts and most green vegetables.

❑ Include in the diet legumes, seeds, and soybeans. These foods contain the amino acid arginine, which is beneficial for the kidneys.

❑ Reduce your intake of potassium and phosphates if your levels of these are elevated. Do not use any salt or potassium chloride, a salt substitute. Also avoid beet greens, chocolate, cocoa, eggs, fish, meat, rhubarb, spinach, Swiss chard, and tea.

❑ If you have symptoms of kidney problems, especially blood in the urine or severe back pain, consult your health care provider promptly. You may need medical treatment.

❑ Drink 6 to 8 ounces of steam-distilled water every waking hour. Quality water is essential for urinary tract function.

❑ Reduce your intake of animal protein, or eliminate it altogether. A diet high in animal protein puts stress on the kidneys. Excess accumulation of protein can result in uremia. Protein is easiest to utilize if it has been broken down into free-form amino acids. Other good protein sources include beans, lentils, millet, peas, soybeans, and whole grains.

❑ Avoid all dairy products except for those that are soured, such as lowfat yogurt, buttermilk, and cottage cheese.

❑ Try a raw goat's milk diet for two weeks, consuming nothing but 4 quarts of raw goat's milk, warmed to body temperature, each day. Add 1 tablespoon of crude blackstrap molasses to each quart. During this period, take 1,000 international units of vitamin E and 75,000 international units of vitamin A in emulsion form.

Note: If you are pregnant, do not take more than 10,000 international units of vitamin A daily.

❑ Try a three-day cleansing and juice fast, and coffee or catnip tea enemas. (*See* ENEMAS and FASTING in Part Three.)

❑ If you are taking antibiotics for a kidney problem, do not take iron supplements as long as the problem exists.

CONSIDERATIONS

❑ To test for kidney failure, a doctor can test your urine for levels of albumin (protein, calcium, creatinine (waste from muscle cells), hemoglobin (if the kidneys are not working properly, hemoglobin levels may fall), phosphorus, potassium, and urea (waste from protein you have eaten).

❑ Lead and other metallic poisons are very harmful to the kidneys. Anyone who works with lead, or who is exposed to lead regularly, should take precautions to protect his or her kidneys from damage. (*See* LEAD POISONING in Part Two.)

❑ If you have diabetes, high blood sugar, high blood pressure, or a family history of kidney disease, you may be at higher risk for kidney disease.

❑ Infectious diseases, such as measles, scarlet fever, and tonsillitis, can damage the kidneys if not treated properly and completely.

❑ A study at the pharmaceutical department of Chiba University in Japan found that spirulina reduced kidney poisoning caused by mercury and drugs. Researchers discovered that adverse effects of certain drugs on the kidneys also may be decreased by the use of spirulina.

❑ Human growth hormone treatment can improve kidney function. (*See* GROWTH HORMONE THERAPY in Part Three.)

❑ Recurrent urinary tract infections indicate the possibility of a serious underlying problem. See your health care provider.

❑ High doses of the painkiller ibuprofen (Advil, Nuprin, and others) can lead to kidney dysfunction.

❑ *See also* BLADDER INFECTION and KIDNEY STONES in Part Two.

Kidney Stones

Kidney stones, medically termed *renal calculi*, are accumulations of mineral salts that can lodge anywhere along the course of the urinary tract, and they can be one of the most painful of all health ailments. Human urine is often saturated to the limit with uric acid, phosphates, and calcium oxalate. Normally, due to the secretion of various protective compounds and natural mechanisms that control the pH of urine, these substances remain suspended in solution. However, if the protective compounds are overwhelmed or immunity becomes depressed, the substances may crystallize and the crystals may begin to clump together, eventually forming stones large enough to restrict urinary flow. These stones can be jagged or smooth. Symptoms of kidney stones include pain radiating from the upper back to the lower abdomen and groin, profuse sweating, frequent urination, pus and blood in the urine, odorous or cloudy urine, absence of urine formation, and sometimes chills and fever. This can be one of the most painful of all health disorders. In milder cases, the symptoms may mimic a bad case of stomach flu or other gastrointestinal ailment.

An estimated 10 percent of Americans develop kidney stones at some point in their lives. They are most common in white men between the ages of thirty and fifty, although if you are prone to kidney stones, they can occur as early as your twenties. Kidney stones are rare in children and in African-Americans. They are more prevalent in the southeastern United States (known to doctors as the "Stone Belt") than in other parts of the country. The reason for this is not known, but it is theorized that the hot climate, which promotes dehydration, and/or regional dietary habits may be to blame. Men are more likely than women to suffer from this ailment, and adult males have a 50-percent rate of recurrence within eight years of the first episode.

Stones can range in size from microscopic specks to the size of a fingertip. There are four kinds of kidney stones: *calcium stones* (composed of calcium oxalate); *uric acid stones;* *struvite stones* (composed of magnesium ammonium phosphate); and *cystine stones*.

About 80 percent of all stones are calcium oxalate stones. High blood calcium levels lead to *hypercalciuria*—excessive absorption of calcium from the intestine—which increases the level of calcium in the urine. This excess calcium eventually forms a stone. High blood calcium levels can also result from malfunctioning parathyroid glands (tiny glands in the neck that regulate blood calcium levels), vitamin D intoxication, and multiple myeloma. The consumption of refined carbohydrates, especially sugar, can help precipitate kidney stones as well, because the sugar stimulates the pancreas to release insulin, which in turn causes extra calcium to be excreted in the urine. Mild chronic or recurrent dehydration can also be a factor in kidney stones; it concentrates the urine, increasing the likelihood of stone formation.

Uric acid stones form when the volume of urine excreted is too low and/or blood levels of uric acid are abnormally high. The latter condition is commonly associated with symptoms of gout. Unlike other types of kidney stones, struvite stones are unrelated to metabolism; these stones are caused by infection. Women often get them with recurrent urinary tract infections. Cystine stones are caused by a condition called cystinuria, a rare congenital defect that can cause stones composed of the amino acid cystine to form in the kidney or bladder.

Calcium stones often run in families because the tendency to absorb too much calcium is hereditary. Also, in people with a family history of kidney stones, there seems to be a stronger than normal correlation between the intake of either vitamin C or oxalic acid and the urinary excretion of oxalate. Apparently, such individuals either absorb more oxalate from their diets or metabolize greater amounts of oxalate precursors. People who have *Crohn's disease* or *irritable bowel syndrome,* or who eat diets high in oxalic acid, may have an increased risk of kidney stones as well, as these factors can cause the excretion of oxalate in the urine to increase. Other risk factors for kidney stones include low urine volume, low bodily pH, heredity, living in a tropical climate, and reduced production of natural urinary inhibitors of crystal formation.

Kidney stones are ten times as common now as they were at the start of the twentieth century. While the consumption of foods high in oxalic acid (mostly eggs, fish, and certain vegetables) has declined markedly in this country in that time, the amount of animal fats and protein in the average American's diet has increased significantly. The ratio of plant to animal protein in the typical diet at the beginning of the twentieth century was roughly 1 to 1. This ratio has since declined to 1 to 2. The consumption of animal protein is strongly associated with oxalate absorption.

NUTRIENTS

SUPPLEMENT	SUGGESTED DOSAGE	COMMENTS
Very Important		
Inositol hexaphosphate (IP6) with inositol	As directed on label.	Has been proven in many studies to prevent and treat kidney stones.
L-Methionine	500 mg daily, on an empty stomach. Take with water or juice. Do not take with milk. Take with 50 mg vitamin B6 and 100 mg vitamin C for better absorption.	Reduces the incidence of kidney stones by destroying free radicals associated with stone formation. (*See* AMINO ACIDS in Part One.)
Magnesium citrate	500 mg daily.	Reduces calcium absorption and can lower urinary oxalate, a mineral salt common in kidney stones.
Vitamin B complex plus extra vitamin B6 (pyridoxine)	50 mg of each major B vitamin 3 times daily, with meals (amounts of individual vitamins in a complex will vary). 50 mg twice daily.	B vitamins work best when all are taken together. Taken with magnesium, reduces oxalate.
Zinc	50–80 mg daily. Do not exceed 100 mg daily.	An important inhibitor of crystallization, which can lead to stone formation. Use zinc gluconate lozenges or OptiZinc for best absorption.
Helpful		
Multivitamin complex	As directed on label.	To maintain a balance of all nutrients.
L-Arginine	500 mg daily. If you are prone to herpes outbreaks, take with L-lysine.	Aids kidney disorders.
Potassium	99 mg daily.	Inhibits crystallization, which can lead to stone formation. Use potassium citrate form.
Proteolytic enzymes	As directed on label. Take between meals.	Aids normal digestion.
Raw kidney glandular	500 mg daily.	Strengthens the kidneys. (*See* GLANDULAR THERAPY in Part Three.)
Vitamin A with mixed carotenoids	25,000 IU daily. If you are pregnant, do not exceed 10,000 IU daily.	Promotes healing of the urinary tract lining, which is often damaged by stones. If you are pregnant, use a natural carotenoid complex such as Betatene in place of vitamin A.
Vitamin C with bioflavonoids	3,000–6,000 mg daily, in divided doses.	Acidifies urine. Most stones will not form in acidic urine.
Vitamin E	600 IU daily.	A powerful antioxidant. Use d-alpha-tocopherol form.

HERBS

❑ Aloe vera juice, taken at levels that do not produce a laxative effect, can be useful in preventing stone formation and in reducing the size of a stone during an acute attack.

❑ Ginkgo biloba and goldenseal, taken in extract form, aid circulation to the kidneys and have anti-inflammatory properties. They are also powerful antioxidants.

Caution: Do not take goldenseal internally on a daily basis for more than one week. Do not use it during pregnancy, and use it with caution if you are allergic to ragweed.

❑ A combination of lobelia tincture (3 to 4 drops) and wild yam tincture (15 drops) in a glass of warm water helps to relax the ureters, relieve pain, and hasten the passing of stones. Sip this mixture throughout the day.

❑ Marshmallow root tea daily helps to cleanse the kidneys and to expel kidney stones. Drink 1 quart daily.

❑ Uva ursi helps to relieve pain and bloating.

❑ Other herbs that may aid in alleviating kidney stones include cleavers, gravel root, horsetail, juniper berries, and pipsissewa (also called Prince's Pine).

RECOMMENDATIONS

❑ For pain relief, drink the juice of half a fresh lemon in 8 ounces of water every half-hour until the pain subsides. You can alternate between lemon juice and fresh apple juice.

❑ To maintain good kidney function, drink plenty of quality water—at least 3 quarts daily. By far the single most important measure one can take to prevent kidney stones from forming is to increase water consumption. Water dilutes urine and helps prevent concentrations of the minerals and salts that can form stones. (Chronic dehydration is a major factor in kidney stone disease in 15 to 20 percent of people.) Also drink unsweetened cranberry juice to help acidify the urine (unless you are prone to uric acid stones). Drinking the juice of a fresh lemon in a glass of warm water first thing each morning can help prevent stones from forming.

❑ Increase your consumption of foods rich in vitamin A. Vitamin A is beneficial to the urinary tract and helps to discourage the formation of stones. Good sources of vitamin A include alfalfa, apricots, cantaloupes, carrots, pumpkin, sweet potatoes, and squash.

❑ Use only distilled water for drinking and cooking. Add trace mineral drops to your drinking water.

❑ Minimize your consumption of animal protein, or eliminate it from your diet altogether. A diet high in animal protein causes the body to excrete calcium, producing excessive amounts of calcium, phosphorus, and uric acid in the kidneys and often resulting in painful kidney stones.

❑ Reduce your intake of potassium and phosphates. Do not use any salt or potassium chloride, a salt substitute, and avoid carbonated soft drinks.

❑ Do not omit calcium from your diet—it is important in lowering your risk of developing osteoporosis, which is a much more common problem than kidney stones, especially for women. Getting extra magnesium can reduce the risk of kidney stones by increasing the solubility of calcium oxalate. Seafood, brown rice, tofu, and soybeans are naturally high in magnesium.

❑ Try drinking a large amount of liquid (preferably pure water), allow twenty minutes for digestion, and then run up and down stairs vigorously. This has been known to allow small, stubborn kidney stones to pass naturally.

❑ If you do not pass the lodged stone, see your physician. He or she may order a urine test and an x-ray for formal diagnosis and proper treatment.

❑ If you have a family history of kidney stones, take calcium supplements *with meals*. When you consume calcium-rich foods with oxalates, they bind together and are expelled in the stool, lessening your risk of kidney stones. Calcium supplements should be avoided only by those with a personal history of kidney stones.

❑ Avoid foods that contain or lead to the production of oxalic acid, including asparagus, beet greens, beets, blueberries, celery, eggs, fish, grapes, parsley, rhubarb, sorrel, spinach, Swiss chard, and vegetables of the cabbage family. Also avoid alcohol, black tea (green tea is a good substitute), chocolate, cocoa, dried figs, nuts, pepper, and poppy seeds.

❑ Avoid all refined sugar and products that contain it. Sugar stimulates the pancreas to release insulin, which in turn causes extra calcium to be excreted in the urine.

❑ Stay active. People who are sedentary tend to accumulate high levels of calcium in the bloodstream. Exercise helps pull calcium from the blood into the bones, where it belongs.

❑ If you have a history of cystine stones, avoid the amino acid L-cystine. If you must take a supplement containing L-cystine, take at least three times as much vitamin C at the same time. Otherwise, cystine can crystallize in the kidneys and form large stones that fill the interior of the kidney.

CONSIDERATIONS

❑ A Harvard University study found that consuming dairy products may actually lower the risk of developing kidney stones, instead of increasing the risk, as was previously thought. They also found that calcium supplements raise the risk slightly unless they are taken with meals.

❑ Drinking coffee, tea, and wine may lower the risk of kidney stones, while grapefruit juice may increase it.

❑ In Japan, the incidence of kidney stones has been rising steadily since the middle of this century, when dietary changes typical of an industrialized nation began to occur. People in Japan who develop kidney stones consume far

more proteins, refined carbohydrates, fats, and oils than did their forebears.

❑ Most kidney stones eventually pass by themselves. Depending on the type and size of stone, your physician may recommend the use of electroshock wave lithotripsy (ESWL) to break up the stones, ureterscope calculus removal, or tunnel surgery (in which the surgeon creates a small tunnel through the skin and inserts an instrument to remove the stone), or the use of a laser or other tiny device that is threaded up the urinary tract to break up stones.

❑ Once kidney stones have formed and have been treated, the risk of recurrence increases; once a person has formed a stone, there is a 20- to 50-percent chance that he or she will form another in the next ten years. Once a second incidence has occurred, the risk increases markedly.

❑ Prescription medications containing sodium cellulose phosphate are effective on calcium-based stones. Potassium citrate (Urocit-K) is effective on stones not of calcium origin. Allopurinol (Lopurin, Zyloprim) and hydrochlorothiazide (Esidrix, HydroDIURIL, and others) are other medications that may help to prevent the occurrence of stones.

❑ Taking up to 100 milligrams of zinc daily can help inhibit the formation of crystals that later accumulate into stones. While the recommended amount of zinc helps to enhance immune function, anything over 100 milligrams per day tends to depress immunity.

❑ To control calcium stones, the pH of the body should be raised, while to control uric acid stones, bodily pH should be lowered. (*See* ACID/ALKALI IMBALANCE in Part Two.)

❑ Diet alone cannot remove kidney stones, but it can be very effective at preventing them. Kidney stones are primarily an affliction of well-fed societies in which people consume large quantities of animal protein. A vegetarian diet can be of great benefit to anyone prone to kidney stones. A strict vegan diet that contains no animal proteins whatsoever, is almost entirely devoid of processed foods, and is low in sodium and high in fiber and water is generally considered conducive to kidney-stone prevention.

❑ Measures used to treat kidney stones and to prevent recurrences depend on the nature of the stone, so it is important to take any stone you pass to your health care provider for analysis.

Lactose Intolerance (Lactase Deficiency)

Lactose intolerance is the inability to digest lactose (milk sugar). It is caused by a lack or deficiency of lactase, an enzyme manufactured in the small intestine that splits lactose into glucose and galactose. When a person with lactose intolerance consumes milk or other dairy products, some or all of the lactose they contain remains undigested, retains fluid, and ferments in the colon, resulting in abdominal cramps, bloating, diarrhea, and gas. Symptoms usually begin between thirty minutes and two hours after consumption of dairy foods.

The degree of lactose intolerance varies from individual to individual. For most of the world's adults, lactose intolerance is actually a normal condition. Only Caucasians of northern European origin generally retain the ability to digest lactose after childhood. In the United States, an estimated 30 to 50 million people are lactose intolerant. Lactase deficiency can also occur as a result of a gastrointestinal disorder that damages the digestive tract, such as celiac disease, irritable bowel syndrome, regional enteritis, or ulcerative colitis. It can also develop on its own. There is no known way to prevent it.

Although far less common, lactose intolerance can occur in children as well as adults. In infants, lactose intolerance can occur after a severe bout of gastroenteritis, which damages the intestinal lining. Symptoms of lactose intolerance in an infant can include foamy diarrhea with diaper rash, slow weight gain and development, and vomiting.

Lactose intolerance can cause discomfort and digestive disruption, but it is not a serious threat to health and it can easily be managed through dietary modification. Unless otherwise specified, the dosages recommended here are for adults. For a child between the ages of twelve and seventeen, reduce the dose to three-quarters of the recommended amount. For a child between six and twelve, use one-half of the recommended dose.

NUTRIENTS

SUPPLEMENT	SUGGESTED DOSAGE	COMMENTS
Very Important		
Acidophilus (Kyo-Dophilis from Wakunaga is a good source)	1 tsp in distilled water twice daily, on an empty stomach.	Replaces lost "friendly" bacteria and promotes healthy digestion. Use a nondairy formula only.
Charcoal tablets	For an acute attack, take 4 tablets every hour with water until symptoms subside. Take separately from other medications and supplements.	Absorbs toxins and relieves diarrhea.
Helpful		
Bone Defense from KAL or Bone Support from Synergy Plus	As directed on label. As directed on label.	To supply necessary calcium and nutrients needed for calcium absorption.
LactAid from Lactaid, Inc.	As directed on label.	To supply the enzyme lactase, needed for digesting milk sugar.
Magnesium	1,000 mg daily.	Needed for calcium uptake. Promotes pH balance.
Multivitamin and mineral complex	As directed on label.	All nutrients are needed for optimal health.
Ultra Clear Sustain from Metagenics	As directed on label.	Promotes favorable bacteria in the digestive tract and provides additional nutritional support for the digestive system. Available only through health care professionals.
Vitamin D$_3$	400 IU daily.	Needed for calcium uptake.
Vitamin E	400–1,000 IU daily.	Protects the cell membranes that line the colon wall. Use d-alpha-tocopherol form.
Zinc plus copper	30 mg 3 times daily. Do not exceed a total of 100 mg daily from all supplements. 3 mg daily.	To maintain immune system and proper mineral balance. Use zinc gluconate lozenges or OptiZinc for best absorption. Needed to balance with zinc.

RECOMMENDATIONS

❑ Avoid milk and all dairy products except yogurt. This is the most important dietary measure for anyone who is intolerant to lactose. Use soymilk or Rice Dream in place of milk and soy cheese instead of dairy cheese. Especially avoid consuming lactose-containing foods on an empty stomach.

❑ Include yogurt in your diet. Yogurt is the one dairy product that can be good for a person with lactose intolerance. The cultures present in yogurt digest the lactose it contains, so it is no longer a problem. They also aid in overall digestion. Be sure to eat only yogurt that contains active live yogurt cultures. Homemade yogurt is best.

❑ Be sure to eat plenty of foods that are high in calcium. Good choices include apricots, blackstrap molasses, broccoli, collard greens, dried figs, kale, calcium-fortified orange juice, rhubarb, salmon, sardines, spinach, tofu, and yogurt. Calcium supplements may be beneficial.

❑ Check with your pharmacist before taking any medications. Many pills are formulated using lactose as filler. Some birth control pills and stomach medications contain lactose.

❑ During an acute attack, do not eat any solid food, but do drink plenty of quality water and replace lost minerals. *See* DIARRHEA in Part Two for dietary suggestions.

❑ Read food product labels carefully, and avoid any that contain lactose or "milk solids." Lactose is added to many different types of processed food, including breads, canned and powdered soups, cookies, pancake mixes, powdered drink mixes such as flavored coffees, processed breakfast cereals, processed meats, and salad dressings.

❑ If you are pregnant and have a family history of lactose intolerance, give serious consideration to breastfeeding your baby. If that is not possible, choose a nondairy baby formula, such as a soy-based product.

CONSIDERATIONS

❑ There are several tests used to measure the absorption

of lactose into the digestive system. The first test is known as the *lactose tolerance test*, in which the person drinks a liquid containing lactose after fasting overnight. Approximately one-half hour later, the amount of glucose (blood sugar) in the blood is measured and the presence of symptoms assessed. If the blood glucose does not rise by at least 20 points, and especially if there are symptoms such as bloating or discomfort, a diagnosis of lactose intolerance is confirmed. The *hydrogen breath test* measures the amount of hydrogen in the breath. Again, the person is given a drink containing a high level of lactose. When lactose is improperly digested in the colon, gases form and are carried through the bloodstream to the lungs and are exhaled. A higher level of hydrogen in the breath indicates faulty digestion of lactose. This test is given to adults and children, but is not recommended for infants and very young children. Young children and infants are tested by the *stool acidity test*, which measures the amount of acid in the stool. This test also assesses the levels of glucose and lactic acid present in the stool.

❑ Lactose intolerance is not the same as milk allergy. Lactose intolerance specifically refers to a syndrome caused by the failure to digest milk sugar; a person with a milk allergy may be able to digest milk normally, but his or her immune system then has an allergic response to one or more of the milk's components. (*See* ALLERGIES in Part Two.)

❑ Hard, aged cheeses, such as Parmesan cheese, are relatively low in lactose, and may be easier to tolerate than other dairy products.

❑ Ice cream is particularly difficult for a person with lactose intolerance to digest. Not only is ice cream made from milk, but many brands add extra lactose to achieve the desired texture, and the cold temperature can be shocking to the digestive system as well.

❑ Consuming small amounts of dairy products with meals may help improve the lactose tolerance level. The large intestine becomes more accustomed to digesting the lactose when it is introduced in small quantities on a regular basis.

❑ The symptoms of lactose intolerance are similar to those of celiac disease, and the two disorders may occur together. (*See* CELIAC DISEASE in Part Two.)

❑ Lactose-free and lactose-reduced products are available in most supermarkets.

Lead Poisoning

Lead is one of the most toxic metal contaminants known. It is a cumulative poison that is retained in the body. Even at low levels, lead that is not excreted through the digestive system accumulates in the body and is absorbed directly from the blood into other tissues. When lead leaves the bloodstream, it is stored, along with other minerals, in the bones, where it continues to build up over a lifetime. Lead from the bones may then reenter the bloodstream at any time as a result of severe biologic stress, such as renal failure, pregnancy, menopause, or prolonged immobilization or illness.

Unlike some metallic elements, lead has no known functions or health benefits for humans. It is considered a metabolic poison, which means that it inhibits some basic enzyme functions. Lead reacts with selenium and sulfur-containing antioxidant enzymes in the cells, seriously diminishing the ability of these substances to protect against free radical damage. When present in toxic amounts, it can damage the heart, kidneys, liver, and nervous system.

The body cannot distinguish between calcium and lead. Once lead enters the body, it is assimilated in the same manner as calcium. Because young children and pregnant women absorb calcium more readily to meet their extra needs, they also absorb more lead than other people. Children absorb 25 to 40 percent more lead per pound of body weight than adults do. People with deficiencies of calcium are more susceptible to lead toxicity as well.

Symptoms of lead poisoning typically come on over the course of several weeks in adults and several days in children. Children's symptoms also tend to be more severe. People with lead poisoning commonly have days of severe gastrointestinal colic. Their gums often turn blue, and they may experience muscle weakness. Other possible symptoms include anxiety, arthritis, confusion, chronic fatigue, diarrhea, gout, insomnia, learning disabilities, loss of appetite, a metallic taste in the mouth, seizures, tremors, and vertigo. Lead poisoning can eventually lead to blindness, loss of memory, mental disturbances, mental retardation, paralysis of the extremities, and even coma and death. Chronic lead poisoning can also cause impotence, infertility and other reproductive disorders, and liver failure.

Lead is one of the most widely used metals in the United States today, and it is estimated that a large number of people have high levels of lead in their bodies. Sources of lead exposure include lead-based paints, ceramic glazes, lead crystal dishes and glassware, leaded gasoline, lead-acid batteries used in automobiles, tobacco, liver, water, some domestic and imported wines, canned fruit (the lead from lead-soldered cans leaches out and is absorbed by fruits), garden vegetables (if grown in lead-contaminated soil), bone meal, and insecticides. Even such innocuous-seeming items as vinyl mini-blinds and porcelain-glazed sinks and bathtubs have been implicated in lead exposure.

Another potential source of lead poisoning is water supplied through lead piping. Lead piping was used in most homes built before 1930. Newer homes use copper pipes; however, even if you have copper pipes in your home, the chances are very good that they were assembled with lead solder, which is 50 percent lead. Solder can leach a significant amount of lead into the water supply, especially in the first few years after installation. Due to mounting concern over the amount of lead leaching into the water, the use of lead solder was banned in 1986.

Lead poisoning first gained widespread public attention when large numbers of children, especially children in inner cities, were found to have been poisoned by chips of lead-based paint that had peeled off the walls. Some children acquired high lead levels from playing in lead-contaminated dirt, which would get on their hands and then into their mouths. Since then, it has been learned that pregnant women who have high levels of lead in their bodies can give birth to babies with high lead levels. An estimated 90 percent of the lead stored in the mother's body is free to cross the placenta to the fetus. Children born to women who have toxic amounts of lead in their bodies generally suffer from growth retardation and nervous system disorders. Even low-level lead exposure in young children may be associated with impaired intellectual development and behavioral problems. Average blood lead levels in the United States have declined dramatically in recent decades, but, according to the U.S. Centers for Disease Control and Prevention (CDC), about 1 million American children under the age of five still have blood lead levels that exceed the acceptable norm.

Unless otherwise specified, the dosages recommended here are for adults. For a child between the ages of twelve and seventeen, reduce the dose to three-quarters of the recommended amount. For a child between six and twelve, use one-half of the recommended dose, and for a child under the age of six, use one-quarter of the recommended amount.

NUTRIENTS

SUPPLEMENT	SUGGESTED DOSAGE	COMMENTS
Essential		
Alpha-lipoic acid (ALA)	As directed on label.	Helps detoxify the body of metal pollutants and works as a powerful antioxidant.
Apple pectin	As directed on label.	Binds toxins and metals, removing them from the body.
Calcium	2,000 mg daily.	Prevents lead from being deposited in the body tissues. Use calcium chelate form. Do not obtain calcium from dolomite, bone meal, or cow's milk, which can contain lead.
and magnesium	1,000 mg daily.	Needed to balance with calcium. Use magnesium chelate form.
Garlic (Kyolic from Wakunaga)	2 tablets 3 times daily, with meals.	Protects the body's immune system. Helps to bind with and excrete lead.
Kelp and/or alfalfa	As directed on label.	Contains essential minerals, especially calcium and magnesium. Also removes unwanted metal deposits. *See under* Herbs, below.

L-Lysine plus	500 mg daily, on an empty stomach.	Assists calcium absorption.
L-cysteine and L-cystine	500 mg each daily, on an empty stomach. Take with water or juice. Do not take with milk. Take with 50 mg vitamin B6 and 100 mg vitamin C for better absorption.	Sulfur-containing amino acids that act as detoxifiers and remove heavy metals. (*See* AMINO ACIDS in Part One.)
Methylsulfonyl-methane (MSM)	As directed on label.	Helps the body detoxify toxic metals.
S-adenosylmethio-nine (SAMe)	As directed on label.	Has antioxidant effects and helps chelate heavy metals out of the body. *Caution:* Do not use if you have manic-depressive or take prescription antidepressants.
Vitamin C with bioflavonoids	5,000–20,000 mg daily, in divided doses. (*See* ASCORBIC ACID FLUSH in Part Three.)	Helps to neutralize the effects of lead.
Zinc	80 mg daily. Do not exceed a total of 100 mg daily from all supplements.	Can displace lead and lower the body burden. Low levels of zinc have been found in people with high lead levels.
Very Important		
Glutathione plus L-methionine	As directed on label, on an empty stomach. Take with water or juice. Do not take with milk. Take with 50 mg vitamin B6 and 100 mg vitamin C for better absorption.	Powerful antioxidants that protect the liver, kidneys, heart, and central nervous system. (*See* AMINO ACIDS in Part One.)
Lecithin granules or capsules	1 tbsp 3 times daily, before meals. 1,200 mg 3 times daily, before meals.	Protects cell membranes.
Selenium	200 mcg daily. If you are pregnant, do not exceed 40 mcg daily.	A potent antioxidant.
Important		
Vitamin B complex	100 mg of each major B vitamin 3 times daily, with meals (amounts of individual vitamins in a complex will vary).	B vitamins work best when taken together.
plus extra vitamin B1 (thiamine) and vitamin B6 (pyridoxine)	100 mg daily. 50 mg daily.	These B vitamins are vital in cellular enzyme function and important in brain metabolism; they help to remove lead from the brain.
Helpful		
Vitamin A with mixed carotenoids plus vitamin E	25,000 IU daily for 2 months. If you are pregnant, do not exceed 10,000 IU daily. Start with 400 IU daily and increase slowly to 800 IU for 2 months.	Potent antioxidants that destroy free radicals and protect the cells from damage due to lead poisoning. Use d-alpha-tocopherol form.
or Micellized Vitamin A emulsion from American Biologics	As directed on label.	An emulsified form of vitamins A and E that enters the system rapidly.

HERBS

❑ Alfalfa is rich in vitamins, minerals, and other valuable nutrients, and has a detoxifying effect on the body.

❏ Try using aloe vera juice. Take $\frac{1}{2}$ cup in the morning and $\frac{1}{2}$ cup before bedtime. This softens bowel movements and aids in removing metals from the digestive tract.

❏ Chlorella and cilantro are helpful for absorbing toxic metals.

RECOMMENDATIONS

❏ Make sure that your diet is high in fiber and that you supplement it with pectin (found in apples).

Note: Always take supplemental fiber separately from other supplements and medications.

❏ Eat beans, broccoli, Brussels sprouts, cauliflower, eggs, garlic, kale, legumes, onions, and spinach. These help to rid the body of lead.

❏ Make sure your diet is low in fat and contains adequate amounts of iron and calcium. The body absorbs lead more easily if it is lacking in calcium or iron, or if it has been exposed to a high-fat diet.

Tips for a Lead-Free Environment

Once lead accumulates in the body, it remains there. Prevention is therefore much better than treatment when it comes to lead poisoning. The following are simple measures you can take to avoid exposure to lead:

• Do not buy foods in cans sealed with lead solder, which leaches into foods. Lead-soldered cans often have remnants of solder and indentations along the seam. If you buy canned foods, look for lead-free cans that have no side seams. Be wary of imported canned foods. Other countries may have no regulations governing the use of lead solder.

• Make sure children's hands are clean before they eat.

• Keep painted surfaces in good repair, so that older layers of paint are not exposed, chipping, or peeling. Although lead-based paints have been banned for use in residences, numerous older homes and public housing units still contain these paints. Do not allow children to eat paint chips. Hire a professional to remove lead-based paint from any surface; people can poison themselves by burning or scraping off layers of paint.

• Have your water tested to ensure a safe level of lead and other minerals. National Testing Laboratories sells a kit for testing impurities in your water. To order one of these kits, call 800–H20–TEST. Your state health department may also conduct tests for water contaminants at a reasonable price. Culligan International provides a WaterWatch Hot Line at 800–285–5442 (Monday through Friday, 8:15 A.M. to 5:00 P.M. Central Standard Time). They will put you in contact with a local Culligan dealer, who will provide a free water-testing service. You may also send away for a free booklet entitled *Water Quality Answers* by writing to the Water Quality Association, 4151 Naperville Road, Lisle, IL 60532. Enclose a stamped, self-addressed envelope.

• Never use the first water drawn from your tap in the morning. Let it run for at least three minutes before you use it. Better yet, use only steam-distilled, filtered, deionized water for drinking and cooking. If safe drinking water is not available, treat water with grapefruit seed extract (available in health food stores) before using it. Add 10 drops of extract per gallon of water and shake or stir vigorously.

• Never boil water longer than necessary. Five minutes is enough. Boiling concentrates contaminants in water, including lead.

• Be careful about buying imported ceramic products. The amount of lead allowable in ceramic ware manufactured in the United States is strictly regulated, but there are often no rules governing the glazing techniques of foreign producers. Standards for acceptable lead levels are relatively strict in countries where many of our dishes are manufactured—Great Britain and Japan, for example—but they are often more lax in other countries, such as Mexico and China. The FDA is unable to check a significant number to insure safety.

• Antiques and other collectibles may look attractive, but this type of dinnerware is more likely to leach lead than dishes made more recently. If you buy such items, use them for decorative purposes only.

• Do not store alcoholic beverages, or acidic foods or beverages such as vinegar, fruit juices, or foods made with tomatoes, in lead crystal glassware for any length of time. The lead that gives fine crystal its sparkle and brilliance leaches into foods and beverages served or stored in it. Babies and children should not be fed from crystal dishes or glassware at all.

• If you are pregnant, avoid drinking hot coffee or other hot acidic beverages, such as tomato soup, from lead-glazed ceramic cups or mugs.

• Do not turn bread bags inside out and use them to store other foods. The ink used to print labels on many bread bags contains considerable amounts of lead. While the lead on the labels doesn't get through the plastic to the bread inside, it can contaminate food if you turn the bags inside out and use them to store other foods.

• If you drink wine, always wipe the mouth of the bottle well (inside and out) with a damp cloth before pouring the wine. The foil wrappers around the corks of wine bottles can deposit lead around the mouth of a bottle and contaminate the beverage. The Bureau of Alcohol, Tobacco, and Firearms analyzed more than 500 samples of wine and found that samples poured directly from bottles often contained more lead than samples drawn from bottles with strawlike instruments.

❏ Drink steam-distilled water only.

❏ Do not smoke, and avoid secondhand smoke.

❏ If you suspect lead poisoning, have a hair analysis done to determine long-term accumulation of lead. Blood tests reveal only the most recent exposure. (*See* HAIR ANALYSIS in Part Three.)

❏ Always check the labels when purchasing foreign-made products such as eye makeup (kajal, surma, or kohl dyes from the Middle East) and over-the-counter remedies (Alarcon, Azarcon, Coral, Greta, Liga, Maria Luisa, or Rueda). Some of these products may contain as much as 99-percent lead oxide.

CONSIDERATIONS

❏ Succimer (Chemet) is a drug that may be prescribed to chelate lead from children. This drug may reduce illness and death from lead poisoning. Succimer has been approved for use only in children who have significantly high blood lead levels (above 45 mg/dl). Succimer may alter immune-system function.

❏ Chelation with EDTA can help prevent accumulation of lead. Chelating agents work by binding to lead in the bloodstream and expediting its elimination from the body in urine. (*See* CHELATION THERAPY in Part Three.)

❏ The CDC recommends routine blood testing for lead in all children at one and two years of age. When small children have blood lead levels above 10 micrograms per deciliter (mg/dl)—the highest level the CDC considers acceptable—their intelligence suffers. Numerous studies show an average decrease of one-quarter point in intelligence quotient (IQ) for each 1-mg/dl increase in blood lead level.

❏ A portable, battery-operated testing system that can analyze lead levels in the blood within three minutes is available. The testing unit was developed by ESA Inc. of Chelmsford, Massachusetts, and Andcare Inc. of Durham, North Carolina.

❏ Hair analysis is another method that can be used to detect heavy metal toxicity. However, results may not be accurate if the sample is contaminated, for example, by hair dye or other possible sources of lead. (*See* HAIR ANALYSIS in Part Three.)

❏ One way to get an indication if your child may be at risk of developing lead poisoning is to have a veterinarian check the lead level in your family dog. Long before children show symptoms of lead poisoning, dogs can get colic, then diarrhea or vomiting, and even seizures. Dogs ingest lead the way small children do—licking toys covered with lead-filled dust, chewing old paint on walls or furniture, or putting things covered with old lead paint flakes in their mouths.

❏ Children with above-average levels of lead in their blood are half an inch shorter, on average, than other children. According to one researcher, lead levels are signifi-

cantly higher in infants who die of sudden infant death syndrome (SIDS) than in infants who die of other causes.

❏ A study reported in *The New England Journal of Medicine* suggested that even low levels of lead in children may lead to lifelong problems, such as severe reading difficulties, learning disabilities, poor eye-hand coordination, retarded growth, and slowed reflexes. High levels of lead in the body have also been implicated in autism, behavioral problems, hyperactivity, and juvenile delinquency.

❏ Even though leaded gasoline has been almost completely replaced with unleaded fuel, there is still an estimated 4 to 5 million metric tons of lead in American soil that accumulated as a result of leaded gasoline use in the past. Anyone who grows crops or garden produce near busy roads or highways should check the lead level in the soil.

❏ Any building fifty years old or older should be inspected by a professional, and if there is lead-based paint on the walls, it should be removed by someone with the proper expertise and equipment. Simply painting over old lead-based paint can release tiny particles containing lead into the air, posing a possible lead hazard.

❏ A previously underreported source of lead poisoning may be lead-based hair colorings used by men. According to the Cosmetic, Toiletry, and Fragrance Association, 80 percent of the hair-coloring products designed for men use so-called progressive coloring agents, which are made of lead acetate. It is known that some lead is absorbed through the scalp, raising questions about the risk of lead poisoning.

❏ The U.S. Food and Drug Administration (FDA) considers children and pregnant women at highest risk for lead poisoning.

❏ An easy way to test dishes for lead is to use LeadCheck Swabs from Hybrivet Systems. The same company also makes a kit for testing for lead in water. (*See* MANUFACTURER AND DISTRIBUTOR INFORMATION in the Appendix.)

❏ More information about lead poisoning is available from the National Lead Information Center. (*See* HEALTH AND MEDICAL ORGANIZATIONS in the Appendix.)

Leg Cramps

See MUSCLE CRAMPS. *See also under* PREGNANCY-RELATED PROBLEMS.

Leg Ulcers

Ulcers are open sores that develop on deteriorated patches of skin. When poor circulation in the legs restricts blood flow, the skin tissue begins to erode; it is thus more susceptible to the development of an open sore. The broken skin can be very slow to heal. Leg ulcers are more likely to develop in people with poor circulation, thrombophlebitis, and/or varicose veins. *Venous ulcers* are leg ulcers related to a condition known as venous stasis, in which leg veins cease to function as they should. Blood pools in the veins, resulting in inflammation of the overlying skin that leads to the development of ulcers. Venous ulcers are usually situated on the lower third of the leg. *Arterial ulcers* occur when an artery or arteries serving the leg fail to deliver an adequate blood supply, which in turn may be caused by atherosclerotic plaque or by an embolism blocking the proper flow of blood. These ulcers usually occur on bony areas around the feet and ankles. *Diabetic ulcers* can be a result of peripheral neuropathy or insufficient blood supply to the surface of the skin. (*See* DIABETES in Part Two.) They normally occur around the feet.

NUTRIENTS

SUPPLEMENT	SUGGESTED DOSAGE	COMMENTS
Important		
Coenzyme Q₁₀	60 mg daily.	Increases resistance to leg ulcers by increasing tissue oxygenation.
plus Coenzyme A from Coenzyme-A Technologies	As directed on label.	Supports the immune system's detoxification of many dangerous substances.
Dimethylglycine (DMG) (Aangamik DMG from FoodScience of Vermont)	As directed on label.	Enhances utilization of oxygen to improve blood flow to the legs.
Garlic (Kyolic from Wakunaga)	2 capsules 3 times daily.	Improves circulation and aids the healing process.
Grape seed extract	As directed on label.	A powerful antioxidant that prohibits free radical damage.
Shark cartilage (Sharkilage from American Biologics)	As directed on label.	To improve blood vessel integrity.
Ultra Connexin from American Biologics	As directed on label.	Supports wound healing and blood-vessel-wall health.
Vitamin C with bioflavonoids	5,000–10,000 mg daily, in divided doses.	Improves circulation and aids in healing process. Also keeps infection in check.
Vitamin E emulsion or capsules	800 IU daily. Start with 400 IU daily and increase slowly to 1,600 IU daily.	Helps the body use oxygen efficiently and speeds healing. Use d-alpha-tocopherol form. Emulsion is preferable to capsules; it provides easier assimilation and greater safety at higher doses.
Helpful		
Colloidal silver	Take orally and apply topically to the affected area as directed on label.	A broad-spectrum antiseptic that promotes rapid healing and subdues inflammation.
Flaxseed oil or Ultimate Oil from Nature's Secret	2 tsp daily. As directed on label.	To minimize clot formation and help keep veins soft and pliable.

Free-form amino acid complex (Amino Balance from Anabol Naturals)	As directed on label. Take on an empty stomach.	Promotes healing and tissue repair.
Iron or Floradix Iron + Herbs from Salus Haus	As directed by physician. Take with 100 mg vitamin C for better absorption. As directed on label.	Important for cell growth and healing. *Caution:* Do not take iron unless anemia is diagnosed. A natural and nontoxic source of iron.
Multivitamin and mineral complex	As directed on label, with meals.	Necessary for proper healing and to remedy and/or prevent nutritional deficiencies.
Vitamin A emulsion with mixed carotenoids	25,000 IU daily for 1 month. If you are pregnant, do not exceed 10,000 IU daily.	Necessary for healing and protection of tissues. Use emulsion form for more rapid and complete assimilation.
Vitamin B complex plus extra vitamin B₁₂ and folic acid	As directed on label. 1,000–2,000 mcg daily. 400 mcg 3 times daily, plus injections (under a doctor's supervision) twice weekly or as prescribed by physician.	B vitamins work best when taken together. Use a high-potency formula. Allows proper tissue enzyme function for healing. Helps prevent anemia. Use a lozenge or sublingual form. Vital for proper utilization of protein during the healing process.
Vitamin K	As directed on label.	Needed for blood clotting and healing.
Zinc	50 mg daily. Do not exceed a total of 100 mg daily from all supplements.	Aids in the healing of ulcers and boosts immune function. Use zinc gluconate lozenges or OptiZinc for best absorption.

HERBS

❑ Alfalfa, in capsule or tablet form, is a good source of vitamin K. Red clover tea or capsules are also beneficial.

❑ Make comfrey tea and use it as a compress; soak a clean cloth in it and apply the cloth to aching, inflamed leg ulcers.
   Note: Comfrey is recommended for external use only.

❑ Echinacea improves immune function and aids healing.

❑ Goldenseal is a natural antibiotic and promotes healing. It can be taken in tea or capsule form. It can also be used as a poultice. Moisten a piece of sterile gauze with alcohol-free goldenseal extract and use this to cover the ulcer.
   Caution: Do not take goldenseal on a daily basis for more than one week at a time, and do not use it during pregnancy. If you have a history of cardiovascular disease, diabetes, or glaucoma, use it only under a doctor's supervision.

RECOMMENDATIONS

❑ Go on a diet of raw foods with lightly steamed vegetables for one month to help the healing process.

❑ Eat dark green leafy vegetables to obtain vitamin K.

❑ Include plenty of fresh garlic and onions in your diet. These promote circulation and healing, and also contain the trace element germanium, which boosts the immune system and improves tissue oxygenation.

❏ *See* FASTING in Part Three and follow the program.

❏ To speed healing, apply vitamin E oil to the sore and bandage it lightly with a sterile gauze pad. Change the bandage daily until the sore is healed.

❏ Keep the ulcer clean and germ-free to prevent infection.

❏ See your physician if you have this medical problem. Sometimes antibiotics are necessary for the sores to heal.

❏ If you must take antibiotics, be sure to take acidophilus liquid or tablets. You can also obtain acidophilus from yogurt and soured-milk products.

CONSIDERATIONS

❏ Dimethylsulfoxide (DMSO) can be applied topically to the sores. It helps to relieve pain and promote healing.

Note: Only DMSO from a health food store should be used. Commercial-grade DMSO found in hardware stores is not suitable for healing. The use of DMSO may result in a temporary garlicky body odor, which is not a cause for concern.

❏ Laser therapy has not proved beneficial for venous leg ulcers. There may be some benefit in combining laser and infrared light therapy, but more research is needed to prove this conclusively.

❏ CircAid Medical Products makes adjustable bands specifically for venous stasis and venous ulcers. (*See* MANUFACTURER AND DISTRIBUTOR INFORMATION in the Appendix.)

❏ Leg ulcers often do not cause much pain, so if you have diabetes or circulatory problems, it is advisable to examine your lower legs and feet often.

❏ *See also* CIRCULATORY PROBLEMS and VARICOSE VEINS in Part Two.

Legionnaires' Disease

This is a serious lung and bronchial tube infection caused by bacteria of the genus *Legionella*, especially *Legionella pneumophila*. It was first identified following an outbreak that affected 182 people attending an American Legion convention in 1976—hence the name. The bacteria live primarily in water and are transmitted through airborne vapor droplets, although they are sometimes found in excavation sites and newly plowed soil. The incubation period is from two to ten days after exposure to the bacteria. The disease does not spread from one person to another.

The first signs of illness may resemble those of the flu—achiness, fatigue, headache, and moderate fever. The disease then progresses to include high fever (up to 105°F), chills, coughing, diarrhea, disorientation, nausea and vomiting, severe chest pain, shortness of breath, and, as a result of inadequate oxygen, a bluish tinge to the lips, nails, or skin. The coughing begins without sputum but eventually produces sputum that is gray or blood-streaked. Laboratory blood studies and cultures of sputum aid in diagnosis.

The risk of contracting Legionnaire's disease increases with chronic illness such as diabetes, emphysema, or kidney failure, and with immune-suppressing lifestyle habits such as smoking and alcohol consumption. Young adults usually recover fully from the disease, whereas elderly people, especially those in poor health, are at greater risk of developing respiratory failure.

NUTRIENTS

SUPPLEMENT	SUGGESTED DOSAGE	COMMENTS
Essential		
Garlic (Kyolic from Wakunaga)	2 capsules 3 times daily, with meals.	Aids in destroying bacteria.
Natural beta-carotene or carotenoid complex (Betatene)	25,000 IU daily. As directed on label.	A precursor of vitamin A that protects the lungs.
Vitamin C plus bioflavonoids	3,000 mg 3 times daily. 100 mg twice daily.	Powerful antioxidants that help to kill bacteria. Intravenous treatment (under a doctor's supervision) may be beneficial.
Very Important		
Coenzyme Q10 plus	60 mg daily.	Increases and regulates immunity. Carries oxygen to the cells.
Coenzyme A from Coenzyme-A Technologies	As directed on label.	Supports and boosts the body's immune system. Works well with coenzyme Q10.
Lactobacillus bulgaricus	As directed on label.	Aids digestion and destroys harmful bacteria.
L-Carnitine plus L-cysteine	500 mg each daily, on an empty stomach. Take with water or juice. Do not take with milk. Take with 50 mg vitamin B6 and 100 mg vitamin C for better absorption.	Important in immune function. Protect lung tissues. (*See* AMINO ACIDS in Part One.)
Vitamin B complex	100 mg of each major B vitamin daily (amounts of individual vitamins in a complex will vary).	A complex of vital coenzymes needed for cellular function and protection.
Important		
Intenzyme from Biotics Research	2 tablets 3 times daily, on an empty stomach.	Stimulates the immune system and reduces inflammation in the body.
Raw thymus glandular and raw lung glandular	As directed on label. As directed on label.	Glandulars that potentiate thymus and lung function and enhance immune function.
Vitamin A with mixed carotenoids	25,000 IU daily. If you are pregnant, do not exceed 10,000 IU daily.	Boosts the immune system and protects and repairs lung tissue. Use emulsion form for easier assimilation and greater safety at high doses.

Vitamin E emulsion or capsules	Up to 400 IU twice daily. 400 IU daily.	An important antioxidant that protects lung tissue. Use d-alpha-tocopherol form. Emulsion form is easier to assimilate.
Zinc	80 mg daily. Do not exceed a total of 100 mg daily from all supplements.	Important for immune response. Zinc gluconate in lozenge form is best.
Helpful		
Aerobic 07 from Aerobic Life Industries or	As directed on label.	To destroy infectious bacteria but not "good" bacteria.
Dioxychlor DC₃ from American Biologics	As directed on label.	A potent antibacterial, antifungal, and antiviral agent.

HERBS

❑ Catnip tea is good for reducing fever.

❑ Clear Lungs from RidgeCrest Herbals is a Chinese herbal formula that protects the lungs. Take 2 capsules three times daily.

❑ Echinacea is a powerful immune stimulant.

❑ Eucalyptus helps to open up air passages.

❑ Goldenseal is a natural antibiotic.

Caution: Do not take goldenseal internally on a daily basis for more than one week at a time, do not use it during pregnancy, and use it with caution if you are allergic to ragweed.

❑ Olive leaf extract helps protect against bacterial and viral infections. It has proven effective against pneumonia and sore throat.

RECOMMENDATIONS

❑ Eat a diet consisting of 75 percent raw foods and very lightly steamed vegetables.

❑ Consume no alcohol, dairy products, fried foods, sugar, or tobacco.

❑ Use a cool mist humidifier to increase the amount of moisture in the air and to thin lung secretions.

❑ Keep warm—do not get chilled, as this will worsen the disease.

❑ Practice deep-breathing exercises. (*See* Breathing Exercises *under* PAIN CONTROL in Part Three.)

❑ Use a heating pad or a hot water bottle on the chest to relieve pain.

❑ Be aware that recovery from Legionnaire's disease takes time. Allow yourself two to four weeks for recovery, and be sure to get adequate rest. Do not push yourself to resume normal activities prematurely.

CONSIDERATIONS

❑ Legionnaire's disease progresses rapidly and can be very dangerous. Hospitalization and aggressive treatment with intravenous antibiotics and oxygen may be necessary.

❑ *Legionella* bacteria may inhabit heating and cooling systems. It is wise to have the heating and cooling systems in both your home and workplace cleaned and inspected regularly, and to change the filters often.

Leukorrhea

See VAGINITIS in Part Two.

Liver Disease

See CIRRHOSIS OF THE LIVER; HEPATITIS.

Lumbago

See under BACKACHE.

Lupus

Lupus is a chronic inflammatory disease that can affect many of the body's organs. It is an autoimmune disease—that is, it occurs when the immune mechanism forms antibodies that attack the body's own tissues. Many experts believe that it is due to an as-yet-unidentified virus. According to this theory, the immune system develops antibodies in response to the virus that then attack the body's own organs and tissues. This produces inflammation of the skin, blood vessels, joints, and other tissues. Heredity and sex hormones are two other possible factors in the development of this illness.

This disease was named *lupus,* which means "wolf," because many people who got it developed a butterfly-shaped rash over the cheeks and nose that was considered to give them something of a wolflike appearance. In fact, rashes may appear elsewhere on the body as well, such as the chest, ears, hands, shoulders, and upper arms. At least 90 percent of those who contract lupus are women, and women of Asian background appear to be at greater risk of developing lupus than other women. Lupus usually develops between the ages of fifteen and thirty-five, although it may occur at any age.

There are two types of lupus: *systemic lupus erythematosus* (SLE) and *discoid lupus erythematosus* (DLE). As the name implies, SLE is a systemic disease that affects many different parts of the body. The severity can range from mild to life threatening. The first symptoms of many cases of SLE resemble those of arthritis, with swelling and pain in the fingers and other joints. The disease may also appear suddenly, with acute fever. The characteristic red rash may appear across the cheeks; there may also be red, scaling lesions elsewhere on the body. Sores may form in the mouth. Other symptoms can include abdominal and chest pains, blood in the urine, fatigue, hair loss, loss of appetite, low-grade fever, nausea, poor circulation in the fingers and toes, shortness of breath, ulcers, vomiting, and weight loss. The lungs and kidneys are often involved. Approximately 50 percent of those with SLE develop nephritis, inflammation of the kidneys. In serious cases, the brain, lungs, spleen, and/or heart may be affected. SLE can cause anemia and inflammation of the surface membranes of the heart and lungs. It can also cause excessive bleeding and increased susceptibility to infection. If the central nervous system is involved, amnesia, deep depression, headaches, mania, paralysis, paranoia, psychosis, seizures, and stroke may be present.

The discoid type of lupus is a less serious disease that primarily affects the skin. The characteristic butterfly rash forms over the nose and cheeks. There may also be lesions elsewhere, commonly on the scalp and ears, and these lesions may recur or persist for years. The lesions are small, soft yellowish lumps. When they disappear, they often leave scars. If these scars form on the scalp, permanent bald patches may result. While DLE is not necessarily dangerous to overall health, it is a chronic and disfiguring skin disease. Some experts have related it to a reaction to infection with the tubercle bacillus.

Both types of lupus follow a pattern of periodic flare-ups alternating with periods of remission. Exposure to the sun's ultraviolet rays can result in a flare-up of DLE and may even induce the first attack. Fatigue, pregnancy, childbirth, infection, some drugs, stress, unidentified viral infections, and chemicals may also trigger a flare-up. Drug-induced cases usually clear up when the drug is discontinued.

According to the American Rheumatism Association, four of the following eight symptoms must occur, either serially or at the same time, before a diagnosis can be made:

1. Abnormal cells in the urine.

2. Arthritis.

3. Butterfly rash on the cheeks.

4. Low white blood cell count, low platelet count, or hemolytic anemia.

5. Mouth sores.

6. Seizures or psychosis.

7. Sun sensitivity.

8. The presence in the blood of a specific antibody that is found in 50 percent of people with lupus.

A kidney biopsy may be needed to diagnose lupus-related nephritis.

NUTRIENTS

SUPPLEMENT	SUGGESTED DOSAGE	COMMENTS
Very Important		
Calcium and magnesium	1,500–3,000 mg daily. 750 mg twice daily.	Necessary for pH balance and for protection against bone loss due to arthritis.
L-Cysteine and L-methionine plus L-lysine	500–1,000 mg each daily, on an empty stomach. Take with water or juice. Do not take with milk. Take with 50 mg vitamin B₆ and 100 mg vitamin C for better absorption.	Assist in cellular protection and preservation; important in skin formation and in white blood cell activity. Aids in preventing mouth sores and offers protection against viruses. (*See* AMINO ACIDS in Part One.)
Proteolytic enzymes	As directed on label. Take with meals.	Powerful anti-inflammatory and antiviral agents.
Important		
Essential fatty acids (black currant seed oil, flaxseed oil, primrose oil, and Kyolic-EPA from Wakunaga are good sources)	As directed on label.	Aids in arthritis prevention, protects skin cells, and needed for reproduction of all body cells.
Glucosamine sulfate or N-acetylglucosamine (N-A-G from Source Naturals)	As directed on label. As directed on label.	Important for healthy skin, bones, and connective tissue. May help to prevent lupus erythematosus.
Garlic (Kyolic from Wakunaga)	2 capsules 3 times daily, with meals.	An immune-system enhancer that protects enzyme systems.
Raw thymus glandular and raw spleen glandular	As directed on label. As directed on label.	Glandulars that enhance thymus and spleen immune function. (*See* GLANDULAR THERAPY in Part Three.)
Vitamin C with bioflavonoids	3,000–8,000 mg daily.	Aids in normalizing immune function.
Zinc plus copper	50–100 mg daily. Do not exceed this amount. 3 mg daily.	Aids in normalizing immune function; protects the skin and organs and promotes healing. Use zinc gluconate lozenges or OptiZinc for best absorption. Needed to balance with zinc.
Helpful		
Acidophilus (Kyo-Dophilus from Wakunaga is a good source)	As directed on label. Take on an empty stomach.	Protects against intestinal bacterial imbalances. Use a nondairy formula.
Herpanacine from Diamond-Herpanacine Associates	As directed on label.	Contains a balance of anti-oxidants, amino acids, and herbs that promote skin health.
Kelp or alfalfa	1,000–1,500 mg daily.	Supplies commonly deficient minerals. *See under* Herbs, below.
Multivitamin and mineral complex with vitamin B complex	50 mg of each major B vitamin 3 times daily, with meals (amounts of individual vitamins in a complex will vary).	To supply commonly deficient nutrients. Use a high-quality, hypo-allergenic formula. Heals mouth sores, protects against anemia, and protects the skin tissues. Important for brain function and digestion.

Pycnogenol or grape seed extract	As directed on label. As directed on label.	Powerful antioxidants and free radical scavengers that protect the cells.
Vitamin A with mixed carotenoids plus natural beta-carotene or carotenoid complex (Betatene)	25,000 IU daily. If you are pregnant, do not exceed 10,000 IU daily. 15,000 IU daily. As directed on label.	Potent antioxidant and free radical scavenger needed for tissue healing. Use emulsion form for easier assimilation. An antioxidant and vitamin A precursor.
Vitamin E	400–800 IU daily.	Powerful antioxidant that helps the body use oxygen more efficiently and promotes healing. Use d-alpha-tocopherol form.

HERBS

❏ Alfalfa capsules or tablets are a good source of minerals needed for healing.

❏ Alcohol-free goldenseal extract is good for mouth sores or inflammation. Place a few drops on a small piece of gauze or cotton before bedtime and leave it on overnight for fast healing.

Caution: Do not take goldenseal internally on a daily basis for more than one week at a time, do not use it during pregnancy, and use it with caution if you are allergic to ragweed.

❏ Other herbs beneficial in treating lupus include feverfew, pau d'arco, and red clover.

Caution: Do not use feverfew during pregnancy.

❏ Try using licorice root as a tea or dilute it to alleviate lupus symptoms. If you are taking immunosuppressive agents such as steroids, you may find licorce root to provide comparable results without being as harmful to your system.

Caution: If overused, licorice can elevate blood pressure. Do not use this herb on a daily basis for more than seven days in a row. Avoid it completely if you have high blood pressure.

❏ Milk thistle cleanses and protects the liver.

❏ Yucca is good for arthritis-type symptoms.

RECOMMENDATIONS

❏ Eat a diet low in fat, salt, and animal protein—this kind of diet keeps the immune system from being overly reactive and is easy on the kidneys. Use only canola or olive oil. Consume sardines often; they are a good source of essential fatty acids.

❏ Eat eggs, garlic, and onions. These foods contain sulfur, which is needed for the repair and rebuilding of bone, cartilage, and connective tissue, and aids in the absorption of calcium.

❏ Include in the diet brown rice, fish, green leafy vegetables, nonacidic fresh fruits, oatmeal, and whole grains.

❏ Eat fresh (not canned) pineapple frequently. Bromelain, an enzyme present in fresh pineapple, is excellent for reducing inflammation.

❏ Use some form of fiber daily.

❏ Do not consume milk, dairy products, or red meat. Also avoid caffeine, citrus fruits, paprika, salt, tobacco, and everything that contains sugar.

❏ Avoid the nightshade vegetables (eggplant, peppers, tomatoes, white potatoes). These foods contain a substance called solanine, which can contribute to inflammation and pain.

❏ Get your iron from food sources, not supplements. Taking iron in supplement form may contribute to pain, swelling, and joint destruction.

❏ Avoid eating alfalfa sprouts. They contain canavain, a toxic substance that is incorporated into protein in place of arginine.

❏ Get plenty of rest and regular moderate exercise that promotes muscle tone and fitness.

❏ Avoid strong sunlight and use protection from the sun. Protect your skin by applying a sunscreen product with an SPF of 15 or higher. Wear a wide-brimmed hat and clothing that will adequately cover exposed skin. Go out in the sun only when absolutely necessary.

❏ Use hypoallergenic soaps and cosmetics. Some deodorant soaps and other toiletry items may contain ingredients that will increase your sensitivity to light.

❏ Try to avoid fluorescent lighting in both the home and the workplace. Exposure to fluorescent lighting can aggravate lupus symptoms. If possible, remove all fluorescent and halogen lighting and replace them with incandescent bulbs.

❏ Avoid large groups of people and those with colds or other viral infections. Autoimmune diseases such as lupus render an individual more susceptible to viral infections.

❏ Avoid using birth control pills. They may cause lupus to flare up.

CONSIDERATIONS

❏ Some researchers believe that faulty genes are the ultimate culprit behind this disorder, but that outside factors can trigger it. Substances that are common contributing factors include chemicals, environmental pollutants, food additives, and some foods.

❏ A test for food allergies is helpful and often very revealing in cases of lupus. (*See* ALLERGIES in Part Two.)

❏ Up to 10 percent of lupus cases are probably caused by drug reactions, according to an article that was published in *The New England Journal of Medicine.* Certain drugs, such as hydralazine (Apresoline), a blood pressure medication, and procainamide (Procan), used for irregular heartbeat, seem to be able to cause lupus in susceptible individuals. Drug-related lupus usually does not affect the kidneys or nervous system. It is likely to be milder, and the condition usually subsides when the drug is stopped.

❏ Many people with lupus also have Raynaud's disease. (*See* RAYNAUD'S DISEASE/RAYNAUD'S PHENOMENON in Part Two.) The condition can lead to false-positive blood-test results for syphilis.

❏ Many different treatments are used for lupus. Anti-inflammatory drugs are usually used first. Antimalarial drugs such as hydroxychloroquine (Plaquenil) may alleviate the skin problems and sun sensitivity that afflict those who have lupus. In severe cases, physicians may have to use cortisone and immunosuppressive agents to induce remission. Corticosteroids, such as prednisone (Deltasone and others) are adrenal hormones that are considered important in the treatment of lupus. Anticonvulsants, drugs used to control seizures, and warfarin (Coumadin), an anticoagulant used to prevent blood clotting and reduce the possibilty of stroke or heart attack, may also be prescribed. All of these drugs, especially the corticosteroids, have potentially serious side effects.

❏ Dehydroepiandrosterone (DHEA) therapy has been found to help in treating lupus. (*See* DHEA THERAPY in Part Three.)

❏ Radiation treatment for lupus is in the experimental stages. It involves using low doses of radiation to the lymph nodes to suppress the immune system. Anticancer drugs are sometimes used to decrease both the immune system's responsiveness and the need for steroids. Anticancer drugs may be toxic to the bone marrow and must be used with caution. Another experimental treatment for lupus involves plasmapheresis, a process in which harmful anti-antigen complexes are filtered out of the blood plasma.

❏ Mild cases of lupus respond well to supplements that build up the immune system. (*See* WEAKENED IMMUNE SYSTEM in Part Two.)

❏ Further information on lupus can be obtained from the Lupus Foundation of America (*see* HEALTH AND MEDICAL ORGANIZATIONS in the Appendix).

❏ *See also* ARTHRITIS in Part Two.

Lyme Disease

This disease takes its name from the town of Old Lyme, Connecticut, where it was first identified in 1975. Since that time, the locations and the number of cases of Lyme disease have continued to increase. In 1983, the year after national surveillance began, 48 cases were reported to the national Centers for Disease Control and Prevention (CDC) in Atlanta. Over 15,000 cases of Lyme disease are reported in the United States every year, according to the CDC, though they say the disease is greatly underreported. Approximately 90 percent of all known cases in the United States have occurred in ten states: California, Connecticut, Maryland, Massachusetts, Minnesota, New Jersey, New York,

Pennsylvania, Rhode Island, and Wisconsin. It also occurs in Europe, Russia, China, Japan, and Australia.

Lyme disease is the most common tick-borne illness in the United States. The bacteria that cause it, spirochetes called *Borrelia burgdorferi*, are transmitted by the deer tick (carried by deer and mice) in most places. In several counties along the northern Pacific coast of California, however, they are transmitted by the closely related black-legged tick, which is also carried by wood rats. Both deer ticks and black-legged ticks are very tiny; an adult tick is less than one-tenth of an inch long, and the nymph is the size of a pinhead. They are hard to spot because they are so much smaller than the common dog tick. Because they are so tiny, they often go undetected. The nymphs and larvae feed primarily on white-footed mice, and the adults on white-tailed deer, although they may feed on many other animals as well, including birds, chipmunks, cows, horses, cats, dogs, lizards, and jackrabbits. The ticks fall off one host animal into grasses in marshes or fields, or into brush in wooded areas, from which they can be picked up by an unsuspecting passerby, whether human or animal, who becomes the next host. Not surprisingly, those most likely to be affected are people who spend time outdoors in or near wooded areas, where the ticks are prevalent, and the majority of cases occur in the summer and fall. Household pets like dogs and cats can pick up ticks and carry them into the home, where they can be transmitted to humans.

After a tick bites, it waits several hours before it begins to feed on the host's blood, and once it does, it feasts for three or four days. As it feeds, it may deposit its infectious cargo in the host's bloodstream. The longer the tick remains attached, the greater the risk of disease.

The symptoms of Lyme disease are extremely variable, as is the incubation period, which may take anywhere from two to thirty-two days. The first sign may be the appearance of a red, circular lesion or rash on the skin, which is known as *erythema migrans* (EM). This is caused by the migration of the infecting organism outward through the skin, and it may appear anywhere from a few days to a few weeks after the bite. The lesion gradually expands in a circular pattern, while the center appears to clear up. For this reason, it is often referred to as a bull's-eye rash. In addition to the rash (or, in some cases, instead of the rash), achiness, backache, difficulty sleeping, fatigue, flulike symptoms, headache, muscle weakness, stiff neck, and, occasionally, nausea and vomiting may occur. The disease then usually progresses through the following three stages, although not everyone experiences all three:

1. Three days to three weeks after a tick bite, small raised bumps on the skin and/or a rash appears and may cover the entire torso, for as little as a day or two or as much as several weeks, and then fade. (If a rash appears immediately at the site of the tick bite, it may be a reaction to the bite itself and not to the bacteria that causes Lyme disease.) Chills, fever, nausea, sore throat, and vomiting may also occur.

2. Facial paralysis that mimics Bell's palsy may occur weeks to months later. An abnormal heart rhythm, enlargement of the heart muscle, enlargement of the spleen and lymph glands, and severe headaches may also occur about this time.

3. Over the long term, persistent backache, stiff neck, joint pains that attack the knees, swelling and pain in other joints, and even degenerative muscle disease may be caused by Lyme disease.

Because these tick bites are usually painless, the incubation period is so long, and the symptoms of Lyme disease are so varied, the disorder may go unrecognized for weeks or even months. A physician may fail to diagnose the disease before it is in its advanced stages. Lyme disease produces symptoms that resemble those of chronic fatigue syndrome, gout, lupus, and multiple sclerosis, and misdiagnosis is not uncommon. Once arthritis appears, the joint pain and stiffness can come and go, recurring even years later. An estimated 10 percent of those with Lyme disease arthritis are left with permanent stiffness in their joints.

Lyme disease is treatable and almost always curable if found in its early stages. If the disease is not treated in the early stages, however, arthritis, enlargement of the spleen and lymph nodes, eye inflammation, hepatitis, irregular heart rhythm, and damage to the cardiovascular and central nervous systems can occur. Some people find that their symptoms slowly subside over two to three years; others develop chronic problems. Often, symptoms leave and recur without another tick bite.

A test has been developed to identify Lyme disease. A blood sample is used to measure the levels of certain antibodies that usually increase in number from three days to three weeks after infection.

Unless otherwise specified, the dosages recommended here are for adults. For a child between the ages of twelve and seventeen, reduce the dose to three-quarters of the recommended amount. For a child between six and twelve, use one-half of the recommended dose, and for a child under the age of six, use one-quarter of the recommended amount.

NUTRIENTS

SUPPLEMENT	SUGGESTED DOSAGE	COMMENTS
Very Important		
Essential fatty acids (Kyolic-EPA from Wakunaga is a good source)	As directed on label.	Reduces inflammation and joint stiffness.
Pancreatin and bromelain or	As directed on label 2–3 times daily, between meals and at bedtime.	To aid protein digestion and reduce inflammation.
Inflazyme Forte from American Biologics	As directed on label.	
Primrose oil	1,000 mg 2–3 times daily.	Helps to combat pain and inflammation by promoting the production of anti-inflammatory prostaglandins.
Helpful		
Garlic (Kyolic from Wakunaga)	2 capsules 3 times daily.	A powerful immune system stimulator; acts as an antibiotic.
Kelp	1,000–1,500 mg daily.	Contains essential vitamins and minerals and aids in detoxifying the body.
Multivitamin and mineral complex	As directed on label.	For necessary vitamins. Use a high-potency formula.
Selenium	200 mcg daily. If you are pregnant, do not exceed 40 mcg daily.	A free radical scavenger.
Taurine Plus from American Biologics	As directed on label.	An important antioxidant and immune system regulator necessary for white blood cell activation and neurological function. Use the sublingual form.
Vitamin A with mixed carotenoids	25,000 IU daily. If you are pregnant, do not exceed 10,000 IU daily.	An important antioxidant.
Vitamin C with bioflavonoids	6,000–10,000 mg daily, in divided doses.	Needed for adequate immune function.
Vitamin E	600 IU daily.	An important antioxidant. Use d-alpha-tocopherol form.
Zinc lozenges	1 15-mg lozenge every 3 waking hours for 4 days. Do not repeat this regimen for at least 30 days.	Necessary for immune function.
plus copper	3 mg daily.	Needed to balance with zinc.

HERBS

❑ Alfalfa supplies needed minerals.

❑ Dandelion root, ginseng, hawthorn, horsetail, and marshmallow root are all good for helping to rebuild the blood and damaged tissues.

❑ Echinacea is an immune enhancer.

❑ Goldenseal is a natural antibiotic. Take 1/2 dropperful of alcohol-free goldenseal extract three times a day for one week. It can be taken under the tongue for fast results, or added to tea.

Caution: Do not take goldenseal internally on a daily basis for more than one week at a time, do not use it during pregnancy, and use it with caution if you are allergic to ragweed.

❑ Milk thistle extract protects the liver.

❑ Red clover cleanses the bloodstream.

RECOMMENDATIONS

❑ Include plenty of garlic in your diet or take garlic supplements. It is a natural antibiotic and immune-booster.

❏ Use barley grass, bee pollen, and/or royal jelly to supply nutrients needed to repair tissue and rebuild the blood.

❏ Use "green drinks" to provide chlorophyll, which aids in detoxification, and other valuable nutrients and enzymes. Kyo-Green from Wakunaga is an excellent choice.

❏ If you develop a bull's-eye-type rash anywhere on your body, see your health care provider as soon as possible, even if you have no memory of being bitten by a tick. Early treatment is essential.

❏ If antibiotics are prescribed, be sure to take some form of acidophilus supplement daily.

❏ Take hot baths or whirlpool treatments. Heat relieves joint pain.

❏ Take precautionary measures to help prevent tick bites:

• When spending time in or near wooded areas, wear long pants and tuck them into your socks. Wear a long-sleeved shirt with a high neck or a scarf, plus a hat and gloves. Wear light-colored clothing so that any ticks will be more visible.

• Use an insect repellent containing diethyl toluamide (deet) on your clothing, your neck, and any other exposed area except your face. Deet lasts longer and is safer when used on clothing than on exposed skin, so cover as much of the body with clothing as you can. Do not use excessive amounts of deet. Follow product label directions carefully, and wash the repellent off as soon as you go indoors.

Caution: Deet is extremely toxic and can be deadly if ingested. Be extremely careful when using it, especially if you are around small children. Do not use it on clothing or other items containing plastic or synthetics such as nylon or polyester, as it can permanently damage such materials (it can even dissolve certain types of paint and nail polish).

• After spending time outdoors, check yourself carefully for any small raised bumps and for pinpoint-sized specks on clothing. Do this right away; the longer a tick is attached, the greater the risk of Lyme disease.

• Check children before they go to bed during the summer if they spend a lot of time outdoors. Look closely at their hair, ears, underarms, trunks, groins, and the backs of their knees. Have them shower when they come in from outdoors, and wash their clothes immediately.

• Dry your laundry in an electric clothes dryer for half an hour to kill any ticks that may be present. Washing clothes, even in hot water and bleach, will not necessarily kill ticks.

• Inspect pets before letting them indoors. They may carry ticks into the house that can fall off and bite family members.

• In a wooded or overgrown area, try to stay near the centers of trails and out of wooded areas, especially in May, June, and July.

• Keep your lawn mowed and remove leaf litter and brush. Move woodpiles away from the house during the summer.

❏ If you find a tick on your body, do the following:

1. Remove the tick with a pair of tweezers. Grasp the tick with the tweezers as close to the skin as possible and pull the tick straight out. Do not twist the tweezers as you pull, and do not squeeze the tick's body, or bacteria may be injected into the skin. If possible, save the tick in a small bottle or jar. *Do not* use a match to try to burn the tick out, or resort to other home remedies like kerosene or petroleum jelly.

2. Once the tick is removed, thoroughly wash your hands and the bite area, and apply rubbing alcohol or another topical antiseptic to the bite. If you suspect the tick may be a deer tick, see your health care provider promptly. Take the tick with you for identification.

3. For the three weeks following a tick bite, be alert for any of the symptoms described in this section. If you have any doubts about your condition, consult your health care provider.

❏ If you are being treated for Lyme disease but are not getting better, consider having yourself tested again. False-positive results are possible, and you may actually have a different problem.

CONSIDERATIONS

❏ Pregnant women need to be especially careful to avoid ticks in Lyme disease areas. The infection can be transferred to the developing fetus and, in rare circumstances, can cause complications such as miscarriage or the birth of a stillborn baby.

❏ Prompt treatment with antibiotics can halt the course of Lyme disease. Many physicians do not like to prescribe antibiotics unless a person develops the characteristic symptoms of Lyme disease—a small red bump at the site of the tick bite, and a bull's-eye rash surrounding it, with flulike symptoms such as fatigue, chills, and joint pain. If treatment is deferred until the onset of more advanced symptoms, such as involvement of the brain, heart, or joints, antibiotic therapy is not as effective.

❏ There is a vaccine available against Lyme disease. It is not 100-percent effective, however, and must be given in three separate doses at specific times of the year. The U.S. Food and Drug Administration advises that the vaccine should not be considered a substitute for standard measures to protect against tick bites, such as wearing protective clothing and using insect repellent.

❏ One study showed that, of 788 people diagnosed with Lyme disease, over half actually had other problems. Physicians blame current laboratory tests for the false-positive results.

❏ Pets can get Lyme disease, too. Call your veterinarian if your pet exhibits any of the following:

• Fever of 103°F to 106°F.

• One or more swollen, hot joints.

- A tendency to sit or lie in one place for longer periods of time than usual.
- Lameness that seems to come and go.
- Reluctance to move.
- Poor appetite.
- A hot, dry nose.

❑ The CDC provides information on Lyme disease to health professionals and the public (*see* HEALTH AND MEDICAL ORGANIZATIONS in the Appendix). The CDC also works with state health departments to track cases of Lyme disease. Your state or local health department can tell you if Lyme disease has been reported in your area.

Macular Degeneration

See under EYE PROBLEMS.

Malabsorption Syndrome

Malabsorption is the failure of the body to properly absorb vitamins, minerals, and other nutrients from food. Even though his or her diet is adequate, an individual with malabsorption develops various nutritional deficiencies. This problem can result from impaired digestion, impaired absorption of nutrients into the bloodstream from the digestive tract (especially the small intestine), or both.

Common symptoms of malabsorption syndrome include constipation or diarrhea, dry skin, fatigue, gas, mental difficulties such as depression or an inability to concentrate, muscle cramps and/or weakness, premenstrual syndrome (PMS), steatorrhea (pale, bulky, fatty stools), a tendency to bruise easily, failure to grow normally, thinning hair, unexplained weight loss, and visual difficulties, especially problems with night vision. Abdominal discomfort may be present as well. A combination of anemia, diarrhea, and weight loss is typical. However, in some individuals, paradoxically, obesity may result, if fats are deposited in the tissues rather than being utilized properly by the body. In addition, in an attempt to get the nutrients it needs but is not absorbing, the body may begin to crave more and more food, often leading to the consumption of many empty and/or fat calories.

Digestive disorders are among the most common health problems in America today. Impaired digestion leads to malabsorption because if food is not broken down properly, the nutrients it contains cannot be absorbed through the lining of the intestines. The intestinal tract, pancreas, liver, and gallbladder all have parts to play in the uptake of nutrients. Consequently, anything that interferes with the proper functioning of any of these can lead to impaired digestion.

Some factors that can contribute to impaired digestion are a lack of adequate levels of digestive enzymes; food allergies; a diet deficient in nutrients, such as the B vitamins, that are needed to produce digestive enzymes; and diseases of the pancreas, gallbladder, liver, and bile ducts that result in a lack of bile and essential enzymes. Although any type of nutrient may be affected by poor digestion, lipids (fats) are affected most often. In addition to causing nutritional deficiencies, the failure to digest food properly causes gastrointestinal problems. Undigested food ferments in the intestinal tract, causing gas, bloating, and abdominal pain and discomfort.

Even if food is properly digested, there may be a problem that prevents nutrients from being taken up by the bloodstream and used to nourish the body tissues. Damage to the intestinal walls, through which nutrients are absorbed, is one such problem. Disorders such as celiac disease, colitis, Crohn's disease, diverticulitis, irritable bowel syndrome, lactose intolerance, parasitic infestation, and excessive consumption of alcohol, antacids, or laxatives can all cause intestinal damage. Chronic constipation and/or diarrhea can have the same result. Another problem is too-rapid intestinal transit time, which results in nutrients being passed out of the body as waste before they can be absorbed. Radiation therapy, digitalis treatment, and surgery that shortens the intestinal tract all reduce the absorptive area, and therefore the absorptive capacity, of the small bowel.

Other factors that can contribute to a malfunction of the absorption mechanism include a poor diet; excess mucus covering the intestinal lining (most commonly a result of the overconsumption of mucus-forming and processed foods); an imbalance in intestinal bacterial flora, such as in candidiasis; the use of certain medications, such as neomycin (an antibiotic), colchicine (an anti-gout drug), and cholestyramine (a cholesterol-lowering drug); food allergies; and illnesses such as cancer and AIDS. People with AIDS are particularly prone to malabsorption problems because of chronic diarrhea, loss of appetite, and an overgrowth of *Candida albicans* in the digestive tract. Obstructions in the lymphatic system may also interfere with nutrient absorption.

Regardless of how good your diet is or how many supplements you take, if you suffer from malabsorption syndrome, you will have nutritional deficiencies. These in turn lead to other problems. The impaired absorption of protein can induce edema (swelling of the tissues due to fluid retention). A lack of potassium can result in muscle weakness and cardiovascular problems. Anemia results from a lack of needed iron and folic acid. Calcium and vitamin D deficiency result in bone loss and tetany, a condition characterized by painful muscular spasms and tremors. Bruising easily results from a lack of vitamin K, night blindness from a deficiency of vitamin A. Malabsorption is also self-perpetuating; the failure to absorb B vitamins and to transfer amino acids across the intestinal lining interferes with the production of needed digestive enzymes and causes further malabsorption, since these nutrients are essential in the absorption process itself. A vicious circle results.

Besides being a serious condition in itself, malabsorption is a factor in other medical and physical problems. The body needs all nutrients in balance because they work in concert. If there is a deficiency in even a single nutrient, the body can no longer function as it should, and all kinds of things can go awry. The result is disease. Malabsorption is a common contributing factor to a wide range of disorders, including cancer, heart disease, osteoporosis, and—because immune function is damaged by a lack of necessary nutrients—all types of infection.

Malabsorption is also a significant factor in the overall aging process, and it may account for the fact that some people seem to age more rapidly than others. As we age, the intestinal tract gets "out of shape" and the lining becomes covered with hard fecal matter and mucus, which makes absorption of nutrients more difficult. This is one reason why older people need to consume greater amounts of nutrients. It is also why it is so important to keep the colon clean. Fecal deposits can irritate the nerve endings in the colon, leading to spastic colon or inflamed colon. Both of these conditions interfere with bowel function and with the proper absorption of nutrients. In addition, the impacted deposits decay after a time, releasing toxins that can seep into the bloodstream, poisoning the organs and tissues.

Those suffering from malabsorption must take in more nutrients than the average person to compensate, and to treat and correct the problem. In supplying these nutrients, it is best to bypass the intestinal tract as much as possible. When choosing supplements, sustained-release and large, hard tablets should be avoided. Many people with malabsorption problems are unable to break down supplements taken in hard pill form; some even discharge pills whole in the stool. Injections, powders, liquids, and lozenges provide nutrients in forms that are more easily assimilated and therefore are preferred.

Unless otherwise specified, the dosages recommended here are for adults. For a child between the ages of twelve and seventeen, reduce the dose to three-quarters of the recommended amount. For a child between six and twelve, use one-half of the recommended dose, and for a child under the age of six, use one-quarter of the recommended amount.

NUTRIENTS

SUPPLEMENT	SUGGESTED DOSAGE	COMMENTS
Very Important		
Acidophilus (Kyo-Dophilus from Wakunaga is a good source)	1 tsp 3 times daily, on an empty stomach.	Needed for uptake and manufacture of many nutrients. Use a nondairy formula.
Dioxychlor DC-3 from American Biologics	As directed on label.	Destroys harmful bacteria in the intestinal tract and cleanses the bloodstream.
Micellized Multiple Vitamin and Mineral from Earth Science	As directed on label.	To supply balanced nutrients in a form that allows for faster, more efficient absorption.
Vitamin B complex injections	2 cc twice weekly, or as prescribed by physician.	To correct deficiencies. B vitamins must be replenished daily. Injections (under a doctor's supervision) are best. Needed for normal digestion and to prevent anemia.
plus extra vitamin B$_{12}$ injections	1 cc twice weekly, or as prescribed by physician.	
and liver extract injections	1 cc twice weekly, or as prescribed by physician.	A good source of B vitamins and other valuable nutrients.
or vitamin B complex plus extra	As directed on label.	If injections are not available, use a lozenge, sublingual, or spray form such as No Shot B-6/B-12/Folic from Superior Source.
vitamin B$_{12}$ and	1,000 mcg 3 times daily, on an empty stomach.	
vitamin B$_6$ (pyridoxine) and	50 mg 3 times daily.	
folic acid	400 mcg 3 times daily.	
Important		
Bioperine (Bioperine from Sabinsa or Bioperine 10 from Nature's Plus)	As directed on label.	Increases the absorption of nutrients and improves digestion.
Calcium	As directed on label.	Necessary for maintaining healthy bones. Use calcium citrate chelate form.
Free-form amino acid complex (Amino Balance from Anabol Naturals)	As directed on label 3 times daily, on an empty stomach.	Needed because protein is not broken down properly into amino acids, which are needed for virtually all life functions.
Garlic (Kyolic from Wakunaga)	As directed on label. Take with meals.	Aids digestion and promotes healing of the digestive tract. Use the liquid form.
Inflazyme Forte from American Biologics	2 tablets with each meal.	A balanced, potent enzyme and cofactor as a powerful inflammatory inhibitor.
Magnesium	As directed on label.	Important for energy production. Assists in calcium and potassium absorption. Use chelate form.
Vitamin C with bioflavonoids	2,000–8,000 mg daily, in divided doses. Take with juice.	Needed to stimulate immune function and to aid uptake of nutrients. Use a buffered powder form.
Vitamin E	As directed on label.	An essential antioxidant, it improves circulation and is necessary for tissue repair. Use d-alpha-tocopherol form.
Helpful		
Essential Fatty Acid Complex from Ecological Formulas	As directed on label.	To repair the cells along the intestinal walls and to assist in proper utilization of fats.
Liquid Liver Extract #521 from Enzymatic Therapy	As directed on label.	Prevents anemia and supplies necessary B vitamins in natural form.
Multivitamin and mineral complex plus	As directed on label.	To replace lost nutrients. Minerals are the key to protein and vitamin utilization. Use a powdered form that is yeast- and allergen-free.
carotenoid complex	As directed on label.	

Proteolytic enzymes	As directed on label 3–6 times daily. Take with meals and between meals.	Needed for protein digestion and breakdown of carbohydrates and fats.
or multienzyme complex with pancreatic enzymes	As directed on label, 3 times daily, with meals.	
Zinc lozenges	1 15-mg lozenge 3 times daily for 1 month. Do not exceed a total of 100 mg	Aids in the manufacture of digestive enzymes and in protein uptake.
plus copper	3 mg daily.	daily from all supplements. Needed to balance with zinc.

HERBS

❑ Alfalfa, dandelion root, fennel seed, ginger, and nettle are rich in minerals and can aid the body in absorbing nutrients.

❑ Aloe vera and peppermint aid digestion.

❑ Black pepper contains piperine, which aids in the digestion and absorption of nutrients.

❑ Buchu decreases inflammation of the colon and mucous membranes.

❑ Goldenseal promotes the functioning capacity of the colon, liver, and pancreas.

Caution: Do not take goldenseal on a daily basis for more than one week at a time, as it may disturb the intestinal flora. Do not use it during pregnancy. If you have a history of cardiovascular disease, diabetes, or glaucoma, use it only under a doctor's supervision.

❑ Irish moss and rhubarb are good for colon disorders.

❑ Yellow dock improves colon and liver function.

RECOMMENDATIONS

❑ Follow the dietary recommendations in this section for at least thirty days to give the colon a chance to heal and to cleanse its walls of hard matter and mucus. After thirty days, you may gradually reintroduce the foods that you have eliminated back into your diet; however, do not add them back too quickly or all at once. Instead, add small amounts of these foods, one at a time, back into your diet.

❑ Eat a diet that is high in complex carbohydrates and low in fats. Include in the diet well-cooked brown rice, millet, oatmeal, and steamed vegetables.

❑ Eat plenty of fruits (except for citrus fruits).

❑ Consume fresh papaya and pineapple often. Chew four to six papaya seeds after meals.

❑ Eat broiled, steamed, or baked white fish three times a week.

❑ Do not eat large meals, as this places too much stress on the digestive system. Instead, eat smaller portions of food throughout the day.

❑ Drink six to eight glasses of liquids daily, including juices, quality water, and herbal teas (*see* Herbs, above, for suggestions). Use barley malt, a small amount of honey, or nut or soymilk for sweeteners, if necessary.

❑ Do not consume wheat products until healing is complete.

❑ Avoid products containing caffeine, which interferes with iron absorption. These include teas, coffee, colas, chocolate, many processed foods, and some over-the-counter medications (read labels).

❑ Keep fats and oils to an absolute minimum. Do not consume any animal products (including butter), fried or fatty foods, or margarine. The fats these foods contain exacerbate malabsorption problems by coating the stomach and small intestines, blocking the passage of nutrients. For the same reason, avoid all dairy products and processed food products, which encourage the secretion of mucus.

❑ Eliminate citrus fruits, shellfish, and white rice from the diet.

❑ Do not eat meat or meat products. Meats are difficult to digest and are acid-forming.

❑ Strictly avoid all junk foods, such as potato chips and candy, as well as other products containing sugar, salt, monosodium glutamate (MSG), and preservatives.

❑ *See* COLON CLEANSING in Part Three and follow the program.

❑ Follow the fasting program once monthly. (*See* FASTING in Part Three.)

❑ Avoid using mineral oil or other laxatives. Especially avoid using them for extended periods, as dependence and damage to the colon may result.

❑ If diarrhea or other symptoms of digestive disturbance occur for longer than three days, call your health care provider. Also consult a professional if you notice black and tarry or bright-red stools, or if digestive problems are accompanied by severe abdominal pain or a fever of over 101°F.

❑ If a change of diet and the correct supplements do not improve your health status in a few months, consult your physician. You may have a malabsorption problem that requires medical attention.

CONSIDERATIONS

❑ Chronic pancreatic insufficiency is a condition in which the pancreas does not secrete enough enzymes for proper digestion. Serious pancreatic disease can lead to malabsorption severe enough to damage the nervous system. Gallbladder and/or liver problems can lead to trouble in the digestion and absorption of essential fatty acids, which are necessary for good health. Impaired absorption of fats in turn can lead to deficiencies of fat-soluble nutrients, such as beta-carotene and vitamins A, D, E, and K.

❑ Treatment of malabsorption requires recognition and, if possible, correction of the underlying cause of the problem, plus a healthful dietary regimen and supplementation. Appropriate medical consultation is needed in cases related to the use of cancer drugs, pancreatic insufficiency, and special problems associated with gastric or intestinal surgery.

❑ Research has found that people who eat food products containing the fat substitute olestra may test false-positive for malabsorption disorder. If you consume foods containing olestra, you should inform your health care practitioner prior to any such testing.

❑ Certain drugs interfere with the absorption of nutrients. Examples include corticosteroids, cholestyramine (Questran), sulfasalazine (Azulfidine), and especially antibiotics. Corticosteroids depress protein synthesis, inhibit normal calcium absorption, and increase the amount of vitamin C lost through excretion. Cholestyramine interferes with the absorption of the fat-soluble vitamins A, D, E, and K. Sulfasalazine inhibits the transport of folate and iron, causing anemia. Antibiotics disrupt the essential bacterial flora of the intestine. All of these drugs increase the need for nutritional supplements.

Malnutrition

See MALABSORPTION SYNDROME; UNDERWEIGHT.

Manic-Depressive Disorder/ Bipolar Mood Disorder

Manic-depressive disorder—medically termed *bipolar mood disorder*—is a variant of classic depression. It typically begins as depression and then develops into alternating periods of depression and mania. A person with severe manic-depressive disorder may go from feeling unrealistically (and dangerously) invincible and elated to being overwhelmed with misery and despair, even suicidal. Some of the symptoms of manic-depressive disorder are changes in sleep pattern, withdrawal from society, extreme pessimism, a sudden loss of interest in and failure to finish projects that were started with enthusiasm, chronic irritability, sudden attacks of rage when crossed, loss of inhibition, and changes in sexual behavior that may range from a complete loss of sex drive to sexual excess. It is estimated that 3 percent of the population of the United States suffers from some form of this disorder.

The course of manic-depressive disorder is highly variable. Both mania and depression can vary in severity, and the length of the cycles, from depression to mania and back again, can occur over the course of a few days or over many months—even, in some cases, years. Low self-esteem and feelings of hopelessness characterize the depressive phase. A person experiencing depression may lack motivation to do anything, even to get out of bed. Some people simply sleep for weeks, withdraw from social activities, avoid re-

lationships with others, and become unable to work. Others may seem to be living normal lives—going to work, interacting with others—but inwardly feel a deadening sadness and are unable to experience genuine pleasure.

The periods of mania often start suddenly and without warning. Some people experience what is called *hypomania,* excitement that does not necessarily appear to be a sign of mental illness—just great enthusiasm and energy. Others experience *full-blown manic psychosis,* in which they have seemingly boundless energy and are ceaselessly active and easily distracted. They may not want to rest or sleep for twenty-four hours or more. Mental activity is sharply accelerated, and delusions of grandeur, persecution, or invincibility are not uncommon. Most people in this condition seem to be utterly elated for no apparent reason, but some become unreasonably irritable and hostile. They may even have hallucinations. Despite all this, a person experiencing full-blown mania generally believes that he or she is functioning at peak efficiency.

The cause of this disorder is not well understood, but there are several theories as to its origin. It may be triggered by extreme stress. Heredity may be a factor in some cases. Some researchers believe that early experiences, such as the loss of a parent or other early childhood trauma, play an important role. Others believe that the manic phase is used (unconsciously) as a kind of psychological compensation for the depression that otherwise engulfs the individual. Biological factors are also possible. There is evidence that concentrations of intracellular sodium increase during the mood swings of manic-depressive disorder, then return to normal after recovery. It is also known that in depressed individuals, brain chemicals called monoamines are depleted.

The symptoms of some childhood psychological disorders such as attention deficit disorder (ADD), attention deficit hyperactivity disorder (ADHD), conduct disorder, and schizophrenia can be similar to those of mania, so a thorough examination is needed to avoid misdiagnosis. It is not uncommon for children who are diagnosed with psychotic depression to be diagnosed with bipolar disorder as adults.

Unless otherwise specified, the dosages recommended here are for adults. For a child between the ages of twelve and seventeen, reduce the dose to three-quarters of the recommended dose. For a child between six and twelve, use one-half of the recommended dose, and for a child under the age of six, use one-quarter of the recommended amount.

NUTRIENTS

SUPPLEMENT	SUGGESTED DOSAGE	COMMENTS
Very Important		
Free-form amino acid complex (Amino Balance from Anabol Naturals)	As directed on label twice daily, on an empty stomach.	To supply protein, needed for normal brain function and to combat depression.

L-Tyrosine	500 mg twice during the day and again at bedtime. Take with water or juice on an empty stomach. Do not take with milk. Take with 50 mg vitamin B_6 and 100 mg vitamin C for better absorption.	Important in treating depression. Stabilizes mood swings. (*See* AMINO ACIDS in Part One.) *Caution*: Do not take this supplement if you are taking an MAO inhibitor drug.
Taurine	500 mg 3 times daily, on an empty stomach.	Deficiency can result in hyperactivity, anxiety, and poor brain function.
Vitamin B complex injections or liver extract injections plus extra vitamin B_6 (pyridoxine) injections and vitamin B_{12} injections or vitamin B complex plus extra vitamin B_{12}	2 cc twice a week or as prescribed by physician. As prescribed by physician. $1/2$ cc twice a week or as prescribed by physician. 1 cc twice a week or as prescribed by physician. 100 mg of each major B vitamin 3 times daily (amounts of individual vitamins in a complex will vary). 1,000–2,000 mcg daily, on an empty stomach.	To supply B vitamins essential for normal brain function and a healthy nervous system. All injectables can be combined in a single injection. Use a hypoallergenic formula. A sublingual form is best. Important in making myelin, the substance of which the sheaths covering the nerves are made. Use a lozenge or sublingual form.
Zinc plus copper	50 mg daily. Do not exceed a total of 100 mg daily from all supplements. 3 mg daily.	Protects the brain cells. Use zinc gluconate lozenges or OptiZinc for best absorption. Needed to balance with zinc.
Important		
Lithium	As prescribed by physician.	A trace mineral that alters the manic-depressive cycles, producing greater mood stability. Available by prescription only.
Helpful		
Essential fatty acids (Kyolic-EPA from Wakunaga is a good source)	As directed on label.	Important for improved cerebral circulation and blood pressure stability.
5-Hydroxytryptophan (5-HTP)	As directed on label.	Increases the body's production of serotonin. *Note*: Do not use this supplement with other antidepressants.
Multivitamin and mineral complex with calcium and magnesium	1,500 mg daily. 750 mg daily.	Mineral imbalances may cause depression. Use a high-potency formula. Has a calming effect; enhances sleep if taken at bedtime.
Nicotinamide adenine dinucleotide (NADH) (Enada NADH from KAL is a good source)	As directed on label.	Enhances production of dopamine and serotonin.
Vitamin C with bioflavonoids	3,000–6,000 mg daily.	To aid in brain function and to protect the immune and nervous systems.

RECOMMENDATIONS

❑ Eat a diet consisting of vegetables, fruits, nuts, seeds, beans, and legumes. Whole grains and whole grain products are recommended, except for those that contain gluten, which should be consumed in moderation only. (*See* CELIAC DISEASE for more information on a gluten-restricted diet.) Eat white fish and turkey twice a week.

❑ Eat fish that are high in omega-3 fatty acids. Tuna, salmon, mackerel, and herring are good choices. Omega-3 fatty acids may stabilize mood swings and have effects similar to those of the medication lithium.

❑ Consume no sugar or sugar byproducts (read food product labels carefully). Also avoid alcohol, dairy products, caffeine, carbonated beverages, and all foods with colorings, flavorings, preservatives, and other additives.

❑ Be aware that food allergies may aggravate mood swings. Use an elimination diet to find which foods may be causing problems, and eliminate them from the diet. (*See* ALLERGIES in Part Two.)

❑ Take high doses of B-complex vitamins, approximately 100 mg of each major B vitamin three times daily (amounts of individual vitamins in a complex will vary). The B complex is very important for all mood disorders. Use injections (under a doctor's supervision) or a sublingual form for best absorption. Persons with manic-depressive disorder do not absorb the B-complex vitamins easily, and often have deficiencies of these vitamins.

❑ Avoid choline and the amino acids ornithine and arginine. These substances may make symptoms worse.

❑ Do not take any drugs except for those prescribed by your doctor.

❑ Establish and maintain a regular routine for your daily activities. A lack of sleep can trigger a relapse.

❑ As much as possible, avoid situations that cause stress, such as a turbulent relationship or a difficult working environment. Stress is a major contributor to serious problems for people with manic-depressive disorder.

CONSIDERATIONS

❑ Injections of vitamin B_{12} and megadoses of the B vitamins often bring about an improvement. The B vitamins have a lithium-like effect on the brain.

❑ Amino acids, especially taurine and tyrosine, are important in the treatment of this disorder.

❑ The trace minerals lithium carbonate and lithium citrate are known to alter the period of the rhythmic cycling of the brain, and help to even out the moods in persons with manic-depressive disorder. Lithium's most important role is to prevent and decrease the occurrence of manic episodes. It is usually taken by mouth in capsule, tablet, or liquid form. The side effects of lithium can include diarrhea, edema, frequent urination, kidney dysfunction, nausea, slight hand tremors, stomach cramps, thirst, thyroid enlargement, weight gain, and worsening of skin conditions such as acne and psoriasis. Toxic levels of lithium in the blood can cause blurred vision, confusion, muscle twitching, nausea, slurred speech, tremors, and vomiting. Lithium levels can be elevated to dangerous levels by changes in the diet, strenuous exercise, surgery, or illness, especially influenza. If you must take lithium, try to keep your weight at a regular level and avoid crash dieting, as lithium levels are elevated by sudden weight loss. Keep your physician informed of any of the above-mentioned circumstances to avoid an imbalance in your dosage. Lithium should not be taken by people with severely impaired kidney function.

❑ Lithium orotate is an organic form of lithium that is sold in health food stores.

❑ For those who cannot tolerate lithium, doctors may prescribe an anticonvulsant drug such as divalproex (Depakote). An antidepressant, such as Paroxetine (Paxil) or bupropion (Wellbutrin), may be prescribed for depressive episodes. To control acute manic episodes, the antipsychotic medications risperidone (Risperdal) and olanzapine (Zyprexa). Stronger medications such as haloperidol (Haldol) or chlorpromazine (Thorazine) are prescribed in rare situations, but these medications can interfere with normal cognitive functioning and have many side effects.

❑ Electroconvulsive therapy (ECT) is sometimes used as a final choice to treat manic-depressive disorder. It is not recommended, as it is traumatic, highly invasive, and can cause identity confusion and memory loss.

❑ Psychotherapy and self-help support groups are very helpful in the treatment of manic-depressive disorder.

❑ According to an article in *The New England Journal of Medicine*, individuals with depression and manic-depressive disorder appear to be hypersensitive to the neurotransmitter acetylcholine. Therefore, choline should not be taken in a dose that exceeds the amount in a multiple vitamin.

❑ Manic-depressive disorder may be aggravated by an overgrowth of yeast in the intestinal tract and by nutritional deficiencies. Food allergies, such as an allergy to wheat products, and the consumption of large amounts of caffeine and/or refined sugar, can make symptoms worse.

❑ According to Richard S. Wilkinson, M.D., of Yakima, Washington, an expert in environmental medicine, environmental sensitivities or allergies may cause manic-depressive disorder.

❑ Certain systemic disorders can cause depression, including Alzheimer's disease, diabetes mellitus, encephalitis, hyper- and hypothyroidism, multiple sclerosis, and Parkinson's disease. Any depression diagnosis should be

made only after a thorough physical examination to rule out an underlying illness.

❑ *See also* DEPRESSION in Part Two.

Mastitis

See under BREASTFEEDING-RELATED PROBLEMS.

Measles

Measles, known to doctors as *rubeola*, is a viral infection that attacks the respiratory tract, eyes, and skin. Although it is typically a childhood disease, adults are also susceptible. Measles is very contagious and is easily spread through the nose, mouth, or throat; secretions on articles or surfaces; or by coughing and sneezing.

Illness usually sets in between seven and fourteen days after exposure to the virus. The first symptoms include fever (temperature of 103°F or higher), cough, sneezing, runny nose, and red eyes that may be sensitive to light. Several days later, Koplik's spots (tiny red spots with white centers) appear in the mouth and throat, the throat becomes sore, and a raised red rash erupts on the forehead and ears. Over a period of five to seven days, the rash spreads to all parts of the body.

In previously healthy children, measles usually runs its course in about ten days. However, it can be followed by a number of complications, some of them potentially serious. These include middle ear infection (especially in children with a history of repeated ear infections), bronchitis, croup, pneumonia, strep throat, and even, in rare cases, encephalitis or meningitis. Adults who develop measles tend to suffer more serious cases of the disease than children do.

Unless otherwise specified, the dosages recommended here are for adults. For a child between the ages of twelve and seventeen, reduce the dose to three-quarters the recommended amount. For a child between six and twelve, use one-half the recommended dose, and for a child under the age of six, use one-quarter the recommended amount.

NUTRIENTS

SUPPLEMENT	SUGGESTED DOSAGE	COMMENTS
Helpful		
Bio-Strath from Nature's Answer	As directed on label.	Acts as a tonic. Contains the vitamin B complex. Use the liquid form.
Calcium and magnesium	As directed on label.	Needed for tissue repair.

Micellized Vitamin A emulsion from American Biologics or	As directed on label.	For adults. Needed to reduce infection and to repair tissues.
vitamin A	10,000 IU twice daily for 1 week, then reduce to 10,000 IU once daily. Do not exceed this dosage. If you are pregnant, do not exceed 10,000 IU daily.	For children.
or cod liver oil	As directed on label.	For children unable to swallow capsules.
Proteolytic enzymes	As directed on label 2–3 times daily, between meals.	Reduces infection and aids digestion.
Raw thymus glandular	500 mg twice daily.	Stimulates the immune system.
Vitamin B complex	100 mg of each major B vitamin 3 times daily or as directed on label (amounts of individual vitamins in a complex will vary).	Important in all bodily functions, including immune response and proper healing. For a child under 8, use a formula designed specifically for children.
Vitamin C with bioflavonoids	For adults: 3,000–10,000 mg daily, in divided doses. For children: 1,000–3,000 mg daily, in divided doses.	Very important for immune function. Controls fever and infection. Has antiviral properties. Use an ascorbate or esterified form.
Vitamin E	200–800 IU daily. For children, do not exceed 200 IU.	Neutralizes harmful free radicals, which can destroy cell membranes. Use d-alpha-tocopherol form.
Zinc lozenges	1 15-mg lozenge 3 times daily for 4 days. Then reduce to 1 lozenge daily.	For immune response and tissue repair. Reduces symptoms and speeds healing. Also relieves itchy throat and coughing.

HERBS

❑ Catnip tea or garlic enemas can be used to help to lower fever if necessary. (*See* ENEMAS in Part Three.)

❑ Lobelia extract helps to relieve pain. Take ½ teaspoon of lobelia extract every four to five hours.

Caution: Do not take lobelia internally on an ongoing basis.

❑ Spirulina is helpful for bolstering the immune system and can help slow replication of the virus.

RECOMMENDATIONS

❑ If you suspect that you or a member of your family has measles, see your health care provider. This is important for a correct diagnosis and to prevent serious complications.

❑ Drink plenty of fluids such as water, juices, herbal teas, and vegetable broths.

❑ Avoid processed foods.

❑ To help relieve coughing, mix 1 tablespoon lemon juice and 2 tablespoons honey with ¼ cup water. Take as needed.

❑ To alleviate itching, place ½ cup of baking soda in a bathtubful of lukewarm water and soak in the bath until the itching decreases. Gently applying witch hazel to the affected area also will help to ease the discomfort and itching associated with the rash.

❑ Try using homeopathic remedies to ease symptoms. *Aconitum napellus* (homeopathic monkshood) is the homeopathic version of vitamin C in that it is helpful in the initial stage of measles. *Ferrum phosphoricum* (homeopathic phosophate of iron) is beneficial for mild infections.

❑ Rest until the rash and fever have disappeared.

❑ Keep the lights dim. Do not read or watch television while your eyes are sensitive to light.

❑ Do not send a child who has had measles to school until seven to nine days after the fever and rash have disappeared.

CONSIDERATIONS

❑ Doctors generally recommend that children receive two measles vaccinations, the first at the age of about fifteen months and the second either before entering school or at approximately twelve years of age. A second vaccination is now considered necessary because there have been outbreaks of measles among college students who received a single immunization in childhood. However, certain individuals should *not* be immunized against measles, including pregnant women and anyone who has cancer or a weakened immune system, is on cortisone or anticancer drugs, is undergoing radiation therapy, or has any type of illness with fever. People who are allergic to eggs should mention this to their physicians prior to having the vaccine. A person who has had and recovered from measles does not require immunization; a single attack of measles gives lifelong immunity to the disease.

❑ Short-term, high doses of vitamin A have been used to lessen the severity and complications of measles. Since high doses of vitamin A can be toxic, high dosages of this vitamin should be taken only for brief periods (two weeks or less) and should be monitored very carefully.

❑ Antibiotics are useless against viruses, so they are not called for unless complications occur.

Melanoma

See under SKIN CANCER.

Memory Problems

Memory is as natural to us as breathing. It is an ability we all have, yet rarely ever think of—unless we perceive that we are losing that ability. Memory lapses are an annoyance in themselves, but worse is the anxiety that often comes along with them. We begin asking ourselves if they are a symptom of some other problem, such as midlife depression or arteriosclerosis. Probably the greatest fear provoked by lapses in memory is that of *Alzheimer's disease,* a progressive and debilitating disease that usually starts in midlife with minor defects in memory and behavior. Although this is a fairly common disorder among older people, it is important to realize that most memory lapses have nothing to do with Alzheimer's disease.

People have come to expect that, as they age, their ability to remember will begin to deteriorate; that their powers of recall will diminish. This is not necessarily true. The aging process itself has little, if any, bearing on the ability to recall information. Occasional memory lapses, such as misplacing the car keys or forgetting something at the grocery store, are a natural, normal part of life at virtually any age, and are not likely to precede serious memory loss. In fact, with proper diet, nutrition, and memory use, the memory should remain sharp and active well into one's nineties or beyond.

One reason many people suffer from memory loss is an insufficient supply of necessary nutrients (especially the B vitamins and amino acids) to the brain. The life of the body is in the blood. It literally feeds and nourishes every cell within our bodies. The brain is surrounded by a protective envelope known as the blood-brain barrier, which allows only certain substances to pass from the bloodstream into the brain. If the blood is "thick" with cholesterol and triglycerides, the amount of nutrient-rich blood that can pass through the blood-brain barrier decreases. Over time, this can result in the brain becoming malnourished.

In addition, the functioning of the brain depends upon substances called neurotransmitters. Neurotransmitters are brain chemicals that act as electrical switches in the brain and, through the functioning of the nervous system, are ultimately responsible for all the functions of the body. If the brain does not have an adequate supply of neurotransmitters, or the nutrients from which to make them, it begins to develop the biochemical equivalent of a power failure or a short circuit. If your mind goes blank when you are trying to recall a specific fact or piece of information, or it begins to plug into some other, irrelevant memory instead, it is likely that such a "short circuit" has occurred.

There are numerous other factors involved in the deterioration of memory. One of the most important is probably exposure to free radicals, which can wreak enormous damage to the memory if unchecked. Alcoholics and drug addicts often suffer a great deal from memory loss. Alcoholics are notorious for "blackouts"—huge memory gaps that occur even though they are conscious. Allergies, candidiasis, stress, thyroid disorders, and poor circulation to the brain may also be contributing factors. Hypoglycemia (low blood sugar) can play a role in memory loss as well, because to function properly, the brain requires that the level of glucose in the blood fall within a very specific narrow range. Wide swings in blood sugar levels affect brain function and memory.

NUTRIENTS

SUPPLEMENT	SUGGESTED DOSAGE	COMMENTS
Essential		
Ultra Brain Power from American Biologics	As directed on label.	Provides nutrients to support memory, concentration, and other higher brain functions.
Very Important		
Acetylcholine	As directed on label.	Most important of the neurotransmitters. Maximizes mental ability and prevents memory loss in adults.
Boron	3–6 mg daily. Do not exceed this amount.	Improves brain and memory function.
Dimethylamino-ethanol (DMAE)	As directed on label.	Aids in learning and memory. *Note:* This supplement is not intended for everyday use. It is best reserved for days when you need to be more focused and alert.
Garlic (Kyolic from Wakunaga)	As directed on label.	May be useful for treating physiological aging and age-related memory deficits. Potent brain cell protector.
Huperzine A or vinpocetine	As directed on label. As directed on label.	Aid the effectiveness of acetylcholine in preventing memory loss.
Lecithin granules or capsules	1 tbsp 3 times daily, before meals. 1,200 mg 3 times daily, before meals.	Needed for improved memory. Contains choline.
Manganese	As directed on label. Take separately from calcium.	Helps nourish the brain and nerves. Aids in the utilization of choline.
Multivitamin and mineral complex with potassium	As directed on label. 99 mg daily.	All nutrients are necessary in balance. Use a high-potency formula. Needed for proper electrolyte balance.
Omega-3 fatty acid complex	As directed on label.	Low levels have been associated with impaired brain function.
Phosphatidyl choline	As directed on label.	Improves memory.
Phosphatidyl serine	300 mg 3 times daily.	Improves memory.
Superoxide dismutase (SOD)	As directed on label.	Known for its ability to eliminate free radicals.
Vitamin A plus carotenoid complex with beta-carotene	15,000 IU daily. If you are pregnant, do not exceed 10,000 IU daily. 25,000 IU daily.	Deficiencies of antioxidants expose the brain to oxidative damage.
Vitamin B complex plus extra pantothenic acid (vitamin B_5) and vitamin B_6 (pyridoxine)	100 mg of each major B vitamin daily (amounts of individual vitamins in a complex will vary). 50 mg 3 times daily. 50 mg 3 times daily.	Needed for improved memory. Injections (under a doctor's supervision) may be necessary. Helps in transformation of the amino acid choline to the neurotransmitter acetylcholine. Needed for proper brain function.

Vitamin B₃ (niacin) and niacinamide	As directed on label.	To promote proper circulation to the brain and aid in brain function. *Caution:* Do not take niacin if you have a liver disorder, gout, or high blood pressure.
Vitamin C with bioflavonoids	3,000–10,000 mg daily.	A powerful antioxidant that also improves circulation.
Vitamin E	Start with 400 IU daily and slowly increase to 1,200 IU daily.	Causes dilation of blood vessels, improving blood flow to the brain. Use d-alpha-tocopherol form.
Zinc	50–80 mg daily. Do not exceed 100 mg daily.	Important in binding toxic substances and removing them from the brain. Use zinc gluconate lozenges or OptiZinc for best absorption.
plus copper	3 mg daily.	Needed to balance with zinc.
Important		
Acetyl-L-carnitine	500 mg twice daily.	May enhance brain metabolism. Slows deterioration of memory and reduces the production of free radicals.
L-Glutamine and L-phenylalanine plus L-aspartic acid	As directed on label, on an empty stomach. Take with water or juice. Do not take with milk. Take with 50 mg vitamin B₆ and 100 mg vitamin C for better absorption.	Amino acids necessary for normal brain function; serve as fuel for the brain and prevent excess ammonia from damaging the brain. *Caution:* Do not take phenylalanine if you are pregnant or nursing, or if you suffer from panic attacks, diabetes, high blood pressure, or PKU.
L-Tyrosine	Up to 100 mg per kg of body weight daily. Take on an empty stomach with 1,000 mg vitamin C and 50 mg vitamin B₆.	Helps sharpen learning, memory, and awareness; elevates mood and motivation; aids in preventing depression. *Caution:* Do not take this supplement if you are also taking an MAO inhibitor drug.
Helpful		
Coenzyme Q₁₀	100 mg daily.	Improves brain oxygenation.
plus Coenzyme A from Coenzyme-A Technologies	As directed on label.	Improves the effectiveness of coenzyme Q₁₀.
Dehydroepiandros-terone (DHEA from Natrol)	As directed on label. Take with vitamins C and E and selenium to prevent oxidative damage to the liver.	May help to improve memory. (*See* DHEA Therapy in Part Three.)
or 7-Keto DHEA (7-Keto from Enzymatic Therapy)	As directed on label.	A metabolite of DHEA that has been found to be superior to DHEA in enhancing memory. Unlike DHEA, it is not converted into estrogen or testosterone in the body.
Diamond Mind from Diamond-Herpanacine Associates	As directed on label.	Combination supplements that can aid with memory-related functions.
or Maximum Living Ginkgo Biloba with DHA from Bay To Bay Distribution or	As directed on label.	

Life Time Brain Support Formula from Life Time Nutritional Specialties or	As directed on label.	
Bacopin & Ginkgo Complex from America's Finest or	As directed on label.	
Cognitex with pregnenolone from Prolongevity	As directed on label.	
Dimethylglycine (DMG) (Aangamik DMG from FoodScience of Vermont)	As directed on label.	Improves brain oxygenation.
Melatonin	2–3 mg daily, taken 2 hours or less before bedtime.	A powerful antioxidant that may prevent memory loss.
Nicotinamide adenine dinucleotide (NADH) (Enada NADH from Kal)	As directed on label.	A coenzyme form of niacin that is essential for the production of certain neurotransmitters and energy. Natural levels decline with age. Supplemental NADH can improve energy production in the brain and nervous system.
Pregnenolone (PREG from TriMedica)	As directed on label.	May improve brain function and enhance memory.
RNA and DNA	As directed on label	Increases energy production for memory transfer in the brain. *Caution:* Do not take this supplement if you have gout.

HERBS

❑ Brahmi, an Ayurvedic herb related to gotu kola, increases circulation in the brain and has been found to improve both short- and long-term memory.

❑ Garlic has been found to possess memory-enhancing properties.

❑ Ginkgo biloba has been attracting attention from researchers because of its ability to increase blood flow to the brain and central nervous system, thereby enhancing memory and brain function. Ginkgo is available in capsule or extract form at most health food stores (Ginkgo Biloba Extract from American Biologics is a good source). For memory enhancement, take capsules as directed on the product label, or place 6 drops of an alcohol-free extract under your tongue and hold it there for a few minutes, then swallow. Do this twice daily.

❑ Other herbs that are helpful for memory include anise, blue cohosh, ginseng, gotu kola, and rosemary.

Caution: Do not use ginseng if you have high blood pressure.

RECOMMENDATIONS

❑ Eat a diet high in raw foods. Consume the following often: brewer's yeast, brown rice, farm eggs, fish, legumes, millet, nuts, soybeans, tofu, wheat germ, and whole grains.

❏ Combine complex carbohydrates with foods containing 10 percent protein and 10 percent essential fats. All-carbohydrate meals have an adverse effect on the memory.

❏ Avoid dairy and wheat products (except for wheat germ) for one month. If there is no memory improvement, slowly add these foods back to your diet.

❏ Eat more blueberries and spinach. Some researchers believe that flavonoids found in these foods may aid in memory retention.

❏ Make certain that you are getting the correct amounts of amino acids, antioxidants, B vitamins, choline, coenzyme Q_{10}, iron, and pregnenolone, either from the diet or through supplementation.

❏ Avoid refined sugars—these "turn off" the brain.

❏ Practice holding your breath for thirty seconds every hour for thirty days. This improves mental alertness.

❏ Consider having a hair analysis done to rule out intoxication by heavy metals such as aluminum and lead. Either of these conditions can lead to impaired mental functioning. (*See* HAIR ANALYSIS in Part Three.)

❏ If you are already taking a multivitamin and mineral supplement, you may wish to try Cognitex from Prolongevity or Fuel for Thought from Nature's Plus. Bee pollen may also be helpful.

Caution: Bee pollen may cause an allergic reaction in some people. Start with a small amount, and discontinue use if a rash, wheezing, discomfort, or other symptom occurs.

❏ Make sure to focus on things that you may wish to remember, and be sure to give them meaning. Often, we blame our inability to recall something on a failing memory when the problem is that we did not really pay attention in the first place.

❏ Keep yourself active mentally by using your brain on a daily basis. Pursue activities such as reading, doing crossword puzzles, surfing the Internet, or playing a mentally challenging game. Research has shown that the more you put your memory to use, the more vital it will be.

❏ Keep yourself physically active. This increases blood flow to the brain.

❏ Be sure to get the proper amount of rest to avoid fatigue, which can have a direct effect on the ability to focus.

CONSIDERATIONS

❏ Human growth hormone (HGH) has been shown to improve brain function. (*See* GROWTH HORMONE THERAPY in Part Three.)

❏ There are conflicting reports on whether or not estrogen can improve memory function.

❏ Some medications may have an adverse effect on memory, including beta-blockers, benzodiazepines (prescribed for anxiety), some painkillers and antihistamines, and anticholinergics (prescribed for incontinence or depression).

❏ Occasional memory loss or forgetfulness is common. However, if you begin to notice certain memory-related problems happening, such as forgetting things much more often than you did before, forgetting how to do something that was commonplace to you before, getting lost in familiar surroundings, or repeating the same conversation over and over again to the same person, there may be cause for concern.

❏ The keys to having a good memory are in attitude and approach. As we age, our attitudes change. Our ability to remember isn't affected as much as we think. It is the change in our motivation to remember things that is probably the larger factor.

❏ *See also* AGING; ALZHEIMER'S DISEASE; ARTERIOSCLEROSIS; HYPOGLYCEMIA; and/or SENILITY, all in Part Two.

Ménière's Disease

Ringing in the ears, variable loss of hearing, loss of balance, vertigo or dizziness, tinnitus (buzzing or ringing in the ears), and a sensation of fullness or pressure are symptoms of the inner ear disturbance known as Ménière's disease. The condition may affect one or both ears. Ménière's disease is rare and the exact cause or causes are unknown, but many experts believe it results from a condition known to researchers as *endolymphatic hydrops,* an excessive swelling of the small, fluid-filled chambers of the inner ear. Eventually, the pressure and severe disruptions within the inner ear cause periodic attacks of vertigo. The attacks can last from ten minutes to several hours. During a severe attack, symptoms can include nausea, sweating, vomiting, and loss of balance. Unsteadiness may last for several days after the attack. Impaired blood flow to the brain from clogged arteries and poor circulation may also be involved. Allergies, consumption of alcohol or caffeine, stress, barometric changes, pregnancy, visual stimuli, experiencing orgasm, sugar, exposure to loud noises, and excessive salt intake may trigger this disorder. Other factors, such as obesity and high blood cholesterol, may contribute to this syndrome. Allergies, spasms of the blood vessels that supply the inner ear, and, for women, fluid retention during the premenstrual period may also be related to Ménière's disease. Drug use, smoking, trauma, and temporomandibular joint (TMJ) syndrome may be involved as well.

Ménière's disease usually affects adults (men more often than women) between the ages of thirty and sixty. For many individuals, Ménière's disease is an unpredictable disorder and the attacks only occur occasionally; for others is it severe and can cause complete deafness and repeated, debilitating vertigo.

Unless otherwise specified, the dosages recommended here are for adults. For a child between the ages of twelve and seventeen, reduce the dose to three-quarters of the recommended amount. For a child between six and twelve, use one-half of the recommended dose, and for a child under the age of six, use one-quarter of the recommended amount.

NUTRIENTS

SUPPLEMENT	SUGGESTED DOSAGE	COMMENTS
Essential		
Manganese	5 mg daily. Take separately from calcium.	Deficiency may be the cause of Ménière's syndrome.
Very Important		
Bio-Strath from Bioforce	As directed on label.	A natural source of the B vitamins. Acts as a tonic and enhances brain function.
Chromium picolinate	200 mcg daily.	Aids in controlling blood sugar levels, which are often high in those with this disorder.
Coenzyme Q_{10} plus	100 mg daily.	Improves circulation.
Coenzyme A from Coenzyme-A Technologies	As directed on label.	Supports and boosts the immune system.
Vitamin B_3 (niacin)	100 mg twice daily. Do not exceed this amount.	Improves circulation. If you are uncomfortable with the flush caused by niacin, use part niacinamide. *Caution:* Do not take niacin if you have a liver disorder, gout, or high blood pressure.
Important		
Vitamin B complex	As directed on label.	Important for the nervous system. Use a high-stress formula.
plus extra vitamin B_6 (pyridoxine)	100 mg twice daily.	Reduces fluid retention.
Vitamin C with bioflavonoids	3,000–6,000 mg daily, in divided doses.	Boosts immune function. Use an esterified or buffered form.
Helpful		
Calcium and	1,500 mg daily.	Needed for stability of the nervous system and for muscle contraction. Chelated forms are the most effective.
magnesium	1,000 mg daily.	
Essential fatty acids (primrose oil, salmon oil, and Kyolic-EPA from Wakunaga are good sources)	As directed on label 3 times daily, with meals.	To correct metabolic disturbances.
Lecithin granules or capsules	1 tbsp 3 times daily, before meals. 1,200 mg 3 times daily, before meals.	For cellular protection and brain function.
Vitamin E	400–800 IU daily. If you have high blood pressure, start with 100 IU daily and increase slowly to 400 IU daily.	Promotes efficient oxygen use. Use d-alpha-tocopherol form.

HERBS

❑ Butcher's broom combats fluid retention and improves circulation.

❑ Ginger is helpful for nausea.

❑ Ginkgo biloba, taken in extract or tablet form, increases circulation to the brain.

❑ St. John's wort can relieve anxiety and depression.

RECOMMENDATIONS

❑ Try a hypoglycemic diet for two weeks. If you experience an improvement, remain on the diet. (*See* HYPOGLYCEMIA in Part Two.)

❑ Do not consume any fats, fried foods, salt, monosodium glutamate (MSG), alcohol, sugar (in any form), or anything containing caffeine.

❑ Check for food allergies. (*See* ALLERGIES in Part Two.)

❑ To help with vertigo attacks, restrict your head movement and keep your eyes fixed on a stationary object at a good distance from you. Also, you can lie down with your unaffected ear against the floor, and look in the direction of the affected ear.

❑ Vertigoheel from Heel Inc. is a homeopathic remedy that may help with the frequency and intensity of vertigo attacks.

❑ As much as possible, reduce the anxiety in your life. Stress is a major trigger in Ménière's disease.

CONSIDERATIONS

❑ Some doctors recommend a high-protein, low-refined-carbohydrate diet because they have found that people with this disorder have high blood insulin levels. High insulin levels impair circulation. (*See* ARTERIOSCLEROSIS and CIRCULATORY PROBLEMS, both in Part Two.)

❑ Doctors prescribe a variety of medications to combat the symptoms of vertigo and nausea. Promethazine (Phenergan) is usually prescribed to treat the nausea, vomiting, and vertigo symptoms. To reduce fluids in the system, diuretics may be prescribed. A low-salt diet may accompany this plan. Diazepam (Valium) is frequently prescribed to lessen anxiety and to sedate the vestibular system. For some people, physicians prescribe antihistamines, and in some cases, steroids.

❑ There may be a correlation between high calcium levels and the incidence of Ménière's disease. Physicians in Europe have prescribed the calcium channel blocker medication flunarizine with positive results in combating vertigo. Flunarizine is not currently available in the United States.

❑ If symptoms are severe and interfere drastically with daily life, surgery may be recommended. Surgical procedure options for Ménière's disease include the insertion of a small tube into the eardrum (a tympanostomy tube), enlarging the endolymphatic sac by drilling the bone surrounding it or draining the fluid to reduce pressure (endolymphatic sac decompression), placing a small tube into the endolymphatic sac to drain excess fluid (endolymphatic sac shunt), removal of the labyrinth or a portion of the labyrinth (surgical labyrinthectomy), cutting the vestibular nerve to destroy the balance function of the ear (vestibular nerve section surgery), placing ototoxic drugs (toxic antibiotics) in the ear to destroy the balance portion of the ear (chemical labyrinthectomy), or inserting drugs into the eardrum with a syringe by laser.

❏ See also HEARING LOSS in Part Two.

❏ For the name and address of an organization that can provide more information about Ménière's disease, see American Academy of Otolaryngology under HEALTH AND MEDICAL ORGANIZATIONS in the Appendix.

Meningitis

Meningitis is an infection of the three membranes, called the meninges, that lie between the brain and the skull. The thin membranes that cover the spinal cord may also be involved. This disorder is more common in children than in adults.

The most common type of meningitis is viral meningitis. This disease causes comparatively mild symptoms, such as headache and malaise, and usually improves on its own in a week or two. Also called *aseptic meningitis,* viral meningitis usually occurs in conjunction with other diseases. Almost 50 percent of cases of viral meningitis infections are caused by intestinal viruses. This condition may also accompany mumps or a herpes outbreak, and it can be carried by mosquitoes as well. The early symptoms of viral meningitis include sore throat, fever, headache, stiff neck, fatigue, and, possibly, a rash and vomiting.

Bacterial meningitis is the more serious infection and it requires prompt, aggressive medical treatment. The bacteria responsible for most outbreaks of bacterial meningitis are *Neisseria meningitidis* (meningococcus), *Streptococcus pneumoniae* (pneumococcus), *Hemophilus influenzae* type B, and group B *Streptococcus. Neisseria* and *Steptococcus* are the leading causes of infection since, after 1990, routine immunization curbed the outbreaks of *H. influenza* type B (Hib). In the case of *N. meningitidis,* at any one time, some 5 to 20 percent of the population carry this bacteria in their saliva without feeling any ill effects—but it can be transmitted through the saliva to other people. The *Streptococcus pneumonia* bacteria is commonly found in the throat and is not contagious. The symptoms of bacterial meningitis include stiff neck, headache, irritability, high fever, chills, nausea, vomiting, delirium, and sensitivity to light. A blotchy, red skin rash may appear. In infants, the signs include fever,

vomiting, poor muscle tone, difficulty feeding, irritability, a high-pitched cry, and a bulging fontanel (soft spot). Changes in temperament and extreme sleepiness signal dangerous changes in the cerebrospinal fluid (the fluid that surrounds and cushions the brain).

The recommendations in this section are designed to support medical treatment, not replace it. Meningitis can progress very quickly and become life threatening in a matter of twenty-four hours for adults, much less for children. If untreated, this disease can cause permanent brain damage and paralysis, even coma and death.

Unless otherwise specified, the dosages recommended here are for adults. For a child between the ages of twelve and seventeen, reduce the dose to three-quarters the recommended amount. For a child between six and twelve, use one-half the recommended dose, and for a child under the age of six, use one-quarter the recommended amount.

NUTRIENTS

SUPPLEMENT	SUGGESTED DOSAGE	COMMENTS
Helpful		
Acidophilus (Kyo-Dophilus from Wakunaga is a good source)	As directed on label. Take on an empty stomach.	Needed to replenish the friendly bacteria antibiotics destroy. Use a nondairy formula.
Colloidal silver	As directed on label.	Taken internally, is effective against many disease causing organisms. Also has antifungal properties.
Dimethylglycine (DMG) (Aangamik DMG from FoodScience of Vermont)	125 mg twice daily.	Carries oxygen to the cells, relieving many symptoms. Use a sublingual form.
Dioxychlor DC-3 from American Biologics	As directed on label.	A potent antibacterial, antifungal, and antiviral agent.
Free-form amino acid complex (Amino Balance from Anabol Naturals)	As directed on label.	Needed for tissue repair and protection of membranes.
Garlic (Kyolic from Wakunaga)	2 capsules 3 times daily, with meals.	An immune system stimulant that also acts as a natural antibiotic.
GE-132 from American Biologics	As directed on label.	An antioxidant and immune stimulator.
Maitake extract or reishi extract or shiitake extract	As directed on label. As directed on label. As directed on label.	To help to build immunity and fight viral infection.
Multivitamin and mineral complex	As directed on label.	All nutrients are needed for tissue protection and healing. Use a high-potency formula.
Raw thymus glandular	500 mg twice daily.	Enhances immune response.
Taurine Plus from American Biologics	As directed on label.	An antioxidant and immune regulator necessary for white blood cell activation and neurological function. Use the liquid form.

Vitamin A emulsion or capsules	50,000 IU daily. 25,000 IU daily for 7 days, then reduce to 15,000 IU daily. If you are pregnant, do not exceed 10,000 IU daily.	A powerful antioxidant and immune booster. Needed for protection and healing of all membranes. Emulsion form is recommended for easier absorption and greater safety at higher doses.
Vitamin C with bioflavonoids	3,000–10,000 mg daily.	Reduces infection and aids in cleansing the bloodstream.
Zinc lozenges	1 15-mg lozenge 3 times daily. Do not exceed a total of 100 mg daily from all supplements.	An immune system booster.

HERBS

❏ For fever, use catnip tea enemas. *See* ENEMAS in Part Three. Catnip tea is also good for sipping.

❏ Echinacea boosts the immune system.

❏ Goldenseal is a natural antibiotic.

Caution: Do not take goldenseal internally on a daily basis for more than one week, as it may disturb normal intestinal flora. Do not use it in large quantities during pregnancy, and use it with caution if you are allergic to ragweed.

❏ Olive leaf extract helps fight viral infections.

❏ St. John's wort is good for viral infections.

RECOMMENDATIONS

❏ If you develop symptoms characteristic of meningitis, see a physician or go to the emergency room of the nearest hospital immediately.

❏ Avoid aspirin, which increases bleeding tendencies.

❏ Once the acute phase of the illness has passed and recovery has begun, eat a well-balanced diet including fresh fruits and vegetables (50 percent of them raw), grains, nuts, seeds, and yogurt and other soured products.

❏ Consume fresh pineapple and papaya frequently. Pineapple reduces inflammation; papaya is good for digestion. Only the fresh forms are effective.

❏ Avoid the following foods, which encourage the formation of mucus: animal protein and its byproducts, caffeine, dairy products (except for yogurt), processed foods, salt, sugar, and white flour products.

❏ Rest in bed in a dimly lit room. Drink plenty of high-quality liquids.

❏ Take cool sponge baths.

CONSIDERATIONS

❏ Diagnosis of meningitis requires microscopic analysis and culture of the cerebrospinal fluid.

❏ If there are no complications, recovery from viral meningitis generally takes three weeks under a physician's care.

❏ Antibiotics do not fight viruses, so they are not appropriate treatment for viral meningitis. Only strains of *bacterial* meningitis can be treated with antibiotics.

❏ For bacterial meningitis, aggressive treatment with antibiotics is necessary. For viral meningitis, antibiotics are ineffective and therefore inappropriate. If meningitis is caused by a fungal infection, treatment with an antifungal drug is used.

❏ Corticosteroids may be prescribed to reduce inflammation. Antinausea and strong pain medication may also be needed.

❏ It is wise to seek prompt treatment for a bacterial infection anywhere in the body, such as strep throat or an ear infection.

❏ Antibiotics may be prescribed as a preventive for those who have been in close contact with a person who has bacterial meningitis.

❏ Adults tend to be immune to *H. influenza* type B, and the Hib vaccine protects most young children. However, if you have been in close contact with someone who has this infection, you may need to see your physician to inquire about antibiotic treatment.

Menopausal and Perimenopausal Problems

Menopause is the point at which a woman stops ovulating and menstruation ceases, indicating the end of fertility. It is important to remember that menopause is *not* a disease. Menopause is as natural a progression in life as puberty.

Many years before a woman stops ovulating, her ovaries slow their production of the hormones estrogen, progesterone, and testosterone. Estrogen and progesterone are commonly thought of as sex or reproductive hormones. While estrogen is indeed essential for reproduction, it also acts on many nonreproductive organs and systems in the body. Cells in the vagina, bladder, breasts, skin, bones, arteries, heart, liver, and brain all contain estrogen receptors, and require this hormone to stimulate these receptors for normal cell function. Estrogen is needed to keep the skin smooth and moist, and the body's internal thermostat operating properly. It is also necessary for proper bone formation. Although estrogen levels drop sharply after menopause, the hormone does not disappear entirely. Other organs take over from the ovaries and continue to produce a less potent form of estrogen. The organs known as endocrine glands secrete some hormones from fatty tissue to maintain bodily functions.

Progesterone works as a counterpart to estrogen. During the second half of the menstrual cycle, it stimulates changes in the lining of the uterus to complete its preparation to act as a "home" for a fertilized egg. If no egg is fertilized, the uterine lining is broken down and expelled. The cycle then begins again. Progesterone too has effects beyond the reproductive system. It has a calming effect on the brain and appears to affect other aspects of nervous system function as well.

Testosterone is the hormone that is most important for sex drive. Women produce much less of this hormone than men do—about 80 percent less—but it is the driving force for maintaining a healthy libido (sexual appetite).

Perimenopause is the period when a woman's body is preparing for menopause. For most women, hormone production begins to slow down when they reach their thirties, and continues to diminish as they age. Many women experience few if any symptoms during this time but others may suffer from some, or all, of the following: anxiety, dry skin, fatigue, feelings of bloating, headaches, heart palpitations, hot flashes, insomnia, irritability, decreased interest in sex, loss of concentration, mood swings, night sweats, reduced stamina, urinary incontinence, vaginal dryness and itching, and weight gain.

Menopause is the time when a woman stops menstruating altogether. By this stage, most of the acute problems a woman may have experienced are actually over and a new balance between all hormones should be established. However, this is the time women become increasingly vulnerable to other, potentially serious health problems. Over the long term, the diminished supply of estrogen increases the likelihood of cardiovascular disease, osteoporosis, and vaginal atrophy. Osteoporosis in particular is a major problem for women after menopause. An estimated 80 percent of the 250,000 hip fractures that occur in the United States every year are due to osteoporosis.

With a proper diet, nutritional supplements, and exercise, most of the unpleasant side effects of menopause can be minimized, if not eliminated.

NUTRIENTS

SUPPLEMENT	SUGGESTED DOSAGE	COMMENTS
Very Important		
Beta-1,3-D-glucan	As directed on label.	Boosts bone marrow production and acts as a powerful stimulant for the immune system.
Cerasomal-cis-9-cetylmyristoleate	As directed on label.	Acts like a lubricant for joints and reduces inflammation. *Caution:* Do not take this supplement if you have liver problems.
Coenzyme Q10 plus Coenzyme A from Coenzyme-A Technologies	As directed on label. As directed on label.	To support the immune system's detoxification of many dangerous substances, streamline metabolism, ease depression and fatigue, increase energy, support adrenal glands, process fats, boost the immune system, and improve overall physical and mental processes.
Dehydroepiandrosterone (DHEA) or 7-keto DHEA	As directed on label. As directed on label.	Increases memory function, reduces stress, and enhances sex drive. *Note:* DHEA is converted into testosterone and estrogens in the body. Use with caution if you are taking HRT. A metabolite of DHEA that is not converted into sex hormones.
Essential fatty acids (primrose oil, black currant seed oil, and Kyolic-EPA from Wakunaga are good sources)	As directed on label.	Act as sedatives and diuretics. Good for hot flashes. Important for production of estrogen.
Lecithin granules or capsules	1 tbsp 3 times daily, before meals. 1,200 mg 3 times daily, before meals.	Important as an emulsifier for vitamin E, which reduces hot flashes and related symptoms.
Multienzyme complex with hydrochloric acid (HCl)	As directed on label. Take with meals.	To aid digestion. HCl production declines with age. *Caution:* Do not use HCl if you have a history of ulcers.
Soy protein	30 grams daily.	Soybeans contain a form of estrogen. Helps relieve hot flashes and protect against heart disease and osteoporosis.
Ultra Osteo Synergy from American Biologics	As directed on label.	Nutritional support for bone renewal.
Vitamin B complex plus extra pantothenic acid (vitamin B5) and vitamin B6 (pyridoxine) and folic acid	As directed on label. 100 mg 3 times daily. 50 mg 3 times daily. As directed on label.	For improved circulation and cellular function. Use a sublingual form for best absorption. Or consider injections (under a doctor's supervision). A powerful anti-stress vitamin needed for adrenal function. Minimizes water retention and eases symptoms. Helps protect against heart disease.
Vitamin D3 (cholecalciferol)	600 IU daily.	Regulates calcium within the body.
Vitamin E	Start with 400 IU daily and slowly increase the dosage until hot flashes are relieved, up to 1,600 IU daily.	Reduces hot flashes and many other symptoms. Use emulsion form for easier assimilation and greater safety at high doses. Use d-alpha-tocopherol form.
Important		
Boron	3 mg daily. Do not exceed this amount.	Enhances calcium absorption.
Calcium and magnesium	2,000 mg daily. 1,000 mg daily.	To relieve nervousness and irritability, and to protect against bone loss. Use chelate forms.
Quercetin Plus from Nature's Plus or Nutrition Now	2 mg daily.	An antioxidant flavonoid that may help with hot flashes.
Silica	As directed on label.	Supplies silicon, needed for connective tissue and for calcium uptake.

Zinc	50 mg daily. Do not exceed a total of 100 mg daily from all supplements.	Aids in protecting against bone loss and reducing symptoms. Use zinc gluconate lozenges or OptiZinc for best absorption.
plus		
copper	3 mg daily.	Needed to balance with zinc.

Helpful		
L-Arginine and	500 mg twice daily.	Detoxifies the liver.
L-lysine	500 mg daily, on an empty stomach. Take with water or juice. Do not take with milk. Take with 50 mg vitamin B$_6$ and 100 mg vitamin C for better absorption.	Aids liver function. (*See* AMINO ACIDS in Part One.)
Meno-Fem from Prevail	As directed on label.	Contains gamma-oryzanol, a component of rice brain oil effective in controlling uncomfortable symptoms of menopause.
Multiglandular complex	As directed on label.	For hormonal stability. (*See* GLANDULAR THERAPY in Part Three.)
Multivitamin and mineral complex with	As directed on label. Take with meals.	All nutrients are needed for normal hormone production and function.
potassium	99 mg daily.	To replace potassium lost through perspiration during hot flashes. Potassium protects the nervous system and encourages a regular heart rhythm.
and selenium	200 mcg daily.	An important trace mineral linked to normal hormonal balance.
Vitamin C plus	3,000–10,000 mg daily.	For hot flashes. Also for heart health.
mixed bioflavonoids	1,000 mg daily.	

HERBS

❑ A paste made from aloe vera gel and slippery elm powder, mixed to the consistency of toothpaste and inserted into the vagina at night, can relieve vaginal dryness.

❑ Damiana enhances sexual desire and pleasure.

❑ Amaranth, chickweed, dandelion greens, nettle, seaweed, and watercress are rich in calcium and can help prevent osteoporosis.

❑ Anise, black cohosh, fennel, licorice, raspberry, sage, sarsaparilla, squawvine, unicorn root, and wild yam root are natural estrogen promoters.

Caution: Do not use licorice on a daily basis for more than seven days in a row, and avoid it completely if you have high blood pressure. Do not use sage if you suffer from any type of seizure disorder.

❑ Chamomile and valerian root help to calm the body and promote restful sleep.

Caution: Do not use chamomile on an ongoing basis, and avoid it completely if you are allergic to ragweed.

❑ Gotu kola and dong quai relieve hot flashes, vaginal dryness, and depression.

❑ St. John's wort is valuable if you suffer from anxiety or depression.

❑ Siberian ginseng aids in relieving depression and in the production of estrogen.

Caution: Do not use this herb if you have hypoglycemia, high blood pressure, or a heart disorder.

RECOMMENDATIONS

❑ Eat a diet consisting of 50 percent raw foods and take a protein supplement to help stabilize blood sugar. Add blackstrap molasses, broccoli, dandelion greens, kelp, salmon with bones, sardines, and white fish to your diet.

❑ Do not consume any animal products except for those recommended in this section. Avoid dairy products—limit your consumption to small amounts of low-fat yogurt or buttermilk. Dairy products and meat promote hot flashes. They also contribute to a loss of calcium from the bones.

❑ Avoid alcohol, caffeine, sugar, spicy foods, and hot soups and drinks; they can trigger hot flashes, aggravate urinary incontinence, and make mood swings worse. They also make the blood more acidic, which prompts the bones to release calcium to act as a buffering agent. This is an important factor in bone loss.

❑ Get regular moderate exercise.

❑ Avoid stress as much as possible.

❑ Substitute garlic or onion powder for salt when cooking. Consuming salt increases urinary excretion of calcium.

❑ Drink 2 quarts of quality water each day to help prevent drying of the skin and mucous membranes.

❑ For itching in the vaginal area, use vitamin E cream (with no fragrance added) or open a vitamin E capsule and apply the oil. Natureworks Marigold Ointment from Abkit stops itching almost immediately.

❑ If sexual intercourse is painful, try using vitamin E oil or aloe vera gel to lubricate the vagina.

CONSIDERATIONS

❑ If a woman has hypoglycemia, her symptoms often become more pronounced during menopause. Stress puts a burden on the adrenal glands, causing them to work harder than they should. The adrenals therefore produce smaller amounts of the hormones that are needed to help reduce the effects of declining estrogen in the body.

❑ Japanese women generally experience far fewer symptoms of menopause than do Western women. An article in the British medical journal *The Lancet* reported that the reason may be that Japanese women consume more phytoestrogens (plant estrogens). These estrogenlike compounds are found in foods such as soybeans, tofu, miso, flaxseeds, pomegranites, and dates. When these substances are eaten, they act like the estrogens produced in the body.

Hormones, Hormone Therapy, and Menopause

Menopause is something all women experience, and as it approaches, they are faced with the decision as to whether or not to opt for some sort of hormone therapy, whether it is hormone replacement therapy (HRT) with estrogen and progesterone, or estrogen replacement therapy (ERT) only. In order to make an informed decision, it is necessary first to understand something about different types of hormones.

Broadly speaking, there are two types of hormone products available: natural and synthetic. Natural hormones are hormones whose molecular structures most closely resemble those of the hormones made by the body. Some doctors argue that natural hormone replacement therapy is not regulated sufficiently. Because the hormones are considered natural, some say, they have not been exposed to the rigorous tests that the synthetic variety has had to undergo. Yet other physicians argue that synthetic hormones carry an additional risk to the health of some, if not all, women. There are no simple answers at present. Much more research into this controversial topic is needed.

ESTROGEN

Three estrogens are naturally made by the body: estradiol, estrone, and estriol. Estradiol is the dominant estrogen produced by the ovaries. Levels of estriol are highest during pregnancy, and this form of estrogen has been shown to have a protective effect against breast cancer. Estrone is formed from estradiol, and appears to be the estrogen responsible for estrogen-dependent breast cancer. Estradiol is available for replacement therapy. Alora, Climara, Estrace, Estraderm, Fempatch, and Vivelle are some of the brand names under which replacement estradiol is sold. Some are taken orally, others are absorbed from skin patches. Both estriol and estrone are also available for replacement therapy.

There are also synthetic versions of estrogen that may be prescribed. These are compounds that have estrogenlike effects in the body, but they are less similar, on a molecular level, to the body's own estrogens. Conjugated or esterified estrogen is manufactured from the purified urine of pregnant mares. Premarin is the synthetic estrogen most prescribed for HRT.

PROGESTERONE

Estrogen dominance is an important concept to understand if you are perimenopausal and/or thinking of hormone replacement. This is a situation that can occur if the correct balance between estrogen and progesterone is not maintained. Symptoms of estrogen dominance can include flagging energy, fluid retention and bloating, and weight gain. Estrogen dominance can also increase certain types of cancer, notably endometrial cancer. This is why, unless you have undergone hysterectomy, HRT regimens usually include both estrogen and progesterone. There are many natural progesterone creams that may be prescribed by your doctor. They are made from diosgenin, a naturally occurring substance contained in yams and fenugreek. That same chemical is used to produce a synthetic form of progesterone, called progestin. Progestins, then, are synthetic progesterones made from a natural source.

TESTOSTERONE

Testosterone is the essential hormone for continuing sexual desire in both sexes. It also supports the skin, muscles, and bones. If sexual desire diminishes, women may want to add this hormone to their replacement therapy. Natural testosterone or methyltestosterone is available for use as part of hormone therapy. There are also synthetic versions of testosterone, but these appear to cause problems more often than the natural hormones. Also, with synthetics, dosage must be carefully controlled, as too much can produce side effects.

TYPES OF REPLACEMENT THERAPY

There are two basic approaches to hormone therapy: ERT and HRT. ERT is suggested for women who have no uterus or ovaries. Estrogen is available in tablets, patches, vaginal creams, vaginal rings, and intervaginal gels. The vaginal creams, rings, or gels are for vaginal dryness or itchiness only, or for urinary problems. These hormones come in various doses. You must discuss the appropriate dose with your doctor.

HRT is normally prescribed for women who have a uterus and ovaries and are approaching, or have reached, menopause. Estrogen is taken every day and progesterone

---

❑ Gamma-oryzanol, a nutrient derived from rice bran, has been shown to be effective in treating symptoms of menopause. A daily dose of 20 milligrams reduced symptoms by 50 percent in 67 percent of the women studied.

❑ Smoking is associated with early menopause.

❑ Frequent sexual intercourse can help relieve vaginal dryness.

❑ Many physicians recommend hormone replacement therapy (HRT) to control severe symptoms caused by estrogen deficiency in menopausal and postmenopausal women. Although hormone therapy appears to be effective, it does have possible serious risks, which should be carefully considered. Be aware that research is ongoing in all aspects of replacement hormones—there is probably more conflicting information on this medical topic than there is is only taken for ten days out of every month to make sure the lining of the uterus is shed. This reduces the risk of developing endometrial cancer as a result of exposure to the stimulating estrogen. There are many different doses and different methods of taking these hormones. You and your doctor need to decide what is right for you.

In addition to ERT and HRT, there is combination estrogen and testosterone therapy. If tests indicate that levels of estrogen and testosterone are low, these hormones are available in combination formulas.

RISKS AND BENEFITS

As with any type of treatment, hormone therapy promises certain benefits but also poses certain risks. Some of the risks and benefits that have been most studied concern the following (it should be noted that most of the studies cited here were conducted with synthetic hormone replacements):

• *Aging.* Most research shows that HRT keeps the skin more supple and the sex organs better lubricated, with less atrophy (thinning of tissues).

• *Alzheimer's disease.* A study conducted between October 1995 and January 1999 and reported in *The Journal of the American Medical Association* indicates that estrogen, taken over the course of one year, does not slow the progression of the disease, nor does it improve the day-to-day ability of people with Alzheimer's disease. This study was conducted with people suffering from mild to moderate cases of the disease.

• *Breast cancer.* According to an article in the January 26, 2000, issue of the *Journal of the American Medical Association,* women who use or have used synthetic estrogen-progestin HRT *recently* (within the last four years), do have a higher risk of developing breast cancer. Estrogen treatment alone entailed less risk, but that finding was not straightforward. It appears that thinner women may well be at *greater* risk than heavier women on an estrogen-only regimen, although the study was not able to draw firm conclusions about heavy women. Heavier women seem to be at more risk from breast cancer anyway, even without any added risk from HRT. With all the conflicting information about breast cancer and hormone therapy, it makes sense to assume that there is indeed some increased risk, however small. The increase appears to be in the 1- to an 8-percent range, depending on all the risk factors added together, including family history of the disease.

• *Colorectal cancer.* Studies suggest that women taking HRT are better protected against colorectal cancer that

those who are not taking HRT. All women over forty should have regular colorectal examinations to test for cancer.

• *Heart disease.* There was a time when research appeared to show a decreased risk of heart disease in menopausal women taking replacement therapy. There is great doubt about this now. Much more research is needed before either argument is proved conclusively. Synthetic estrogens do not appear to have the same protective benefits as the estrogen produced by the body. Heart disease kills more women than all types of cancer put together, so it is important to take measures to protect yourself against heart disease whether you opt for hormone therapy or not. (*See* HEART ATTACK in Part Two.)

• *Hot flashes and mood swings.* Hormone therapy, whether ERT or HRT should eliminate hot flashes. It may also alleviate mood swings—although that depends on exactly what causes them.

• *Osteoporosis.* Estrogen replacement does appear to protect women from severe bone loss and osteoporosis. For osteoporosis prevention, experts recommend taking estrogen with about 1,000 milligrams of calcium a day. (*See* OSTEOPOROSIS in Part Two.)

MAKING THE DECISION

This decision to take—or not to take—hormone therapy is not an easy one for many women, and there are no easy answers. Everyone must weigh her own particular risk factors and decide whether the potential benefits outweigh those risks. You also need to decide whether to use synthetic or natural hormones, or approach any discomfort you may have with a more holistic approach that makes use of the nutrients and other remedies outlined elsewhere in this section.

There are also the questions of when to begin hormone therapy and how long to continue. Some doctors think that women should be introduced to HRT during perimenopause, but there are many others who think that this is unnecessary and, with the correct diet, stress management, and exercise, women do not need to opt for replacement therapy at this early stage unless there are profound reasons for doing so. Discuss this issue with your doctor. Also discuss how long you should continue taking HRT. The uncomfortable symptoms of menopause and perimenopause often last for only a short time, so you may not need to remain on the therapy for a prolonged period. On the other hand, if you are taking hormone therapy because of long-term concerns such as osteoporosis prevention, a different duration may be necessary.

about any other condition. It is essential to work with a good physician who can advise you about which of the vast array of products available may help you overcome any discomforts you may be experiencing. (*See* Hormones, Hormone Therapy, and Menopause, page 514.)

❑ Conventional treatment for a problematic perimenopause is to prescribe a low-dose contraceptive. However,

natural progesterone rather than estrogen may be the answer during this period, because symptoms are often a result of estrogen dominance (see the discussion of estrogen dominance in Hormones, Hormone Therapy and Menopause, page 514).

❑ After menopause, a reduction in the amount of the sex hormone estrogen can cause shrinkage of urethral and

Male Menopause

The term "male menopause" is often used in a joking way, sometimes as a dismissive substitute for "midlife crisis." But while men do not face the end of fertility in midlife as women do, they too undergo important physical and hormonal changes at that time. Men should not take male menopause—sometimes called andropause—lightly. During male menopause, sex drive may weaken, anxiety may increase, and depression and moodiness may accompany a sense of failure. These symptoms can occur because of falling levels of testosterone. Men's testosterone levels begin to decline by the age of forty—earlier in some cases—and this may cause a loss of sexual desire, mood swings, and irritability, and may even increase the risk of heart disease. If low testosterone levels are a problem, testosterone replacement therapy may be prescribed. Before a man makes a decision about testosterone replacement, he should undergo a prostate specific antigen (PSA) test to look for signs of prostate cancer, and he should have a frank discussion with his physician about potential side effects. It is advisable also to check DHEA and estrogen levels (estrogen is a male as well as a female hormone) so that if therapy is needed, it can be tailored to the individual's particular needs.

Many of the supplements mentioned in this section can help men also as they deal with some of the uncomfortable features of moving from one period of their lives to another.

---

vaginal membranes, promoting incontinence. There may be a continuous dribbling of urine. Urethral dilation helps stretch a contracted urethra.

❏ It may be more important to replace progesterone than estrogen. Natural progesterone cream is a good way to do this.

❏ Hypothyroidism is common in menopausal women. Many symptoms ascribed to menopause may be due to improper thyroid function. (*See* HYPOTHYROIDISM in Part Two.)

❏ Symptoms of perimenopause are often mistaken for those of premenstrual syndrome (PMS). Both PMS and perimenopausal symptoms are a result of an imbalance between estrogen and progesterone—specifically, rising estrogen and diminishing progesterone. If your menstrual cycles have changed—for example, if your periods are lasting for a longer or shorter time than they used to, or if they are irregular when they were not irregular before—it is more likely that you are perimenopausal rather than premenstrual. A blood test to determine your level of a hormone called follicle-stimulating hormone (FSH) is also helpful in determining whether you are experiencing perimenopause. FSH levels increase as estrogen diminishes.

❏ It is important for menopausal and postmenopausal women to take measures to protect themselves against heart disease. (*See* HEART ATTACK in Part Two.) Many women have been led to believe that taking estrogen protects against this disease, but there is very reasonable doubt about the protective benefits of synthetic estrogen against heart attacks. (*See* Hormones, Hormone Therapy, and Menopause on page 514.)

❏ *See also* HYPOGLYCEMIA and HYSTERECTOMY-RELATED PROBLEMS in Part Two.

Menstrual Cramps

See under PREMENSTRUAL SYNDROME.

Mercury Toxicity

Mercury is one of the most toxic metals—even more so than lead. This poison is found in our soil, water, and food supply, as well as in sewage sludge, fungicides, and pesticides. Some grains and seeds are treated with methyl mercury chlorine bleaches, which seep into the food supply. Because methyl mercury contaminates our waters, large amounts are found in fish, particularly larger ones that are farther up in the food chain. Mercury is also present in a wide variety of everyday products, including cosmetics, dental fillings, fabric softeners, batteries, industrial instruments, inks used by printers and tattooists, latex, some medications, some paints, plastics, polishes, solvents, and wood preservatives.

Mercury is a cumulative poison. There is no barrier that prohibits mercury from reaching the brain cells, and it is retained in the pain center of the brain and in the central nervous system. Its presence there can prevent both the normal entry of nutrients into the cells and the removal of wastes from the cells. It can bind to immune cells, distorting them and interfering with normal immune responses. This may be one factor behind autoimmune disorders. Mercury can cause permanent kidney, cardiac, and respiratory problems. Significant amounts of mercury in the body can produce arthritis, depression, dermatitis, dizziness, fatigue, gum disease, nausea, vomiting, hair loss, insomnia, headaches, joint pain, slurred speech, memory loss, diarrhea, muscle weakness, and excessive salivation. High levels can also interfere with enzyme activity, resulting in blindness and paralysis. The symptoms of mercury poisoning can mimic those of multiple sclerosis and amyotrophic lateral sclerosis (ALS, also known as Lou Gehrig's disease). Many food and environmental allergies may be directly attributable to mercury poisoning. The U.S. Environmental Protection Agency has linked exposure to mercury vapor to menstrual disorders and spontaneous abortion (miscarriage) as well. Mercury exposure in pregnant women can cause neurological damage, such as lowered intelligence and delayed development in infants. In addition, the mortality rate for infants is significantly increased when mothers are exposed to mercury. Children who have severe mercury poisoning can experience acrodynia, a syndrome characterized by peeling and pinkness of the skin on the hands, nose, and feet; blindness; increased heart rate; agitation; and pain in the arms and legs.

Signs that indicate the presence of toxic mercury levels include behavioral changes, depression, confusion, irritability, and hyperactivity. People with this toxicity may also experience allergic reactions or asthma. They may complain about a metallic taste in the mouth, and their teeth may loosen. These symptoms can occur within a few minutes, or they can take as long as thirty minutes to appear.

According to the World Health Organization, amalgam dental fillings are a prime source of mercury exposure. More than 180 million Americans have mercury amalgam dental fillings. When dentists refer to "silver" fillings, they are usually referring to amalgams, which are silver in color but actually contain approximately 50 percent mercury, 25 percent silver, and 25 percent other materials, such as copper, tin, and nickel. While all the metals used in fillings can be toxic, none is as harmful as the mercury. One amalgam filling can release 3 to 17 micrograms of mercury each day. The mercury vapor released from dental amalgams combines with chemicals in the mouth to create minute amounts of toxic methyl mercury, which is absorbed through the tissues of the mouth and air passages and transported in the blood to the brain and other body tissues. Many people have suffered for years from various health problems—including candidiasis, muscle spasms, chronic fatigue, and recurring infections—that cleared up after they had their amalgam dental fillings removed.

Unless otherwise specified, the dosages recommended here are for adults. For a child between the ages of twelve and seventeen, reduce the dose to three-quarters of the recommended amount. For a child between six and twelve, use one-half of the recommended dose, and for a child under the age of six, use one-quarter of the recommended amount.

NUTRIENTS

SUPPLEMENT	SUGGESTED DOSAGE	COMMENTS
Essential		
Glutathione plus L-methionine and L-cysteine	As directed on label, on an empty stomach. Take with water or juice. Do not take with milk. Take with 50 mg vitamin B$_6$ and 100 mg vitamin C for better absorption.	Needed for sulfur. Also helps to detoxify harmful metals and toxins. (*See* AMINO ACIDS in Part One.)
Selenium	200 mcg daily, in divided doses. If you are pregnant, do not exceed 40 mcg daily.	Neutralizes the effects of mercury.
Vitamin E	400–800 IU daily.	Works with selenium to neutralize mercury. Use d-alpha-tocopherol form.
Very Important		
Apple pectin	As directed on label.	Aids in removing toxic metals from the body.
Garlic (Kyolic from Wakunaga)	2 capsules 3 times daily.	Acts as a detoxifier.
Kelp or alfalfa	1,000–1,500 mg daily.	Aids the body in removing toxins. See under Herbs, below.
Vitamin A plus carotenoid complex with beta-carotene	25,000 IU daily. If you are pregnant, do not exceed 10,000 IU daily. 15,000 IU daily.	A powerful antioxidant; destroys free radicals. Powerful free radical scavengers.
Vitamin C with bioflavonoids	4,000–10,000 mg daily.	Helps remove metals and strengthens the immune system.
Important		
Vitamin B complex	100 mg of each major B vitamin twice daily (amounts of individual vitamins in a complex will vary).	Important for the functioning and protection of the brain.
Helpful		
Brewer's yeast	As directed on label.	A good source of B vitamins.
Hydrochloric acid (HCl)	As directed on label.	To aid digestion. Take this supplement if you are over 40 and deficient in HCl (*see* INDIGESTION in Part Two).
Lecithin granules or capsules	1 tbsp 3 times daily, before meals. 1,200 mg 3 times daily, before meals.	Protects brain cells from mercury poisoning.

HERBS

❑ Alfalfa contains valuable nutrients and helps the body to eliminate toxins.

RECOMMENDATIONS

❑ Eat organically grown foods, especially beans, onions, and garlic, for added sulfur, which helps protect the body against toxic substances.

❑ Drink water only if it is steam-distilled. Drink plenty of pure fresh fruit and vegetable juices.

❑ Supplement your diet with plenty of fiber (oat bran is a good source) and pectin (found in apples).

Note: Always take supplemental fiber separately from other supplements and medications.

❑ Eat fish in moderation, and always broil it; do not baste it in its juices. While some fish may contain mercury, fish also contains compounds called alkylglycerols, which help to remove mercury from the body. If there is mercury in the fish, it is primarily stored in the fat. By broiling the fish and draining the juices, you will get rid of much of the fat and retain the beneficial alkylglycerols.

❑ If you suspect mercury toxicity, have a hair analysis performed. This can detect toxic levels of mercury. Mercury does not show up in urine or blood samples. (*See* HAIR ANALYSIS in Part Three.)

❑ Do not rush to have amalgam dental fillings removed until you have tests done that show elevated levels of mercury. Removal of the fillings should be tried only after other measures, such as the program outlined in this section, have been tried.

CONSIDERATIONS

❑ Chelation therapy removes toxic metals from the body. (*See* CHELATION THERAPY in Part Three.)

❑ Hal A. Huggins, D.D.S., has done extensive research on the toxic effects of mercury from dental amalgams. He has found links between mercury toxicity and many debilitating and degenerative diseases, including multiple sclerosis, Alzheimer's disease, Parkinson's disease, arthritis, and lupus. Dr. Huggins has written an informative book describing the dangers of dental amalgams called *It's All in Your Head* (Avery Publishing Group, 1993).

❑ In response to concern about the health hazards of mercury amalgam fillings, the Swedish government has taken steps to ban their use.

❑ High mercury levels have been linked to candidiasis. (*See* CANDIDIASIS in Part Two.)

❑ The U.S. Consumer Product Safety Commission (CPSC) has issued a warning to consumers to inform them of the dangers of inhaling mercury vapors. Certain ethnic and religious customs involve using a product called *azogue*, which in reality is metallic mercury. This product is sold in herb shops, or *botanicas*. Azogue is sprinkled throughout the home for religious purposes. The CDC suggests *immediate* removal of the mercury if it has been sprinkled in the home, but removal must be done in the proper way to avoid making the danger worse. Call your local health department for information on the correct procedure for mercury removal.

❑ *See also* CHEMICAL ALLERGIES and ENVIRONMENTAL TOXICITY in Part Two.

Migraine

Migraines are severe, throbbing headaches that may or may not be accompanied by nausea, visual disturbances, and other symptoms. An estimated 28 million people in the United States suffer from migraine headaches. Many more women than men suffer from this condition. Migraines are one of the most severe types of headache.

Traditional research has described migraines as vascular headaches involving excessive dilation or contraction of the brain's blood vessels. More recent current research gives other clues. Single photon emission computerized tomography (SPECT) scanning indicates that the inflammation involved in migraines is most noticeable in the meninges. These are three membranes—the dura, the arachnoid, and the very inner layer of membrane separated from the other two by cerebrospinal fluid, called the pia—that surround the brain and spinal cord. However, it is not the inflammation that leads to the pain, but rather abnormal nerve activity. Stimulation of the trigeminal nerve, which goes from the brain to the head and face, appears to trigger the release of substances known as calcitonin gene-related peptides (CGRP), which both induce inflammation and send messages to pain receptors in the meninges. Some researchers liken migraines in many ways to meningitis, another condition affecting the meninges, noting that with meningitis, the symptoms are very similar—headache, nausea, and sensitivity to light. Meningitis, however, is caused by viral or bacterial infection, while much more research needs to be conducted before the underlying cause of migraines is known.

Migraines may occur anywhere from once a week to once or twice a year, and they often run in families. One factor behind the higher incidence of migraine in women may be fluctuations in the level of the hormone estrogen; women typically get migraines around the time of menstruation, when estrogen levels are low. Migraines occur most often in people between the ages of twenty and thirty-five, and tend to decline with age. However, children too can suffer from migraines. In children, migraine pain tends to be more diffuse, rather than localized. Migraine can first show up in childhood not as headaches, but as colic, periodic abdominal pains, vomiting, dizziness, and severe motion sickness. There are usually five phases in a migraine:

1. A day before the onset of a headache, there may be detectable changes in mood, problems with memory, an alteration in one or all of the five senses, or speech problems.

2. Just before the headache begins, some people see flashes or patterns of light and/or experience numbness of the hands or mouth. This is called an aura, much like auras

that affect many people with epilepsy before a seizure. A migraine preceded by an aura is called a *classic migraine*. Migraines without auras are called *common migraines*.

3. The headache starts, with severe, throbbing pain. It may occur on one side or on both sides of the head. The pain can also move from side to side. Nausea may set in, along with tenderness in the neck and scalp. The eyes may be very sensitive to light, and the person may be almost immobilized by the pain.

4. The headache dissipates. Nausea may linger, however.

5. The person may feel tired and lethargic and may simply want to sleep.

Any number of things can trigger a migraine in a susceptible individual, including allergies, constipation, stress, liver malfunction, too much or too little sleep, emotional changes, hormonal changes, sun glare, flashing lights, lack of exercise, and changes in barometric pressure. Dental problems may also be a factor. Low blood sugar is frequently associated with migraine; studies have shown that blood sugar levels are low during a migraine attack, and the lower the blood sugar level, the more severe the headache.

Unless otherwise specified, the dosages recommended here are for adults. For a child between the ages of twelve and seventeen, reduce the dose to three-quarters the recommended amount. If a child under twelve experiences severe headache pain, especially if it is accompanied by nausea or visual disturbances, contact a physician promptly. (*See* MENINGITIS in Part Two.)

NUTRIENTS

SUPPLEMENT	SUGGESTED DOSAGE	COMMENTS
Very Important		
Calcium and magnesium	2,000 mg daily. 1,000 mg daily.	Minerals that help to regulate muscular tone and to transmit nerve impulses throughout the body and to the brain. Use chelate forms.
Coenzyme Q10 plus Coenzyme A from Coenzyme-A Technologies	60 mg daily. As directed on label.	Increases blood flow to the brain and improves circulation. Works with coenzyme Q10.
Dimethylglycine (DMG) (Aangamik DMG from FoodScience of Vermont) and trimethylglycine (TMG)	125 mg twice daily. As directed on label.	Improve brain oxygenation.
DL-Phenylalanine (DLPA)	As directed on label.	Taken with care, and after consulting a physician, DLPA can relieve pain and elevate mood.
Essential fatty acid complex or primrose oil	As directed on label. As directed on label.	Needed for brain cells and for fat metabolism. An anti-inflammatory agent to keep the blood vessels from constricting.
5-Hydroxytryptophan (5-HTP)	As directed on label.	Increases the body's production of serotonin, a neurotransmitter involved in blood-vessel regulation.
Multivitamin and mineral formula	As directed on label.	All nutrients are necessary in balance.
Rutin	200 mg daily.	Removes toxic metals, which may cause migraines.
Vitamin B complex plus extra vitamin B2 (riboflavin) and vitamin B3 (niacin) and niacinamide and pantothenic acid (vitamin B5) or royal jelly and vitamin B6 (pyridoxine)	As directed on label. 400 mg daily. 200 mg 3 times daily. Do not exceed this amount. 800 mg daily. 100 mg twice daily. 1 tsp twice daily. As directed on label.	Needed for a healthy nervous system. Use a hypoallergenic form. Injections (under a doctor's supervision) may be necessary. Necessary for cell respiration and growth. Increase blood flow to the brain. *Caution:* Do not take niacin if you have a liver disorder, gout, or high blood pressure. Needed by the adrenal glands when the body is under stress. Royal jelly is high in pantothenic acid. Use royal jelly from a natural source. Required for normal brain function. Use a hypoallergenic form.
Helpful		
Garlic (Kyolic from Wakunaga)	2 capsules 3 times daily, with meals.	A potent detoxifier.
Quercetin and bromelain or Activated Quercetin from Source Naturals	500 mg daily, before meals. As directed on label.	Helps control food allergies. Needed for a variety of enzyme functions. Contains quercetin plus bromelain and vitamin C to aid absorption.
Taurine Plus from American Biologics	10–20 drops daily.	An important antioxidant and immune regulator, needed for white blood cell activation and neurological function. Use the sublingual form.
Vitamin C with bioflavonoids	3,000–6,000 mg daily.	Aids in producing anti-stress adrenal hormones and enhances immunity. A buffered or esterified form is best.

HERBS

❑ Bio-Rizin from American Biologics contains liquid licorice extract, which improves energy levels and helps to relieve allergy symptoms that can trigger migraines.

Caution: Do not use this herb on a daily basis for more than seven days in a row. Avoid it completely if you have high blood pressure.

Distinguishing Migraine Headaches

Just because a headache is very painful, that does not mean it is a migraine. Migraines have certain distinct characteristics that set them apart from other types of headaches. The following table will help you to determine whether you have a true migraine or one of the two types most commonly confused with migraine—a tension or cluster headache.

Characteristic	Migraine	Tension Headache	Cluster Headache
Site of pain	One or both sides of the head.	Both sides of the head.	One side of the head.
Duration of pain	4 to 72 hours.	2 hours to days.	30 to 90 minutes per episode, but episodes can recur multiple times daily.
Severity of pain	Usually severe, but may be mild.	Mild or moderate.	Very severe.
Accompanied by nausea, sensitivity to light, sound or smells	Common.	No.	No.
Accompanied by red or watery eyes or runny nose	Sometimes.	No.	No.

❑ Cordyceps is a Chinese herb that may, through its ability to reduce anxiety and stress and promote sound sleep, help people who suffer from migraines.

❑ Feverfew helps to alleviate pain.
Caution: Do not use feverfew during pregnancy.

❑ Ginkgo biloba extract enhances cerebral circulation.

❑ Other herbs effective for the treatment of migraines include cayenne (capsicum), chamomile, ginger, peppermint, rosemary, valerian, willow bark, and wormwood.
Caution: Do not use wormwood during pregnancy. It is not recommended for long-term use.

RECOMMENDATIONS

❑ Adopt a diet that is low in simple carbohydrates and high in protein. *See* HYPOGLYCEMIA in Part Two and follow the dietary guidelines.

❑ Include almonds, almond milk, watercress, parsley, fennel, garlic, cherries, and fresh pineapple in the diet.

❑ Omit from the diet foods that contain the amino acid tyramine, including aged meats, avocados, bananas, beer, cabbage, canned fish, dairy products, eggplant, hard cheeses, potatoes, raspberries, red plums, tomatoes, wine, and yeast. Also avoid alcoholic beverages, aspirin, chocolate, monosodium glutamate (MSG), and nitrites (preservatives found in hot dogs and luncheon meats). Through the process of elimination, try to see if you have a particular allergy to some, or all, of these foods.

❑ Get regular moderate exercise.

❑ Massage your neck and back of your head daily.

❑ Avoid salt and acid-forming foods such as meat, cereal, bread, and grains. Also avoid fried foods and fatty and greasy foods.

❑ Eat small meals, and eat small, nutritious snacks between meals if needed, to help stabilize wide swings in blood sugar that may precipitate a migraine. Especially avoid missing meals.

❑ Take only hypoallergenic supplements.

❑ See your dentist for treatment of any tooth problems, such as gum disease, tooth decay, bacterial infection, temporomandibular joint syndrome (TMJ), or tooth-grinding, that may be contributing to the problem.

❑ Do not smoke, and avoid secondhand smoke.

❑ Avoid loud noises, strong odors, and high altitudes.

❑ Call a doctor if you have a headache that is triggered by, accompanied by, or linked to, any of the following:

• Exertion (including sexual exertion), bending, or coughing.

• Stiff neck and fever.

• Head injury.

• Vomiting.

• Slurred speech, distorted vision, or numbness or tingling in part of the body.

These can be signs of more serious disorders.

CONSIDERATIONS

❏ Researchers believe many migraine attacks are caused by chemical imbalances in the brain. Levels of the brain chemical serotonin drop during a headache. This triggers an impulse along the trigeminal nerve to blood vessels in the meninges, the brain's outer covering. In the meninges, the blood vessels become inflamed and swollen. The result is a headache.

❏ Migraine headaches in women may result from hormonal changes during the menstrual cycle. After menopause, the headaches usually decrease.

❏ Women who suffer from migraines may benefit from the use of natural progesterone cream.

❏ A study reported in the British medical journal *The Lancet* found that when allergenic foods were eliminated from the diets of migraine sufferers, as many as 93 percent of them found relief. (*See* ALLERGIES in Part Two.)

❏ Caffeine has been found to be a very safe and effective method for increasing pain relief. Caffeine taken with over-the-counter pain relievers has been shown to reduce headache pain by up to 40 percent.

❏ Researchers in France have identified a gene linked to a rare, severe type of migraine called *familial hemiplegic migraine*.

❏ Music has a calming effect and can help to relieve migraines. (*See* MUSIC AND SOUND THERAPY in Part Three.)

❏ Some find migraine relief by taking lecithin (a soybean derivative). In one study, those who took between three and six 1,200-milligram capsules when they felt a headache coming on had fewer, milder migraine attacks.

❏ Acupuncture and acupressure have helped many people control the pain of migraines.

❏ A study on the herb feverfew conducted at the University of Nottingham in England found that participants who took the herb got an average of 24 percent fewer migraines than those who did not, and they also found that vomiting was reduced, with no side effects.

❏ The drug sumatriptan (Imitrex) relieves acute migraine attacks by increasing the amount of serotonin in the brain. In clinical studies, 82 percent of people with migraines who took sumatriptan improved within two hours of treatment. This drug may be administered by injection, orally, or as a nasal spray. It can be effective, but it can also cause side effects, including dizziness, drowsiness, anxiety, and malaise. Naratriptan (Amerge), rizatriptan (Maxalt), and zolmitriptan (Zomig) are drugs that are similar to sumatriptan. Dihydroergotamine (DHE or Migranal) is a different type of migraine drug available in spray form. Midrin, a combination drug, and nonsteroidal anti-inflammatory drugs (NSAIDs) are also prescribed for migraine. These drugs are not appropriate for everyone. Because they have the potential to cause coronary artery constriction, they should not be taken by people with ischemic heart disease (angina or a history of heart attack). Treatment with sumatriptan may result in a rise in blood pressure, so people with uncontrolled hypertension should not use it. You should always discuss potential side effects of any prescription medication with your physician.

❏ Antidepressants are sometimes prescribed for people who get migraines. These include amitriptyline (Elavil, Endep) and nortriptyline. They are used as a preventive rather than as therapy for an acute attack. Other medications sometimes used as preventives include diazepam (Valium), methysergide (Sansert), and propranolol (Inderal).

❏ For names and addresses of organizations that offer information about how to deal with headaches, see HEALTH AND MEDICAL ORGANIZATIONS in the Appendix.

❏ *See also* HEADACHE in Part Two and PAIN CONTROL in Part Three.

Miscarriage

See under PREGNANCY-RELATED PROBLEMS.

Mononucleosis

Mononucleosis ("mono") is an infectious viral disease. The vast majority of cases (85 percent) are caused by the Epstein-Barr virus (EBV). More rarely, it may be caused by cytomegalovirus (CMV). Both of these viruses are members of the herpes family. Once the virus enters the body, it multiplies in lymphocytes (white blood cells). Mono affects the respiratory system, the lymphatic tissues, and glands in the neck, groin, armpits, bronchial tubes, spleen, and liver. Symptoms include depression, extreme fatigue, fever, generalized aching, headache, jaundice, loss of appetite, sore throat, pain on the upper left side of the abdomen, puffy eyelids, swollen glands, and, sometimes, a bumpy red rash. The spleen may become enlarged, and liver function may be affected. Meningitis, encephalitis (inflammation of the brain), or rupturing of the spleen are very rare complications that can develop from mono.

The viruses that cause mono are contagious and can be transmitted from person to person by close contact such as kissing (mono is often referred to as the "kissing disease") or by sharing food or utensils, although they can also spread during sexual contact or through the air like the common cold. The incubation period is about ten days in children and thirty to fifty days in adults. Many of the cases occur in the military and in colleges, where living conditions are crowded and sleeping patterns are inadequate. High school students also have a high incidence of this disease. Mono is most common among children and adolescents. Nearly 90 percent of people over age thirty-five have mono antibodies in their blood, indicating that they had the disease at some point in their lives—although many do not even know they had it.

Because the symptoms are often so similar to those of influenza, mononucleosis is often mistaken for it. However, with mono, the symptoms tend to be more persistent. The acute symptoms usually last from two to four weeks, and fatigue can persist for three to eight weeks after the other symptoms disappear. In some individuals, the disease lingers for a year or more, producing recurring, but successively milder, attacks. If the immune system is weakened due to an organ transplant, HIV/AIDS, or other viruses, the mononucleosis symptoms can be serious and chronic.

A diagnosis of mono is made through a blood test called a mononucleosis spot test. This reveals the presence of specific viral antibodies and confirms the presence of mono. A liver function test may aid in diagnosis.

Unless otherwise specified, the dosages recommended here are for adults. For a child between the ages of twelve and seventeen, reduce the dose to three-quarters of the recommended amount. For a child between six and twelve, use one-half of the recommended dose, and for a child under the age of six, use one-quarter of the recommended amount.

NUTRIENTS

SUPPLEMENT	SUGGESTED DOSAGE	COMMENTS
Very Important		
Acidophilus (Kyo-Dophilus from Wakunaga and Bio-Dophilus from American Biologics are good sources)	As directed on label.	"Friendly" bacteria are important. Use a nondairy formula.
Proteolytic enzymes	As directed on label 3–4 times daily, between meals and at bedtime, on an empty stomach.	Reduces inflammation and aids in absorption of nutrients.
Vitamin A with mixed carotenoids and vitamin E	25,000 IU daily for 2 weeks, then slowly reduce to 15,000 IU daily. If you are pregnant, do not exceed 10,000 IU daily. 400–800 IU daily for 4 weeks, then slowly reduce to 400 IU daily.	Essential for the immune system. Use emulsion forms for easier assimilation and greater safety at high doses. Use d-alpha-tocopherol form.
Vitamin C with bioflavonoids	5,000–10,000 mg daily, in divided doses.	Destroys the virus and boosts the immune system. A buffered or esterified form is best.
Important		
Dimethylglycine (DMG) (Aangamik DMG from FoodScience of Vermont)	125 mg twice daily.	An immune stimulant that enhances oxygenation.
Free-form amino acid complex	1/4 tsp 2–3 times daily, on an empty stomach.	To provide protein, necessary for healing and to rebuild tissues. Use a powdered form.
Garlic (Kyolic from Wakunaga)	2 capsules 3 times daily, with meals.	A powerful immune booster. Acts as a natural antibiotic.
Vitamin B complex plus extra vitamin B₁₂	100 mg of each major B vitamin 3 times daily, with meals (amounts of individual vitamins in a complex will vary). 2,000 mcg twice daily.	B vitamins increase energy and are needed for every bodily function, including proper digestion and brain function. Use a high-stress, hypoallergenic formula. A sublingual form is recommended. Injections (under a doctor's supervision) may be necessary. Required for proper digestion and to prevent anemia. Use a lozenge or sublingual form.
Zinc lozenges	As directed on label.	A powerful antioxidant that helps fight free radicals.
Helpful		
Maitake extract or reishi extract or shiitake extract	As directed on label. As directed on label. As directed on label.	Mushroom extracts with immune-boosting and antiviral properties.
Multivitamin and mineral complex with calcium and magnesium and potassium	1,000 mg daily. 75–1,000 mg daily. 99 mg daily.	All nutrients are necessary for normal cellular function and repair. Use a high-potency formula.
Raw thymus glandular plus multiglandular complex (Multi-Glandular from American Biologics)	500 mg 3 times daily. As directed on label.	To enhance immune response. (*See* GLANDULAR THERAPY in Part Three.)

The vitamin B complex subscripts: plus extra vitamin B_{12}.

HERBS

❏ Astragalus and echinacea boost the immune system.

❏ Cat's claw has immune-enhancing properties and acts against viral infection.

❏ Dandelion and milk thistle protect the liver.

❏ Goldenseal fights infection. If a sore throat is present, place a dropperful of alcohol-free goldenseal extract in the mouth and hold it there for a few seconds, then swallow. Do this every four hours for three to five days.

Caution: Do not take goldenseal internally on a daily basis for more than one week at a time, do not use it during pregnancy, and use it with caution if you are allergic to ragweed.

❏ Olive leaf extract appears to help inhibit the growth of viruses that cause diseases such as mononucleosis.

❏ Pau d'arco balances the bacteria in the colon.

❏ Spirulina contains phytonutrients that appear to boost the immune system.

RECOMMENDATIONS

❏ Eat a diet composed of at least 50 percent raw foods.

Consume as much of your food raw as possible. Also emphasize wholesome soups, root vegetables, and whole grains, including brown rice.

❏ Each day, drink eight 8-ounce glasses of distilled water, plus fresh juice.

❏ Do not consume any coffee, fried foods, processed foods, soft drinks, stimulants, sugar, tea, or white flour products. These depress immune function.

❏ Eat four to six small meals daily. Avoid overeating at any one meal.

❏ Get plenty of rest. Round-the-clock bed rest is a good idea during the acute phase of the disorder.

❏ Gargle with a glass of warm salt water to relieve sore throat. Add ½ teaspoon of salt to a glass of warm water and gargle several times a day.

❏ Use a protein supplement from a vegetable source. Spirutein from Nature's Plus is a good protein drink for between meals.

❏ Use chlorophyll in tablet form, or in a liquid form such as "green drinks" made from leafy green vegetables or wheatgrass. Kyo-Green from Wakunaga is a highly concentrated natural barley and wheatgrass source of amino acids, vitamins, minerals, carotene, chlorophyll, and enzymes. It is also available in powder form containing chlorella, kelp, and brown rice.

❏ Do not strain when having a bowel movement, as this may injure an enlarged spleen.

❏ Do not give aspirin to a child or adolescent with mononucleosis, as it may lead to complications such as Reye's syndrome. (See REYE'S SYNDROME in Part Two.)

❏ Avoid close physical contact with others as much as possible. Flush all tissues after use, and do not share food, eating utensils, or towels. Wash your hands frequently.

❏ Avoid strenuous exercise and competitive sports until you are completely recovered.

❏ If you have a fever over 102°F, or if you develop severe pain in the upper left abdomen that lasts for five minutes or more, or if breathing and/or swallowing becomes difficult as a result of throat inflammation, consult your health care provider promptly. These can be signs that a more serious condition is developing.

CONSIDERATIONS

❏ Once contracted, both EBV and CMV remain in the body for life, but the acute illness eventually runs its course in nearly all cases. Because there is no cure for mononucleosis, a proper diet and supplements, plus adequate rest, are especially important for this disorder.

❏ Antibiotics are of no use unless there is a secondary infection such as ear infection or strep throat. However, in approximately 20 percent of cases, strep throat is also present, and antibiotic therapy may be prescribed. The antibiotic ampicillin (Omnipen, Polycillin) should be *avoided,* as this drug often causes skin rashes and intensifies the complications associated with mononucleosis.

❏ Adequate rest, exercise, and nutrition are essential for the maintenance of general health and the prevention of mononucleosis.

❏ Protein is needed to stimulate the formation of antibodies that protect against complications such as hepatitis and jaundice.

❏ *See also* CHRONIC FATIGUE SYNDROME in Part Two.

Morning Sickness

See under PREGNANCY-RELATED PROBLEMS.

Motion Sickness

Motion sickness occurs when motion causes the eyes, the sensory nerves, and the vestibular apparatus of the ear to send conflicting signals to the brain, causing a loss of equilibrium or a sense of vertigo. It usually is experienced in a car, airplane, train, boat, elevator, or swing. Anxiety, genetics, overeating, poor ventilation, and traveling immediately after eating are common contributing factors. A susceptibility to things such as offensive odors, sights, or sounds can often precede an attack of motion sickness. Women are affected by this condition more frequently than men are. Elderly people and children under the age of two usually are not affected.

People suffering from motion sickness experience symptoms that range from severe headache to queasiness to nausea and vomiting while flying, sailing, or traveling in automobiles or trains. Other symptoms of motion sickness include cold sweats, dizziness, excessive salivation and/or yawning, fatigue, loss of appetite, pallor, severe distress, sleepiness, weakness, and, occasionally, breathing difficulties that can make you feel as though you are suffocating. If severe, an attack can make you completely uncoordinated, and sometimes injury can occur from loss of balance. Once the stimulus is removed, the motion sickness usually goes away; however, it can persist for hours or days. If you suffer from motion sickness for a prolonged amount of time, you may experience depression, dehydration, or low blood pressure. It can also worsen any other illness you may already have.

Natural remedies have been used with great success for motion sickness. Prevention is the key; motion sickness is far easier to prevent than it is to cure. Once excessive salivation and nausea set in, it is often too late to do anything but wait for the trip to be over so recovery can begin.

Unless otherwise specified, the dosages recommended here are for adults. For a child between the ages of twelve and seventeen, reduce the dose to three-quarters of the recommended amount. For a child between six and twelve, use one-half of the recommended dose, and for a child under the age of six, use one-quarter of the recommended amount.

NUTRIENTS

SUPPLEMENT	SUGGESTED DOSAGE	COMMENTS
Important		
Charcoal tablets	5 tablets 1 hour before travel. Take separately from other medications and supplements.	A detoxifier.
Magnesium	500 mg 1 hour before trip.	Acts as a nerve tonic.
Vitamin B₆ (pyridoxine)	100 mg 1 hour before trip, then 100 mg 2 hours later.	Relieves nausea.

HERBS

❑ Black horehound can reduce nausea.

❑ Butcher's broom, kudzu, and motherwort help to relieve vertigo.

❑ Ginger is an excellent treatment and preventive for nausea and upset stomach. Studies have shown that it may be more effective than dimenhydrinate (Dramamine) without the side effects. Take 2 ginger capsules (approximately 1,000 milligrams) every three hours, starting one hour before the beginning of the trip.

❑ Peppermint tea soothes and calms the stomach. A drop of peppermint oil on the tongue provides excellent relief from nausea and motion sickness. Peppermint can also be taken in lozenge form.

RECOMMENDATIONS

❑ When traveling, take whole-grain crackers with you on trips. Olives can help ward off nausea because they have the effect of decreasing salivation.

❑ Try sipping green or ginger tea during long trips. Sucking on a fresh lemon may also calm the stomach.

❑ Pay special attention to your diet. If a certain dish disagrees with you at home, it will most certainly disagree with you on the road.

❑ Do not eat spicy, salty, sugary, heavy, or fatty foods, especially fried foods, before or during travel. Also avoid dairy products and processed and junk foods. These can contribute to nausea or cause digestive imbalances.

❑ Also avoid large meals when traveling. Instead, eat smaller, more frequent meals so that your stomach is never empty.

❑ Avoid alcohol. Alcohol disrupts the delicate operations that occur in the inner ear. If you are prone to motion sickness, alcohol consumption will only aggravate the problem by further disrupting communication between the eyes, the inner ears, and the brain.

❑ Avoid odors and aromas that can bring about nausea. Aside from obvious things such as smoke and engine exhaust, certain food odors can make you ill, as can paint fumes, nail polish, or animal waste. Even otherwise pleasant smells, such as those from perfume or after-shave, can cause a problem if you are prone to motion sickness.

❑ Sit still and breathe deeply. Your brain is already thoroughly confused without extra motion on your part. Especially try to keep your head still. Rest in a reclined position in an area where there is the least amount of motion (in the center of a ship or in the wing area of an airplane). Focus your eyes on a distant object and try not to allow your eyes to drift to either side. Or close your eyes and take deep breaths. If possible, lie down in a dark place with a cool, damp cloth over your eyes.

❑ Stay cool, if possible. Fresh air can assist in battling motion sickness. If in a car, roll down a window. If on a ship, standing on deck and taking in the sea breezes may help. In an airplane, open the overhead vent.

❑ When you begin to feel sick, rub or press on your wrist, about three fingers' width down from the line that separates the hand from the arm. Massaging this acupressure point often stops motion sickness.

❑ Do not read while traveling.

❑ Limit or eliminate visual input. This will cut down on the conflicting information assaulting the brain. Traveling at night helps many people, simply because visual acuity is diminished, so that they do not perceive motion to the same degree as during the day.

CONSIDERATIONS

❑ Symptoms of nausea may indicate that the liver needs attention.

❑ A homeopathic liver remedy may help reduce nausea.

❑ Chewable papaya tablets can be helpful.

❑ There are numerous over-the-counter products available that may help to prevent motion sickness, including cyclizine (Marezine), dimenhydrinate (Dramamine), and meclizine (Antivert, Bonine). These drugs are not always effective, however, and can cause side effects, especially drowsiness. Motion sickness medication should not be taken with alcohol, sleep aids, or any type of tranquilizers. It is important to use extreme caution and carefully follow the dosage instructions for children.

❑ If motion sickness is debilitating, and herbal, homeopathic, and over-the-counter medications do not bring relief, a physician can prescribe scopolamine (which is a component of the herb belladonna) to be applied in a patch (Transderm-Scop) that delivers the drug through the skin for up to three days. Possible side effects of scopolamine include dry mouth, drowsiness, blurred vision, and a dilated pupil on the side the patch is worn. This drug should not be used by anyone with glaucoma, as it raises pressure within the eye. If you are pregnant or nursing, talk to your doctor before using scopolamine. It is not recommended for use by children.

❑ To a certain extent, motion sickness is psychological. In many cases, it can be prevented if you consciously tell yourself that you *will not* get sick. If you travel frequently and are prone to motion sickness, you may benefit from psychotherapy or counseling.

Mouth and Gum Disease

See HALITOSIS; PERIODONTAL DISEASE. *See also* Bleeding Gums *under* PREGNANCY-RELATED PROBLEMS.

Multiple Sclerosis

Multiple sclerosis (MS) is a progressive, degenerative disorder of the central nervous system, including the brain, the optic nerve, and the spinal cord. It is characterized by many areas of inflammation and scarring of the myelin sheaths in the brain and spinal cord. These are wrappings, composed of a fatty substance, that insulate the nerve fibers throughout the body. *Sclerosis* means hardening of tissue; *multiple* simply indicates many regions of tissue hardening. It seems that the body's immune system malfunctions and produces antibodies that attack the myelin sheaths. Consequently, the sheaths are damaged, and the damaged areas develop scarring that leads to either distorted communication or lack of communication between the nerve endings. This may produce a multiplicity of symptoms, from slurred speech to vision problems to loss of mobility.

Some 350,000 people in the United States have multiple sclerosis. Symptoms vary from individual to individual, depending on which portion or portions of the nervous system are most affected. In the earlier stages, the primary symptoms may include episodes of dizziness; extreme fatigue; eye problems such as blurred or double vision; a feeling of tingling and/or numbness, especially in the hands and feet; loss of balance and/or coordination; muscular stiffness; slurred speech; tremors; or bowel and bladder dysfunction. Secondary symptoms, which are problems that arise because of the primary symptoms rather than because of the underlying illness itself, may include bone loss, muscle wasting, paralysis, sexual dysfunction, urinary tract infections, and weak respiration. Many of these secondary conditions occur as a result of decreased mobility if the disease progresses.

The disease typically follows a pattern of periodic flare-ups, called *exacerbations,* followed by periods in which symptoms diminish or even disappear called *remissions.* MS is variable in its rate of progression. It can be relatively benign, with only a few minor attacks spread over decades, or it can be rapidly and completely disabling. Most commonly, it progresses slowly, disappearing for periods of time but returning intermittently, often in progressively more severe attacks.

The underlying cause of MS is not known, but it is widely believed to be an autoimmune disease in which white blood cells attack the myelin sheaths as if they were a foreign substance. Stress and malnutrition, whether from poor absorption or poor diet, often precede the onset of the disease. Some experts suspect that an as-yet-unidentified virus may be involved. Heredity may also be a factor. Another theory is that this condition may be caused by food intolerances or allergies, especially allergies to dairy products and gluten.

Chemical poisoning of the nervous system by pesticides, industrial chemicals, and heavy metals may also play a part in the development of MS. Environmental toxins can cause disturbances in the body's normal metabolic pathways that result in damage to the nerves' protective myelin sheaths. Even substances that are not necessarily toxic to everyone can be a problem for susceptible individuals. Toxins such as those produced by bacteria and fungi in the body have been known to produce symptoms like those of MS.

Many experts suspect that mercury poisoning is behind many cases of MS. Mercury has been shown to bind to the DNA of cells and cell membranes, causing cellular distortion and inhibited cell function. The installation of mercury amalgam dental fillings (the chief source of mercury exposure for most people in the United States) has been known to produce symptoms indistinguishable from those of multiple sclerosis in some people. Further, the levels of mercury in people with MS have been found to be an average of seven times higher than those in healthy people.

Finally, diet may play a key role in the development of MS. This is suggested by the fact that MS is fairly common in the United States and Europe and almost unheard of in some other countries, such as Japan, Korea, and China. The consumption of saturated fats, cholesterol, and alcohol, so common in Western countries, leads to the production of a hormonelike substance called prostaglandin 2 (PG2), which promotes the inflammatory response and worsens symptoms of multiple sclerosis. People in Asian countries typically consume much less fat than people in North America and northern Europe do. Their diets are also rich in marine foods, seeds, and fruit oils, which are high in essential fatty acids, including the omega-3 essential fatty acids, which have an inhibitory effect on the inflammatory response.

MS is usually diagnosed between the ages of twenty-five and forty. Women are affected nearly twice as often as men are. MS is rarely diagnosed in children and in people over sixty years of age. In the United States, MS occurs much more often in states north of the thirty-seventh parallel (an imaginary line stretching approximately from Newport News, Virginia, to Santa Cruz, California) than in other parts of the country.

Diagnosing MS is not a simple task, so the illness often goes undiagnosed for some time. Tests that can be used to detect the disease include magnetic resonance imaging (MRI), to look for signs of plaques or lesions; lumbar puncture (spinal tap), to detect abnormalities in the levels of white blood cells and/or immune-system proteins in the cerebrospinal fluid; a visual evoked potential (VEP) test, done to assess the connection between the retina and the visual area of the brain; an audio evoked potential (AEP) test, which may help to detect lesions in the brain; and electrodiagnostic tests that measure the rate at which nerve impulses travel (this may be slower than normal in people with MS).

There is no known cure for this disease, but the supplement and dietary programs outlined in this section have been shown to be helpful. Long-term sufferers of MS may not benefit as much, but younger people who are just starting to exhibit symptoms may find that the correct supplements slow or even stop the progression of the disease.

NUTRIENTS

SUPPLEMENT	SUGGESTED DOSAGE	COMMENTS
Very Important		
Coenzyme Q$_{10}$	90 mg daily.	Needed for improved circulation and tissue oxygenation. Strengthens the immune system.
plus Coenzyme A from Coenzyme-A Technologies	As directed on label.	Supports the immune system's detoxification of many dangerous substances. Can ease depression and fatigue, increase energy, process fats, remove toxins from the body, and boost the immune system.
Methylsulfonyl-methane (MSM)	As directed on label.	Helps keep cell walls permeable, allowing water and nutrients to freely flow into cells and allowing wastes and toxins to properly flow out. With vitamin C, is used by the body to build healthy new cells.
Gamma-linolenic acid (GLA) or flaxseed oil or primrose oil or omega-3 essential fatty acid complex	As directed on label 3 times daily, with meals. As directed on label 3 times daily, with meals. As directed on label 3 times daily, with meals. As directed on label 3 times daily, with meals.	An essential fatty acid needed to control symptoms. Deficiency is common in people with MS. If GLA is not available, use one of these supplements for essential fatty acids.
Garlic (Kyolic from Wakunaga)	2 capsules 3 times daily.	An excellent source of sulfur.
Oxy-5000 Forte from American Biologics	As directed on label.	A potent nutritional antioxidant formula.
Vitamin B complex	100 mg of each major B vitamin 3 times daily (amounts of inidividual vitamins in a complex will vary).	Aids immune system function and maintains healthy nerves. Use hypoallergenic formulas for all the B vitamins.
plus extra vitamin B$_6$ (pyridoxine)	50 mg 3 times daily.	Promotes red blood cell production; aids the nervous system and immune function. Deficiency may cause MS in susceptible persons.
and vitamin B$_{12}$	1,000 mcg twice daily.	Aids in cellular longevity and helps prevent nerve damage by maintaining the protective myelin sheaths. Use a lozenge or sublingual form.
and choline and inositol	As directed on label.	To stimulate the central nervous system and aid in protecting the myelin sheaths from damage.
Important		
Acidophilus (Kyo-Dophilus from Wakunaga is a good source)	1 tsp twice daily, on an empty stomach.	Helps to detoxify harmful substances, enhances absorption of nutrients, and aids digestion. Use a powdered nondairy form.
Amino-VIL from Carlson Labs	1/4 tsp twice daily, on an empty stomach.	A combination of the branched-chain amino acids, which aid in use of nutrients by the muscles. (*See* AMINO ACIDS in Part One.)
plus L-glycine	500 mg twice daily, on an empty stomach.	Aids in supporting the myelin sheaths.
Calcium	2,000–3,000 mg daily.	Deficiency may create a predisposition to developing MS. Use chelate form for best assimilation.
and magnesium	1,000–1,500 mg daily.	Needed for calcium absorption and for proper muscular coordination.
Creatine	As directed on label. Do not take with fruit juice, as this combination produces creatinine, which is difficult for the kidneys to process. Do not exceed the recommended dose.	May help counteract muscle depletion. Should be used in combination with a balanced diet.
Free-form amino acid complex	As directed on label 3 times daily, between meals.	Helps maintain good absorption of nutrients needed for proper brain function.
Grape seed extract	As directed on label.	A powerful antioxidant and anti-inflammatory.
Multienzyme complex or Inflazyme Forte from American Biologics	As directed on label. Take with meals. As directed on label.	For proper breakdown of foods. To reduce inflammation and aid digestion.
Multiglandular complex	As directed on label.	Needed for the endocrine, hormonal, and enzyme systems. (*See* GLANDULAR THERAPY in Part Three.)
Nicotinamide adenine dinucleotide (NADH)	As directed on label.	Important in the creation and transfer of chemical energy, especially during breathing.
Parasitin+ from Växa International or ParasiVeda from Solaray	As directed on label. As directed on label.	To detoxify the body of parasites.

Potassium	300–1,000 mg daily.	Needed for normal muscle function.
Raw thymus glandular	500 mg twice daily.	Enhances immune function.
Selenium	150–300 mcg daily.	An antioxidant and immune system stimulant.
7-Keto DHEA	As directed on label.	Slows overall body deterioration. Enhances fat loss and lean muscle mass development. Preferable to ordinary DHEA because it is not converted into sex hormones in the body.
Ultra Osteo Synergy from American Biologics	As directed on label.	To provide nutritional support for bone renewal.
Vitamin A plus carotenoid complex (Betatene)	25,000 IU daily. If you are pregnant, do not exceed 10,000 IU daily. As directed on label.	Important antioxidants. Use emulsion forms for easier assimilation.
Vitamin C with bioflavonoids	3,000–5,000 mg daily.	Promotes production of the antiviral protein interferon in the body. Also an antioxidant and immune stimulant. Use buffered ascorbic acid or an esterified form such as Ester C Plus Bioflavonoids from Natrol.
Vitamin D₃	800 IU daily.	Aids in calcium absorption.
Vitamin E	Begin with 400 IU daily and increase slowly to 1,800 IU daily.	Important for circulation, destroys free radicals, and protects the nervous system. Use d-alpha-tocopherol form. Emulsion form is recommended for easier assimilation and greater safety at high doses.
Vitamin K or alfalfa	200 mcg 3 times daily, with meals.	Helps prevent nausea and vomiting. See under Herbs, below.
Helpful		
Brewer's yeast	Start with ¼ tsp daily and slowly increase to 2 tsp daily	Improves blood sugar metabolism when taken with chromium. Aids in lowering cholesterol and improving HDL/LDL ratio.
Kyo-Green from Wakunaga	1 tsp in liquid 3 times daily.	A good source of organic chlorophyll, live enzymes, vitamins, and minerals plus amino acids.
Lecithin granules or capsules	1 tbsp 3 times daily, before meals. 1,200 mg 3–4 times daily, before meals.	Protects the cells. Needed for normal brain function.
Manganese	5–10 mg daily. Take separately from calcium.	An important mineral often deficient in people with MS.
Multimineral complex	As directed on label.	Needed for all enzyme systems in the body and to supply needed nutrients. Use a high-potency formula.
Phosphorus	900 mg daily.	Needed for transfer of energy within cells.

HERBS

❑ Alfalfa is a good source of vitamin K. It can be taken in liquid or tablet form.

❑ Burdock, dandelion, echinacea, goldenseal, pau d'arco, red clover, St. John's wort, sarsaparilla, and yarrow are effective detoxifiers.

Caution: Do not take goldenseal internally on a daily basis for more than one week at a time, do not use it during pregnancy, and use it with caution if you are allergic to ragweed.

❑ Cordyceps is a Chinese herb that improves memory, helps you assimilate nutrients more efficiently, and increases energy.

❑ Lobelia, skullcap, and valerian root relax the nervous system. Taken at bedtime, they aid in preventing insomnia. Lobelia is good for daytime use also.

Caution: Do not take lobelia internally on an ongoing basis.

RECOMMENDATIONS

❑ Eat only organically grown foods with no chemical treatments or additives, including eggs, fruits, gluten-free grains, raw nuts and seeds, vegetables, and cold-pressed vegetable oils. The best diet for people with this disorder is totally vegetarian.

❑ Eat plenty of raw sprouts and alfalfa, plus foods that contain lactic acid, such as sauerkraut and dill pickles. Also good are "green drinks" that contain plenty of chlorophyll.

❑ Eat plenty of dark leafy greens. These are good sources of vitamin K.

❑ Drink at least eight 8-ounce glasses of quality water each day to prevent toxic buildup in the muscles.

❑ Do not consume any alcohol, barley, chocolate, coffee, dairy products, fried foods, highly seasoned foods, meat, oats, refined foods, rye, salt, spices, sugar, tobacco, wheat, or processed, canned, or frozen foods.

❑ Take a fiber supplement. Fiber is important for avoiding constipation. Periodically take warm cleansing enemas with the juice of a fresh lemon. A clean colon is important for keeping toxic waste from interfering with muscle function. (*See* COLON CLEANSING and ENEMAS in Part Three.)

❑ Never consume saturated fats, processed oils, oils that have been subjected to heat (either in processing or in cooking), or oils that have been stored without refrigeration.

❑ Have yourself tested for possible food allergies. (*See* ALLERGIES in Part Two.) We believe that food allergies are a major factor in the development and progression of multiple sclerosis. Unfortunately, all too often the allergies are not discovered until irreversible nerve damage has occurred. Early detection is therefore vital. Eliminating offending foods from your diet may slow down the progression of the disease and help you avoid further damage.

❏ Avoid stress and anxiety. Attacks of MS are often precipitated by a trauma or a period of emotional distress.

❏ Avoid exposure to heat, such as hot baths, showers, sunbathing, and overly warm surroundings, and avoid becoming overheated when working or exercising. Avoid exhaustion and viral infections. All of these may trigger an attack or worsen symptoms.

❏ Get periodic massages and regular exercise, and keep mentally active. These are extremely valuable in maintaining muscle function and bringing about remission of symptoms. However, exercises that may increase body temperature can decrease the function of the nerves involved and make symptoms worse. Swimming is the best activity. Doing other exercises in cool water is good as well because body temperature is kept lower and the body's weight is supported by the water. Stretching exercises help to prevent muscle contractures. Physical therapy is often needed.

❏ When an exacerbation begins, take at least two days of complete bed rest. This can often stop a mild attack.

❏ Educate yourself and your family about the disease, and seek out sources of emotional support. For names and addresses of organizations that can help, see HEALTH AND MEDICAL ORGANIZATIONS in the Appendix.

CONSIDERATIONS

❏ A strong immune system may help to prevent multiple sclerosis by helping the body avoid infection, which often precedes the onset of this disease.

❏ While the effects of MS on pregnancy seem to be minimal, slightly more flare-ups occur during the six months following childbirth.

❏ Gluten intolerance may make a person more susceptible to MS.

❏ Recent studies point to a possible link between MS and candida infection. A significant proportion of people with MS show evidence of imbalanced bowel flora, which is characteristic of candidiasis. Further, chronic fatigue is a symptom of candidiasis, and it is also one of the most common complaints of people with multiple sclerosis. Treatments to reduce candida activity have been found to reduce the fatigue experienced by many people with MS. (See CANDIDIASIS in Part Two.)

❏ The symptoms of Lyme disease may mimic those of multiple sclerosis. (See LYME DISEASE in Part Two.)

❏ Chlamydia pneumoniae, a very common type of bacteria, has been cited as a possible cause of MS. In an article in the July 1999 issue of Annals of Neurology, researchers reported that C. pneumoniae were found in all MS patients in their study group. It may be, however, that this was a result of MS, not a cause.

❏ A 1997 study concentrated on the ability of hypericin, a chemical found naturally in St. John's wort, to destroy viruses and cancer cells when exposed to light. Hypericin has shown promise as a disease-fighting agent, and research is continuing.

❏ Researchers in Scandinavia have long used essential fatty acid supplementation to treat MS and to reduce the frequency of new events.

❏ Some people with MS have experienced relief of symptoms by using honeybee venom. Bee venom apparently acts as an anti-inflammatory and immune-system stimulant. Aerobic Life Industries manufactures a bee venom cream for topical application.

❏ Although its use is considered controversial by many physicians in the United States, hyperbaric oxygen therapy has been used with success for people with multiple sclerosis in some other countries. (See HYPERBARIC OXYGEN THERAPY in Part Three.)

❏ There are three drugs that doctors sometimes prescribe to treat MS: interferon-beta-1a and -1b (Avonex and Betaseron, respectively) and glatiramer acetate (Copaxone, also known as copolymer-1). Possible side effects of interferon include flulike symptoms and depression. Vitamin C promotes the production of natural interferon in the body.

❏ Oral corticosteroids, such as prednisone (Deltasone and others), are often used to hasten remission and to reduce the severity of attacks. Giving cortisone intravenously for a short period (five days) eliminates the side effects that come with the use of oral medication. The same drugs now used by transplant patients to keep their bodies from rejecting donated organs can be used to control symptoms. These immunosuppressant drugs are not without side effects, however; people who take them commonly experience nausea, vomiting, and hair loss, and they run a greater risk of cancer as well.

❏ There are many drugs that doctors prescribe to treat the accompanying conditions of MS. Always ask your physician about all available medications, and especially about possible side effects, so that you can make informed decisions about which (if any) to take.

❏ According to the New Jersey College of Medicine, x-ray irradiation to the lymph glands and the spleen may halt the progress of MS in some cases. However, radiation exposure depresses the immune system.

❏ Because there are so many conditions that can occur over time with MS—including bowel and bladder problems, chronic fatigue, depression, headaches, impotence, pain, problems with vision and hearing loss, seizures, urinary tract infections, and vertigo—it is advisable to read the sections that cover these individual conditions in this section of this book. Consult the Table of Contents to look for sections that may be relevant for you.

Mumps

Mumps is a common viral illness, mostly of childhood, caused by a type of virus known as a paramyxovirus that infects the parotid glands—the salivary glands located at the jaw angles below the ears. Symptoms include swelling of one or both glands plus headache, fever, chills, decreased appetite, sore throat, and pain when swallowing or chewing, especially when swallowing acidic substances such as citrus juices. Often, one of the parotid glands swells before the other, and as swelling in one gland subsides, the other begins to swell.

Mumps is transmitted from person to person by means of infected droplets of saliva or direct contact with contaminated materials. It can be contracted through sneezing, coughing, kissing, talking, breathing, drinking out of the same glass as an infected person, and sharing utensils. The incubation period of the virus can vary from fourteen to twenty-four days (the average is eighteen days). A person with mumps is contagious any time from forty-eight hours before the onset of symptoms to six days after the symptoms have started. This illness is not as contagious as measles or chickenpox, and one attack usually affords lifetime immunity. Mumps is most common in children between the ages of three and ten, although it can occur through teenage years and, in rare cases, in adulthood. If it does occur after puberty, the ovaries or testes may become involved and sterility may result. If the testicles are affected, they become swollen and painful; if the ovaries or pancreas is affected, abdominal pain results. Other organs that can be affected in rare, severe cases include the brain, pancreas, and kidneys—possibly with serious complications.

Unless otherwise specified, the dosages recommended here are for adults. For a child between the ages of twelve and seventeen, reduce the dose to three-quarters the recommended amount. For a child between six and twelve, use one-half the recommended dose, and for a child under the age of six, use one-quarter the recommended amount.

NUTRIENTS

SUPPLEMENT	SUGGESTED DOSAGE	COMMENTS
Very Important		
Lactobacillus bifidus	As directed on label.	"Friendly" bacteria contain antibiotic substances that inhibit pathogenic organisms.
Vitamin C with bioflavonoids	500 mg every 2 hours until improvement is noted, up to 3,000–10,000 mg daily.	Destroys the virus and eliminates toxins. For children, use sodium ascorbate form to lessen diarrhea.
Zinc lozenges (ImmunActinZinc lozenges from Nature's Plus)	1 15-mg lozenge every 4–6 hours. Do not exceed a total of 100 mg daily.	Aids healing. Lozenges are fast acting. Do not chew them, but allow them to dissolve slowly in the mouth.
Important		
Acidophilus (Kyo-Dophilus from Wakunaga and Bio-Dophilus from American Biologics are good sources)	As directed on label.	For adults and children. Contains antibiotic substances that inhibit pathogenic organisms. Use a nondairy formula.
Free-form amino acid complex plus	As directed on label.	Important for tissue repair and healing.
vitamin B complex	100 mg of each major B vitamin 3 times daily (amounts of individual vitamins in a complex will vary).	Needed for healing.
plus potassium	99 mg daily.	To restore electrolytes depleted by fever. Potassium levels are depressed by fever over 101°F.
Vitamin A with mixed carotenoids and	For children under 12, 15,000 IU daily. For adults, 50,000 IU daily. If you are pregnant, do not exceed 10,000 IU daily.	Vitamins A and E potentiate immune function. Use emulsion forms for easier assimilation.
vitamin E	For children, 200 IU daily for 1 week. For adults, 400–800 IU daily for 1 week.	Use d-alpha-tocopherol form.
Helpful		
Kelp	1,000–1,500 daily.	Contains essential minerals, iodine, and vitamins.

HERBS

❑ Catnip and chamomile teas are good calming agents and help to induce sleep. Catnip tea enemas help reduce fever. (*See* ENEMAS in Part Three.)

❑ Taken as a tea, dandelion cleanses and supports the liver. Ground into a powder and combined with a little aloe vera gel in a poultice, it helps to reduce swelling.

❑ Echinacea helps to reduce swelling and cleanses the blood and lymphatic system. Take it in tea form, mixed with a little juice, four times a day or more.

❑ Elder flower tea helps to reduce fever.

❑ Lobelia extract is good for pain. Take ¹/₂ teaspoon every three to four hours.

Caution: Do not take lobelia internally on an ongoing basis.

❑ Mullein poultices are good for relieving pain and swelling of the salivary glands. (*See* USING A POULTICE in Part Three.)

❑ Peppermint tea soothes an upset stomach and helps to flush infection from the body.

❑ Adding powdered slippery elm bark to barley water makes a drink that is nourishing and soothing to the throat and digestive tract. (*See* THERAPEUTIC LIQUIDS in Part Three.)

❑ Yarrow reduces fever and inflammation and is a good lymphatic cleanser.

RECOMMENDATIONS

❑ As long as the glands are swollen, eat mostly raw fruits and vegetables that are juiced or softened. Sticking to a diet of soft foods helps to minimize the pain of chewing.

❑ Drink plenty of pure water and fresh juices to keep the body well hydrated and to flush the system clean.

❑ Do not consume coffee, dairy products, tobacco, or white flour or sugar. Avoid acidic foods, such as pickles and citrus fruits or juices, as they are likely to cause discomfort.

❑ Follow a fasting program to detoxify the body. (*See* FASTING in Part Three.)

❑ Stay warm and dry, and get plenty of rest.

❑ Intermittently apply warmth or cold, whichever feels best, to the swollen glands and around the neck. Use hot towels, hot water bottles, and ice packs with caution.

❑ If testicular swelling and pain occurs, support the scrotum by means of an adhesive tape "bridge" between the thighs and use cool compresses to help relieve pain.

CONSIDERATIONS

❑ Complete recovery from mumps usually can be expected in about ten days if no complications occur. If any of the following symptoms develop, you should see your doctor as soon as possible: tenderness or swelling of the testicles, severe vomiting (this may indicate infection that has spread to the pancreas), a fever over 104°F, lethargy, or a stiff neck accompanied by a severe headache (this may be a sign of developing meningitis).

❑ Because complications are more common when this disease is contracted in adulthood, immunization should be considered for any adult who has not had mumps or who has not already been vaccinated against it.

❑ The mumps virus may be contagious even during incubation. Anyone who has come in contact with a person who had or who developed mumps should be on the lookout for symptoms for a fourteen- to twenty-eight-day period following exposure, and should minimize his or her contact with persons who may be susceptible during this period.

❑ There is no medication that can cure mumps. Treatment focuses on bed rest and measures to support the body as the virus runs its course. Your doctor may recommend acetaminophen (Tylenol, Datril, and others) or ibuprofen (Advil, Nuprin, and others) if fever causes significant discomfort.

❑ A doctor may advise the use of corticosteroids to diminish testicular pain and swelling. These are powerful drugs, and should be used with caution.

❑ If nausea and/or pain on swallowing is so severe that a person with mumps becomes unable to eat, intravenous administration of dextrose and fluids may be required.

❑ Swelling of the parotid and/or other salivary glands can also be caused by a number of other factors, including cirrhosis of the liver; bulimia, a bacterial infection such as strep throat; poor oral hygiene; a salivary gland tumor or a calcium-based stone in one of the salivary ducts; and Mikulicz's syndrome, which is characterized by swelling (usually painless) of the parotid glands and, sometimes, the tear glands, and which can occur in people with a number of different diseases, including leukemia, lupus, non-Hodgkin's lymphoma, and tuberculosis. Swollen salivary glands can also be related to the use of certain drugs. Consequently, an isolated case of mumps (a case not associated with a local outbreak of the disease) warrants extra care in diagnosis.

❑ In most U.S. states, immunization against mumps is required before a child can be admitted into public kindergarten.

Muscle Cramps

Ordinarily, a muscle contracts when it is used, then stretches out when the motion is completed or another muscle moves it in the opposite direction. If a muscle contracts with great intensity without stretching out again, you feel the pain of a muscle cramp. Many people experience muscle cramps during the night. This type of cramp generally affects the legs, especially the calf muscles, and the feet. They occur more frequently in older adults than in younger people. Children sometimes experience a type of crampy muscle and leg pain often called "growing pains."

Muscle cramping is often caused by an imbalance in the body's levels of electrolytes—minerals such as potassium, calcium, and magnesium—and/or a deficiency of vitamin E. Another common cause is unaccustomed physical overexertion. Sitting, standing, or lying for a long time in one position; anemia; the use of tobacco; inactivity; fibromyalgia; hormone imbalances; allergies; arthritis; and even arteriosclerosis can also result in cramping, as can dehydration, heat stroke, hypothyroidism, or varicose veins, or, more rarely, the early stages of amyotrophic lateral sclerosis (ALS, or Lou Gehrig's disease).

The use of diuretic drugs for high blood pressure or heart disorders may lead to electrolyte imbalances, causing muscle cramps. Poor circulation also contributes to leg cramps.

Unless otherwise specified, the dosages recommended here are for adults. For a child between the ages of twelve and seventeen, reduce the dose to three-quarters of the recommended amount. For a child between six and twelve, use one-half of the recommended dose, and for a child under the age of six, use one-quarter of the recommended amount.

NUTRIENTS

SUPPLEMENT	SUGGESTED DOSAGE	COMMENTS
Essential		
Calcium and magnesium	1,500 mg daily. 750 mg daily and up.	Deficiencies are most often the cause of cramping in the legs and feet at night. Use chelate or citrate forms.
Vitamin E	Start with 400 IU daily and increase slowly to 1,000 IU daily.	Improves circulation. Deficiency may cause leg cramps while standing or walking. Especially good if cramping is related to varicose veins. Use d-alpha-tocopherol form.
Very Important		
Bone Support from Synergy Plus or	As directed on label.	Contains minerals that aid in absorption of calcium.
Ultra Osteo Synergy from American Biologics	As directed on label.	Provides nutritional support for bone renewal.
Malic acid and magnesium	As directed on label.	Malic acid is involved in the production of energy in muscle cells; magnesium is a cofactor in cellular energy production.
Potassium	99 mg daily.	Needed for proper calcium and magnesium metabolism; aids in relieving muscle cramps.
Silica	As directed on label.	Supplies silicon, which aids in calcium absorption.
Vitamin B complex	50 mg of each major B vitamin 3 times daily, with meals (amounts of individual vitamins in a complex will vary).	For improved circulation and cellular function.
plus extra vitamin B$_1$ (thiamine) and	50 mg 3 times daily, with meals.	Enhances circulation and may aid in maintaining proper muscle tone.
vitamin B$_3$ (niacin)	50 mg 3 times daily, with meals. Do not exceed this amount	Increases circulation. *Caution:* Do not take niacin if you have a liver disorder, gout, or high blood pressure.
Vitamin C with bioflavonoids	3,000–6,000 mg daily.	Improves circulation.
Vitamin D$_3$	400 IU daily.	Needed for calcium uptake.
Important		
Dimethylglycine (DMG) (Aangamik DMG from FoodScience of Vermont)	As directed on label.	Improves tissue oxygenation.
Helpful		
Coenzyme Q$_{10}$ plus	100 mg daily.	Improves heart function and circulation. Lowers blood pressure.
Coenzyme A from Coenzyme-A Technologies	As directed on label.	Improves the effectiveness of coenzyme Q$_{10}$.
Lecithin granules or capsules	1–2 tbsp 3 times daily, before meals. 1,200–2,400 mg 3 times daily, before meals.	Reduces cholesterol levels.
Multivitamin and mineral complex	As directed on label.	All nutrients are necessary for healthy muscles.
Zinc	50 mg daily. Do not exceed a total of 100 mg daily from all supplements.	Needed for absorption of calcium and action of B vitamins. Use zinc gluconate lozenges or OptiZinc for best absorption.

HERBS

❑ Alfalfa, bayberry, blessed thistle, cayenne, dong quai, echinacea, elder flower, elderberry extract, garlic, ginkgo biloba, horsetail, and saffron are good for circulation.

❑ Horsetail, meadowsweet, valerian, and skullcap help to relieve muscle cramps.

❑ Rubbing lobelia extract on the affected area helps to relieve muscle spasms.

❑ Taking valerian root at bedtime helps to relax the muscles.

RECOMMENDATIONS

❑ Eat alfalfa, brewer's yeast, plenty of dark-green and leafy vegetables, cornmeal, and kelp.

❑ Drink a large glass of quality water (preferably steam-distilled) to flush out toxins stored in the muscles. Do this every three hours throughout the day.

❑ Massage the muscles and use heat to relieve pain.

❑ If you are on diuretic medication for high blood pressure or a heart disorder, be sure to take supplemental potassium daily.

Note: Do not take supplemental potassium if you are taking a potassium-sparing diuretic (discuss this with your doctor).

❑ Rub pure, unprocessed olive or flaxseed oil into your muscles before and after strenuous exercise. Add 25 drops of oil to a hot bath and soak. Canola oil is also good for this purpose.

❑ Take a hot bath using mineral salts before bedtime to increase blood flow to the muscles.

❑ If you have cramps during the day, while you are active, consult your health care provider. This can be a sign of impaired circulation or arteriosclerosis. (*See* CIRCULATORY PROBLEMS in Part Two.)

❑ If cramping occurs after walking and is relieved when you stop, suspect impaired circulation. *See* ARTERIOSCLEROSIS/ATHEROSCLEROSIS in Part Two and take the artery function self-test.

CONSIDERATIONS

❑ Creatine, a popular supplement with athletes and body builders, may increase the likelihood of muscle cramps.

❑ Hydrotherapy (the therapeutic use of water, steam, and ice) or massage therapy (manipulation of muscles and other soft tissue) may be useful in controlling muscle cramps. (*See* HYDROTHERAPY and MASSAGE *under* PAIN CONTROL in Part Three.)

❑ Gabapentin (Neurontin), a drug used in the treatment of epilepsy, is under study for its ability to relieve muscle cramps.

Muscle Injuries

See SPRAINS, STRAINS, AND OTHER INJURIES OF THE MUSCLES AND JOINTS.

Myocardial Infarction

See HEART ATTACK.

Nail Problems

The nails protect the nerve-rich fingertips and tips of the toes from injury. Nails are a substructure of the epidermis (the outer layer of the skin) and are composed mainly of keratin, a type of protein. The nail bed is the skin on top of which the nails grow. Nails grow from 0.05 to 1.2 millimeters (approximately $1/500$ to $1/20$ inch) a week. If a nail is lost, it takes about seven months to grow out fully.

Healthy nail beds are pink, indicating a rich blood supply. Changes or abnormalities in the nails are often the result of nutritional deficiencies or other underlying conditions. The nails can reveal a great deal about the body's internal health. Nail abnormalities on either the fingers or the toes can indicate an underlying disorder.

The following are some of the changes that nutritional deficiencies can produce in the nails:

• A lack of protein, folic acid, and vitamin C causes hangnails. White bands across the nails are also an indication of protein deficiency.

• A lack of vitamin A and calcium causes dryness and brittleness.

• A deficiency of the B vitamins causes fragility, with horizontal and vertical ridges.

• Insufficient intake of vitamin B_{12} leads to excessive dryness, very rounded and curved nail ends, and darkened nails.

• Iron deficiency may result in "spoon" nails (nails that develop a concave shape) and/or vertical ridges.

• Zinc deficiency may cause the development of white spots on the nails.

• A lack of sufficient "friendly" bacteria (lactobacilli) in the body can result in the growth of fungus under and around nails.

• A lack of sufficient hydrochloric acid (HCl) contributes to splitting nails.

The following table lists supplements that promote healthy nail growth.

NUTRIENTS

SUPPLEMENT	SUGGESTED DOSAGE	COMMENTS
Very Important		
Acidophilus (Kyo-Dophilus from Wakunaga)	As directed on label.	Taken internally, inhibits the harmful bacteria that causes fungal infection. Use a nondairy formula.
Free-form amino acid complex (Amino Balance from Anabol Naturals) plus extra L-cysteine and L-methionine	As directed on label, on an empty stomach. Take with water or juice. Do not take with milk. Take with 50 mg vitamin B_6 and 100 mg vitamin C for better absorption.	The building materials for new nails. Also supplies sulfur, which is necessary for skin and nail growth. (*See* AMINO ACIDS in Part One.)
Silica or horsetail or oat straw	As directed on label.	Supplies silicon, needed for hair, bones, and strong nails. *See under* Herbs, below. *See under* Herbs, below.
Vitamin A emulsion or capsules plus carotenoid complex	50,000 IU daily. If you are pregnant, do not exceed 10,000 IU daily. 25,000 IU daily. As directed on label.	The body cannot utilize protein without vitamin A. Emulsion form is recommended for easier assimilation and greater safety at higher doses.
Helpful		
Black currant seed oil	500 mg twice daily.	Helpful for weak, brittle nails.
Calcium and magnesium and vitamin D_3	As directed on label. As directed on label. As directed on label.	Necessary for nail growth. Needed to balance with calcium. Enhances calcium absorption.
Iron (ferrous fumarate from Freeda Vitamins) or Floradix Iron + Herbs from Salus Haus	As directed by physician. Take with 100 mg vitamin C for better absorption. *Do not* take with vitamin E. As directed on label.	Deficiency produces "spoon" nails and/or vertical ridges. *Caution:* Do not take iron unless anemia is diagnosed. A natural source of iron.
Ultimate Oil from Nature's Secret	As directed on label.	A combination of essential fatty acids necessary for the health of skin, hair, and nails.
Ultra Nails from Nature's Plus	As directed on label.	Contains calcium, gelatin, amino acids, magnesium, iron, and other nutrients important for healthy nails.
Vitamin B complex plus extra vitamin B_2 (riboflavin) and vitamin B_{12} and biotin and folic acid	As directed on label. 50 mg 3 times daily. 1,000 mcg 3 times daily. 300 mg 3 times daily for 9 months. 400 mcg 3 times daily.	Deficiencies result in fragile nails. Useful for treating brittle nails. Reduces splitting and other nail irregularities.

Vitamin C with bioflavonoids	3,000–6,000 mg daily.	Hangnails and inflammation of the paronychia (the tissue surrounding the nail) may be linked to vitamin C deficiency.
Zinc	50 mg daily. Do not exceed a total of 100 mg daily from all supplements.	Affects absorption and action of vitamins and enzymes. Use zinc gluconate lozenges or OptiZinc for best absorption.
plus copper	3 mg daily.	Needed to balance with zinc.

HERBS

❑ Alfalfa, black cohosh, burdock root, dandelion, gotu kola, and yellow dock are rich in minerals, including silica and zinc, as well as B vitamins—all of which strengthen the nails. Horsetail and oat straw also are good sources of silica.

❑ Borage seed, flaxseed, lemongrass, parsley, primrose, pumpkin seed, and sage are all good sources of essential fatty acids, which nourish the nails.

Caution: Do not use sage if you suffer from any kind of seizure disorder.

❑ Butcher's broom, chamomile, ginkgo biloba, rosemary, sassafras, and turmeric are good for circulation, which nourishes the nails.

RECOMMENDATIONS

❑ For healthy nails, be sure to get plenty of quality protein, and take a protein supplement. Eat grains, legumes, oatmeal, nuts, and seeds. Eggs also are a good source of protein, as long as your blood cholesterol levels are not too high.

❑ Avoid refined sugars and simple carbohydrates.

❑ Eat a diet composed of 50 percent fresh fruits and raw vegetables to supply necessary vitamins, minerals, and enzymes. Eat foods that are rich in sulfur and silicon, such as broccoli, fish, onions, and sea vegetables. Also include in the diet plenty of foods that are high in biotin, such as brewer's yeast, soy flour, and whole grains.

❑ Drink plenty of quality water and other liquids. Cuts and cracks in the nails may indicate a need for more liquids.

❑ Drink fresh carrot juice daily. This is high in calcium and phosphorus and is very good for strengthening the nails.

❑ Consume citrus fruits, salt, and vinegar in moderation, if at all. Excessive intake of these foods can result in a protein/calcium imbalance that may adversely affect the health of the nails.

❑ Supplement your diet with royal jelly, a good source of essential fatty acids, and spirulina or kelp, which are rich in silica, zinc, and B vitamins, and help to strengthen nails.

❑ For splitting nails and/or hangnails, take 2 tablespoons of brewer's yeast or wheat germ oil daily.

❑ To restore color and texture to brittle, yellowed nails, make a mixture of equal parts of honey, avocado oil, and egg yolk, and add a pinch of salt. Rub the mixture into your nails and cuticles. Leave it on for half an hour, then rinse it off. Repeat this treatment daily. You should begin to see results after about two weeks.

❑ To strengthen the nails, try soaking them in warm olive oil or cider vinegar for ten to twenty minutes daily.

❑ Treat your nails gently. Using them to pry, pick, scrape, or perform tasks such as removing staples can damage them.

❑ Keep your nails relatively short. Nails longer than one-quarter inch beyond the fingertip break and bend easily.

❑ Do *not* cut the cuticles. Uncovering the nails this way is harsh and irritating, and may cause infection. Use baby oil or cream and gently push the cuticles back.

❑ Soak your nails before trimming them. Nails are most likely to split and peel when they are dry. Apply hand cream each morning and evening to prevent nails from drying out.

❑ Do not repeatedly immerse your hands in water that contains detergents or chemicals such as bleach or dish soap; this results in split nails. Wear cotton-lined gloves when doing housework such as dishes and laundry or when using furniture polish. This protects your hands and nails against harsh chemicals. Wearing gloves is especially important for people who work in jobs where their hands are exposed to chemicals. Not only does this damage the nails, but it causes the skin surrounding the nail bed to dry out and crack. This can lead to bleeding and can be quite painful.

❑ Do not pull at hangnails. Cut them with sharp clippers or scissors. Keep your hands moisturized to help prevent hangnails.

❑ If you are diabetic, see your health care provider if your cuticles become inflamed, because the infection can spread.

❑ If you wear nail polish, use a base coat underneath it to prevent yellowing.

❑ Use nail polish removers as little as possible. They contain solvents that leach lipids from the nails and make them brittle. These solvents are also potentially highly toxic and can be absorbed through the skin. If you need to use a polish remover, use one that contains acetate instead of acetone.

❑ Never apply artificial nails over your own. They may look nice for a while, but they destroy the underlying nail. The chemicals and glue used are dangerous to the body, and are readily absorbed through the damaged nail and nail bed. The use of artificial nails has also been known to contribute to the development of fungal infection of the fingernails.

❑ Many professional manicure businesses have been cited for not meeting health codes. If you have professional manicures, always insist on sterile instruments or bring your own to ensure they are free from bacteria and disease. Use isopropyl alcohol to sterilize your instruments.

Disorders That Show Up in the Nails

Nail changes may signify a number of disorders elsewhere in the body. These changes may indicate illness before any other symptoms do. Seek medical attention if any of the following symptoms are suspected.

• **Black, splinterlike bits under the nails** can be a sign of infectious endocarditis, a serious heart infection; other heart disease; or a bleeding disorder.

• **Black bands** from the cuticle outward to the end of the nail can be an early sign of melanoma.

• **Brittle, soft, shiny nails without a moon** may indicate an overactive thyroid.

• **Brittle nails** signify possible iron deficiency, thyroid problems, impaired kidney function, and circulation problems.

• **Crumbly, white nails** near the cuticle are sometimes an indication of AIDS.

• **Dark nails and/or thin, flat, spoon-shaped nails** are a sign of vitamin B_{12} deficiency or anemia. Nails can also turn gray or dark if the hands are placed in chemicals such as cleaning supplies (most often bleach) or a substance to which one is allergic.

• **Deep blue nail beds** show a pulmonary obstructive disorder such as asthma or emphysema.

• **Downward-curved nail ends** may denote heart, liver, or respiratory problems.

• **Flat nails** can denote Raynaud's disease.

• **Greenish nails,** if not a result of a localized fungal infection, may indicate an internal bacterial infection.

• **A half-white nail with dark spots at the tip** points to possible kidney disease.

• **An isolated dark-blue band in the nail bed,** especially in light-skinned people, can be a sign of skin cancer.

• **Lindsay's nails** (sometimes known as "half–and–half" nails), nails in which half of the top of the nail is white and the other half is pink, may be a sign of chronic kidney disease.

• **Nail beading** (the development of bumps on the surface of the nail) is a sign of rheumatoid arthritis.

• **Nails raised at the base with small white ends,** show a respiratory disorder such as emphysema or chronic bronchitis. This type of nail may also simply be inherited.

• **Nails separated from the nail bed** may signify a thyroid disorder (this condition is known as onyholysis) or a local infection.

• **Nails that broaden toward the tip and curve downward** are a sign of lung damage, such as from emphysema or exposure to asbestos.

• **Nails that chip, peel, crack, or break easily** show a general nutritional deficiency and insufficient hydrochloric acid and protein. Minerals are also needed.

• **Nails that have pitting resembling hammered brass** indicate a tendency toward partial or total hair loss.

• **Pitted red-brown spots and frayed and split ends** indicate psoriasis; vitamin C, folic acid, and protein are needed.

• **Red skin around the cuticles** can be indicative of poor metabolism of essential fatty acids or of a connective tissue disorder such as lupus.

• **Ridges** can appear in the nails either vertically or horizontally. Vertical ridges indicate poor general health, poor nutrient absorption, and/or iron deficiency; they may also indicate a kidney disorder. Horizontal ridges can occur as a result of severe stress, either psychological or physical, such as from infection and/or disease. A horizontal indentation in the nail (Beau's line) can occur as a result of a heart attack, major illness, or surgery. Ridges running up and down the nails also indicate a tendency to develop arthritis.

• **Spooning** (upward-curling) **or pitting nails** can be caused by disorders such as anemia or problems with iron absorption.

• **Thick nails** may indicate that the vascular system is weakening and the blood is not circulating properly. This may also be a sign of thyroid disease.

• **Thick toenails** can be a result of fungal infection.

• **Thinning nails** may signal lichen planus, an itchy skin disorder.

• **Two white horizontal bands that do not move as the nail grows** are a sign of hypoalbuminemia, a protein deficiency in the blood.

• **Unusually wide, square nails** can suggest a hormonal disorder.

• **White lines** show possible heart disease, high fever, or arsenic poisoning.

• **White lines across the nail** may indicate a liver disease.

• **If the white moon area of the nail turns red,** it may indicate heart problems; **if it turns slate blue,** then it can indicate either heavy metal poisoning (such as silver poisoning) or lung trouble.

• **White nails** indicate possible liver or kidney disorders and/or anemia.

• **White nails** with pink near the tips are a sign of cirrhosis.

• **Yellow nails or an elevation of the nail tips** can indicate internal disorders long before other symptoms appear. Some of these are problems with the lymphatic system, respiratory disorders, diabetes, and liver disorders.

CONSIDERATIONS

❏ If you expose your hands to too much water and soap, the nail may become loose from the nail bed. Water causes the nails to swell. They then shrink as they dry, resulting in loose and brittle nails.

❏ Discolored nails can be caused by prolonged illness, stress, nicotine, allergies, or diabetes. If your nails are green, you may have a bacterial infection or a fungal infection between the nail and the nail bed. If you have a fungal or bacterial infection, and especially if you are taking antibiotics, acidophilus is needed.

❏ Fungal infections can be treated by using a cotton swab to apply a mixture of equal parts of vinegar and water.

❏ Physicians often prescribe a regimen of 250 milligrams of griseofulvin (Fulvicin), four times daily, for a fungal infection of the nails. The white blood cell count must be monitored during this treatment. Another prescription antifungal agent is ketoconazole (Nizoral), which is available as a cream or shampoo, as well as in tablet form.

❏ Anticancer medications can cause bands and streaks of color to appear in the nails. These conditions disappear when the medication is stopped.

❏ A recent study found that hospital nurses with artificial nails had twice as much bacteria on their hands than those nurses who had natural nails. The area around and underneath the fingernails is one of the easiest places for germs to collect. The best way to prevent this is to thoroughly wash your hands for at least fifteen seconds using antiseptic soap under hot water. Make sure you wash the area underneath the nail and around the cuticle area. Use a clean towel to dry your hands. Use disposable towels if they are available.

❏ Poor thyroid function may be reflected in the nails. (*See* HYPOTHYROIDISM in Part Two.)

Narcolepsy

Narcolepsy is a rare neurological disorder that may affect as many as 250,000 Americans. There are four classic symptoms that define this syndrome: sleep attacks, cataplexy, sleep paralysis, and hypnagogic (sleep-related) hallucinations. A person with narcolepsy may experience any or all of these classic phenomena.

The best known symptom of narcolepsy is the sleep attack. A person with narcolepsy can suddenly fall into a sleep state with almost no warning whatsoever. Sleep attacks can occur at any time, even in mid-conversation, as many as ten times a day (even more, in some cases). These periods of sleep usually last only a matter of minutes, but in some cases sleep can continue for an hour or more. Afterwards, the person may feel refreshed, yet he or she may fall asleep again in a few minutes.

While the sleep that results from narcolepsy looks like ordinary sleep, researchers have found at least one key difference. Normal sleep is a cyclical process that alternates between periods of rapid-eye-movement (REM) and non-rapid-eye-movement (NREM) sleep. During the NREM part of the cycle, the entire body slows down—pulse, breathing, blood pressure, and brain wave activity are all lowered. When the REM cycle begins, the body remains asleep, but the brain becomes significantly active; brain waves as recorded by an electroencephalograph (EEG) more closely resemble those of the waking brain. It is during REM sleep that most dreaming occurs.

In healthy individuals, sleep begins with the NREM phase. After sixty minutes or so of NREM sleep, REM sleep begins. A short time later, the entire cycle begins again. In a narcoleptic sleep attack, in contrast, researchers have found that REM sleep begins almost instantly, with no introductory NREM sleep. The precise significance of this is not yet understood, but it does provide a useful diagnostic tool as well as a clue for researchers to pursue in trying to understand this mysterious disorder.

The second classic symptom of narcolepsy is cataplexy. This is a type of paralysis that usually occurs in response to some type of heightened emotion, such as anger, fear, or excitement. The individual does not lose consciousness, but experiences a sudden and temporary loss of muscle tone. Often, only the legs and/or arms are affected. These episodes normally last less than a minute, and they seem to be most likely to occur if the person is surprised in some way.

Sleep paralysis is the third classic symptom of narcolepsy. Just as you are falling asleep, or as you are beginning to awaken, you try to move or say something but find that you cannot, even though you are fully conscious. This lasts for only a second or two, but it can be frightening, especially the first time it happens. These episodes usually end either on their own or when someone touches or speaks to you. Many doctors feel that sleep paralysis is similar to cataplexy and to the state that accompanies REM sleep, in which motor activity is inhibited even though the brain is active. This phenomenon is not strictly limited to people with narcolepsy; many otherwise healthy people may experience it occasionally.

Like sleep paralysis, sleep-related hallucinations—medically termed *hypnagogic phenomena*—usually occur just prior to sleep, or sometimes upon awakening. The affected individual may hear sounds that aren't there and/or see illusions. These visual and auditory illusions are very vivid. This phenomenon also can occur in individuals who do not suffer from narcolepsy, particularly in children.

Because the symptoms of narcolepsy vary from individual to individual (it is estimated that only 10 percent of people with narcolepsy experience all four of the classic symptoms), this disorder is frequently misdiagnosed. Further compounding the problem is the fact that other sleep disorders, such as sleep apnea, also can produce spells of marked daytime drowsiness. Narcolepsy is not a particularly dangerous problem, unless one experiences a sleep attack while operating a motor vehicle or other machinery. It can, however, be embarrassing and extremely inconvenient. The cause or causes of this disorder are unknown, but brain infection, head trauma, or brain tumors may be behind some cases. It is known that narcolepsy is almost never the result of insomnia or sleep deprivation. There is currently no cure for this disorder, so the focus must be on treating the symptoms.

Unless otherwise specified, the dosages recommended here are for adults. For a child between the ages of twelve and seventeen, reduce the dose to three-quarters the recommended amount. For a child between six and twelve, use one-half the recommended dose, and for a child under the age of six, use one-quarter the recommended amount.

NUTRIENTS

SUPPLEMENT	SUGGESTED DOSAGE	COMMENTS
Essential		
Calcium and magnesium	2,000 mg daily, at bedtime. 400 mg twice during the day and at bedtime.	Needed for energy production and the nervous system.
Choline or lecithin granules or capsules	300 mg daily. 1 tbsp 3 times daily, before meals. 1,200 mg 3 times daily, before meals.	Acts as a neurotransmitter and is important for brain function. A good source of choline.
Chromium picolinate	100 mcg daily.	Boosts energy and regulates sugar metabolism.
Coenzyme Q_{10} plus Coenzyme A from Coenzyme-A Technologies	As directed on label. As directed on label.	Promotes circulation to the brain.
Free-form amino acid complex (Amino Balance from Anabol Naturals)	As directed on label.	Increases energy levels; needed for proper brain function. Use a formula that contains all the essential amino acids.
L-Glutamine	As directed on label, on an empty stomach. Take with water or juice. Do not take with milk. Take with 50 mg vitamin B_6 and 100 mg vitamin C for better absorption.	Promotes mental ability. Known as brain fuel because it can pass the blood-brain barrier freely. (*See* AMINO ACIDS in Part One.)
L-Tyrosine	As directed on label. Take at bedtime.	Important in thyroid function. Low levels have been associated with narcolepsy. *Caution:* Do not take tyrosine if you are taking an MAO inhibitor drug.
Multivitamin and mineral complex	As directed on label.	All nutrients are needed to balance body functioning.
Nicotinamide adenine dinucleotide (NADH)	As directed on label.	Important in the creation and transfer of chemical energy, especially during breathing.
Octocosanol	100 mg daily.	Increases oxygen utilization and boosts endurance.
Omega-3 essential fatty acids (fish oil and flaxseed oil are good sources)	As directed on label.	To protect cell membranes.
Vitamin B complex (Coenzymate B Complex from Source Naturals) plus extra vitamin B_6 (pyridoxine)	150 mg of each major B vitamin daily (amounts of individual vitamins in a complex will vary). 200 mg daily.	B vitamins boost metabolism and are essential for increased energy levels and normal brain function.
Vitamin C with bioflavoinoids	2,000–6,000 mg daily, in divided doses.	Increases energy and promotes production of interferon in the body to protect against free radical damage.
Vitamin D_3	400 IU daily.	Essential for calcium absorption.
Vitamin E	400–600 IU daily.	Increases circulation and protects heart functioning and brain cells. Use d-alpha-tocopherol form.

HERBS

❏ Ephedra, gotu kola, and St. John's wort boost energy levels and possess antioxidant properties as well.

❏ Ginkgo biloba improves circulation to the brain and is a powerful antioxidant for protecting cells.

RECOMMENDATIONS

❏ Eat a low-fat diet high in cleansing foods such as leafy green vegetables and sea vegetables. Also eat foods high in the B vitamins, such as brewer's yeast and brown rice.

❏ Eat foods high in protein (meats, poultry, cheese, nuts, seeds, and soy products) in the middle of the day, and save the complex carbohydrates (fresh fruits and vegetables, legumes, natural whole grains, and pasta) for the evening meal. High-protein foods increase alertness, whereas carbohydrates have a calming effect and can promote sleepiness.

❏ Include in the diet foods rich in the amino acid tyrosine. Good choices include eggs, oats, poultry, and wheat germ.

Caution: If you are taking an MAO inhibitor drug, *avoid* foods containing tyrosine, as drug and dietary interactions can cause a sudden, dangerous rise in blood pressure. Discuss food and medicine limitations thoroughly with your health care provider or a qualified dietitian.

❏ Avoid alcohol and sugar. They may seem stimulating initially, but will only make you tired later.

❏ Exercise daily to improve circulation and oxygenate tissues.

❏ Napping can rejuvenate you when you have lost sleep. Take up to a forty-five-minute nap in the early afternoon.

❏ Make sure your home and workplace are well lit, either by natural sunlight or overhead lighting. Light suppresses the production of melatonin, which is the hormone that produces drowsiness. Full-spectrum light bulbs are best.

CONSIDERATIONS

❏ Narcolepsy and sleep apnea are the leading causes of tiredness during the day.

❏ A diagnosis of narcolepsy may involve a *multiple sleep latency test* (MSLT), usually conducted in a sleep disorders clinic.

❏ Irregular sleep patterns are just as likely to cause drowsiness as lack of sleep. Jet lag, shift work, inconsistent bedtimes, and weekend partying can all disturb our natural sleep/wake cycles. America is a nation of sleep-starved yawners fighting a daily battle against the sandman. We live in a world where people drive themselves on relentless schedules that leave insufficient time for quality sleep.

❏ There have been some documented cases in which persons who suffered from narcolepsy were cured by eliminating allergenic foods from the diet. One person, for instance, was found to have an allergy to potatoes. When he removed potatoes from his diet, he no longer experienced the symptoms. (*See* ALLERGIES in Part Two.)

❏ There is some evidence that the immune systems of people who suffer from narcolepsy may react abnormally to the chemical processes in the brain that cause sleep.

❏ Certain dogs, mainly Doberman pinschers, have been observed to sleep excessively and to collapse when overstimulated. Research has revealed a withering away of axons (the "communication cables" that convey signals between nerve cells) in the brains of these animals, especially in three regions of the brain that have been linked to sleep inhibition, motor control, and the processing of emotions. If similar degeneration can be demonstrated in human brains, this may offer further clues as to the causes of narcolepsy.

❏ Doctors have traditionally prescribed stimulants (amphetamines) and antidepressants for people with narcolepsy. A newer drug, modafinil (Provigil), acts on the hypothalamus, a part of the brain responsible for wakefulness, and may reduce sleep attacks. This drug should not be used by people with heart conditions, liver dysfunction, or a history of mental illness, and it can reduce the effectiveness of certain birth control methods.

❏ *See also* the discussion of sleep apnea *under* INSOMNIA in Part Two.

Nausea and Vomiting

See under FOODBORNE/WATERBORNE DISEASE; INDIGESTION. *See also under* INFLUENZA.

Nephritis

See under KIDNEY DISEASE.

Nervousness

See ANXIETY DISORDER; STRESS.

Nickel Toxicity

Nickel is a silver-white metal used to produce steel, nickel-cadmium batteries, nickel plating, heating fuel, and ceramics. It has been described as a trace mineral and is present in many cells within the human body. Small amounts of nickel are useful in certain bodily functions. For example, minute amounts of nickel are important in DNA and RNA stabilization. Nickel may play a role in the metabolism of glucose and hormonal functions. It also helps to activate certain important enzymes, such as trypsin and arginase. A nickel deficiency may affect iron and zinc metabolism.

Too much nickel can be toxic, however. Nickel carbonyl is the most toxic form of this metal. Lethal exposure to nickel through inhalation causes nausea, dizziness, diarrhea, headache, vomiting, chest pain, weakness, and coughing. Contact with the vapor can lead to brain and liver swelling; degeneration of the liver; irritation to the eyes, throat, and nose; and cancer. Although toxic levels of nickel have not been established, it is known that the presence of excess amounts of nickel can cause dermatitis (skin rash and inflammation), also called "nickel itch," and respiratory illness, and can interfere with the Kreb's cycle, a series of enzymatic reactions necessary for cellular energy production. Significant levels of nickel may also contribute to thyroid malfunction, or myocardial infarction (heart attack). Environmental exposure to nickel can occur by contact with automobile exhaust, cigarette smoke, manufacturing emissions, and airborne dust. Skin absorption can come from coins, hairpins, jewelry, prosthetic joints and heart valves, and nickel plating.

Many foods naturally contain some amount of nickel. These include bananas, barley, beans, buckwheat, cabbage hazelnuts, legumes, lentils, oats, pears, soybeans, and walnuts. Nickel can also be present in hydrogenated fats and oils, refined and processed foods, baking powder, cocoa powder, superphosphate fertilizers, and tobacco smoke. Using cooking utensils containing nickel may add unnecessarily to your dietary intake of nickel.

NUTRIENTS

SUPPLEMENT	SUGGESTED DOSAGE	COMMENTS
Important		
Apple pectin	As directed on label.	Binds toxic metals and removes them from the body.
Garlic (Kyolic from Wakunaga)	As directed on label.	Acts as a detoxifier and aids in removing harmful metals.

Kelp	1,000–1,500 mg daily.	Supplies minerals and iodine to aid in removing toxic metals.
L-Cysteine and L-methionine	As directed on label, on an empty stomach. Take with water or juice. Do not take with milk. Take with 50 mg vitamin B$_6$ and 100 mg vitamin C for better absorption.	Helps to detoxify the body, including the liver, of harmful metals. (*See* AMINO ACIDS in Part One.)
Selenium	200 mcg daily. If you are pregnant, do not exceed 40 mcg daily.	A powerful free radical destroyer.
Vitamin A with mixed carotenoids plus	25,000 IU daily. If you are pregnant, do not exceed 10,000 IU daily.	A powerful antioxidant that destroys free radicals.
natural beta-carotene	15,000 IU daily.	A free radical scavenger.
Vitamin C with bioflavonoids including rutin	4,000–10,000 mg daily.	Helps to remove metals from the body and strengthens immunity.
Vitamin E	400 IU daily.	A powerful free radical scavenger that also improves circulation. Use d-alpha-tocopherol form.

RECOMMENDATIONS

❑ If you suspect you may have symptoms of metal toxicity, have a hair analysis done to detect toxic levels of nickel and other minerals. (*See* HAIR ANALYSIS in Part Three.)

❑ Avoid processed food products, as well as any products containing hydrogenated fats and oils.

❑ Do not smoke, and avoid those who do.

❑ Beware of metal cookware, especially when preparing acidic foods, such as tomato sauce. Use glass cookware instead. Also avoid using metal cooking utensils. Use utensils made from plastic or wood instead (wood is best).

❑ Ask your dentist about the metal content of the materials he or she uses. Nickel toxicity can result from nickel alloys used in dental surgery and appliances.

❑ If your job or hobby involves using nickel to plate metals, use a face mask while working. Inhalation of nickel can cause pulmonary edema (accumulation of fluid in the lungs).

CONSIDERATIONS

❑ Chelation can remove toxic metals from the body. (*See* CHELATION THERAPY in Part Three.)

❑ Aside from being potentially toxic, nickel is often allergenic. The nickel in watchbands, zippers, bra closures, pierced earrings, and other everyday items has been associated with many allergic reactions. A high incidence of allergic reactions to nickel in pierced earrings has been reported among children. Many earrings and posts contain nickel. Gold (14-karat or higher) is probably the safest metal for pierced earrings. (*See* CHEMICAL ALLERGIES in Part Two.)

Nosebleed

Any injury to the tissues inside the nose can cause a nosebleed. Injury can result from a blow to the nose; the intrusion of foreign objects (including fingers); a sudden change in atmospheric pressure; or simply blowing the nose too forcefully. Winter often brings about nosebleeds because heated air tends to be dry. Excessive dryness can cause the nasal membranes to crack, form crusts, and bleed.

In some cases, nosebleeds—medically termed *epistaxis*—can be associated with an underlying illness. Arteriosclerosis, high blood pressure, malaria, scarlet fever, sinusitis, and typhoid fever are all known to cause nosebleeds, some of which can be serious and result in significant blood loss. Conditions that cause increased bleeding tendencies, such as hemophilia, leukemia, thrombocytopenia (a below-normal concentration of platelets in the blood), aplastic anemia, or liver disease, also may be implicated in nosebleeds.

Nosebleeds are much more common in children than in adults. This is no doubt largely due to the fact that children are prone to inserting their fingers and other objects into their nostrils. In addition, children's tissues, including the mucous membranes lining the nose, are thinner than those of adults and therefore more susceptible to damage.

There are two classifications of nosebleeds, depending on where in the nose the blood is coming from. *Posterior nosebleeds* primarily afflict elderly people and those with high blood pressure. In this type of nosebleed, blood comes from the rear of the nose and runs down the back of the mouth into the throat, no matter what position the person is in. The blood is usually dark red in color, although it can be bright red. If the bleeding is severe, blood can flow from the nostrils as well.

The overwhelming majority of nosebleeds are *anterior nosebleeds,* in which bright-red blood flows from the front part of the nose. Most often they are the result of some type of trauma to the nasal tissues. If the person stands or sits, the flow of blood comes out of one or both nostrils. If the person lies on his or her back, the blood may flow backward, into the throat. This type of nosebleed can be frightening, and it may look as if there is a lot of blood, but in reality it is not usually serious and very little blood is actually lost.

NUTRIENTS

SUPPLEMENT	SUGGESTED DOSAGE	COMMENTS
Helpful		
Bioflavonoid complex with rutin	As directed on label.	Deficiencies have been linked to nosebleeds.
Vitamin C with bioflavonoids	3,000 mg when bleeding starts and 1,000 mg every hour thereafter until bleeding has completely stopped.	Promotes healing.

HERBS

❑ If your nasal membranes become sore from dryness, use aloe vera gel, calendula ointment, or comfrey ointment as needed.

❑ A snuff made from finely ground oak bark is soothing and healing.

❑ To promote healing, rub a small amount of Calendula Ointment from Natureworks into each nostril once the bleeding subsides. Repeat as needed.

RECOMMENDATIONS

❑ To stop an anterior nosebleed, do the following:

1. Sit up in a chair and lean forward (*do not* tilt your head back). Do not put your head between your legs or lie flat on your back.

2. Pinch all the soft parts of the nose together between your thumb and index finger for approximately ten minutes. The pressure should be firm but not painful. Breathe through your mouth.

3. Apply crushed ice or cold washcloths to your nose, neck, and cheeks. This can be done both as you apply pressure (*see* No. 2, above) and afterwards.

4. Then lie back until the bleeding subsides. Refrain from any physical activity for a few hours and any vigorous exercise for at least two days.

5. If the bleeding does not stop, place a cloth or piece of cotton moistened with water or an over-the-counter decongestant spray into the nasal cavity. Hold your nostrils together tightly for about five minutes.

❑ To help stop a nosebleed, try rolling a piece of cotton or gauze and place it in the top part of your upper lip, under the gum. An artery supplying blood to the nose is located in this region. Applying pressure in this manner may help constrict the blood flow.

❑ If you suspect a posterior nosebleed, consult your doctor. This type of nosebleed requires the care of a physician.

❑ Do not blow your nose for at least twelve hours after a nosebleed stops. Doing so may dislodge the blood clots that stanch bleeding.

❑ Once bleeding is controlled and healing has begun, apply a small amount of vitamin E to the affected tissues— open a capsule and *gently* apply the oil inside the nose. If vitamin E is unavailable, use a little petroleum jelly or A&D Ointment. If you wish, pack the nose with gauze to prevent leakage.

❑ While healing, eat plenty of foods high in vitamin K, which is essential for normal blood clotting. Good sources include alfalfa, kale, and all dark green leafy vegetables.

❑ Avoid foods high in salicylates, aspirinlike substances found in tea, coffee, most fruits, and some vegetables. Foods to avoid include apples, apricots, almonds, all ber-ries, cloves, cherries, cucumbers, currants, grapes, mint, oil of wintergreen, bell peppers, peaches, pickles, plums, raisins, tangelos, and tomatoes.

❑ To counteract dryness in the nasal passages, especially during the winter, use nasal irrigation. Spray inside the nostrils with plain warm water or a saline mist spray from time to time.

❑ To prevent nosebleeds, increase the environmental humidity, especially in winter. Use a cool mist humidifer, a vaporizer, or even a pan of water placed near a radiator.

❑ When you sneeze, keep your mouth open.

❑ If you have frequent nosebleeds, see your doctor. The cause of frequent nosebleeds is often an underlying problem such as hypertension, which should be treated.

❑ If you are prone to nosebleeds, an iron supplement may help to rebuild the blood. Iron is an important component in hemoglobin, which is a vital element in red blood cells.

Caution: Do not take iron supplements unless anemia has been diagnosed.

CONSIDERATIONS

❑ If packing the nose with gauze or cotton is necessary to stem the flow of blood, some medical authorities recommend moistening the packing material with white vinegar. They contend that the acid in white vinegar gently cauterizes broken blood vessels and aids in stopping the bleeding.

❑ Sometimes the use of drugs that thin the blood, such as the anticoagulants warfarin (Coumadin) or heparin, may cause nosebleeds. Even aspirin can act as an anticoagulant and interfere with blood clotting, which is necessary in stopping nosebleeds.

❑ High estrogen levels increase the flow of blood from the mucous membranes in the nose. This is why nosebleeds are more common during pregnancy. Oral contraceptives also can contribute to nosebleeds.

❑ The risk of serious nosebleeds increases with hemophilia, Hodgkin's disease, rheumatic fever, vitamin C deficiency, or the prolonged use of nose drops or nasal sprays.

❑ Nosebleeds are common among alcoholics. As alcohol dilates blood vessels, including those in the nasal cavities, the vessels bleed more easily. Heavy alcohol use can also create problems with blood clotting because of the toxic effects of alcohol on the liver and bone marrow.

❑ People with hypertension are especially prone to nosebleeds. A low-fat, low-cholesterol diet is recommended for keeping blood pressure under control. (*See* HIGH BLOOD PRESSURE in Part Two.)

❑ If you have recurring nosebleeds, your doctor may recommend surgical or chemical treatment. In some situations, topical chemical solutions are applied to the blood vessels to constrict the blood flow. If topical applications are unsuccessful, nasal blood vessels can be constricted through cauterization (surgical burning of tissues), using either a chemical solution or an electrical heating tool. If all of the above measures fail, both sides of the nasal cavity may be packed with a spongelike or gauze material. Nasal packing is almost always a standard procedure when an anterior nosebleed will not stop bleeding. Your physician may not remove the packs for two to five days.

☐ *See also under* PREGNANCY-RELATED PROBLEMS in Part Two.

Obesity

Obesity is, quite simply, an excess of body fat. Usually, anyone who is 20 percent over the normal weight for his or her age, sex, build, and height is considered obese. According to the Mayo Clinic in Rochester, Minnesota, a person's weight is healthy if it falls within the acceptable range for his or her height and age; if the pattern of fat distribution does not place the person at increased risk for certain diseases; and if the person has no medical problem for which a physician recommends that he or she lose weight.

Being overweight is a contributing cause of many preventable illnesses. How much a person weighs is only part of the story, however. Perhaps more important than weight is the percentage of fat in the body. For healthy women, fat can account for as much as 25 percent of body weight; 17 percent is a healthy percentage for men. Women's bodies are designed to carry a higher proportion of fat tissue to ensure that there is plenty of fuel for pregnancy and nursing, even if food is scarce.

The average human body has 30 to 40 billion fat cells. Most of the extra calories we eat that we do not need for immediate energy are stored as fat. If we were still "hunter/ gatherers" like our early ancestors, the fat would provide a needed food store for times when no food is readily available. In fact, some researchers believe that our seemingly innate love of high-calorie (especially fatty) foods may be a remnant of a survival tactic from ancient times, when we needed to store food for energy. But in modern society, storing energy as fat is no longer necessary for most people. Most Americans wait no more than four hours between meals and snacks. So instead of being a valuable survival mechanism, the body's ability to store fat now is more likely to have a profoundly negative effect on health. As fat accumulates, it crowds the space occupied by the internal organs. Obesity—even moderate overweight—puts an undue stress on the back, legs, and internal organs, and this can eventually exacerbate many physical problems and compromise health. Obesity increases the body's resistance to insulin and susceptibility to infection, and puts one at a higher risk for developing coronary artery disease, diabetes, gallbladder disease, high blood pressure, kidney disease, stroke, and other serious health problems that can

result in premature death. Complications of pregnancy and liver damage also are more common in overweight individuals. Obese persons suffer psychologically as well as physically, because our society tends to equate beauty, intelligence, and even success with thinness.

The most common causes of obesity are poor diet and/or eating habits and a lack of exercise. Other factors that can lead to obesity include glandular malfunctions, diabetes, hypoglycemia, hyperinsulinemia, emotional tension, boredom, and a simple love of food. Obesity has also been linked to food sensitivities and/or allergies. It is strongly suggested that heredity is another causal factor for obesity. The discovery of the "obesity gene" was a major breakthrough in the study of obesity. Ironically, poor nutrition may be an important factor in obesity. When there is inadequate intake of certain essential nutrients, fat is not easily or adequately burned and can accumulate in the body.

Obesity is a serious health problem and, according to the U.S. Centers for Disease Control and Prevention, it is on the rise in the United States. At least one third of Americans are 20 percent or more overweight. Even though this country has gone through several fitness crazes in recent years, Americans today are fatter, more stressed out, and no likelier to get regular exercise than we were ten years ago. And if we are getting fatter, it isn't because we have stopped trying to lose weight. National surveys estimate that at any given time, 25 to 50 percent of adult Americans are on some sort of diet, and we spend more than $30 billion each year on diet aids and remedies. Unfortunately, even those who lose weight often put it back on. It is estimated that two-thirds of those who lose weight regain the lost pounds within three to five years.

Traditionally, there are three basic approaches to weight management through nutritional supplementation. The first is the use of diuretic herbs and nutrients to reduce water retention. The second is the use of lipotropic vitamins, which have the ability to reduce cholesterol and fat. Third is the use of natural appetite suppressants. Permanent weight loss, however, requires a lifetime commitment to a healthier lifestyle in general.

NUTRIENTS

SUPPLEMENT	SUGGESTED DOSAGE	COMMENTS
Very Important		
Aerobic Bulk Cleanse from Aerobic Life Industries or psyllium husks	As directed on label. Always take supplemental fiber separately from other supplements and medications. 1 tbsp ¹/₂ hour before meals with a large glass of liquid. Drink it quickly.	Especially good for high or low blood sugar problems and also provides fiber. Gives a full feeling, cutting down hunger pangs.
Chromium picolinate	200–600 mcg daily.	Reduces sugar cravings by stabilizing the metabolism of simple carbohydrates (sugars).

Dimethylamino-ethanol (DMAE)	As directed on label.	Increases vitality.
Essential fatty acids (flaxseed oil, primrose oil, and salmon oil are good sources)	As directed on label.	Use these with a low-fat diet to provide essential fatty acids, needed by every cell in the body and for appetite control.
Kelp	1,000–1,500 mg daily.	Contains balanced minerals and iodine. Aids in weight loss.
Lecithin granules or capsules	1 tbsp 3 times daily, before meals. 1,200 mg 3 times daily, before meals.	A fat emulsifier; breaks down fat so it can be removed from the body.
Spirulina or Spiru-tein from Nature's Plus	As directed on label 3 times daily. Take between meals.	Excellent sources of usable protein. Contains needed nutrients and stabilizes blood sugar. Can replace a meal.
Vitamin C with bioflavonoids	3,000–6,000 mg daily.	Necessary for normal glandular function. Speeds up a slow metabolism, prompting it to burn more calories.

Helpful

Calcium	1,500 mg daily.	Involved in activation of lipase, an enzyme that breaks down fats for utilization by the body.
Choline and inositol	As directed on label.	Helps the body burn fat.
Coenzyme Q_{10} plus	As directed on label.	Necessary for energy.
Coenzyme A from Coenzyme-A Technologies	As directed on label.	Improves the effect of coenzyme Q_{10}, metabolizes fat, and may aid in weight loss.
Dehydroepiandro-sterone (DHEA)	As directed on label.	Inhibits an enzyme that is involved in fat production.
Gamma-amino-butyric acid (GABA)	As directed on label.	Suppresses cravings and has antidepressant qualities. (See AMINO ACIDS in Part One.)
5-Hydroxy L-tryptophan (5-HTP)	As directed on label.	Suppresses appetite. Caution: Do not use if you are pregnant or nursing.
L-Arginine and L-ornithine plus L-lysine	500 mg each or as directed on label, before bedtime. Take on an empty stomach with water or juice. Do not take with milk. Take with 50 mg vitamin B_6 and 100 mg vitamin C for better absorption.	These amino acids decrease body fat. (See AMINO ACIDS in Part One.) Caution: Do not take these supplements if you have diabetes. Do not take arginine or ornithine without lysine.
L-Carnitine	500 mg daily.	Has the ability to break up fat deposits and aids in weight loss.
L-Glutamine	As directed on label.	Lessens carbohydrate cravings.
L-Methionine	As directed on label.	Assists in the breakdown of fat.
L-Phenylalanine	As directed on label, on an empty stomach.	An appetite suppressant that tells the brain you are not hungry. (See AMINO ACIDS in Part One.) Caution: Do not take this supplement if you are pregnant or nursing, or suffer from panic attacks, diabetes, high blood pressure, or PKU.

L-Tyrosine	As directed on label. Take at bedtime.	Suppresses cravings and has antidepressant qualities. (See AMINO ACIDS in Part One.) Caution: Do not take tyrosine if you are taking an MAO inhibitor drug.
Maitake extract	As directed on label.	Aids in weight loss.
Multivitamin and mineral complex with potassium	As directed on label. 99 mg daily.	Obesity and nutritional deficiency are parts of the same syndrome. Important in the production of energy. Sodium and potassium levels must be balanced.
Pyruvate	As directed on label.	Promotes weight loss and may aid in reducing body fat.
Taurine	As directed on label.	Taurine is the building block for all other amino acids; aids in the digestion of fats.
Vitamin B complex plus extra vitamin B_2 (riboflavin) and vitamin B_3 (niacin) and vitamin B_6 (pyridoxine) and vitamin B_{12} and para-aminobenzoic acid (PABA)	50 mg of each major B vitamin 3 times daily. (amounts of individual vitamins in a complex will vary.) 50 mg 3 times daily. 50 mg 3 times daily. Do not exceed this amount. 50 mg 3 times daily. 1,000 mcg 3 times daily. As directed on label.	Needed for proper digestion. Required for efficiency in burning calories. Lessens sugar cravings. Caution: Do not take niacin if you have a liver disorder, gout, or high blood pressure. Boosts metabolism. Needed for proper digestion and absorption. A sublingual form is best. Aids in carbohydrate and protein utilization.
Zinc plus copper	80 mg daily. Do not exceed a total of 100 mg daily from all supplements. 3 mg daily.	Enhances the effectiveness of insulin and boosts immune function. Use zinc gluconate lozenges or OptiZinc for best absorption. Needed to balance with zinc.

HERBS

❑ Alfalfa, corn silk, dandelion, gravel root, horsetail, hydrangea, hyssop, juniper berries, oat straw, parsley, seawrack, thyme, uva ursi, white ash, and yarrow can be used in tea form for their diuretic properties.

❑ Aloe vera juice improves digestion and cleanses the digestive tract.

❑ Amla is an Ayurvedic herb that helps to increase lean body mass and reduce fat.

❑ Astragalus increases energy and improves nutrient absorption.

Caution: Do not use this herb in the presence of a fever.

❑ Borage seed, hawthorn berry, licorice root, and sarsaparilla stimulate the adrenal glands and improve thyroid function.

Caution: If overused, licorice can elevate blood pressure. Avoid it completely if you have high blood pressure. Do not use this herb on a daily basis for more than seven days in a row.

❑ Butcher's broom, cardamom, cayenne, cinnamon, ephedra (ma huang), *Garcinia cambogia*, ginger, green tea (which has gained a great deal of attention for its ability to aid in weight loss), and mustard seed are thermogenic herbs that improve digestion and aid in the metabolism of fat.

Caution: Do not use cinnamon in large quantities during pregnancy. Use extreme caution when taking any products containing ephedra. It has been known to cause adverse side effects, including nausea, irregular heartbeat, anxiety, chest pains, heart palpitations, high blood pressure, insomnia, and, in rare cases, even death. Do not use it at all if you suffer from anxiety, glaucoma, heart disease, high blood pressure, irregular heart rhythm, or insomnia, or if you are taking a monoamine oxidase (MAO) inhibitor drug for depression.

❑ Chlorella, gudmar, schizandra, and suma aid in glucose utilization, hormone, neural regulation, and digestion.

❑ Citrin is a trademarked name for a standardized herbal extract from the fruit of the *Garcinia cambogia* plant, also known as Indian berry. Tests have shown it to be a safe and effective method of inhibiting the synthesis of fatty acids in the liver, promoting the burning of body fat as fuel, and suppressing the appetite. It may also prevent or slow the development of atherosclerosis and heart disease.

❑ Fennel removes mucus and fat from the intestinal tract and is a natural appetite suppressant.

❑ Fenugreek is useful for dissolving fat within the liver.

❑ Gotu kola aids in reducing body mass and aids in adrenal processes that facilitate carbohydrate metabolism. It also increases energy.

❑ Guarana and kola nut are appetite suppressants.

❑ Guggul, an ancient Ayurvedic herbal remedy, helps to normalize blood cholesterol and triglyceride levels. It also has a mildly stimulating effect on the thyroid.

❑ Siberian ginseng aids in moving fluids and nutrients throughout the body and reduces the stress of adjusting to new eating habits.

Caution: Do not use this herb if you have hypoglycemia, high blood pressure, or a heart disorder.

❑ Trifala is an Ayurvedic herbal remedy that rejuvenates glandular balance and stimulates thyroid hormones with long-term use.

❑ Turmeric strengthens digestion, increases energy, and cleanses the blood.

RECOMMENDATIONS

❑ Do not worry as much about the number of calories you consume as about eating the proper foods. Rotate your foods, and be sure to eat a variety of foods. Eat meals that consist of a balance of proteins, complex carbohydrates,

and some fat. Proteins can increase your metabolic rate by as much as 30 percent and help to balance the release of insulin by prompting secretion of the pancreatic hormone glucagon. Protein-induced glucagon mobilizes fats from the tissues in which it is stored, thus aiding in weight loss. By eating balanced meals you get more steady blood sugar levels and the ability to burn stored body fat for long-term weight loss.

❑ Eat more complex carbohydrates that also offer protein, such as tofu, lentils, plain baked potatoes (no toppings, except for vegetables), sesame seeds, beans, brown rice, whole grains, skinless turkey or chicken breast, and white-fish (no shellfish). Poultry and fish should be broiled or baked, never fried.

❑ Eat fresh fruits and an abundance of raw vegetables. Have one meal each day that consists entirely of vegetables and fruits. Use low-calorie vegetables such as broccoli, cabbage, carrots, cauliflower, celery, cucumbers, green beans, kale, lettuce, onions, radishes, spinach, and turnips. Low-calorie, low-carbohydrate fruits include apples, cantaloupe, grapefruit, strawberries, and watermelon. The following are higher in calories and should be consumed in moderation: bananas, cherries, corn, figs, grapes, green peas, hominy, pears, pineapple, sweet potatoes, white rice, and yams.

❑ Eat foods raw, if possible. If foods are heated, they should be baked, broiled, steamed, or boiled. Never consume fried or greasy foods.

❑ Drink six to eight glasses of liquids daily. Herbal teas and steam-distilled water with trace minerals (such as ConcenTrace from Trace Minerals Research) added are good. Taken before meals, they help to reduce your appetite. They are nonfattening fillers that also help to dilute toxins and flush them out of the body. Herbal teas mixed with unsweetened fruit juice are very satisfying low-calorie drinks and are also very filling. Use these between meals and when a desire for sweets hits you. Drink sparkling water mixed with fruit juice in place of sodas.

❑ Pay particular attention to the fat in your diet. Some fat is necessary, but it must be the right kind. Avocados, olives, olive oil, raw nuts and seeds, and wheat and corn germ are sources of "good" fats that contain essential fatty acids. Use these foods in moderation—no more than twice a week. Eliminate saturated fats from the diet completely. Avoid animal fat, found in butter, cream, gravies, ice cream, mayonnaise, meat, rich dressings, and whole milk. Do not eat any fried foods.

❑ Consume the following foods in moderation: apples, brown rice, buckwheat, chestnuts, corn, grapes, oatmeal, white potatoes, and yellow vegetables. These foods contain small amounts of essential fatty acids, but they should not be overused.

❑ If you must eat snacks occasionally to ward off hunger, make sure they are healthy. Good choices include:

- Celery and carrot sticks.

- Low-fat cottage cheese topped with fresh applesauce and walnuts.

- Unsweetened gelatin made with fruit juice in place of sugar and water.

- Natural sugar-free whole-grain muffins.

- Freshly made unsalted popcorn.

- Rice cakes topped with nut butter (but not peanut butter).

- Watermelon, fresh fruit, or frozen fruit popsicles.

- Unsweetened low-fat yogurt topped with granola or nuts and fresh fruit.

❑ Do not eat any white flour products, salt, white rice, or processed foods. Also, avoid fast food restaurants and all junk foods.

❑ Do not consume sweets such as soda, pastries, pies, cakes, doughnuts, or candy. Omit all forms of refined sugar (including white sugar, brown sugar, and corn sweetener) from the diet. Sugar triggers the release of insulin, which then activates enzymes that promote the passage of fat from the bloodstream into the fat cells.

❑ Follow a fasting program once monthly. (*See* FASTING in Part Three.)

❑ Spirulina aids in fighting obesity. Take it thirty minutes before meals to decrease your appetite. Spirulina also sustains energy, aids in detoxification, and aids in maintaining proper bowel function.

❑ Avoid eating before bedtime and during the night. Supplementation with melatonin may help with this. "Night eaters" often have low melatonin levels.

❑ Use wheatgrass to calm the appetite. This is a very nutritious fuel from whole food that assists metabolic functions. Kelp is also beneficial.

❑ Do not consume alcohol in any form, including beer and wine. Alcohol not only adds calories, but it inhibits the burning of fat from fat deposits. It can also interfere with your judgment, so you may find yourself eating things you ordinarily would not.

❑ Use powdered barley malt sweetener (found in health food stores) instead of sugar. This is highly concentrated but not dangerous. It contains only 3 calories per gram (approximately 2 teaspoons). This sweetener is also beneficial for people with diabetes or hypoglycemia.

❑ Use extra fiber daily. Guar gum and psyllium husks are good sources. Take fiber with a large glass of liquid one-half hour before meals.

Note: Always take supplemental fiber separately from other supplements and medications.

❑ Move your bowels daily. A clean colon is important in stabilizing your weight. (*See* COLON CLEANSING in Part Three.)

❑ Keep a diet diary to help you keep track of what you eat, the caloric and fat content of what you eat, and what triggers your eating. This can help you to pinpoint and eliminate trigger factors (such as allergies or depression), as well as let you see if you are eating too much of the wrong types of foods. (*See under* ALLERGIES in Part Two.)

❑ Be active. Take a brisk walk every day before breakfast or dinner to burn off fat. Make a habit of using the stairs instead of the elevator. Walk or ride a bicycle instead of driving whenever possible. Exercise increases the metabolic rate as well as burning off calories.

❑ Be sure to get regular aerobic exercise, such as walking, running, bicycling, or swimming, *and* do exercises for strength and flexibility, such as yoga or stretching exercises. Exercise is better than an overly strict diet for maintaining your health and controlling your weight. It is the best way to rid the body of fat and to maintain good muscle tone. Be sure to drink water during exercise to prevent dehydration and muscle cramps.

Caution: If you are over thirty-five and/or have been sedentary for some time, consult your health care provider before beginning an exercise program.

❑ If you have been sedentary for some time, try exercising in water. Water aerobics are excellent for those who are overweight or who find running or walking difficult. They are also good for arthritis sufferers. Water aerobics tone the body and strengthen the heart without straining the joints. Start by taking a class at a local fitness center or YMCA. Sedentary individuals should consult their health care providers before starting an exercise program.

❑ Change your eating habits. This is extremely important not only for losing weight, but for maintaining weight loss. Begin with the following:

- Always eat breakfast. It jump-starts the metabolism at the beginning of the day. Eat small but nutrient-dense meals every three to four hours throughout the day to keep your metabolism stable, to maintain a full feeling, and to avoid wide swings in blood sugar. Good choices might include a 2-ounce portion of protein food (beans, an egg, poultry) with $\frac{1}{2}$ cup fresh salad dressed with apple cider vinegar; or $\frac{1}{2}$ cup of a steamed vegetable with some type of grain ($\frac{1}{2}$ cup brown rice or a piece of whole- or multi-grain bread).

- Don't skip meals. This only intensifies hunger and food cravings.

- Make your main meal lunch, not dinner. Some people have had excellent results consuming no food after 3:00 P.M.

- At meals, put less food on your plate. Chew slowly. Stop eating as soon as you are no longer hungry—don't wait until you feel full.

❑ Try eating a small amount (200 calories or so) of complex carbohydrate prior to having a high-protein meal. This will help supply tryptophan to the brain, which in turn helps to reduce food cravings.

❑ If you get the urge to eat, put on a tight belt. This will make you uncomfortable and remind you that you want to lose that excess fat.

❑ Learn to ride out your food cravings. They peak and subside like ocean waves. When you get an urge to eat, tell yourself that you can satisfy the craving if you *really* want to. Then wait ten minutes. This ensures that your eating is conscious, not compulsive. Keep in mind that most cravings last only a few minutes. Try doing something to distract yourself. Also remember that food addiction is the same as any other addiction: That first bite only makes you want more. If you ultimately decide that you really do want that food, then decide how much is reasonable and enjoy it. *Really* enjoy it. Take one bite and savor the taste. Eat slowly.

❑ Find out what causes your cravings. A craving for salt, chocolate, or sugar may actually be an indication of an underlying condition such as a mineral deficiency, food allergy, hypoglycemia, or hypothyroidism. If you get a strong urge to snack while you're watching television, try reading a book, drinking a large glass of liquid, or taking a walk instead. If your cravings are triggered by where you are, move. If you're in the kitchen, go outside to relax, take a walk, or do yard work. If you're in the mall, avoid the food court.

❑ If you are always tired in midmorning or midday, are always craving carbohydrates, and are always hungry, you may be consuming too many simple carbohydrates. Simple carbohydrates include refined sugars and sweet fruits; complex carbohydrates, which include whole grains, peas, and beans, provide more long-term energy. (*See* Carbohydrates *under* NUTRITION, DIET, AND WELLNESS in Part One.) Protein is another long-term source of energy.

❑ Frequent bloating and water retention may be a result of excess insulin production, which makes it almost impossible to burn fat. Try lowering your carbohydrate intake and increasing your consumption of protein and fat. Excess sodium intake can also cause water retention.

❑ Consider having yourself tested for food allergies. Many people who have eliminated allergenic foods from their diets have stabilized their weight quickly.

❑ Do not chew gum. Chewing gum starts the digestive juices flowing and makes you feel hungry.

❑ Do not grocery shop on an empty stomach. You will be tempted to buy forbidden foods and will often buy more food than you need or can use before it loses its freshness.

❑ Avoid crash dieting. A very low calorie diet causes the metabolism to slow down, resulting in fewer calories being burned. Instead, increase your activity level. This will raise your metabolic rate, burn fat, and help prevent the loss of lean tissue.

❑ To maintain weight loss, calculate how many calories you need daily by multiplying your weight by 10. Then add 30 percent (about one-third) of that amount to the result. Assuming a moderate activity level, consuming anything less than that number of calories should allow you to lose weight. This is the number of calories you can consume daily without gaining the weight back.

CONSIDERATIONS

❑ The basic arithmetic of weight loss is that each pound of body fat is worth 3,500 calories. Thus, to lose 1 pound a week (a safe, reasonable goal), you must tip the calorie consumption/expenditure balance in your favor by 500 calories each day. To do this, you can, for example, lose 250 calories by drinking a glass of water flavored with lemon or lime juice instead of a can of regular soda and leaving the cheese off your sandwich at lunch, and then make up the other 250 calories by walking two and a half miles.

❑ The best way to lose weight—and virtually the only way to maintain weight loss—is to adopt a healthier, more active lifestyle. A lifestyle that includes a natural, healthy diet and regular exercise will keep you healthy; give you more energy; lower your risk of heart disease, stroke, and cancer; and still allow you to lose weight. Those who choose fad diets over such a lifestyle can count on gaining back their lost weight and more. Almost 95 percent of all dieters regain their lost weight within a year and have to diet all over again.

❑ Fad diets may produce some results, but the fact is that not only can these diets be unhealthy (particularly if you jump from one diet to the next), but once you go off the diet, the weight often returns—along with some added pounds. Much of the rapid weight loss you see with some of the diets and/or products available can be attributed to loss of water weight.

❑ Losing weight too quickly can suppress the immune system. One popular diet today, the high-protein, low-carbohydrate diet, is controversial because it can produce a state of excess *ketosis* (a process whereby the body burns stored fat for fuel) due to the absence of carbohydrates. Vital electrolytes, especially potassium, can be dangerously depleted, placing you at high risk for heart arrhythmia or heart attack. In excess, ketosis is thought by some experts to put the body in a state of starvation—it turns to its own tissues for fuel, robbing even vital internal organs. Another dieting method that is popular with many actors, actresses, and models is the starvation diet, which can have the same effect on the body. To ensure good health, any type of diet you follow should be closely monitored by a health care professional and/or a nutritionist.

❑ Repeated crash dieting is not healthy and can increase the risk of heart disease. Quick weight loss tends to come back rapidly. This rapid weight gain often results in elevated cholesterol levels and can also damage vital organs. In one study, a third of people who had gone on crash diets of 500 calories or less per day were found to have developed gallstones. The fourteen-year Framingham Heart Study showed that those whose weight changed a lot or changed often had higher death rates than other people. They also ran a greater risk of coronary heart disease. The study showed that weight fluctuation seemed to pose as great a risk of heart disease and premature death as being overweight.

❏ Thermogenesis is a term used to describe the body's natural process for burning calories. Scientists studying thermogenesis are focusing on understanding and improving the thermogenic process, which may aid in weight loss. Many new weight loss products focus on thermogenesis. Many of these products contain ephedrine, a derivative of the herb ephedra (ma huang). It is important to exercise caution when using ephedra because it can raise blood pressure and speed up the heart rate.

❏ A study by the U.S. Department of Agriculture showed that one of every four teenagers carries enough excess weight to put him or her at high risk of heart attack, stroke, colon cancer, gout, and other health problems later in life—regardless of whether the individual slims down as an adult.

❏ The American Cancer Society has found that people who regularly use artificial sweeteners tend to gain, not lose, weight. These substances seem to increase the appetite and slow down the digestive process.

❏ Researchers at Rockefeller University in New York discovered a gene in mice that, if defective, leads to obesity. When activated, the gene (called the "obesity gene" or "ob gene") apparently produces a hormonelike protein called leptin that is secreted by the fat cells into the bloodstream. The mouse gene is said to be 85 percent identical to its human counterpart. Its discovery may eventually lead to the development of effective drugs to battle obesity. It also lends credence to the theory that some people truly are predisposed to put on more weight than others.

❏ A person whose body has a high ratio of muscle to fat will have a higher metabolic rate than a person of the same weight with a lower muscle-to-fat ratio, and therefore will require more calories. This is because it takes more calories to maintain muscle tissue than fat tissue. Conversely, obese persons tend to have lower than normal metabolic rates. Unfortunately, this can make the battle to lose weight that much more difficult and frustrating.

❏ The body mass index (BMI) is what most experts look at to determine whether or not a person is overweight. This is a calculation that uses your weight and height to determine your total body fat. (See the table on page 546.)

❏ Calories derived from fat are more easily converted into flab than calories from other sources. Only 3 percent of fat calories are burned in the digestive process. By contrast, 25 percent of calories from complex carbohydrates (fruits, vegetables, whole grains) are burned in the course of digestion.

❏ Many people feel the need to eat something sweet after meals, but this is an acquired habit and it *can* be broken. In many cultures, sweetened foods are reserved only for rare special occasions (and even then are less sweet-tasting than many of the foods Americans eat every day). It may take some time to break the cycle, but if you stick with it you will eventually realize that you no longer even want sweets very often. You will also probably find that virtually all other foods taste much better. In fact, once your taste buds recover from years of overexposure to sugar, you will be surprised to discover just how heavily sweetened many food products are.

❏ Eating a low-fat diet that is high in complex carbohydrates does *not* mean eating tasteless, bland foods. There are many delicious and healthy foods available that can be eaten. The goal is to reduce the total fat, saturated fat, and cholesterol in the diet and to increase the amount of complex carbohydrates. Potatoes, pasta, breads, corn, rice, and other complex-carbohydrate-rich foods are not the cause of obesity, as some people think. They are the cure. The exception to this rule involves people who are addicted to carbohydrates. Carbohydrate addicts respond to carbohydrates the way alcoholics respond to alcohol. When they consume carbohydrates, it results in a release of insulin that is even greater than is needed, which in turn leads to even less of a feeling of satisfaction, so the urge to eat sets in again. Because of this, carbohydrate addicts end up trying to satisfy their hunger by eating more and more carbohydrates. People who are addicted to carbohydrates should limit their intake of foods high in complex carbohydrates and avoid *all* simple carbohydrates. They should consume two low-carbohydrate meals each day and save all of their carbohydrate-rich foods for a third "reward" meal. Keeping a daily record of what you eat and when, and how you feel afterward, is a simple way to reveal possible carbohydrate addiction.

❏ Hydroxycitric acid (HCA), a substance extracted from the rind of fruit of the *Garcinia cambogia* tree, is proving very effective for weight management. Not only does it suppress hunger, but it helps to prevent the body from turning carbohydrate calories into fat by inhibiting the action of an enzyme called ATP-citrate lyase. HCA is available in supplement form and is an ingredient in various diet products.

❏ Gamma-linolenic acid (GLA), the active ingredient in borage oil, black currant seed oil, flaxseed oil, and primrose oil, helps to control the metabolism of fats. Taking at least 250 IU of GLA a day helps to control the appetite.

❏ Diet Esteem Plus from Esteem Products is a diet product that contains many of the nutrients recommended in this section plus the herbal extract HCA. Along with good nutrition and regular exercise, this product has helped many people to lose weight and maintain weight loss.

Body Mass Index

The body mass index (BMI) is a figure that represents the percentage of your body weight that is due to fat. It is determined by looking at your weight in combination with your height. The following table will give you a rough idea of your BMI.

Height	Healthy Weight (lbs) BMI = 19–25	Moderate Overweight (lbs) BMI = 25–29	Severe Overweight (lbs) BMI = 25 or over
4'10"	91–118	119–137	138 +
4'11"	94–123	124–143	144 +
5'0"	97–127	128–147	148 +
5'1"	101–131	132–152	153 +
5'2"	104–136	137–157	158 +
5'3"	107–140	141–162	163 +
5'4"	111–145	146–168	169 +
5'5"	114–149	150–173	174 +
5'6"	118–154	155–178	179 +
5'7"	121–159	160–184	185 +
5'8"	125–163	164–189	190 +
5'9"	129–168	169–195	196 +
5'10"	132–173	174–201	202 +
5'11"	136–178	179–206	207 +
6'0"	140–183	184–212	213 +
6'1"	144–188	189–218	219 +
6'2"	148–194	195–224	225 +
6'3"	152–199	200–231	232 +
6'4"	156–204	205–237	238 +

Source: U.S. Department of Agriculture and Department of Health and Human Services.

❑ A study sponsored by the U.S. Department of Agriculture revealed that the trace mineral boron may speed the burning of calories. Raisins and onions are good food sources of boron.

❑ In human studies, the hormone dehydroepiandrosterone (DHEA) has led to a loss of body fat by blocking an enzyme that is known to produce fat tissue. (See DHEA THERAPY in Part Three.)

❑ A weight-loss diet research center in England reported on using one part vegetable oil to two parts apple cider vinegar in massage to rid the body of fat. We recommend using pure virgin olive oil because it needs no refrigeration. Knead lightly but firmly over the fat areas at least three times weekly. This treatment is also good for sore and stiff joints.

❑ Obesity has been linked to causing a number of other conditions, including asthma, diabetes, gallbladder disease, heart disease, high blood pressure, hyperlipidemia (high blood fats), infertility, stroke, and certain types of cancer.

❑ Researchers have found that weight reduction can be improved with the use of a combination of the amino acids L-ornithine and L-arginine, enhanced by L-lysine (see the Nutrients table in this entry for recommended dosages). L-Ornithine helps to release growth hormone, normally lacking in adults, which burns fat and builds muscle. This combination works best while the body is at rest.

Note: Never take an amino acid that contains L-arginine but not L-lysine. Too much L-arginine without L-lysine can cause an imbalance of amino acids, possibly causing an outbreak of cold sores or previously dormant herpes.

❑ Numerous ongoing studies using genetically engineered human growth hormone (HGH) have been effective in causing weight reduction in animals. An injection or capsule for humans is years away, however. The long-term consequences of using HGH are yet unknown.

❏ Phenylpropanolamine, a common ingredient in over-the-counter appetite suppressants (and many commercial cold remedies), acts on the central nervous system and increases blood pressure. Persons with diabetes, high blood pressure, hyperthyroidism, or who have difficulty urinating, should consult a doctor before using a product containing this drug.

❏ In rare cases, if obesity is deemed to be life threatening, stomach surgery may be recommended. This is done either to restrict the amount of food consumed by creating a small pouch at the top of the stomach with a small opening to the stomach, or to bypassing the normal digestive process by creating a very small pouch and connecting it directly to the small intestine. Obviously, this is a drastic measure. It should be considered only in extreme cases, if one cannot lose enough weight by any other means to be in a healthy weight range.

❏ The U.S. Food and Drug Administration has approved the use of a synthetic fat called olestra in snack foods. A synthetic compound of fatty acids and sugar, olestra is neither absorbed nor digested by the body and therefore contributes no calories. For the same reason, however, it can cause indigestion, gas, and diarrhea. Scientists have also raised concerns over its safety because it may inhibit the absorption of necessary fat-soluble vitamins.

❏ There are many drugs on the market today that doctors may prescribe to fight obesity. All of these drugs have side effects, some of them potentially dangerous. If you are considering prescription weight-loss medication, do as much research as possible on the drugs available, and discuss with your doctor how these medications could affect your health.

❏ There are many nutritional products available today that may aid in weight reduction, including the following:

• Calorad from Enhanced Fitness, a liquid food supplement designed to help the body lose fat without losing lean muscle tissue. The primary ingredient is hydrolyzed collagen. Other ingredients are extracted from plants.

• Cell Pill from Nature's ScienCeuticals is designed to support the circulatory system in its fight to reduce the appearance of cellulite.

• CellaFree from Bodyonics is an herbal product intended to reduce the appearance of cellulite. Ingredients include uva ursi to reduce water retention and chitosan to inhibit the absorption of dietary fat.

• Cellasene from Rexall Sundown is an herbal product intended to reduce the appearance of cellulite. Ingredients include grape seed extract, sweet clover extract, bladder-wrack, and ginkgo.

• Cell-U-Lite from Växa International is designed to battle cellulite.

• CelluRid from BioTech Corporation is an herbal product

intended to reduce the appearance of cellulite. Ingredients include kelp, uva ursi, juniper berries, lecithin, milk thistle, and cayenne.

• Cravex from Natrol contains the herb *Gymnema sylvestre*, chromium picolinate, L-glutamine, and other nutrients intended to reduce food cravings, especially cravings for sweets.

• Diamond Trim from Diamond-Herpanacine Associates is intended to help appetite, reduce cravings, cleanse the system, burn calories, and increase energy.

• Diet Chrome-Care from Bluebonnet inhibits the synthesis of fats and cholesterol. This product is a combination of L-carnitine, CitriMax (a trademarked extract of *Garcinia cambogia*), and chromium picolinate.

• Diet System 6 Cellulite Removal Program from Omni Nutraceuticals is an herbal product intended to reduce the appearance of cellulite. Ingredients include gotu kola, horsetail, ginkgo, horse chestnut, and hawthorn. This supplement helps to reduce water retention.

• Tonalin 1000-CLA and Tonalin 750-CLA from Natrol is intended to promote loss of body fat without muscle loss and to increase energy. The primary ingredient is conjugated linoleic acid (CLA).

❏ More detailed information and dietary suggestions helpful for weight loss, including nutritional information and recipes, may be found in *Prescription for Dietary Wellness* by Phyllis A. Balch, C.N.C.

Oily Skin

Oily skin occurs when the sebaceous (oil-secreting) glands produce more oil than is needed for proper lubrication of the skin. This excess oil can clog pores and cause blemishes. Oily skin is probably largely a matter of heredity, but it is known to be affected by factors such as diet, hormone levels, pregnancy, birth control pills, and the cosmetics you use. Humidity and hot weather also stimulate the sebaceous glands to produce more oil. Because skin tends to become dryer with age, and because of the hormonal shifts of adolescence, oily skin is common in teenagers, but it can occur at any age. Many people have skin that is oily only in certain areas and dry or normal in others, a condition known as combination skin. In general, the forehead, nose, chin, and upper back tend to be oilier than other areas.

Oily skin has its positive aspects. It is slow to develop age spots and discoloration, fine lines, and wrinkles. It often doesn't freckle or turn red in the sun—on the contrary, it tans evenly and beautifully. On the negative side, oily skin is prone to "breakouts" well past adolescence and has a chronically shiny appearance, an oily or greasy feeling, and enlarged pores.

Unless otherwise specified, the dosages recommended here are for adults. For a child between the ages of twelve and seventeen, reduce the dose to three-quarters of the recommended amount.

NUTRIENTS

SUPPLEMENT	SUGGESTED DOSAGE	COMMENTS
Very Important		
Flaxseed oil capsules or	1,000 mg daily.	Supplies needed essential fatty acids. A good healer for most skin disorders.
liquid or	1 tsp daily.	
primrose oil	Up to 500 mg daily.	Contains linoleic acid, which is needed by the skin.
Vitamin A with mixed carotenoids	25,000 IU daily for 3 months, then reduce to 15,000 IU daily. If you are pregnant, do not exceed 10,000 IU daily.	Necessary for healing and construction of new skin tissue.
Vitamin B complex plus extra vitamin B₁₂	As directed on label. 1,000–2,000 mcg daily.	B vitamins are important for healthy skin tone.
Important		
Kelp	1,000–1,500 mg daily.	Supplies balanced minerals needed for good skin tone.
Vitamin E	Start with 400 IU daily and increase slowly to 800 IU daily.	Protects against free radicals. Use d-alpha-tocopherol form.
Zinc plus copper	50 mg daily. Do not exceed a total of 100 mg daily from all supplements. 3 mg daily.	For tissue repair. Enhances immune response. Use zinc gluconate lozenges or OptiZinc for best absorption. Needed to balance with zinc.
Helpful		
GH3 cream from Gero Vita	Apply topically as directed on label.	Good for acne. Also good for any discoloration of the skin.
Grape seed extract	As directed on label.	A powerful antioxidant that protects skin cells.
Herpanacine from Diamond-Herpanacine Associates	As directed on label.	Contains antioxidants, amino acids, and herbs that promote overall skin health.
L-Cysteine	500 mg daily, on an empty stomach. Take with water or juice. Do not take with milk. Take with 50 mg vitamin B₆ and 100 mg vitamin C for better absorption.	Contains sulfur, needed for healthy skin. (*See* AMINO ACIDS in Part One.)
Lecithin granules or capsules	1 tbsp 3 times daily, before meals. 1,200 mg 3 times daily, before meals.	Needed for better absorption of the essential fatty acids.
Superoxide dismutase (SOD)	As directed on label.	A free radical destroyer.
Tretinoin (Retin-A)	As prescribed by physician.	Acts as a gradual chemical peel; unclogs pores and speeds up sloughing off of top layers of skin, exposing new, fresh skin. Available by prescription only.

HERBS

❏ Aloe vera has excellent healing properties. Apply aloe vera gel topically, as directed on product label or as needed.

❏ Burdock root, chamomile, horsetail, oat straw, and thyme nourish the skin.

❏ Lavender is very good for oily skin. Mist your skin with lavender water several times daily.

❏ A facial sauna using lemongrass, licorice root, and rosebuds is good for oily skin. Two or three times a week, simmer a total of 2 to 4 tablespoons of dried or fresh herbs in 2 quarts of water. When the pot is steaming, place it on top of a trivet or thick potholder on a table, and sit with your face at a comfortable distance over the steam for fifteen minutes. You can use a towel to trap the steam if you wish. After fifteen minutes, splash your face with cold water and allow your skin to air dry or pat it dry with a towel. After the sauna, you can allow the herbal water to cool and save it for use as a toning lotion to be dabbed on your face with a cotton ball after cleansing.

❏ Try a steam facial using the herbal laxative Swiss Kriss twice a week to remove excess oils from the skin. Add about two tablespoons per two quarts of water.

❏ Witch hazel applied to the skin is excellent for absorbing oil.

RECOMMENDATIONS

❏ Drink plenty of quality water to keep the skin hydrated and flush out toxins.

❏ Reduce the amount of fat in your diet. Consume no fried foods, animal fats, or heat-processed vegetable oils such as those sold in supermarkets. Do not cook with oil, and do not eat any oils that have been subjected to heat, whether in processing or cooking. If a little oil is necessary, such as in salad dressing, use cold-pressed canola or olive oil only.

❏ Do not drink soft drinks or alcoholic beverages. Avoid sugar, chocolate, and junk food.

❏ Keep your skin very clean. Wash your face two or three times in the course of a day—no more, because too much washing will stimulate your skin to produce more oil. Use your hands instead of harsh scrubs or washcloths. Sterile gauze pads are also good for cleaning the skin. (Do not use a pad more than once.) Do not use harsh soaps or cleansers. Use a pure soap with no artificial additives, such as E•Gem Skin Care Soap from Carlson Laboratories. Do not use cleansers or lotions that contain alcohol. After cleansing, apply a natural *oil-free* moisturizer to keep the skin supple.

❏ Use hot water when washing your face. Hot water dissolves skin oil better than lukewarm or cold water.

❏ Try using a clay or mud mask. White or rose-colored clays are best for sensitive skin.

❑ Choose cosmetic and facial care products specifically designed for oily skin.

❑ Alpha-hydroxy acids are a group of naturally occurring acids (found mostly in fruits) that help to stimulate cell renewal, aid the skin in retaining water, and give it a smoother, less oily appearance. Oily skin can benefit from the use of products containing alpha-hydroxy acids because they aid in removal of the top layer of dead skin cells, which stimulates healthy skin growth and may diminish large pores. Glycolic acid is probably the best of the alpha-hydroxy acids for this purpose. If you decide to try an alpha-hydroxy acid product, begin with a product containing 5 percent alpha-hydroxy acid (not more), and apply it at night only. First wash your face, then wait five minutes before applying a small amount of the product. After two or three weeks of nighttime application, you can begin applying the product in the morning as well. As your skin becomes accustomed to the effects of alpha-hydroxy acids, you may wish to work your way up to higher-concentration products.

❑ Products containing benzoyl peroxide are effective for oily skin. Start with a mild-strength formula to minimize possible irritation.

❑ Choose an astringent that contains acetone, which is known for dissolving oil.

❑ Two or three times a week, use a loofah sponge for the face (available in health food stores) and warm water to boost circulation, remove dead skin cells, and remove many of the impurities found in oily skin. Avoid using the loofah around your eyes, and do not use it on areas with open sores.

❑ To clear away excess oil, use a clay or mud mask. Blend together well 1 teaspoon green clay powder (available in health food stores) and 1 teaspoon raw honey. Apply the mixture to your face, avoiding the eye area. Leave it on for fifteen minutes, then rinse well with lukewarm water. Do this at least three times a week—or more often if necessary. White or rose-colored clays are best for sensitive skin.

❑ Once or twice daily, mix equal parts of lemon juice and water together. Pat mixture on your face and allow it to dry, then rinse with warm water. Follow with a cool-water rinse.

❑ Look for facial powder that contains talcum powder. It is oil-free and blots the oil on your skin.

❑ For combination skin, simply treat the oily areas as oily skin and the dry areas as dry skin. (See DRY SKIN in Part Two.)

❑ Do not smoke. Smoking promotes enlargement of the pores and impairs the overall health of the skin.

CONSIDERATIONS

❑ Caring for oily skin does *not* mean trying to dry the skin out. Despite having excess oil, skin may still lack moisture. Moisture is a term that is used to refer to the amount of water inside the skin cells, not the amount of oil on the surface of the skin. While oil and moisture levels are related (the oil helps prevent loss of moisture through evaporation), the two are not the same. There are products available that help to supply and protect moisture without adding oil. Vitamin A Moisturizing Gel from Derma-E Products is a good nongreasy moisturizer. Using such a moisturizer may help prevent the development of wrinkles in the long run.

❑ Many companies that specialize in skin care have developed foil-wrapped packets of wipes saturated in alcohol for skin care away from home. These can be placed in your briefcase or purse for cutting through the oil and freshening up the skin.

❑ Although it is a common myth, oily skin doesn't actually cause acne. Although there is an association between the severity of acne and the amount of oil a person's skin produces, not all people with oily skin have acne.

❑ See also ACNE in Part Two.

Osteoarthritis

See under ARTHRITIS.

Osteomalacia

See RICKETS/OSTEOMALACIA.

Osteoporosis

Osteoporosis is a progressive disease in which the bones gradually become weaker and weaker, causing changes in posture and making the individual extremely susceptible to bone fractures. The term *osteoporosis*, derived from Latin, literally means "porous bones." Because of the physiological, nutritional, and hormonal differences between males and females, osteoporosis affects many more women than men. However, men also suffer from bone loss, often as a side effect of certain medications, such as chemotherapy drugs, thyroid hormone, corticosteroids, and anticonvulsants, or as a result of other illnesses. Fully half of all women between the ages of forty-five and seventy-five show signs of some degree of osteopenia (low bone mass) or osteoporosis.

Bone is constantly restoring itself. Cells called osteoblasts are responsible for making bone, and other cells, called osteoclasts, are needed to remove old bone as its minerals are absorbed for use elsewhere in the body. If the osteoclasts break down the bone more quickly than it is replaced, then bone tends to become less dense and is therefore likely to break more easily.

Bone is at its strongest when a person is around age thirty, and thereafter begins to decline. In women, this decline begins to accelerate at menopause. If you have not accumulated sufficient bone mass during those formative times in childhood, adolescence, and early adulthood, or if you lose it too quickly in later years, you are at increased risk of osteoporosis.

A diagnosis of osteoporosis is reached by measuring bone density. The standard of measurement for that diagnosis has been determined by the World Health Organization (WHO) and was obtained by measuring the bone mass of people who have not had fractures related to low bone mass. The standard measurement is therefore the bone density of a thirty-year-old premenopausal woman. The bone density measurement is referred to as a T-score or a SD (standard deviation) score. T-scores of less than 1 standard deviation (SD) indicate a low risk of fracture, T-scores of 1 to 2 are considered to indicate osteopenia, T-scores of more less 2.5 standard deviation from the norm confirm a diagnosis of osteoporosis. But the T-score alone is not the only determinant of fracture risk. Heavy women are less likely to fracture a bone in a fall than thin women; women taking medications that may cause disturbances in balance are more likely to fall and suffer from a fracture. So two women with the same T-score may have a different fracture risk. Many women, then, can be diagnosed with osteoporosis yet suffer few, if any, ill effects from the condition. The T-score is based on a comparison with the bone of a thirty-year-old, so the standard is set very high. Moreover, it is possible to have osteoporosis in one area of the skeleton and not in another. The spine and hips are the areas that cause most concern because hip fractures in older adults take a long time to heal and osteoporosis in the spine may lead to loss of height and curvature of the spine. With the techniques now being used to diagnose this condition early, so that treatment can begin before fractures occur, many people will probably discover the beginnings of osteoporosis before it is diagnosed due to a fracture. Osteoporosis is not a curable condition as yet, but there are various methods that may slow down the process of bone loss.

Many people have the impression that osteoporosis is caused solely by a dietary calcium deficiency and that it therefore can be remedied by taking calcium supplements. This is not quite correct. It is the way calcium is absorbed and used by the body that seems to be the important factor, not necessarily the amount of calcium consumed. Also, the *type* of calcium consumed is important.

While calcium supplementation is important in dealing with osteoporosis, there are other considerations as well.

The correct balance of magnesium, boron, potassium, folic acid, and vitamins C, D, E, and K, all play vital roles in battling osteoporosis, as does protein. There is some debate on the subject of osteoporosis and dietary protein. Some research has indicated that consuming large quantities of protein may cause an acid imbalance in the body, which the body attempts to counteract by releasing minerals from the bone—including calcium. A contrary point of view holds that protein consumption increases the production of insulinlike growth factor (IGF-1), which is responsible for maintaining muscle and bone strength.

In the United States alone, 25 million people—80 percent of them women—are affected by osteoporosis. It is estimated that the cost of treating osteoporosis and related illnesses such as bone fractures is over $10 billion a year. There are three basic types of osteoporosis. Type I is believed to be caused by hormonal changes, particularly a loss of estrogen, which causes the loss of minerals from the bones to accelerate. Type II is linked to dietary deficiency, especially a lack of sufficient calcium and of vitamin D, which is necessary for the absorption of calcium. Type III occurs in men and women at any age and is caused by drug treatment for other illnesses or other diseases unconnected with osteoporosis. Many women mistakenly believe that osteoporosis is something they need be concerned about only after menopause. However, recent evidence indicates that osteoporosis often begins early in life and is *not* strictly a postmenopausal problem. Although bone loss accelerates after menopause as a result of the drop in estrogen levels, it begins much earlier. A number of factors are known to influence an individual's risk of developing osteoporosis. The first, and probably the most important, is the peak bone mass achieved in adulthood; the larger and denser the bones are to begin with, the less debilitating bone loss is likely to be. Small, fine-boned women therefore have more reason for concern than women with larger frames and heavier bones. Race and ethnicity also appear to play a role. Women of northern European or Asian ancestry are more likely to develop osteoporosis, while women of African descent are less likely to be affected.

Dietary and lifestyle habits are important as well. Insufficient calcium intake is one factor, but equally important are other dietary practices that affect calcium metabolism. Caffeine, alcohol, and many other drugs appear to have a detrimental effect on calcium absorption. Bone density also depends on exercise. When the body gets regular weight-bearing exercise (such as walking), it responds by depositing more mineral in the bones, especially the bones of the legs, hips, and spine. Conversely, a lack of regular exercise accelerates the loss of bone mass. Other factors that make one more likely to develop osteoporosis include smoking, late puberty, early menopause (natural or artificially induced), a family history of the disease, hyperthyroidism, chronic liver or kidney disease, and the long-term use of corticosteroids, antiseizure medications, or anticoagulants.

NUTRIENTS

SUPPLEMENT	SUGGESTED DOSAGE	COMMENTS
Essential		
Bone Defense from KAL or	As directed on label.	Contains calcium, magnesium, phosphorus and other valuable bone-reinforcing nutrients.
Bone Support from Synergy Plus or	As directed on label.	A complex containing many of the nutrients listed in this section.
Calcitite Hi-Strength from Metagenics or	As directed on label.	Useful for enhancing bone health and warding off osteoporitis.
Osteo-B-Plus from Biotics Research	As directed on label.	Contains calcium, magnesium, zinc, and other vitamins and minerals.
Boron	3 mg daily. Do not exceed this amount.	Improves calcium absorption. *Note*: If you are taking a complex containing boron, omit this supplement.
Calcium	For women under 50 and men under 65: 1,200 mg daily. For women over 50 and men over 65: 1,500–2,000 mg daily.	Necessary for maintaining strong bones. (Injections under a doctor's supervision) may be needed. (*See* Calcium and Osteoporosis on page 553.)
Copper	3 mg daily.	Aids in the formation of bone.
Floradix Iron+ Herbs from Salus Haus	As directed on label.	Provides organic iron and other nutrients needed for optimum health.
Glucosamine plus chondroitin	As directed on label. As directed on label.	Nutrients necessary for the development of bone and connective tissue.
Magnesium	1,000 mg daily.	Important in calcium uptake.
Phosphorus	As directed on label.	Works with calcium to increase bone strength.
Silica	As directed on label.	Supplies silicon, for calcium utilization and bone strength.
Soy isoflavones	As directed on label.	Have an estrogenic effect on the body. Estrogen promotes bone mass.
Ultra Osteo Synergy from American Biologics	As directed on label.	To support bone renewal.
Vitamin B complex plus extra vitamin B_6 (pyridoxine) and vitamin B_{12}	As directed on label. 200 mg daily. Do not exceed this amount. 1,000–2,000 mcg daily.	Provides strength to protein in bone tissue and promotes the production of progesterone.
Vitamin D_3	As directed on label.	Needed for the absorption of calcium.
Vitamin K	As directed on label.	Essential for the production of bone protein.
Very Important		
L-Lysine and L-arginine	As directed on label, on an empty stomach. Take with water or juice. Do not take with milk. Take with 50 mg vitamin B_6 and 100 mg vitamin C for better absorption.	Aid calcium absorption and connective tissue strength. (*See* AMINO ACIDS in Part One.)
Methylsulfonyl-methane (MSM) (MSM With Glucosamine from the American Council for Natural Pain Relief or OptiMSM from Cardinal Nutrition)	As directed on label. Do not exceed the recommended dose.	A natural sulfur compound found in foods and present in body tissues It is used by the body to build healthy new cells. MSM provides the flexible bond between the cells and provides support for tendons, ligaments, and muscles. Use a capsule form for easier absorption.
Multienzyme complex with betaine hydrochloride (HCl) plus proteolytic enzymes	As directed on label. Take with meals. As directed on label. Take between meals	Needed for proper absorption of calcium and all nutrients. *Note*: Do not use a formula containing HCl if you have an ulcer or suffer from stomach acidity.
Vitamin A with mixed carotenoids and vitamin E	25,000 IU daily. If you are pregnant, do not exceed 10,000 daily. 400 IU daily.	Important in retarding the aging process. Use emulsion forms for easier assimilation. Aids in the use of vitamin A and protects it from destruction by oxygen. Use d-alpha-tocopherol form.
Zinc plus copper	50 mg daily. Do not exceed a total of 100 mg daily from all supplements. 3 mg daily.	Important for calcium uptake and immune function. Use zinc gluconate lozenges or OptiZinc for best absorption. Needed to balance with zinc.
Helpful		
Chromium picolinate	400–600 mcg daily.	Improves insulin efficiency, which improves bone density.
DL-Phenylalanine (DLPA)	As directed on label, on an empty stomach. Take with water or juice. Do not take with milk. Take with 50 mg vitamin B_6 and 3,000 mg vitamin C for better absorption.	Good for bone pain. (*See* AMINO ACIDS in Part One.) *Caution*: Do not take this supplement if you suffer from panic attacks, diabetes, high blood pressure, or PKU.
Kelp	2,000–3,000 mg daily.	A rich source of important minerals.
Manganese	As directed on label. Take separately from calcium.	Vital in mineral metabolism.
Multivitamin and mineral complex	As directed on label.	To supply essential minerals. Use a high-potency formula.
Trace mineral complex (Trace Supreme from International Health Products)	As directed on label.	Trace (also called micro) minerals are important for healthy bone formation.
Vitamin C with bioflavonoids	3,000 mg and up daily.	Important for collagen and connective tissue formation.

HERBS

❑ Feverfew is good for pain relief and acts as an anti-inflammatory.

Caution: Do not use feverfew during pregnancy.

❑ Alfalfa, barley grass, black cohosh, boneset, dandelion root, nettle, parsley, poke root, rose hips, and yucca help to build strong bones.

Caution: Do not use boneset on a daily basis for more than one week, as long-term use can lead to toxicity.

❑ Horsetail and oat straw contain silica, which helps the body absorb calcium.

RECOMMENDATIONS

❑ Eat plenty of foods that are high in calcium and vitamin D. Good sources of easily assimilable calcium include broccoli, chestnuts, clams, dandelion greens, most dark green leafy vegetables, flounder, hazelnuts, kale, kelp, molasses, oats, oysters, salmon, sardines (with the bones), sea vegetables, sesame seeds, shrimp, soybeans, tahini (sesame butter), tofu, turnip greens, and wheat germ.

❑ Consume whole grains and calcium foods at different times. Whole grains contain a substance that binds with calcium and prevents its uptake. Take calcium at bedtime, when it is best absorbed and also aids in sleeping.

❑ Include garlic and onions in the diet, as well as eggs (if your cholesterol level is not too high). These foods contain sulfur, which is needed for healthy bones.

❑ If you are a menopausal or postmenopausal woman with osteoporosis, include plenty of soy products in your diet. Soy is rich in phytoestrogens, which may, to some extent, substitute for your body's own estrogen if it is manufacturing too little. The latter effect is very important for osteoporosis. Estrogen depletion is strongly associated with osteoporosis.

❑ Avoid phosphate-containing drinks and foods such as soft drinks and alcohol. Avoid smoking, sugar, and salt. Limit your consumption of citrus fruits and tomatoes; these foods may inhibit calcium intake.

❑ Avoid yeast products. Yeast is high in phosphorus, which competes with calcium for absorption by the body.

❑ If you are over fifty-five, include a calcium lactate (if you are not allergic to milk) or calcium phosphate supplement in your daily regimen, and take hydrochloric acid (HCl) supplements. In order for calcium to be absorbed, there must be an adequate supply of vitamin D as well as sufficient HCl in the stomach. Older people often lack sufficient stomach acid.

❑ If you take thyroid hormone or an anticoagulant drug, increase the amount of calcium you take by 25 to 50 percent.

❑ If you take a diuretic, consult your physician before beginning calcium and vitamin D supplementation. Thiazide-type diuretics increase blood calcium levels, and complications may result if these drugs are taken in conjunction with calcium and vitamin D supplements. Other types of diuretics increase calcium requirements, however.

❑ Keep active, and exercise regularly. A lack of exercise can result in the loss of calcium, but this can be reversed with sensible exercise. Walking is probably the best exercise for maintaining bone mass.

CONSIDERATIONS

❑ Manganese may help prevent osteoporosis, according to a report presented at an American Chemical Society meeting in Anaheim, California. Biologist Paul Saltman of the University of California–San Diego found that rats on a low-manganese diet developed porous bones.

❑ Many people prefer to take a single supplement rather than many separate ones. JCTH from Bio-Metabolic Nutrition is a formula that contains almost all of the nutrients mentioned in the Nutrients table.

❑ For people who find it difficult to swallow pills, Osteo Solutions from Neways is a calcium and magnesium supplement in liquid form.

❑ Both men and women slowly lose bone as they age. A woman may lose 30 to 50 percent of her cortical bone thickness over a lifetime.

❑ A study conducted by *The Journal of Clinical Nutrition* reported that women who are vegetarians experience significantly less bone loss than women who consume meat. Soy, beans, peas, and lentils supply proteins, and green vegetables are all very rich in calcium, as well as containing abundant amounts of other vitamins and minerals.

❑ Klinefelter's syndrome, which results in low testosterone levels in men, also leads to osteoporosis.

❑ A study reported in the *Journal of the American Medical Association* revealed that senior citizens who took tranquilizers suffered 70 percent more hip fractures than did other people their age. Very often, medications can affect balance. You should discuss this particular side effect with your physician before taking any medication.

❑ Caffeine has been linked to calcium loss. In one study, adults given 300 milligrams of caffeine excreted more than the normal amount of calcium in their urine. Another study revealed that caffeine is associated with decreased bone minerals in women.

❑ Carbonated soft drinks contain high amounts of phosphates. These cause the body to eliminate calcium as the phosphates themselves are excreted, even if calcium must be taken from the bones to do this.

❑ Bone disintegration with pain in the hips, lower back, or legs and vertebral fractures (usually affecting people over fifty years old) is common.

❑ The use of sodium fluoride, which was once thought to be helpful in building bone, has been shown to be ineffective for the treatment of osteoporosis. While sodium fluoride does increase bone mass in the vertebral column, the bone itself is of inferior quality. Women participating in a study at the Mayo Clinic in Rochester, Minnesota, were three times as likely to suffer from a fracture of the arm, leg, or hip if they took sodium fluoride than if they took a placebo. Some of the participants also suffered from unusual lower leg pain, perhaps due to stress fractures.

Calcium and Osteoporosis

People in the United States consume more dairy products and other foods high in calcium per capita than the citizens of any other two nations on earth put together. We even have orange juice and antacids that are fortified with calcium. Yet we eat far less total food, take in less calcium, and get less exercise that stimulates bone growth than our grandparents did. At the same time, we consume more animal protein and phosphate-containing foods such as soft drinks. Perhaps not surprisingly, therefore, we also have the world's highest rates of osteoporosis and bone fractures among elderly people. Obviously, we need to eat more of the right foods and take high-quality supplements in some form as well.

If you are depending on your diet to supply your calcium requirements, it is useful to know that one cup of low-fat yogurt contains about 300 milligrams of calcium and that one cup of broccoli supplies about 180 milligrams of calcium. Green vegetables, sardines, salmon (including the bones), beans, and almonds are also calcium rich. In addition to supplying enough calcium, your diet needs to be balanced with the correct amounts of other vitamins and minerals that allow the calcium to be absorbed and used to nourish bone. Among these are magnesium, potassium, and vitamin K. Magnesium and potassium are found in all fruits and vegetables. Vitamin K is found in dark leafy vegetables including, broccoli, collard greens, kale, and spinach. If you find that you cannot meet the suggested requirements and other nutrients from your diet, then you should consider a supplement.

Drugstores and health food stores carry a bewildering array of vitamin and mineral supplements in a variety of brands and forms. There can be significant nutritional differences between the various supplements available. Where calcium is concerned, the number on the label does not necessarily reflect the amount of calcium you can expect to absorb from the product. For example, if a label says "calcium lactate 600 milligrams," this may mean that each tablet weighs 600 milligrams—but out of 600 milligrams of calcium lactate, only 60 milligrams are actually calcium that is available for absorption. This is because minerals cannot be turned into tablets in their pure state; they must be combined with some other substance or substances to make a stable compound. The important information to look for is the amount of *elemental* calcium that is present in the supplement. It is the elemental calcium that is absorbed by the body. Then, too, some supplements may contain large amounts of calcium, but in a form that is not absorbed, or is not well absorbed, by the body. The letters *USP* (US Pharmacopeia) on the label are an indication that the standard for absorbability has been met.

The following are some of the common forms of calcium found in calcium supplements:

• Calcium carbonate usually contains a relatively large percentage of elemental calcium, but is not easily absorbed by the body. It contains 40 percent elemental calcium by weight.

• Calcium citrate is easily absorbed by the body. However, many calcium citrate products contain lower amounts of elemental calcium. Calcium citrate can be used if you have low stomach acid levels, which is common in postmenopausal women and people who those take antacid medications. This type of supplement contains 21 percent elemental calcium by weight.

• Calcium gluconate contains 9 percent elemental calcium. This form of calcium can sometimes cause diarrhea and nausea.

• Calcium lactate contains 13 percent elemental calcium, along with lactic acid.

• Calcium lactate gluconate contains 13 percent elemental calcium.

• Calcium phosphate contains phosphorus and vitamin D in addition to calcium. This helps the body absorb the calcium. This type of supplement contains 30 percent elemental calcium. (Tums contains calcium phosphate.)

For men, problems with calcium appear to be more complex than was originally thought. Research conducted over ten years by the Physician's Health Study—the group that discovered aspirin's effect on heart attack risk—found that men who consumed two and a half servings of dairy products per day were 30 percent more likely to develop prostate cancer than men who did not. Calcium is known to lower body levels of 1,25-dihydroxyvitamin D. This is the most active form of vitamin D and is not the same form of vitamin D that is sometimes added to milk. Low levels of this vitamin may protect men against prostate cancer. In a previous study, the same group of researchers found that men who consumed high amounts of dairy foods had 70 percent increased risk of prostate cancer, and that calcium supplements increased the risk of prostate cancer by 30 percent. Fortunately, men are not nearly as likely to develop osteoporosis as women, so forgoing calcium supplementation is less of a problem for them.

If you are in doubt about your calcium tablets, you can do a home test to determine whether the supplement will dissolve readily in your body. Place a tablet in a cup of vinegar and stir it every few minutes. The tablet should be completely dissolved within half an hour. If it isn't, it will not dissolve in your stomach either, and you should choose another supplement.

❏ A number of different prescription drugs are sometimes prescribed for people with osteoporosis, including:

• Alendronate (Fosamax) is a type of drug known as a bisphosphonate. It inhibits the resorption of bone.

• Calcitonin (sold under the brand names Calcimar, Cibacalcin, and Miacalcin) is said to prevent further loss of bone mass in 70 percent of the people who take it. It should not be taken by anyone with a history of kidney stones.

• Raloxifene (Evista) is selective estrogen receptor modulator (SERM)—a drug that acts *like* an estrogen in some respects but is not estrogen.

All of these drugs have potential side effects. They are not suitable for everyone.

❑ Hormone replacement therapy is often prescribed for people who have osteoporosis. There are risks attached to this treatment. Before agreeing to it, you need to consider whether the risks outweigh the benefits. (*See* Hormones, Hormone Therapy, and Menopause on page 514.)

❑ Alendronate is now being tested for use in men with osteoporisis.

❑ For corticosteroid-induced osteoporosis—that is, osteoporosis that develops as a result of taking corticosteroids for a major illness such as arthritis—treatment with biphosphonates appears to prevent bone loss.

❑ Dehydroepiandrosterone (DHEA) and human growth hormone (HGH) are two hormones whose production progressively declines with age. Research suggests that supplementation with either of these hormones may help increase bone strength and treat osteoporosis. (*See* DHEA THERAPY and GROWTH HORMONE THERAPY in Part Three.)

❑ Research conducted by the World Health Organization concluded that people who were given a protein supplement recovered more quickly from hip fractures than those who were not. In addition, they found that people who took protein supplements were less likely to suffer a hip fracture in the first place.

❑ A study reported in the March 2000 issue of *The Journal of Family Practice* found that taking vitamin C can help to prevent nerve pain after a fracture.

❑ Tests for bone loss are very easy and noninvasive. Dual energy x-ray absorptiometry (DEXA) is probably the most reliable method of determining osteoporosis. Exposure to radiation from this test is less than in other methods used to detect this condition.

❑ *See also* RICKETS in Part Two.

Paget's Disease of Bone

Paget's disease of bone (named for Sir James Paget, who first described it) is a chronic disorder characterized by excessive bone degeneration combined with the creation of new bone that is deficient in calcium and therefore more fragile than normal bone. The result is enlarged and deformed bones in one or more sections of the skeleton, bone degeneration, bone pain, arthritis, noticeable deformities, and an increased susceptibility to fractures.

Paget's disease most often affects the bones of the pelvis, the spine, the thighs, the skull, the hips, the shins, and the upper arms. It affects over 3 percent of Americans over the age of forty and about 10 percent of those over the age of eighty, although in rare instances it has been reported in young adults. It affects men and women nearly equally.

In the early stages, the disease usually causes no symptoms, although there may be mild pain in the affected bones. As it progresses, bone pain tends to become more severe and persistent, especially at night, and to worsen with exertion. Paget's disease can also lead to neck and/or back pain; pain and/or stiffness in affected joints; warming of the skin over the area of the affected bones; unexplained bone fractures; hearing loss; headaches; dizziness; ringing in the ears; and impaired mobility. If the pelvis or a thighbone is involved, there may be hip pain. The disease follows a pattern of alternating remissions and flare-ups. Over time, the flare-ups gradually become worse. Sometimes joints adjacent to the affected bone become involved, and osteoarthritis may develop. Over time, deformities such as bowed legs, an increasingly barrel-shaped chest, a bent spine, and/or an enlarged forehead may develop as well. Other possible late complications include kidney stones (caused by immobilization), congestive heart failure, deafness or blindness (caused by the skull pressing on the brain), high blood pressure, and gout. In approximately 5 percent of cases, the affected bone undergoes malignant changes, leading to osteosarcoma (bone cancer). High-output cardiac failure can occur from prolonged increased blood flow. The life expectancy of individuals with Paget's disease is somewhat reduced, but most live with the disease for at least ten to fifteen years.

Because this disease usually does not cause significant symptoms, especially in the early stages, most cases go undetected unless discovered accidentally when x-rays or blood tests are taken for another reason. The cause is unknown, although some researchers suspect a slowly progressing viral infection of the bone is involved. Multiple cases of the disease within families have been reported. However, Paget's disease does not appear to be transmitted from one generation to another, a finding more consistent with an infectious disorder than with a hereditary condition.

Paget's disease is often confused with hyperthyroidism and other disorders that cause bone lesions, such as bone cancer, fibrous dysplasia, and multiple myeloma. To diagnose Paget's disease, doctors may use bone scans or x-rays to detect bone changes characteristic of the disease. Blood tests may detect elevated levels of alkaline phosphatase, an enzyme produced by bone-building cells. Urine tests and CT scans also may be used to arrive at a diagnosis of Paget's disease.

NUTRIENTS

SUPPLEMENT	SUGGESTED DOSAGE	COMMENTS
Essential		
Calcium plus	1,500 mg daily.	For the formation of strong bones. Use a chelate form. Nutrients that are needed for calcium absorption.
boron and	3 mg daily. Do not exceed this amount.	
magnesium and	750 mg daily.	
vitamin D₃	400 IU daily.	
Copper	3 mg daily.	Aids in the formation of bone.
Glucosamine Plus from FoodScience of Vermont plus	As directed on label.	Contains nutrients necessary for healthy development of bone and connective tissues.
chondroitin and	As directed on label.	Helpful for pain.
methylsulfonyl-methane (MSM)	As directed on label.	
Kyolic-EPA from Wakunaga	As directed on label.	Supplies essential fatty acids. Vital for proper growth and cell formation.
Liquid Kyolic with B₁ and B₁₂ from Wakunaga	As directed on label.	Aids in red blood cell formation and energy production.
Manganese	2 mg daily.	Required for normal bone growth.
Phosphorus	1,200 mg daily.	Required for bone formation.
Primrose oil or	As directed on label.	To supply essential fatty acids vital for proper growth and cell formation.
Ultimate Oil from Nature's Secret	As directed on label.	
Silica	As directed on label.	Necessary for bone formation.
Vitamin A with mixed carotenoids including natural beta-carotene	10,000 IU daily.	To improve immune function and promote proper bone growth.
Vitamin B complex	50 mg of each major B vitamin 3 times daily, with meals (amounts of individual vitamins in a complex will vary).	Involved in energy production.
plus extra vitamin B₁₂ and	1,000–2,000 mcg daily.	Assists in nutrient absorption and aids in cell formation.
folic acid	400 mcg daily.	Needed for energy production.
Vitamin C with bioflavonoids	3,000–6,000 mg daily, in divided doses.	Enhances immunity and aids in proper bone growth.
Zinc	30 mg daily. Do not exceed a total of 100 mg daily from all supplements.	Promotes a healthy immune system. Use zinc gluconate lozenges or OptiZinc for best absorption.
Helpful		
Bone Builder from Ethical Nutrients	As directed on label.	Contains minerals and the organic matrix that makes up bone.
DL-Phenylalanine (DLPA)	As directed on label.	Alleviates chronic pain. *Caution:* Do not take this supplement if you are pregnant or nursing, or suffer from panic attacks, diabetes, high blood pressure, or PKU.
Floradix Iron+ Herbs from Salus Haus	As directed on label.	Provides organic iron and other nutrients needed for optimum health and fitness.
Reishi extract or	As directed on label.	To help reduce inflammation.
shiitake extract	As directed on label.	

HERBS

❏ Alfalfa and horsetail contain minerals needed for proper bone formation and that help to reduce inflammation.

❏ Angelica, cayenne (capsicum), feverfew, hops, passionflower, skullcap, valerian root, and white willow bark work well for pain.
Caution: Do not use feverfew during pregnancy.

❏ Black cohosh and St. John's wort help both to reduce inflammation and to alleviate pain.
Caution: Do not use black cohosh during pregnancy.

❏ Boneset, dandelion root, nettle, parsley, poke root, rose hips, and yucca help to build strong bones.
Caution: Do not use boneset on a daily basis for more than one week, as long-term use can lead to toxicity.

❏ Echinacea, goldenseal, and licorice aid in reducing inflammation.
Caution: Do not take goldenseal internally on a daily basis for more than one week at a time, and do not use it during pregnancy. Use with caution if you are allergic to ragweed. Do not use licorice on a daily basis for more than seven days in a row, and avoid it if you have high blood pressure.

RECOMMENDATIONS

❏ Eat plenty of calcium-rich foods. These include brewer's yeast, buttermilk, carob, goat's milk, all leafy greens, salmon (with the bones), sardines, seafood, tofu, whey, and yogurt.

❏ Include plenty of garlic in the diet. Garlic is beneficial for circulation and helps to keep inflammation down.

❏ Eat fresh papaya and pineapple frequently. These fruits contain enzymes that help to reduce inflammation.

❏ Avoid nightshade vegetables. These include tomatoes, potatoes, eggplant, cayenne peppers, chili peppers, sweet peppers, paprika, and pimiento. These vegetables are high in alkaloids, chemical substances with strong physiological effects. They affect the metabolism of calcium and, through a mechanism not yet understood, cause calcium from the bones to be deposited in other areas of the body where it does not belong, such as the arteries, joints, and kidneys.

❏ Use barley grass and/or kelp to supply valuable minerals and other nutrients needed for bone formation.

❏ Use heat to alleviate pain. Hot soaks, hot compresses, and heat lamps are all effective.

❑ Follow an exercise program recommended by your health care provider to combat immobility.

❑ Sleep on a very firm mattress or use a bed board. This will lessen the chance of developing spinal deformities.

❑ During active phases of the disease, rest in bed and move or turn often to prevent pressure sores.

❑ Accident-proof your home to help prevent fractures. Remove throw rugs and avoid slippery flooring. Install hand rails next to the bathtub and toilet.

❑ Avoid placing extreme physical stress on the bones.

❑ Get regular medical checkups to screen for early bone cancer and to detect hearing loss. If hearing loss occurs, consider a hearing aid.

CONSIDERATIONS

❑ There is no known cure for Paget's disease. However, most patients never develop symptoms and so do not require treatment. For those who do, drug treatment can relieve and manage symptoms. Drug therapy for Paget's disease may include:

• *Analgesics* can be useful in relieving pain.

• *Calcitonin (Calcimar, Cibacalcin, Miacalcin)*, a natural hormone given by injection, and *etidronate (Didronel)*, a calcium regulator, which both slow the progression of the disease.

• *Diphosphonates* impair bone mineralization, which is linked to bone pain and fractures.

• *Fluoride*, which is sometimes used to correct deformities, relieve pinched nerves, and prevent or reduce fractures.

• *Pliamycin (Mithracin)*, an anti-tumor drug, which can produce a remission of symptoms within two weeks, and further improvement in two months. However, this drug can also cause kidney damage and destruction of red blood cells.

❑ For names and addresses of organizations that can provide more information on Paget's Disease, *see* HEALTH AND MEDICAL ORGANIZATIONS in the Appendix.

Paget's Disease of the Nipple

See under BREAST CANCER.

Pancreatitis

Pancreatitis is an inflammation of the pancreas, a five- to six-inch-long leaf-shaped gland situated behind the lower part of the stomach and extending downward toward the spleen and left kidney. It has two primary functions: to produce digestive enzymes that break down proteins, fat, and carbohydrates in the small intestine; and to release the hormones glucogen and insulin, which regulate blood sugar levels. The pancreas can become inflamed if digestive enzymes build up inside it and begin to attack it.

The disease can be either acute or chronic. In 80 percent of cases, acute pancreatitis is due to excessive alcohol use or gallstones. This condition can also come about as a result of infection (such as with hepatitis A or D or Epstein-Barr virus) or the use of certain drugs (such as divalproex [Depakote], used to prevent seizures and treat bipolar mood disorder; azathioprine [Imuran], sometimes used for rheumatoid arthritis; and 6–MP, a cancer chemotherapy agent). In very rare cases, acute pancreatitis may be caused by injury to the abdomen.

Acute pancreatitis usually causes severe pain that comes on suddenly, starting in or around the area of the navel and radiating to the back. The pain is typically exacerbated by movement and relieved by sitting, and may be accompanied by nausea and vomiting, sometimes severe. Other symptoms include upper abdominal swelling and distension, excessive gas, upper abdominal pain described as burning or stabbing, fever, sweating, hypertension, muscle aches, and abnormal, fatty stools.

Chronic pancreatitis is a condition in which the inflammation has caused irreversible changes in the microscopic structure of the gallbladder tissue. Repeated episodes of gallbladder infection and gallstones are often involved. (*See* GALLBLADDER DISORDERS in Part Two.) The symptoms of chronic pancreatitis may be hard to distinguish from those of acute pancreatitis, except that the pain tends to be chronic rather than coming on suddenly. In addition, chronic pancreatitis may be punctuated with periodic episodes of acute disease. In the majority of cases, chronic pancreatitis is caused by long-term alcohol use.

Because the pancreas is the gland that produces the hormones insulin and glucagon, which regulate blood sugar levels, pancreatitis—especially if chronic—often leads to glucose intolerance (diabetes) and digestive difficulties.

NUTRIENTS

SUPPLEMENT	SUGGESTED DOSAGE	COMMENTS
Essential		
Chromium picolinate	300–600 mcg daily.	Important in maintaining stable blood sugar levels.
Garlic (Kyolic from Wakunaga)	As directed on label.	Powerful antiviral and antioxidant.
Very Important		
Calcium and	1,500 mg daily.	Works closely with magnesium.
magnesium	1,000 mg daily.	Counteracts glandular disorders. Use chelate forms.

Digestive enzymes with ox bile (D.A. #34 from Carlson Labs)	As directed on label.	Needed for proper digestion and gallbladder function. Important if gallbladder has been removed.
Pancreatin	As directed on label. Take with food.	Pancreatic enzyme deficiency is common in people with pancreatitis.
Probiata from Wakunaga or Kyo-Dophilus from Wakunaga	As directed on label. As directed on label.	To replace the friendly bacteria and aid in digestion.
Proteolytic enzymes	As directed on label. Take between meals and at bedtime, on an empty stomach.	Aids in reducing inflammation; reduces strain on the pancreas by aiding protein digestion. *Caution:* Do not give this supplement to a child.
Raw pancreas glandular	As directed on label.	Contains certain proteins needed to repair the pancreas. (*See* GLANDULAR THERAPY in Part Three.)
Vitamin B complex plus extra vitamin B$_3$ (niacin) and pantothenic acid (vitamin B$_5$)	50 mg of each major B vitamin 3 times daily (amounts of individual vitamins in a complex will vary). 50 mg 3 times daily. Do not exceed this amount. 100 mg 3 times daily.	Anti-stress vitamins. Niacin and pantothenic acid are important in fat and carbohydrate metabolism. *Caution:* Do not take niacin if you have a liver disorder, gout, or high blood pressure.

Important		
Choline and inositol and/or lecithin and/or lipotropic factors	As directed on label. As directed on label. As directed on label.	Fat emulsifiers that aid in fat digestion.
Vitamin C with bioflavonoids	1,000 mg 4 times daily.	Potent free radical scavengers. Use a buffered form.

Helpful		
Coenzyme Q$_{10}$ plus Coenzyme A from Coenzyme-A Technologies	75 mg daily.	A powerful antioxidant and oxygen carrier. Works well with coenzyme Q$_{10}$ and increases energy, supports adrenal glands, processes fats, removes toxins from the body, and boosts the immune system.
CTR Support from PhysioLogics	As directed on label.	Helps diminish damage caused by inflammation and protects against future damage.
DL-Phenylalanine (DLPA)	As directed on label.	To relieve pain in acute cases. *Caution:* Do not take this supplement if you are pregnant or nursing, or if you suffer from panic attacks, diabetes, high blood pressure, or PKU.
Grape seed extract	As directed on label.	A powerful anti-inflammatory and antioxidant.
L-Cysteine	As directed on label.	Protects the liver.

OmegaBrite by CX Research	As directed on label.	Contains essential fatty acids that act as anti-inflammatory agents and also lower triglycerides.
Vitamin E	Start with 200 IU daily and increase slowly to 400–800 IU daily.	A powerful antioxidant and oxygen carrier. Important in tissue repair. Use d-alpha-tocopherol form.
Zinc	50 mg daily. Do not exceed a total of 100 mg daily from all supplements.	Facilitates proper enzyme activity for cell division, growth, and repair. Plays a role in the manufacture of insulin. Use zinc gluconate lozenges or OptiZinc for best absorption.

HERBS

❑ Burdock root, milk thistle, and red clover aid in cleansing the bloodstream and liver, reducing the burden on the pancreas.

❑ Cedar berries, echinacea, gentian root, and goldenseal stimulate and strengthen the pancreas.

Caution: Do not take goldenseal internally on a daily basis for more than one week at a time, do not use it during pregnancy, and use it with caution if you are allergic to ragweed.

❑ Dandelion root stimulates bile production and improves the health of the pancreas.

❑ Detoxygen from Nature's Plus is an herbal formula that detoxifies the body and oxygenates cells.

❑ Licorice root supports all glandular functions.

Caution: If overused, licorice can elevate blood pressure. Do not use this herb on a daily basis for more than seven days in a row. Avoid it if you have high blood pressure.

❑ Olive leaf extract acts as an anti-inflammatory agent and is helpful if you have an infection.

RECOMMENDATIONS

❑ If you develop symptoms of pancreatitis, call your physician. This is an extremely serious condition that requires medical attention.

❑ Eat a diet low in fat and sugar. This is very important for recovery. High levels of sugar and fats in the blood are common in pancreatitis. *See* DIABETES in Part Two and follow the dietary guidelines.

❑ Consume no alcohol in any form.

❑ If antibiotics are prescribed, be sure to consume kefir, and yogurt, and add some form of acidophilus to the program.

❑ If you smoke, stop, and try to avoid secondhand smoke. Recent studies point to a distinct link between chronic pancreatitis and cigarette smoking.

❑ *See* FASTING in Part Three and follow the program. Fasting can improve the health of all organs, including the pancreas.

CONSIDERATIONS

❏ Pancreatic cancer is the fourth leading cause of cancer deaths in the United States. Pancreatitis can lead to the development of this type of cancer. Improving the health of the pancreas may help to prevent it.

❏ A high level of triglycerides (fat) in the blood is a factor in pancreatitis.

Panic Attack

See under ANXIETY DISORDER.

Parkinson's Disease

Parkinson's disease (PD) is a degenerative disease affecting the nervous system. The underlying cause is unknown, but symptoms appear when there is a lack of dopamine in the brain. Dopamine is a neurotransmitter that carries messages from one nerve cell to another. In healthy persons, it exists in balance with another neurotransmitter, acetylcholine. In people with what is called primary Parkinson's disease, the *substantia nigra*—the area of the brain containing cells that manufacture dopamine, noradrenaline, and serotonin—are damaged or dying, and the brain loses the ability to manufacture these chemicals.

The disease may start almost imperceptibly, with a mild to moderate tremor of the hand or hands while at rest, a general slow and heavy feeling, muscular stiffness, bradykinesia (slowness of movement), and a tendency to tire more easily than usual. Later symptoms may include muscular rigidity; drooling; loss of appetite; a stooped, shuffling gait; tremors, including a characteristic "pill-rolling" movement in which the thumb and forefinger rub against each other; impaired speech; and a fixed facial expression. The body gradually becomes rigid and the limbs stiffen. Depression and/or dementia may accompany the physical symptoms.

Parkinson's disease is one of the most common debilitating diseases in the United States. It affects men more often than women. Recent statistics indicate that 1 in every 200 persons over the age of sixty is affected.

While the cause of the loss of brain cells that causes Parkinson's disease remains unknown, a number of different theories have been developed. One hypothesis is that the cells are destroyed by toxins within the body that the liver is unable to filter out, metabolize, or detoxify because as the body ages, the liver loses its ability to work as effectively and as efficiently as it once did. Another theory is that

exposure to environmental toxins, such as herbicides and pesticides that leach into ground water, is responsible.

NUTRIENTS

SUPPLEMENT	SUGGESTED DOSAGE	COMMENTS
Essential		
Calcium	As directed on label.	People with PD often develop porous bones and are in danger of fractures. Calcium also supports the nervous system. Use calcium citrate form.
and magnesium	As directed on label.	Important for the function of nerves and muscles.
and potassium	As directed on label.	Aids nerve-impulse transmission and muscle contraction.
Coenzyme Q_{10} plus	As directed on label.	Allows cells to produce energy.
Coenzyme A from Coenzyme-A Technologies	As directed on label.	Works well with coenzyme Q_{10} to streamline metabolism, ease depression and fatigue, and increase energy.
Creatine	As directed on label. Never exceed the recommended dose.	Normally used by body builders to increase muscle stamina. Research is ongoing in the use of creatine in muscle depleting illnesses.
5-Hydroxy-L-tryptophan (5-HTP)	As directed on label.	Increases serotonin levels in the brain, which helps overcome insomnia and depression.
Glutathione	As directed on label.	Often depleted in people with PD. Found in the *substantia nigra* in the brain, where cells are dying.
L–Phenylalanine and	As directed by physician.	Amino acids that are converted into dopamine.
L–tyrosine	As directed by physician.	*Caution:* Do not take these supplements if you are pregnant or nursing; if you take an MAO inhibitor drug or levodopa, or if you suffer from panic attacks, diabetes, high blood pressure, or PKU.
Vitamin B complex	50 mg of each major B vitamin 3 times daily, with meals (amounts of individual vitamins in a complex will vary).	Extremely important in brain function and enzyme activity. Use a high-potency sublingual formula. Consider injections (under a doctor's supervision). A lack of this vitamin causes depression, nerve damage, and a reduction in neurotransmitter levels.
plus extra vitamin B_2 (riboflavin) and	50 mg 3 times daily, with meals.	
vitamin B_3 (niacin) or niacinamide and	50 mg 3 times daily, with meals. Do not exceed this amount.	Helps maintain a strong immune system and overcome depression and irritability. Flushing may occur from niacin use—this is normal. Niacinamide does not cause flushing. *Caution:* Do not take niacin if you have a liver disorder, gout, or high blood pressure.

vitamin B₆	50–75 mg 3 times daily, with meals.	Dopamine production depends on adequate supplies of this vitamin. Consider injections (under a doctor's supervision). *Caution:* Do not take this supplement if you are taking a levodopa preparation.
Vitamin C and vitamin E plus selenium	3,000–6,000 mg daily, in divided doses. Start with 400 IU daily and increase gradually to 1,200 IU daily. 200 mcg daily. Do not exceed this amount.	Antioxidants that may slow progression of the disease and postpone the need for drug therapy. A powerful antioxidant.
Very Important		
Aangamik DMG from FoodScience of Vermont	50 mg twice daily.	Enhances tissue oxygenation.
Bone Support from Synergy Plus	As directed on label.	Contains calcium, magnesium, zinc, phosphorus, and other nutrients.
Dimethylamino-ethanol (DMAE)	As directed on label.	Stimulates the production of choline for brain function. Improves memory and learning ability.
Floradix Iron + Herbs from Salus Haus	As directed on label.	Contains iron derived from natural food sources, beneficial in the treatment of Parkinson's disease.
Gamma-amino-butyric acid (GABA)	As directed on label.	Functions as a neurotransmitter that stabilizes neuron activity. (*See* AMINO ACIDS in Part One.)
Grape seed oil (Salute Santé Grapeseed Oil from Lifestar International)	As directed on label.	Contains a high level of vitamin E as well as the essential fatty acid linoleic acid.
Lecithin granules or capsules and/or phosphatidyl choline	1 tbsp 3 times daily, before meals. 1,200 mg 3 times daily, before meals. As directed on label.	To supply choline, important in transmission of nerve impulses.
Nicotinamide adenine dinucleotide (NADH) (Enada NADH from Kal)	10 mg daily.	A form of vitamin B₃ that is important in the creation and transfer of chemical energy, especially during breathing.
Pycnogenol or grape seed extract	As directed on label. As directed on label.	Potent bioflavonoids and free radical scavengers.
Superoxide dismutase (SOD)	As directed on label.	An enzyme that retards oxidation, protecting neurons and sparing neurotransmitters like dopamine.
Trimethylglycine (TMG)	As directed on label.	A natural phytochemical extracted from sugar beets that has been shown in laboratory tests to increase muscle mass, reduce body fat, and increase bone density. Reduces levels of homocysteine.
Helpful		
Multienzyme complex (Novenzyme from International Health Products)	As directed on label.	To aid digestion and assimilation of all nutrients, especially the B vitamins.

Multivitamin and mineral complex with potassium	As directed on label. 99 mg daily.	To correct nutritional deficiencies, common in people with Parkinson's disease.
Primrose oil or omega-3 essential fatty acid complex	2,000–4,000 mg daily, in divided doses.	May reduce the severity and frequency of tremors.
Raw brain glandular	As directed on label.	A glandular extract that improves brain function. (*See* GLANDULAR THERAPY in Part Three.)

HERBS

Degenerative disease is often facilitated by the accumulation of toxins in the body. The following herbs have detoxifying properties.

❑ Burdock root, dandelion root, ginger root, and milk thistle detoxify the liver.

❑ Cayenne (capsicum), goldenseal, mullein, Siberian ginseng, and yarrow stimulate the thymus and lymphatic system.

Caution: Do not take goldenseal internally on a daily basis for more than one week at a time, do not use it during pregnancy, and use it with caution if you are allergic to ragweed. Do not use Siberian ginseng if you have hypoglycemia, high blood pressure, or a heart disorder.

❑ Hawthorn, licorice, red clover, and sarsaparilla cleanse the blood.

Caution: Do not use licorice on a daily basis for more than seven days in a row. Avoid it completely if you have high blood pressure.

❑ Yellow dock cleanses the blood and detoxifies the liver.

❑ Black cohosh, catnip, lemon balm, passionflower, skullcap, and valerian root have antistress properties and can help nourish the nervous system.

Caution: Do not use black cohosh during pregnancy.

❑ Ginkgo biloba helps to improve memory and brain function. Source Naturals offers an excellent extract.

RECOMMENDATIONS

❑ Eat a diet consisting of 75 percent raw foods, with seeds, grains, nuts, and raw milk.

❑ Include in the diet foods containing the amino acid phenylalanine, such as almonds, Brazil nuts, fish, pecans, pumpkin, sesame seeds, lima beans, chickpeas, and lentils.

❑ Reduce your intake of animal protein, especially if you are taking levodopa (*see under* Considerations, below). This can help with control of coordination and muscle movements. Try to limit your protein consumption to 7 grams per day, consumed mostly at dinner. Eat barley, tofu, yogurt, beans, lentils, and other sources of protein instead of meat and poultry.

❑ If you must take the drug levodopa, consume the following foods in moderation only: bananas, beef, fish, liver, oatmeal, peanuts, potatoes, and whole grains. These foods contain vitamin B_6, which interferes with the drug's potency. *Do not* take supplemental vitamin B_6, as it counteracts the drug's therapeutic effects (be careful with multivitamin supplements). Also, because some of the amino acids contained in food proteins can prevent this drug from reaching the brain, where it is needed, eat protein foods only in the evening, and not at the same time as the drug is taken. Once on medication, discuss with your physician any dietary change you plan to make, as dosage adjustments may be needed.

❑ If your work or a hobby exposes you to chemicals or metals such as lead or aluminum, always wear protective clothing, including gloves and a face mask.

CONSIDERATIONS

❑ Hand tremors are common in middle age and later. There are different types of tremors. *Parkinsonian tremors* are most pronounced during rest, can be aggravated by tension or fatigue, and disappear during sleep. *Intention tremors* occur only when a muscle is being used, rather than at rest. *Essential tremors* are more or less continuous up-and-down tremors that seem to run in families. These usually affect both hands and become milder with rest, more severe with activity and/or stress. Attempts to stop this type of tremor through willpower often seem to make the trembling worse. Any persistent or recurrent tremor deserves investigation, especially if it interferes with normal activity, but it should be kept in mind that most tremors are *not* an indication of Parkinson's disease.

❑ Some people with Parkinson's disease have been found to have high levels of lead in their brains. Chelation therapy is the only way to remove lead from the body. (*See* CHELATION THERAPY in Part Three.)

❑ Because there are no definitive tests for Parkinson's disease, people with hypoglycemia are sometimes misdiagnosed as having the condition. (*See* HYPOGLYCEMIA in Part Two.)

❑ Fasting and chelation are both beneficial and may help to halt the progression of Parkinson's disease. (*See* FASTING and CHELATION THERAPY in Part Three.)

❑ Physical therapy, including active and passive range-of-motion exercises, plus daily moderate exercise like walking, can help to maintain normal muscle tone and function.

❑ "Green drinks" may significantly reduce symptoms. (*See* JUICING in Part Three.)

❑ Octocosanol, a substance found in wheat germ oil, has been shown to have beneficial effects on neuron membranes, and may make it possible to reduce the dosage of levodopa required.

❑ Iron supplementation appears to be beneficial to some people with Parkinson's disease. The production of tyrosine hydroxylase, an enzyme involved in the production of dopa (the precursor of dopamine), apparently can be stimulated by iron supplementation.

❑ A study published in *The New England Journal of Medicine* concluded that when the drug selegiline (Eldepryl), also known as deprenyl, is taken in the early stages of the disease, the onset of the more disabling symptoms seems to be delayed. The drug's mechanism of action is unclear, however, and it has not been proved that it can actually delay or slow the disease process, as opposed to easing symptoms.

❑ Treatment with the hormone dehydroepiandrosterone (DHEA) may help to prevent Parkinson's disease. (*See* DHEA THERAPY in Part Three.)

❑ The use of antioxidant supplements may delay the need for the levodopa therapy in people with Parkinson's disease, in some cases by as much as two to three years. In one study, people with Parkinson's disease were given 3,000 milligrams of vitamin C and 3,200 international units of vitamin E daily. The results strongly suggested that the progression of the disease can be slowed significantly by the administration of high dosages of antioxidants. If Parkinson's disease is related to free radical damage of dopamine-producing brain cells, in theory, a person who takes antioxidants while still healthy might never develop Parkinson's disease. Other research is exploring the role of a naturally occurring substance, glial-cell-line-derived neutrotrophic factor (GDNF), which nourishes the neurons that produce dopamine.

❑ There is no known cure for Parkinson's disease. Treatment is focused on relieving the symptoms and maintaining independence as long as possible. Drug therapy, physical therapy, and surgery are among the treatment methods used.

❑ The drug first used to treat this disease was levodopa (sold under the brand names Dopar and Larodopa). This drug is not effective alone, however, and can have serious side effects, including paranoia and hallucinations. A combination of levodopa and a drug called carbidopa (Sinemet) is also used. This drug also reduces stiffness. Other drugs that may be prescribed for people with Parkinson's disease are bromocriptine (Parlodel), entacapone (Comtan), pergolide (Permax), pramipexole (Mirapex), ropinirole (Requip), and tolcapone (Tasmar). Some of these drugs can be used either on their own or with levodopa; others must be used with levodopa. All of these medications can cause side effects.

❑ Pallidotomy is a surgical procedure sometimes recommended for people with Parkinson's disease. In this technique, the surgeon uses targeted electrical current to destroy the area in the brain that is causing involuntary movements. Although this has become safer and more accurate, it is still a high-risk operation.

❏ The transplantation of brain tissue from an animal that is still manufacturing dopamine into the brains of people with Parkinson's disease have proved successful in relieving symptoms in some cases.

❏ Brain stimulators to curb involuntary movements are much like pacemakers for the heart. They can be implanted in the brain and operated by the individual when needed.

❏ Additional information is available from the National Parkinson's Foundation (*see* HEALTH AND MEDICAL ORGANIZATIONS in the Appendix).

Peptic Ulcer

A peptic ulcer is a spot where the lining of the stomach or small intestine and the tissues beneath—and sometimes part of the stomach muscle itself—have been eroded, leaving an internal open wound. The surrounding tissue is usually swollen and irritated. Ulcers can occur anywhere along the gastrointestinal tract, but are most common in the stomach (gastric ulcers) and duodenum (duodenal ulcers), the portion of the small intestine closest to the stomach. Peptic ulcers affect approximately 5 million Americans each year, and it is estimated that they will affect approximately 10 percent of Americans at some point in their lives.

The symptoms of a peptic ulcer include chronic burning or gnawing stomach pain that usually begins forty-five to sixty minutes after eating or at night, and that is relieved by eating, taking antacids, vomiting, or drinking a large glass of water. The pain may range from mild to severe. It may cause the individual to awaken in the middle of the night. Other possible symptoms include lower back pain, headaches, a choking sensation, itching, and possibly nausea and vomiting.

An ulcer results when the lining of the stomach fails to provide adequate protection against the effect of digestive acids and enzymes, which, in effect, start to digest the stomach itself.

It was once believed that stress and anxiety were the main cause of ulcers. However, evidence has shown ulcers to be the result of infection with *Helicobacter pylori* bacteria combined with the presence of stomach acid. *H. pylori* can live on the lining of the stomach and small intestine, where it can cause damage to the lining and also to the mucous layer that protects the lining from digestive acids. Many health care professionals believe that the bacteria are transmitted from person to person through close contact. However, many health care professionals still consider stress to be a risk factor for peptic ulcers, as it increases stomach acid production. Certain drugs and supplements also may increase acid production. Taking aspirin or nonsteroidal anti-inflammatory drugs, especially over a long period of time, can increase stomach acidity and lead to ulcers. Steroids,

such as those taken for arthritis, can contribute to stomach ulcers. Having a family history of peptic ulcer disease also increases your risk, as does alcohol consumption. Heavy smokers are more prone to developing ulcers, and have greater trouble getting ulcers to heal. African-Americans and Latinos are twice as likely as Caucasians to have ulcers. If left untreated, ulcers can cause internal bleeding or puncture of the stomach or small intestine.

STOMACH ACID SELF-TEST

If you suffer from stomach pain, you can determine whether the problem is caused by excess stomach acid with this simple test. When you have the pain, swallow a tablespoon of apple cider vinegar or lemon juice. If this makes the pain go away, you most likely have too little stomach acid, not too much. If it makes your symptoms worse, then you may have an overly acidic stomach. The suggestions in this section should help to correct the problem.

NUTRIENTS

SUPPLEMENT	SUGGESTED DOSAGE	COMMENTS
Important		
Acid-Ease from Prevail	As directed on label.	Balances acidity in the body, reducing symptoms. For some people, may be able to replace ulcer medications such as ranitidine (Zantac).
L-Glutamine	500 mg daily, on an empty stomach. Take with water or juice. Do not take with milk. Take with 50 mg vitamin B_6 and 100 mg vitamin C for better absorption.	Important in the healing of peptic ulcers. (*See* AMINO ACIDS in Part One.)
Pectin	As directed on label.	Helps relieve duodenal ulcers by creating a soothing protective coating in the intestines.
Vitamin E	400–800 IU daily.	A potent antioxidant that aids in reducing stomach acid and in relieving pain. Helps promote healing. Use d-alpha-tocopherol form.
Helpful		
Acidophilus (Kyo-Dophilus from Wakunaga is a good source)	2–3 capsules, 1–3 times daily.	To provide flora for the small intestine that improve assimilation of nutrients and aid in digestion. Use a nondairy, nonrefrigeration formula.
Bromelain	250 mg 3 times daily.	An enzyme from pineapple that improves digestion and relieves symptoms. Chewable papaya tablets are also good.
Curcumin	250–500 mg 2–3 times daily, between meals.	Promotes healing.
Essential fatty acids (MaxEPA, primrose oil, and salmon oil are good sources)	As directed on label.	Protects the stomach and intestinal tract from ulcers.

Iron or Floradix Iron + Herbs from Salus Haus	As directed by physician. Take with 100 mg buffered or esterified vitamin C for better absorption. As directed on label.	Helps prevent anemia, which may occur with bleeding ulcers. Use ferrous chelate or ferrous fumarate form. *Caution:* Do not take iron unless anemia is diagnosed. A nontoxic form of iron from food sources.
Multivitamin and mineral complex	As directed on label.	To provide a balance of essential nutrients.
Proteolytic enzymes or Inflazyme Forte from American Biologics or Wobenzym N from Marlyn Nutraceuticals	As directed on label. Take between meals. As directed on label. As directed on label.	Works on undigested food remaining in the colon, and helps reduce inflammation. *Caution:* Do not use a formula containing HCl.
Pycnogenol or grape seed extract	As directed on label. As directed on label.	Powerful free radical scavengers that also act as anti- inflammatories and strengthen tissues.
S-Adenosylmethio- nine (SAMe)	200 mg twice a day, in the morning and in the evening.	Aids in relief of stress and depression, eases pain, and produces antioxidant effects. *Caution:* Do not use if you have manic-depressive disorder or take prescription antidepressants. A very small number of people taking high doses have reported gastrointestinal disturbances. If this happens, discontinue the supplement.
Vitamin A emulsion or capsules	50,000 IU daily for 1 month; then 25,000 IU daily for 1 month; then reduce to 10,000 IU daily. 25,000 IU daily. If you are pregnant, do not exceed 10,000 IU daily.	Needed for healing. Protects the mucous membranes of the stomach and intestines.
Vitamin B complex plus extra vitamin B$_6$ (pyridoxine)	50 mg of each major B vitamin 3 times daily (amounts of individual vitamins in a complex will vary.) Do not exceed a total of 25 mg vitamin B$_3$ (niacin) daily from all sources. 50 mg 3 times daily.	Needed for proper digestion. A sublingual type is best. Needed for enzyme production and wound healing.
Vitamin C	3,000 mg daily.	Promotes wound healing and protects against infection. Use a buffered or esterified form.
Vitamin K	100 mcg daily.	Needed for healing and to prevent bleeding; promotes nutrient absorption and has a neutralizing effect on the intestinal tract. Deficiency is common in those with digestive disorders.
Zinc	50–80 mg daily. Do not exceed a total of 100 mg daily from all supplements.	Promotes healing. Use zinc gluconate lozenges or OptiZinc for best absorption.

HERBS

❏ Alfalfa is a good source of vitamin K.

❏ Aloe vera aids in pain relief and speeds healing. Take 4 ounces of aloe vera juice or gel daily. Be sure to buy a food-grade product.

❏ Bupleurum, used in combination with angelica and licorice root, is good for treating ulcers.

❏ Cat's claw is cleansing and healing to the digestive tract. Cat's Claw Defense Complex from Source Naturals is a combination of cat's claw and other herbs, plus anti-oxidant nutrients such as beta-carotene, N-acetylcysteine, vitamin C, and zinc.

Caution: Do not use cat's claw during pregnancy.

❏ Comfrey is beneficial for treating ulcers.

Caution: Do not take this herb internally for more than one month, and use it only under the close supervision of a health care professional.

❏ Garlic is an antimicrobial and may aid in eradicating ulcers.

❏ Hops, passionflower, skullcap, and valerian root are good for promoting a restful sleep. These supplements can be found in a single complex.

❏ Kava kava and St. John's wort have calming effects and reduce stress.

❏ Licorice promotes healing of gastric and duodenal ulcers. Take 750 to 1,500 milligrams of deglycyrrhizinated licorice (DGL) two to three times daily, between meals, for eight to sixteen weeks. Studies have shown that DGL may be as effective as the pharmaceutical drug cimetidine (Tagamet) or ranitidine (Zantac) in treating peptic ulcers.

Caution: Do not substitute ordinary licorice root for the deglycyrrhizinated variety. Ordinary licorice can elevate blood pressure if used on a daily basis for more than seven days in a row, and should be avoided completely by persons with high blood pressure. Deglycyrrhizinated licorice has had a component known as glycyrrhizinic acid removed, which should eliminate this side effect.

❏ Malva tea calms the stomach and reduces intestinal irritation.

❏ Marshmallow root and slippery elm soothe irritated mucous membranes.

❏ Rhubarb, taken in juice or tablet form, is good for treating intestinal bleeding, which sometimes accompanies peptic ulcers.

❏ Other beneficial herbs include bayberry, catnip, chamomile, goldenseal, myrrh, and sage. All of these can be taken in tea form.

Caution: Do not use chamomile on an ongoing basis, as ragweed allergy may result. Avoid it completely if you are allergic to ragweed. Do not take goldenseal on a daily basis for more than one week at a time, as it may disturb normal intestinal flora. Do not use it during pregnancy, and use it with caution if you are allergic to ragweed. Do not use sage if you suffer from any type of seizure disorder.

RECOMMENDATIONS

❑ Eat plenty of dark green leafy vegetables. These contain vitamin K, which is needed for healing and is likely to be deficient in people with digestive problems.

❑ Do not consume coffee (even decaffeinated) or alcoholic beverages.

❑ Drink freshly made cabbage juice daily. Drink it immediately after juicing. (See JUICING in Part Three.)

❑ If symptoms are severe, eat soft foods such as avocados, bananas, potatoes, squash, and yams. Put vegetables through a blender or food mill. Eat vegetables like broccoli and carrots occasionally—well steamed.

❑ Eat frequent small meals; include well-cooked millet, well-cooked rice, raw goat's milk, and soured milk products such as yogurt, cottage cheese, and kefir. Drink barley, wheat, and alfalfa juice. They contain chlorophyll, making them potent anti-ulcer treatments.

❑ If you have a bleeding ulcer, consume organic baby foods or steamed vegetables blended in a blender or mashed. Add nonirritating fiber such as guar gum and/or psyllium seed. These foods are easy to digest and nutritious, and they contain no chemicals.

❑ For rapid relief of pain, drink a large glass of water. This dilutes the stomach acids and flushes them out through the stomach and duodenum.

❑ Avoid fried foods, tea, caffeine, chocolate, animal fats of any kind, and carbonated drinks. Instead of drinking soda, sip distilled water with a bit of lemon juice added.

❑ Avoid salt and sugar. They have been linked to increased stomach acid production.

❑ Reduce your intake of refined carbohydrates, as they have been linked to peptic ulcers.

❑ Do not drink cow's milk. Even though it neutralizes existing stomach acid, the calcium and protein it contains actually stimulate the production of more acid, and it is known to be associated with the occurrence of ulcers. Almond, rice, or soy milk are good substitutes.

❑ Chew your food thoroughly. This improves digestion. Taking bitters also improves digestion. Place 10 to 15 drops under your tongue before meals.

❑ Allow teas and other hot beverages to cool before drinking them. Otherwise, they may trigger gastric discomfort.

❑ Keep the colon clean. Make sure the bowels move daily, and take cleansing enemas periodically. (See COLON CLEANSING and ENEMAS in Part Three.)

❑ Do not smoke. Smoking can delay or even prevent healing, and makes relapse more likely.

❑ Avoid painkillers such as aspirin. Aspirin is present in many over-the-counter remedies; read labels carefully. Also avoid ibuprofen (in Advil, Nuprin, and other products).

❑ Try to avoid stressful situations. Learn stress management techniques. (See STRESS in Part Two and Meditation under PAIN CONTROL in Part Three.) Music therapy may be helpful. (See MUSIC AND SOUND THERAPY in Part Three.)

CONSIDERATIONS

❑ Physicians can use two procedures to locate a peptic ulcer: an upper gastrointestinal (GI) series, in which you drink a chalky barium liquid and have a series of x-rays taken of the stomach and duodenum; and an endoscopy, in which a physician inserts a thin lighted tube attached to a camera down through your throat and into the stomach or duodendum.

❑ While prescription and over-the-counter drugs may temporarily relieve the symptoms of ulcers, they do not get to the root of the problem, which is damaged tissue. They offer short-term relief by temporarily decreasing stomach acid. In the long run, they may make the problem worse because they create the illusion that the ulcer has been cured. They also disrupt the normal digestive processes and alter the structure and functioning of the tissues that line the digestive tract.

❑ With treatment, most peptic ulcers heal, but it may take eight weeks or longer for healing to be complete.

❑ Antacids are often recommended for people with ulcers. If you must take antacids, avoid products containing aluminum, which has been linked to Alzheimer's disease. (See ALZHEIMER'S DISEASE in Part Two.) Maalox has been known to cause a gray film on the tongue in rare instances. Discontinue use if this occurs.

❑ People who take cimetidine (Tagamet) or ranitidine (Zantac) for ulcers should be cautious about ingesting alcohol. These drugs can magnify the effects of alcohol on the brain.

❑ A simple procedure using Kool-Aid to test for the presence of stomach ulcers has been developed by the Cabrini Medical Center in New York City. The person being tested is given two glasses of Kool-Aid made with extra sugar. After a short period, he or she takes a urine test. In people with ulcers, the sugar leaks across the stomach wall and shows up in the urine as undigested sugar. If there is no ulcer, the sugar is broken down normally by the body.

❑ Infection with *H. pylori* is very common. For reasons unknown, only about one out of six infected people develops ulcers. Your physician can test for *H. pylori* by a direct biopsy of the stomach lining, a blood test, or a breath test. If you test positive for *H. pylori*, there are several antibiotic treatments available for your physician to prescribe.

❑ Peptic ulcers were once thought to be a chronic illness that one "just has to live with." However, it is now known that 90 percent of peptic ulcers can be cured with appropriate treatment.

❑ If an ulcer does not heal, your physician may perform a biopsy to rule out cancer.

❑ The combination of two prescription medications, omeprazole (Prilosec, an ulcer medication) and clarithromycin (Biaxin, an antibiotic), may be prescribed for people with with *H. pylori* infection and duodenal ulcer. These drugs should not be used for an extended period of time, as they have known side effects.

❑ Gastroesophagaeal reflux disease (GERD) and peptic ulcers cause very similar symptoms. However, GERD is both more common and, usually, less serious than a peptic ulcer. (*See* HEARTBURN/GASTROESOPHAGEAL REFLUX DISEASE (GERD) in Part Two.)

❑ Many experts believe that food allergies may be a cause of ulcers. *See* ALLERGIES in Part Two and follow the self-test program to identify possible problem foods.

Periodontal Disease

Periodontal disease is second only to the common cold as the most prevalent infectious ailment in the United States. It affects 75 percent of Americans over the age of thirty-five and is the major cause of adult tooth loss. The rate of periodontal disease increases with age.

Periodontal means "located around a tooth." *Periodontal disease* therefore can refer to any disorder of the gums or other supporting structures of the teeth. *Gingivitis* (inflammation of the gums) is the early stage of periodontal disease. It is caused by plaque—sticky deposits of bacteria, mucus, and food particles—that adheres to the teeth. The accumulation of plaque causes the gums to become infected and swollen. As the gums swell, pockets form between the gums and the teeth that act as a trap for still more plaque. Other factors that contribute to the development of gingivitis include breathing through the mouth, badly fitting fillings and prostheses that irritate surrounding gum tissue, and a diet consisting of too many soft foods that rob the teeth and gums of much needed "exercise." The gums become red, soft, and shiny, and they bleed easily. In some cases, there is pain, but gingivitis can also be essentially painless.

If left untreated, gingivitis can lead to a condition called *pyorrhea* or *periodontitis*. This is an advanced stage of periodontal disease in which the bone supporting the teeth begins to erode as a result of the infection. Abscesses are common. Pyorrhea causes halitosis, with bleeding and often painful gums. Poor nutrition, improper brushing, wrong foods, sugar consumption, chronic illness, glandular disorders, blood disease, smoking, drugs, and excessive alcohol consumption make an individual more likely to develop pyorrhea. It is often related to a deficiency of vitamin

C, bioflavonoids, calcium, folic acid, or niacin. Smokers are more susceptible than nonsmokers to periodontitis and tooth loss. Periodontal disease can be made worse by missing teeth, food impaction, malocclusion, tongue-thrusting, tooth-grinding, and toothbrush trauma.

Stomatitis is inflammation of the oral tissues and may affect the lips, palate, and insides of the cheeks. It often occurs as part of another disease. Stomatitis produces swollen gums that bleed easily. Sores may develop in the mouth and eventually become blisterlike lesions that can affect the gums. Two common types of stomatitis are *acute herpetic stomatitis* (better known as oral herpes) and *aphthous stomatitis* (canker sores).

Problems in the mouth often are reflections of deficiencies or underlying disorders in the body. Bleeding gums may signal a vitamin C deficiency; dryness and cracking at the corners of the mouth may indicate a deficiency of vitamin B_2 (riboflavin). Both conditions may also signal a generalized nutritional deficiency. Dry or cracked lips can be the result of an allergic reaction. Raw, red mouth tissue may be a sign of stress; a smooth, reddish tongue can indicate anemia or poor diet. Sores under the tongue can be an early warning sign of mouth cancer. Regular dental checkups can help detect these conditions early.

NUTRIENTS

SUPPLEMENT	SUGGESTED DOSAGE	COMMENTS
Essential		
Coenzyme Q10	100 mg daily.	Provides energy needed for gum cell growth and healing of gum tissue.
plus Coenzyme A from Coenzyme-A Technologies	As directed on label.	Works effectively with coenzyme Q10 to support the immune system's detoxification of many dangerous substances.
Vitamin C with bioflavonoids	4,000–10,000 mg daily, in divided doses throughout the day.	Promotes healing, especially of bleeding gums. Bioflavonoids retard plaque growth.
Very Important		
Bone Support from Synergy Plus	As directed on label.	Contains calcium, magnesium, phosphorus, zinc, and other nutrients that are easily absorbed by the body to rebuild bone.
or calcium and	1,500 mg daily.	Helps prevent bone loss around the gums.
magnesium	750 mg daily.	Works with calcium. Use a chelate form.
Methylsulfonyl-methane (MSM)	As directed on label.	Has remarkable therapeutic properties.
Vitamin A plus carotenoid complex (Betatene)	25,000 IU daily for 1 month, then reduce to 10,000 IU daily. If you are pregnant, do not exceed 10,000 IU daily. As directed on label.	Needed for healing of gum tissue. Emulsion form is recommended for easier assimilation and greater safety at high doses. Antioxidants used by the body to manufacture vitamin A as needed.

Vitamin E	Start with 400 IU daily and increase slowly to 1,000 IU daily. Also open a capsule and rub the oil on the gums 2–3 times daily.	Needed for healing of gum tissue. Use d-alpha-tocopherol form. Do *not* use the dl-form.
plus selenium (E-Sel from Carlson Labs)	200 mcg daily. If you are pregnant, do not exceed 40 mcg daily.	A powerful antioxidant that works with vitamin E to ward off cancer.
Important		
Grape seed extract	As directed on label.	A powerful antioxidant and anti-inflammatory.
Proteolytic enzymes with pancreatin	As directed on label. Take between meals and also at bedtime.	Aids in keeping down inflammation and aids proper digestion.
Quercetin	As directed on label.	Has anti-inflammatory properties.
Vitamin B complex	50 mg of each major B vitamin 3 times daily, with meals (amounts of individual vitamins in a complex will vary).	Needed for proper digestion and healthy mouth tissues.
Zinc	50–80 mg daily. Do not exceed a total of 100 mg daily from all supplements.	Enhances immune function. Needed to prevent infection and promote healing. Use zinc gluconate lozenges or OptiZinc for best absorption.
plus copper	3 mg daily.	Needed to balance with zinc.

HERBS

❑ Applying aloe vera gel directly to inflamed gums eases discomfort and soothes the tissues.

❑ Strained chamomile tea and calendula flower tea are both soothing and help to heal gum tissues.

❑ Clove oil is good for temporary relief of tooth and/or gum pain. Simply rub a drop or two of clove oil on the affected area. If the oil is too strong in its pure form, it can be diluted with a drop or two of olive oil.

❑ Echinacea, hawthorn berries, myrrh gum, and rose hips help to keep down inflammation and enhance immune function. You can apply these herbs directly to the inflamed areas as a poultice or drink them in tea form.

❑ Goldenseal destroys the bacteria that cause periodontal disease. Take 3,000 milligrams daily. Or place a dropperful of alcohol-free goldenseal extract in your mouth, swish it around for three minutes, then swallow. For inflamed gums, place 5 drops of alcohol-free goldenseal extract on a piece of gauze or pure cotton and place this on the inflamed area. Do this immediately whenever mouth sores or inflammation starts, and you will be amazed at the results. In severe cases, it may take three to five nights for sores to heal. Be sure to pack the gauze or cotton tightly under the inside of the front of the mouth between the lips and gum.

Caution: Do not take goldenseal internally on a daily basis for more than one week at a time, as it may disturb normal intestinal flora. Do not use it during pregnancy, and use it with caution if you are allergic to ragweed.

❑ Sage is good for its anti-inflammatory properties. Boil 2 tablespoons of dried, crushed sage leaves in one cup of water, steep for twenty minutes, strain, and rinse your mouth several times daily.

❑ Tea tree oil, rubbed on the gums, helps to prevent and treat gum disease.

Caution: Do not take tea tree oil internally.

❑ Thyme is a natural antiseptic that reduces the level of bacteria in the mouth.

RECOMMENDATIONS

❑ Eat a varied diet of fresh fruits, green leafy vegetables, meat, and whole grains to provide the teeth and gums with needed exercise and supply the body with the vitamins and minerals that are essential for dental health. Although all vitamins and minerals are essential for the proper formation and continued health of the teeth, adequate vitamin C intake is particularly important for the prevention of gingivitis and pyorrhea. Vitamin A seems to control the development and general health of the gums; a lack of this vitamin often results in gum infection. Vitamin A is also necessary for healthy tooth development in children. Minerals important for healthy teeth include sodium, potassium, calcium, phosphorus, iron, and magnesium.

❑ Eat plenty of high-fiber foods, such as whole grains, vegetables, and legumes.

❑ Avoid sugar and all refined carbohydrates. Sugar causes plaque buildup and inhibits the ability of white blood cells to fight off bacteria.

❑ Brush your teeth with goldenseal powder every day for at least one month. You can open up a capsule of goldenseal and mix the contents with toothpaste, or use a liquid extract in the same way. After one month, change brands of toothpaste. Don't stay with the same brand; some brands may irritate the gums.

❑ Change toothbrushes every month to keep the disease in check, and keep your toothbrush clean between uses. Bacteria live on toothbrushes. There are special devices that kill bacteria that you can keep your toothbrush in when not in use.

❑ Floss your teeth at least once a day. Unwaxed dental floss is good for getting under the gumline.

❑ Scrape your tongue each morning after you brush and floss to remove bacteria. Use a tongue scraper (available in health food stores and some pharmacies) or the back of a spoon. This is important because bacteria thrive on a moist tongue.

❑ Stim-U-Dent, found in drug stores, is beneficial for keeping the gums massaged and clean between brushing. Make sure you soak it in water or hold in the mouth until it softens, so as not to damage the gums. Massage between each tooth between meals. This also helps to remove plaque and should be used daily after eating.

❏ Use your fingertips to massage your gums to increase circulation.

❏ Interdental-space brushes are good for cleaning the spaces between teeth.

❏ Try using a dental rinse called Plax to help loosen plaque. Unlike mouthwashes, this is designed to be used before brushing. Listerine also helps to remove plaque.

❏ Use a *very* soft natural-bristle toothbrush. Be sure to brush your gums and tongue as well as your teeth at least twice a day. The most effective way to get under the gum line is to tilt the toothbrush so that the bristles are at a 45-degree angle to the gum, and brush in a forward and backward motion using short strokes across the gums to remove bacteria.

❏ If inflammation is present, run very hot water over the toothbrush to soften it before brushing, and be gentle until healing is complete.

❏ Open a capsule of vitamin E and rub the oil on inflamed gums. This is very healing and helps to alleviate soreness.

❏ For relief of toothache pain until you can get to your dentist, apply ice to the gums. Clove oil can also be helpful (*see under* Herbs, above).

❏ Avoid taking antibiotics. The mouth is the hardest place for them to work, and they destroy needed friendly bacteria in the colon. Try goldenseal first (*see under* Herbs, above).

❏ In addition to the products described above, we recommend the following tooth and gum products. Most of these can be bought at health food stores.

• *Nature de France (Pierre Cattier).* Contains a clay base for healing.

• *Nature's Gate.* Contains baking soda and sea salt, which is effective against plaque and gum disease. Also contains vitamin C.

• *Peelu.* Contains a natural tooth whitener derived from the small peelu tree, native to the Middle East and Asia. People have chewed its branches for centuries to keep their teeth white. Also contains natural flavor, fruit pectin, sodium lauryl sulfate (from coconut oil), and vegetable glycerine. Unlike many over-the-counter tooth-whitening products, this does not irritate or damage gums.

• *Herbal Toothpaste and Gum Therapy with Baking Soda* from The Natural Dentist. Fights plaque and gingivitis.

• *Herbal Crème de Anise.* Another good product found in health food stores.

• *Herbal Mouth and Gum Therapy Mouth Wash.* Good for rinsing the mouth between brushes.

• *Tom's Natural Toothpaste.* Contains a natural calcium base. Features myrrh (an astringent herb) and propolis.

• *Weleda Salt Toothpaste.* Contains baking soda and salt formulation with medicinal herbs and silica.

• *Vicco Pure Herbal Toothpaste.* Contains extracts from plants, bark, roots, and flowers used in Ayurvedic medicine.

❏ Be sure your dentist is taking the proper steps to avoid transmitting disease. The dentist's office and waiting room should be clean. Dentists, hygienists, and dental assistants should wash their hands and change gloves between patients. Every reusable instrument should be sterilized between patients, and large equipment and all surfaces in the treatment room should be cleaned and disinfected periodically. If you have questions about your dentist's procedures, do not hesitate to ask.

CONSIDERATIONS

❏ Periodontal disease should ideally be treated by a periodontist, a dentist who specializes in this area of dentistry.

❏ The process of periodontal disease is easier to reverse if it is caught early. It is important to know the symptoms and get regular dental check-ups for periodontal disease.

❏ Severe cases of periodontal disease may necessitate surgery to remove the infected tissue from the gum and reshape the bone.

❏ Certain illnesses, such as diabetes and several kinds of blood disorders, create a higher risk for developing gum disease.

❏ Research suggests that people who have severe periodontal disease may be at greater risk of heart disease, lung disease, stroke, ulcers, poor control of diabetes, and giving birth prematurely. Studies are ongoing regarding the effect periodontal disease has on the health of the body. It is suspected that bacteria that exist in periodontal pockets may easily enter the bloodstream. So by caring for your teeth, you may also be caring for whole-body health.

❏ A simple blood test can detect gum disease up to eight months before symptoms appear, according to Dr. Jeffrey Ebersole, associate professor of periodontics at the University of Texas Health Science Center. A dentist can draw a drop of blood from a finger and have it analyzed for the bacteria that cause gum disease.

❏ Regular intimate contact with an infected person can transmit the bacteria that cause periodontal disease.

❏ Smoking is a major factor in irritating the gums and mouth. It has also been linked to mouth and esophagus cancer.

❏ Some people appear to be more susceptible than others to the bacteria that cause gum disease because of a genetic predisposition.

❏ Dry mouth, a condition in which there is not enough saliva in the mouth, can promote tooth decay and periodontal disease. Saliva is essential for ridding the mouth of plaque, sugar, and debris. Dry mouth problems increase with age; more than half of people over the age of fifty-five are affected by it. It can also be caused by alcohol consumption or by prescription or over-the-counter drugs, especially those for high blood pressure, depression, colds, and allergies. Diabetes is also associated with dry mouth. The best treatment for dry mouth is to draw more moisture from the salivary glands by chewing carrots, celery, or sugar-free gum; drinking 8 to 10 cups of water a day, chewing ice chips; and/or breathing through the nose.

❏ Dental implants look more natural than dentures, and many people are opting for them. Unfortunately, improperly inserted dental implants can cause or exacerbate periodontal disease. If you are interested in implants, consult an implant specialist.

❏ Researchers are studying a possible link between hormone replacement therapy (HRT) and a decrease in tooth loss. Researchers at Harvard Medical School and Brigham and Women's Hospital in Boston found a 24-percent decrease in tooth loss among woman using HRT. It is suspected that this may be because HRT aids in protecting against loss of bone-mineral density in the jaw. HRT is not without its risks, however, some of them potentially serious (*see* MENOPAUSAL AND PERIMENOPAUSAL PROBLEMS in Part Two).

❏ Air abrasion technology, a dental technique that painlessly removes tooth decay without drilling, allows dentists to make smaller fillings and save more of the natural tooth. The new technique, considered to be a major breakthrough, does not necessitate numbing drugs or anesthesia.

❏ Regular dental checkups are important in detecting oral cancer, a disease that strikes 30,000 Americans each year. If oral cancer is caught early, nine out of ten people survive.

❏ One advantage (perhaps the only one) to having allergies is that people who suffer from allergies are less likely to lose teeth to periodontal disease. The reason apparently is that the allergy sufferer's overactive immune system is better at fighting off the bacteria that cause periodontal disease.

❏ There is a tablet you can purchase at most drugstores that shows areas your toothbrush missed. Chew a tablet after brushing, then brush until the color is gone.

❏ Electric toothbrushes, such as the Braun or Oral B systems, help to remove plaque.

❏ An automatic toothbrush sanitizer has been proven effective in keeping toothbrushes free of bacteria. The device automatically turns on every half-hour for two minutes to sanitize the bristles twenty-four hours a day. As an alternative, you can store your toothbrush in hydrogen peroxide or grapefruit seed extract to kill germs (if using hydrogen peroxide, rinse it well before brushing).

❏ Fluoride is a mineral that strengthens the underlying structure supporting the teeth—especially important for menopausal women who have lost density in their jawbones. Fluoride also helps to protect root surfaces that become exposed as gums recede with age from decay. There is debate among health care professionals regarding the use of fluoride. Some believe in using it, while others do not.

❏ *See also* CANKER SORES and HERPESVIRUS INFECTION, both in Part Two.

❏ *See also* Bleeding Gums *under* PREGNANCY-RELATED PROBLEMS in Part Two.

Phlebitis

See THROMBOPHLEBITIS.

Photophobia

See under EYE PROBLEMS.

Pinkeye

See under EYE PROBLEMS.

Plantar Fasciitis

See under HEEL OR BONE SPUR.

PMS

See PREMENSTRUAL SYNDROME.

Pneumonia

Pneumonia is a serious infection of the lungs that can be caused by any of a number of different infectious agents, including viruses, bacteria, fungi, protozoa, and mycoplasma. The infection causes tiny air sacs in the lung area to become inflamed and filled with mucus and pus, inhibiting oxygen from reaching the blood. *Lobar pneumonia* affects only a section, or lobe, of one lung. *Bronchial pneumonia* affects portions of both lungs. Although symptoms can vary in intensity, they usually include fever, chills, cough, bloody sputum, muscle aches, fatigue, sore throat, enlarged lymph glands in the neck, cyanosis (a bluish cast to the skin and nails), pain in the chest, and rapid, difficult respiration.

Pneumonia is typically preceded by an upper respiratory infection such as a cold, influenza, or measles. Factors that increase the risk of pneumonia include being either under one year or over sixty years of age, a weakened immune system, cardiovascular disease, diabetes, HIV infection, seizure or stroke, aspiration under anesthesia, alcoholism, smoking, kidney failure, sickle cell disease, malnutrition, foreign bodies in the respiratory passages, exposure to chemical irritants, and even allergies.

Bacterial pneumonia can be very dangerous and may come on either suddenly or gradually, usually as a complication of some other health problem such as respiratory disease, a weakened immune system, or viral infection. Older adults, young children, alcoholics, and people who have just undergone surgery are also at risk. *Streptococcus pneumoniae* is the most common cause of bacterial pneumonia. Symptoms usually include shaking, chills, and a high temperature. The cough is dry at first. Then a rust-colored sputum is produced, and breathing becomes rapid and labored. Chest pain that worsens upon inhalation, abdominal pain, and fatigue are also common. This type of pneumonia is unlikely to spread from one person to another.

Viral pneumonia is more variable in course and severity. It can come on suddenly or gradually, and symptoms—which are much the same as those of bacterial pneumonia—can be mild, severe, or anywhere in between. It is less serious than bacterial pneumonia, but if not cared for properly, a second, bacterial pneumonia infection can set in.

Fungal pneumonia, especially *Pneumocystis carinii* pneumonia (PCP), is much less common than either the bacterial or viral variety, and is often associated with a weakened or suppressed immune system. People with HIV, AIDS, or certain types of cancer, or who are taking immunosuppressive drugs following organ transplantation, are most likely to be affected.

Mycoplasma pneumonia, or "walking pneumonia," is caused by an agent that is unclassified but appears to be both bacterium and virus. This form of pneumonia usually affects people under forty. The symptoms tend to be less severe than those of viral or bacterial pneumonia and include a cough that is spasmodic, along with chills and a fever.

Infants can contract pneumonia due to a *Chlamydia trachomatis* infection transferred to the child during birth. Childhood pneumonia can also be caused by the same bacteria that cause whooping cough.

Young children (especially infants), older adults, and people who have compromised immune systems are very vunerable to the potentially life-threatening effects of this illness. Pneumonia is now the fifth leading cause of death in the United States. No matter what the cause, pneumonia usually leaves the sufferer with weakness that persists for four to eight weeks after the acute phase of the infection has resolved.

Unless otherwise specified, the dosages recommended here are for adults. For a child between the ages of twelve and seventeen, reduce the dose to three-quarters the rec-ommended amount. For a child between six and twelve, use one-half the recommended dose, and for a child under the age of six, use one-quarter the recommended amount.

NUTRIENTS

SUPPLEMENT	SUGGESTED DOSAGE	COMMENTS
Essential		
Colloidal silver	As directed on label.	Reduces inflammation and promotes healing of lesions in lung tissue.
Garlic (Kyolic from Wakunaga)	As directed on label.	Protects against respiratory infections and destroys unwanted bacteria in the body.
Liquid oxygen supplement	As directed on label.	Increases oxygen intake and aids the body in eliminating toxins.
Nicotinamide adenine dinucleotide (NADH) (ENADA NADH from Kal)	10 mg daily.	Important in the creation and transfer of chemical energy, especially during breathing.
Vitamin A with mixed carotenoids	Up to 25,000 IU daily. If you are pregnant, do not exceed 10,000 IU daily.	Enhances immunity and promotes repair of lung tissue. Use emulsion form for easier assimilation and greater safety at high doses. Do not take such high doses in capsule form.
Vitamin C plus bioflavonoids	5,000–20,000 mg daily, in divided doses. (*See* ASCORBIC ACID FLUSH in Part Three.) 100 mg twice daily.	Very important for immune response and for reducing inflammation. Needed to activate vitamin C.
Very Important		
Free-form amino acid complex (Amino Balance from Anabol Naturals)	As directed on label.	To supply protein, important in tissue repair.
L-Carnitine plus L-cysteine plus glutathione	As directed on label, on an empty stomach. Take with water or juice. Do not take with milk. Take with 50 mg vitamin B₆ and 100 mg vitamin C for better absorption.	To protect the lungs from free radical damage and break down mucus in the respiratory tract.
Pycnogenol and/or grape seed extract	50 mg 4 times daily. As directed on label.	Boost the immune system and protect lung tissue; reduce the frequency and severity of colds and flu.
Vitamin B complex	100 mg of each major B vitamin 3 times daily (amounts of individual vitamins in a complex will vary).	Needed for normal digestion, production of antibodies and formation of red blood cells, and for healthy mucous membranes. Use a sublingual form.
Important		
Raw thymus glandular and raw lung glandular	500 mg each twice daily.	Stimulates immune response and promotes healing of lung tissue. (*See* GLANDULAR THERAPY in Part Three.)
Vitamin E emulsion or capsules	1,500 IU daily. 400 IU twice daily, before meals.	A potent antioxidant that protects the lung tissues and enhances oxygen utilization. Emulsion form is recommended. Use d-alpha-tocopherol form.

Zinc	80 mg daily. Do not exceed a total of 100 mg daily from all supplements.	Needed for tissue repair and immune function. Zinc gluconate lozenges are very effective.
Helpful		
Coenzyme Q10 plus Coenzyme A from Coenzyme-A Technologies	100 mg daily.	Enhances cellular oxygen utilization. Works well with coenzyme Q10 and supports the immune system's detoxification of many dangerous substances.
Essential fatty acids (flaxseed oil, primrose oil, salmon oil, and Ultimate Oil from Nature's Secret are good sources)	As directed on label.	Needed to build new lung tissue and to reduce inflammation. Improves stamina, speeds recovery, and boosts immunity.
Maitake extract or reishi extract or shiitake extract	As directed on label. As directed on label. As directed on label.	Mushroom extracts that help to build immunity and fight infection.
Melatonin	1.5–5 mg daily, taken 2 hours or less before bedtime.	To improve sleep. This is a natural hormone produced by the pineal gland that controls the body's sleep/wake cycle. *Caution:* This supplement is not suitable for children.
Multivitamin and mineral complex	As directed on label.	To maintain a balance of all necessary nutrients in the body.
Proteolytic enzymes (Novenzyme from International Health Products)	As directed on label 3 times daily, on an empty stomach.	Aids in absorption of nutrients and reduces inflammation.

HERBS

❏ Astragalus enhances the immune system.

❏ Clear Lungs from RidgeCrest Herbals is an herbal combination that helps provide relief from shortness of breath, tightness in the chest, and wheezing due to bronchial congestion. It is available in two formulas: one with ephedra and the other without. They appear to be equally effective.

❏ Echinacea enhances immunity.

❏ Ginger is an effective antimicrobial agent and is helpful for fever.

❏ Goldenseal and licorice root are natural antibiotics.

Caution: Do not take goldenseal internally on a daily basis for more than one week at a time, do not use it during pregnancy, and use it with caution if you are allergic to ragweed. Do not use licorice on a daily basis for more than seven days in a row, and avoid it completely if you have high blood pressure.

❏ Lung Tonic from Herbs, Etc. contains a variety of herbs that support the lungs.

RECOMMENDATIONS

❏ See your health care provider if you suspect pneumonia. This is a potentially dangerous disease.

❏ Eat a diet consisting of raw fruits and vegetables.

❏ Take a protein supplement from a vegetable source, such as a free-form amino acid complex. Amino acids are the building block of proteins. Soy is an excellent source of nondairy protein.

❏ Drink plenty of fresh juices. Liquids help to thin the lung secretions. Fast on pure juices, fresh lemon juice, and distilled water. (*See* FASTING and JUICING, both in Part Three.)

❏ Include "green drinks" in your diet or take chlorophyll in tablet form. Earth Source Greens & More from Solgar is a good green-drink product.

❏ If you are taking antibiotics, take acidophilus in capsule or liquid form three times each day.

❏ Exclude dairy products, sugar, and white flour products from your diet.

❏ Do not smoke.

❏ Use a cool mist from a humidifier or vaporizer to help ease breathing.

❏ Place a heating pad or a hot water bottle on your chest to relieve pain.

❏ Consider using a device called Air Supply from Wein Products. This is a personal air purifier that is worn around the neck. It kills and deactivates airborne viruses, bacteria, molds, and spores.

❏ To avoid passing the infection along to others, dispose of secretions properly. Sneeze and/or cough into disposable tissues. Flush used tissues to discard them.

❏ Children with pneumonia have to be carefully monitored. If you suspect that your child might have pneumonia, seek medical advice immediately.

CONSIDERATIONS

❏ Vitamin A is necessary for maintaining the health of the lining of the respiratory passages. A deficiency of this vitamin increases susceptibility to respiratory infections, which in turn can lead to pneumonia.

❏ Pneumococcal vaccine provides protection against more than twenty different strains of microorganisms that can cause pneumonia. It is recommended for anyone without a spleen, anyone with a chronic disease (especially diseases that affect the lungs), and everyone over the age of sixty-five.

❏ A urine test for *Streptococcus pneumoniae* takes fifteen minutes to perform. It is more efficient than diagnosis from mucus, blood, or saliva.

❏ The use of antibiotics for minor infections such as colds may lead to the development of antibiotic-resistant bacteria in the upper airway, which can cause pneumonia.

❏ *See also* INFLUENZA and COMMON COLD, both in Part Two.

Poison Ivy/Poison Oak/ Poison Sumac

Poison ivy, poison oak, and poison sumac are probably the most common allergenic plants in the United States. These plants grow in every state except Alaska and are common along roadsides, in forests and pastures, and along streams—even, in the case of poison ivy, in suburban backyards.

Poison ivy and poison oak are members of the same botanical family. Poison ivy is more prevalent east of the Rocky Mountains; poison oak is more common to the west and southwest. Poison sumac is common in southern swamps and northern wetlands. All three plants produce similar symptoms, and as a result all three are often referred to simply as poison ivy.

It is estimated that 65 percent of Americans are sensitive to these plants, and about 2 million people each year have a reaction from contact with them. Sensitivity to poison ivy is acquired and is at its peak during childhood. Most susceptible are people who are sensitive to sunlight. The irritating substance in poison ivy is urushiol, a substance present in the oily sap in the leaves, flowers, fruit, stem, bark, and roots. Urushiol is one of the most potent toxins on earth; less than 1 ounce would be enough to affect every living person. The blisters, swelling, and itching are caused by an immune system response to this poisonous sap. The plant is poisonous even long after it has dried out, but it is particularly irritating in the spring and early summer, when it is full of sap. Every part of these plants is toxic.

The first symptom of poison ivy is a burning and itching sensation. This is followed by the development of a red, intensely itchy rash, often accompanied by swelling, oozing, and crusting blisters. A mild case may involve only a few small blisters, while a severe case may cause many large blisters, acute inflammation, fever, and/or inflammation affecting the face or genitals. Symptoms can appear anywhere from a few hours to seven days after contact and tend to be at their worst between the fourth and seventh days. The rash often forms a linear pattern. Exposed parts of the body, such as the hands, arms, and face, are the areas most likely to be affected. Scratching can then spread the inflammation to other parts of the body. Itching, redness, and swelling begin to heal by the second day after the appearance of the rash, and most people are completely healed within seven to fourteen days.

Direct contact with the plant is the most common means of contracting poison ivy, but the poisons can be conveyed to the skin in other ways. Some people have contracted poison ivy by petting an animal that has been in contact with it. It can also be transmitted by clothing or objects that have come in contact with the plant. People who are highly sensitive to poison ivy can develop a reaction if the plant is

burned and they inhale the smoke. Severe cases of mouth poisoning have occurred in children who have eaten the plant's leaves or grayish berries.

Unless otherwise specified, the dosages recommended here are for adults. For a child between the ages of twelve and seventeen, reduce the dose to three-quarters the recommended amount. For a child between six and twelve, use one-half the recommended dose, and for a child under the age of six, use one-quarter the recommended amount.

NUTRIENTS

SUPPLEMENT	SUGGESTED DOSAGE	COMMENTS
Important		
Vitamin C with bioflavonoids	3,000–8,000 mg daily.	To prevent infection and spreading of the rash. A natural antihistamine that reduces swelling.
Helpful		
All-Purpose Bactericide Spray from Aerobic Life Industries	Apply topically as directed on label.	Destroys bacteria. Prevents spreading of the rash.
Calamine lotion	Apply topically as directed on label.	Contains calamine, phenol, and zinc oxide. Has drying properties for faster healing.
Shark cartilage (BeneFin)	1 gram per 15 lbs of body weight daily, divided into 3 doses.	Reduces inflammation.
Vitamin A with mixed carotenoids	25,000 IU daily. If you are pregnant, do not exceed 10,000 IU daily.	Needed for healing of skin tissue. Also boosts the immune system.
Vitamin E oil or cream	Apply topically as directed on label. Apply topically as directed on label.	To aid in healing and prevent scarring.
Zinc	80 mg daily. Do not exceed a total of 100 mg daily from all supplements.	Needed for repair of skin tissues. Use zinc gluconate lozenges or OptiZinc for best absorption.

HERBS

❑ Aloe vera gel helps relieve burning and itching. Apply pure aloe vera gel as directed on the product label or as needed.

❑ A strong tea made of equal parts lime water and white oak bark is very good for poison ivy, poison oak, or poison sumac. Apply a compress wet with this solution. Replace the compress with a fresh one as often as it becomes dry.

❑ Marshmallow root both soothes and heals skin.

❑ Tea tree oil disinfects and heals skin conditions.

❑ Witch hazel helps stop itching and aids in healing.

❑ The following herbs can be used topically as remedies for poison ivy, poison oak, or poison sumac: black walnut extract, bloodroot, echinacea, goldenseal, and myrrh. Black walnut has antiseptic properties and helps to fight infection; bloodroot reduces swelling; echinacea promotes healing of skin wounds; goldenseal is good for skin inflammation; myrrh is a powerful antiseptic. Echinacea can also be taken internally to boost the immune system.

Caution: Do not use bloodroot during pregnancy. Use goldenseal with caution if you are allergic to ragweed.

RECOMMENDATIONS

❑ Treat a mild case of poison ivy with one or more of the following:

• Apply compresses made with very hot plain water for brief intervals.

• Apply compresses soaked in a diluted Burow's solution (use 1 pint to 15 pints of cool water). You can purchase Burow's solution at most drugstores.

• Soak the affected skin in cool water with colloidal oatmeal (Aveeno) added, available at most drugstores.

• For relief of itching, apply a paste made from water, cornstarch, baking soda, oatmeal, or Epsom salts. Use 1 teaspoon of water to 3 teaspoons of the dry ingredient.

• Apply aloe vera juice, tofu, or watermelon rind to the area for cooling relief. Using 1 pint of buttermilk with 1 tablespoon of sea salt added may be helpful.

• Use an herbal preparation suggested under Herbs, above.

• Try homeopathic remedies. *Rhus toxicodendron* is the classic homeopathic remedy for poison ivy. It relieves itching and promotes healing. Poison Ivy/Oak Tablets from Hyland's is a homeopathic combination remedy for poison ivy.

❑ For a severe case of poison ivy, consult a physician. Symptoms that warrant medical attention include an extensive rash that covers more than half of the body; extreme swelling and redness; and fever. You should also consult your health care provider if poison ivy occurs near the eyes, mouth, or genitals.

❑ Stay cool. Sweating and heat can make itching worse.

CONSIDERATIONS

❑ Oral prednisone is sometimes prescribed to relieve itching and reduce swelling. However, this treatment should be reserved only for very severe cases involving fever, difficulty urinating, dangerous facial or genital swelling, or other symptoms of acute illness. Oral steroids are extremely powerful drugs and can cause serious side effects.

❑ Topical steroids are not helpful for poison ivy and should be avoided.

❑ The toxin urushiol does not affect dogs or cats, but they can bring the irritating substance home on their fur and pass it to you. If you suspect your pet may have walked through poison ivy or poison oak, wash the animal thoroughly (wear rubber gloves and protective clothing).

❑ Prevention is better than treatment when it comes to poison ivy, poison oak, and poison sumac. When spending time outdoors, keep the following in mind:

• Lightweight fabrics do not provide adequate protection against poison ivy or oak, because the sap can easily penetrate them. Wear gloves and heavier clothing if you might be exposed to the plant.

• Everyone, even children, should learn to recognize, and avoid, these harmful plants. Poison ivy usually grows as a vine, but it can also take the form of a shrub, growing anywhere from two to seven feet high. Its leaves always grow in clusters of three, one at the end of the stalk, the other two opposite each other. Poison oak grows as a shrub exclusively, and its leaves are lobed, like oak leaves. Like those of poison ivy, they grow in threes. Poison sumac grows as a shrub or small tree that has multiple leaflets growing on both sides of a stem. The number of leaflets may range from seven to thirteen, but it is always an odd number.

• Appropriate protective clothing should be worn for activities that take you into forests or through thick underbrush—long pants, a long-sleeved shirt, shoes, socks, and gloves. These items should be washed after they are worn; if they come into contact with poison ivy, they are not safe to wear again until they have been laundered or dry-cleaned.

• If you know or suspect that you may have come in contact with poison ivy, remove all clothing and shoes, and *immediately* scrub your skin using brown or yellow laundry soap (such as Fels Naptha) and water or alcohol to remove the irritating oil. Lather several times and rinse in running water after each sudsing. This procedure is useless if not done within ten minutes; after that time, the oil will have penetrated the skin and cannot be washed off. Wash clothing, gear, or pack material in plenty of hot, soapy water, with chlorine bleach added, if possible. Stubborn cases of poison ivy that do not respond to proper treatment are often due to repeated contact with contaminated clothing.

Poisoning

There are literally thousands of substances, both natural and synthetic, that can cause poisoning. Many of these are present in everyday items and products, including drugs, cleaning products, pesticides, paints and varnishes, hobby and art supplies, batteries, cosmetics, and house plants. Some are poisonous only if ingested; others can cause problems if inhaled or absorbed through the skin or eyes.

Most cases of accidental poisoning involve young children, especially children under the age of five. Young chil-

Poison Control Centers

The following are telephone numbers for local Poison Control Centers in the United States and Canada. It is a good idea to post the number of your local center near your telephone, especially if you have young children. If you can program your telephone for automatic dialing, you may wish to add the number to your phone's programming as well. Please note that all phone numbers are subject to change.

UNITED STATES

ALABAMA
800–462–0800 (AL only)
205–345–0600
Children's Hospital
800–292–6678 (AL only)
205–939–9201
205–933–4050

ALASKA
800–478–3193
907–261–3193

ARIZONA
Statewide
800–362–0101 (AZ only)
520–626–6016
Phoenix Area
602–253–3334
Tucson Area
602–626–6016

ARKANSAS
800–376–4766
 (Emergency)
800–641–3805

CALIFORNIA
Sacramento and Madera
 Area
800–876–4766
(No. CA only)
San Diego Area
800–876–4766
San Francisco/Bay Area
800–876–4766

COLORADO
800–332–3073
(CO only/outside metro
Denver area)
303–739–1123
(Denver metro area)

CONNECTICUT
800–343–2722 (CT only)
860–679–3456

DELAWARE
800–722–7112
215–368–2100

DISTRICT OF COLUMBIA
202–625–3333
202–362–8563 (TTY)

FLORIDA
Jacksonville area
813–253–4444
904–549–4480
Miami area
800–282–3171 (FL only)
305–585–5253
Tampa area
800–282–3171
813–253–4444

GEORGIA
404–589–4400
800–282–5846 (GA only)
404–616–9000
404–616–9287 (TDD/TTY)

HAWAII
808–941–4411

IDAHO
800–860–0620 (ID only)

ILLINOIS
800–942–5969 (IL only)

INDIANA
317–929–2323
800–382–9097 (IN only)
317–929–2336 (TTY)

IOWA
800–352–2222
800–272–6477 (IA only)
712–277–2222

KANSAS
800–332–6633 (KS only)
913–588–6633
913–588–6639 (TDD/TTY)

KENTUCKY
502–589–8222

LOUISIANA
800–256–9822 (LA only)

MAINE
800–442–6305 (ME only)
207–871–2950

MARYLAND
Statewide
410–528–7701
800–492–2414 (MD only)
410–706–1858 (TDD/TTY)
DC Suburbs
202–625–3333
202–362–8563 (TTY)

MASSACHUSETTS
617–232–2120
800–682–9211 (MA only)

MICHIGAN
Statewide
800–764–7661 (MI only)
313–745–5711
800–356–3232 (TTY)

MINNESOTA
Statewide
800–POISON1
(MN and SD only)
612–347–3141
612–904–4691
 (TDD/TTY)

MISSISSIPPI
601–354–7660

MISSOURI
800–366–8888
816–234–3430
314–772–5200

MONTANA
800–525–5042 (MT only)

NEBRASKA
Statewide
800–955–9119 (NE & WY
only)
402–354–5555

NEVADA
503–494–8968
800–466–6179 (NV only)

NEW HAMPSHIRE
603–650–8000
800–562–8236 (NH only)

NEW JERSEY
800–POISON1 (NJ only)

NEW MEXICO
800–432–6866 (NM only)
505–272–2222

NEW YORK
Central New York State
800–252–5655 (NY only)
315–476–4766
Eastern NY (from NYC
 to Canada)
800–336–6997
914–366–3030
Finger Lakes Region
800–333–0542
716–275–3232
716–273–3854 (TDD/TTY)
Long Island
516–542–2323
516–663–2650
516–924–8811 (TDD/TTY)
New York City
212–340–4494
212–764–7667
Western New York
800–888–7655 (NY
 western regions only)
716–878–7654

NORTH CAROLINA
800–848–6946
 (NC only)
704–355–4000

NORTH DAKOTA
800–732–2200 (ND, MN,
 and SD only)
701–234–5575

OHIO

Statewide
800–682–7625 (OH only)
800–762–0727 (Dayton,
   OH only)
614–228–2272 (TDD/TTY)

Cincinnati Area
513–558–5111
800–872–5111 (OH only)
888–231–4455 (OH only)
216–231–4455

OKLAHOMA

800–764–7661 (OK only)
405–271–5454

OREGON

503–494–8968
800–452–7165 (OR only)

PENNSYLVANIA

Hershey/Central PA
800–521–6110
717–531–6111
717–513–8335 (TDD/TTY)

Western Pennsylvania
412–681–6669

Southeastern Pennsylvania/
   Lehigh Valley
800–722–7112
215–386–2100

PUERTO RICO

787–726–5674
787–726–5660

RHODE ISLAND

401–444–5727

SOUTH CAROLINA

803–922–1117 (SC only)
803–777–1117

SOUTH DAKOTA

800–POISON1 (MN &
   SD only)
612–347–3141
612–904–4691 (TDD/TTY)

TENNESSEE

Statewide
800–288–9999 (TN only)
615–936–2034 (Greater
   Nashville)
615–936–2047 (TDD/TTY)

Western & Eastern
   Tennessee
800–288–9999 (TN only)
901–528–6048

TEXAS

Central Texas
254–724–7401
800–POISON1 (TX only)

North Texas
800–764–7661 (TX only)

South Texas
800–764–7661

Southeast Texas
800–764–7661

Texas Panhandle
800–764–7661

West Texas
800–764–7661

UTAH

801–581–2151
800–456–7707 (UT only)

VERMONT

877–658–3456 (toll free)
802–658–3456

VIRGINIA

Central & Western Virginia
800–451–1428
804–924–5543

DC Suburbs
202–625–3333
202–362–8563 (TDD/TTY)

Eastern & Central Virginia
800–552–6337
804–828–9123

WASHINGTON

800–732–6985 (WA only)
206–526–2121
206–517–2394 (TDD/TTY)

WEST VIRGINIA

800–642–3625 (WV only)

WISCONSIN

Madison/Southwestern and
   Northern WI
800–815–8855
608–262–3702

WYOMING

800–955–9119 (WY only)
402–354–5555

CANADA

ALBERTA

800–332–1414
403–670–1414

BRITISH COLUMBIA

800–567–8911
604–682–5050

MANITOBA

204–787–2591
   (emergency)
204–787–2444 (general)

NEW BRUNSWICK

Fredericton
506–857–5555
   (emergency)
506–857–5353 (general)

St. John
506–648–6222

NEWFOUNDLAND

709–722–1110

NOVA SCOTIA

902–428–8161 (local)
800–565–8161 (toll free
   from P.E.I.)

ONTARIO

Provincewide
800–267–1373 (ON only)
613–737–1100
   (emergency)
613–738–2320
800–268–9017 (toll free)
416–598–5900 (local)

PRINCE EDWARD ISLAND

800–565–8161 (toll free
   from P.E.I.)

QUEBEC

800–463–5060 (QB only)
418–656–8090

SASKATCHEWAN

Provincewide
800–667–4545
306–359–4545

Saskatoon
800–363–7474
306–966–1010

YUKON TERRITORY

403-667-8726

TTY= teletype (for the hearing impaired)
TDD= telecommunications device for the deaf

---

dren are very curious, and their preferred method of exploring often involves putting things in their mouths. However, there are also many cases of poisoning every year among elderly people and hospital patients (most commonly the result of overmedication or drug mix-ups), as well as adolescents, who may experiment with the ingestion of toxic substances, including recreational drugs. Other causes of poisoning include exposure to environmental pollutants and toxic substances used in the workplace. Toxins in food can also cause poisoning. (*See* FOODBORNE AND WATERBORNE DISEASE in Part Two.)

RECOMMENDATIONS

❏ Keep the telephone number of your local Poison Control Center posted near your telephone (*see* Poison Control Centers on page 572). This is particularly important if you have children. Also, keep a bottle of syrup of ipecac and charcoal tablets, available in drugstores and health food stores, on hand at all times. However, *do not* use syrup of ipecac unless specifically directed to do so by a physician or your Poison Control Center. For some poisonous substances, it is not advisable to take anything by mouth—for example if the poison contains an acid that will create more internal burning. If advised to do so by the Poison Control Center, take 5 charcoal tablets immediately. This will help to absorb the poison. Do not use charcoal tablets that are not made for internal use.

❑ If you suspect that you or another have been poisoned, call your local Poison Control Center and follow their directions. The appropriate measures to take depend on the toxin involved and the method of ingestion. The professionals who staff these centers will be able to tell you what to do.

❑ If you are directed to go to the nearest hospital emergency room, take the container of the suspected poison with you, if possible. This can help medical personnel to deal with the situation and save precious time.

CONSIDERATIONS

❑ When dealing with suspected poisoning, it is better to rely on the advice of a Poison Control Center staff rather than the information on product packaging. Poison Control Centers keep up to date with the latest knowledge and practices; information provided by manufacturers may not be as current or reliable.

❑ *See also* ALUMINUM TOXICITY; ARSENIC POISONING; CADMIUM TOXICITY; CHEMICAL POISONING; COPPER TOXICITY; ENVIRONMENTAL TOXICITY; FOODBORNE/WATERBORNE DISEASE; LEAD POISONING; MERCURY TOXICITY; and/or NICKEL TOXICITY, all in Part Two.

Polyps

Polyps are benign (noncancerous) growths of various sizes that are found on stalklike structures growing from the epithelial lining of the large intestine, cervix, bladder, nose, and other body structures. They are most common in the rectum and sigmoid colon, and usually occur in groups.

Most polyps of the colon and/or rectum cause no symptoms at all and are discovered only during routine physical examinations that include examination of the colon, or during examination or treatment of other disorders. If they are very large, however, they may cause rectal bleeding, cramping, or abdominal pain. The relationship between polyps and cancer is not fully understood. Some physicians believe most colon cancers begin as polyps. However, most polyps probably do not turn into cancer. On the other hand, it is true that many people who have a cancerous growth in the colon also have multiple polyps surrounding that growth, and it does appear that the larger a polyp grows, the greater the chance that it will become malignant.

Familial polyposis is a hereditary disease in which large numbers of growths (100 or more) develop in the colon. If removed, they grow back. Rectal bleeding and mucous drainage are common symptoms. This disorder is more closely linked to cancer than ordinary polyps are; unless it is treated, it virtually always leads to colon cancer.

Cervical polyps line the inside of the cervix, the passage from the vagina into the uterus. Symptoms indicative of cervical polyps include a heavy, watery, bloody discharge from the vagina. Bleeding may occur after sexual intercourse, between periods, and after menopause. The growth of cervical polyps may be caused by infection, injury to the cervix, or hormonal changes during pregnancy. Polyps are more common in women who have not had children. Women with diabetes also have a higher than normal chance of developing polyps. A pap smear may or may not detect cervical polyps. They rarely return once removed.

Bladder polyps produce blood in the urine. Unless they are removed, cancer of the bladder may follow.

Nasal polyps usually form in the back of the nose, near the openings into the sinuses. They too can bleed and can interfere with normal breathing. People with hay fever and other nasal allergies are most prone to nasal polyps, as are people who overuse nose drops and nasal sprays.

Polyps on the vocal cords are caused by abuse (such as from repeated and prolonged episodes of screaming or, among singers especially, improper vocal technique), usually in the presence of an infection. People who smoke or have allergies are more susceptible. Vocal cord polyps usually cause painless hoarseness.

NUTRIENTS

SUPPLEMENT	SUGGESTED DOSAGE	COMMENTS
Essential		
Multivitamin and mineral complex	As directed on label.	Provides a balance of necessary nutrients.
plus extra calcium	1,000–1,500 mg daily.	Protects against colorectal polyps and colon cancer.
and magnesium	750 mg daily.	Assists in the absorption of calcium.
Vitamin A with mixed carotenoids	25,000 IU daily. If you are pregnant, do not exceed 10,000 IU daily.	Protects the membranous linings. Use emulsion form for easier assimilation.
Vitamin C with bioflavonoids	5,000–10,000 mg daily, in divided doses.	Can reduce the number of polyps, and may eliminate them altogether.
Very Important		
Vitamin E	Start with 400 IU daily and increase slowly to 800 IU daily.	A potent antioxidant. Protects against the effects of lipid peroxidation; if deficiency occurs, cells are vulnerable to damage. Use d-alpha-tocopherol form.
Important		
Aerobic Bulk Cleanse (ABC) from Aerobic Life Industries	As directed on label. Take with aloe vera juice.	Cleanses the colon, assisting in normal stool formation to aid in removing harmful toxins.

Helpful		
Coenzyme Q$_{10}$ plus Coenzyme A from Coenzyme-A Technologies	60 mg daily. As directed on label.	An important antioxidant. Increases cellular oxygen levels. Works well with coenzyme Q$_{10}$ to support adrenal glands, from the body, and boost the immune system.
ConcenTrace trace mineral drops from Trace Minerals Research	As directed on label.	Normalizes electrolytes after bowel cleansing.
Garlic (Kyolic from Wakunaga)	2 capsules 3 times daily, between meals.	Acts as a natural antibiotic and enhances immune function.
Homozon from Aerobic Life Industries	As directed on label.	Supplies oxygen to the intestines to cleanse the colon.
Superoxide dismutase (SOD) or Cell Guard from Biotec Foods	As directed on label. As directed on label.	An important antioxidant and free radical destroyer. An antioxidant complex that contains SOD.

HERBS

❏ Aloe vera juice improves digestion and cleanses the digestive tract.

❏ Butcher's broom, cardamom, cayenne, cinnamon, *Garcinia cambogia,* ginger, green tea, and mustard seed are thermogenic herbs that improve digestion.

Caution: Do not use cinnamon in large quantities during pregnancy.

❏ Cascara sagrada is a colon cleanser and laxative.

❏ Coloklysis from PhysioLogics contains herbs and a blend of soluble and insoluble fiber to support healthy digestion.

RECOMMENDATIONS

❏ A high-fiber diet with no animal fats is important. Include in your diet apricots, broccoli, brown rice, cabbage, cantaloupe, carrots, cauliflower, garlic, oatmeal, onions, green peppers, sweet potatoes, sesame seeds, spinach, sunflower seeds, and whole grains. Fruits with edible seeds, such as figs, raspberries, strawberries, and even bananas, tend to contain lots of fiber. *See* CANCER in Part Two and follow the diet recommended there.

❏ Take some form of supplemental fiber daily. Barley, legumes, oat bran, psyllium husks (in Aerobic Bulk Cleanse), and rice bran are good sources of fiber.

Note: Always take supplemental fiber separately from other supplements and medications.

❏ Be sure to increase your water intake when increasing fiber consumption. If you do not, it may result in bloating, gas, pain, and constipation.

❏ Exclude from your diet fried foods, highly processed foods, caffeine, and alcohol. Do not use tobacco.

❏ Regular physical examinations are important, particularly after age forty. A digital rectal exam is easily performed in the physician's office and can quickly determine if there are any abnormalities along the colon wall.

❏ If you experience rectal bleeding, or if blood appears in the stool, consult your physician. A fecal occult blood test (FOBT) should be done to identify the source of the blood. Bleeding can be a symptom of polyps, but it also can be a sign of cancer.

CONSIDERATIONS

❏ The treatment of choice for most polyps, regardless of location, is surgical removal. In most cases this is a relatively minor procedure, often performed on an outpatient basis.

❏ Vocal cord polyps may be treated with humidification, speech therapy, and rest. Surgical removal of the polyps may be necessary.

❏ For familial polyposis, a surgical procedure called a colectomy (removal of the colon) may be necessary. In some cases, the rectum is left in place and connected to the small intestine to allow for bowel evacuation. However, in most cases, polyps return in the rectum.

❏ Research has found that men with the highest consumption of saturated fat were twice as likely to develop potentially malignant polyps as men who limited their fat intake.

Pregnancy-Related Problems

Many women find being pregnant a thoroughly enjoyable experience and suffer very few unpleasant symptoms, but there are those who discover that being pregnant can lead to some uncomfortable effects. Very few of these incidental discomforts threaten either the fetus or the expectant mother—but the more enjoyable a pregnancy, the better for both mother and child.

Pregnancy lasts for approximately forty weeks. This time is commonly divided into three periods, or trimesters: from the first day of the last menstrual period to week 12; from week 12 to week 28; from week 28 until delivery.

Most of the discomforts that occur during pregnancy are the result of hormonal changes within the body, nutritional deficiencies, and profound anatomical changes. This section addresses some of the most common pregnancy-related problems and offers natural remedies as well as helpful hints and suggestions for maintaining maximum health during pregnancy. For a healthy pregnancy and birth, it is necessary to consult and work with a qualified health care professional, be it a physician, nurse practitioner, or midwife. It is also wise to work with your health care practitioner on a birth plan. This allows you to decide in advance what you want and what you would choose from among your options before, during, and after labor. (*See* BIRTH PLAN on page 586.)

PREGNANCY SELF-TEST

Over-the-counter pregnancy test kits are sold in most drugstores. You should always see your health care provider to confirm a positive result.

ANEMIA

During pregnancy, blood volume (the amount of blood circulating in the body) increases by about 40 percent. The increase in volume is largely due to an increase in plasma (the liquid part of blood) rather than in red (or white) blood cells. Plasma volume, then, is increasing faster than red blood cell volume. The protein hemoglobin, which carries oxygen to the body's cells, inhabits red blood cells. Because there is a decreased proportion of red blood cells in the blood, there is also a decreased proportion of hemoglobin, and the result can be anemia.

Anemia is most likely to develop in the second trimester of pregnancy. It can cause fatigue, a rapid heartbeat, and paleness of the skin, gums, and around the inside of the eye. There may also be cravings to eat substances other than food, such as coal, dirt, ice, starch, or hair. This is called *pica* and is normally the sign of a nutritional deficiency.

Anemia is unlikely to affect the developing baby. The fetus depletes the mother's iron resources and does not suffer any deficiency itself.

Recommendations

❑ Make sure you have enough folic acid, vitamin B$_{12}$, and the other B-complex vitamins in your diet. (See the Nutrients table on page 583).

❑ Eat foods rich in iron, such as green leafy vegetables, prunes, raisins, organically raised red meat and liver, and bread and pastas made from whole grain flour.

❑ If your health care provider prescribes iron supplements, take them with vitamin C to help the absorption of this mineral. Iron supplements can also cause constipation, so eat plenty of high-fiber foods and increase your fluids intake.

Note: Do not take iron supplements unless anemia has been diagnosed.

ASTHMA

Many women who have asthma reduce their use of asthma medication when they become pregnant to avoid harming the fetus—and as a result, their asthma symptoms become worse. It currently appears that there is more danger to a developing fetus from frequent asthma attacks than from taking asthma medications. Inhaled medications are normally preferred during this time because they are more localized in action. Asthma sufferers should be checked at least every four to six weeks by a physician during pregnancy. You should discuss your medication in detail with your physician.

Recommendations

❑ Avoid anything that might trigger an attack. Keep your bedroom, at least, as a place you can go to relax and get away from any airborne pollutants that can trigger an attack.

❑ The Air Supply personal air purifier from Wein Products is a miniature unit that is worn around the neck. It sets up an invisible, pure air shield against microorganisms (such as viruses, bacteria, and mold) and microparticles (including dust, pollen, and pollutants) in the air. It also eliminates vapors, smells, and harmful volatile compounds in the air. The Living Air XL-15 unit from Alpine Industries is an ionizing unit that is good for purifying the air in the home or workplace.

BACKACHE

Backache is common during pregnancy due to the considerable anatomical changes and stresses in the body. The increase in body weight, the muscle-relaxing effects of the hormone progesterone, and the shift in one's center of gravity contribute to the problem.

Recommendations

❑ To minimize back pain during pregnancy, do not stay in any one position for a long period of time.

❑ Pay attention to your posture. Keep your shoulders relaxed and your back as straight as possible at all times.

❑ Swimming is a good way to relieve the strain on the back and on all other parts of the body.

❑ Include two to three minutes of gentle stretching exercises in your daily routine. Do not strain—stretch only to your comfort level.

❑ Make sure your mattress is firm enough to support you, and sleep with a pillow supporting your back. Sleep on your side, not on your back.

❑ Do not wear high-heeled shoes. High heels throw your body off balance and put extra strain on your back. Instead, wear well-fitting, well-padded flat or low-heeled shoes that support your feet and provide ample room for your toes. Be aware that you may require larger shoes than normal while you are pregnant.

❑ Teach your partner or friends how to massage your back. You can use liniments or herbal oils.

❑ Learn how to lift correctly, putting less pressure on the back.

❑ When your back hurts, try soaking a small towel in cider vinegar. Squeeze off any excess and lie down on your side in bed. Spread the towel directly across your back. Relax this way for fifteen to twenty minutes.

❏ *See also* BACKACHE in Part Two.

BLADDER DISCOMFORT/INFECTION

During pregnancy, the bladder is pressed upon by an expanding uterus and must, in general, deal with far more fluids. You may need to urinate more frequently. However, the bladder may not always empty fully, so infections of the bladder are very common. These should always be treated.

Recommendations

❏ Avoid sugary foods. Infectious bacteria thrive on sugar.

❏ Increase your fluid intake. Drink quality bottled or filtered water rather than tap water. *Do not* cut back on liquids because of urinary frequency.

❏ Eat plain natural yogurt every day. This helps to maintain the correct balance of natural "friendly" bacteria in the system.

❏ Wear cotton underwear. Avoid wearing anything tight or containing synthetic material next to your skin.

❏ Do not douche.

❏ *See also* BLADDER INFECTION (CYSTITIS) and CANDIDIASIS in Part Two.

BLEEDING GUMS

During pregnancy, increasing estrogen levels causes the gums to swell and become somewhat softer than normal, and the circulation of blood to them increases. This makes the gums more prone to bleeding and infection, especially if good oral hygiene is not maintained.

Recommendations

❏ Be sure your diet contains enough calcium and high-quality, complete proteins such as soy products.

❏ Increase your intake of foods rich in vitamin C, as a deficiency in this vitamin can contribute to bleeding gums.

❏ If you smoke, quit—preferably *before* you get pregnant. Cigarette smoking reduces the oxygen supply to the developing fetus and also drains vitamin C from the body.

❏ Brush your teeth three to four times daily (remembering to rinse your mouth well), and massage your gums with clean fingers when necessary. Floss your teeth daily.

❏ See your dentist at least once during the pregnancy, and be sure to inform the dentist that you are pregnant. *Do not* permit him or her to take any dental x-rays while you are pregnant.

CONSTIPATION

Hormonal changes during pregnancy have a relaxing effect on the muscles, including those of the digestive tract. The increasing level of progesterone in your system makes the bowels less efficient. The normal rhythmic contractions of the intestines slow down, and the result can be constipation. This happens most often in the third trimester.

Recommendations

❏ Eat fresh and dried fruit such as prunes, raisins, and figs.

❏ Eat fresh vegetables and salads containing a variety of raw green and colored vegetables daily.

❏ Increase the amount of fiber in your diet. Whole-grain breads, cereals, and bran are helpful. Begin by taking 2 teaspoons of bran in a glass of apple juice twice daily. The bran may cause some gas until your system is used to it, but after that you should not have any difficulty.

❏ Drink six to eight 8-ounce glasses of liquid, including water, each day.

❏ Walk at least a mile a day.

❏ Set a regular time each day for a bowel movement. This is very helpful for digestion and elimination. Elevate your feet and legs during elimination to relax the anal muscles.

❏ If your health care provider prescribes iron supplements, be aware that they can cause constipation. Increase your fluid intake and eat a diet high in fiber.

❏ *Do not* take over-the-counter laxatives unless specifically recommended by your health care provider.

❏ *See also* CONSTIPATION in Part Two.

❏ *See* Hemorrhoids later in this section.

COUGHS AND COLDS

Coughs and colds are more common during pregnancy and are often more difficult than usual to shake off. Once you have a cold, there is little you can do but let it run its course, so prevention is most important.

Recommendations

❏ Eat a healthy diet and increase your consumption of foods containing vitamin C.

❏ For congestion, make a steam inhaler using essential oil of eucalyptus, lavender, or lemon.

❏ *See* COMMON COLD in Part Two for additional recommendations. You can use any of the external remedies mentioned, but consult your health care provider before taking any nutrients or other supplements internally.

DEPRESSION

Depression is fairly common during pregnancy. It can come and go, but because of shifting hormone levels, it is not uncommon to experience at least one bout of depression at some point during the forty weeks of pregnancy. Mood swings are common too. It is not unusual to find that you are more emotional and volatile during pregnancy. It helps if people around you are sympathetic to this and know what to expect.

Recommendations

❑ Do not continue to feel depressed without seeking help. Having someone to talk to and knowing that you are not alone in experiencing these feeling can help you to cope during times of depression.

❑ Acupuncture has been used successfully for hundreds of years to treat depression.

❑ Exercise can help to lessen depression.

❑ Be open about your fears and concerns relating to having a child. Pregnancy and childbirth are profound experiences, and many women experience feelings of anxiety about the responsibilities attached to this event. Pregnancy is a complicated emotional experience, and you should be aware that it is normal not to be happy all the time.

❑ If you become pregnant while taking antidepressants, consult your physician about the possible effect on the development of the fetus. Research has not found that tricyclic antidepressants such as amitriptyline (Elavil, Endep) or imipramine (Tofranil) cause birth defects, but antianxiety drugs such as alprazolam (Xanax) and diazepam (Valium) and monoamine oxidase (MAO) inhibitors may increase the incidence of cleft palate and cleft lip. A report in *The New England Journal of Medicine* in January 1997 stated that the children of mothers who took fluoxetine (Prozac) while pregnant appeared to suffer no ill effects. The children were monitored until they were seven years old. You should not stop taking your medication without discussing it with your physician.

DIABETES, GESTATIONAL

This is a form of diabetes that occurs only during pregnancy. It affects 3 to 5 percent of women. It occurs because insulin, which regulates blood sugar, does not work as efficiently during pregnancy due to hormones secreted by the placenta. Blood sugar can become high, and although this condition rarely causes harm to the mother, the baby's birth weight often increases, and the baby may be born with a low blood sugar level. A problem may arise if the baby's birth weight is excessive enough to make delivery complicated. *Macrosomia* (heavy birth weight), a potential complication, is defined as a birth weight over 9 pounds 14 ounces.

Women are normally tested for blood sugar levels around the twenty-eighth week of pregnancy. The 50-gram screen (gestational diabetes screening) involves drinking a glass of very sweet liquid containing 50 grams of sugar and testing the blood sugar level one hour later to see how your body has processed the sugar. Symptoms of gestational diabetes may include frequent urination, excessive thirst, and increased fatigue, but it is also likely that there will be no symptoms at all.

Recommendations

❑ Eat little and often. Do not miss meals, even if you are experiencing nausea.

❑ Discuss your dietary intake with your health care provider.

❑ Avoid foods rich in sugar, and remember that some carbohydrates increase blood sugar levels more than sugar. (*See* DIABETES in Part Two.)

Considerations

❑ If a baby is born with a low blood sugar, sweet drinks can alleviate the condition. The baby's blood sugar level should return to normal within hours. The mother's blood sugar also should return to normal after delivery.

❑ If the baby is too large, your health care provider may recommend delivering the baby early, possibly by Cesarean section.

DIZZINESS

During pregnancy, especially during the second trimester, blood pressure often drops as the expanding uterus presses on major blood vessels. The blood supply also has extra work to do, and at times the blood may pool in the lower part of the body, leaving the brain a bit short of oxygen for brief moments. These factors can cause dizziness.

Recommendations

❑ Do not change positions quickly. Always go from lying down to sitting to standing slowly. Take your time and focus on what you are doing.

❑ If you have to stand for long periods, keep moving and flexing your muscles to make sure the blood is circulating properly.

❑ Do not take hot baths.

❑ If you feel dizzy, sit down somewhere safe. Try lowering your head to your knees until the feeling passes.

❑ If you have diabetes, make sure your blood sugar level is well controlled. (*See* DIABETES in Part Two.)

ECLAMPSIA AND PREECLAMPSIA

Preeclampsia is a complication of pregnancy characterized by high blood pressure, edema (swelling due to fluid retention), and an excess of protein in the urine. It may develop in the second half of pregnancy or later. The cause is not known, but if you have suffered from this complaint during a prior pregnancy, you are at increased risk of having it again in following pregnancies. Other risk factors include multiple births, kidney disease, diabetes, lupus, long-term high blood pressure, and heredity. A small percentage of women who develop preeclampsia go on to develop eclampsia, with seizures and/or coma.

It was once thought that eclampsia and preeclampsia were a result of toxemia—the presence of some sort of toxin or poison in the bloodstream—but it is now known that this is not the case. If you develop *any* of the symptoms of preeclampsia, you must be monitored constantly by your health care provider.

NUTRIENTS

SUPPLEMENT	SUGGESTED DOSAGE	COMMENTS
Essential fatty acids (black currant seed oil, flaxseed oil, Kyolic-EPA from Wakunaga, olive oil, and primrose oil are good sources)	As directed on label or by your physician.	Improves circulation, lowers blood pressure, and thins the blood. *Caution:* If you have blood-clotting problems, do not take this supplement.
Garlic (Kyolic from Wakunaga)	As directed on label.	Effective in lowering blood pressure.
Vitamin E	As directed on label or by your physician.	Improves circulation. Use d-alpha-tocopherol form.

Recommendations

❏ Get adequate rest. Rest is vitally important if you develop this condition.

❏ Make sure that your physician or midwife is aware of any risk factors you may have for preeclampsia.

Considerations

❏ If you develop high blood pressure without any of the other symptoms of preeclampsia, your physician may recommend treatment for high blood pressure.

❏ Because the cause is not known, there is no specific treatment for eclampsia except delivery of the baby.

ECTOPIC PREGNANCY

An ectopic pregnancy, sometimes called a tubal pregnancy, is a situation in which a fertilized egg becomes implanted in a fallopian tube rather than in the uterus. The result is that the pregnancy is not viable because there is not room for the fetus to grow. This can happen if the fallopian tube is blocked due to inflammation, scar tissue, or endometriosis, making it impossible for the egg to pass into the uterus. Other possible causes for ectopic pregnancy include anatomical abnormalities such as a misshapen fallopian tube.

The easiest way to diagnose an ectopic pregnancy, after a pelvic examination, is to measure levels of chorionic gonadotropin (hCG), a hormone produced by the placenta that increases in quantity until the end of the first trimester. If the hCG level is *not* increasing, a physician may decide than the pregnancy is not proceeding as it should and order more tests, such as an ultrasound, to find out where the fetus is growing.

Considerations

❏ There is no known way to salvage an ectopic pregnancy. The fetus must be removed to preserve the life of the woman. This is usually done surgically and laparoscopically.

❏ You are more at risk for this condition if you have had a previous ectopic pregnancy. Discuss this risk with your health care provider.

EDEMA (SWELLING) OF THE HANDS AND FEET

The rise in estrogen in the body during pregnancy increases the tendency to retain fluids. This can cause some swelling of the hands and feet, and is considered normal—but it must be monitored continually because it may be an indication of a more serious condition called preeclampsia.

Recommendations

❏ Early in the pregnancy, remove any rings you wear on a regular basis. Do not wait, or the rings may have to be cut off.

❏ As soon as you notice your hands, legs, or feet getting puffy or larger than usual, tell your health care provider. While some swelling is acceptable, the condition should nevertheless be evaluated by a professional, as edema can also be the first sign of preeclampsia, a potentially serious complication of pregnancy.

❏ Avoid salt and all highly processed foods, while maintaining a well-balanced high protein diet. *Do not* take diuretics (water pills).

❏ Wear loose, comfortable clothing and properly fitting shoes. You may require larger shoes than normal. Once the baby arrives, your feet will return to normal.

❏ When you are relaxing, sit with your feet elevated.

❏ Walk one mile each day. This helps to keep edema under control.

❏ *See also* EDEMA in Part Two.

GAS (FLATULENCE)

Gas, like other digestive upsets, is a common complaint during pregnancy. Even foods that cause no difficulties at other times may begin to cause trouble.

Recommendations

❏ Keep a food diary to help you determine which foods, or combinations of foods, seem to be causing the gas. Avoid any suspect foods.

❏ You may have to adapt your usual diet during pregnancy. Many foods you liked before may suddenly seem unappealing.

❏ Eat four to five small meals a day, instead of three big meals. Chew your food slowly and well. Do not overtax your digestive system.

❑ Eat four or more servings of fresh fruits and vegetables every day.

❑ Cook vegetables quickly using a perforated steamer instead of boiling them for long periods of time.

❑ Drink as much quality water (not tap water) as you can.

❑ Get adequate exercise. Walking is an excellent way to alleviate gas.

❑ To reduce gas-causing sulfur compounds in beans (garbanzo, pinto, navy, and so on), use the following cooking method: Place 1 cup of beans in 5 cups of water and bring them to a boil. Boil the beans for one minute. Then drain them and add 5 cups of fresh water. Bring the water to a boil and continue cooking the beans according to directions. Cabbage, cauliflower, and broccoli can also cause flatulence.

❑ When eating potentially gas-inducing foods, take the enzyme product Beano with the first bite. This should help to eliminate the problem.

GROIN SPASM, STITCH, OR PRESSURE

When the round ligaments connecting the corners of the uterus to the pubic area kink and go into spasm, it feels like a "stitch" on the right side. In the later months of pregnancy, lower groin pressure may develop.

Recommendations

❑ Exercise daily, using exercises recommended by your health care provider. This can help alleviate this condition.

❑ During spasms, breathe deeply and bend toward the point of pain in order to allow the ligament to relax. Rest in bed on one side until the spasm is over.

HEARTBURN

Heartburn occurs more often than normal during pregnancy. This is because the expanded size of the uterus promotes the reentry of stomach fluids into the esophagus, and hormones present during pregnancy tend to soften the sphincter muscles.

Recommendations

❑ To prevent heartburn, do not consume spicy or greasy foods, alcohol, coffee, baking soda, or antacids containing sodium bicarbonate (such as Alka-Seltzer).

❑ Remain active and upright, especially after meals.

❑ To relieve discomfort, try using Acid-Ease from Prevail Corporation or chewable papaya tablets. These products, found in health food stores, contain natural plant enzymes and can be taken with meals and/or between meals, as needed. They are safe and effective for reducing heartburn.

❑ When heartburn strikes, try drinking a glass of warm soymilk or rice milk.

❑ Do not eat or drink anything except water for a few hours before going to bed or taking a nap.

Considerations

❑ A high-carbohydrate diet can help if heartburn is a problem.

❑ *See also* HEARTBURN/GASTROESOPHAGEAL REFLUX DISEASE (GERD) in Part Two.

HEMORRHOIDS

Hemorrhoids are common during pregnancy. A number of factors contribute to the development of hemorrhoids, including constipation and the pressure exerted by the uterus as the fetus gains in size and weight.

Recommendations

❑ Increase your intake of roughage. Eat plenty of raw vegetables, fruits, dried fruits, bran, and whole-grain breads. These fiber-rich foods helps to soften stools and make elimination easier. Hard stools can be very painful to pass and can cause bleeding.

❑ Drink six to eight 8-ounce glasses of liquid each day, including water, juices, and herbal teas.

❑ Use cold witch hazel compresses to help shrink hemorrhoids.

❑ Walk one mile a day to help digestion and elimination.

❑ Do not strain to have a bowel movement if you are constipated. (*See* CONSTIPATION in Part Two.)

❑ *See also* HEMORRHOIDS in Part Two.

INSOMNIA

Insomnia is very common during the last weeks of pregnancy when finding a comfortable sleeping position is difficult. Needing to get up to urinate can disrupt a night's sleep. Deficiencies of the B vitamins also can cause insomnia. The emotional changes that accompany pregnancy often contribute to sleep difficulties as well.

Recommendations

❑ Increase your intake of foods rich in the B vitamins. (*See* VITAMINS in Part One.)

❑ Take a warm (not hot) bath with a soothing oil (such as lavender) added to the water.

❑ Consider taking up yoga or some other form of meditation. These can help you to relax and may be useful during and after labor. (*See* Breathing Exercises; Guided Imagery; Meditation; and Relaxation Techniques *under* PAIN CONTROL in Part Three. *Also see* YOGA in Part Three.)

❑ Do not force yourself to sleep if you are not really tired. Read, meditate, or do something else nonstrenuous until you feel sleepy.

❏ Try drinking a cup of hot herbal tea with honey or lemon before bed or in the middle of the night. Herbal teas such as chamomile, marjoram, lemon balm, and passion-flower are known for their sleep-inducing qualities.

Caution: Do not use chamomile on an ongoing basis, as ragweed allergy may result. Avoid it completely if you are allergic to ragweed.

❏ Avoid stimulants.

❏ Do not eat heavy meals before bedtime.

❏ Arrange pillows behind or under your abdomen to relieve breathlessness.

❏ *See also* INSOMNIA in Part Two.

LEG CRAMPS

Leg cramps during pregnancy are often a result of nutritional deficiencies, electrolyte imbalances, and/or circulatory changes, in addition to the strain placed on the legs by the extra weight.

Recommendations

❏ Increase your calcium and potassium intake by eating foods such as almonds, bananas, grapefruit, low-fat cottage cheese, oranges, salmon, sardines, sesame seeds, soy products (such as tofu), and low-fat yogurt to help avert leg cramps. Adequate calcium is also needed to help prevent high blood pressure and for fetal development.

❏ While sleeping or sitting, elevate your legs so that they are higher than your heart.

❏ Do not stand in one place for too long. Shift your weight from one leg to the other every few minutes.

❏ Do not point your toes.

❏ Walk at least a mile every day to stimulate the circulation of blood through the legs.

❏ Make sure your levels of calcium, magnesium, and potassium are correctly balanced. It is often easier to take a single formula that contains all three minerals in the correct proportions.

❏ To relieve cramps, flex your feet, with your toes pointing upward.

❏ When experiencing a cramp, apply a hot water bottle or heating pad to the cramping area and apply pressure with your hands.

❏ *See also* MUSCLE CRAMPS in Part Two.

MISCARRIAGE (SPONTANEOUS ABORTION)

Some pregnancies are not carried to full term, resulting in a miscarriage. *Spontaneous abortion* is the technical term for a miscarriage. It is defined as the loss of a pregnancy before twenty weeks. The most likely reason for a miscarriage is a chromosomal abnormality in the fetus that makes it unlikely the fetus would survive. Other reasons for a miscarriage include cervical incompetence (the cervix opens and

thins before the pregnancy has reached full term), ectopic pregnancy (implantation of the fertilized egg outside the uterine cavity, most commonly in one of the fallopian tubes), infection, glandular disorders, diabetes, and pregnancy-induced hypertension (high blood pressure). Miscarriages generally are *not* caused by exercise, sexual activity, heavy lifting, or falls.

Herbs

❏ Taking raspberry leaf tea during the last few months of pregnancy is thought to help strengthen the uterus and minimize the risk of miscarriage.

Recommendations

❏ If you experience bleeding or cramping during pregnancy, contact your health care provider immediately and follow his or her advice.

❏ Do not minimize any feelings of grief, depression, or guilt you may experience after having a miscarriage. Your health care provider can refer you to a grief counselor or someone who will understand how you feel. It is also important to talk to your doctor about the possible reason for the miscarriage so that he or she can reassure you about the outcome of a following pregnancy. It is also quite normal to be able to cope with a miscarriage without experiencing any emotional trauma.

Considerations

❏ Bleeding is not necessarily a sign of impending miscarriage, but it should always be taken seriously. A pelvic examination will probably be necessary to determine if your cervix has started to dilate and if the membranes surrounding the fetus have broken. If both of these conditions are present, it is certain that you will have a miscarriage.

❏ Premature labor is the onset of rhythmic uterine contractions before fetal maturity. It usually occurs between the twentieth and thirty-seventh weeks of gestation.

❏ Decaffeinated coffee, rather than regular coffee, is thought to be a contributing cause of spontaneous abortion during the first trimester.

MORNING SICKNESS

Approximately 50 percent of all pregnant women experience some degree of nausea and vomiting between the sixth and twelfth weeks of pregnancy. This is normal. Although it is commonly called morning sickness, it can occur at any time of day.

Abnormal vomiting—severe, continual nausea and vomiting after the twelfth week—occurs in approximately 1 in 300 pregnancies. This is called *hyperemesis gravidarum*, and it can result in dehydration, acidosis, malnutrition, and substantial weight loss. If the condition persists, it can endanger the fetus. The reason for abnormally severe nausea is not clear, but an association has been made between it and very high levels of the hormones estrogen and chorionic gonadotropin (hCG), a hormone produced by the placenta that increases in quantity until the end of the first trimester. Other possible causes of abnormal vomiting include bile duct disease, drug toxicity, pancreatitis, low blood sugar, a molar pregnancy (a rare condition in which an abnormal mass rather than a fetus grows inside the uterus), problems with the thyroid, and inflammatory bowel disorders.

NUTRIENTS

SUPPLEMENT	SUGGESTED DOSAGE	COMMENTS
L-Methionine	1,000 mg daily.	Effective in preventing nausea.
Vitamin B$_6$ (pyridoxine) plus	50 mg every 4 hours when experiencing nausea.	A combination of nutrients that helps to prevent and alleviate nausea.
magnesium	400 mg daily, upon arising.	Caution: Do not take this combination for longer than 6 weeks.

Herbs

❏ Ginger, taken in capsule or tea form, is helpful for relieving nausea. Other beneficial herbs include catnip, dandelion, peppermint, and red raspberry leaf.

Recommendations

❏ Keep crackers or whole wheat toast near your bed and eat some before arising.

❏ Eat small, frequent meals and snack on whole-grain crackers with nut butters (but not peanut butter) or cheese. It helps to keep some food in the stomach at all times.

❏ Do not go without food or drink because of the nausea.

❏ Do not sit up or get out of bed too quickly.

❏ Try using *Nux vomica,* a homeopathic remedy that is good for nausea.

❏ Keep in mind that morning sickness usually does not last beyond the first thirteen weeks of pregnancy. If you suffer from persistent nausea or vomiting later in pregnancy, consult your health care provider. With appropriate treatment, the prognosis is good.

NOSEBLEEDS AND NASAL CONGESTION

During pregnancy, increased blood volume often causes some of the tiny capillaries in the nasal passages to rupture, causing a nosebleed. Inner nasal passages normally swell as well. A lack of vitamin C and the bioflavonoids may be a contributing factor. These conditions disappear with the birth of the baby.

Recommendations

❏ Increase your intake of foods rich in vitamin C, including broccoli, cabbage, grapefruits, lemons, oranges, peppers, and strawberries.

❏ If congestion is a problem, eat fewer dairy products and supplement your diet with calcium and magnesium. Dairy products tend to stimulate the secretion of mucus.

❏ Use a humidifier to help keep nasal tissues moisturized.

❏ Do not use nasal sprays or nose drops. Instead, use an empty nasal spray container filled with warm water to spray into the nostrils. This helps to moisten the nose and shrink the membranes.

❏ See also NOSEBLEED in Part Two.

SCIATICA

The sciatic nerve is the longest nerve in the body. It arises from the sacral plexus, in the lower back, threads downward through the pelvis through an opening called the greater sciatic foramen and runs through the hip joint and down the back of the thigh. Irritation of this nerve is common during pregnancy and usually disappears with the birth of the baby.

Recommendations

❏ Ask your health care provider to recommend a registered physical therapist or a chiropractor who has been specially trained to deal with pregnancy problems. A competent practitioner is best able to deal with this problem.

SKIN PROBLEMS

Common skin problems during pregnancy include pimples, acne, red marks, and mask of pregnancy (dark blotches on the skin of the face). These skin changes usually disappear with the birth of the baby.

Recommendations

❏ Keep your skin clean.

❏ If you wear makeup, use only water-based, hypoallergenic cosmetics if your skin is broken out.

Considerations

❏ Folic acid, one of the most essential nutrients during pregnancy, should also help with skin problems.

❏ See also ACNE and OILY SKIN, both in Part Two.

SORENESS IN THE RIB AREA

Soreness in the rib area during pregnancy is common. It is caused by the pressure of the expanding uterus.

Recommendations

❏ Change positions frequently.

❏ Keep in mind that this problem is temporary. It often disappears in the last six weeks of pregnancy, once the baby drops into position to be born.

STRETCH MARKS

Stretch marks are wavy stripes appearing on the abdomen, buttocks, breasts, and thighs. They start out reddish in color and gradually turn white. They are caused by rapid weight gain such as that typically associated with pregnancy and appear when the skin becomes overstretched and the fibers in the deep layers tear. Once they appear, they are permanent, but they do become much less noticeable with time.

Recommendations

❏ Try the following recipe for preventing stretch marks:

$1/2$ cup virgin olive oil
$1/4$ cup aloe vera gel
liquid from 6 capsules vitamin E
liquid from 4 capsules vitamin A

1. Mix all the ingredients together in a blender.

2. Pour the mixture into a jar and store it in the refrigerator.

Once a day, apply the oil externally all over the abdomen, hips, and thighs—the places where stretch marks commonly appear. If you do this diligently, every day, you may be able to prevent stretch marks.

❏ Apply cocoa butter and/or elastin cream topically as directed on the product label. These substances are very good for stretch marks.

SWEATING

While you are pregnant, your body makes sure that its temperature is perfect for your baby's development. In addition, as your size increases, the amount of effort it takes to walk, climb stairs, and do many everyday things also increases. As a result, you may find yourself sweating more than you did before.

Recommendations

❏ Wear loose, light, comfortable clothing. Choose clothing made of "breathable" natural fibers such as cotton or linen.

❏ Do not use a hot tub during pregnancy. This increase in body temperature can cause fetal distress. For the same reason, be careful about strenuous exercise, especially in hot weather.

VARICOSE VEINS

Varicose veins are enlarged veins close to the surface of the skin that often emerge during pregnancy. In some cases they disappear after the baby's birth.

Recommendations

❏ As often as possible, sit with your feet elevated, higher than your heart.

❏ Change positions frequently. Do not stand for long periods of time or sit in cross-legged positions.

❏ Wear support hose if your health care provider recommends them. Keep them near your bed and put them on before you get out of bed.

❏ Walk one mile each day to promote circulation.

❏ Do not wear elastic-topped knee socks, garters, belts, or high-heeled shoes.

❏ See also VARICOSE VEINS in Part Two.

NUTRITIONAL HEALTH IN PREGNANCY

During pregnancy, it is more important than ever to have a balanced diet that is high in nutrients and fiber and low in bad fats and cholesterol. The following are recommendations for maintaining health in pregnancy.

NUTRIENTS

SUPPLEMENT	SUGGESTED DOSAGE	COMMENTS
Very Important		
Iron	30 mg daily, or as directed by physician. Take with 100 mg vitamin C for better absorption.	Extra iron is needed during pregnancy. Increase fiber consumption, as iron supplements may cause constipation.
or Floradix Iron + Herbs from Salus Haus	As directed on label.	A natural, nontoxic source of iron.
Protein supplement	As directed on label.	A lack of protein has been linked to birth defects. Use protein from a vegetable source, such as soy.
Quercetin	500 mg daily.	A valuable bioflavonoid that promotes proper circulation.
Vitamin B complex plus extra	As directed on label.	To prevent deficiencies.
folic acid	400 mcg daily.	Adequate levels of folic acid reduce the chance of birth defects such as spina bifida. Recommended for women throughout the childbearing years, and especially in the first 6 weeks of pregnancy.
Vitamin C with bioflavonoids	2,000–4,000 mg daily, in divided doses.	Larger doses taken before delivery may help reduce labor pain.
Zinc	15–25 mg daily. Do not exceed 75 mg daily.	Insufficient zinc intake may be a cause of low birth weight. Use zinc gluconate lozenges or OptiZinc for best absorption.
Helpful		
Acidophilus or Kyo-Dophilus from Wakunaga	As directed on label. Take on an empty stomach. As directed on label.	To provide necessary "friendly" bacteria to prevent candidiasis (yeast infection), protect the baby at birth, and ensure proper assimilation of nutrients.
Bifa-15 from Eden Foods	As directed on label.	An natural intestinal bacteria supplement that aids in the production of folic acid, enzymes, and B vitamins.

Tests Performed During Pregnancy

Your health care provider may do a number of different tests when you become pregnant—or before pregnancy, if you are planning to have a child. If you believe that some of these tests are inappropriate or unnecessary, you can, of course, decline to have them. Discuss this with your physician.

There are also tests that can be performed during pregnancy to assess the health and development of the fetus. However, some of these tests involve an element of risk for both mother and child. Therefore, they should be done only when medically indicated. and not used routinely or for the mother's or the health care provider's convenience. If a test is suggested, be sure that you are fully aware of why it is needed and of any dangers that may be involved before deciding to have it done.

ROUTINE TESTS

The routine tests most health care providers recommend during pregnancy include the following:

• Blood pressure. This is taken to test for preeclampsia. It is usually taken at each visit.

• Blood sugar level. This is a urine test for gestational diabetes. It is usually taken at the first visit and on further visits if you are considered to be at high risk for the condition.

• Blood type. This is taken in case a blood transfusion becomes necessary and to see if there are blood-type incompatibilities (Rh-factor) between you and your baby. It is usually done during your first visit.

• Drug test. This is a urine test for illicit drug use. It may be taken on your first visit.

• Hemoglobin level. This is a blood test to check for anemia. It is usually done at your first visit.

• Pap smear. This is an internal swab test of the cervix to check for cancer cells. It is usually done on the first visit.

• Protein (albumin). This is another urine test for preeclampsia. It is usually done at each visit.

• Rubella antibody test. This is done to determine whether you have achieved immunity to rubella (German measles), which can be dangerous to a developing fetus in the first twelve weeks of pregnancy. It is usually taken on the first visit.

• Sexually transmitted disease testing. Genital swabs may be taken to test for signs of diseases such as chlamydia, gonorrhea, and syphilis. This is usually done during the first visit and, possibly, in later visits.

• Urinalysis. This is done to test for urinary tract infection. It is usually done at the first visit and, possibly, on subsequent visits.

AMNIOCENTESIS

This medical procedure is sometimes performed during pregnancy to determine the health of the fetus. It is rarely carried out unless there is a possibility of fetal abnormality. Routine amniocentesis is recommended only for women over thirty-five, women who are more at risk for having a Down syndrome child, or for couples who have an increased risk of passing on a genetic abnormality to their child. A local anesthetic is administered and then a long, hollow needle is inserted through the mother's abdomen into the uterus to remove amniotic fluid for cellular analysis. The needle can be seen on ultrasound, which allows a three-dimensional real-time view of the uterus and fetus. The amniotic fluid contains fetal cells that can be cultivated and tested. Although it has become fairly common as women are choosing to have children in later years, this procedure entails risks for both the pregnant woman and the fetus. There may be some danger of blood exchange between the mother and the fetus, infection of the amniotic fluid, peritonitis, the development of blood clots, placental hemorrhage, and premature labor. Therefore, great care must be taken in recommending, and then in performing, amniocentesis.

Amniocentesis can be done only during the sixteenth to eighteenth week of pregnancy, and the results are not known for two weeks. This test should be performed only if you plan to terminate the pregnancy if an abnormality is found or if knowledge of any problem is necessary for proper prenatal care.

CHORIONIC VILLUS SAMPLING (CVS)

This test is performed rarely and carries a greater risk than amniocentesis. The chorionic villi are fingerlike projections of the embryonic sac that contain cells with the same genetic composition as the embryo. In this test, a small sample of this chorionic tissue is taken and analyzed to determine genetic abnormalities in the fetus. It can be performed earlier than amniocentesis, usually in about the twelfth week of pregnancy, and takes about a half-hour to complete.

Possible dangers from CVS include infection, maternal or fetal bleeding, spontaneous abortion, Rh immunization, birth defects, and perforation of the membrane surrounding the embryo. The chief advantage is that it can be performed earlier in pregnancy, when termination, if deemed necessary, is a simpler and less dangerous procedure. As with all tests, you should weigh all the pluses and minuses carefully before making a decision.

ULTRASOUND

Ultrasound scanning is a commonly used technique in which high-frequency sound waves are bounced off objects to create images of those objects.

An outline of the fetus, placenta, and other body structures involved in pregnancy is transmitted to a video screen. In this way, the physician can determine fetal size and position, estimate the maturity of the fetus, confirm a multiple pregnancy, find signs of fetal abnormalities, find the location of the placenta, check the fetal heart rate, and estimate the baby's due date and sex. Ultrasound has become a sophisticated diagnostic tool and is frequently used during pregnancy. The usual schedule for ultrasound examination is the following:

• At around seven weeks, it is done to determine that you are indeed pregnant and to rule out ectopic or molar pregnancies. At this time, the fetus is measured and the heartbeat is confirmed.

• Between eighteen and twenty weeks, a second scan may be taken to see if the fetus is growing normally and to look for any abnormalities that may be present.

• At thirty-four weeks, a third scan may be done to look at the growth of the fetus.

The number of scans your health care provider may want to perform will depend on how necessary he or she thinks it is. It is not normally done more often than three times during any pregnancy unless there is a problem with the developing fetus.

Like all tests, it should be used only when medically indicated.

ESTRIOL EXCRETION STUDIES, NONSTRESS TEST, OXYTOCIN CHALLENGE TEST

These tests are also used to determine the health of the fetus. The estriol excretion study determines the best time for delivery of the baby in cases of diabetes or other difficulties in pregnancy. The nonstress test determines fetal well-being, and the oxytocin challenge test helps to predict how well the baby will fare during the stress of labor.

If it is determined that any of these tests is necessary, your health care provider should discuss it with you in depth. When considering any type of prenatal testing, always remember that it is your body and your baby. You should be fully informed of all the advantages and all the risks of any procedure before agreeing to it.

Supplement	Suggested Dosage	Comments
Body Language Essential Green Foods from OxyFresh	As directed on label.	Promotes health and protects the intestinal tract and blood cells.
Calcium	1,500 mg daily.	Necessary for formation of healthy bones and teeth. May prevent hypertension and premature birth.
and magnesium	750 mg daily.	Needed to balance with calcium.
Carotenoid complex with beta-carotene	10,000 IU daily.	Precursor of vitamin A. *Caution:* Do not substitute vitamin A for beta-carotene. Excessive intake of vitamin A during pregnancy has been linked to birth defects.
Coenzyme Q_{10}	As directed on label.	Helps the body convert food to energy, enhances circulation, and protects the heart.
Kelp	As directed on label.	Rich in necessary minerals.
Multimineral and trace mineral complex	As directed on label.	For optimal health and to provide a balance of nutrients needed for fetal development.
Vitamin D_3	1,000 IU daily.	Needed for calcium absorption and bone formation.
Vitamin E	400 IU daily.	Premature and low birth weight infants are often deficient in vitamin E. Use d-alpha-tocopherol form. *Caution:* Do not take vitamin E during the last month of pregnancy.
Vitamin K or alfalfa	As directed on label.	Take for excessive bleeding. *See under* Herbs, below.

Herbs

❑ Alfalfa is a good source of vitamins and minerals, especially vitamin K, which is essential for normal blood clotting.

❑ Blue cohosh, false unicorn root, and squawvine are beneficial taken in the last four weeks of pregnancy. They help to prepare the body for an easier birth and aid contractions.

Caution: These herbs should *not* be taken in the first two trimesters of pregnancy.

❑ Burdock root, dandelion, ginger, and nettle help to enrich a mother's milk.

❑ Red raspberry leaf tea helps the uterus contract more effectively. It also helps to enrich mother's milk. Drink no more than 1 cup per day until the last four weeks of pregnancy. Then drink 1 quart daily.

❑ St. John's wort and shepherd's purse help uterine contractions at birth.

❑ Avoid the following herbs during pregnancy: aloe vera (internally), angelica, arnica, barberry, black cohosh, bloodroot, cat's claw, celandine, cottonwood bark, dong quai, ephedra, feverfew, ginseng, goldenseal, lobelia, myrrh, Oregon grape, pennyroyal, rue, sage, saw palmetto, tansy, and turmeric. Use caution when taking any herbs during pregnancy, especially in the first twelve weeks.

Recommendations

❑ Eat a well-balanced, nutritious diet and be sure to get moderate exercise, fresh air, and plenty of rest.

❑ Do not consume junk food, fried foods, or too much coffee.

❑ Avoid eating rare or undercooked meat, poultry, or fish. Do not eat grilled meats. Grilling has been shown to produce carcinogens in meat.

❑ Do not use any medications while you are pregnant

without consulting your health care provider. The first trimester is arguably the most important stage of development for your child. There are many drugs that may affect that development, so if you are planning to become pregnant—or if you are already pregnant—consult your physician about the possible consequences of any drug, prescription or otherwise, that you may be taking. If it is possible and does not harm your health, you should not take *any* medications during the first trimester of pregnancy.

❏ Do not smoke, consume alcohol in any form, or use drugs, except as prescribed by your health care provider.

❏ Do not take supplements containing the amino acid phenylalanine. Phenylalanine may alter brain growth in the fetus. Also avoid food products containing the sweetener aspartame (Equal, NutraSweet), which contains high levels of phenylalanine. (*See* Is Aspartame a Safe Sugar Substitute? on page 10.)

❏ Do not take mineral oil, which blocks the absorption of the fat-soluble vitamins. Consult your health care provider about the use of any supplements and over-the-counter medications.

❏ Avoid activities that may endanger the abdomen, or that involve jarring, bouncing, or twisting movements. Also avoid activities involving rapid starts and stops, because the body's center of gravity changes during pregnancy and it is easy to lose your balance.

❏ Do *not* take any preparations containing shark cartilage

Birth Plan

Formulating a birth plan while you are pregnant is a good way to ensure that your wishes regarding labor and childbirth are clearly stated and respected. It allows you to decide in advance what you want and what you would choose from among the options you may face during the birth of your child. It is a good idea to work with your health care provider and your partner in drawing up the plan. The following are a number of things you should ask about, and decide upon, in developing a birth plan:

• Where will you have your child, and what options are open to you in that facility? For example, do you wish to simply stay in a bed during labor, or would you rather walk around or take a shower or sit in a tub?

• If you have chosen to have the baby in a private home, who will be there and what additional facilities might you need?

• If you are in hospital, can you wear your own clothes? Listen to music? Watch a video?

• How many people will be allowed to stay with you? How many people do you want to be with you? Do you want them to take photographs or videotape the birth?

• Do you want an intravenous (IV) line inserted during labor? In many places, this is considered routine procedure. However, it often is not necessary.

• Do you want to be given drugs (usually oxytocin [Pitocin]) to speed up labor? Oxytocin is often given through the IV and can make labor more painful.

• What type of medication (if any) do you want? If you decide against any pain medication at the time you write your birth plan, will it still be available should you change your mind at any time during labor?

• If you do decide to use drugs for any pain you might experience, what are the potential side effects? Is it safe for the baby if you breastfeed immediately after using pain medication? Does your physician or midwife use homeopathic and/or natural remedies for pain?

• What methods will be used to monitor the baby during labor?

• Do you have to have your baby in the lithotomy position (flat on your back with your feet in stirrups)?

• Will you have an episiotomy? (This is an incision made to enlarge the vaginal opening either so that forceps can be used or to hasten delivery or to prevent tearing in this area, which takes longer to heal than an incision does.)

• Probably the most important question: Are you willing to have a cesarean section, and under what emergency circumstances do they perform this operation? If you had a cesarean for a previous delivery, will you be supported through a vaginal birth after cesarean (VBAC) this time? Over 24 percent of American women who give birth in hospitals undergo cesarean sections. The World Health Organization (WHO) has stated that no area in the world is justified in having a cesarean rate greater than 10 to 15 percent. Cesarean births cost more than twice as much as vaginal births. It takes much longer for the mother to recover, and she has to remain in the hospital for an extra two days, on average. The most common reason for performing a cesarean is that the mother had one for a previous delivery. But VBAC is possible, and this is something you should discuss with your physician or midwife. The risk of rupturing the previous incision is very small. The reasons for *emergency* cesarean usually fall into the following categories: The umbilical cord presents before the baby; the baby is a breech presentation (coming down the birth canal feet first, buttocks first, or sideways, instead of head down); the placenta breaks up before the baby is born; or the baby's head is too big to fit through the pelvis (a very unusual event). Many problems can be corrected before or during labor without resorting to a major operation such as a cesarean section.

during pregnancy. Shark cartilage inhibits the formation of new blood vessels, which is essential during pregnancy.

❑ Do not use an electric blanket. Several experts warn that the invisible electromagnetic field emanating from an electric blanket may increase the risk of miscarriage and developmental problems.

❑ Take warm, rather than hot, showers or baths. Anything that increases the core body temperature for any length of time may cause neural tube defects in babies such as anencephaly and spina bifida. Anencephalic babies do not develop a brain and rarely survive. Spina bifida is a defect of the spinal column that can affect the baby to varying degrees, depending on the severity of the condition.

CONSIDERATIONS

❑ Lack of zinc, manganese, and folic acid, as well as amino acid imbalances, have been linked to fetal deformities and mental retardation.

❑ All women of childbearing age who are thinking of becoming pregnant should take a daily supplement of 400 micrograms of folic acid and a B-vitamin complex. Folic acid deficiency is linked to such neurologic birth defects as spina bifida and anencephaly. To prevent these disorders, this B vitamin must be present in the body during the first six weeks following conception, a crucial early phase in fetal neurological development. Since most women do not know they have conceived until several weeks afterward, the best way to prevent these birth defects is for women who are planning to become pregnant to have an adequate supply of this nutrient at all times. Supplementation is recommended because many women do not get enough folic acid from dietary sources. Folic acid also helps alleviate hemorrhaging in childbirth and improves milk production. Men too should be as healthy as they possibly can before they conceive children.

❑ Both partners should give up alcohol, cigarettes, and drugs—legal or otherwise—at least three to six months before they decide to conceive. Marijuana, heroin, morphine, and tobacco all reduce levels of male sex hormones and increase the risks of birth defects.

❑ Men should make sure to have an adequate intake of selenium, zinc, vitamins C and E, and the carotenoids.

❑ Taking the drug phenytoin (Dilantin) or phenobarbital, used to control epileptic seizures, creates four times the usual risk of producing a baby with heart defects. In addition, the antibiotics ampicillin (Omnipen, Polycillin) or tetracycline may cause heart malformations. Ask your physician for a *detailed* list of teratogenic agents and drugs (chemicals that cause birth defects). These include, but are not limited to, the following:

- Some ACE inhibitors.
- Some acne medications.
- Some antibiotics.
- Some blood thinning medications.
- Some cancer drugs.
- Some hormone preparations.
- Some seizure medications.
- Some thyroid treatment drugs.
- Chronic (long-term) alcohol intake.
- Cocaine.

These teratogens which affect the development of the baby, include drugs taken by men during the time of conception.

❑ Excessive intake of vitamin A has been linked with cleft palate, heart defects, and other congenital defects. Foods rich in vitamin A may also cause problems. Foods containing natural beta-carotene, however, are not harmful because the body converts beta-carotene to vitamin A only as needed, and not in amounts that may be toxic to the body.

❑ One of the best things you can do for your child is to breastfeed your baby for at least the first three months of life—longer if possible. Mother's milk is not only the most nutritious food for a baby, but it also provides crucial disease-fighting agents. A new mother should consume 500 more calories per day when nursing than she ate during pregnancy. The diet should include a substantial amount of liquids and extra portions of calcium-rich foods. If nursing is not possible and you must bottlefeed, use a well-balanced soy-based product. Cow's milk does not supply a human infant with enough iron, linoleic acid, or vitamin E, and babies who are fed cow's milk have a greater chance of developing allergies to milk and dairy products later in life.

Premenstrual Syndrome

Premenstrual syndrome (PMS) is a disorder that affects many women during the one to two weeks before menstruation begins. Symptoms can include any or all of the following: abdominal bloating, acne, anxiety, backache, breast swelling and tenderness, cramps, depression, food cravings, fainting spells, fatigue, headaches, insomnia, joint pain, nervousness, skin eruptions, water retention, and personality changes such as drastic mood swings, outbursts of anger, violence, and, sometimes, even thoughts of suicide. The symptoms are so numerous and various that diagnosing and treating this condition is often difficult.

While there are no hard statistics, it is estimated that as many as 80 percent of all women experience some premenstrual symptoms at one time or another. Approximately 5 percent of women have symptoms so severe as to be incapacitating, and 30 to 40 percent report symptoms severe enough to interfere with their day-to-day lives.

For many years, PMS was dismissed as a psychological problem. We now know that this is a physically based problem, although it is still far from clear what causes all the symptoms. It is possible, of course, that there is more than one cause of PMS and that there may be different causes of symptoms in different people. One of the reasons for PMS may be hormonal imbalance—excessive levels of estrogen and inadequate levels of progesterone—as well as sensitivity to fluctuating hormones. Diet may be an important contributing factor for some women. Unstable blood sugar levels are an important factor as well. PMS has also been linked to food allergies, changes in carbohydrate metabolism, hypoglycemia, and malabsorption. Other suspected causes of PMS symptoms include erratic levels of beta-endorphin (a narcoticlike substance produced by the body), vitamin and/or mineral deficiencies (especially calcium deficiency), and an inability to metabolize fatty acids. All of these may play a part in PMS.

Unless otherwise specified, the dosages recommended here are for adults. For a girl between the ages of twelve and seventeen, reduce the dose to three-quarters of the recommended amount.

NUTRIENTS

SUPPLEMENT	SUGGESTED DOSAGE	COMMENTS
Very Important		
Acidophilus (Kyo-Dophilus from Wakunaga is a good source)	As directed on label.	Breaks down metabolites of estrogen.
Black currant seed oil *or* flaxseed oil *or* primrose oil	As directed on label 3 times daily. / As directed on label 3 times daily. / 1,000 mg 3 times daily.	To supply gamma-linolenic acid (GLA), an essential fatty acid that is important in relieving symptoms and aiding proper glandular function.
Calcium *and* magnesium *and* vitamin D$_3$	1,500 mg daily. / 1,000 mg daily. / As directed on label.	Studies have shown that calcium supplements can reduce many symptoms of PMS by as much as 30 percent. Use a citrate or chelate form. Deficiency may be associated with PMS. Should be taken with calcium. Use magnesium chloride or chelate form. Needed for the uptake of calcium and magnesium.
Gamma-amino-butyric acid (GABA)	750 mg daily.	Assists in controlling anxiety and restlessness by increasing levels of serotonin in the brain.
Melatonin	As directed on label.	Important for regulating hormone levels. Helps combat insomnia.
Natural progesterone cream (Pro-G + from TriMedica)	As directed on label.	A progesterone supplement that has proved helpful for some women.

SUPPLEMENT	SUGGESTED DOSAGE	COMMENTS
Pregnenolone *or* DHEA *or* 7 keto-DHEA	10–100 mg daily (increase the dose for the 5 days before your period, but never exceed more than 100 mg daily for 5 days). / 10 mg daily. / As directed on label.	Made from diosgenin, a compound found in some plants, this is a precursor to DHEA. In the body, it is converted into progesterone, cortisone, testosterone, DHEA, and estrogen. Is converted into estrogen and testosterone. Enhances memory and the immune system. Unlike ordinary DHEA, is not converted into hormones.
S-Adenosylmethio-nine (SAMe)	200 mg twice daily.	Aids in prevention of depression.
Ultimate Cleanse from Nature's Secret	As directed on label.	A cleansing program that enhances the liver's ability to metabolize estrogen.
Vitamin B complex *plus extra* pantothenic acid (vitamin B$_5$) *and* vitamin B$_6$ (pyridoxine) *and* vitamin B$_{12}$	100 mg of each major B vitamin 3 times daily (amounts of individual vitamins in a complex will vary). / 100–200 mg daily. / 50 mg 3 times daily. / 1,000–2,000 mcg daily.	B vitamins work best when taken together. Reduces stress and is needed by the adrenal gland. Reduces water retention and increases oxygen flow to the female organs. Also aids in restoring estrogen levels to normal. Reduces stress, prevents anemia, and is needed for all bodily functions. Use a lozenge or sublingual form.
Vitamin E	Start with 400 IU daily and increase slowly to 800 IU daily.	Good for sore breasts and other PMS symptoms; improves oxygen utilization and limits free radical damage. Also helps to relieve nervous tension, irritability, and depression. Use d-alpha-tocopherol form.
Helpful		
Choline *and* inositol *or* lecithin	1,000 mg each daily. / As directed on label.	To aid in nerve impulse transmission and help prevent estrogen-related cancers.
Chromium picolinate	200 mcg daily.	Stabilizes blood sugar levels.
DL-Phenylalanine (DLPA)	375 mg 3–4 times daily.	Helpful for alleviating headaches and pain. *Caution:* Do not take this supplement if you suffer from panic attacks, diabetes, high blood pressure, or PKU.
Floradix Iron + Herbs from Salus Haus	As directed on label. Do not take at the same time as vitamin E; iron depletes vitamin E in the body.	To supply iron in easily assimilable natural formula. Women with heavy menstrual flow are often anemic.
Kelp	1,000–1,500 mg daily.	A good source of needed minerals. Helps protect thyroid function.
L-Tyrosine	500 mg twice daily, on an empty stomach. Take with water or juice. Do not take with milk. Take with 50 mg vitamin B$_6$ and 100 mg vitamin C for better absorption.	Reduces anxiety, depression, and headache. *Caution:* Do not take this supplement if you are taking an MAO inhibitor drug.

Multivitamin and mineral complex	As directed on label.	All nutrients are needed for relief of symptoms.
Vitamin A plus	10,000 IU daily.	Deficiency has been linked to PMS.
carotenoids complex with natural beta-carotene	15,000 IU daily.	Antioxidants and precursors of vitamin A.
Vitamin C with bioflavonoids	3,000–6,000 mg daily, in divided doses.	Aids in relief of discomfort and breast swelling. Also boosts the immune system.
Zinc plus	50 mg daily. Do not exceed a total of 100 mg daily from all supplements.	Needed for proper immune function. Diuretics deplete zinc. Use zinc gluconate lozenges or OptiZinc for best absorption.
copper	3 mg daily.	Needed to balance with zinc.

HERBS

❑ Angelica root, cramp bark, kava kava, and red raspberry have antispasmodic properties and may alleviate cramps.

❑ Black cohosh, blessed thistle, dong quai, false unicorn root, fennel seed, sarsaparilla root, and squawvine are hormone-balancing herbs effective in the treatment of PMS.

Caution: Do not use black cohosh if you are pregnant or have any type of chronic disease.

❑ Black haw and rosemary are good for cramps and help to calm the nervous system.

❑ Corn silk or an herbal combination such as SP-6 Cornsilk Blend from Solaray aids in releasing excess water from the tissues and relieves many premenstrual symptoms. Dandelion and hawthorn also act as natural diuretics.

❑ Feverfew is good for migraines.

❑ Milk thistle cleanses the liver and helps improve liver function, thus enhancing the liver's ability to metabolize estrogen. For best results, this herb should be taken on a daily basis for a period of three months.

❑ Pau d'arco tea is good for protecting against candidiasis (yeast infection).

❑ Peppermint, strawberry leaf, and valerian root help to stabilize mood swings and tone the nervous system.

❑ Wild yam extract contains natural progesterone and has proved effective in alleviating many symptoms of PMS, including cramps, headache, mood swings, depression, irritability, and insomnia.

RECOMMENDATIONS

❑ Eat plenty of fresh fruits and vegetables, whole-grain cereals and breads, beans, peas, lentils, nuts and seeds, and broiled chicken, turkey, and fish. Have high-protein snacks between meals.

❑ Include in your diet foods that are high in complex carbohydrates and rich in fiber. These can help the body to get rid of excess estrogen if high estrogen levels are your problem.

❑ Drink 1 quart of distilled water daily, starting a week before the menstrual period and ending one week after.

❑ Do not consume salt, red meats, processed foods, or junk or fast foods. At the very least, omit these foods from the diet for at least one week before the expected onset of symptoms. Eliminating sodium (principally salt and foods that contain it) is especially important for preventing bloating and water retention.

❑ Eat fewer dairy products. Dairy products block the absorption of magnesium and increase its urinary excretion. Refined sugars also increase magnesium excretion.

❑ Avoid caffeine. Caffeine is linked to breast tenderness and is a central nervous system stimulant that can make you anxious and jittery. It also acts as a diuretic and can deplete many important nutrients.

❑ Do not consume alcohol or sugar in any form, especially during the week before symptoms are expected. These foods cause valuable electrolytes, particularly magnesium, to be lost through the urine.

❑ Fast on fresh juices and spirulina for several days before the anticipated onset of menstruation to help minimize symptoms. (*See* FASTING in Part Three.)

❑ Get regular exercise. Walking, even if only one-half to one mile per day, can be very helpful. Exercise increases the oxygen level in the blood, which helps in nutrient absorption and efficient elimination of toxins from the body. It also helps to keep hormone levels more stable.

❑ See a physician to rule out an underlying medical condition that may be causing symptoms, such as abnormal thyroid function, endometriosis, or a genuine psychological problem such as clinical depression. A food allergy test and a hair analysis to rule out heavy metal intoxication are also recommended. (*See* ALLERGIES in Part Two and HAIR ANALYSIS in Part Three.)

❑ Do not smoke.

CONSIDERATIONS

❑ PMS is a syndrome with many causes, and there may not be one answer to the problem that fits every woman. It may be best to try altering your diet, using natural progesterone cream, avoiding certain foods and drinks, taking up meditation, or trying acupuncture, and seeing which one suits you best and gives you optimum relief from your particular symptoms.

❑ Premenstrual depression may be due to a miscue of the biological clock that results in lower than normal levels of certain brain chemicals. Research at the University of California–San Diego suggests that some women who suffer from PMS may be deficient in melatonin, a hormone secreted at night by the pineal gland.

❑ Studies have shown that women who regularly consume caffeine are four times more likely than others to have severe PMS.

❑ Some physicians recommend oral contraceptives for women with PMS, especially if they also are interested in reliable birth control. If you take oral contraceptives, be aware that their effectiveness at preventing pregnancy can be sharply reduced if you also take antibiotics. Oral contraceptives and other preparations containing estrogen-type substances should *not* be used if you are pregnant or if you have breast cancer, abnormal vaginal bleeding, or phlebitis (inflammation of leg veins).

❑ Proper diet is extremely important in treating PMS. Meals high in complex carbohydrates have been found to help in dealing with stress. Researchers speculate that such a diet may increase the body's production of serotonin, a brain chemical with antidepressant properties. Conversely, eating red meat and dairy products promotes the type of hormonal imbalance that causes PMS—excessive estrogen levels and inadequate progesterone levels.

❑ Wild yam cream, which contains a natural form of the hormone progesterone, has been helpful for many women. You rub the cream into the skin on your chest, inner arms, thighs, and abdomen just after ovulation, and the active ingredient is absorbed through the skin.

❑ The amino acid L-glutamine, either alone or in combination with DL-phenylalanine (DLPA), may help to reduce food cravings.

❑ Research has discovered that many women with PMS also suffer from some form of immune system disorder or frequently suffer from some variety of yeast infection. (*See* CANDIDIASIS in Part Two.)

❑ A significant number of women who suffer from PMS have some sort of thyroid dysfunction. (*See* HYPOTHYROIDISM in Part Two.)

❑ Clinics specializing in the treatment of PMS are springing up all over the country. Experience and expertise can vary greatly among these establishments, however. Ask your health care provider for a referral or recommendation, or look for a clinic that is affiliated with a major local hospital. Beware of clinics that promote only one type of treatment or a quick-fix approach to this complicated disorder.

Prolapse of the Uterus

Uterine prolapse (sometimes called a pelvic floor hernia or a pudendal hernia) is a condition that develops when muscular support for the uterus is lost. The uterus is normally held in place by the pelvic muscles and supporting ligaments. When these muscles become weakened or injured, uterine prolapse can occur. In mild cases, a portion of the uterus descends into the top of the vagina. In more serious cases, the uterus may even protrude through the vaginal opening and can be accompanied by a cystocele (a bladder that bulges into the front wall of the vagina) or a ureterocele (a urethra that does the same). In some instances, the rectum may bulge into the back wall of the vagina, a condition known as rectocele.

Symptoms of prolapse of the uterus can include backache, abdominal discomfort, a feeling of heaviness, and urinary incontinence, especially stress incontinence (the involuntary passage of urine when straining, sneezing, or otherwise putting pressure on the abdomen). Other symptoms can include excessive menstrual bleeding, abnormal vaginal discharge or bleeding, painful intercourse, and constipation. However, a woman with a prolapsed uterus may not exhibit any symptoms at all.

Women who have borne several children and/or who have gone through difficult and prolonged labor are more prone to prolapse. Other factors that can increase the likelihood of uterine prolapse include obesity, uterine cancer, diabetes, chronic bronchitis, asthma, heavy lifting or straining (particularly if the pelvic muscles are already weakened), and a retroverted uterus (a uterus that is tilted toward the back of the body). Two-thirds of all women who prolapse do so before the age of fifty-five.

NUTRIENTS

SUPPLEMENT	SUGGESTED DOSAGE	COMMENTS
Important		
Calcium and	1,500 mg daily.	Essential minerals needed for muscle tone and metabolism.
magnesium or	1,000 mg daily.	
Bone Defense from KAL	As directed on label.	A good source of necessary minerals and other nutrients.
L-Carnitine plus	500 mg twice daily, on an empty stomach.	Improves muscle strength in the uterus.
L-glycine	500 mg twice daily, on an empty stomach. Take with water or juice. Do not take with milk. Take with 50 mg vitamin B_6 and 100 mg vitamin C for better absorption.	Retards muscle degeneration.
plus branched-chain amino acid complex	As directed on label.	Promotes healing of muscle tissue.
Methylsulfonyl-methane (MSM) (MSM With Glucosamine from the American Council for Natural Pain Relief or OptiMSM from Cardinal Nutrition)	As directed on label.	A natural sulfur compound found in foods and present in body tissues that is used by the body to build healthy new cells. MSM provides the flexible bond between the cells and provides support for tendons, ligaments, and muscles.
Multivitamin and mineral complex with mixed carotenoids and vitamin B complex	As directed on label.	All nutrients work together for healing and tissue repair.
Vitamin C with bioflavonoids	3,000–5,000 mg daily, in divided doses.	Important for keeping bladder infections under control and to enhance immune function. Use an esterified form for best absorption.

Zinc	50 mg daily. Do not exceed a total of 100 mg daily from all supplements.	Needed for proper immune function, bone support, and all bodily enzyme systems. Use zinc gluconate lozenges or OptiZinc for best absorption.

HERBS

❑ Buchu has anti-inflammatory properties and aids in controlling bladder problems.

❑ Cranberry aids in bladder function and helps to prevent urgency incontinence. It can be taken in capsule form. Pure, unsweetened cranberry juice is good also.

❑ Damiana helps provide oxygen to the genital area and balances female hormones.

❑ Ginger can help with bowel disorders.

RECOMMENDATIONS

❑ Eat a diet consisting of 75 percent raw fruits and vegetables plus whole grains such as brown rice and millet.

❑ Use a fiber supplement daily to prevent constipation.

❑ Do not strain during bowel movements or urination.

❑ Drink 8 to 10 full glasses of quality water daily.

CONSIDERATIONS

❑ Doing Kegel's exercises to tone the pelvic floor muscles when prolapse is beginning may prevent the condition from getting worse. These exercises can be done in two ways:

1. Tighten and squeeze the vagina and rectum by drawing the muscles inward and upward. Hold this position for five to ten seconds, then relax. Repeat as many times as possible, preferably at least 100 times a day.

2. When urinating, start and stop the flow of urine as many times as possible. This form of the exercise is particularly useful for stress incontinence.

❑ If the prolapse causes no symptoms, no treatment is needed, other than perhaps adopting an exercise program designed for the individual problem and situation.

❑ Natural progesterone replacement may be more beneficial than estrogen therapy.

❑ A vaginal device (a ring-shaped pessary) can be inserted to hold the uterus in place. This approach can have undesirable results, however. It can interfere with sexual intercourse and may also cause an irritating discharge with an unpleasant odor and even infection.

❑ It is possible to surgically resuspend the uterus into its normal position. This procedure is usually performed on women who wish to bear children in the future. For women who have completed childbearing, or who do not wish to have children, vaginal hysterectomy is a viable option for this condition. Women pondering a hysterectomy should give the matter close and careful consideration. (*See* HYSTERECTOMY-RELATED PROBLEMS in Part Two.)

Prostate Cancer

The prostate is a walnut-sized gland at the base of the bladder that encircles the urethra, the tube through which urine is voided. The prostate produces prostatic fluid, which makes up the bulk of the male ejaculate and nourishes and transports the sperm. Cancer of the prostate gland is the second leading cause of cancer death among men. It is primarily a disease of aging. Men in their thirties and forties rarely develop prostate cancer, but the incidence increases steadily after the age of fifty. Approximately 80 percent of all cases occur in men over the age of sixty-five, and by the age of eighty, 80 percent of all men have prostate cancer to some degree. The American Cancer Society estimates that more than 180,400 new cases of prostate cancer are diagnosed annually, and 31,900 men die from the disease. A male baby born today has a 13 percent chance of developing prostate cancer at some time in his life, and a 3 percent chance of dying from the disease. Many experts feel that every man will eventually develop prostate cancer if he lives long enough. Prostate cancer deaths have been declining for the past several years, which many experts believe to be the result of better screening and earlier diagnosis.

Although it is relatively common, in most cases prostate cancer is, fortunately, a slow-growing cancer. Most prostate cancers arise in the rear portion of the prostate gland; the rest originate near the urethra. Lymphatic vessels leading from the prostate gland to the pelvic lymph nodes provide a route for prostate cancer to spread to other areas of the body. Prostate cancers double in mass every six years, on average (by comparison, breast cancers commonly double every three and a half years). Possible symptoms of prostate cancer can include one or more of the following: pain or a burning sensation during urination, frequent urination, a decrease in the size and force of urine flow, an inability to urinate, blood in the urine, and continuing lower back, pelvic, or suprapubic discomfort. However, the disease often causes no symptoms at all until it reaches an advanced stage and/or spreads outside the gland. In addition, these symptoms most often are caused not by cancer, but by an enlarged prostate, *benign prostatic hyperplasia* (BPH).

The exact cause or causes of prostate cancer are not known. However, there are certain risk factors that have been linked to its development. Men aged sixty-five and older, African-American men, and men who have a first-degree relative (parent or sibling) with prostate cancer are at increased risk. The incidence is higher among married men than it is among unmarried men. Also at increased risk are men who have had recurring prostate infections, those with a history of venereal disease, and those who have taken testosterone. Exposure to cancer-causing chemicals increases risk as well. Researchers have also found a link between a high-fat diet that is low in fruits and vegetables and prostate cancer. This may be due to the fact that heavy fat consumption raises testosterone levels, which could then stimulate growth of the prostate, including any cancer cells it may be harboring. Some studies have suggested that vasectomy may increase the risk of developing prostate cancer, although other studies contradict this hypothesis.

There is no known way to prevent this disease, but early detection can make it possible to catch the cancer before it spreads to other sites in the body. A careful digital rectal exam of the prostate is the simplest and most cost-effective approach for detecting prostate cancer. The American Cancer Society recommends that every man have an annual exam beginning at age forty; the American Urological Association suggests beginning at age fifty. A blood test to detect elevated levels of a protein called prostate-specific antigen (PSA) is an excellent screening test for prostate cancer. PSA is currently the most valuable "tumor marker" available to diagnose and evaluate the effectiveness of therapy for prostate cancer. A PSA test result between 0 and 4 is considered to be within the normal range. A level between 4 and 10 may raise a doctor's suspicion, and scores above 50 may indicate a tumor that has spread to elsewhere in the body. High PSA levels can be caused by factors other than cancer, including benign enlargement or inflammation of the prostate, an activity as innocuous as bicycle riding, or even the rectal exam itself. If a man's PSA level is found to be high, the test should always be repeated, because it does yield false-positive or false-negative results an estimated 10 to 20 percent of the time. Having the test repeated every year may help a physician to better interpret the results; in healthy men, PSA levels tend to remain relatively stable, rising only gradually from year to year, while cancer causes the levels to rise more dramatically.

Ultrasound scanning of the prostate is often done to follow up on an abnormal rectal exam or PSA test. Other diagnostic tests, including computerized tomography (CT) scans, bone scans, and magnetic resonance imaging (MRI) may be necessary, but are costly. Ultimately, if test results point consistently to the presence of cancer, a tissue diagnosis must be done to confirm it. This can be done only by microscopic examination of a needle biopsy, preferably directed under ultrasound control. Repeated biopsies may be needed in some cases. This invasive procedure may itself cause complications. Bleeding, urinary retention, impotence, and sepsis ("blood poisoning") have been reported. Another important measure, the Gleason score, gauges the probable aggressiveness of a tumor based on the cellular characteristics of the cancer. Tumor cells that look more similar to normal cells tend to be less aggressive, while those that are distributed randomly with uneven edges are likely to spread rapidly.

NUTRIENTS

SUPPLEMENT	SUGGESTED DOSAGE	COMMENTS
Essential		
Coenzyme Q$_{10}$ plus	100 mg daily.	Improves cellular oxygenation.
Coenzyme A from Coenzyme-A Technologies	As directed on label.	Works effectively with coenzyme Q$_{10}$ to support the immune system's detoxification of many dangerous substances.
Colostrum (New Life Colostrum from Symbiotics [original and high-Ig] and Colostrum Specific from Jarrow Formulas are good sources)	As directed on label.	Has been shown to boost the immune system, burn fat, build lean muscle, and have an anti-aging effect.
Dimethylglycine (DMG) (Aangamik DMG from FoodScience of Vermont)	As directed on label.	Enhances oxygen utilization.
Garlic (Kyolic from Wakunaga)	2 capsules 3 times daily.	Enhances immune function. Helps to break down testosterone. Has been shown to slow cancer cell growth.
Proteolytic enzymes	As directed on label. Take with meals.	To keep down inflammation and destroy free radicals.
Selenium	200 mcg daily.	Needed for proper prostate function. The incidence of prostate cancer has been shown to be substantially lower in men with higher selenium levels.
Shark cartilage (BeneFin)	1 gm per 2 lbs of body weight daily, divided into 3 doses. If you cannot tolerate taking it orally, it can be administered rectally in a retention enema.	Inhibits tumor growth and stimulates the immune system.
Superoxide dismutase (SOD)	As directed on label.	Destroys free radicals. Consider injections (under a doctor's supervision).
Vitamin A	50,000–100,000 IU daily for 10 days or as long as on the program.	Powerful antioxidants that destroy free radicals. Use emulsion forms for easier assimilation, and greater safety at higher doses.
plus carotenoid complex with extra lycopene	As directed on label.	Lycopene has been shown to lower risk of developing prostate cancer.
plus vitamin E	Up to 1,000 IU daily.	Protects against prostate cancer. Use d-alpha-tocopherol form.
Vitamin B complex	100 mg of each major B vitamin daily (amounts of individual vitamins in a complex will vary).	B vitamins necessary for normal cell division and to improve circulation, build red blood cells, and aid liver function. *Caution:* Do not take niacin if you have a liver disorder, gout, or high blood pressure.
plus extra vitamin B$_3$ (niacin)	100 mg daily. Do not exceed this amount.	
and choline	500–1,000 mg daily.	
and folic acid	400 mcg daily.	
plus vitamin B$_6$ (pyridoxine) and	100 mg daily.	Enhances the efficacy of zinc.

vitamin B$_{12}$	2,000 mcg daily.	Prevents anemia. Use a lozenge or sublingual form. Consider injections (under a doctor's supervision).
Vitamin C with bioflavonoids	5,000–20,000 mg daily, in divided doses. (*See* ASCORBIC ACID FLUSH in Part Three.)	Powerful anticancer agent. Has been shown in laboratories to inhibit the spread of prostate cancer.
Vitamin D$_3$	As directed on label.	Low levels may be linked to higher prostate cancer incidence.
Important		
Maitake extract	4,000–8,000 mg (4–8 gm) daily.	Inhibits the growth and spread of cancerous tumors. Also boosts immune response.
Helpful		
Aerobic 07 from Aerobic Life Industries	As directed on label.	An antimicrobial agent.
Berry Seeds Complex from International Health Products	1–2 tablets after each meal.	Has a regulating effect on cell function and a suppressive effect on cancer cells.
Glutathione plus	As directed on label.	Protects against environmental toxins.
L-cysteine and L-methionine	As directed on label, on an empty stomach. Take with water or juice. Do not take with milk. Take with 50 mg vitamin B$_6$ and 100 mg vitamin C for better absorption.	Sulfur-containing amino acids that act as detoxifiers and protect the liver and other organs. (*See* AMINO ACIDS in Part One.)
Kelp or seaweed	1,000–1,500 mg daily.	For mineral balance.
Kyo-Dophilus from Wakunaga	As directed on label. Take on an empty stomach.	Has an antibacterial effect on the body. Use a non-dairy, nonrefrigeration formula.
L-Carnitine	As directed on label.	Protects against free radical damage and toxins. Use a form from fish liver (squalene).
Multienzyme complex	As directed on label. Take with meals.	To aid digestion.
Multiglandular complex plus	As directed on label.	To stimulate glandular function, especially that of the thymus, site of T lymphocyte production. (*See* GLANDULAR THERAPY in Part Three.)
raw thymus glandular	As directed on label.	
Multimineral complex with	As directed on label.	Essential for normal cell division and function.
calcium and	1,500 mg daily.	
magnesium and	750–1,000 mg daily.	
potassium	99 mg daily.	
Multivitamin complex	As directed on label.	Many nutrients in this table may be found in a combination multivitamin. Do not use a sustained-release formula. Choose a product that is iron-free.
Taurine	As directed on label.	An amino acid that functions as foundation for tissue and organ repair.
Zinc	50–100 mg daily. Do not exceed this amount.	Plays a role in the prevention of prostate cancer. Use zinc gluconate lozenges or OptiZinc for best absorption.

HERBS

❑ Black radish, dandelion, milk thistle, and red clover are good for cleansing the liver and the blood.

❑ Buchu, Carnivora, echinacea, goldenseal, pau d'arco, and suma have all shown anticancer properties. Take them in tea form, using two at a time and alternating among them.

❑ Damiana and licorice root have the ability to balance hormones and glandular function.

❑ Gravel root, hydrangea, oat straw, parsley root, uva ursi, and yarrow are diuretics that also dissolve sediment.

❑ A plant substance in green tea has been found by researchers at the Mayo Clinic to be a potent killer of prostate cancer cells. Many studies have linked green tea consumption to a reduced risk for prostate cancer.

❑ Modified citrus pectin has shown to substantially inhibit the growth of cancer cells and is especially effective in combating prostate cancer.

❑ Pygeum and saw palmetto are helpful. European studies suggest pygeum may prevent prostate cancer.

❑ Turmeric is a spice that contains curcumin, an antioxidant that may be effective in controlling prostate cancer cells.

RECOMMENDATIONS

❑ Maintain a whole-foods diet. Eat plenty of whole grains, raw nuts and seeds, and unpolished brown rice. Millet cereal is a good source of protein. Eat wheat, oats, and bran. Also eat plenty of cruciferous vegetables, such as broccoli, Brussels sprouts, cabbage, and cauliflower, and yellow and deep orange vegetables, such as carrots, pumpkin, squash, and yams. This type of diet is important for the prevention of cancer as well as for healing.

❑ Include in the diet apples, fresh cantaloupe, all kinds of berries, especially blueberries and strawberries; Brazil nuts; cherries; grapes; legumes, including chickpeas, lentils, and red beans; plums; and walnuts. All of these foods help to fight cancer.

❑ Consume freshly made vegetable and fruit juices daily. Carrot and cabbage juices are good choices.

❑ Eat plenty of grapefruit, watermelon, and tomatoes and tomato products such as tomato juice and tomato-based sauces. These contain lycopene, which has been shown to protect against prostate cancer.

❑ Include in your diet foods that are high in zinc, such as mushrooms, pumpkin seeds, seafood, spinach, sunflower seeds, and whole grains. Zinc nourishes the prostate gland and is vital for proper immune function.

❏ Eat salmon, mackerel, sardines, or herring. Regular consumption of these sources of omega-3 fatty acids may lower the risk of prostate cancer.

❏ Drink at least eight 8-ounce glasses of water a day. This hydrates the body, keeps the prostate working efficiently, and helps to eliminate toxins from the body.

❏ Restrict your intake of dairy products. Moderate consumption of soured products such as low-fat yogurt and kefir is acceptable.

❏ If you experience difficulty urinating or notice an increasing trend toward waking up to urinate during the night, consult your health care provider. This may indicate prostatic obstruction.

❏ Use cold-pressed organic oils such as sesame, safflower, or olive oil to obtain essential fatty acids.

❏ Do not eat red meat. There is a definite correlation between high red meat consumption (five servings a week or more) and the development of prostate cancer.

❏ Eliminate from the diet alcoholic beverages, coffee, and all teas except for caffeine-free herbal teas.

❏ Strictly avoid the following foods: junk foods, processed refined foods, salt, saturated fats, polyunsaturated vegetable oils, sugar, and white flour. Instead of salt, use a kelp or potassium substitute. If necessary, a small amount of blackstrap molasses or pure maple syrup can be used as a natural sweetener in place of sugar. Use whole wheat or rye instead of white flour.

❏ Unless otherwise recommended in the table above, take vitamins and other supplements daily with meals, with the exception of vitamin E, which should be taken before meals.

❏ Try to avoid *all* known carcinogens. Eat only organic foods, if possible. Avoid tobacco smoke, polluted air, polluted water, noxious chemicals, and food additives. Use only distilled water or reverse-osmosis-filtered water. Municipal and well water can contain chlorine, fluoride, and agricultural chemical residue.

❏ Try following a macrobiotic diet.

❏ Get regular physical activity. Active men maintain better health and have lower risk of developing prostate cancer.

❏ Enjoy regular sexual activity. Regular ejaculation activates the prostate gland, keeping it from getting stagnant and inflamed.

❏ Do not take any drugs except those that are prescribed by your physician. Always seek counsel and alternative opinions before deciding which treatments, if any, you will pursue.

CONSIDERATIONS

❏ Diet and nutrition are important not only for treatment, but for prevention. An anticancer diet is composed primarily of brown rice, fresh raw fruits and vegetables, fresh juices, legumes, raw nuts and seeds, and whole grains, and *excludes* alcohol, coffee, refined carbohydrates, and strong tea. Regular intake of zinc (50 milligrams daily) and essential fatty acids (in supplement form or from cold-pressed sesame, safflower, or olive oil) in later life also may help to prevent the development of problems.

❏ A high-fat, low-fiber diet is linked not just to heart disease, but also to prostate cancer. Chemical reactions occur when fat is cooked, leading to the production of free radicals, which play a major role in certain cancers. It is logical to assume that the accelerating increase in prostate cancer since the 1950s must be attributable at least in part to a parallel increase in fat consumption in the United States. According to the *Journal of the National Cancer Institute,* men who eat red meat five times a week may have a risk of prostate cancer that is nearly three times higher than that for men who eat red meat less than once a week. Butter consumption also appears to contribute to this disease. Researchers theorize that a diet high in fat raises the levels of testosterone and other hormones in the body, which stimulates the prostate—and any cancerous cells in it—to grow. A high intake of milk and coffee may also increase the risk of developing prostate cancer.

❏ Research has shown that soybeans and soy products, such as tofu, tempeh, soy flour, and soymilk, have cancer-fighting powers due to the presence of a protein called genistein. Genistein apparently retards tumor growth by preventing the growth of new blood vessels to feed the tumor. It appears to be particularly effective against prostate cancer, but also works against breast cancer in women and colon cancer in both sexes.

❏ Berries help protect DNA from damage and mutation that may result in cancer.

❏ Excess dietary calcium may increase the risk of prostate cancer. This may be because calcium can reduce the levels of vitamin D, which has been shown to be prostate-protective.

❏ Men who have higher levels of the enzyme 5-alpha-reductase may be at greater risk for prostate cancer. This is an enzyme that transforms testosterone into dihydrotestosterone (DHT), a form of the hormone that promotes the growth of prostate cells.

❏ Prolactin is another hormone that may alter the cells of the prostate gland. Studies have shown that it may promote the growth of prostate cancer. If you have prostate cancer, you may want to consider having your prolactin levels checked. If they are elevated, the drugs bromocriptine (Parlodel), cabergoline (Dostinex), and pergolide (Permax) are effective in suppressing the release of prolactin from the pituitary gland.

❏ Researchers are looking into the role of angiogenesis (the formation of new blood vessels from existing microvessels) in prostate cancer.

❏ *The New England Journal of Medicine* published a study in September 1998 about a study on PC Spes, an herbal formula that diminished PSA levels in men with advanced prostate cancer in clinical trials. Researchers are currently studying PC SPES in an effort to determine dosage and effects, as it may cause serious side effects.

❏ Research is ongoing on genes that may be related to inherited prostate cancer. Some researchers believe that mutated BRCA genes (the gene implicated in some cases of breast cancer) may slightly increase the risk of prostate cancer.

❏ Although the American Cancer Society, the American Urological Association, and the National Comprehensive Cancer Network believe that PSA test screening for prostate cancer can save lives, there are major scientific and medical organizations that do not advocate mass screening or routine screening for prostate cancer. These organizations recommend that physicians offer men fifty years or older the option of testing for early detection of prostate cancer. They also recommend discussing the potential benefits, side effects, and questions regarding early prostate cancer detection and treatment, so that men can make informed decisions about testing.

❏ With the numerous treatment methods available today, if you are diagnosed with prostate cancer, it is imperative to be educated about your treatment options. You should include your partner in your decisions.

❏ If the disease is caught while the cancer is still localized (confined to the prostate gland), the five-year survival rate is approximately 100 percent. If the cancer has spread beyond the prostate, however, it is difficult to treat and cure. The American Cancer Society estimates that in 58 percent of men diagnosed with prostate cancer, the cancer is localized, 31 percent have spread locally (in close vicinity of the prostate gland), and 11 percent have spread to other parts of the body. If the cancer has spread locally, the survival rate over the next five years is about 94 percent. If the disease spreads to the lymph nodes, bones, or other organs, the chances of survival drop to 31 percent.

❏ If the cancer has spread into the capsule of the gland, the standard approach is some form of radiation therapy. Radiation therapy results in impotence about 50 percent of the time. It can also adversely affect the bladder and rectum.

❏ If the disease is confined to the prostate and a man is healthy and under seventy years old, removal of the gland (radical prostatectomy) is often recommended. About 50 percent of men who have radical prostatectomy, even with the new "nerve sparing" techniques, become impotent. Significant incontinence occurs in up to 25 percent of cases. "Watchful waiting," an option that involves no specific treatment, but close monitoring plus nutritional support and lifestyle changes, is becoming the preferred approach if the cancer is in the early stages. If symptoms develop or if tests indicate that symptoms are likely to develop, treatment is usually started. The primary benefit of watchful waiting is that the adverse effects of the existing treatment options are avoided. This may be advantageous for older men who have other serious health problems and for men who have non-aggressive, early-stage cancers.

❏ If the cancer has spread outside the gland, treatment is aimed at trying to block production of testosterone, which fuels the cancer. This can be done by means of orchiectomy (surgical removal of the testes) or through the use of hormone therapy to suppress the production and action of hormones. For the latter, either goserelin (Zoladex) or leuprolide (Lupron) is given by monthly injections (they are fundamentally the same drug). In addition, bicalutamide (Casodex), flutamide (Eulexin), or nilutamide (Nilandron) can be taken orally. Together, these agents effectively shut down testosterone production and use by the body. Both orchiectomy and hormone suppression result in impotence in nearly 100 percent of the cases. Side effects of hormone therapy can include loss of sex drive, hot flashes, and sexual dysfunction.

❏ Cryosurgery (also called cryotherapy or cryoablation) is a treatment method for localized prostate cancer. In this technique, the cancerous cells are frozen by means of a metal probe. This type of treatment is less invasive than radical surgery and there is less blood loss. Brachytherapy (a form of radiation treatment in which tiny pellets containing radioactive material are implanted directly into the prostate) and neoadjuvant therapy (a combination of radiation and hormonal treatment) are other approaches that may be recommended for fighting prostate cancer.

❏ The effect of the drug finasteride (Proscar) on prostate cancer risk is under study.

❏ Estrogens have been used effectively for the treatment of prostate cancer for sixty years. However, they can cause breast growth and other feminizing effects, as well as cardiac complications.

❏ Dr. Hans Nieper, a German cancer specialist, used Carnivora, a substance derived from a South American plant, to treat prostate cancer.

❏ Fresh cabbage and carrot juice are used in alternative clinics worldwide in cancer therapy.

❏ Studies from Israel indicate shark cartilage may be effective in treating prostate cancer. Its antiangiogenic potential seems to inhibit new blood vessel formation, especially in highly malignant vascular cancers.

❏ The hormone dehydroepiandrosterone (DHEA) is believed to help prevent cancer by blocking an enzyme that promotes cancer cell growth. 7-keto DHEA is a form of DHEA that appears not to be converted into testosterone or estrogens in the body. It may be a better option for those at high risk for prostate cancer. (*See* DHEA THERAPY in Part Three.)

❑ S-allyl-mercaptocysteine (SAMC), a compound derived from aged garlic, appears to diminish the growth of human prostate cancer cells. Researchers from Memorial Sloan Kettering Cancer Center in New York City found that the SAMC causes cancer cells to break down testosterone two to four times more quickly than normal—and through a route that does not produce dihydrotestosterone (DHT), a form of the hormone strongly associated with the multiplication of prostate cells. SAMC can be found only in garlic extract that is aged.

❑ A man with prostate cancer needs support and understanding from family members, friends, and physicians. Besides coming to grips with cancer and its treatments, he also has to deal with the possible loss of sexual potency, which can be very difficult. A book entitled *Coping With Prostate Cancer* by Robert H. Phillips, Ph.D. (Avery Publishing Group, 1994) provides a great deal of detailed information and practical advice to help the man with prostate cancer and his family to deal with the many different aspects of this disease.

❑ A man who is impotent as a result of treatment for prostate cancer may be able to remain sexually active through penile prostheses and other devices. (*See* IMPOTENCE in Part Two.)

❑ *See also* PROSTATITIS/ENLARGED PROSTATE in Part Two.

❑ *See also* PAIN CONTROL in Part Three.

❑ For names and addresses of organizations that can provide more information on prostate cancer, *see* HEALTH AND MEDICAL ORGANIZATIONS in the Appendix.

Prostatitis/Benign Prostatic Hypertrophy (BPH)

The prostate is a doughnut-shaped male sex gland, positioned beneath the urinary bladder. It encircles the urinary outlet, or urethra. Contraction of the muscles in the prostate squeeze fluid from the prostate into the urethral tract during ejaculation. Prostatic fluid makes up the bulk of semen.

The prostate is the most common site of disorders in the male genitourinary system. Generally speaking, there are three conditions that can cause problems with the prostate: prostatitis, which is inflammation of the prostate; benign prostatic hypertrophy (BPH), which is an enlarged prostate with no signs of cancer; and prostate cancer.

Prostatitis, common in men of all ages, is the inflammation of the prostate gland. The usual cause is infectious bacteria that invade the prostate from another area of the body. Hormonal changes associated with aging may also be a cause. The inflammation can result in urine retention. This causes the bladder to become distended, weak, tender, and itself susceptible to infection. Infection in the bladder is in turn easily transmitted up the ureters to the kidneys.

There are three types of prostatitis: acute infectious prostatitis, chronic infectious prostatitis, and noninfectious prostatitis. Acute infectious prostatitis is usually caused by bacteria. The onset is sudden. Symptoms may include pain between the scrotum and rectum, fever, frequent urination accompanied by a burning sensation, a feeling of fullness in the bladder, and blood or pus in the urine. Chronic (long-term) prostatitis is also a bacterial infection. Symptoms may include nothing more than a recurring bladder infection. Noninfectious prostatitis is, as the name suggests, not caused by a bacterial infection. The cause for this inflammation is not known. Symptoms can include frequent urination possibly accompanied by pain; pain after ejaculation; and lower abdominal pain. All types of prostatitis, if untreated, can lead to impotence and difficulty with urination.

Benign prostatic hypertrophy is the gradual enlargement of the prostate. It occurs in approximately half of all men over the age of fifty and three quarters of men over seventy years of age—a total of about 10 million American men—and is largely attributable to hormonal changes associated with aging. After the age of fifty or so, a man's testosterone and free testosterone levels decrease, while the levels of other hormones, such as prolactin and estradiol (a type of estrogen) increase. This creates an increase in the amount of dihydrotestosterone—a very potent form of testosterone—within the prostate. This causes a hyperplasia (overproduction) of prostate cells, which ultimately results in prostate enlargement.

While not cancerous, an enlarged prostate can nevertheless cause problems. If it becomes too large, it obstructs the urethral canal, interfering with urination and the ability to empty the bladder completely. Because the bladder cannot empty completely, the kidneys also may not empty as they should. Dangerous pressure on the kidneys can result. In severe cases, the kidneys may be damaged both by pressure and by substances in the urine. Bladder infections are associated with both prostatitis and enlarged prostate.

The major symptom of enlargement of the prostate is the need to pass urine frequently, with frequency increasing as time passes. A man may find himself rising several times during the night to urinate. There can also be pain, burning, and difficulty in starting and stopping urination. The presence of blood in the urine is not uncommon.

Testing for prostatitis and enlarged prostate usually involves a digital rectal exam plus a blood test that screens for levels of prostate-specific antigen (PSA), a protein secreted by the prostate.

NUTRIENTS

SUPPLEMENT	SUGGESTED DOSAGE	COMMENTS
Essential		
Acidophilus (Kyo-Dophilus from Wakunaga is a good source)	As directed on label.	Breaks down metabolites of estrogen. Use a nondairy source.

Quercetin	1,200–2,000 mg daily.	An anti-inflammatory and antitumor flavonoid.
Selenium	As directed on label. Do not take more than the prescribed amount. Overdoses can cause toxicity.	Has antioxidant properties that help protect cells from toxin damage linked to prostatitis. Particularly effective when taken with vitamin E.
Vitamin B complex	50 mg of each major B vitamin 3 times daily (amounts of individual vitamins in a complex will vary).	Necessary for all cellular functions. Anti-stress vitamins.
plus extra vitamin B₆ (pyridoxine)	50 mg twice daily.	Has anticancer properties.
Zinc	80 mg daily. Do not exceed a total of 100 mg daily from all supplements.	Deficiency has been linked to BPH, prostatitis, and even prostate cancer. Use zinc gluconate lozenges or OptiZinc for best absorption.
plus copper	3 mg daily.	Needed to balance with zinc.

Very Important

Essential fatty acids (fish oil and flaxseed oil are good sources)	As directed on label 3 times daily.	Important in prostate function.
Garlic (Kyolic from Wakunaga)	2 capsules 3 times daily.	Acts as a natural antibiotic.
L-Alanine and L-glutamic acid and L-glycine	As directed on label, on an empty stomach. Take with water or juice. Do not take with milk. Take with 50 mg vitamin B₆ and 100 mg vitamin C for better absorption.	Amino acids needed for maintaining normal prostate function. (See AMINO ACIDS in Part One.)
Methylsulfonyl-methane (MSM)	As directed on label.	Relieves pain and inflammation.
Raw prostate glandular	As directed on label.	To normalize prostate function.
Vitamin A plus carotenoid complex	5,000–10,000 IU daily. As directed on label.	Potent antioxidants and immune system enhancers.
Vitamin E	600 IU daily.	Potent antioxidant and immune system enhancer. Use d-alpha-tocopherol form.

Helpful

Berry Seeds Complex from International Health Products	1–2 tablets after each meal.	Has shown anti-inflammatory effects on benign prostatic hyperplasia.
Kelp	1,000–1,500 mg daily.	Supplies necessary minerals for improved prostate function.
Lecithin granules or capsules	1 tbsp 3 times daily, before meals. 1,200 mg 3 times daily, before meals.	For cellular protection.
Magnesium plus calcium	As directed on label. As directed on label.	Necessary minerals for improved prostate function.
Vitamin C with bioflavonoids	1,000–5,000 mg daily.	Promotes immune function and aids healing.

HERBS

❏ Teas made from the diuretic herbs buchu and corn silk are helpful. Juniper berries, parsley, slippery elm bark, and uva ursi are also natural diuretics and urinary tract tonics.

❏ Bilberry and birch are urinary tract antiseptics.

❏ Chinese ginseng is beneficial for prostate health and sexual vitality.

❏ Echinacea and goldenseal have antiviral and antibacterial properties that can help to alleviate infection.

❏ Goldenseal root is a diuretic and antiseptic.

Caution: Do not take goldenseal internally on a daily basis for more than one week at a time, and use it with caution if you are allergic to ragweed.

❏ A decoction of equal quantities of gravel root, hydrangea root, and sea holly helps to ease inflammation and reduce the discomfort of urination. Take 3 to 4 teaspoonfuls three times daily. Marshmallow leaves may be added to this mixture for their demulcent properties if burning persists.

❏ Olive leaf extract contains anti-inflammatory agents.

❏ Nettle and turmeric are anti-inflammatory agents. Combined extracts of nettle root and saw palmetto have proved effective for BPH.

❏ Horsetail is astringent and can be used if small amounts of blood are passed, as well as for frequent urination at night. Combine it with hydrangea for even greater effect.

❏ Pygeum (*Pygeum africanum*) has been proven effective in the treatment and prevention of BPH and prostatitis in many worldwide studies. It has become a primary therapy for these conditions in Europe.

❏ Saw palmetto has been used to treat prostate enlargement and inflammation, painful ejaculation, difficult urination, and enuresis (the inability to control urination). It reduces prostatic enlargement by reducing the amount of hormonal stimulation of the prostate gland.

❏ Siberian ginseng is a tonic for the male reproductive organs.

Caution: Do not use Siberian ginseng if you have hypoglycemia, high blood pressure, or a heart disorder.

❏ Other herbs beneficial for the prostate include cayenne (capsicum) and false unicorn root.

RECOMMENDATIONS

❏ Drink more cranberry juice. This can protect against urinary tract infections, which have been linked to some forms of prostatitis.

❏ *See* Herbs, above, and try one or more of the recommended combinations. Acute inflammation or enlargement of the prostate gland often responds to certain herbal teas. If no improvement takes place or if the symptoms recur, consult a urologist.

❏ Take steps to reduce your blood cholesterol level. (*See* HIGH CHOLESTEROL in Part Two.) Studies have shown a connection between high cholesterol and prostate disorders. Cholesterol has been shown to accumulate in enlarged or cancerous human prostates.

❏ Use hydrotherapy to increase circulation in the prostate region. One method involves sitting in a tub that contains the hottest water tolerable for fifteen to thirty minutes once or twice a day. Another form of hydrotherapy involves spraying the lower abdomen and pelvic area with warm and cold water, alternating between three minutes of hot water and one minute of cold. Still another technique involves sitting in hot water while immersing the feet in cold water for three minutes, and then sitting in cold water while immersing the feet in hot water for one minute.

❏ Eat 1 to 4 ounces of raw pumpkin seeds every day. Pumpkin seeds are helpful for almost all prostate troubles because they are rich in zinc. As an alternative, pumpkin seed oil can be taken in capsule form.

❏ Eliminate from your lifestyle such items as tobacco, alcoholic beverages (especially beer and wine), caffeine (especially coffee and tea), chlorinated and fluoridated water, and spicy and junk foods. Limit your exposure to pesticides and other environmental contaminants.

❏ If you have prostatitis, increase your fluid intake. Drink two to three quarts of spring or distilled water daily to stimulate urine flow. This helps to prevents cystitis and kidney infection as well as dehydration.

❏ Get regular exercise. Do not ride a bicycle, however; this may put pressure on the prostate. Walking is good exercise.

❏ If your prostate is enlarged, be cautious about using over-the-counter cold or allergy remedies. Many of these products contain ingredients that can inflame the condition and cause urinary retention.

❏ Avoid exposure to very cold weather.

CONSIDERATIONS

❏ It is important that prostatitis be diagnosed correctly because the appropriate treatment depends on the cause. For bacterial prostatitis, the conventional treatment involves antibiotics. Antibiotics do not work with the noninfectious type of this condition.

❏ Prostate Enzyme Formula from Prevail Corporation, Prostate R$_x$ from Biotec Corporation and Prost-Actin from Nature's Plus are complexes designed to promote prostate health.

❏ If the prostate is infected, treatment with antibiotics and analgesics may be necessary.

❏ Enlarged prostate may be treated surgically with a procedure called transurethral resection of the prostate (TURP). This procedure is twice as likely to provide long-term relief than drugs or other treatments are. Side effects of the procedure include retrograde ejaculation (in which the semen is pumped back up into the bladder) and, in some cases, impotence or incontinence. About 15 percent of men who have the procedure need another operation within eight years. Transurethral vaporization of the prostate (TVP) is an advance on TURP. TVP uses an electrical current to bombard tissue and vaporize it causing less bleeding. Transurethral incision of the prostate (TUIP), usually done on an outpatient basis, consists of making a few small incisions in the urethra to relieve the pressure. A lower incidence of retrograde ejaculation is reported with this procedure.

❏ The drug finasteride (Proscar) may be used to treat moderate prostate enlargement. It blocks an enzyme that converts the male hormone testosterone into dihydrotestosterone, which promotes the growth of prostate tissue. The drug has been shown to increase urine flow in 30 percent of test cases and to reduce the size of the prostate by 20 percent in more than half the test cases. But it also causes impotence and reduced libido in many cases. In addition, because it reduces the amount of prostate tissue, it can skew the results of the blood test used to detect prostate cancer.

❏ Alpha-blockers such as prazosin (Minipress), terazosin (Hytrin), and doxazosin (Cardura) can be used to reduce the size of an enlarged prostate.

❏ Engaging in sexual intercourse while the prostate is infected and irritated may further irritate the prostate and delay recovery.

❏ Some people believe that prostatitis is caused by an inability to process uric acid, a condition that can lead to gout. (*See* GOUT in Part Two.)

❏ Vasectomy for sterilization has been linked to prostate disorders and even cancer.

❏ Although antibiotics are often used to treat prostatitis, the long-term use of such drugs can lead to bacterial resistance, which in turn necessitates more potent drugs, more expense, and more medical complications.

❏ Zinc deficiency is linked to enlargement of the prostate. Soil used for farming is often deficient in zinc, and unless you eat husks of cereals or brewer's yeast, it is difficult to get enough zinc in the diet. Alcohol causes a deficiency of zinc and other serious nutritional deficiencies. However, too much zinc (over 100 milligrams a day) can depress immune function.

❏ The injectable drug leuprolide (Lupron) may shrink an enlarged prostate. Side effects that can occur with the use of leuprolide include impotence, decreased libido, and even hot flashes. You should take this drug only if you are not concerned with potency. It is available by a doctor's prescription only.

❏ All men aged forty or over should have a yearly rectal examination, during which the prostate gland is checked.

Psoriasis

Psoriasis appears as patches of skin on the legs, knees, arms, elbows, scalp, ears, and back that are red to brown in color and covered with silvery-white scales. Toes and fingernails can lose their luster and develop ridges and pits. Often hereditary, this condition is linked to a rapid growth of cells in the skin's outer layer. These growths on the epidermis never mature. Whereas a normal skin cell matures and passes from the bottom layer of the skin to the epidermis in about twenty-eight days, psoriatic cells form in about eight days, causing scaly patches that spread to cover larger and larger areas. The result of this disorder is the production of excessive numbers of skin cells in a very short time. The condition is not contagious.

Psoriasis generally follows a pattern of periodic flare-ups alternating with periods of remission, most commonly beginning between the ages of fifteen and twenty-five. Among other things, attacks can be triggered by nervous tension, stress, illness, injury, surgery, cuts, poison ivy, viral or bacterial infection, sunburn, overuse of drugs or alcohol, or the use of nonsteroidal anti-inflammatory drugs, lithium, chloroquine (Aralen), and beta-blockers, a type of medication frequently prescribed for heart disease and high blood pressure. Some people experience an associated arthritis (psoriatic arthritis) that is similar to rheumatoid arthritis and difficult to treat.

The underlying cause of the condition is not known, but it may result from a faulty utilization of fat; psoriasis is rare in countries where the diet is low in fat. Current research points also to an immune system role in psoriasis. People with HIV or AIDS often have severe psoriasis. The buildup of toxins in an unhealthy colon also has been linked to the development of psoriasis.

NUTRIENTS

SUPPLEMENT	SUGGESTED DOSAGE	COMMENTS
Essential		
Flaxseed oil or	As directed on label 3 times daily.	To supply essential fatty acids, important for all skin disorders.
primrose oil or	As directed on label 3 times daily.	Aids in preventing dryness.
Ultimate Oil from Nature's Secret	As directed on label.	
Vitamin A with mixed carotenoids plus	25,000 IU daily. If you are pregnant, do not exceed 10,000 IU daily.	Protects the skin tissue. *Note:* If you have diabetes, omit these supplements. People with diabetes often cannot utilize beta-carotene.
natural beta-carotene	As directed on label.	
Vitamin D₃	As directed on label.	A hormone vital for healthy skin.
Zinc	50–100 mg daily. Do not exceed this amount.	Protein metabolism depends on zinc. Protein is needed for healing. Use zinc gluconate lozenges or OptiZinc for best absorption.
plus copper	3 mg daily.	Needed to balance with zinc.

Very Important		
Proteolytic enzymes	As directed on label. Take between meals.	Stimulates protein synthesis and repair.
Selenium	200 mcg daily. Do not exceed this amount. If you are pregnant, do not exceed 40 mcg daily.	Has powerful antioxidant properties.
Shark cartilage (BeneFin)	1 gm per 15 lbs of body weight daily, divided into 3 doses. If you cannot tolerate taking it orally, it can be administered rectally, in a retention enema.	Inhibits the growth of blood vessels to stop the spread of psoriasis. Itching and scaling clear first, then redness gradually fades. Allow 2–3 months to see results.
Vitamin B complex	50 mg of each major B vitamin 3 times daily. (amounts of individual vitamins in a complex will vary).	Necessary for all cellular functions; anti-stress vitamins that help to maintain healthy skin.
plus extra vitamin B₁ (thiamine) and	50 mg 3 times daily.	Needed for repair and healing of skin tissue.
pantothenic acid (vitamin B₅) and	100 mg 3 times daily.	Aids in proper adrenal function, relieving stress on this organ.
vitamin B₆ (pyridoxine) and	50 mg 3 times daily.	Aids in reducing fluid retention, keeping down infection.
vitamin B₁₂ and	2,000 mcg daily.	Use a lozenge or sublingual form.
folic acid	400 mcg daily.	
Vitamin C with bioflavonoids	2,000–10,000 mg daily.	Important for formation of collagen and skin tissue, and for enhancing the immune system.
Vitamin E	Start with 400 IU daily and increase the dosage every 4 days to a maximum of 1,200 IU daily.	Neutralizes free radicals that damage the skin. Use an emulsion form for and easier assimilation. Use d-alpha-tocopherol form.
Important		
Kelp	1,000–1,500 mg daily.	Supplies balanced minerals. A good source of iodine.
Methylsulfonyl-methane (MSM)	As directed on label.	Needed for tissue repair. Often deficient in this disorder.
Helpful		
Glutathione	500 mg twice daily, on an empty stomach.	A powerful antioxidant that inhibits the growth of psoriatic cells.
Herpanacine from Diamond-Herpanacine Associates	As directed on label.	Contains antioxidants, amino acids, and herbs that promote overall skin health.
Lecithin granules or	1 tbsp 3 times daily, with meals.	Fat emulsifiers. Lecithin also protects the cells.
capsules or	1,200 mg 3 times daily, with meals.	
lipotrophic factors	200–500 mg daily.	
Multivitamin and mineral complex with	As directed on label.	Needed for basic vitamins and minerals.
calcium and	1,500 mg daily.	
magnesium	750 mg daily.	
VitaCarte from Phoenix Biolabs	As directed on label.	Contains pure bovine cartilage, which has been shown to be effective in improving psoriasis.

HERBS

❑ Burdock root and red clover cleanse the blood.

❑ Poultices made from chaparral, dandelion, and yellow dock can help psoriasis. (*See* USING A POULTICE in Part Three.)

❑ Add 2 teaspoons of ginger to bath water.

❑ To reduce redness and swelling, lightly brush off scales with a loofah and apply alcohol-free goldenseal extract.

❑ Lavender is good to use in a sauna or steam bath. It fights inflammation and soothes and heals irritated skin.

Note: If you are pregnant or have heart disease or high blood pressure, do not use heat treatments.

❑ Sarsaparilla, and yellow dock are good detoxifiers.

❑ Silymarin (milk thistle extract) increases bile flow and protects the liver, which is important in keeping the blood clean. Take 300 milligrams three times daily.

RECOMMENDATIONS

❑ Eat a diet that is composed of 50 percent raw foods and includes plenty of fruits, grains, and vegetables. Include fish in the diet as well.

❑ Get plenty of dietary fiber. Fiber is critical for maintaining a healthy colon. Many fiber components, such as apple pectin and psyllium husks, are able to bind to bowel toxins and promote their excretion in the feces. Also follow the program for colon cleansing. (*See* COLON CLEANSING in Part Three.) A clean colon is very important.

❑ Use fish oil, flaxseed oil, or primrose oil supplements. They contain ingredients that interfere with the production and storage of arachidonic acid (AA), a natural substance that promotes the inflammatory response and makes the lesions of psoriasis turn red and swell. Red meat and dairy products contain AA. Avoid these foods.

❑ Apply seawater to the affected area with cotton several times a day.

❑ Use cold-pressed flaxseed, sesame, or soybean oils.

❑ Do not consume citrus fruits, fried foods, processed foods, saturated fats (found in meat and dairy products), sugar, or white flour.

CONSIDERATIONS

❑ There is no known cure for psoriasis. Treatment is aimed at reducing the symptoms and includes the use of ointments and creams to soften the scales combined with gentle scrubbing to remove them. Sometimes ultraviolet light (UVL) therapy is used to retard the production of new skin cells. UVL therapy is sometimes combined with tar therapy; tar is applied to the scaly patches, which are then exposed to the UV light. A similar treatment involves using a drug called anthralin (Drithocreme, Dritho-Scalp) instead of tar in tandem with the UV light. Only the scales and skin debris, which can be quite itchy, can be removed. Psoralen plus ultraviolet light A (PUVA) is a therapy recommended for people who have not benefitted from other therapies.

❑ Outbreaks of psoriasis seem to lessen during the summer months. It may even go away on its own, but once you have had psoriasis, it is always possible that it will return.

❑ Recent research has led some to believe that rapid growth of psoriatic cells can be attributed to problems with prostaglandin regulation and a deficiency of sulfur and fatty acids. In a study at Marselisborg Hospital in Denmark, Dr. Knud Kragballe used a mixture of omega-3 and omega-6 essential fatty acids to treat people with psoriasis. At the end of the twelve-week test, there was a moderate improvement of the skin condition in most cases. Some researchers disagree, but we have found fatty acid supplementation to benefit skin disorders.

❑ The freezing of moderately sized psoriatic lesions using liquid nitrogen has been tested with good results.

❑ Cortisone creams, which discourage skin cells from multiplying, are often prescribed for psoriasis, but long-term use makes the skin thin and delicate.

❑ The drug methotrexate (also sold as Rheumatrex) is effective for severe psoriasis. However, this drug can cause liver damage, especially with long-term use. Another drug, hydroxyurea (Hydrea), and drugs called retinoids, are under study. Cyclosporine (Sandimmune) therapy has been tested with good results. A study by Boston University of a drug called calcitriol (Rocaltrol) found it resulted in improvement when applied directly to the skin. All of these drugs have potentially serious side effects.

❑ Acitretin (Soriatane) is another drug that may be prescribed for people with severe psoriasis. This drug should not be used by women who may become pregnant in the three years following treatment.

❑ A skin patch called Actiderm, manufactured by Conva-Tec/Squibb, can be applied over most topical psoriasis medications, especially steroid (cortisone) ointments, to make them more effective. The patch allows one to achieve better results with milder steroids and fewer doses.

❑ Activated vitamin D_3 ointment (Dovonex), available by prescription only, has produced good results for many people with severe forms of psoriasis.

❑ The drug etretinate (Tegison), a retinoid used for stubborn cases of psoriasis, can cause bone spurs in the knees and ankles. One study found that 84 percent of those who used this drug for five years had bony buildups causing stiffness and restriction of movement.

❑ Long-wave ultraviolet light has been effectively used to treat psoriasis, but it may increase the likelihood of skin cancer. Exposure to the sun for fifteen minutes to half an hour (not longer) may reduce the scaling and redness. A liquid drug called methoxsalen (Oxsoralen-Ultra) is also widely used.

❑ Further study must be done on the subject, but researchers believe that shark cartilage may be very effective for the treatment of psoriasis, without the risk of toxicity that standard drugs entail.

❏ For names and addresses of organizations that can provide more information about psoriasis, *see* HEALTH AND MEDICAL ORGANIZATIONS in the Appendix.

Pyelonephritis

See under KIDNEY DISEASE.

Pyorrhea

See under PERIODONTAL DISEASE.

Radiation Exposure

In today's environment, we worry not so much about nuclear war and fallout from atomic testing, but about radioactive pollution from nuclear reactors, plutonium disposal, and uranium mining. Cellular telephones, x-rays, nuclear medicine, computer monitors, television sets, smoke detectors, and microwave ovens are among the common items that are sources of radiation exposure. Radiation is around us all the time in both natural and artificially introduced forms. The sun is a natural source of radiation exposure, and so is radon, a naturally occurring radioactive gas that is reported to be the second leading cause of lung cancer in the United States. The human body itself is a source of some radiation.

Radioactive elements are made up of unstable atoms that give off energy as the result of spontaneous decay of their nuclei. If the energy released by a radioactive element is strong enough to dislodge electrons from other atoms or molecules in its path, it can damage or even kill living tissue. This type of radiation is called ionizing radiation. Even if only one cell is exposed to radiation, the radiation can destroy, damage, or alter the makeup of that cell. The alteration of cell structure by radioactive particles can lead to the development of cancer. If a cell's DNA is damaged, this can cause genetic mutations that can be passed down to offspring.

The National Council on Radiation Protection and Measurements (NCRP) estimates that radiation exposure in the United States come primarily from the following sources, in order:

• Radon: 55 percent.

• Other natural sources: 27 percent.

• Medical sources: 27 percent.

• Other manmade sources: 3 percent.

Radiation exposure is measured in units called *rem*. The U.S. Environmental Protection Agency (EPA) and the NCRP estimate that the average American is exposed to about 360 millirem (a millirem is equal to $1/_{1,000}$ rem) of radioactivity per year. Our bodies naturally produce about 39 millirem of radiation per year. Flying across the United States exposes you to about 5 millirem of radiation (the high altitude eliminates some natural protection from the sun's rays). A dental x-ray exposes you to about around 3 millirem; a chest x-ray, 20 to 50 millirem. Living in a home with a smoke detector increases exposure by under 1 millirem a year.

The risk of dying from radiation-induced cancer increases by 8 percent for each exposure exceeding 10 rem (or 10,000 millrem). The least amount of exposure it would take to kill a person is 200 rem, but with aggressive treatment, people can survive 1,000 rem of exposure. Acute radiation sickness is induced by exposure to doses of 100 rem or more. This can be a consequence of some types of cancer treatment or events such as nuclear power plant accidents.

Radioactive elements are structurally similar to their nonradioactive counterparts, differing only in the number of neutrons the atoms contain. This is why nutrition is important in preventing or blocking damage from exposure to radioactive elements. If you do not obtain sufficient amounts of calcium, potassium, and other minerals in your diet, your body may absorb radioactive elements that are similar in structure to these nutrients. For example, if you do not obtain enough calcium, your body will absorb radioactive strontium 90 (SR-90) or other elements that are similar in structure to calcium, if they are available. Similarly, if you obtain sufficient potassium from your diet, your body will be less likely to retain any radioactive cesium 137 it encounters, as this element is similar to potassium. If the cells are able to obtain all nutrients they need from your diet, they will be less likely to absorb radioactive substitutes, which are then more likely to be discarded from the body.

The effects of radiation exposure can be acute, following a single, relatively high-intensity exposure, or they can be delayed or chronic. Acute reactions to radiation are extremely dangerous. They cause symptoms of listlessness, nausea, vomiting, weakness, and loss of coordination, leading to dehydration, convulsions, shock, and even death. Fortunately, the amount and type of exposure that causes such serious reactions is extremely rare.

Radiotherapy treatment for cancer involves the administration of fairly high doses of radiation specifically targeted at cancerous cells. The idea underlying this treatment is that the radiation kills the cancer, but healthy tissue, which is not targeted, is only minimally affected. Not surprisingly, the major side effect of this type of treatment is radiation sickness, with the classic symptoms of nausea, vomiting, headache, weakness, loss of appetite, and hair loss.

Dental checkups today often include x-rays to locate cavities. Physicians take x-rays to determine whether a bone is broken, to check cardiovascular and respiratory health, and to locate tumors and areas of dysfunction. Women are urged to have regular mammograms, or breast x-rays, for early detection of breast cancer. Cancer research indicates that a significant percentage of women in the United States have inherited a gene, dubbed *oncogene AC*, that is sensitive to x-ray exposure. For these women, even short periods of x-ray exposure can lead to the development of cancer.

Fruit and vegetables—in fact, all foods—contain some level of radioactive material. Milk is checked in some states for the presence of strontium 90 (Sr-90), an element that is present as a result of above-ground nuclear testing (though above-ground testing now banned in the United States). Sr-90 has a half-life of twenty-nine years.

There is nothing that can protect a person against radioactive substances such as radon except detection and eradication of the problem. But good nutrition and a good supplement program will provide support and protection for your immune system. It is advisable to buy your fruit, vegetables, meat, and grains from sources that employ organic methods of farming to exclude further toxins from your diet.

NUTRIENTS

SUPPLEMENT	SUGGESTED DOSAGE	COMMENTS
Very Important		
Calcium and magnesium	1,500 mg daily. 750 mg daily.	To help prevent the body from absorbing radioactive materials.
Coenzyme Q10 plus Coenzyme A from Coenzyme-A Technologies	100 mg daily.	Protects the body from harmful radiation. Works with coenzyme Q10 to support the immune system and detoxify the bloodstream.
Glutathione plus L-cysteine and L-methionine	500 mg each daily, on an empty stomach. Take with water or juice. Do not take with milk. Take with 50 mg vitamin B6 and 100 mg vitamin C for better absorption.	To detoxify harmful substances and protect against the harmful effects of radiation.
Kelp	1,000–1,500 mg daily.	Protects against radiation. Take kelp in tablet form or eat sea vegetables.
Important		
Garlic (Kyolic from Wakunaga)	2 capsules 3 times daily.	Stimulates and protects the immune system.
Grape seed extract	As directed on label.	A powerful antioxidant.
Oxy-5000 Forte from American Biologics	As directed on label.	This antioxidant is high in superoxide dismutase (SOD), a powerful antioxidant.
Pantothenic acid (vitamin B5)	200 mg before and after x-ray exposure; 50 mg daily thereafter.	Protects against the harmful effects of radiation.
Selenium	200 mcg daily. If you are pregnant, do not exceed 40 mcg daily.	A free radical scavenger that protects against cancer.
Vitamin C with bioflavonoids including rutin	5,000–20,000 mg daily in divided doses. (See ASCORBIC ACID FLUSH in part Three.)	A powerful free radical scavenger. A vitamin C complex that contains 200 mg of rutin per capsule is best.
Helpful		
Brewer's yeast	As directed on label.	A natural source of pantothenic acid, as well as the other B vitamins.
Lecithin granules or capsules	1 tbsp 3 times daily, with meals. 1,200 mg 3 times daily, with meals.	Protects cell membranes from radiation.
Vitamin A with mixed carotenoids including beta-carotene	25,000 IU daily. If you are pregnant, do not exceed 10,000 IU daily.	Protects and strengthens the immune system, especially in combination with vitamin E.
Vitamin B complex plus extra inositol	50 mg of each major B vitamin 3 times daily (amounts of individual vitamins in a complex will vary). 100 mg daily.	Helps to protect against the harmful effects of radiation.
Vitamin E	Start with 400 IU daily and increase every 4 days to a maximum of 1,200 IU daily.	Protects and strengthens the immune system, especially in combination with vitamin A. Use d-alpha-tocopherol form.
Zinc	50–80 mg daily. Do not exceed a total of 100 mg daily from all supplements.	Helps increase immunity. Use zinc gluconate lozenges or OptiZinc for best absorption.

HERBS

❑ The herb chaparral helps protect against harmful radiation.

Caution: Do not use this herb on a regular basis, and do not take it daily for longer than one week. Long-term use may be harmful to the liver.

RECOMMENDATIONS

❑ Include apples in the diet; they are a good source of pectin, which binds with radioactive particles. Pectin is also available in supplement form.

❑ Eat buckwheat, which is high in rutin, a bioflavonoid that protects against radiation.

❑ Consume avocados, lemons, and cold-pressed safflower and olive oils. These supply essential fatty acids.

❑ Drink plenty of steam-distilled water.

❑ If you use a cellular telephone, guard against possible contamination by purchasing an earpiece or phone guard. Use the phone only for short calls and only when needed. No link between brain cancer and cell phone use and illness has yet been proved, but it makes sense to be cautious. The electromagnetic waves from a cell phone are supposed to meet government guidelines, but this is uncharted territory. It is best to err on the side of caution. There is a product on the market called "NoDanger." This is an earpiece that allows you to keep the telephone some distance from your body.

❑ If you use a computer and sit in front of a monitor all day, use a radiation/glare filter screen. Monitors are much better than they used to be, but it is wise to be cautious.

❑ Have your home tested for radon. This is a radioactive gas that occurs naturally in the soil in some places. It has no smell. The biggest danger is from exposure to radon inside the home, where the gas can accumulate and escape detection. People who smoke are at even greater risk from the damaging effects radon has on the lungs. Radon detection kits are available in most hardware stores and home centers. They may also be available from your local department of health and some drugstores.

❑ If there is even a chance you might be pregnant, do not let your doctor or dentist do any x-ray testing. Women exposed to x-rays in the first three to five weeks of pregnancy are at a higher risk of having a miscarriage or delivering a baby with birth defects. Exposure between the eighth and fifteenth week can cause the baby to suffer from brain damage. Childhood leukemia can occur if a fetus is exposed to x-rays during the first trimester of pregnancy.

CONSIDERATIONS

❑ As technology improves and more becomes known about how cancer cells work, the part that radiation therapy has to play in cancer treatment has been reduced. Radiation exposure is also more carefully monitored than it was in the past.

❑ A study at the University of Medicine and Dentistry of New Jersey in Newark showed that rats given orange juice before exposure to low-level radiation (1 to 50 rads) suffered two times less damage than rats given water before exposure.

❑ See also WEAKENED IMMUNE SYSTEM in Part Two.

Rash

See SKIN RASH.

Raynaud's Disease/ Raynaud's Phenomenon

Raynaud's disease is a circulatory disorder that results in

the hands, and sometimes the feet, being hypersensitive to the cold. When the hands are exposed to cold temperatures, the small arteries that supply the toes and fingers suddenly contract and go into spasm. As a result, the fingers and toes are deprived of adequate amounts of oxygenated blood, and become whitish or bluish in color. Over time, the condition may result in a general shrinkage of the affected area. Ultimately, ulcers may form, damaging the tissues and resulting in chronic infection under and around the fingernails and toenails. In severe cases, gangrene may result from prolonged and persistent contraction of the arteries. This condition is more common in women than in men. Raynaud's phenomenon is a similar condition that is caused by complications of surgery, injury, frostbite, autoimmune diseases such as lupus or rheumatoid arthritis, or some other underlying condition.

Certain drugs that affect the blood vessels—such as calcium channel blockers, ergot preparations, and alpha- and beta-adrenergic blockers—have been known to produce symptoms similar to those of Raynaud's as a side effect. Recent research has also linked Raynaud's with other conditions involving abnormal constriction of blood vessels, including migraine and Prinzmetal's angina, a type of angina caused by spasms in the coronary arteries. (See CIRCULATORY PROBLEMS in Part Two.)

NUTRIENTS

SUPPLEMENT	SUGGESTED DOSAGE	COMMENTS
Essential		
Coenzyme Q$_{10}$ plus	100–200 mg daily.	Improves tissue oxygenation.
Coenzyme A from Coenzyme-A Technologies		Works well with coenzyme Q$_{10}$ in supporting the immune system's detoxification of many dangerous substances.
Vitamin E	Start with 200 IU daily and increase slowly to 1,000 IU daily.	Improves circulation; acts as an anticoagulant, dissolving clots in the legs, heart, and lungs. Use d-alpha-tocopherol form. Use emulsion form for easier assimilation and greater safety at higher doses.
Very Important		
Calcium and magnesium and zinc	1,500 mg daily, at bedtime. 750 mg daily. 50 mg daily. Do not exceed a total of 100 mg daily from all supplements.	To protect the arteries from stress caused by sudden blood pressure changes.
Chlorophyll or Kyo-Green from Wakunaga	As directed on label. As directed on label.	Helps to fight infection and enhance blood flow. A fresh "green drink" made from leafy greens that supplies chlorophyll and other nutrients.
Choline and inositol	As directed on label.	Lowers cholesterol and helps circulation.

603

Dimethylglycine (DMG) (Aangamik DMG from FoodScience of Vermont)	1 tablet 3 times daily.	Improves tissue oxygenation.
Lecithin granules or capsules	1 tbsp 3 times daily, with meals. 1,200 mg 3 times daily, with meals.	Lowers blood lipid levels.
Vitamin B complex	100 mg of each major B vitamin daily (amounts of individual vitamins in a complex will vary).	B vitamins are necessary for metabolism of fat and cholesterol. Use a high-potency formula.
plus extra vitamin B$_6$ (pyridoxine) and	50 mg daily.	
folic acid plus	400 mcg daily.	
vitamin B$_3$ (niacin)	100 mg daily. Do not exceed this amount.	Dilates small arteries, improving circulation. *Caution:* Do not take niacin if you have a liver disorder, gout, or high blood pressure.
Important		
Aerobic 07 from Aerobic Life Industries	As directed on label.	Improves tissue oxygenation.
Bee propolis or royal jelly	As directed on label. As directed on label.	To strengthen the cardiovascular system and act as a natural antibiotic.
Flaxseed oil or primrose oil or salmon oil	1,000 mg daily. 1,000 mg daily. As directed on label.	To supply essential fatty acids, which are necessary for circulation and help prevent hardening of the arteries.

HERBS

❏ Black cohosh aids circulation and lowers cholestrol levels.

Caution: Do not take this herb if you are pregnant.

❏ Butcher's broom, cayenne (capsicum), ginkgo biloba, and pau d'arco can be used separately or in combination to improve circulation and strengthen blood vessels.

❏ Hyssop may prove helpful for problems affecting the circulation.

RECOMMENDATIONS

❏ Eat a diet composed of 50 percent raw foods. *See* NUTRITION, DIET, AND WELLNESS in Part One, and follow the dietary guidelines.

❏ Avoid fatty and fried foods.

❏ Avoid caffeine. This stimulant constricts the blood vessels.

❏ Keep your hands and feet warm. A warm climate is best. Wear comfortable shoes and do not go barefoot outdoors. Always wear gloves in cold weather.

❏ Avoid stress as much as possible.

❏ Avoid drugs that constrict the blood vessels, such as birth control pills and migraine headache medicine.

❏ Do not smoke. Nicotine constricts the blood vessels.

CONSIDERATIONS

❏ The calcium channel blocker nifedipine (Adalat, Procardia) is a generally accepted treatment for Raynaud's phenomenon. Like all drugs, this can have side effects.

❏ *See also* CIRCULATORY PROBLEMS in Part Two.

Repetitive Motion Injury

See CARPAL TUNNEL SYNDROME.

Retinitis Pigmentosa

See under EYE PROBLEMS.

Reye's Syndrome

Reye's syndrome is a rare, serious disease that affects many internal organs, particularly the brain and liver. It primarily strikes children between the ages of four and twelve. Most cases of Reye's syndrome occur in children who were given aspirin or aspirin-containing medications for a viral infection such as the flu or chickenpox. Reye's syndrome has also been associated with Epstein-Barr virus, influenza B, and enteroviruses (viruses that infect mainly the gastrointestinal tract).

Four to six days after the onset of the viral illness, the child suddenly develops a fever and severe vomiting. Other symptoms include mental and personality changes that may manifest themselves as confusion, drowsiness, lethargy, memory lapses, and/or unusual belligerence and irritability. In addition, the child may experience weakness and paralysis in the arms or legs, double vision, palpitations, speech impairment, impaired skin integrity, and/or hearing loss. Convulsions, coma, brain damage, and even death may follow, usually the result of cerebral edema or respiratory failure. Fortunately, due to increased awareness of the disease, and especially of the importance of early detection and prompt treatment, the mortality rate has declined to about 20 to 30 percent in recent years.

The exact cause of Reye's syndrome is unknown, but as a result of research conducted in the early 1980s, it is known that the combination of aspirin and viral illness dramatically increases the risk of developing this dangerous disorder. This is why aspirin is no longer recommended for routine use as a pain reliever for children.

The following supplements are designed for use once appropriate medical measures, including hospitalization, have been taken and recovery has begun. Discuss any supplements with a health care professional before using them. Unless otherwise specified, the doses recommended here are for persons age eighteen and over. For a child between twelve and seventeen, use three-quarters the recommended dose; for a child between six and twelve, use one-half the recommended dose; and for a child under six, use one-quarter the recommended dose.

NUTRIENTS

SUPPLEMENT	SUGGESTED DOSAGE	COMMENTS
Important		
Branched-chain amino acid complex	As directed on label.	Prevents muscle depletion. (*See* AMINO ACIDS in Part One.)
Flaxseed oil	As directed on label.	To supply essential fatty acids.
Garlic (Kyolic from Wakunaga)	As directed on label.	Increases energy and enhances immune function.
Lecithin granules or capsules or phosphatidyl choline	1 tbsp 3 times daily. 1,200 mg 3 times daily. As directed on label.	To supply choline, important in transmission of nerve impulses and in energy production.
L-Methionine plus glutathione	As directed on label. As directed on label.	Powerful antioxidants that protect and detoxify the liver.
Raw brain glandular	As directed on label.	To improve brain function.
Vitamin A plus carotenoid complex with beta carotene	5,000 IU daily. 15,000 IU daily.	Helps in formation of healthy skin cells. Used by the body to make vitamin A as needed.
Vitamin B complex	50–100 mg of each major B vitamin daily (amounts of individual vitamins in a complex will vary).	Needed for all enzyme systems and to support healing.
Vitamin E	400 IU daily.	To protect against free radical damage. Use d-alpha-tocopherol form.

HERBS

❏ The following are herbal remedies that can be useful once the acute phase of the illness has passed and recovery has begun:

• Alfalfa, hawthorn berry, hyssop, milk thistle, pau d'arco, Siberian ginseng, and wild yam help to rebuild and strengthen the liver.

Caution: Do not use Siberian ginseng if you have hypoglycemia, high blood pressure, or a heart disorder.

• A lotion containing aloe vera, calendula, and/or chamomile can be used to nourish and heal the skin.

• Catnip or chamomile tea helps to reduce anxiety.

Caution: Do not use chamomile on an ongoing basis, and avoid it completely if you are allergic to ragweed.

• Ginger and peppermint are good for relief of nausea.

• Gravel root, hydrangea, oat straw, parsley root, and uva ursi have diuretic properties.

• Korean (or Chinese) ginseng (*Panax ginseng*) helps to reduce fatigue.

Caution: Do not use this herb if you have high blood pressure.

❏ Before administering them, discuss any herbal remedies you wish to use with your health care provider.

❏ Because the main component of the herbs meadowsweet and white willow bark are related to aspirin, these should *not* be given to a child with a fever that may be due to viral illness, including colds, flu, measles, or chickenpox.

RECOMMENDATIONS

❏ Be alert for the following warning signs any time your child is recovering from a viral infection such as a cold, the flu, an ear infection, or chickenpox:

• Prolonged and heavy vomiting, followed by drowsiness.

• Agitation, disorientation, and delirium.

• Fatigue, lethargy, and lapses in memory.

If you have *even a suspicion* that you (or your child) may be developing the disease, seek professional help at once. Reye's syndrome progresses rapidly and is extremely dangerous. Go to the nearest hospital emergency room immediately and explain the situation.

❏ Be sure that any supplements your child is taking do not contain glutamine, as it can lead to an accumulation of ammonia in the blood. Be aware that although the names glutamine, glutamic acid (also sometimes called glutamate), glutathione, gluten, and monosodium glutamate sound similar, these are all different substances.

❏ If Reye's syndrome is diagnosed, follow your health care provider's recommendations regarding treatment and care, both during the period of hospitalization and afterwards, at home.

❏ *Never* give aspirin to a child with a fever or other sign of viral illness. To be safe, many experts recommend against giving children aspirin for any reason. Use acetaminophen (Tylenol, Datril, and others) or ibuprofen (Advil, Nuprin, and others) instead.

CONSIDERATIONS

❏ There is no cure for Reye's syndrome. Treatment focuses on balancing chemical levels in the blood, while monitoring and supporting the functions of the lung, liver, heart, and brain. The measures that may be taken depend upon the stage of the disease, but treatment almost always involves hospitalization. Typical hospital care includes the administration of intravenous fluids to restore blood electrolytes and glucose levels, and sometimes a diuretic to reduce inflammation and help eliminate waste and excess fluid. In some cases, surgery may be performed to reduce swelling and pressure on the brain.

❑ One way that Reye's syndrome can be detected is through a spinal tap, a procedure that involves inserting a needle into the spinal canal, usually at the lower back, to withdraw a sample of cerebrospinal fluid for examination.

❑ If a person with Reye's syndrome receives an intravenous solution of glucose (sugar) and electrolytes (mineral salts) within twelve to twenty-four hours after the heavy vomiting starts, the chance of recovery is excellent. This treatment is safe.

❑ The British aspirin industry withdrew all children's aspirin products from the British market a number of years ago in response to the discovery of the link with Reye's syndrome.

❑ A study done by the U.S. Centers for Disease Control and Prevention found that 96 percent of the children who had Reye's syndrome had been given aspirin in the presence of a viral illness. The study also indicated a direct correlation between the amount of aspirin taken and the severity of the disease. The makers of aspirin are now required to alert users to the link between aspirin and this potentially life-threatening condition.

❑ *See also* CHICKENPOX, COMMON COLD, and INFLUENZA, all in Part Two.

Rheumatic Fever

Rheumatic fever is a complication of a streptococcal infection. It typically develops following strep throat, tonsillitis, scarlet fever, or ear infection. It most often affects children aged three to eighteen. Rheumatic fever develops as a result of the buildup of antibodies that have been produced to fight off the strep infection—only the antibodies end up attacking the body's own tissues. This disorder may affect one or several parts of the body, among them the heart, brain, and joints. If the heart is affected, permanent damage to one or more heart valves may result.

The first signs of rheumatic fever are typically pain, inflammation, and stiffness in a large joint such as the knee, accompanied by fever. The pain and swelling can travel from one joint to another. There may be an accompanying skin rash. Other symptoms may include bumps or nodules over a joint or joints, fatigue, and uncontrollable jerky movements of the arm, leg, or facial muscles. After one occurrence, the disease tends to recur.

Long-term effects of rheumatic fever can include heart failure, skin disorders, anemia, endocarditis (inflammation of the heart lining), heart arrhythmias, pericarditis (inflammation of the sac surrounding the heart), Sydenham's chorea (a disorder of the nervous system), and arthritis.

Unless otherwise specified, the following recommended dosages are for persons over the age of eighteen. For a child between twelve and seventeen years old, reduce the dose to three-quarters the recommended amount. For a child between six and twelve, use one-half the recommended dose, and for a child under six years old, use one-quarter the recommended amount.

NUTRIENTS

SUPPLEMENT	SUGGESTED DOSAGE	COMMENTS
Important		
Acidophilus (Kyo-Dophilus from Wakunaga is a good source)	As directed on label.	Especially important if antibiotics are prescribed. Use a nondairy formula.
Chondroitin sulfate	500–1,000 mg daily.	To provide nutritional support for strengthening joints, ligaments, and tendons.
Garlic (Kyolic from Wakunaga)	2 capsules 3 times daily.	A natural antibiotic that boosts immune function and fights infection. Destroys free radicals.
L-Carnitine	500 mg twice daily, on an empty stomach.	Protects the heart.
L-Methionine	500 mg daily, on an empty stomach. Take with water or juice. Do not take with milk. Take with 50 mg vitamin B_6 and 100 mg vitamin C for better absorption.	An important free radical fighter. (*See* AMINO ACIDS in Part One.)
Vitamin C with bioflavonoids	5,000–20,000 mg daily, in divided doses. (*See* ASCORBIC ACID FLUSH in Part Three.)	Boosts immune function and aids in reducing pain and swelling.
Helpful		
Calcium plus magnesium	1,500 mg daily. 1,000 mg daily.	Important nutrients that work together. Use chelate forms.
Coenzyme Q_{10} plus Coenzyme A from Coenzyme-A Technologies	100 mg daily. As directed on label.	Boosts immune function. Enhances the effectiveness of coenzyme Q_{10}.
ConcenTrace from Trace Minerals Research	As directed on label.	To supply trace minerals needed for bone and joint health. Increases energy.
Dimethylsulfoxide (DMSO)	Apply topically as directed on label.	To relieve joint pain. Should be used by adults only. Use only DMSO from a health food store.
Flaxseed oil	As directed on label.	Reduces pain and inflammation.
Free-form amino acid complex (Amino Balance from Anabol Naturals)	As directed on label.	To supply protein, needed to strengthen body and for tissue repair. Use a formula containing all essential amino acids.
Kelp	1,000–1,500 mg daily.	Contains essential nutrients.
Multivitamin and mineral complex	As directed on label.	To maintain a balance of all necessary nutrients.
Proteolytic enzymes	As directed on label. Take between meals.	An important antioxidant.

Raw thymus glandular	An important antioxidant.	Stimulates immune response.
S-Adenosylmethio-nine (SAMe) (SAMe Rx-Mood from Nature's Plus)	As directed on label.	Deficiency results in inability to maintain cartilage properly. Aids in reducing pain and inflammation. *Caution:* Do not use if you have manic-depressive disorder or take prescription antidepressants. Do not give this supplement to a child under 12.
Vitamin A plus carotenoid complex with beta-carotene	10,000 IU daily. As directed on label.	Important antioxidants. Use emulsion forms for easier assimilation.
Vitamin B complex	50 mg of each major B vitamin 3 times daily (amounts of individual vitamins in a complex will vary).	For healing and improved immune function.
Vitamin D₃ or cod liver oil	400 IU or more daily. As directed on label.	Needed for healing and absorption of minerals, especially calcium.
Vitamin E emulsion or capsules	800 IU daily. Start with 200 IU daily and increase slowly to 800 IU daily.	Increases tissue oxygenation and reduces fever. Emulsion form is recommended for easier assimilation.

HERBS

❏ Bayberry bark, burdock root, milk thistle, nettle, pau d'arco, sage, and yellow dock purify the blood, fight infection, and aid in recuperation after the trauma of illness.

Caution: Do not use sage if you suffer from any kind of seizure disorder.

❏ Birch leaves and lobelia both help to reduce pain.

Caution: Do not take lobelia internally on an ongoing basis.

❏ Catnip tea is a nerve tonic. It can also be used as an enema to reduce fever. (*See* ENEMAS in Part Three.)

❏ Cordyceps, a Chinese herb, is beneficial for the heart. It can slow the heart rate, increase blood supply to the arteries and heart, and lower blood pressure.

❏ Dandelion has a long history in the treatment of fever.

❏ Ginkgo biloba can benefit the cardiovascular system by preventing the formation of free radicals. Use a ginkgo extract containing 24 percent ginkgo flavone glycosides.

❏ Goldenseal is a natural antibiotic.

Caution: Do not take goldenseal internally on a daily basis for more than one week at a time, do not use it during pregnancy, and use it with caution if you are allergic to ragweed.

❏ Hawthorn leaf, myrrh gum, and red clover detoxify and de-acidify the blood.

❏ Wintergreen oil can be applied to the chest in compress form to relieve pain.

RECOMMENDATIONS

❏ Drink plenty of fresh juices and distilled water.

❏ Eat no solid food until the fever subsides and joint pain begins to ease. Then keep to a light diet, including fresh fruits and vegetables, yogurt, cottage cheese, and fruit juices.

❏ Do not consume any caffeine, carbonated soft drinks, fried foods, processed or refined foods, salt, or sugar in any form during the recovery period. These foods slow healing.

❏ Get plenty of bed rest. This is vital for recovery.

❏ If antibiotics are prescribed, take acidophilus following antibiotic treatment to replace the needed "friendly" bacteria. Antibiotics may be necessary to combat the underlying *Streptococcus* infection and help prevent permanent heart damage. Do not take the acidophilus at the same time as the antibiotics, however, or the antibiotics will kill the friendly bacteria.

❏ Do not give aspirin to a child with a fever. Use acetaminophen or ibuprofen instead.

❏ If you (or your child) are experiencing symptoms of strep throat, see a physician to be tested and, if appropriate, treated. Symptoms of strep throat include a severe sore throat accompanied by a fever of over 101ºF without any other cold symptoms, or a mild sore throat that does not dissipate after several days.

❏ Use homeopathic treatments to ease symptoms. Homeopathic remedies that have been used to treat rheumatic fever include *Aconite, Bryonia, Pulsatilla,* and *Rhus toxicodendron.*

CONSIDERATIONS

❏ Massage therapy and mild exercise such as yoga can be helpful for preventing muscle atrophy during bed rest. (*See* MASSAGE THERAPY in Part Three.)

❏ If you develop rheumatic heart disease, you may need surgery to repair the damage to the heart.

❏ *See also* ARTHRITIS; FEVER; and/or SORE THROAT, all in Part Two.

Rheumatoid Arthritis

See under ARTHRITIS.

Rickets/Osteomalacia

Rickets and osteomalacia are two terms for the disorder caused by vitamin D deficiency. In children, this disease is called rickets, and results either from inadequate intake of vitamin D or from too little exposure to sunlight (sunlight causes vitamin D to be synthesized in the skin). The lack of vitamin D in turn affects the body's ability to absorb calcium and phosphorus. Early signs include nervousness, painful muscle spasms, leg cramps, and numbness in the extremities. Ultimately, bone malformations may develop due to softening of the bones—bowed legs, knock-knees, scoliosis (abnormal curvature of the spine), a narrow rib cage, a protruding breastbone, and/or beading at the ends of the ribs—as well as decaying teeth, delayed walking, irritability, restlessness, and profuse sweating. Rickets is now very rare in the United States. It is most often seen in children aged six to twenty-four months old.

In adults, vitamin D deficiency disease is referred to as osteomalacia and is usually related to the body's inability to absorb phosphorus and calcium properly. It is most likely to occur in pregnant women and nursing mothers, whose nutritional requirements are higher than normal, or in people with malabsorption problems. It may also affect individuals who do not get enough exposure to sunshine or those whose diets are so low in fat that adequate bile cannot be manufactured and vitamin D cannot be absorbed. This condition can be caused by chronic renal failure. Osteomalacia is difficult to diagnose and is often misdiagnosed as osteoporosis.

Unless otherwise specified, the dosages recommended in this section are for adults. For a child between the ages of twelve and seventeen, reduce the dose to three-quarters the recommended amount. For a child between six and twelve, use one-half the recommended dose, and for a child under the age of six, use one-quarter the recommended amount.

NUTRIENTS

SUPPLEMENT	SUGGESTED DOSAGE	COMMENTS
Essential		
Boron	3 mg daily. Do not exceed this amount.	Enhances calcium absorption.
Calcium	1,500 mg daily.	Necessary to remineralize bone. Do not use bone meal or dolomite as a source of calcium, as these may contain lead.
Phosphorus	As directed on label.	Needed for bone and tooth formation.
Silica	500 mg daily.	Supplies silicon, which strengthens bones and connective tissue. Aids calcium absorption.
Vitamin D$_3$	400–600 IU daily. Do not exceed this amount.	Necessary for utilization of calcium and phosphorus.
Important		
Betaine hydrochloride (HCl)	As directed on label.	May be needed for proper digestion.
Cod liver oil	As directed on label.	A good source of vitamins A and D.
Multivitamin and mineral complex plus extra vitamin B$_{12}$	As directed on label. 1,000–2,000 mcg daily.	If malabsorption is a problem, take higher amounts of all vitamins and minerals.
Proteolytic enzymes	As directed on label. Take between meals.	Important in digestion.
Vitamin A with mixed carotenoids	10,000 IU daily.	Necessary for growth.
Zinc	30 mg daily.	Needed for calcium absorption. Use zinc gluconate lozenges or OptiZinc for best absorption.

HERBS

❏ Dandelion root, horsetail, nettle, and oat straw promote bone building and are all good sources of calcium and magnesium.

RECOMMENDATIONS

❏ Change your diet. Eat more raw fruits and vegetables, raw nuts and seeds, yogurt, and cottage cheese. A diet high in calcium is essential.

❏ Do not consume sugar, junk foods, or carbonated beverages.

❏ Have a hair analysis done to check for mineral deficiencies. (See HAIR ANALYSIS in Part Three.)

❏ Be watchful if a child has severe allergies, celiac disease, asthma, bronchitis, or colon disturbances. These conditions can result in absorption problems. This may be difficult to detect at first because growth and weight are usually normal with these conditions.

CONSIDERATIONS

❏ Food allergy testing may be beneficial.

❏ There are a number of combination supplement products available that contain many of the nutrients recommended in the table above. Bone Builder from Ethical Nutrients, Bone Defense from KAL, Bone Support from Synergy Plus, and Cal Apatite from Metagenics are good products for promoting proper bone growth.

❏ See also OSTEOPOROSIS in Part Two.

Ringworm

See under FUNGAL INFECTION.

Rosacea

Rosacea is a chronic skin disorder that most often affects the forehead, nose, cheekbones, and chin. Groups of capillaries close to the surface of the skin become dilated, resulting in blotchy red areas with small bumps and, sometimes, pimples. The redness can come and go, but eventually may become permanent if blood vessels under the skin become dilated, a phenomenon known as telangiectasia. The skin tissue can swell and thicken, and may be tender and sensitive to the touch.

The inflammation of rosacea can look a great deal like acne, but it tends to be more chronic, blackheads and whiteheads are almost never present. It is a fairly common disorder—about one in every twenty Americans has it to some degree—but many never realize they have it. Rosacea usually begins with frequent flushing of the face, particularly the nose and cheeks. The flushing is caused by the swelling of the blood vessels under the skin. This "red mask" can serve as a flag for attention. Inflammation can then spread across the face and small bumps may appear. Later, swelling of the nose may occur. However, it can take years from the beginnings of this condition before the later stages develop. Rosacea can also cause a persistent burning and feeling of grittiness in the eyes or inflamed and swollen eyelids. In severe cases, vision can be impaired.

The underlying cause or causes of rosacea are not understood, but certain factors are known to aggravate the condition, including the consumption of alcohol, hot liquids, and/or spicy foods; exposure to sunlight; humidity; extremes of temperature; and the use of makeup and skin care products containing alcohol. Stress, vitamin deficiencies, and infection can be contributing factors. The things that aggravate one person's rosacea may have no effect on another person.

Rosacea is most common in white women between the ages of thirty and fifty. When it does occur in men, rosacea tends to be more severe, and is usually accompanied by rhinophyma (a nose that becomes chronically red and enlarged). Fair-skinned individuals seem to be more susceptible to this condition than darker skinned people. People who flush easily seem to be more prone than others to develop rosacea.

In rare cases, rosacea may affect the skin in other parts of the body as well as the face. It is not a dangerous condition, but it is chronic and can be distressing for cosmetic reasons. Without proper care, it can develop into a disfiguring condition.

NUTRIENTS

SUPPLEMENT	SUGGESTED DOSAGE	COMMENTS
Very Important		
Primrose oil	500 mg 3 times daily.	A good healer for many skin disorders. Contains linoleic acid, which is needed by the skin.
Pycnogenol	As directed on label.	Powerful antioxidant that moderates allergic and inflammatory responses by reducing histamine production.
Vitamin A with mixed carotenoids	25,000 IU daily for 3 months, then reduce to 15,000 IU daily. If you are pregnant, do not exceed 10,000 IU daily.	Necessary for healing and construction of new skin tissue.
Vitamin B complex	100 mg of each major B vitamin 3 times daily (amounts of individual vitamins in a complex will vary).	Anti-stress vitamins that are necessary in all cellular functions and help to maintain healthy skin.
plus extra vitamin B₂ (riboflavin) and vitamin B₁₂	50 mg daily.

1,000–2,000 mcg daily. | B vitamins that have been shown to be particularly useful in the treatment of rosacea. |
Important		
Kelp	1,000–1,500 mg daily.	Supplies balanced minerals needed for good skin tone.
Multivitamin and mineral complex	As directed on label.	To ensure optimum nutrition and guard against deficiencies.
Vitamin E	Start with 400 IU daily and increase slowly to 800 IU daily.	Protects against free radicals. Use d-alpha-tocopherol form.
Zinc	50 mg daily. Do not exceed a total of 100 mg daily from all supplements.	For tissue repair. Enhances immune response. Use zinc gluconate lozenges or OptiZinc for best absorption.
Helpful		
Ageless Beauty from Biotec Foods	As directed on label.	Protects the skin from free radical damage.
Chlorophyll

or
alfalfa | As directed on label. | Aids in cleansing the blood, preventing infections. Also supplies needed balanced minerals. *See under* Herbs, below. |
| Flaxseed oil capsules or liquid | 1,000 mg daily.

1 tsp daily. | To supply needed essential fatty acids. |
| Herpanacine from Diamond-Herpanacine Associates | As directed on label. | Contains antioxidants, amino acids, and herbs that promote skin health. |
| L-Cysteine | 500 mg daily, on an empty stomach. Take with water or juice. Do not take with milk. Take with 50 mg vitamin B₆ and 100 mg vitamin C for better absorption. | Contains sulfur, needed for healthy skin. (*See* AMINO ACIDS in Part One.) |
| Lecithin granules or capsules | 1 tbsp 3 times daily, before meals.
1,200 mg 3 times daily, before meals. | Aids absorption of the essential fatty acids. |
Proteolytic enzymes	As directed on label. Take between meals.	Helps to reduce inflammation.
Selenium	200 mcg daily. Do not exceed this dose.	Encourages tissue elasticity and is a powerful antioxidant.
Superoxide dismutase (SOD)	As directed on label.	A free radical destroyer.
Vitamin C with bioflavonoids	3,000–5,000 mg daily, in divided doses.	Promotes immune function, strengthens capillaries, and acts as a mild anti-inflammatory.

HERBS

❑ Alfalfa is a good source of chlorophyll, which has detoxifying properties. It also supplies many needed vitamins and minerals.

❑ Aloe vera has excellent healing properties. Apply pure aloe vera gel topically to dry skin as directed on the product label or as needed.

Note: Some people with rosacea may experience irritation as a result of using aloe. If this occurs, discontinue use.

❑ Borage seed, dandelion root, dong quai, parsley, sarsaparilla, and yellow dock root improve skin tone.

❑ Bromelain and turmeric (curcumin) help to control inflammation.

❑ Burdock root and red clover are powerful blood cleansers. Burdock also helps to improve skin tone.

❑ Calendula, cayenne (capsicum), fennel seed, ginger, marshmallow root, sage, and slippery elm nourish the skin and promote healing.

Caution: Do not use sage if you suffer from any kind of seizure disorder.

❑ Milk thistle aids the liver in cleansing the blood.

❑ Nettle and rosemary improve skin tone, nourish the skin, and promote healing.

RECOMMENDATIONS

❑ Eat a diet that emphasizes raw vegetables and grains, organically grown if possible.

❑ Avoid fats, especially saturated fats, and all animal products. Saturated fats promote inflammation. Also avoid alcohol, caffeine, cheese, chocolate, cocoa, dairy products, eggs, fat, fish, salt, sugar, and spicy foods.

❑ Do not drink hot beverages such as coffee or tea. Allow your food to cool to room temperature before eating it.

❑ Investigate the possibility of food allergies. Keep a food diary for one month to see which foods may be aggravating the condition. Then avoid those foods. (*See* ALLERGIES in Part Two for further information.)

❑ Once a month, follow a fasting program. (*See* FASTING in Part Three.)

❑ Keep the skin scrupulously clean, but treat it gently. Use a mild natural soap and lukewarm to cool (never cold or hot) water for cleansing. Pat the skin dry after washing—do not rub it. Avoid touching the skin except when cleansing it.

❑ Avoid extremes of temperature, especially heat. Keep baths and showers short, and use water that is as cool as you can tolerate comfortably. Avoid saunas (including the type used for facials and steam inhalations), steam baths, and hot tubs. If you need to increase the humidity in your home, use only a cool mist humidifier.

❑ As much as possible, avoid wearing makeup. If you do use cosmetics, choose all-natural, water-based products.

❑ *Do not* use topical steroid creams. These only make the condition worse.

❑ Friction is extremely irritating, so avoid wearing tight clothing such as turtlenecks that can rub against the skin. Be careful about anything that comes close to or into contact with your face. Even holding the telephone receiver against your face for a while can raise the local temperature and irritate sensitive skin.

❑ In severe cases, a laser or electrical device can be used to remove the excess tissue. Dermabrasion also has helped some people with rosacea.

CONSIDERATIONS

❑ There is no known cure for rosacea. Topical and/or oral antibiotics, usually tetracycline, are often prescribed to keep the inflammation under control. As with any drug, these can have side effects, especially with long-term use. Moreover, if you stop taking the antibiotics, the condition may rebound.

❑ An underlying vascular disorder may be involved in the development of rosacea. Several findings support this theory. First, there are structural abnormalities in the small blood vessels in the facial skin of people with rosacea. Second, the condition is exacerbated by the use of drugs that dilate blood vessels, such as theophylline and nitroglycerin. Finally, people with rosacea are more likely than most to suffer from migraines, a type of headache also linked to vascular malfunction.

❑ *Demodex folliculorum,* a type of microscopic mite that lives on cast-off skin cells and is normally present on human skin, has been found in significantly higher than normal numbers in skin samples taken from people with rosacea. Researchers speculate that this organism, or some type of reaction to it, may be involved in rosacea.

Scabies

Scabies is a parasitic infection that causes a persistent, itchy rash. It is caused by a tiny mite that burrows into the top layer of the skin to lay its eggs. This results in groups of small red lumps. The scabies skin mite, so small it can hardy be seen without a microscope, infects over 300 million people worldwide every year. When the rash first appears, you may see fine, wavy lines emanating from some of the lumps if you look closely. The skin may then become dry and scaly, and the itching can be intense, especially at night. Scratching can set the stage for a bacterial infection as well.

Scabies can be a particular problem in institutional settings such as nursing homes and day care centers. It is spread primarily by skin-to-skin contact, and it is highly contagious. The areas most commonly affected are the buttocks, genitals (in men), nipples (in women), wrists, and armpits, as well as the skin between the toes and fingers.

To diagnose the condition, a physician usually takes a scraping of skin from the affected area and examines it under a microscope. It is easily spread from one person to another by close contact, so if one family member develops scabies, all the members of the household should be checked and, if necessary, treated. Children under the age of fifteen have the highest incidence of scabies and are usually the first in the family to contract it. It is also considered to be a sexually transmitted disease.

Unless otherwise stated, the dosages recommended here are for adults. For a child between the ages of twelve and seventeen, reduce the dose to three-quarters of the recommended amount. For a child between the ages of six and twelve, use one-half the recommended dose, and for a child under six, use one-quarter of the recommended amount.

NUTRIENTS

SUPPLEMENT	SUGGESTED DOSAGE	COMMENTS
Very Important		
Garlic (Kyolic from Wakunaga)	2 capsules 3 times daily, with meals.	Has antiparasitic and antibiotic properties.
ParasiVeda from Solaray	As directed on label.	Helps rid the body of parasitic infections.
Primrose oil	1,000 mg 3 times daily.	A good healer for most skin disorders.
Vitamin A with mixed carotenoids	25,000 IU daily for 3 months, then reduce to 15,000 IU daily. If you are pregnant, do not exceed 10,000 IU daily.	Necessary for healing and for construction of new skin tissue.
Important		
Kelp	1,000–1,500 mg daily.	Supplies balanced minerals.
Zinc	50 mg daily. Do not exceed a total of 100 mg daily from all supplements.	For tissue repair. Enhances immune response. Use zinc gluconate lozenges or zinc methionate (OptiZinc) for best absorption.
Helpful		
Colloidal silver	Apply topically as directed on label.	To prevent secondary infection.
Vitamin E	600 IU daily.	Promotes healing. Use d-alpha-tocopherol form.

HERBS

❑ Aloe vera has excellent healing properties. Apply gel topically to the affected area as directed on the product label.

❑ Balsam of Peru, goldenseal, and/or tea tree oil can be applied topically to fight the infection. Goldenseal can also be taken internally to bolster the immune system.

Caution: Do not take goldenseal internally on a daily basis for more than one week at a time, as it may disturb

normal intestinal flora. Do not use it during pregnancy, and use it with caution if you are allergic to ragweed.

❑ Black walnut, garlic, and wormwood are useful for parasitic infections.

❑ Comfrey and/or calendula salve helps to soothe itching and irritation.

Note: Do not take comfrey internally.

❑ Rhubarb helps the body to rid itself of parasitic infections.

RECOMMENDATIONS

❑ Diet alone cannot cure scabies. To get rid of the mites, apply permethrin cream (Elemite) or 25-percent benzyl benzoate topically to the entire body from the neck down, as directed on the label or prescribed by your physician.

❑ Thoroughly wash all bed linens used by infected individuals in hot water. A product called Rid spray, which also contains permethrin, may be recommended for treating infested clothes and bedding.

❑ Practice scrupulous personal hygiene. Avoid contact with infested persons or their clothing.

❑ To promote healing, eat plenty of foods high in zinc, such as soybeans, sunflower seeds, wheat bran, whole-grain products, yeast, and blackstrap molasses.

❑ Do not drink soft drinks or alcoholic beverages. Consume no sugar, chocolate, or junk foods.

❑ Drink at least eight 8-ounce glasses of clean water a day.

❑ Avoid fried foods and all animal products. Use cold-pressed vegetable oils only.

CONSIDERATIONS

❑ A topical scabicide called lindane (gamma benzene hexachloride, found in the product Kwell) was once considered a standard treatment for scabies. In recent years, however, it has largely been replaced by permethrin, which is believed to be safer and cause fewer side effects.

❑ Scabicides are not recommended for children under the age of six or for pregnant women. In such cases, a milder sulfur solution is usually recommended.

❑ It may take one to two weeks for the itching to subside, even after treatment. An antihistamine or a cortisone cream may be recommended to provide relief. Calendula salve, cool compresses, and cool oatmeal baths are natural alternatives to those medications.

❑ Crowded, unsanitary, or institutional living conditions are conducive to the spread of scabies.

Schizophrenia

Schizophrenia is a disorder that makes it impossible to differentiate between what is imagined and what is real. The characteristic symptoms include disordered thinking, speech, and perception; a lack of curiosity; diminishing emotional contact with others; lethargy; emotional changes such as tension and/or depression; and more dramatic behavioral disturbances, ranging from catatonia to violent outbursts and delusions. People with schizophrenia lose, to some degree, their hold on reality, and many seem to withdraw into their own worlds. Hallucinations are not uncommon.

There are four basic types of schizophrenia:

• *Catatonic schizophrenia* is characterized by unusual rigid postures, lack of movement, or frenzied movement.

• *Disorganized schizophrenia*, which used to be called hebephrenic schizophrenia, is characterized by a lack of the normal range of emotions along with speech that displays a disorganized way of thinking.

• *Paranoid schizophrenia* is characterized by hallucinatory and delusional symptoms.

• *Undifferentiated schizophrenia* involves a mixture of symptoms.

While the onset of the disorder is often related to a stressful life event, the underlying cause or causes of schizophrenia are not known. There are many theories, however. Some researchers believe that schizophrenia is hereditary, and there is evidence that some cases of schizophrenia are the result of an inherited defect in body chemistry in which brain chemicals called neurotransmitters function abnormally. Others theorize that schizophrenia results from external factors, such as complications during birth, head injury, a reaction to a virus, including the influenza virus, or environmental poisons that reach and damage the brain. There is a high incidence of childhood head injuries and birth complications among people with schizophrenia. A wide range of drugs also can cause schizophrenic-type symptoms.

Yet another theory focuses on nutritional factors. There is some indication that schizophrenia may be associated with high copper levels in body tissues. When copper levels are too high, the levels of vitamin C and zinc in the body drop. A zinc deficiency may result in damage to the pineal area of the brain, which normally contains high levels of zinc, which in turn may make an individual vulnerable to schizophrenia or other psychoses. Evidence indicates that male babies are particularly susceptible to gestational zinc deficiencies. Other clues come from the seasonality of the disorder. The incidence of schizophrenic episodes tends to peak in cold-weather months, when zinc intake tends to be lower. As many as 2 million Americans suffer from schizophrenia. In general, men appear to become more disabled by this condition than women, which has given rise to a hypothesis that the hormone estrogen may protect the brain. When women reach the age of diminishing estrogens in their late forties, the incidence and severity of schizophrenic episodes appears to increase.

Magnesium deficiency may also be a factor. Some research has shown that magnesium levels in the blood of people with active schizophrenia are lower than normal and that the levels are higher in persons whose schizophrenia is in remission. It has been hypothesized that a type of vicious cycle may be at work here; the high level of stress experienced by those with severe psychiatric disorders may lead to magnesium deficiency, which in turn would exacerbate symptoms such as anxiety, fear, hallucinations, weakness, and physical complaints.

Levels of, and the balance between, the neurotransmitters dopamine, serotonin, epinephrine, and norepinephrine, and the way in which the brain responds to these substances, is thought to play a profound role in the development of schizophrenia.

Unless otherwise specified, the dosages recommended here are for adults. For a child between the ages of twelve and seventeen, reduce the dose to three-quarters the recommended amount.

NUTRIENTS

SUPPLEMENT	SUGGESTED DOSAGE	COMMENTS
Essential		
5-Hydroxytryptophan (5-HTP)	As directed on label.	Increases the body's production of serotonin, a vital brain chemical.
Flaxseed oil	As directed on label.	To supply essential fatty acids, needed for proper brain and nerve function.
Folic acid	2,000 mcg daily.	Deficiency has been found in approximately 25 percent of those hospitalized for psychiatric disorders.
and vitamin B_{12}	1,000 mcg twice daily.	Folic acid works best when taken with vitamin B_{12} and vitamin C.
and vitamin C with bioflavonoids	5,000 mg daily.	
Gamma-aminobutyric acid (GABA)	As directed on label, on an empty stomach. Take with water or juice. Do not take with milk. Take with 50 mg vitamin B_6 and 100 mg vitamin C for better absorption.	Essential for brain metabolism. Aids in proper brain function. (*See* AMINO ACIDS in Part One.)
Garlic (Kyolic from Wakunaga)	As directed on label.	Enhances brain function.
Glutathione	As directed on label.	Deficiency can affect the nervous system.
or cysteine	As directed on label.	Nutrients used to synthesize glutathione.
and glutamic acid	As directed on label.	
and glycine	As directed on label.	
L-Asparagine	As directed on label.	Maintains balance in the central nervous system.
L-Glutamic acid	As directed on label.	Important in brain metabolism. Acts as an excitory neurotransmitter.

L-Methionine	As directed on label.	Helps to counteract histamine, which is found in high levels in people with schizophrenia.
L-Phenylalanine	As directed on label.	An amino acid that is converted into tyrosine, which is important for synthesis of both dopamine and norepinephrine.
Pycnogenol or grape seed extract	As directed on label. As directed on label.	Antioxidants useful for dementia and other syndromes of the brain.
Zinc plus manganese	Up to 80 mg daily. Do not exceed 100 mg daily from all supplements. Take separately from calcium.	Balances copper, often found in high concentrations in people with this disorder. Enhances action of B vitamins necessary for brain function.

Very Important		
Free-form amino acid complex	As directed on label. Take on an empty stomach.	Needed for normal brain function. Use a formula containing all the essential amino acids.
Raw liver extract injections or vitamin B complex injections plus extra vitamin B$_6$ (pyridoxine) and vitamin B$_{12}$ or vitamin B complex	1 cc 3 times weekly for 3 weeks, then twice weekly for 3 months. Then reduce to 1 cc once weekly. 1 cc 3 times weekly for 3 weeks, then twice weekly for 3 months. Then reduce to 1 cc once weekly. ^{1}/$_2$ cc 3 times weekly for 3 weeks, then twice weekly for 3 months. Then reduce to ^{1}/$_2$ cc once weekly. 1 cc 3 times weekly or as prescribed by physician. 100 mg of each major B vitamin 3 times daily (amounts of individual vitamins in a complex will vary).	To supply B vitamins and other valuable nutrients. B vitamin deficiencies are related to brain malfunction. Many people with brain disorders have found this program helpful. All injectables can be combined in a single shot. If injections are not available, use a sublingual form.
plus extra vitamin B$_6$ (pyridoxine) plus vitamin B$_3$ (niacin) or niacinamide	100 mg twice daily. 100 mg 3 times daily. Do not exceed this amount. 1,000 mg daily.	Required by the nervous system; necessary for normal brain function. Deficiency has been linked to schizophrenia. Injections (under a doctor's supervision) are best. *Caution:* Do not take niacin if you have a liver disorder, gout, or high blood pressure.
Vitamin E emulsion or capsules	800 IU daily. Start with 200 IU daily and slowly increase to 1,000 IU daily.	An antioxidant that improves brain circulation. Emulsion form is recommended for easier assimilation and greater safety at high doses.

Important		
Dimethylglycine (DMG) (Aangamik DMG from FoodScience of Vermont)	As directed on label.	Enhances cerebral oxygen utilization.
Essential fatty acids (black currant seed oil and primrose oil are good sources)	As directed on label 3 times daily.	Helps cerebral circulation.

Lecithin granules or capsules	1 tbsp 3 times daily, before meals. 1,200 mg 3 times daily, before meals.	Improves brain function. Contains choline and inositol. Works well with vitamin E.
L-Glutamine	1,000–4,000 mg daily, on an empty stomach. Take with water or juice. Do not take with milk. Take with 50 mg vitamin B$_6$ and 100 mg vitamin C for better absorption.	Needed for normal brain function. (*See* AMINO ACIDS in Part One.)

Helpful		
Kelp	1,000–1,500 mg daily.	Contains balanced essential minerals.
Multivitamin and mineral complex with calcium and magnesium	As directed on label.	All nutrients are needed for normal brain function.
Raw thyroid glandular	As directed on label.	Reduced thyroid function results in poor cerebral function. (*See* HYPOTHYROIDISM in Part Two and GLANDULAR THERAPY in Part Three.)

HERBS

❏ Ginkgo biloba improves brain function and cerebral circulation, and enhances memory.

❏ Kava kava and passionflower are good for relief of stress and depression.

RECOMMENDATIONS

❏ Eat a high-fiber diet including plenty of fresh raw vegetables and quality protein, and try eating more frequent small meals rather than three larger ones each day. This helps to keep blood sugar levels stable, which in turn has a stabilizing influence on mood and behavior. *See* HYPOGLYCEMIA in Part Two for additional suggestions.

❏ Include the following in your diet: breast of chicken or turkey, brewer's yeast, halibut, peas, sunflower seeds, and tuna. Also eat foods rich in niacin, such as broccoli, carrots, corn, eggs, fish, potatoes, tomatoes, and whole wheat.

❏ Do not consume caffeine. It promotes the release of unwanted norepinephrine, a stimulating neurotransmitter.

❏ Avoid alcohol. Alcohol consumption depletes the body of zinc. Many psychological disorders are known to be adversely affected by zinc deficiencies.

❏ Keep environmental pressures under control. Overstimulation from strong emotions or an excessive workload can exacerbate symptoms. Also avoid understimulation.

CONSIDERATIONS

❏ A study reported in the August 29, 1992, issue of the British medical journal *The Lancet* linked city-dwelling, winter birth, and prenatal exposure to influenza to schizophrenic disorders. In addition, these factors appear to compound one another; city-born people with schizophrenia are much more likely to have been born in winter than their non-city-born counterparts.

❏ Sometimes extremely high doses of certain vitamins are needed to keep the mind functioning well.

❏ Hair analysis reveals mineral imbalances that may contribute to mental difficulties. (*See* HAIR ANALYSIS in Part Three.)

❏ Some experts believe that many suicides among the young may be related to undiagnosed schizophrenia.

❏ Psychiatrists found a link between schizophrenia and pellagra (vitamin B₃ [niacin] deficiency). Taking several grams of niacinamide daily (under a doctor's supervision) has been tried with good results.

❏ Undiagnosed celiac disease, caused by an intolerance to gluten, can cause symptoms similar to those of schizophrenia. Gluten intolerance can also cause severe depression. (*See* CELIAC DISEASE in Part Two.)

❏ Drug therapy is usually the medical treatment of choice for schizophrenia. However, there is no single medication that is effective in all cases. It may be necessary to try several different drugs in order to find the one that works best to keep symptoms under control.

❏ If you are taking prescription drugs for schizophrenia, do not stop taking your medication without first consulting a physician. Do not take any of the supplements listed above that might affect dopamine, serotonin, or norepinephrine synthesis without consulting a physician.

❏ Some cases of schizophrenia have been linked to food allergies. Many people find their symptoms improve after they fast. (*See also* ALLERGIES in Part Two and FASTING in Part Three.)

Sciatica

See under BACKACHE.

Scotoma

See under EYE PROBLEMS.

Seasonal Affective Disorder (SAD)

See under DEPRESSION.

Sebaceous Cyst

Sebaceous cysts are skin growths that contain a mixture of sebum (oil) and skin proteins. They generally appear as small, slowly growing swellings on the face, scalp, or back. A whitehead is actually a tiny sebaceous cyst.

These nodules feel firm but movable and rarely hurt unless they become infected. If infection sets in, there may be redness and swelling, and the area may become sensitive to the touch. Sebaceous cysts are benign, but they can become a site of chronic, usually bacterial, infection. With chronic infection, an abscess may form.

NUTRIENTS

SUPPLEMENT	SUGGESTED DOSAGE	COMMENTS
Very Important		
Primrose oil	1,000 mg 3 times daily.	A good healer for most skin disorders.
Vitamin A	25,000 IU daily for 3 months, then reduce to 15,000 IU daily. If you are pregnant, do not exceed 10,000 IU daily.	Necessary for healing and construction of new skin tissue.
plus carotenoid complex with beta carotene	As directed on label.	Used by the body to make vitamin A as needed.
Vitamin B complex plus extra	As directed on label.	Anti-stress and anti-aging vitamins.
vitamin B₁₂	1,000–2,000 mcg daily.	Needed for healthy skin.
Important		
Garlic (Kyolic from Wakunaga)	2 capsules 3 times daily, with meals.	Has anti-infective properties.
Kelp	1,000–1,500 mg daily.	Supplies balanced minerals needed for good skin tone.
Zinc	50 mg daily. Do not exceed a total of 100 mg daily from all supplements.	For tissue repair. Enhances immune response. Use zinc gluconate lozenges or OptiZinc for best absorption.
Helpful		
Superoxide dismutase (SOD)	As directed on label.	A free radical destroyer.

HERBS

❏ Aloe vera is soothing and healing. Apply pure aloe vera gel to the affected area as directed on the product label.

❏ Burdock root and red clover are powerful blood cleansers.

❏ Goldenseal extract or tea tree oil can be applied topically to fight infection.

❏ Milk thistle aids the liver in cleansing the blood.

❏ Witch hazel, applied to the skin, is excellent for absorbing oil.

RECOMMENDATIONS

❏ Avoid fats, especially saturated fats, and all fried foods. Also avoid alcohol, caffeine, chocolate, cocoa, dairy products, eggs, fat, fish, meat, salt, and sugar.

❏ Follow a fasting program. (*See* FASTING in Part Three.)

❏ Apply warm compresses several times daily.

❏ Use hot water when washing your skin. This helps to dissolve skin oil.

CONSIDERATIONS

❏ Drugs often prescribed for acne, including topical and oral antibiotics such as tetracycline and erythromycin, and tretinoin (Retin-A), a derivative of vitamin A that comes in cream, gel, or liquid form, may be prescribed for severe and/or extensive infection. Another acne drug, isotretinoin (Accutane), also derived from vitamin A, has serious side effects.

❏ If an antibiotic is prescribed, be sure to take an acidophilus supplement to replace necessary "friendly" bacteria. Do not take acidophilus at the same time of day as the antibiotic.

❏ If you develop an inflamed or infected sebaceous cyst, you physician may suggest surgical drainage, a procedure that is performed in the doctor's office.

❏ *See also* OILY SKIN in Part Two.

Seborrhea

Seborrhea, or seborrheic dermatitis, is characterized by scaly patches of skin that result from a disorder of the sebaceous (oil-secreting) glands. Seborrhea most often occurs on the scalp, face, and chest, but can appear on other parts of the body as well. It may or may not be itchy.

Seborrheic skin may be yellowish and/or greasy or dry and flaky. The scaly bumps may coalesce to form large plaques or patches. Seborrheic dermatitis can occur at any age, but is most common in infancy ("cradle cap") and middle age. The exact cause is not known, but it may be linked to nutritional deficiencies (especially a lack of biotin and vitamin A) or the effects of a yeast organism, *Pityrosporum ovale*, which normally lives in the hair follicles. Heredity and climate probably also play a role. Adult seborrheic dermatitis, which usually affects the scalp and face, is often associated with stress and anxiety. Other factors associated with an increased chance of developing seborrhea include infrequent shampooing, oily skin, obesity, Parkinson's disease, AIDS, and other skin disorders, such as acne, rosacea, and psoriasis.

Unless otherwise specified, the dosages recommended here are for adults. For a child between the ages of twelve and seventeen, reduce the dose to three-quarters the recommended amount. For a child between six and twelve, use one-half the recommended dose, and for a child under the age of six, use one-quarter the recommended amount.

NUTRIENTS

SUPPLEMENT	SUGGESTED DOSAGE	COMMENTS
Essential		
Essential fatty acids (primrose oil and Ultimate Oil from Nature's Secret are good sources)	As directed on label.	Important for many skin disorders; contains needed linoleic acid.
Vitamin B complex plus extra vitamin B₆ (pyridoxine)	As directed on label. 50 mg 3 times daily.	The B vitamins, especially vitamin B₆, are needed for protein metabolism, which is essential for healing and repair. Use a super-high-potency formula. A sublingual form is recommended for best absorption. Consider injections (under a doctor's supervision).
and biotin	300–400 mcg 3 times daily.	Deficiency has been linked to seborrhea.
Zinc	50 mg daily. Do not exceed a total of 100 mg daily from all supplements.	Important for healing. Enhances immunity. Use zinc gluconate lozenges or OptiZinc for best absorption.
Important		
ConcenTrace from Trace Minerals Research	As directed on label.	Contains essential trace minerals to nourish the skin.
Herpanacine from Diamond-Herpanacine Associates	As directed on label.	Amino acids, vitamins, and herbs that promote skin health and remove toxins.
Methylsulfonyl-methane (MSM)	As directed on label.	Possesses healing and nutritional properties for the skin.
Panoderm I from American Biologics	As directed on label.	Contains squalene, a substance found in healthy skin. Acts as a natural antioxidant and prevents damage to the skin due to cosmetics, wind, sun, and pollutants.
Pycnogenol or grape seed extract	As directed on label. As directed on label.	Powerful antioxidants that strengthen the skin to resist disease.
Vitamin A plus carotenoid complex with beta-carotene	Up to 50,000 IU daily. If you are pregnant, do not exceed 10,000 IU daily. As directed on label.	Deficiency may cause or contribute to seborrhea.
plus vitamin E or	400–800 IU daily.	Speeds healing. Increases oxygen intake.
AE Mulsion Forte from American Biologics	As directed on label.	Supplies vitamins A and E in emulsion form for easier assimilation and greater safety at higher doses.

Helpful		
Acidophilus (Kyo-Dophilus from Wakunaga is a good source)	As directed on label. Take on an empty stomach.	To replenish "friendly" bacteria. Especially important if antibiotics are prescribed. Use a nondairy formula.
Coenzyme Q$_{10}$	60 mg daily.	An important free radical scavenger that supplies oxygen to the cells.
plus Coenzyme A from Coenzyme-A Technologies	As directed on label.	Works effectively with coenzyme Q$_{10}$ to support the immune system's detoxification of many dangerous substances.
Dimethylglycine (DMG) (Aangamik DMG from FoodScience of Vermont)	As directed on label.	Increases oxygenation of tissues.
Free-form amino acid complex	As directed on label.	For healing and repair of tissues.
Kelp	1,000–1,500 mg daily.	Contains balanced minerals. A good source of iodine.
Lecithin granules or capsules	1 tbsp 3 times daily, with meals. 1,200 mg 3 times daily, with meals.	For cellular protection.
Multivitamin and mineral complex	As directed on label.	All nutrients are necessary in balance.

HERBS

❑ Dandelion, goldenseal, and red clover, taken internally, are good for most skin disorders.

Caution: Do not take goldenseal internally on a daily basis for more than one week at a time, do not use it during pregnancy, and use it with caution if you are allergic to ragweed.

❑ Emu oil, applied topically, has an anti-inflammatory effect on skin tissues.

❑ Oat straw may be used in a bath to reduce symptoms, especially inflammation and itching.

❑ Olive leaf extract has healing properties for the skin.

❑ Tea tree oil is a natural antiseptic and antifungal that can be applied directly to the affected area. If it is too strong, it can be diluted with an equal amount of jojoba oil (available in health food stores) or distilled water.

RECOMMENDATIONS

❑ Eat a diet composed of 50 to 75 percent raw foods and soured products such as low-fat yogurt.

❑ Avoid chocolate, dairy products, white flour, fried foods, seafood, nuts, and anything containing sugar.

❑ Do not eat any foods containing raw eggs. Egg whites contain high levels of avidin, a protein that binds biotin and prevents it from being absorbed. Biotin is needed for healthy hair and skin. Eating uncooked eggs also poses a risk of *Salmonella* poisoning (*see* FOODBORNE/WATERBORNE DISEASE in Part Two).

❑ If antibiotics are prescribed, take extra B-complex vitamins and an acidophilus supplement to replace the "friendly" bacteria destroyed by the antibiotics.

❑ Try changing your hair products. Choose products without chemicals. Sometimes this helps.

❑ To minimize the frequency and severity of flare-ups, dry your skin thoroughly after bathing, and wear loose-fitting clothing made of natural fibers that "breathe."

❑ *Echinacea purpurea*, a homeopathic preparation, can be used to reduce symptoms.

❑ Avoid using over-the-counter ointments to treat seborrhea. This can cause an overload on the skin.

❑ Do not pick at or squeeze the affected skin.

❑ Avoid using irritating soaps, but make sure you keep the affected areas clean. Avoid greasy ointments and creams. Keep your hair clean and make sure you use a non-oily shampoo.

❑ If dietary changes and nutritional supplementation do not produce an improvement, seek the advice of a qualified health care professional.

❑ Follow a fasting program once a month. (*See* FASTING in Part Three.)

CONSIDERATIONS

❑ Dermatologists usually prescribe cleansing lotions containing a drying agent with sulfur and resorcinol and/or Diprosone cream from Schering-Plough.

❑ Cradle cap has been associated with food allergies. For infants, controlling food allergies plus giving supplemental biotin (if there is a deficiency) is most effective. For a child over six months old, adding liquid vitamin B complex to juice is a good way to administer the needed biotin. Discuss any nutritional supplementation for a very young child with your health care practitioner.

❑ An absence of intestinal flora may be responsible for biotin deficiency in infants. Studies have shown that treating both the nursing mother and her infant with biotin can be successful in resolving cradle cap. For adults, treatment with biotin alone does not appear to be effective, but supplementation with biotin combined with the whole vitamin B complex and essential fatty acids produces improvement in many cases.

❑ Consumption of raw egg whites has produced seborrheic dermatitis in laboratory tests.

❑ Colloidal silver is a natural antibiotic that has been known to fight skin conditions such as seborrhea.

❑ Some findings suggest that many skin disorders, including eczema and psoriasis, may be related to gluten allergy. A gluten-free diet may be helpful. *See* CELIAC DISEASE in Part Two for dietary suggestions.

❑ Taking supplemental vitamin B complex has been shown to be the most effective treatment in many cases.

❑ *See also* DANDRUFF and DERMATITIS in Part Two.

Seizure

See under EPILEPSY.

Senility (Dementia)

Senility was once considered an inevitable consequence of aging. However, we now know that it is a physically based disease resulting from a loss of brain cells. Brain function, or certain aspects of brain function, decline to the point that mental disability results. Forgetfulness, fearfulness, depression, agitation, difficulty absorbing new information, loss of normal emotional responses, and an ability to remember things that happened years ago, but not things that took place a few minutes ago, are typical. Other signs include mood swings, jealousy, paranoia, frustration, anger, insensitivity to the feelings of others, fear of being alone, repeating conversations, inability to make decisions or complete a task, lack of a sense of time, hoarding, failure to recognize people, and self-neglect. The disorder usually gets progressively worse. Complications that may occur include injuries (primarily due to falls), inadequate nutrition, constipation, and a variety of infections.

Dementia can be caused by several diseases affecting brain function. It can also result from nutritional deficiency (especially deficiencies of vitamins B_1 [thiamin], B_3 [niacin], B_6 [pyridoxine], and B_{12}), alcoholism, Alzheimer's disease, kidney or liver failure, hypothyroidism, multiple strokes, atherosclerosis, multiple sclerosis, AIDS, or diabetes, to name a few.

Many people diagnosed as senile actually suffer from *pseudodementia*—symptoms that mimic dementia but that are actually caused by depression, deafness, brain tumors, thyroid problems, liver or kidney problems, the use of certain drugs, or other disorders. A thorough medical and psychological examination by a qualified professional, preferably a specialist in the field, is necessary for an accurate diagnosis.

Dementia is considered incurable. However, because generally declining health contributes to the problem, proper diet and nutritional supplements can help. The following supplements are helpful for improving brain function. When choosing supplements, avoid heavily coated or sustained release products. These are difficult to break down. Instead, choose liquids, powders, or sublingual forms.

NUTRIENTS

SUPPLEMENT	SUGGESTED DOSAGE	COMMENTS
Essential		
Dimethylglycine (DMG) (Aangamik DMG from FoodScience of Vermont)	As directed on label.	Helps to maintain mental acuity and enhances immune function.
Essential fatty acids (flaxseed oil and primrose oil are good sources)	As directed on label.	Promotes brain and nerve function as well as a healthy immune system.
Free-form amino acid complex	As directed on label.	To supply protein, needed for normal brain function. Protein deficiency is common among elderly people.
Gamma-amino-butyric acid (GABA)	As directed on label, on an empty stomach. Take with water or juice. Do not take with milk. Take with 50 mg vitamin B_6 and 100 mg vitamin C for better absorption.	Essential for brain function and metabolism. Has a calming effect. (*See* AMINO ACIDS in Part One.)
Garlic (Kyolic from Wakunaga)	As directed on label.	Enhances brain function; helps to reduce stress and anxiety.
L-Asparagine	As directed on label, on an empty stomach.	To maintain balance in the brain and central nervous system.
L-Phenylalanine	As directed on label, on an empty stomach.	Promotes alertness, aids memory, and helps overcome depression. *Caution:* Do not take this supplement if you are taking an MAO inhibitor drug, or if you suffer from panic attacks, diabetes, high blood pressure, or PKU.
L-Tyrosine	As directed on label, on an empty stomach.	Promotes brain function and helps fight depression. *Caution:* Do not take tyrosine if you are taking an MAO inhibitor drug, commonly prescribed for depression.
Melatonin	2–3 mg daily, taken 2 hours or less before bedtime.	Aids sleep, helps maintain equilibrium, and strengthens the immune system.
Nicotinamide adenine dinucleotide (NADH)	As directed on label.	A coenzyme form of niacin that is essential for production of energy and various neurotransmitters.
Phosphatidyl choline	As directed on label.	Aids in treating neurological disorders, memory loss, and depression. Is safe and effective. However, if you have manic-depressive disorder, you should not take large amounts.
Phosphatidyl serine	As directed on label.	Has been known to reverse depression and symptoms of Alzheimer's disease, and to enhance memory and learning abilities. The brain normally produces it, but production dwindles with age.

Pregnenolone	As directed on label.	May treat symptoms of aging, increase brain function, and enhance mood, memory, and thinking.
Vitamin B complex injections	1 cc once weekly or as prescribed by physician.	All B vitamins are necessary for brain and nerve health. Older adults often have deficiencies because the ability to absorb the B vitamins declines with age. Injections (under a doctor's supervision) are best.
plus extra vitamin B_6 (pyridoxine) injections and	$1/2$ cc once weekly or as prescribed by physician.	Vital for mental health and for maintaining proper electrolyte balance in the body.
vitamin B_{12} injections plus	As prescribed by physician.	
liver extract injections or vitamin B complex	1 cc once weekly or as prescribed by physician. 100 mg of each major B vitamin 3 times daily (amounts of individual vitamins in a complex will vary).	A good source of B vitamins and other valuable nutrients. If injections are not available, use a sublingual form.
plus extra vitamin B_3 (niacin)	100 mg daily. Do not exceed this amount. Take with 100 mg niacinamide to reduce flushing.	Improves cerebral circulation and lowers cholesterol levels. *Caution:* Do not take niacin if you have a liver disorder, gout, or high blood pressure.
and vitamin B_6 (pyridoxine) and	50 mg daily.	
vitamin B_{12}	2,000 mcg daily.	Needed to prevent anemia. Also prevents nerve damage and may assist memory and learning. Use a lozenge or sublingual form.

Very Important

S-Adenosylmethio-nine (SAMe)	400 mg 2 times daily.	Aids in relieving stress and depression, eases pain, and produces antioxidant effects. *Caution:* Do not use if you have manic-depressive disorder or take prescription antidepressants.
Trimethylglycine (TMG)	500–1,000 mg in the morning.	Assists the body in utilizing vitamin B_6, vitamin B_{12}, and folic acid. Also helps to rid the body of toxic elements (such as homocysteine) and increases levels of the natural mood elevator S-adenosylmethionine.
Vitamin C with bioflavonoids	3,000–10,000 mg daily.	Reduces blood clotting tendency, improving cerebral circulation.
Vitamin E	Start with 200 IU daily and increase slowly to 600–1,000 IU daily.	Improves cerebral circulation and boosts immunity, which declines with age. Use d-alpha-tocopherol form.

Important

GH3 from Gero Vita	As directed on label.	Helps to promote brain function. Consider injections (under a doctor's supervision). *Caution:* Do not use GH3 if you are allergic to sulfites.

Helpful

Coenzyme Q_{10} plus	100–200 mg daily.	Free radical scavenger and immunostimulant. Increases cellular oxygen levels.
Coenzyme A from Coenzyme-A Technologies	As directed on label.	Works effectively with coenzyme Q_{10} to support the immune system's detoxification of many dangerous substances.
Kelp	As directed on label.	Reported to be very beneficial to brain tissue, the membranes surrounding the brain, the sensory nerves, and the spinal cord.
Lecithin granules or capsules	1 tbsp 3 times daily, before meals. 1,200 mg 3 times daily, before meals.	For brain cell protection and function.
L-Glutamine	As directed on label, on an empty stomach. Take with water or juice. Do not take with milk. Take with 50 mg vitamin B_6 and 100 mg vitamin C for better absorption.	Needed for normal brain function. (*See* AMINO ACIDS in Part One.)
Multivitamin complex	As directed on label.	For necessary vitamins. Use a high-potency formula.
Zinc	50–80 mg daily. Do not exceed a total of 100 mg daily from all supplements.	Aids in heavy metal detoxification and enhancing immunity. Use zinc gluconate lozenges or OptiZinc for best absorption.

HERBS

❏ Anise, blessed thistle, and blue cohosh appear to sharpen brain power.

❏ Ginkgo biloba improves cerebral circulation, enhances brain function and memory, and destroys free radicals to protect brain cells. Three times a day, place $1/2$ dropperful of alcohol-free liquid extract under your tongue and hold it there for a few minutes before swallowing. Or take 400 milligrams in capsule form three times daily.

❏ Gotu kola, ginseng, and mullein oil all aid with memory function.

❏ Kava kava and St. John's wort help to calm people who anger easily.

❏ The Chinese herb qian ceng ta (*Huperzia serrata*), increases memory retention. It is the source of the compound huperzine A. Pure standardized extracts of this compound have been shown to increase clearheadedness, language ability, and memory in a significant percentage of people with Alzheimer's disease. It is a potent blocker of acetylcholinesterase, an enzyme that regulates the activity of acetylcholine, which is an important brain chemical involved in maintaining healthy learning and memory functions.

❏ Valerian root promotes better sleep patterns when taken at bedtime.

RECOMMENDATIONS

❏ Eat a diet consisting of 50 to 75 percent raw foods, along with seeds, whole-grain cereals and breads, raw nuts, and low-fat yogurt and soured products. Eat Swiss cheese, brown rice, and plenty of fiber daily.

❏ Drink plenty of liquids, even if you are not thirsty—as we grow older, our "thirst system" does not work as well.

❏ Move the bowels daily. Oat bran, rice bran, and a high-fiber diet are important. Aerobic Bulk Cleanse (ABC) from Aerobic Life Industries, a colon cleanser, is very helpful. Enemas may be needed. (See ENEMAS in Part Three.)

❏ Keep active. Exercising, walking, engaging in mental activity, and doing things you enjoy, like pursuing a hobby, are important. Seek out companionship and new experiences. Some people withdraw and keep to themselves as they get older because it seems easier and/or safer, but this can lead to loneliness and depression. If getting out and about is a problem, consider investing in and learning to use a computer. There are a number of on-line services geared to seniors that can serve as a source of companionship as well as information.

❏ Be sure to maintain a safe environment at home.

❏ Protect against head injury by wearing your seat belt and by wearing protective headgear when participating in activities such as bicycle riding.

❏ Have a complete physical examination to rule out the possibility of underlying illness as a cause of symptoms.

CONSIDERATIONS

❏ To make an accurate diagnosis of senile dementia, a physician needs to be thoroughly informed about symptoms—exactly what they are, how often they occur and under what circumstances, and any factors that have been noted to improve or worsen them. He or she will also need to know about any medical conditions you may have and what types of medications (prescription and over-the-counter) and supplements you are taking, as these can have an effect on memory. To rule out other conditions, the doctor may perform a number of tests, including blood tests, memory testing, an electrocardiogram (EKG) to measure heart activity, an electroencephalogram (EEG) to measure brain waves, brain scans, and/or a spinal tap.

❏ There is no cure for most types of dementia. Often, treatment is aimed at controlling anger, depression, delusions, and other symptoms that are present as a result of the condition. Antidepressants and tranquilizers are some of the types of medications that may be recommended.

❏ Evidence suggests that many cases of dementia may be prevented by "stroke reduction" measures—not smoking, controlling high blood pressure, pursuing chelation therapy to remove toxic metals from the body, adhering to a proper diet, and taking appropriate nutritional supplements.

❏ Ultimately, a person with long-term dementia is unable to live independently, and often requires nursing care.

❏ Feelings of isolation, loneliness, frustration, anger, fatigue, and loss of a social life often accompany this condition—and this can be overwhelming. Frequent time spent with family members and friends, along with psychological care, can help to alleviate these feelings.

❏ Smoking may increase your chance of getting dementia.

❏ Persons with atherosclerosis and high blood pressure have a higher risk of developing senility. (See ARTERIOSCLEROSIS/ATHEROSCLEROSIS and HIGH BLOOD PRESSURE in Part Two.)

❏ Food allergies can cause mental as well as physical symptoms. (See ALLERGIES in Part Two.)

❏ Toxic metals in the body can produce symptoms similar to those of senility. A hair analysis can reveal whether the body is incurring damage due to the presence of toxic levels of metals like aluminum and lead. (See HAIR ANALYSIS in Part Three.)

❏ See also ALUMINUM TOXICITY; ALZHEIMER'S DISEASE; and PARKINSON'S DISEASE, all in Part Two.

Sexually Transmitted Disease (STD)

There are numerous diseases that are passed on either exclusively or primarily through intimate sexual contact. These include acquired immune deficiency syndrome (AIDS), chancroid, chlamydia, genital herpes, gonorrhea, lymphogranuloma venereum (LGV), granuloma inguinale, some types of hepatitis, syphilis, and trichomoniasis. Genital candidiasis also can be transmitted through sexual contact. Crabs (pubic lice) and scabies also are sexually transmitted, but are considered parasitic infestations rather than infectious diseases. This section deals primarily with two of the more common sexually transmitted diseases, gonorrhea and syphilis.

Gonorrhea is caused by a microorganism called *Neisseria gonorrhoeae*. These bacteria are commonly referred to as gonococci. This is not a common infection in the United States—the infection rate is approximately 123 per 100,000 people. In women, gonorrhea often causes no symptoms. When it does, they include frequent and painful urination, vaginal discharge, abnormal menstrual bleeding, acute inflammation in the pelvic area, and rectal itching. Men with gonorrhea usually do experience symptoms, including a yellow discharge of pus and mucus from the penis and slow, difficult, and painful urination. Symptoms usually appear between two and twenty-one days after sexual contact. If not treated, the infection can travel through the bloodstream and go into the bones, joints, tendons, and other tissues, causing a systemic illness with mild fever, achiness, inflamed joints, and, occasionally, skin lesions. At this stage, the organism is difficult to detect, and the condition is often misdiagnosed as simple arthritis. In men, complications of gonorrhea can include sterility and urethral stricture.

Syphilis also is rare in the United States. It affects 3 in every 100,000 people nationwide. Syphilis is caused by a type of bacteria called *Treponema pallidum.* This disease is occasionally contracted through close physical contact such as kissing, as well as through sexual intercourse. If not treated, this illness progresses, usually over the course of many years, through three basic stages. In the first stage, ten to ninety days after contact, a chancre—a red, painless ulcer—appears at the spot where the bacteria entered the body. In the second stage, perhaps four to ten weeks after contact, a rash and patches of flaking tissue appear in the mouth, palms of the hands, soles of feet, or genital area. There may be systemic symptoms, usually mild, as well—headache, nausea, and general discomfort. If the disease progresses to its third stage (which is quite rare in the United States), a year or more after the initial infection,

brain damage, hearing loss, heart disease, and/or blindness can occur. This disease can remain dormant for up to twenty years.

Unless otherwise stated, the dosages recommended here are for adults. For a child between the ages of twelve and seventeen, reduce the dose to three-quarters of the recommended amount.

NUTRIENTS

SUPPLEMENT	SUGGESTED DOSAGE	COMMENTS
Very Important		
Acidophilus (Kyo-Dophilus from Wakunaga is a good source)	As directed on label 3 times daily, on an empty stomach.	To restore "friendly" bacteria. Important when taking antibiotics, which are usually prescribed for STDs. Use a nondairy formula.
Free-form amino acid complex	As directed on label.	Needed for tissue repair. Use free-form amino acids for quicker absorption and assimilation.
Garlic (Kyolic from Wakunaga)	2 capsules 3 times daily.	A natural antibiotic and immune system stimulant.

Early Symptoms of Sexually Transmitted Diseases

It is important to detect sexually transmitted diseases in their early stages so that prompt treatment can begin and, in the case of some diseases, irreparable damage to the body can be prevented. Use the table below to familiarize yourself with the beginning stages of various STDs.

Disease	First Symptoms
AIDS (Acquired Immune Deficiency Syndrome)	Headache, night sweats, unexplained weight loss, fatigue, swollen lymph glands, persistent fever, oral thrush (a heavy, whitish coating on the tongue and the insides of the mouth), recurrent vaginal yeast infections, persistent diarrhea, lung infections.
Candidiasis	Itching in the genital area, pain when urinating, a thick odorless vaginal discharge.
Chlamydia	For women: a white vaginal discharge that resembles cottage cheese, a burning sensation when urinating, itching, painful intercourse. For men: a clear, watery urethral discharge. Often, however, there are no symptoms at all.
Genital herpes	Itching, burning in the genital area, discomfort while urinating, a watery vaginal or urethral discharge, weeping, fluid-filled eruptions in the vagina or on the penis.
Genital warts	Soft, cauliflower-like growths appearing either singly or in clusters in and around the vagina, anus, penis, groin, and/or scrotal area.
Gonorrhea	For women: frequent and painful urination, a cloudy vaginal discharge, vaginal itching, inflammation of the pelvic area, rectal discharge, abnormal uterine bleeding. For men: a yellowish, pus-filled urethral discharge. Often, however, there are no symptoms, especially in women.
Pelvic Inflammatory Disease (PID)	A pus-filled vaginal discharge with fever and lower abdominal pain.
Syphilis	A sore on the genitalia, rash, patches of flaking tissue, fever, sore throat, sores in the mouth or anus.
Trichomoniasis	For women: vaginal itching and pain, with a foamy, greenish or yellow foul-smelling discharge. For men: a clear urethral discharge.

Vitamin C with bioflavonoids	750–2,500 mg 4 times daily.	Boosts immune function and is an antiviral agent.
Zinc	100 mg daily. Do not exceed this amount.	Important for the health of the reproductive organs. Promotes wound healing and boosts immune function to fight a broad range of microbes. Use zinc gluconate lozenges or OptiZinc for best absorption.

Important		
Colloidal silver	Use sublingually or topically as directed on label.	An antiseptic that rapidly reduces inflammation and promotes healing of lesions.
Kelp	1,000–1,500 mg daily.	Supplies balanced vitamins and minerals.
Vitamin B complex	50 mg of each major B vitamin 3 times daily (amounts of individual vitamins in a complex will vary).	Necessary in all cellular enzyme system functions.

Helpful		
Coenzyme Q$_{10}$	30–60 mg daily.	A powerful free radical scavenger.
Multivitamin and mineral complex	As directed on label.	All nutrients are necessary in balance. Use a high-potency formula.
Raw glandular complex plus raw thymus glandular	As directed on label. As directed on label.	Promotes immune function.
Vitamin K or alfalfa	100 mcg daily.	Antibiotics destroy the intestinal bacteria that produce vitamin K, which is necessary for blood clotting. *See under* Herbs, below.

HERBS

❑ Alfalfa is a good source of vitamin K, which is needed for blood clotting and healing. This vitamin is depleted by antibiotics.

❑ Astragalus helps to protect the immune system.

❑ Echinacea, goldenseal, pau d'arco, and suma may alleviate symptoms. Alternate among two or more of these herbs. Consume three cups of herbal tea daily or take herbs in capsule or extract form as directed on the product label.

Caution: Do not take goldenseal internally on a daily basis for more than one week at a time, do not use it during pregnancy, and use it with caution if you are allergic to ragweed.

❑ Hops helps to relieve pain and stress.

❑ Red clover acts as an antibiotic and anti-inflammatory agent, and aids relaxation.

❑ Suma enhances the immune system and helps prevent stress. This herb is sometimes referred to as Brazilian ginseng.

RECOMMENDATIONS

❑ Use a latex (not sheepskin) condom for any sexual activity until the infection has cleared completely. These diseases are highly contagious. Be aware, however, that even the use of a condom does not guarantee protection against STDs. Abstinence is the only way to avoid any chance of transmitting the infection.

❑ If you are taking penicillin or another antibiotic for a sexually transmitted disease, be sure to add some form of acidophilus to your diet to replace lost "friendly" bacteria.

CONSIDERATIONS

❑ Antibiotics are the usual treatment for both syphilis and gonorrhea. It is important to take any prescribed antibiotic for the full course, even if symptoms abate. Do not stop taking the medication early.

❑ Many health care providers consider cervical dysplasia (a precancerous condition of the cervix characterized by the formation of abnormal tissue in the cervix) to be a sexually transmitted disease. They believe that it is caused by papillomaviruses, the same viruses that cause venereal warts.

❑ Many STDs that were in decline are becoming more common. Many experts link this rise to the AIDS epidemic; because the immune system is compromised, AIDS increases susceptibility to disease of every kind.

❑ *See also* AIDS; CANDIDIASIS; CHLAMYDIA; HERPESVIRUS INFECTION; WARTS; and/or YEAST INFECTION, all in Part Two.

Shingles (Herpes Zoster)

Shingles, also known as herpes zoster, is a disease caused by the varicella-zoster virus, the same virus that causes chickenpox. It affects the nerve endings in the skin. Shingles can appear anywhere on the body; however, it is most commonly found on the skin of the abdomen underneath the ribs, leading toward the navel. Other commonly affected areas are the vaginal tissues and the inside of the mouth.

Most adults have already contracted chickenpox. This common childhood disease causes a fever and a rash that itches maddeningly, but rarely does any permanent damage. However, once the varicella-zoster virus enters the body and has caused chickenpox, it doesn't go away. It may lie dormant in the spinal cord and nerve ganglia for years until activated, usually by a weakening (temporary or permanent) of the immune system. Then the varicella-zoster infection spreads to the very ends of the nerves, causing them to send impulses to the brain that are interpreted as severe pain, itching, or burning, and rendering the overlying skin much more sensitive than usual. An estimated 90 percent of people who have had chickenpox are at risk of developing shingles. Those who have never had chicken-pox have very little chance of developing shingles because it is not very contagious.

An attack of shingles is often preceded by three or four days of chills, fever, and achiness. There may also be pain in the affected area. Then crops of tiny fluid-filled blisters surrounded by a red rim appear. The affected area becomes excruciatingly painful and sensitive to the touch. Other symptoms can include numbness, fatigue, depression, tingling, shooting pains, swollen and painful lymph nodes, fever, and headache. This phase of shingles lasts seven to fourteen days. The blisters eventually form crusty scabs and drop off. Scarring can occur in severe cases.

The chance of an attack of shingles can be increased by many factors, including stress; cancer; the use of anticancer drugs; spinal cord injuries; and conditions that suppress the immune system, such as the human immunodeficiency virus (HIV); or the use of medications such as corticosteriods or cyclosporin. However, serious illness is not required to activate the virus. Any type of physical or emotional stress can make one susceptible. Often, something as innocuous as a minor injury or a mild cold can lead to an attack in an otherwise healthy person. In most cases, it is never determined just what the trigger is.

Shingles strikes some 750,000 Americans each year. It can appear at any age, but is most common in people over the age of fifty, when immune function naturally begins to decline as a result of aging. Most cases of shingles run their course within a few weeks. More severe cases may last longer and require aggressive treatment. In some cases, the pain continues for months, even years, after the blisters have disappeared. This syndrome, called postherpetic neuralgia, is more likely to occur in older people. If shingles develop near the eyes, the cornea may be affected and blindness may result. About 20 percent of persons who get shingles go on to suffer a recurrence of the disease.

For people with immune deficiencies, shingles and its aftermath can be devastating. The disease is capable of affecting the internal organs, attacking even the lungs, kidneys, and liver. Disseminated shingles can cause permanent injury—including blindness, deafness, or paralysis, depending upon the area of the body that is served by the infected nerves—if it goes unchecked. Death can occur as the result of a secondary bacterial infection or viral pneumonia brought on by shingles.

NUTRIENTS

SUPPLEMENT	SUGGESTED DOSAGE	COMMENTS
Essential		
L-Lysine	500 mg twice daily, on an empty stomach. Take with water or juice. Do not take with milk. Take with 50 mg vitamin B6 and 100 mg vitamin C for better absorption.	Important for healing and for fighting the virus that causes shingles. (See AMINO ACIDS in Part One.) Caution: Do not take this supplement for longer than 6 months at a time.
Vitamin C with bioflavonoids	2,000 mg 4 times daily.	Aids in fighting the virus and boosting the immune system.
Very Important		
Beta-1,3-D-Glucan	As directed on label.	Useful for treating bacterial, viral, and fungal infections.
Vitamin B complex plus extra vitamin B12	100 mg of each major B vitamin 3 times daily (amounts of individual vitamins in a complex will vary). 1,000 mcg twice daily.	Needed for nerve health and to counteract deficiencies. Injections (under a doctor's supervision) may be necessary. Use a lozenge or sublingual form.
Zinc	80 mg daily for 1 week, then reduce to 50 mg daily. Do not exceed a total of 100 mg daily from all supplements.	Enhances immunity and protects against infection. Use zinc chelate lozenges or zinc picolinate in sublingual form for faster absorption.
Important		
Calcium plus magnesium	1,500 mg daily. 750 mg daily.	For nerve function and healing, and to combat stress. Use chelate forms.
Garlic (Kyolic from Wakunaga)	2 capsules 3 times daily, with meals.	Excellent for building the immune system.
S-Adenosylmethionine (SAMe) (SAMe Rx-Mood from Nature's Plus)	As directed on label.	Aids in reducing pain and inflammation. A natural antidepressant. Caution: Do not use if you have manic-depressive disorder or take prescription antidepressants. Do not give this supplement to a child under 12.
Vitamin A emulsion or capsules plus carotenoid complex with beta-carotene	50,000 IU daily for 2 weeks, then reduce to 25,000 IU daily. If you are pregnant, do not exceed 10,000 IU daily. 10,000 IU daily. As directed on label.	Boosts the immune system and protects against infection. Emulsion form is recommended for easier assimilation and greater safety at higher doses. To protect immune function and enhance healing.
Vitamin D3	1,000 IU twice daily for 1 week, then reduce to 400 IU daily.	Aids in tissue healing and is needed for calcium absorption.
Vitamin E	400–800 IU daily. Can also open a capsule and apply the oil directly to the affected areas of skin.	Helps prevent formation of scar tissue. Also alleviates pain from long-term cases of shingles. Use d-alpha-tocopherol form.
Helpful		
Acidophilus (Kyo-Dophilus from Wakunaga is a good source)	As directed on label.	Provides "friendly" bacteria to the intestines and stimulates immune function. Use a nondairy formula.
Coenzyme Q10 plus Coenzyme A from Coenzyme-A Technologies	60 mg daily. As directed on label.	A free radical scavenger that boosts immune function. Works effectively with coenzyme Q10 to support the immune system's detoxification of many dangerous substances.
Colloidal silver	As directed on label.	A natural antibiotic that has shown effectiveness in treating shingles. Can be taken internally and used topically.

Essential fatty acids (flaxseed oil and primrose oil are good sources)	As directed on label.	Promotes healing of skin and nerve tissue.
Grape seed extract	As directed on label.	A powerful antioxidant that protects skin cells and decreases the number of outbreaks of blisters.
Herpanacine from Diamond-Herpanacine Associates	As directed on label.	Builds the immune system and fights infection.
Inflazyme Forte from American Biologics	4 tablets 3 times daily, with meals.	Has antioxidant properties and aids in proper breakdown of proteins, fats, and carbohydrates.
Maitake extract or reishi extract or shiitake extract	As directed on label. As directed on label. As directed on label.	Has immune-boosting and antiviral properties.
Multivitamin and mineral complex	As directed on label.	All nutrients are necessary in balance.
Wobenzym N from Marlyn Nutraceuticals	3–6 tablets 2–3 times daily, between meals.	Destroys free radicals and aids in proper breakdown and absorption of foods. Also good for inflammation.

HERBS

❑ Alfalfa, chamomile, and dandelion promote healing by helping to restore the body's normal acid/alkaline balance. Dandelion also helps to detoxify and support the liver. A cool chamomile compress can aid in soothing the blisters.

Caution: Do not use chamomile on an ongoing basis, and avoid it completely if you are allergic to ragweed.

❑ Astragalus root and echinacea boost immune function.

Caution: Do not use astragalus in the presence of a fever.

❑ Bi phaya yaw (*Clinacanthus nutans*), an herb used in traditional Thai medicine, has been shown in clinical studies to shorten the time it takes to recover from shingles in some cases. It is applied in cream form.

❑ Burdock and red clover cleanse both the lymph nodes and the bloodstream.

❑ Cayenne (capsicum) contains a substance called capsaicin, which relieves pain and aids in healing. It also acts as a detoxifier. Cayenne is available in tablet and capsule form.

❑ Goldenseal has powerful antibiotic properties and reduces infection.

Caution: Do not take this herb internally on a daily basis for more than one week at a time, do not use it during pregnancy, and use it with caution if you are allergic to ragweed.

❑ Green tea has antiviral, anti-inflammatory, and antioxidant properties. The polyphenols it contains have been found to fight herpesviruses.

❑ Licorice extract can be used topically to treat shingles and postherpetic neuralgia. It appears to interfere with the growth of the virus.

❑ Milk thistle protects the liver and promotes healthy liver function.

❑ A combination of oat straw, St. John's wort, and skullcap helps to reduce stress and itching. Mix equal amounts of oat straw, St. John's wort, and skullcap tinctures together, and take 1 teaspoon of this mixture four times daily.

❑ Olive leaf extract aids in fighting the virus.

❑ Rose hips are high in vitamin C and are good for preventing infections on the skin.

❑ Valerian root calms the nervous system. Taken at bedtime, it acts as a sleep aid.

RECOMMENDATIONS

❑ Include in the diet brewer's yeast, brown rice, garlic, raw fruits and vegetables, and whole grains.

❑ Eat plenty of foods that contain vitamin B_6, including bananas, nuts, potatoes, and sweet potatoes.

❑ Go on a cleansing fast. (*See* FASTING in Part Three.)

❑ Use bee pollen or propolis, chlorophyll, and/or kelp to fight the virus and promote healing.

Caution: Bee pollen may cause an allergic reaction in some individuals. Start with a small amount, and discontinue use if a rash, wheezing, discomfort, or other symptoms occur.

❑ Keep stress to a minimum. Stress reduces the immune system's effectiveness in fighting off infection. Studies have found that people with shingles report having recently been through stressful periods more often than other people.

❑ Avoid drafts. Allow the affected area to be exposed to sunlight for fifteen minutes each day. Wash the blisters gently when bathing, and otherwise avoid touching or scratching them.

❑ If you are suffering from a rash or blisters of an unknown origin, see a dermatologist—he or she can administer a test that only takes a few minutes.

❑ See an ophthalmologist if the shingles appear on the forehead, near the eyes, or on the tip of the nose. Untreated ophthalmic herpes zoster can lead to vision loss.

❑ Try using essential oils. Bergamot oil, calophyllum oil (related to St. John's wort), eucalyptus oil, geranium oil, goldenseal oil, and lemon oil can be used singly or in combination. These highly concentrated plant essences have strong antiviral properties. The best way to use them is to add a few drops of essential oil to a tablespoon of a carrier oil such as almond, peanut, or olive oil, and apply the mixture directly to the lesions at the first sign of an outbreak. In most instances, the lesions dry up and disappear completely within three to five days after this treatment.

❑ Consider using homeopathic remedies to alleviate symptoms. *Apis mellifica, Arsenicum album, Clematis erecta,*

Iris versicolor, and *Rhus toxicodendron* are homeopathic remedies that may be helpful.

CONSIDERATIONS

❏ There is no known cure for shingles. Treatment focuses on shortening the acute phase of pain and rash, minimizing pain and discomfort, and attempting to prevent or minimize possible complications. Physicians often prescribe an antiviral medication called acyclovir (Zovirax), which is also used for herpes. Acyclovir often helps minimize pain as well as prevent some complications, particularly for people with compromised immune systems. If acyclovir treatment is not begun within the first few days of the onset of shingles, however, it is not usually effective. This can be a problem because early diagnosis is often difficult. Acyclovir is also relatively expensive.

❏ Pain medication, such as acetaminophen (Tylenol, Datril, and others) or nonsteroidal anti-inflammatory drugs (NSAIDs) may be used to control inflammation and mild or moderate pain. Narcotics may be needed for severe pain.

❏ Adenosine monophosphate (AMP), a compound that occurs naturally in the body, has been found to be effective against shingles.

❏ Capsaicin has been attracting attention for its ability to relieve pain in persons suffering from postherpetic neuralgia. Capsaicin is not a product of chemical engineering, but a component found in plants of the same family as red peppers. Researchers in Toronto found that 56 percent of people with postherpetic neuralgia who were treated with capsaicin cream (Zostrix) for four weeks experienced significant relief of pain, and that 78 percent had at least some improvement in pain. Clinical studies suggest that capsaicin directly reduces the amount of substance P, a neurotransmitter responsible for the transmission of pain impulses. If there is a deficiency of substance P, the nerves are unable to transmit sensations of pain. Capsaicin is easy to adminster—it is simply applied topically to the affected area three or four times a day. In addition, capsaicin does not interact with any other drugs or medications, which makes it an especially attractive option for elderly people, who are often taking one or more drugs on a regular basis. Capsaicin cream is sold over the counter in most drug stores and health food stores. It should not be applied until the blisters caused by shingles have healed completely, however, or extreme burning pain may result.

❏ Topical lidocaine (Lidoderm) may be prescribed for the pain of postherpetic neuralgia. Possible side effects of this drug include redness and swelling. However, this is usually mild and does not last long.

❏ People with compromised immune systems may be given serum or other biological products obtained from the pooled blood of people who have recently recovered from shingles to assist their own immune systems in resisting the virus. However, in this age of AIDS, such treatment has become riskier and more expensive due to screening procedures to assure safety. Physicians are now more likely to administer huge doses of antiviral drugs to try to destroy or cripple the virus.

❏ Orthomolecular physicians often administer injections of vitamin B_{12} combined with adenosine monophosphate (AMP) for shingles. This treatment, together with applications of zinc oxide and plain yogurt along the path of the affected nerve two to three times daily, can bring relief.

❏ Dimethylsulfoxide (DMSO) has been used with success to relieve the pain of shingles and promote healing of the lesions.

❏ While shingles itself is not very contagious, a person with shingles may infect previously uninfected persons, particularly children, with chickenpox.

❏ If conservative measures are not effective, an antidepressant such as amitriptyline (Elavil, Endep) may be prescribed. These drugs not only ease the emotional impact of unrelenting pain, but they seem to alleviate the pain itself. They appear to do this by causing an increase in the production of endorphins, the body's own natural painkillers.

❏ Experiments are being conducted in which live chickenpox vaccine is given intravenously in an attempt to prevent shingles. Since you cannot develop shingles if you never contract chickenpox, researchers theorize that a vaccine that prevents chickenpox would therefore also prevent shingles. Detractors argue that while this approach may produce immunity in those who have never had chickenpox, the virus in the vaccine may also take refuge in the central nervous system and cause shingles years or decades later.

❏ One of the biggest obstacles to researchers in learning more about the varicella-zoster virus is the fact that there are no animals in which it can be studied; chickenpox and shingles occur only in humans, and the virus grows poorly in laboratory cultures. Nonetheless, research continues into the biology of varicella-zoster, with the hope of developing a better understanding of how the immune system controls it and perhaps finding ways to ease the suffering caused by shingles and postherpetic neuralgia.

❏ *See also* PAIN CONTROL in Part Three.

❏ For names and addresses of organizations that can offer further information about shingles, *see* HEALTH AND MEDICAL ORGANIZATIONS in the Appendix.

Sinusitis

Sinusitis is an inflammation of the nasal sinuses. There are sinuses located above the eyes (frontal sinuses); to either side of the nose, inside the cheekbones (maxillary sinuses); behind the bridge of the nose (sphenoid sinuses); and in the upper nose (ethmoid sinuses). Sinuses are air-filled pockets in the skull that are connected to the nose and throat by passages designed to drain away mucus. The sinuses are the first line of defense in protecting the lungs against infection. Most cases of sinusitis affect the frontal and/or maxillary sinuses, but any or all of the sinuses may be involved, and each individual tends to have problems with a particular set of sinuses. If the sinuses are too small or poorly positioned to handle the volume of mucus produced, they can become clogged. Pressure in the sinuses increases, causing pain. Sinuses that are clogged for a long time seem to invite infection.

Sinusitis can be either acute or chronic. Acute sinusitis is frequently caused by bacterial or viral infections of the nose, throat, and upper respiratory tract, such as the common cold. More than 50 percent of all cases of sinusitis are caused by bacteria. Air travel also can lead to acute inflammation of the sinuses, because of changes in air pressure. Chronic sinusitis problems may be caused by small growths in the nose, injury of the nasal bones, air pollution, dental complications, emotional stress, smoking, and exposure to irritant fumes and smells. Allergic sinusitis may be caused by hay fever or food allergies, especially allergies to milk and dairy products. People with compromised immune systems are susceptible to fungal sinusitis, a potentially dangerous condition that requires aggressive treatment.

Symptoms of sinusitis include fever (usually low-grade, but higher in some cases), cough, headache, earache, toothache, facial pain, cranial pressure, difficulty breathing through the nose, loss of the sense of smell, and tenderness over the forehead and cheekbones. If tapping the forehead just over the eyes, the cheekbones, or the area around the bridge of the nose causes pain, the sinuses may be infected. Sometimes sinusitis produces facial swelling followed by a stuffy nose and thick discharge of mucus. The symptoms suffered by those with sinusitis can have other unpleasant effects. Postnasal drip can cause a sore throat, nausea, and bad breath; difficulty breathing can cause snoring and loss of sleep.

Unless otherwise stated, the dosages recommended here are for adults. For a child between the ages of twelve and seventeen, reduce the dose to three-quarters of the recommended amount. For a child between the ages of six and twelve, use one-half the recommended dose, and for a child under six, use one-quarter of the recommended amount.

NUTRIENTS

SUPPLEMENT	SUGGESTED DOSAGE	COMMENTS
Very Important		
Acidophilus (Kyo-Dophilus from Wakunaga is a good source)	As directed on label.	Replaces good bacteria in the colon. Important if antibiotics are prescribed. Use a nondairy formula.
Bee pollen	Start with 1/2 tsp daily and increase slowly to 1 tbsp daily, taken in juice.	Increases immunity and speeds healing. *Caution:* Bee pollen may cause an allergic reaction in some individuals. Discontinue use if at any time a rash, wheezing, discomfort, or other symptoms occur.
Flaxseed oil	As directed on label.	Reduces pain and inflammation. Enhances all body functions.
Multivitamin and mineral complex	As directed on label.	To improve overall health and assure proper nutrition.
Quercetin plus	As directed on label.	Protects against allergens and increases immunity.
bromelain or	As directed on label.	Enhances the effectiveness of quercetin.
AntiAllergy formula from Freeda Vitamins	As directed on label.	Contains quercetin, calcium pantothenate, and calcium ascorbate to provide nutritional support and reduce allergic response.
Raw thymus glandular	500 mg twice daily.	Protects immune function and health of the mucous membrane cells.
SinuCheck from Enzymatic Therapy	2 capsules 4 times daily.	A natural decongestant to help clear blocked nasal passages due to colds and sinusitis.
Vitamin A with mixed carotenoids	10,000 IU daily.	Enhances the immune system; protects against colds, flu, and other infections. Helps maintain the health of the mucous membranes.
including natural beta-carotene	15,000 IU daily.	Precursor of vitamin A.
Vitamin B complex	75–100 mg of each major B vitamin 3 times daily, with meals. (amounts of individual vitamins in a complex will vary).	Helps to maintain healthy nerves and reduce stress. A sublingual form is best. Aids in the formation of antibodies.
plus extra pantothenic acid (vitamin B5) and	100 mg 3 times daily, with meals.	Aids immune system function.
vitamin B6 (pyridoxine) and	50 mg 3 times daily, with meals.	
vitamin B12	1,000 mcg 3 times daily.	
Vitamin C with bioflavonoids	3,000–10,000 mg daily, in divided doses.	Boosts immune function and aids in preventing infection and decreasing mucus.
Vitamin E	400–1,000 IU daily.	Improves circulation and speeds healing. Use d-alpha-tocopherol form.
Helpful		
Coenzyme Q10	60 mg daily.	Valuable immune system stimulant. Increases cellular oxygenation.
Colloidal silver	As directed on label.	A natural antibiotic.
Dimethylsulfoxide (DMSO)	As directed on label.	Relieves pain and strengthens the immune system. Use only DMSO from a health food store.
Garlic (Kyolic from Wakunaga)	2 capsules 3 times daily.	An immune system stimulant that helps to keep infection in check.
Methylsulfonyl-methane (MSM)	As directed on label.	Use for pain relief and to reduce inflammation.

Proteolytic enzymes (Novenzyme from International Health Products)	As directed on label. Take with meals and between meals.	Destroys free radicals. Also aids in digestion of foods.
Pycnogenol or grape seed extract	As directed on label. As directed on label.	Powerful antioxidants that reduce inflammation and the frequency of colds and flu, and neutralize allergic reactions.
Sea mussel	As directed on label.	Provides needed amino acids and aids in the functioning of the mucous membranes. Reduces inflammation.
Zinc lozenges	1 15-mg lozenge every 2–4 waking hours for 1 week. Do not exceed this amount.	Antiviral agent and immunity booster.

HERBS

❑ Anise, fenugreek, marshmallow, and red clover help to loosen phlegm and clear congestion.

❑ Bayberry is a decongestant and astringent.

❑ Bitter orange oil can be used to swab nasal passages for local relief.

❑ Cat's Claw Defense Complex from Source Naturals contains a combination of herbs designed to strengthen the body and help the body deal with outside elements.
Caution: Do not use cat's claw during pregnancy.

❑ ClearLungs from RidgeCrest Herbals contains Chinese herbal ingredients to restore free breathing, ease mucus accumulation, and enhance tissue repair. Echinacea boosts the immune system and fights viral infection.

❑ Fenu-Thyme from Nature's Way Products relieves nasal and sinus congestion. Take 2 capsules three times daily. P.S.I. from Terra Maxa is also good.

❑ Ginger root can be crushed and applied as a poultice to the forehead and nose to stimulate circulation and drainage.

❑ Goldenseal is effective in combating sinusitis. Its benefits can be enhanced by combining it with 250 to 500 milligrams of bromelain, an enzyme present in fresh pineapple. Goldenseal can be taken as a tea, or the tea can be used as an intranasal douche. Or put a dropperful of alcohol-free goldenseal extract in your mouth, swish it around for a few minutes, then swallow. Do this three times daily.
Caution: Do not take goldenseal internally on a daily basis for more than one week at a time, do not use it during pregnancy, and use it with caution if you are allergic to ragweed.

❑ Horehound helps to relieve symptoms.

❑ Mullein reduces inflammation and soothes irritation.

❑ Nettle is good for all types of allergies and respiratory problems.

❑ Olive leaf extract has antibacterial and anti-inflammatory properties.

❑ Rose hips are a good source of vitamin C.

RECOMMENDATIONS

❑ Eat a diet consisting of 75 percent raw foods.

❑ Drink plenty of distilled water and fresh vegetable and fruit juices. Also consume plenty of hot liquids such as soups and herbal teas. These help the mucus to flow, relieving congestion and sinus pressure. Adding cayenne pepper, garlic, ginger, horseradish, and raw onion to soups or teas may bring even faster relief.

❑ Eliminate sugar from your diet. Reduce your salt intake.

❑ Do not eat dairy foods, except for low-fat soured products like yogurt and cottage cheese. Dairy products increase mucus formation.

❑ Go on a cleansing fast. (*See* FASTING in Part Three.)

❑ Mix a solution of 1 cup warm water, 1/2 teaspoon of sea salt, and a pinch of bicarbonate of soda. Use a squeeze spray bottle (available over the counter in drugstores) or an eyedropper to instill the solution in the nostrils, one side at a time. Repeat this procedure three or four times a day as necessary for relief from stuffiness.

❑ Try using a menthol or eucalyptus pack applied over the sinuses to relieve pain and swelling. Stop if the packs cause irritation.

❑ Use a vaporizer to ease breathing and clear secretions.

❑ Use steam inhalations to promote drainage and ease pressure. Boil a pot of water and add a few drops of eucalyptus oil or rosemary oil. Remove the pot from the heat and lean your face over it at a distance of about 6 inches to inhale the steam. (Be careful not to get so close that irritation or scalding results.) Place a towel over your head to capture the steam and breathe in deeply. Do this several times daily for five to ten minutes at a time. Or simply take a hot shower to help relieve the pain and pressure of sinusitis.

You can also use a Neti pot, a small teapot-like device especially designed for nasal irrigation. They are available in many health food stores. Fill the pot with sea salt and water (2 teaspoons salt to one pint water) and rinse out your nose with this solution. This should reduce inflammation and congestion.

❑ Use warm compresses or ice packs to help relieve pain (experiment to see which works best for you).

❑ Try homeopathic remedies to alleviate symptoms. *Belladonna* is good for infections accompanied by fever and pain in the face and forehead. *Kali bichromicum* is useful if there is an overabundance of mucus in the throat.

❑ If you are taking antibiotics for a sinus infection, be sure to add an acidophilus supplement to your program. Do not take the acidophilus and the antibiotic at the same time.

❑ If you use decongestants, use them only as directed and

for the prescribed amount of time. If possible, avoid using nose drops and sprays. These can become addictive and interfere with normal sinus function. In addition, drops and sprays, as well as inhalers, can shrink blood vessels in the nose, eventually causing the vessels to weaken. Moreover, withdrawal from decongestants can cause a rebound effect, in which the swelling becomes worse after use is discontinued than it was to begin with. They can also cause dangerous elevations in blood pressure. Do not use these medications if you have high blood pressure or heart problems.

❏ If sinusitis causes your eyes to become swollen, red, or itchy, or to begin tearing, try a product called OcuDyne. Made by NutriCology, this is a complex containing vitamins, minerals, antioxidants, key amino acids, active bioflavonoids, and the herbs bilberry and ginkgo biloba to protect the eyes and boost immune function.

❏ Do not use force when blowing your nose, as this forces mucus back into the sinus cavities. Instead, draw secretions to the back of the throat by sniffing, then expel them.

❏ Do not smoke, and avoid secondhand smoke. If you live in a smoggy area, consider getting an air purifier or moving to a less polluted area. The Living Air XL-15 from Alpine Industries is an air purification unit for home use. Air Supply from Wein Products is a personal air purifier. Worn around the neck, it sets up a defensive shield against microorganisms and microparticles in the air wherever you go.

❏ If you notice swelling around the eyes, consult your physician. This is a serious sign.

❏ Have regular dental examinations. Infections in the mouth can easily spread to the sinuses.

CONSIDERATIONS

❏ If nasal secretions turn clear after a week, you probably do not have an infection; if the mucus is greenish or yellowish, you probably do. If secretions are clear and you have no other symptoms of a cold, you probably have allergies.

❏ Antibiotics may be necessary to clear a bacterial infection. Always take antibiotics for the full course prescribed, even if symptoms seem to improve earlier. Stopping prematurely can lead to antibiotic-resistant bacteria and a worse infection.

❏ Sometimes physicians prescribe antibiotics even if they cannot confirm a bacterial infection. The reasoning for this is that it is very difficult to ascertain whether bacteria are causing the sinusitis, and that it may be worth it to prevent a bacterial infection from appearing later. As with any medication, it is important to know the benefits, risks, and costs of using and of not using an antibiotic.

❏ If sinus trouble is chronic and severe, and medication fails to relieve it, surgery may be needed to drain the si-

nuses, not only to relieve discomfort but to guard against serious consequences.

❏ Endoscopic surgery, a treatment sometimes recommended for chronic, severe sinusitis, clears nasal passages without external incisions or scars. The procedure can be performed using local anesthesia and results in minimal pain and swelling.

❏ While they are uncommon, polyps and benign cysts that retain mucus can develop in the sinuses, especially in the large maxillary or frontal sinuses. Intrusive or malignant growths require surgical removal.

❏ Anyone suffering from unremitting sinusitis should consult a health care provider to rule out an underlying immune dysfunction. In a University of Miami study, 50 percent of chronic sinusitis patients were found to be suffering from immunological disorders.

Skin Cancer

Skin cancer affects more people in the United States than any other form of cancer. It is estimated that 600,000 Americans are diagnosed with skin cancer every year. There are several different types of skin cancer. The two most common skin cancers are *basal cell carcinoma* and *squamous cell carcinoma*. Both are highly curable if treated early. The third major type of skin cancer is *malignant melanoma*, which is a more serious disease.

Basal cell carcinoma is the most common of the three major types of skin cancer. It is most prevalent in blond, fair-skinned people. Unlike many other malignant growths, it does not spread until it has been present for a long period of time. The cell damage results in an ulcerlike growth that spreads slowly as it destroys tissue. A large pearly-looking lump, most often on the face by the nose, neck, or ears, is usually the first sign. About six weeks after it appears, the lump becomes ulcerated, with a raw, moist center and a hard border that may bleed. Scabs continually form over the ulcer and then come off, but the ulcer never really heals. Sometimes basal cell carcinomas show up on the back or chest as flat sores that grow slowly. Basal cell carcinomas do not usually spread thoughout the body and generally are curable. However, recurrences are common. If they are not treated, they can do substantial damage to the lower layers of skin and bone.

In squamous cell carcinoma, the underlying skin cells are damaged, and this leads to the development of a tumor or lump under the skin, most often on the ears, hands, face, or lower lip. The lump may resemble a wart or a small ulcerated spot that never heals. This type of skin cancer occurs most frequently in fair-skinned people over fifty years old. The risk is higher for those who have had long-term outdoor employment and for those who reside in sunny climates. This is a very treatable type of skin cancer if it is detected and dealt with in the early stages.

Malignant melanoma is rarer than either squamous cell or basal cell carcinoma, but is much more serious. With this type of skin cancer, a tumor arises from the pigment-producing cells of the deeper layers of the skin. It is estimated that as many as half of all cases of melanoma originate in moles. People in some families seem to have a genetically based higher risk of developing melanoma. They often have odd moles, called *dysplastic nevi,* that are irregular in shape and color and can be as large as half an inch in diameter. Dysplastic nevi may be precursors to skin cancer. This cancer can also appear in the form of a new mole. In men, melanomas tend to occur anywhere from the neck to the waist; in women, the arms and legs seem to be affected most.

If not treated at an early stage, melanoma can be life threatening, spreading through the bloodstream and lymphatic vessels to the internal organs. However, if the disease is treated early, the chances of recovery are quite good.

There are four types of melanoma, each with slightly different characteristics:

• *Superficial spreading melanoma* (SSM) is the most common type. It occurs primarily in Caucasians and more often in women than in men. An SSM lesion typically begins as a flat mole, most often on the lower legs or upper back, that develops a raised, irregular surface. As it grows, its borders usually become asymmetrical and notched.

• *Acral lentiginous melanoma* is most common among people of African and Asian descent. The lesions have flat dark-brown areas with bumpy portions that are brown-black or blue-black in color. They are most likely to appear on the palms of the hands, the soles of the feet, the nailbeds of fingers and toes, and the mucous membranes.

• *Lentigo maligna melanoma* is more common in women than in men. The lesions usually occur on the face, neck, ears, or other areas that have been heavily sun-exposed for a long period of time. This type of melanoma rarely occurs before the age of fifty, and it is usually preceded by a precancerous stage called *lentigo maligna* that appears years in advance of the melanoma.

• *Nodular melanoma* is a type of disease that attacks the underlying tissue without first spreading across the surface of the skin. It is more common in men than in women. The lesions may resemble blood blisters, and they may range in coloration from pearly white to blue-black. Nodular melanoma tends to metastasize (spread to other sites in the body) sooner than the other types of melanoma.

Melanoma tends to progress through four different stages of melonoma. The so-called *TNM system* is often used to describe these stages: T stands for the existence of a *t*umor; N represents the fact that the tumor has spread to the lymph *n*odes; and M stands for *m*etastasis, or spread of the cancer to other places in the body. The four stages are the following:

• *Stage one.* The cancer is found in the top of the inner layer of skin but has not spread.

• *Stage two.* The cancer has spread into the inner layer of skin but not yet into the lymph nodes.

• *Stage three.* The tumor has spread to body tissue beneath the skin's outer and inner layers. There may be additional tumors near the site of the original tumor. The cancer may have spread to the lymph nodes near the tumor.

• *Stage four.* The cancer has spread to other parts of the body, away from the original site of the melonoma.

Overexposure to the sun's ultraviolent (UV) rays is the major factor in basal cell carcinoma, squamous cell carcinoma, and melanoma. These rays disrupt the genetic material in the skin cells, causing tissue damage. They also harm the skin's normal repair mechanism. Normally, after UV exposure, this mechanism causes damaged cells to immediately cease reproducing, die, and be sloughed off to be replaced by new, healthy skin cells—this is why skin peels after a sunburn. If this repair system is impaired, damaged cells may continue to reproduce, and the skin becomes increasingly vulnerable to injury from subsequent exposure to UV rays. Sun exposure is not only the major cause of wrinkles; it is responsible for 90 percent of most forms of skin cancer. People who have had severe or blistering sunburns, especially in childhood, are twice as likely to develop the disease later in life. People with blond or red hair, blue or green eyes, and fair skin, who sunburn or freckle easily, are at the greatest risk for skin cancer, because they have less protective pigment in their skin. One sign that cumulative sun damage may have reached dangerous levels is the development of spots called *actinic* or *solar keratoses.* Considered precancerous lesions, these appear most often in and around the face, neck, and head, and take the form of rough bumps or flat patches that may be itchy or tingly. Later, these spots may become hard to the touch and grayish or brown in color. Although these abnormalities may not be dangerous in themselves, they should be evaluated and, if need be, treated, as they can develop into more serious skin cancers.

In addition to the three major types of skin cancer, there are a number of other, less common types of cancer that affect the skin. *Mycosis fungoides* is technically a type of lymphoma (lymphatic cancer), but its main effects are on the skin. Initially, it appears as an itchy rash that may last for several years. Over time, the lesions spread, become firmer, and ulcerate. Eventually, if untreated, the disease may spread to the lymph nodes and other internal organs. Mycosis fungoides is a rare, slow-growing cancer that can be difficult to diagnose, especially early in the disease. A skin biopsy should make correct diagnosis possible.

A type of skin cancer that has become increasingly common in recent years is *Kaposi's sarcoma.* This type of cancer causes raised lesions that may be pink, red, brown, or purplish in color. They may appear anywhere on the body, but the most common sites are the legs, toes, upper torso, and mucous membranes. Kaposi's sarcoma was once a rare, very slowly progressing disease seen primarily in older men of Mediterranean descent. Since the AIDS epidemic began, however, it is no longer uncommon and is primarily associated with a poorly functioning immune system. People with AIDS tend to get a more aggressive variety of this cancer that eventually affects the lymph nodes and other internal organs.

In recent years, the incidence of skin cancer has been rising steadily, and the average age of people with skin cancer has been getting lower. Women under forty are developing the disease twice as fast as men in the same age group. Fortunately, skin cancer is quite curable when treated early. More than 90 percent of all cases of skin cancer are completely cured.

NUTRIENTS

SUPPLEMENT	SUGGESTED DOSAGE	COMMENTS
Essential		
Beta-1,3-D-glucan	As directed on label.	Can stimulate immune cells to digest cellular debris.
Coenzyme Q₁₀ plus Coenzyme A from Coenzyme-A Technologies	100 mg daily.	Improves cellular oxygenation.
Dimethylglycine (DMG) (Aangamik DMG from FoodScience of Vermont)	As directed on label.	Improves cellular oxygenation.
Essential fatty acids (primrose oil)	As directed on label 3 times daily, before meals.	For cellular protection.
Garlic (Kyolic from Wakunaga)	2 capsules 3 times daily.	Enhances immune function.
Histidine	As directed on label.	Is said to increase the skin's immunity to damage from the sun's rays.
Proteolytic enzymes or Wobenzym N from Marlyn Nutraceuticals	As directed on label. Take with meals. 3–6 tablets 2–3 times daily, between meals.	Powerful free radical scavengers that also reduce inflammation and aid in proper breakdown from foods.
Quercetin	As directed on label.	A flavonoid that has antioxidant properties.
Selenium	200 mcg daily. If you are pregnant, do not exceed 40 mcg daily.	Powerful free radical scavenger. Protects against UV damage.
Superoxide dismutase (SOD)	As directed on label.	Destroys free radicals. Consider injections (under a doctor's supervision).
Vitamin A plus natural beta-carotene and carotenoid complex (Betatene)	10,000–50,000 IU daily for 10 days or for as long as you are on the program. If you are pregnant, do not exceed 10,000 IU daily. 15,000 IU daily. As directed on label.	Powerful antioxidants that destroy free radicals. Use emulsion form for easier assimilation and greater safety at high doses. Precursor of vitamin A.

SUPPLEMENT	SUGGESTED DOSAGE	COMMENTS
Vitamin B complex and/or brewer's yeast	100 mg of each major B vitamin daily (amounts of individual vitamins in a complex will vary). 2 20-grain tablets 3 times daily.	Necessary for normal cell division and function. A good source of B vitamins.
Vitamin C with bioflavonoids	5,000–20,000 mg daily, in divided doses. (*See* ASCORBIC ACID FLUSH in Part Three.)	Powerful anti-cancer agent. Boosts immunity.
Vitamin E	Up to 1,000 IU daily.	Promotes healing and tissue repair. Use d-alpha-tocopherol form.
Important		
Maitake extract or reishi extract or shiitake extract	4,000–8,000 mg daily. As directed on label. As directed on label.	These mushrooms contain substances that inhibit the growth and spread of cancerous tumors and also boost immune response.
Phytocharged nutritional supplements from Schiff	As directed on label.	Dietary supplements that protect against damage from sunlight and promote health.
Pycnogenol or grape seed extract	As directed on label. As directed on label.	Antioxidants that protect against UV-induced oxidative changes in skin.
Shark cartilage (BeneFin)	1 gm per 2 lbs of body weight daily, divided into 3 doses. If you cannot tolerate taking it orally, it can be administered rectally in a retention enema.	Has been shown to inhibit and even reverse the growth of some types of tumors. Also stimulates the immune system.
Zinc	As directed on label.	Important in activity of enzymes; cell division, growth, and repair; and proper immune function. Use zinc gluconate lozenges or zinc methionate (OptiZinc) for best absorption.
Helpful		
Acidophilus	As directed on label. Take on an empty stomach.	Has an antibacterial effect on the body. Use a nondairy formula.
Aerobic 07 from Aerobic Life Industries or Dioxychlor from American Biologics	As directed on label. As directed on label.	Antimicrobial agents.
ConcenTrace from Trace Minerals Research	As directed on label.	To nourish skin and hair.
Dimethylsulfoxide (DMSO)	Apply topically as directed on label.	Promotes healing. Use only DMSO from a health food store.
Herpanacine from Diamond-Herpanacine Associates	As directed on label.	Contains antioxidants, amino acids, and herbs that promote skin health.
Kelp	1,000–1,500 mg daily.	For mineral balance. Use kelp in tablet form and/or eat sea vegetables.
L-Cysteine and L-methionine	As directed on label, on an empty stomach. Take with water or juice. Do not take with milk. Take with 50 mg vitamin B₆ and 100 mg vitamin C for better absorption.	To detoxify harmful substances. (*See* AMINO ACIDS in Part One.)

Multienzyme complex	As directed on label. Take with meals.	To aid digestion.
Multivitamin and mineral complex	As directed on label, with meals.	All nutrients are necessary in balance. Do not use a sustained-release formula.
N-A-G from Source Naturals	As directed on label.	Supplies glucosamine, which helps in the formation of mucous membrane and connective tissues.
Para-aminobenzoic acid (PABA)	25 mg daily.	Helps to protect against skin cancer.
Raw glandular complex plus raw thymus glandular	As directed on label. As directed on label.	Stimulates glandular function, especially the thymus, an important component of the immune system.
Taurine	As directed on label.	Functions as foundation for tissue and organ repair.
Vitamin B$_3$ (niacin) plus choline and folic acid	100 mg daily. Do not exceed this amount. 500–1,000 mg daily. 400 mcg daily.	B vitamins that improve circulation, build red blood cells, and aid liver function. Caution: Do not take niacin if you have a liver disorder, gout, or high blood pressure.
Vitamin B$_{12}$ injections or vitamin B$_{12}$	As prescribed by physician. 1,000 mcg 3 times daily.	To prevent anemia. Injections (under a doctor's supervision) are best. If injections are not available, use a lozenge or sublingual form.

HERBS

❏ Alfalfa, burdock, dandelion root, horsetail, Irish moss, marshmallow root, oat straw, rose hips, and yellow dock are all beneficial for tissue repair. Rose hips are also a good source of vitamin C.

❏ Astragalus generates anticancer cells in the body and boosts the immune system.

❏ Bilberry, cayenne (capsicum), ginger, goldenseal, nettle, sarsaparilla, and turmeric stimulate the liver and help to stabilize blood composition, and may retard the proliferation of cancer cells.

❏ Burdock root and red clover aid in cleansing the blood and lymph nodes.

❏ The seeds and peel of the Chinese cucumber inhibit cancer cells.

❏ Skin cancers may respond to treatment with poultices combining comfrey, pau d'arco, ragwort, and wood sage. (See USING A POULTICE in Part Three.)

❏ Ginkgo biloba, pau d'arco, and curcumin (a naturally occurring pigment isolated from turmeric) are powerful antioxidants with immune-enhancing capabilities.

❏ Studies have shown that green tea has anticancer properties. Drink 4 cups daily.

❏ Tea tree oil cream, applied topically, is a natural antiseptic and antifungal that enhances healing.

RECOMMENDATIONS

❏ Eat a diet that is low in fat and high in antioxidants, such as beta-carotene–rich carrots, sweet potatoes, squash, and spinach; cruciferous vegetables such as broccoli, Brussels sprouts, cabbage, kale, and turnips; and citrus fruits.

❏ Be aware of the warning signs of skin cancer:

• An open sore that bleeds, crusts over, and does not heal properly.

• A reddish, irritated spot, usually on the chest, shoulder, arm, or leg. It may itch or hurt, or cause no discomfort.

• A smooth growth with an elevated border and an indented center. As it becomes bigger, tiny blood vessels develop on the surface.

• A shiny scarlike area that is white, yellow, or waxy, with a shiny, taut appearance.

• An enlarging, irregular, "angry-looking" lesion on the face, lips, or ears.

❏ Examine your skin regularly. The Skin Cancer Foundation recommends performing a full-body self-examination every three months. To do this, you need a full-length mirror, a hand-held mirror, and ample lighting. Look for any changes in any moles or marks on your body, using the following A-B-C-D checklist:

• **A**ssymetry. Both sides of the mole should be shaped similarly.

• **B**order. The edges of moles should be smooth, not blurred or ragged.

• **C**olor. Tan, brown, and dark brown are normal. Red, white, blue, and black are not.

• **D**iameter. Any mole that is larger than $\frac{1}{4}$ inch in diameter, or whose diameter seems to be increasing, is suspicious.

In addition to keeping track of moles, look carefully for other unusual spots or growths. Any irregularities you find should be evaluated by a dermatologist.

❏ Stay away from tanning salons. Their equipment is sometimes said to be safer than the sun because tanning beds emit ultraviolet-A (UVA) rays, the so-called cool rays, rather than the ultraviolet-B (UVB) rays, which are most often implicated in sunburn. It has been established, however, that UVA rays can cause skin cancer as well as UVB rays can. Do not be misled by claims to the contrary. The essential differences between UVA and UVB rays are that UVA rays are more likely to penetrate deeper into the skin, and are more likely to lead to skin damage such as wrinkling and collagen damage and, perhaps, melanoma. UVB rays are more likely to burn the top layer of skin and cause skin cancers such as basal and squamous cell cancers, are at their strongest at low and high altitudes, and have a shorter wavelength than UVA rays.

❏ Beware of new moles that appear after age forty, as well as any mole that appears unusual; is irregularly shaped or changes in size or color; is pearly white, translucent, black, or multicolored; has a ridge around the edge; spreads, bleeds, or itches; or is constantly irritated by clothing. Check for discharge from moles. Have any suspicious mole evaluated by a professional.

❏ See your health care provider if you find a growth that fits any of the descriptions in this section. Early detection is the key to successful treatment of skin cancer.

❏ Include in the diet plenty of foods that are high in vitamin E. A diet rich in vitamin E may protect your skin against damage from UV rays. Good food sources of vitamin E include asparagus, green leafy vegetables, raw nuts, wheat germ, and organic, cold-pressed vegetable oils.

❏ To protect against skin cancer, take protective measures while in the sun. The sun's ultraviolet rays are strongest between 10:00 A.M. and 3:00 P.M. Stay out of the sun as much as possible between these hours. When spending time outdoors, wear light-colored clothing made of tightly woven material (you can buy clothing made of materials that act as a sun block) plus a hat and sunglasses that block ultraviolet rays. Always use sunscreen. Choose a product with a sun protection factor (SPF) of 15 or higher and that specifies *broad-spectrum* protection. Even if a sunscreen is water-resistant, you should reapply it every three or four hours for as long as you are outside—more often if you go swimming or if you are perspiring heavily. (Sunscreens can claim only to be water *resistant*, not water*proof*.) Wear sunscreen on cloudy days; nearly 85 percent of the sun's UV rays penetrate through clouds. Apply sunscreen to all exposed skin, and reapply it every three or four hours while you are outside. Be sure to protect your lips with a lip balm that has an SPF of 15, too.

❏ If you have a family history of melanoma, avoid the sun as much as possible and use a sun block every day. Keep a close watch on any moles or other skin lesions and have them checked regularly by a physician.

❏ Avoid exposure to halogen lighting at close range. Halogen lights also emit UV radiation. The National Foundation for Cancer Research advises maintaining a distance of at least 20 inches from a 20-watt halogen bulb and 3 to 6 feet from 35- to 50-watt bulbs.

CONSIDERATIONS

❏ Skin cancer often originates in moles, but moles are not necessarily a cancer risk. They are extremely common (most people have them), and the overwhelming majority of them do *not* become cancerous.

❏ Medical treatment for skin cancer often involves surgery. Excisional biopsy (removal of the growth for analysis) cures skin cancer in its early stages in about 95 percent of cases. More radical surgery may be necessary if excision is delayed, and if the growth is large, a skin graft may be necessary. Other treatments sometimes used for skin cancer include:

• *Chemical peeling*, in which an acid (either trichloroacetic or phenolic acid) is used to burn off the top layer of the skin. It is used to remove cancers confined to this top skin layer.

• *Cryosurgery*, a method that uses liquid nitrogen to freeze and kill the diseased tissue, which later flakes away. This type of treatment is used frequently for people with bleeding disorders and for those who cannot tolerate anesthesia.

• *Electrosurgery*, in which the cancer is scooped out with a curette (a circular blade) and an electric current burns a border around the site to kill remaining cancer cells.

• *Laser surgery*, in which a laser is used to cut away the damaged tissue and seal off surrounding blood vessels as it goes.

• *Moh's microsurgery*, in which a surgeon shaves off cancerous tissue one thin layer at a time until healthy tissue is reached. Each layer is then examined under a microscope so that the doctor can be assured he or she has gotten all the cancer while taking a minimum of healthy skin. This surgery is most effective for recurrent cancers and for cases in which the tumor is large or the extent of the cancer is unknown.

• *Radiation therapy*, which involves training an x-ray or an electron beam on the diseased area to kill cancerous tissue. This alternative is good for cases in which surgery poses particular risks.

❏ Actinic keratoses may be treated by curettage/electrodesiccation, in which the lesion is scraped and a biopsy is taken, or shave removal or dermabrasion to remove the upper layers of skin.

❏ Seborrheic keratoses are slightly raised, brownish spots on the skin that may appear waxy, scaly, or wartlike. They seem to be stuck on the skin and are most often found on the chest and back. They are harmless—neither cancerous nor precancerous—and appear normally as people age. They result from irregular clumping together, rather than even distribution, of skin pigment. The tendency to develop seborrheic keratoses is inherited. Laypeople can mistake these growths for melanomas. If there is any doubt as to the nature of a spot on the skin, a dermatologist should take a scraping of the area and examine the sample for cancer cells. Treatment, if any is necessary, can include curettage, cryosurgery, chemosurgery, or electrosurgery. Actinic keratoses are flatter and redder than seborrheic keratoses, and are considered a precursor of cancer. They tend to appear on areas of skin that are normally exposed to the sun.

❏ With early detection and treatment, most people recover from skin cancer, but regular checkups are advised for at least the next five years.

❏ The average person incurs between 50 and 80 percent of all sun exposure prior to the age of eighteen. Thus, even though skin cancer is rare in children, the childhood years have a major influence on a person's tendency to develop skin cancer later in life. An infant under the age of six months should never be exposed to direct sunlight or have sunscreen applied to his or her skin. Infants should always be dressed in protective clothing when they are outside. Sunscreen can be used on a baby over six months old (choose a PABA-free formula, preferably one meant for young children), but sun exposure should still be limited, and the child should still be dressed in protective clothing. For toddlers and young children, limit time in the sun and apply sunscreen regularly whenever they are outdoors. Older children should be taught the importance of applying sunscreen regularly—an important lifelong habit.

❏ Certain medications may make the skin more susceptible to sun damage. These include antibiotics, antidepressants, diuretics, antihistamines, sedatives, estrogen, and acne medications such as retinoic acid. Ask your health care provider or pharmacist if any medication that you take might have such an effect.

❏ A study reported in the *Journal of the American Academy of Dermatology* found that well-educated white-collar men have the highest risk of developing melanoma. Researchers surmise that a pattern of many months of little sun exposure (a result of working indoors) with occasional overexposure and sunburn (such as that acquired at sunny resort vacations) may be responsible.

❏ The prescription medication tretinoin (Retin-A) may be able to reverse precancerous sun damage in skin. Skin care products containing alpha-hydroxy acids, which are available over the counter, may have a similar effect, although they are less potent.

❏ The U.S. Food and Drug Administration has approved for marketing as a sun protectant a line of clothing produced by Sun Precautions, Inc., of Seattle. The clothing, which carries an SPF rating of 30, is sold under the brand name Solumbra.

❏ Preliminary research into the potential of beta-carotene, folic acid, retinoic acid, vitamin C, vitamin E, and minerals as inhibitors of skin cancer is encouraging.

❏ Garlic may be effective in fighting basal cell carcinoma by boosting the body's immune response.

❏ There is some doubt about the protective value of sunscreen. Skin cancer rates are still rising, despite steady sunscreen sales. One reason may be that people think that they are adequately protected and stay in the sun too long. Another is that all sunscreens protect against UVB rays, but only some protect against UVA rays. UVB rays are the "burning" rays, so a sunscreen that protects only against UVB takes away an important warning sign. Consequently, people may be overexposing themselves to UVA rays, which do not cause sunburn but have been linked to skin cancer.

❏ A worldwide rise in the incidence of skin cancer has been linked to the destruction of the earth's ozone layer. The ozone layer acts as a protective atmospheric sunscreen. As it becomes thinner and holes develop in it, more of the sun's harmful rays reach the earth.

❏ To increase awareness of the damaging potential of UV radiation, the U.S. Environmental Protection Agency and the National Weather Service have developed the following UV index and exposure guidelines for use in weather reports to help individuals evaluate the level of danger from sun exposure on any given day:

UV Index Number	Danger Level
0–2	minimal
3–4	low
5–6	moderate
7–8	high
9–10+	very high

❏ More information about skin cancer is available from the American Cancer Society (*see* HEALTH AND MEDICAL ORGANIZATIONS in the Appendix).

Skin Problems

See ACNE; AGE SPOTS; ATHLETE'S FOOT; BEDSORES; BOIL; BRUISING; BURNS; CANKER SORES; COLD SORES (FEVER BLISTERS); CORNS AND CALLUSES; DANDRUFF; DERMATITIS; DRY SKIN; HIVES; INSECT BITE; LEG ULCERS; OILY SKIN; PSORIASIS; ROSACEA; SCABIES; SEBACEOUS CYST; SEBORRHEA; SKIN CANCER; SKIN RASH; SUNBURN; VITILIGO; WRINKLES. *See also under* FUNGAL INFECTION; PREGNANCY-RELATED PROBLEMS.

Skin Rash

The skin is the body's largest organ. It consists of three layers—the epidermis (outer layer), the dermis (middle layer), and the subcutaneous layer (inner layer). The skin acts as a shield between the body and the millions of foreign substances that exist in our environment. It also functions as a means of excreting toxins and other substances from the body, as the kidneys and bowels do. As a result, the skin is subject to the development of various bumps and blisters, as well as to changes in color, cracking, dryness, flaking, itching, redness, roughness, scaling, thickening, and a host of other problems.

There are many reasons for skin reactions. Some of the most common include allergies to molds, foods, chemicals, cosmetics, and other substances; insect bites; reactions to plants, such as poison ivy, or fungi; diaper rash; reactions to the sun and wind; reactions to drugs or alcohol; reactions to detergents; reactions to jewelry and fragrances; food allergies; nervous tension; and friction, either from two parts of the body rubbing against each other or from contact with an external agent, such as ill-fitting clothing or shoes.

A rash should not be taken lightly, as it can sometimes be

Common Types of Rashes

The best way to approach treatment for a rash is to eliminate the underlying cause. Following are descriptions of some of the conditions most often responsible for skin rashes. This list is not exhaustive, and it is not meant as a substitute for diagnosis by a qualified health care practitioner. Any rash that persists for longer than one week, that seems to be getting worse, or that is accompanied by other symptoms, such as fever, should be evaluated by a professional.

Cause of Rash	Characteristic Features
Athlete's foot	Inflammation, scaling, cracking, and blisters on the feet, especially between the toes. Burning and/or itching may be severe.
Chickenpox	Crops of small round blisterlike pimples that crust over as they heal. Usually appears first on the torso, following a day or so of fever and headache, and then spreads to the face and extremities. Extremely itchy. Most common in children.
Dermatitis (eczema)	There are several types of dermatitis, including atopic dermatitis, nummular dermatitis, seborrheic dermatitis, and hand dermatitis. General features include patches of scaling, flaking, and thickening skin that may appear anywhere on the body. Skin color in the affected area may change. Itching is common. One type of dermatitis causes round lesions on the limbs.
Food or drug allergy	A flat pink or red rash, with possible swelling and/or itching.
Fungal infection (candida)	Moist, possibly itchy, red patches that may appear anywhere on the body, but are most common in areas where skin surfaces rub together. In babies, an inflamed, shiny diaper rash.
Herpesvirus infection	Painful fluid-filled blisters that erupt periodically around the mouth and/or genitals.
Hives	A rash that usually appears suddenly and can take the form of patches of tiny, goosebump-like spots or red, itchy welts that cover significant areas of the body—or anything in between.
Lyme disease	A red, circular lesion that gradually expands as the center appears to clear up. This may be followed by a rash composed of small raised bumps on the torso. The rash may or may not be accompanied by flu-like symptoms of fever, chills, and nausea.
Measles	A raised red rash that usually begins on the forehead and ears and spreads to the rest of the body. The rash usually follows several days of viral symptoms including fever, cough, sneezing, runny nose, and possibly conjunctivitis. There may be tiny red spots with white centers in the mouth as well.
Mononucleosis	A bumpy red rash accompanied by headache, achiness, low-grade fever, sore throat, and persistent fatigue.
Poison ivy/poison oak/poison sumac	A red, intensely itchy rash with swelling and oozing blisters. If scratched, the rash can spread.
Psoriasis	Silvery, scaly patches that may appear anywhere on the body, but are most common on the scalp, ears, arms, legs, knees, elbows, and back. The rash follows a pattern of periodic flare-ups followed by healing. It may or may not be itchy.
Ringworm	Small, itchy round red spots that grow to be approximately $1/4$ inch in diameter, with scaly, slightly raised borders. They tend to clear in the center as they expand.
Rosacea	Reddening, small bumps, and pimples, usually affecting the nose and the center of the face. It resembles acne, but is chronic and is more common in middle-aged and older individuals.
Scabies	A persistent itchy rash with small red lumps that may become dry and scaly. Fine, wavy dark lines may emanate from some lumps. Most often occurs between the fingers, on the wrists and/or forearms, and on the breasts and/or genitals.
Seborrhea	Greasy yellowish, flaky patches of skin that form scales and crusts. It can appear anywhere on the body, but most often affects the scalp, face, and/or chest. It may or may not be itchy.
Shingles	Crops of tiny blisters that are extremely painful and sensitive to the touch and that eventually crust, scab, and are shed. Most common on the abdomen below the ribs, but it can occur anywhere on the body. May be preceded and/or accompanied by flu-like symptoms of chills, fever, and achiness.

an indication of an underlying illness—sometimes a potentially serious illness. Certain types of rashes can be valuable as early warning signals.

Unless otherwise stated, the dosages recommended here are for adults. For a child between the ages of twelve and seventeen, reduce the dose to three-quarters of the recommended amount. For a child between the ages of six and twelve, use one-half the recommended dose, and for a child under six, use one-quarter of the recommended amount.

NUTRIENTS

SUPPLEMENT	SUGGESTED DOSAGE	COMMENTS
Bee pollen	As directed on label.	Has antioxidant properties that can aid in healing.
Beta 1,3-D glucan	As directed on label.	Can attack organisms that do not belong on the body, including bacteria, viruses, and fungi.
Colloidal silver	As directed on label.	A powerful antibiotic that has been shown to be effective in fighting many skin rashes.
Grape seed extract	As directed on label.	Has antioxidant properties that can aid in healing.
Vitamin A and	As directed on label.	Vitamins that are thought to improve the health of the skin.
vitamin C and	As directed on label.	
vitamin E plus	As directed on label.	
niacinamide and	As directed on label.	
panthenol	As directed on label.	

HERBS

❏ Aloe vera gel, ginkgo biloba extract, and green tea extract have antioxidant properties that can aid in healing.

❏ Calendula, chamomile, elder flower, and tea tree oil can be used externally as a soothing wash on rashes.

❏ A poultice made with chaparral, dandelion, and yellow dock root benefits many types of skin rashes. (See USING A POULTICE in Part Three.)

❏ Itch Relief Lotion from Derma-E Products contains chamomile, tea tree oil, and vitamin E. It offers quick relief of skin irritation.

❏ Soak a washcloth in malva tea and apply it as a warm compress to the infected area to reduce inflammation.

❏ Oat straw may be used topically in a bath to reduce symptoms, especially inflammation and itching.

❏ Olive leaf extract has healing properties for the skin.

RECOMMENDATIONS

❏ For quick relief of itching and inflammation, soak a clean cloth in cool water (or, for even greater soothing effect, in comfrey tea that has cooled), wring it out, and apply it to the affected area for ten minutes. Repeat this procedure as often as necessary for relief.

❏ Take lukewarm showers instead of baths, and try not to shower every day during the duration of the rash. Also avoid using the same washcloth, sponge, or shower pouf each time you shower, as bacteria and fungi can grow in these moist areas.

❏ Whenever possible, use hypoallergenic skin care products, deodorants, shaving creams, soaps, hair products, cosmetics, household products, and laundry detergents. Keep in mind, however, that *hypoallergenic* means only that a product *is not likely to* cause allergies; not that it *will not*. Also, when choosing products, look for "fragrance-free" formulas rather than an "unscented" one.

❏ Wear cool, loose clothing. Next to the skin, cotton is best.

❏ Avoid prolonged contact with known skin irritants including chemicals, dust, direct sunlight, and water.

❏ Radiation and chemotherapy treatments can cause skin to become more sensitive to allergens and irritants. Occasionally, radiation can also cause the skin to thin, lose elasticity, and become lighter or darker in color. Emollients and high-SPF sunscreens should be used generously on affected areas.

❏ Many medications cause skin rashes in people when they are exposed to sunlight. If your medication causes photosensitivity, ask your doctor if there are any alternatives.

❏ *See* Common Types of Rashes on page 633 to help you identify possible causes of a rash, and refer to the appropriate sections in Part Two for advice on treatment.

CONSIDERATIONS

❏ Four of the most serious diseases in which skin rash is an early warning signal are Rocky Mountain spotted fever, meningococcal disease, staphylococcal toxic shock syndrome, and streptococcal toxic shock syndrome.

❏ Skin rashes in children are often caused by food allergies, especially to chocolate, dairy products, eggs, peanuts, milk, wheat, fish, chicken, pork, or beef. Some experts estimate that allergies to eggs, peanuts, and milk account for as many as 75 percent of all skin rashes in children.

❏ Many doctors recommend hydrocortisone cream for minor irritations, poison ivy, itchy insect bites, and diaper rash. The use of antihistamines and antibiotics are also common treatments prescribed by doctors for various types of rashes. In severe cases, a doctor may prescribe an oral steroid (such as prednisone, prednisolone, or hydrocortisone) or the use of phototherapy (procedures involve the use of ultraviolet radiation).

❏ Allergy testing is advised, particularly for persistent rashes. (*See* ALLERGIES in Part Two.)

❏ *See also* ACNE; ALLERGIES; ATHLETE'S FOOT; CANDIDIASIS; CHEMICAL ALLERGIES; CHICKENPOX; DERMATITIS; ENVIRONMENTAL TOXICITY; FUNGAL INFECTION; GANGRENE; HER-

PESVIRUS INFECTION; HIVES; INSECT BITE; LUPUS; LYME DISEASE; MEASLES; MONONUCLEOSIS; POISON IVY/POISON OAK/POISON SUMAC; PSORIASIS; RHEUMATIC FEVER; ROSACEA; SCABIES; SEBORRHEA; SHINGLES (HERPES ZOSTER); VITILIGO; and/or WARTS, all in Part Two.

Sleep Problems

See under INSOMNIA; NARCOLEPSY.

Smoking Dependency

Every time a person smokes, he or she inhales over 4,000 different chemicals, including nicotine. Nicotine, which is extremely addictive, increases levels of the pleasure-inducing brain chemicals serotonin, dopamine, and norepinephrine. Tobacco has been used as a mood-altering substance for centuries. It has been ingested by various means, including chewing, sniffing, and smoking. Today it is most commonly consumed by smoking cigarettes.

Nicotine acts as a stimulant on the central nervous system; when nicotine is ingested, adrenaline production increases, raising the blood pressure and heart rate. Nicotine also affects the overall metabolic rate, the regulation of body temperature, the degree of tension in the muscles, and the levels of certain hormones. These and other metabolic changes create a pleasurable sensation in the user that often—and paradoxically—is experienced as a feeling of relaxation. This pleasurable sensation is one of the factors that makes tobacco so addictive. Another is the fact that tolerance to the effects of nicotine develops quite rapidly. That is, the dose needed to achieve the desired effect begins to rise almost immediately, encouraging you to increase the amount you smoke—which in turn increases the likelihood of addiction. Once you become addicted, your body depends on the presence of nicotine. If you then refrain from smoking, withdrawal symptoms occur. These include irritability, frustration, anger, anxiety, difficulty concentrating, restlessness, increased appetite, headache, stomach cramps, a slowed heart rate, a rise in blood pressure, and, most of all, an intense craving for nicotine.

Once the smoking habit has been acquired, it is difficult to break. Some authorities have stated that addiction to tobacco may be harder to overcome than addiction to heroin or cocaine. This is because smoking creates both physical *and* psychological dependency. It may be easier to overcome the physical addiction than the psychological dependency. Acute physical withdrawal, while unpleasant, lasts for a limited period of time, usually no more than several weeks. Long-term cravings are more likely a matter of

psychological dependency, and require an ongoing effort to master. By the time an individual has become addicted to nicotine, the act of smoking itself has become a source of pleasure, and it may be so intertwined in your mind with other activities—having your morning coffee, reading the newspaper, working, socializing, whatever—that you find yourself unable to imagine engaging in these activities without a cigarette in hand. In addition, smoking provides a convenient excuse for taking a momentary break, especially during times of stress, and may help to smooth over awkward moments. Many smokers also are afraid of what might happen if they stopped; they fear withdrawal symptoms, weight gain, or a decreased ability to concentrate. All of these factors combine to make quitting difficult.

Even though it can be difficult to stop smoking, many people do it every day. There is certainly no shortage of reasons to quit. Cigarettes are a factor in approximately 17 percent of all deaths in the United States annually—that's 350,000 to 400,000 people a year. This is more than the number of deaths from alcohol, illegal drugs, traffic accidents, suicide, and homicide combined. Tobacco smoking causes an estimated 33 percent of all cancer deaths, 25 percent of fatal heart attacks, and 85 percent of deaths from chronic obstructive pulmonary disease. It accounts for at least 85 percent of lung cancer cases. Many other health problems have been linked to smoking as well, including angina, arteriosclerosis, cataracts, chronic bronchitis, circulatory ailments, colorectal cancer, diarrhea, emphysema, heartburn, high blood pressure, impotence, peptic ulcers, respiratory ailments, urinary incontinence, and cancers of the mouth and throat, especially among cigarette smokers who also consume alcohol and/or use mouthwash containing alcohol. Smoking increases the risk of catching colds and lengthens recovery time. Tobacco smoke paralyzes the cilia (hairlike protrusions lining the nose and throat), reducing their capacity to clear the passages by moving mucus—and the cold viruses trapped within it—to the outside.

Nicotine has long been known to be a deadly toxin. A single pinhead-sized drop of liquid nicotine, introduced directly into the bloodstream, would be fatal. At the doses normally ingested by smokers, nicotine makes the heart pump faster and work harder, increasing the likelihood of heart disease. It also constricts the peripheral blood vessels, contributing to circulatory disorders such as Raynaud's phenomenon and hardening of the arteries. And nicotine is not the only ingredient in cigarettes that poses a danger to health. In all, over 4,000 chemical substances have been identified as constituents of cigarette smoke, and at least 43 of these substances are known to cause cancer in humans. Cigarette smoke contains carbon monoxide, benzene, cyanide, ammonia, nitrosamines, vinyl chloride, radioactive particles, and other known irritants and carcinogens. Carbon monoxide binds to hemoglobin, interfering with the transport of oxygen throughout the body. Carbon monoxide also promotes the development of cholesterol deposits on artery walls. These two factors increase the risk of heart attack and stroke. Hydrogen cyanide causes bronchitis by inflaming the lining of the bronchi. Over the long term, smoking dramatically reduces flow of blood to the brain. Men who have smoked for years are more likely to have abnormally low penile blood pressure, which contributes to impotence. This is probably because smoking damages the blood vessels, including the tiny blood vessels that supply the penis. It also contributes to sterility; the sperm of men who smoke have less ability than that of nonsmokers to penetrate, and thus to fertilize, an egg.

Female cigarette smokers tend to experience menopause earlier, face a greater risk of osteoporosis after menopause, and have a much higher risk of developing cervical or uterine cancer. They also appear less fertile and have more difficulties during pregnancy. Smokers tend to have more miscarriages, stillbirths, and premature deliveries. Their babies often are smaller and have more health problems than babies of nonsmokers. Infants whose mothers smoke both during pregnancy and after childbirth appear to be three times as likely to die of sudden infant death syndrome (SIDS) as infants of nonsmokers.

Children whose fathers smoke also face an increase in health problems. Children of male smokers have been shown to be at a higher than normal risk of developing brain cancer and leukemia.

Smoking has a detrimental effect on nutrition. Smokers break down vitamin C about twice as fast as nonsmokers. This can deprive the body of adequate amounts of one of the most powerful and versatile antioxidants at our disposal. Other antioxidant vitamins are depleted as well. Cigarette smoke contains high concentrations of nitrogen dioxide ozone, a compound that oxidizes the antioxidant vitamins and is also known to do damage to DNA. The accelerated antioxidant usage, in combination with the DNA damage, speeds the aging process.

Finally, smoking is increasingly a social problem. More and more nonsmokers are becoming concerned about the effects of "secondhand" smoke on their own health, and justifiably so. There is a growing body of evidence that secondhand smoke may be even more dangerous than the smoke the smoker breathes. Smoking is now prohibited in many workplaces and public buildings.

The dangers of smoking are well known today, yet people continue to smoke. Why? Some people started smoking before the hazards were widely known; others start in adolescence, when people generally feel invulnerable and are more likely to engage in risk-taking behavior—especially if it seems "adult," helps them fit in with a particular social group, and/or provokes their parents. However, surveys consistently show that no matter when or why they started, most current smokers do not smoke because they want to (well over 50 percent say they wish they had never started), but because they are addicted.

The good news is that this addiction can be overcome, and that health benefits begin almost immediately. In just twenty-four hours after your last cigarette, your blood pressure and pulse rate should return to normal, as should the levels of oxygen and carbon monoxide in your blood. Within a week, your risk of heart attack begins to decrease, your senses of smell and taste improve, and breathing becomes easier.

The nutrients and dietary suggestions below are recommended to correct probable smoking-related deficiencies and damage while you work to kick the habit. They are recommended also if you cannot avoid being a passive smoker.

Unless otherwise stated, the dosages recommended here are for adults. For a child between the ages of twelve and seventeen, reduce the dose to three-quarters of the recommended amount.

NUTRIENTS

SUPPLEMENT	SUGGESTED DOSAGE	COMMENTS
Essential		
Coenzyme Q$_{10}$	200 mg twice daily.	Aids oxygen flow to the brain; protects heart tissue. Also acts as an antioxidant to protect cells and the lungs.
plus Coenzyme A from Coenzyme-A Technologies	As directed on label.	Works well with coenzyme Q$_{10}$ to rid the body of toxic substances.
Oxy-5000 Forte from American Biologics	2 tablets 3 times daily.	A powerful antioxidant. Destroys free radicals produced in the smoke.
Pycnogenol or grape seed extract	As directed on label.	Helps to protect and repair the lungs.
Vitamin B complex	100 mg of each major B vitamin daily (amounts of individual vitamins in a complex will vary).	Necessary in cellular enzyme systems often damaged in smokers. Use sublingual form.
plus extra vitamin B$_{12}$	1,000 mcg twice daily.	Increases energy; needed for liver function. Use a lozenge or sublingual form.
and folic acid	400 mcg daily.	Needed for the formation of red blood cells; important for healthy cell division and replication.
Vitamin C with bioflavonoids	5,000–20,000 mg daily. (*See* ASCORBIC ACID FLUSH in Part Three.)	Important antioxidant that protects against cell damage. Smoking drastically depletes the body of vitamin C.
Vitamin E	Start with 200 IU daily and increase by 200 IU each month, up to 800 IU daily.	One of the most important antioxidants, needed to protect cells and organs from damage by the smoke. Use d-alpha-tocopherol form.
Very Important		
Vitamin A	25,000 IU daily. If you are pregnant, do not exceed 10,000 IU daily.	Antioxidants that aid in the healing of mucous membranes. Important for lung protection.
and natural beta-carotene	15,000 IU daily.	
plus carotenoid complex (Betatene)	As directed on label.	
Zinc	50–80 mg daily. Do not exceed a total of 100 mg daily from all supplements.	Important in immune function. Use zinc gluconate lozenges or OptiZinc for best absorption.

Helpful		
Body Language Super Antioxidant from Oxyfresh	As directed on label.	Contains antioxidant vitamins and herbs to protect against free radical damage.
Cell Guard from Biotec Foods	As directed on label.	Provides high levels of antioxidant enzymes for cellular health.
Dimethylglycine (DMG) (Aangamik DMG from FoodScience of Vermont)	As directed on label.	Detoxifies the body and helps the body maintain high energy levels.
Herpanacine from Diamond-Herpanacine Associates	As directed on label.	Detoxifies the body, balances the nervous system, and boosts immunity.
L-cysteine and L-methionine and L-cysteine plus	As directed on label, on empty stomach. Take with water or juice. Do not take with milk. Take with 50 mg vitamin B_6 and 100 mg vitamin C for better absorption.	Potent detoxifiers that protect the lungs, liver, brain, and tissues from cigarette smoke.
glutathione	As directed on label.	Protects the liver.
Maitake extract	1,000–4,000 mg daily.	Inhibits carcinogenesis and protects against metastasis through the lungs.
Multivitamin and mineral complex with selenium	As directed on label. 200 mcg daily.	Necessary for immune function. Helps to prevent cell damage.
Raw thymus glandular	As directed on label.	A glandular that improves immune function.

HERBS

❏ Burdock root and red clover help to cleanse the bloodstream of toxins.

❏ Cayenne (capsicum) desensitizes respiratory tract cells to irritants from cigarette smoke.

❏ Catnip, hops, lobelia, skullcap, and/or valerian root can be used to help reduce the nervousness and anxiety that may accompany nicotine withdrawal.

Caution: Do not take lobelia internally on an ongoing basis.

❏ Dandelion root and milk thistle protect the liver against harmful toxins from cigarette smoke.

❏ Ginger causes perspiration, which helps the body to shed some of the poisons ingested through smoking. It also soothes stomach irritation occasionally experienced with the use of cayenne or lobelia.

❏ Slippery elm relieves lung congestion and coughs.

RECOMMENDATIONS

❏ Consume more asparagus, broccoli, Brussels sprouts, cabbage, cauliflower, spinach, sweet potatoes, and turnips. Eat plenty of grains, nuts, seeds, and unpolished brown rice. Millet cereal is a good source of protein. Eat wheat, oat,

and bran. Also consume yellow and deep-orange vegetables such as carrots, pumpkin, squash, and yams. Apples, berries, Brazil nuts, cantaloupe, cherries, grapes, legumes (including chickpeas, lentils, and red beans), and plums are also helpful.

❏ Eat onions and garlic, or take garlic in supplement form.

❏ Drink fresh carrot juice daily as a preventive measure against lung cancer. Also drink fresh beet juice (made from both the roots and the greens) and asparagus juice. All dark-colored juices are good, as are black currants. Also beneficial is apple juice, if it is fresh. Drink fruit juices in the morning and vegetable juices in the afternoon.

❏ Cook all sprouts slightly except for alfalfa sprouts, which should be eaten raw.

❏ *Do not* consume junk foods, processed refined foods, saturated fats, salt, sugar, or white flour. Instead of salt, use a kelp or potassium substitute. If you must, use a *small* amount of blackstrap molasses or pure maple syrup as a natural sweetener in place of sugar. Use whole wheat or rye instead of white flour. Eliminate alcohol, coffee, and all teas except for herbal teas.

❏ Do not eat any animal protein except for broiled fish (up to three servings per week). *Never* eat luncheon meat, hot dogs, or smoked or cured meats. Limit your consumption of dairy products to a little low-fat yogurt, kefir, or raw cheese on an occasional basis.

❏ Do not eat any peanuts. Limit, but do not eliminate altogether, your intake of soybean products; they contain enzyme inhibitors.

❏ Keep in mind that the acute craving for a cigarette usually lasts only three to five minutes. Focusing on this fact may make it easier to wait it out. Also remember that it gets easier and easier as time goes by. When cravings strike, try taking a walk, doing some sit-ups, or engaging in any activity that can momentarily take your mind off cigarettes.

❏ To accelerate toxin elimination, *see* FASTING in Part Three, and follow the program.

❏ Take coffee enemas daily. Use cleansing enemas with lemon and water or garlic and water two or three times weekly. (*See* ENEMAS in Part Three.)

❏ Drink spring or steam-distilled water only.

❏ As much as possible, avoid stress.

❏ If you take any medications, consult with your physician about the possible need for an adjustment in dosage after you quit smoking. Tobacco alters the absorption and utilization of many medications, including insulin, asthma drugs, and certain antidepressants, blood pressure medications, and painkillers.

CONSIDERATIONS

❏ The difficulty of quitting appears to be related less to

how many packs a day you smoke than to how early in life you started smoking.

❏ Many people have been successful in the quest to stop smoking by going on a fast using only live juices and quality steam-distilled water. A live juice fast can quickly remove nicotine and other damaging chemicals from the body. Adhering to a five-day live juice fast can have amazing effects.

❏ There are several natural products on the market that may help you deal with withdrawal symptoms, such as Smoking Withdrawal from Natra-Bio Homeopathic.

❏ A lack of beta-carotene and the B-complex vitamins has been linked to lung and throat cancer.

❏ A study cosponsored by the British and Norwegian governments found that DNA taken from the lungs of female smokers showed significantly more damage than that taken from men. DNA damage is a marker of increased cancer risk.

❏ Research at the University of Indiana found that people who drank six cups of tea a day were protected from the toxic effects cigarette smoke has on the lungs by up to 50 percent.

❏ Research at the University of Toronto suggests that a drug called methoxsalen (8-MOP, Oxsoralen-Ultra), sometimes used to treat psoriasis, may help a smoker reduce the number of cigarettes he or she smokes by blocking an enzyme that causes the body to metabolize nicotine more quickly.

❏ Smoking a pack of cigarettes a day or more triples the risk of needing surgery for a herniated disk, but quitting smoking reduces that risk, according to researchers at the Medical College of Wisconsin.

❏ According to a study reported in the *Archives of Internal Medicine,* smoking increases the risk of developing leukemia by 30 percent.

❏ There are alternative sources of nicotine for those who wish to quit smoking. They are available either in transdermal patch form, as chewing gum, and as nasal sprays and inhalers. Some of these are available over the counter, while others require a prescription.

❏ Buproprion (Zyban) is an antidepressant that acts on the brain in the same manner as nicotine. It can help some people to stop smoking. If you are concerned about gaining weight after you quit, buproprion may help limit the amount of weight you put on.

❏ A diagnostic procedure called a sputum cytology test can sometimes detect the presence of cancer before there are symptoms and before other tests show the disease. In this test, sputum coughed up from the lungs and the bronchial tubes is examined for signs of tumor cells.

❏ There are many different strategies for overcoming smoking dependency. The secret to success may be finding the approach that is right for you. *No If's, And's or Butts, The*

Smoker's Guide to Quitting, by Harlan M. Krumholz and Robert H. Phillips (Avery Publishing Group, 1993), is a comprehensive and detailed guide to the many and varied strategies that have helped people to break the smoking habit. There are also a number of organizations that can provide valuable information and programs to help you quit smoking. Two of the most highly recommended are the American Cancer Society and the American Lung Association (*see* HEALTH AND MEDICAL ORGANIZATIONS in the Appendix).

Snakebite

There are four types of poisonous snakes in the United States: copperheads, coral snakes, cottonmouths (or water moccasins), and rattlesnakes. Approximately 7,000 Americans are bitten by snakes each year, most commonly in the summer months, in grassy or rocky environments. The toxicity of snake venom, which varies from species to species, can kill local tissue and release toxins into the body that can cause serious problems with blood pressure, heart rate, and pain. A person who has been bitten by a poisonous snake may exhibit mild to severe symptoms, which can include swelling or discoloration of the skin in the area of the bite, a racing pulse, weakness, shortness of breath, nausea, and vomiting. In extreme cases, pain and swelling can be severe, the pupils may dilate, and shock and convulsion may occur. The person may twitch and his or her speech may become slurred. In the most severe cases, paralysis, unconsciousness, and death can result.

It is worth emphasizing that the majority of snakes are *not* poisonous. Nevertheless, anyone who has been bitten by a snake should be seen by a professional immediately, because the severity of initial symptoms does not always reflect the seriousness of the bite. After appropriate medical care has been administered, taking the nutrients and following the suggestions outlined here should help alleviate pain and hasten healing. Unless otherwise stated, the dosages recommended here are for adults. For a child between the ages of twelve and seventeen, reduce the dose to three-quarters of the recommended amount. For a child between the ages of six and twelve, use one-half the recommended dose, and for a child under six, use one-quarter of the recommended amount.

NUTRIENTS

SUPPLEMENT	SUGGESTED DOSAGE	COMMENTS
Helpful		
Calcium	500 mg every 4–6 hours until pain begins to ease.	To relieve pain. Acts as a sedative. Use calcium gluconate form.
and magnesium	1,000 mg with the first 500 mg of calcium.	Works with calcium.

Charcoal tablets	8 tablets every 3 hours. Take with a large glass of water. If possible, take immediately after being bitten.	A powerful detoxifying agent.
Colloidal silver	Apply topically as directed on label.	An antiseptic that reduces inflammation and promotes healing of skin sores.
L-Serine	As directed on label, on an empty stomach. Take with water or juice. Do not take with milk. Take with 50 mg vitamin B$_6$ and 100 mg vitamin C for better absorption.	Helps maintain a healthy immune system and aids in the production of antibodies.
Multivitamin and mineral complex	As directed on label.	All nutrients work together to promote health.
Pantothenic acid (vitamin B$_5$)	500 mg every 4 hours for 2 days.	The anti-stress vitamin.
Ultimate Cleanse from Nature's Secret	As directed on label.	A 2-part body cleansing program that detoxifies the organs, blood, and the channels of elimination.
Vitamin A with mixed carotenoids including beta-carotene	10,000 IU daily.	Enhances immunity and promotes tissue healing.
Vitamin C with bioflavonoids	2,000 mg every hour for 5–6 hours, up to a total of 15,000 mg.	A powerful detoxifier. Relieves pain and discomfort and fights infection.
Vitamin E	600 IU daily.	Promotes healing and reduces blood pressure. Use d-alpha-tocopherol form.
Zinc	30 mg daily.	Boosts immune function. Use zinc gluconate lozenges or OptiZinc for best absorption.

HERBS

❑ Black cohosh syrup helps to relieve pain. Take ½ to 1 tablespoon of the syrup three times daily.

❑ Poultices of comfrey, slippery elm, or white oak bark leaves and bark can be used. (*See* USING A POULTICE in Part Three.) Comfrey salve, plantain poultice, or plantain salve can also be used.

❑ Echinacea, taken in tea and/or capsule form, boosts the immune system.

❑ Olive leaf extract has antibacterial properties.

❑ Yellow dock can be used to alleviate symptoms. Drink a cup of yellow dock tea or take 2 capsules of yellow dock every hour until the symptoms are gone.

RECOMMENDATIONS

❑ Call for emergency medical help or go to the nearest hospital emergency room immediately. Until you can get professional help, remain as still as possible, preferably with the injured area just below heart level. Keep warm. Remove any constricting items such as rings and watches in case significant swelling occurs. Place a cool, clean com-

press and damp dressing over the bite to reduce swelling and pain. Monitor the person who has been bitten to be sure that he or she is breathing. If you suspect the person may be going into shock, lie him or her down on a flat surface, elevate his or her feet approximately twelve inches above the level of the head, and cover the person with a blanket or clothing to keep him or her warm.

❑ If possible, bring the snake (if dead) to the emergency room for identification.

❑ If medical help is not available, apply a constricting band two to four inches above the bite. Keep calm and immobilize the affected area, keeping it below heart level if possible. If rapid swelling or severe pain develops, an incision can be made directly below the fang marks and suction performed. The cut should be made along the long axis of the limb with a sharp, sterilized blade. Cut just through the skin (about an eighth of an inch deep), making an incision about one-half-inch long, and then apply suction for at least thirty minutes with a suction cup, snakebite kit, or with the mouth (spit out the blood).

Caution: This procedure should be performed *only* in an extreme situation, only if the bite occurred less than five minutes ago, and only if you have had some training in how to do it. Otherwise, it can cause more problems than it solves. *Never* make cuts on the head, neck, or trunk. Do not perform this procedure if the snake was a coral snake.

❑ If possible, splint the wounded area to immobilize it. This helps to prevent muscle contractions from spreading the poison faster.

❑ Do not apply cold therapy, such as an ice pack. This can cause tissue damage.

❑ To reduce the possibility of snakebite, always remain on paths and hiking trails when in wooded areas. Wear leather boots and long pants if walking in tall grass. Be alert. If you see a snake, do not approach it. Stay at least six feet away. If you come across a log, step onto the log and then over it. Never step directly over it. If you are walking in a tall grassy area, use a long stick or other object to tap the ground in front of you before you step. Take special caution when walking near or through a wet marshy area, as water moccasins can occupy these areas.

CONSIDERATIONS

❑ A poisonous snakebite is a medical emergency. In the United States, treatment is a complex process that may include the administration of antivenin plus fluid and electrolyte replacement, the administration of oxygen, and other supportive measures. If possible, it is wise to call ahead to the emergency room and alert them of the situation before your arrival so that the proper antivenin can be ready for treatment as soon as possible.

❑ If you spend much time outdoors, a snakebite kit is a good investment. Sawyer Products of Safety Harbor,

Florida, makes a kit called The Extractor that is available in many outdoor supply and camping equipment stores.

❏ Snakebite is more likely to be life threatening for children and for elderly people.

❏ In a life-threatening situation, massive doses of vitamin C may save the victim's life. (*See* ASCORBIC ACID FLUSH in Part Three.)

❏ Most cases of snakebite occur between sunrise and sunset. Snakes are cold-blooded and are more likely to be out then, basking in the warmth of the day.

❏ Nonpoisonous snakebites are usually treated with antibiotics in order to prevent infection.

Sore Throat

Sore throats are one of the most common health complaints. They are characterized by a raw, burning, and/or scratchy feeling at the back of the throat. Most sore throats are caused by viral infections such as the common cold. Bacterial infection, especially *Streptococcus* infection, can also be responsible. In addition, a sore throat can be caused by anything that irritates the sensitive mucous membranes at the back of the throat and mouth. Some irritants include medications, surgery, radiation therapy, dust, smoke, fumes, extremely hot foods or drinks, tooth or gum infections, dental work, and abrasions. Chronic coughing and excessive loud talking also irritate the throat.

An acute sore throat usually runs its course within a few days to a few weeks. Sore throats are seldom serious, but quite often are the first symptom of another disorder. Sore throats can signal a cold, flu, mononucleosis, Epstein-Barr virus, herpes simplex, as well as many childhood illnesses such as measles and chickenpox. More rarely, a sore throat may indicate chronic fatigue syndrome, diphtheria, epiglottitis, gingivitis, laryngeal cancer, or an abscess around the tonsils.

Unless otherwise stated, the dosages recommended here are for adults. For a child between the ages of twelve and seventeen, reduce the dose to three-quarters of the recommended amount. For a child between the ages of six and twelve, use one-half the recommended dose, and for a child under six, use one-quarter of the recommended amount.

NUTRIENTS

SUPPLEMENT	SUGGESTED DOSAGE	COMMENTS
Helpful		
Acidophilus (Kyo-Dophilus from Wakunaga is a good source)	As directed on label. Take on an empty stomach.	To replenish "friendly" bacteria. Especially important if antibiotics are prescribed. Use a nondairy formula.
Bee propolis	As directed on label.	Protects mucous membranes of the mouth and throat.
Colloidal silver	As directed on label. Gargle before swallowing.	A powerful antibiotic with no known side effects.
Garlic (Kyolic from Wakunaga) or	2 capsules 3 times daily, with meals.	For improved immune function.
Kyo-Green from Wakunaga	As directed on label.	Contains live enzymes, amino acids, vitamins, minerals, and chlorophyll for healing.
Maitake extract or	As directed on label.	To boost immunity and fight viral infection.
reishi extract or	As directed on label.	
shiitake extract	As directed on label.	
Multivitamin and mineral complex	As directed on label.	To maintain a balance of all necessary nutrients.
Vitamin A emulsion or capsules plus carotenoid complex with beta carotene	100,000 IU daily for 1 week, then 50,000 IU daily for 1 week, then reduce to 25,000 IU daily. If you are pregnant, do not exceed 10,000 IU daily. 25,000 IU daily for 1 week; then reduce to 10,000 IU daily. If you are pregnant, do not exceed 10,000 IU daily. As directed on label.	Aids healing and potentiates immune function. Emulsion form is recommended for easier assimilation and greater safety at high doses. Provides important antioxidant protection. Enhances immunity.
Vitamin C with bioflavonoids	5,000–20,000 mg daily, in divided doses. (See ASCORBIC ACID FLUSH in Part Three.)	Has antiviral properties.
Vitamin E	600 IU daily.	Promotes healing and tissue repair. Use d-alpha-tocopherol form.
Zinc lozenges	As directed on label.	For pain relief, healing, and improved immune function.

HERBS

❏ Bee pollen, blackberry, calendula, and cayenne all have been known to soothe or heal a sore throat.

❏ Catnip tea enemas help to reduce fever. (*See* ENEMAS in Part Three.)

❏ Echinacea and goldenseal fight bacterial and viral infection.

Caution: Do not take goldenseal internally on a daily basis for more than one week at a time, do not use it during pregnancy, and use it with caution if you are allergic to ragweed.

❏ Fenugreek used as a gargle can relieve a sore throat and reduce the pain of swollen glands. Add 20 drops of extract to 1 cup water and gargle with the mixture three times daily.

❏ Licorice soothes a sore, hoarse throat. Lungwort soothes throat irritation. Slippery elm is very soothing for a painful, scratchy sore throat and for mouth irritation. Licorice and slippery elm can be found in lozenge form.

Caution: Do not use licorice on a daily basis for more than seven days in a row. Avoid it if you have high blood pressure.

❏ Marshmallow root tea soothes a scratchy, itchy throat. Raspberry leaf tea is good for easing the pain of a sore throat as well as fever blisters.

❏ Hot mullein poultices are soothing to sore throats. (*See* USING A POULTICE in Part Three.)

❏ Olive leaf extract has been found to be a good remedy for a sore throat.

❏ Singer's Saving Grace from Herbs Etc. is a soothing throat spray containing several herbs, including echinacea, licorice, and ginger.

RECOMMENDATIONS

❏ Be sure to cook all your food until it is tender. Poaching and steaming are good methods of cooking to retain moisture.

❏ Cut your food into very small pieces—or, if necessary, grind or purée it. This will cause less irritation to the throat. Be sure to chew your food well before swallowing.

❏ Use frozen popsicles, ice cream, yogurt, and sherbet to soothe a sore throat.

❏ Avoid eating foods that are spicy, hot, salty, or acidic. These can be irritating to the throat.

❏ If you are having an especially difficult time swallowing and are not able to get the proper intake of nutrients, try drinking an instant breakfast drink.

❏ If your physician prescribes antibiotics for a bacterial throat infection, eat yogurt and take an acidophilus supplement to replace the "friendly" bacteria. Do not take the acidophilus at the same time of day as the antibiotic, however.

❏ Liquid vitamin C, made by dissolving vitamin C powder in water or juice, is good to sip. Allow it to drip down the throat slowly.

❏ Gargle alternately with chlorophyll liquid and sea salt (½ teaspoon in a glass of warm water) every few hours.

❏ Drink plenty of liquids. Fresh juices are best.

❏ Sip tea made from chamomile or sage, or some chicken or vegetable broth to keep your throat lubricated.

❏ Use a mixture of raw honey and lemon juice to coat and soothe the throat.

❏ Try using homeopathic remedies to relieve symptoms. *Aconite, Belladonna, Ferrum phosphoricum,* and *Gelsemium* are some of the homeopathic remedies that have been used to treat sore throat.

❏ *See* FASTING in Part Three, and follow the program.

❏ If you smoke, stop. Smoking is a major cause of sore throats. (*See* SMOKING DEPENDENCY in Part Two.)

❏ Snoring can make a sore throat much more painful. If you snore, try sleeping on your side or using adhesive strips that hold the nostrils open. These can be found in drugstores and many supermarkets.

❏ Seek a physician's care if your sore throat is accompanied by any of the following:

• High or persistent fever. A fever that is higher than 102°F should be evaluated by a physician.

• Rash. This can be a sign of strep throat or other potentially serious conditions.

• Severe headache and stiff neck. This can be a symptom of meningitis.

• Prolonged hoarseness. This may indicate an underlying medical problem such as throat cancer or oral cancer.

CONSIDERATIONS

❏ A constant tickle or chronic irritating cough can be an indication of food allergies. (*See* ALLERGIES in Part Two.)

❏ If sore throat recurs or lasts for longer than two weeks, you may have an underlying illness such as mononucleosis.

❏ Many sore throats and infections are contracted from bacteria on toothbrushes. Toothbrushes should be replaced once monthly and after any type of infectious illness. Between uses, store your toothbrush in hydrogen peroxide or grapefruit seed extract to kill germs (if you use hydrogen peroxide, rinse the toothbrush well before brushing).

❏ Breathing in dry air can sometimes worsen the soreness. A humidifier or vaporizer can help by adding more moisture to the air.

❏ *See also* COMMON COLD; MONONUCLEOSIS; SINUSITIS; and TONSILLITIS, all in Part Two.

Spider Bite

The bites of spiders can be poisonous and painful. However, most spiders are not big enough to cause serious harm. Infants, older adults, and people of any age who have allergies are at greatest risk of having more serious reactions. However, a bite from a poisonous spider may produce a wide variety of symptoms, including intense pain, numbness, redness, and swelling in the affected area, as well as generalized convulsions, difficulty breathing, dizziness, fever or chills, headache, impaired speech, itching, joint pain, muscle spasms, muscular cramping, nausea, stiffness, sweating, vomiting, and weakness.

Two types of spider—the black widow and the brown recluse—are more poisonous than most and can cause a serious reaction. The bite of the black widow spider can cause abdominal pain similar to that of appendicitis, spastic muscle contractions, and localized tissue death. In about 4 percent of cases, black widow bites lead to anaphylactic shock and death. This spider has a black body with a red hourglass shape on the main body segment. The venom of the brown recluse spider usually creates a blister encircled by red and white rings. This "bull's-eye" appearance is used to distinguish it from other spider bites. Death from this type of bite is even more rare than from black widow bites.

If you suspect you have been bitten by a poisonous spider, seek medical help immediately. After appropriate medical care has been administered, taking the following nutrients should help alleviate pain and hasten healing. Unless otherwise stated, the dosages recommended here are for adults. For a child between the ages of twelve and seventeen, reduce the dose to three-quarters of the recommended amount. For a child between the ages of six and twelve, use one-half the recommended dose, and for a child under six, use one-quarter of the recommended amount.

NUTRIENTS

SUPPLEMENT	SUGGESTED DOSAGE	COMMENTS
Helpful		
Calcium and magnesium	1,000–2,000 mg daily until the wound heals. 500–1,000 mg daily until the wound heals.	Helps relieve pain. Use calcium gluconate form. Needed to balance with calcium.
Charcoal tablets	6–10 capsules as soon as possible after the bite, with a large glass of water.	A powerful detoxifying agent. Take immediately after being bitten if possible.
Colloidal silver	Apply topically as directed on label.	An antibiotic that reduces inflammation, promotes healing, and inhibits infection.
Dimethylglycine (DMG) (Aangamik DMG from FoodScience of Vermont)	As directed on label.	Enhances immunity and detoxifies the body.
Flaxseed oil	As directed on label.	Reduces pain and inflammation and aids recovery.
Herpanacine from Diamond-Herpanacine Associates	As directed on label.	Promotes good skin health and detoxifies the body.
Multivitamin and mineral complex	As directed on label.	To maintain a balance of all essential nutrients.
Pycnogenol or grape seed extract	As directed on label. As directed on label.	Protect the skin, reduce inflammation, and enhance immunity.
Ultimate Cleanse from Nature's Secret	As directed on label.	Stimulates and detoxifies the organs, blood, and channels of elimination.
Vitamin A plus carotenoid complex with beta-carotene	10,000 IU daily. As directed on label.	Enhances immunity and protects the body from bacteria. Powerful antioxidants that boost the immune system.
Vitamin B complex plus extra pantothenic acid (vitamin B$_5$)	As directed on label. 500 mg daily.	Maintains healthy nerves and skin. A sublingual form is recommended. Has anti-allergenic and anti-stress properties.
Vitamin C with bioflavonoids	1,000 mg every hour until pain and swelling subside.	Aids in detoxifying the venom and eliminating it from the body. Very important in crisis allergy situations.
Vitamin E oil	Apply topically 3–4 times daily.	Aids healing and relieves discomfort. Purchase in oil form or cut open a capsule to release the oil.
Zinc	60–90 mg daily. Do not exceed a total of 100 mg daily from all supplements.	Boosts immune response. Also acts as a natural insect repellent. Use zinc gluconate lozenges or OptiZinc for best absorption.

HERBS

❑ Any of the following poultices may be beneficial (*see* USING A POULTICE in Part Three):

• A combination of dandelion and yellow dock relieves itchy skin.

• Fenugreek and flaxseed mixed with slippery elm bark is useful for treating inflammation.

• Goldenseal is good for inflammations of all kinds.

• A mixture of lobelia and crushed charcoal tablets is beneficial for insect bites and most wounds.

❑ A tincture made from calendula buds and alcohol should be on hand for stings and other "surface" injuries. A poultice made from the fresh flower heads is also good. (*See* USING A POULTICE in Part Three.)

❑ A cream containing 5 percent tea tree oil helps to heal insect bites, sunburn, cuts, rashes, and other skin irritations.

❑ Echinacea, taken in tea or capsule form, boosts the immune system.

❑ Ginkgo biloba helps to relieve muscle pains.

❑ Yellow dock purifies the blood and is beneficial for many problems affecting the skin. Drink as much yellow dock tea as you can, or take 2 capsules of yellow dock every hour until symptoms are relieved.

RECOMMENDATIONS

❑ If you suspect you have been bitten by a poisonous spider, seek medical help immediately. In the meantime, try to remain calm. If there is swelling or pain, apply a constricting band two to four inches *above* the bite. Immobilize the affected area, keeping it below heart level if possible. Lie down and keep warm. If you have been bitten by a black widow spider, pack ice around the wound to relieve pain and to slow down the spread of the poison. *Do not* apply ice to the wound if you have been bitten by a brown recluse spider.

❑ If medical help is not available, try to rid the body of as much poison as possible by encouraging bleeding. This can be done by suction. (*See* SNAKEBITE in Part Two.)

❑ Use essential oils of basil, cinnamon, lavender, lemon, sage, savory, or thyme for their antitoxic and antivenomous properties. Apply a drop of essential oil on the sting.

CONSIDERATIONS

❏ In life-threatening cases of spider bite, injections of vitamin C and pantothenic acid (vitamin B₅), administered by a medical professional, may be invaluable.

❏ For bites that do not appear to be life threatening, a doctor may administer calcium gluconate to relieve muscle soreness and an antianxiety medication for muscle spasms.

❏ Hydrocortisone ointment, calamine lotion, or a paste made from baking soda may be used to soothe the wound.

❏ Bites from scorpions, especially those found in the southwestern United Statets, require emergency medical care. Scorpions can be identified by their elongated bodies and curled tails.

❏ Rattlesnake and black widow venom are similar in many respects. Treatment for a black widow bite is therefore similar to that for snakebite.

❏ If you have been bitten by any type of spider, it is important to be sure that your tetanus immunization is current.

❏ *See also* BEE STING; INSECT ALLERGY; and/or SNAKEBITE in Part Two.

Sprains, Strains, and Other Injuries of the Muscles and Joints

A sprain is not the same thing as a strain. If a muscle is stressed beyond its capability, it becomes *strained*. Putting undue weight on the muscles and using the muscles for prolonged periods without rest can create muscle strain. A strained muscle may go into spasms or knot up instead of relaxing normally. Localized pain (during movement), swelling, and loss of mobility occur.

If one of the ligaments, the tissues that connect bones to muscles, is wrenched or stretched excessively, the ligament may tear, causing a *sprain*. There is likely to be a brief sharp pain followed by rapid swelling. Soft tissue surrounding the joint may be sore and bruised. Sprains can result from unexpected movement or twisting of the affected area, or from a hard fall. The joints most often sprained are the ankle, back, finger, knee, and wrist.

These types of injuries are common in athletes. In most cases, they heal on their own. The following supplement program can help these injuries heal. Unless otherwise stated, the dosages recommended here are for adults. For a child between the ages of twelve and seventeen, reduce the dose to three-quarters of the recommended amount. For a child between the ages of six and twelve, use one-half the recommended dose, and for a child under six, use one-quarter of the recommended amount.

NUTRIENTS

SUPPLEMENT	SUGGESTED DOSAGE	COMMENTS
Very Important		
Chondroitin sulfate	500–1,000 mg daily.	Nutritional support for strengthening joints, ligaments, and tendons.
Glucosamine sulfate (GS-500 from Enzymatic Therapy) or N-Acetylglucosamine (N-A-G from Source Naturals)	As directed on label.	Very important for the formation of bones, tendons, ligaments, cartilage and synovial (joint) fluid.
Inflazyme Forte from American Biologics or Wobenzym N from Marlyn Nutraceuticals	As directed on label. Take between meals. / As directed on label. Take between meals.	To destroy free radicals released during injury.
Methylsulfonyl-methone (MSM)	500–1,000 mg 3 times daily.	A sulfur compound needed for reducing pain and inflammation; also for joint and tissue repair.
Helpful		
Bromelain	400 mg 3 times daily between meals.	An enzyme that helps to stimulate production of prostaglandins and reduces inflammation.
Calcium and magnesium	1,500–2,000 mg daily. / 750–1,000 mg daily.	Needed for repair of connective tissue. Use both calcium chelate and calcium gluconate forms to assure assimilation. Very important for the skeletal system.
Curcumin	600 mg 3 times daily.	Reduces inflammation and aids in healing.
Desiccated liver	As directed on label.	Aids in building healthy blood cells.
Dimethylglycine (DMG) (Aangamik DMG from FoodScience Labs)	As directed on label.	Increases tissue oxygenation.
Essential fatty acids (flaxseed oil and Ultimate Oil from Nature's Secret are good sources)	As directed on label.	Promotes cellular and cardiovascular health; improves stamina and speeds recovery.
Free-form amino acid complex	As directed on label, on an empty stomach.	To help repair and strengthen connective tissue, reduce body fat, and help increase energy.
Grape seed extract	As directed on label.	A powerful anti-inflammatory.
L-Leucine plus L-isoleucine and L-valine	As directed on label, on an empty stomach. Take with water or juice. Do not take with milk. Take with 50 mg vitamin B₆ and 100 mg vitamin C for better absorption.	Branched-chain amino acids that promote the healing of bones, skin, and muscle tissue. (*See* AMINO ACIDS in Part One.)
Manganese	15 mg daily.	Strengthens wounded ligaments and/or tendons.
Multivitamin and mineral complex	As directed on label.	To promote good health, nutritional balance, and tissue repair.

Neonatal Multi-Gland from Biotics Research or B Cell Formula from Ecological Formulas	As directed on label. As directed on label.	To stimulate healing of connective tissue.
Potassium	99 mg daily.	Vital for tissue repair.
S-Adenosylmethio-nine (SAMe) (SAMe Rx-Mood from Nature's Plus)	400 mg 2 times daily.	A deficiency results in the inability to maintain cartilage properly. Aids in reducing pain and inflammation. *Caution:* Do not use if you have manic-depressive disorder or take prescription antidepressants.
Silica	500 mg daily.	Supplies silicon, needed for connective tissue repair and calcium absorption.

Vitamin A plus carotenoid complex with beta-carotene	10,000 IU daily. As directed on label.	Enhances immunity and aids in protein utilization. Powerful antioxidants that boost the immune system.
Vitamin B complex plus extra pantothenic acid (vitamin B$_5$)	100 mg of each major B vitamin daily (amounts of individual vitamins in a complex will vary). 500 mg daily.	All the B vitamins are important during stressful situations. Use a high-potency formula. The most important anti-stress vitamin.
Vitamin C with bioflavonoids	5,000–20,000 mg daily, in divided doses. (*See* ASCORBIC ACID FLUSH in Part Three.)	An antioxidant required for tissue growth and repair. Calcium ascorbate is the best source of vitamin C to use for these injuries.
Vitamin E	400–1,000 IU daily.	A free radical scavenger. Use d-alpha-tocopherol form.

Sports Nutrition for the Serious Bodybuilder

Nutrition and dietary supplements have become a focus of serious attention from athletes of all types, especially body-builders. Many of them have found that the combination of proper diet, appropriate supplements, and a good comprehensive workout plan work together to help them achieve their personal goals. There are three basic approaches to the use of supplements to build muscle: providing the body with protein that it can use to make the muscle; promoting the body's production of androgenic hormones such as testosterone so that it is inclined to build itself up in response to exercise; and providing nutrients that increase endurance, so that more—and more strenuous—exercise is possible. The following is a sports nutrition and supplementation plan developed in collaboration with Tom Witman, owner of Vintage Whole Foods Market in Indianapolis, Indiana, who has specialized in sports nutrition for over a decade.

Note: This program is an advanced supplementation program intended for the serious bodybuilder who has some knowledge of sports nutrition, not for the person who has just begun to exercise or tone his or her muscles.

SUPPLEMENT	SUGGESTED DOSAGE	COMMENTS
Beta-hydroxy-beta-methylbutyrate (HMB) (HMB from EAS)	As directed on label.	Potent cortisol inhibitor. Cortisol is an anti-anabolic agent released as a result of strenuous physical exertion. *Caution:* Do not use if you are suffering from joint problems.
Calcium D-gluconate	200–400 mg. daily.	Blocks conversion of testosterone to estrogen.
Calcium pyruvate	2,000–6,000 mg daily, with meals.	Enhances endurance by as much as 20–50 percent. Increases metabolism, resulting in fat loss of up to 48 percent. Increases protein uptake.
Chrysin	500–2,000 mg daily with meals.	Prevents excess testosterone precursors from being converted to estrogen in the body. This increases lean muscle mass development.
Colostrum	2,000–3,000 mg daily.	Helps stimulate growth, regeneration, and repair of muscle, skin, bone, and cartilage. Stimulates body to catabolize adipose (fat) tissue rather than lean muscle tissue.
Conjugated linoleic acid (CLA)	750–1,500 mg daily, with meals.	Decreases body fat and improves muscle tone, and increases lean muscle mass gain and exercise tolerance.
Creatine	During loading phase: 30 g daily. For maintenance: 5 g daily.	Use micronized effervescent or micronized creatine monohydrate form. These are more easily digested than ordinary creatine. Avoid products from Asia due to quality issues.
Cross-flow micro-filtered whey protein isolates (CytoPro from Cytodyne, Perfect IsoPure from Nature's Best, and Pro Complex from Optimum Nutrition are good sources)	1 g for every 2.2 lbs of body weight.	To promote protein synthesis. Provides glycomacropeptides, low molecular weight oligopeptides, and branched-chain amino acids.
D-Ribose	2,200 mg daily. Can be taken with creatine to boost its effectiveness.	Increases effectiveness of creatine monohydrate. A precursor to ATP (the cellular energy source). Complements creatine monohydrate in its ability to generate lean muscle mass, endurance, and muscular energy.

5-Androstenediol	As directed on label, or 50–100 mg daily.	Prohormone to maximize lean muscle mass development, increase strength and endurance, and enhance recovery, energy, and growth from resistance and cardiovascular exercise. *Note:* To reduce spike effect on testosterone levels, use transdermal solution.
4-Androstenedione	As directed on label, or 50–100 mg daily.	Prohormone to maximize lean muscle mass development, increase strength and endurance, and enhance recovery, energy, and growth from resistance and cardiovascular exercise. Increases testosterone levels for approximately 3 hours. Available in capsules, sublingual liquid, or transdermal solution.
Glucosamine sulfate	1,500–4,000 mg daily.	To improve joint integrity, function, and range of motion.
Human growth hormone (HGH) (Humagro or Testatropinol from ASN Inc.)	As directed on label.	Homeopathic growth hormone 4c impacts testosterone, growth hormone, adrenalin, adrenocorticotropic hormone, luteinizing hormone, FSH, TSH hormones.
GH Stak from Muscle-Link Regenesis Pro from Regenesis	As directed on label.	Increase lean muscle mass, reduce adipose (fat tissue), support cardiac output, increase libido, increase energy. Improves blood lipid levels, slows down overall body deterioration associated with aging. Use effervescent or sublingual forms only.
Methylsulfonyl-methane (MSM)	1,000–4,000 mg daily.	To improve tissue integrity in the joints.
19-Norandrostenediol (products from ASN, AST Sports Science, Euthenics, Human Development Technologies [HDT], MedLean, and MuscleTech are good sources)	As directed on label.	Prohormone to maximize lean muscle mass development, increase strength and endurance, and enhance recovery, energy, and growth from resistance and cardiovascular exercise. Is not converted to testosterone in the body and does not raise testosterone levels. Is converted to nandrolone, a powerful hormonal anabolic agent. Available in capsule, sublingual liquid, or transdermal solution.
19-Norandrostenedione (products from ASN, AST Sports Science, Euthenics, Human Development Technologies [HDT], MedLean, and MuscleTech are good sources)	As directed on label.	Prohormone to maximize lean muscle mass development, increase strength and endurance, and enhance recovery, energy, and growth from resistance and cardiovascular exercise. Is not converted to testosterone in the body and does not raise testosterone levels. Is converted to nandrolone, a powerful hormonal anabolic agent. Available in capsule, sublingual liquid, or transdermal solution.
Ornithine alpha-ketoglutarate (OKG)	1,300–2,600 mg daily, before exercise or at bedtime.	Helps prevent muscle tissue breakdown. Aids in muscle growth and stimulates growth hormone release.
7 Keto-DHEA	50–150 mg daily.	The best form of DHEA—it is not converted into estrogens in the body. Slows overall body deterioration. Enhances fat loss and lean muscle mass development.
Sodium phosphate and potassium bicarbonate (Phos Fuel from Twinlab)	As directed on label.	Delays onset of muscular fatigue by buffering lactic acid, improving muscular power and endurance.

HERBS

❑ *Tribulus terrestris* (an herb whose common name is puncture vine) increases production of luteinizing hormone and testosterone in men, thereby increasing strength and lean muscle mass.

❑ Yohimbe is a central nervous system stimulant that increases testosterone levels. It is used to increase strength and lean muscle mass, as well as to enhance libido.

RECOMMENDATIONS

❑ For bruises, muscle strain, and other workout-related injuries, use homeopathic *Arnica montana.*

CONSIDERATIONS

❑ Research performed at the University of Toronto in Canada demonstrated that by mixing a specified amount of water with a creatine monohydrate mixture containing creatine and carbohydrates, you can vastly increase the speed at which the creatine and carbohydrates enter the bloodstream, thus enhancing your training. This is known as the osmotic acceleration principle. The following schedule applies:

Body Weight	Creatine mix	Water
0–170 lbs	9 g creatine 65 g carbohydrate	10 oz, followed by 10 oz 10 minutes later.
170–220 lbs	10 g creatine 75 g carbohydrate	20 oz, followed by 10 oz 10 minutes later.
220–300 lbs	12 g creatine 85 g carbohydrate	20 oz, followed by 12 oz 10 minutes later.

Cell-Tech from MuscleTech is a premade creatine product that can be used for this purpose.

Zinc	50 mg daily. Do not exceed a total of 100 mg daily from all supplements.	Important in tissue repair. Use zinc gluconate lozenges or OptiZinc for best absorption.

HERBS

❑ Boswellia, an Ayurvedic herb, is good for reducing inflammation. Choose a product standardized to contains 150 milligrams of boswellic acids per dose. Boswellia cream can be good for relieving pain as well. Boswellin Cream from Nature's Herbs is a good product.

❑ Fenugreek and flaxseed powder can be combined with slippery elm bark to make a poultice for swelling. (*See* USING A POULTICE in Part Three.)

❑ Feverfew and ginger are good for pain and soreness. Ginger is also a powerful antioxidant that has anti-inflammatory effects.

❑ Green tea and nettle leaf have anti-inflammatory properties.

❑ Goldenseal poultices are good for reducing inflammation.

❑ Horse chestnut extract gel, applied topically to the injured area, can reduce swelling and inflammation.

❑ Mustard poultices are good for swelling and can relax tense muscles.

❑ After the initial treatment of applying ice to the injury, combine turmeric and a little hot water to make a paste. Apply this mixture to the injured area with a gauze dressing. This treatment helps to reduce swelling. It is also good for bruising.

RECOMMENDATIONS

❑ Immediately after the injury, raise the affected area—above heart level if possible—and apply ice for no longer than twenty minutes. *Do not* use heat immediately following an injury. Apply ice intermittently every four hours for the first one to two days. Then, after the inflammation has subsided, apply heat for twenty-minute periods two or three times a day. If possible, use a splint or sling to immobilize and protect the injured area.

❑ If there is significant swelling, call your physician right away or go to a hospital emergency room to have the injury evaluated. Especially with injuries to the wrists and ankles, it is wise to have x-rays taken to make sure no bones have been broken.

❑ Consume plenty of juices made from fresh raw vegetables, including beets, garlic, and radishes. Raw vegetables are high in valuable vitamins and enzymes.

❑ Use homeopathic remedies to ease the discomfort. Homeopathic remedies used to treat symptoms of sprains, strains, and other types of injuries include *Aconitum napellus, Arnica montana, Hypericum, Rhus toxicodendron, Ruta graveolens,* and *Symphytum officinalis.*

❑ To prevent sprains and strains, do stretching exercises both before and after exercise and other physical activity.

CONSIDERATIONS

❑ Minor sprains can usually be treated at home. However, anytime an injury becomes painful and swollen, you should see a medical professional—especially if you hear a popping sound and find that you cannot use the injured joint normally.

❑ Aromatherapy can be helpful. Cold compresses made with essential oils of camphor, chamomile, eucalyptus, lavender, and/or rosemary are good. Add 10 drops or so of essential oil to 1 quart of cool water and use the mixture to make the compresses.

❑ Clay poultices can be used to treat sprains and fractures. (*See* USING A POULTICE in Part Three.)

❑ The risk of injury to the muscles and joints is higher in contact sports than in other types of activity.

❑ *See* Sports Nutrition for the Serious Bodybuilder on page 644.

❑ *See also* BRUISING and FRACTURE, both in Part Two.

❑ *See also* PAIN CONTROL in Part Three.

Stress

The term "stress" refers to any reaction to a physical, mental, social, or emotional stimulus that requires a response or alteration to the way we perform, think, or feel. Change is stressful—whether the change is good or bad. Worry produces stress. Indeed, stress is an unavoidable part of life. It can result from many things, both physical and psychological. Pressures and deadlines at work, problems with loved ones, the need to pay the bills, and getting ready for the holidays are obvious sources of stress for many people. Less obvious sources include everyday encounters with crowds, noise, traffic, pain, extremes of temperature, and even welcome events such as starting a new job or the birth or adoption of a child. Overwork, lack of sleep, and physical illness put stress on the body. Excessive alcohol consumption and smoking are usually increased as a reaction to stress and yet create more stress for the body. Some people create their own stress; whether there is anything objectively wrong in their lives or not, they find things to worry about. For such people, stress becomes almost an addiction.

Some people handle stress well, and it has little impact on their emotional or physical health. Others are very negatively influenced by it. Stress can cause fatigue, chronic headaches, irritability, changes in appetite, memory loss, low self-esteem, withdrawal, tooth-grinding, cold hands, high blood pressure, shallow breathing, nervous twitches, lowered sexual drive, insomnia or other changes in sleep patterns, and/or gastrointestinal disorders. Stress creates an excellent breeding ground for illness. Researchers estimate that stress contributes to as many as 80 percent of all major illnesses, including cardiovascular disease, cancer, endocrine and metabolic disease, skin disorders, and infectious ailments of all kinds. Many psychiatrists believe that the majority of back problems—one of the most common adult ailments in the United States—are related to stress. Stress is also a common precursor of psychological difficulties such as anxiety and depression.

Stress is viewed as a psychological problem, but it has very real physical effects. The body responds to stress with a series of physiological changes that include increased secretion of adrenaline, elevation of blood pressure, acceleration of the heartbeat, and greater tension in the muscles. Digestion slows or stops, fats and sugars are released from stores in the body, cholesterol levels rise, and the composition of the blood changes slightly, making it more prone to clotting. This in turn increases the risk of stroke or heart attack. Almost all body functions and organs react to stress. The pituitary gland increases its production of adrenocorticotropic hormone (ACTH), which in turn stimulates the release of the hormones cortisone and cortisol. These have the effect of inhibiting the functioning of disease-fighting white blood cells and suppressing the immune response. This complex of physical changes is called the "fight or flight" response and is apparently designed to prepare one to face an immediate danger. Today, most of our stresses are not the result of physical threats, but the body still responds as if they were.

The increased production of adrenal hormones is responsible for most of the symptoms associated with stress. It is also the reason that stress can lead to nutritional deficiencies. Increased adrenaline production causes the body to step up its metabolism of proteins, fats, and carbohydrates to quickly produce energy for the body to use. This response causes the body to excrete amino acids, potassium, and phosphorus; to deplete magnesium stored in muscle tissue; and to store less calcium. Further, the body does not absorb ingested nutrients well when under stress. The result is that, especially with prolonged or recurrent stress, the body becomes at once deficient in many nutrients and is unable to replace them adequately. Many of the disorders that arise from stress are the result of nutritional deficiencies, especially deficiencies of the B-complex vitamins, which are very important for proper functioning of the nervous system, and of certain electrolytes, which are depleted by the body's stress response. Stress also promotes the formation of free radicals that can become oxidized and damage body tissues, especially cell membranes.

Anxiety, panic attacks, obsessive-compulsive disorder, post-traumatic stress disorder (PTSD), dissociative disorders, and phobic disorders are among the more serious emotional manifestations of stress. They are often a result of an event that the individual was unable to deal with at the time.

Many people attribute their stress-related symptoms to "nerves," and in fact stress usually does affect the parts of the body that are related to the nervous system first, especially through the digestive organs. Symptoms of stress-related digestive disorders may be a flare-up of an ulcer or irritable bowel syndrome. If stress that produces such symptoms is not handled properly, then more serious illnesses may result.

Stress can be either acute or long-term. Long-term stress is particularly dangerous. A state of continual stress eventually wears out the body. Because of its effect on immune response, stress increases susceptibility to illness and slows healing.

NUTRIENTS

SUPPLEMENT	SUGGESTED DOSAGE	COMMENTS
Essential		
ACES + Zn from Carlson Labs	2 capsules daily.	Contains beta-carotene, selenium, and vitamins C and E, which work together as antioxidants to disarm damaging free radicals caused by stress.
Gamma-amino-butyric acid (GABA) (GABA Plus from Twinlab)	750 mg twice daily. Take with 50 mg inositol and 500 mg niacinamide to enhance effectiveness.	Acts as a tranquilizer and is important for proper brain function. (*See* AMINO ACIDS in Part One.)
Glutathione	As directed on label.	An antioxidant that protects the cells against damage.
Nicotinamide adenine dinucleotide (NADH)	10 mg daily first thing in the morning.	Important in the creation and transfer of chemical energy, especially during breathing.
S-Adenosylmethionine (SAMe)	As directed on label.	Can ease depression. *Caution:* Do not use if you have manic-depressive disorder or take prescription antidepressants.
Taurine (Taurine Plus from American Biologics)	As directed on label.	Essential amino acid for brain and heart protection. Use a sublingual form.
Trimethylglycine (TMG)	As directed on label.	Reduces homocysteine levels in the blood and acts like SAMe to ease depression.
Vitamin B complex injections	1 cc weekly or as prescribed by physician.	All B vitamins are necessary for health and proper functioning of the nervous system. Intramuscular injections (under a doctor's supervision) give fast results.
plus extra vitamin B6 (pyridoxine) injections	1/2 cc weekly or as prescribed by physician.	
and vitamin B12 injections	1 cc weekly or as prescribed by physician.	
and/or vitamin B complex	100 mg of each major B vitamin daily (amounts of individual vitamins in a complex will vary).	Take oral supplements either in addition to injections or alone, if injections are unavailable. Use a sublingual form.
plus extra pantothenic acid (vitamin B5)	500 mg daily.	An anti-stress vitamin needed by the thymus gland.
Vitamin C with bioflavonoids	3,000–10,000 mg daily.	Essential to adrenal gland function. Stress depletes the adrenal gland hormones, the anti-stress hormones.

Very Important		
Anti-Stress Enzymes from Biotec Foods	As directed on label.	Enzymes that remove toxic wastes and restore balance and equilibrium to the system.
Calcium and magnesium	2,000 mg daily. 1,000 mg daily.	Lost when stress is present. Use calcium chelate form. Deficiency is common in highly stressed individuals, and can result in anxiety, fear, and even hallucinations.
Coenzyme Q$_{10}$ plus Coenzyme A from Coenzyme-A Technologies	As directed on label. As directed on label.	Both these coenzymes work to increase energy and protect the heart and immune system.
L-Tyrosine	500 mg twice daily, during the day and at bedtime. Take with water or juice on an empty stomach. Do not take with milk. Take with 50 mg vitamin B$_6$ and 100 mg vitamin C for better absorption.	Helps reduce stress on the body. An effective and safe sleeping aid. Also good for depression. (See AMINO ACIDS in Part One.) Caution: Do not take this supplement if you are taking an MAO inhibitor drug.
Melatonin	Start with 1.5 mg daily, taken 2 hours or less before bedtime. If this is not effective, gradually increase the dosage until an effective level is reached (up to 5 mg at night).	A natural hormone that promotes sound sleep; helpful if stress leads to occasional sleeplessness.

Helpful		
Fiber (oat bran and psyllium husks are good sources)	As directed on label. Take separately from other supplements and medications.	For bowel cleansing and improved bowel function. Stress often causes diarrhea and/or constipation.
Free-form amino complex (Amino Balance from Anabol Naturals)	As directed on label.	To supply protein, which is used rapidly by the body at stressful times. Use a formula containing both essential and nonessential amino acids.
Lecithin granules or capsules	1 tbsp 3 times daily, with meals. 2,400 mg 3 times daily, with meals.	For cellular protection and brain function.
L-Lysine	As directed on label. Take with 50 mg vitamin C and 1 15-mg zinc gluconate lozenge.	For cold sores, often an early indicator of stress. Reduces stress so it is better handled. Caution: Do not take for longer than 6 months at a time.
Maitake extract or reishi extract or shiitaki extract	As directed on label. As directed on label. As directed on label.	Adaptogens that help the body adapt to stress and normalize body functions.
Multivitamin and mineral complex with natural beta-carotene and potassium and selenium	25,000 IU daily. 99 mg daily. 200 mcg daily.	Especially necessary during stress. An important antioxidant. To replace potassium lost due to excretion during stress. A potent antioxidant that decreases anxiety attacks.

Raw adrenal glandular and raw thymus glandular	As directed on label. As directed on label.	To stimulate the adrenal and thymus glands, important in the body's stress reaction.
Vitamin E	400–600 IU daily. Take with meals.	Needed for immune function. A powerful antioxidant. Use d-alpha-tocopherol form.
Zinc	50 mg daily. Do not exceed a total of 100 mg daily from all supplements.	Needed for immune function and to protect the cells from free radical damage. Use zinc gluconate lozenges or OptiZinc for best absorption.

HERBS

❑ Ashwagandha is an Ayurvedic herb that acts as a sedative and nerve tonic.

❑ Bilberry prevents destruction, mutation, and premature death of cells throughout the body.

❑ Ginkgo biloba aids in proper brain function and good circulation.

❑ Milk thistle cleanses and protects the liver, and has antioxidant properties.

❑ Many plants produce their own antioxidants, which they use as protection against environmental stresses. Specific herbs tend to protect specific parts of the body. However, because of their strong antioxidant properties, most have important influences on other parts of the body as well. For a robust anti-stress tonic, mix 1/2 teaspoon of any three of the herbs listed below and steep in 2 cups of almost-boiling distilled water, or use alcohol-free extracts mixed in water.

❑ Catnip is an effective anti-stress herb that also causes drowsiness.

❑ Chamomile is a gentle relaxant. It is a good nerve tonic, soothing to the digestive tract, and a pleasant sleep aid.

Caution: Do not use this herb on an ongoing basis and avoid it completely if you are allergic to ragweed.

❑ Dong quai, rehmannia, and schizandra support the kidneys, adrenal glands, and central nervous system. These organs are among the most susceptible to the effects of stress.

❑ Hops helps to ease nervousness, restlessness, and stress. It also decreases the desire for alcohol.

❑ Kava kava relaxes the mind as well as the entire body.

❑ Passionflower is calming and is a potent addition to any anti-stress formula.

❑ Polygala root and sour jujube seed are powerful Chinese herbs known to soothe and calm the spirit.

❑ St. John's wort is good for depression and nerve pain.

❑ Siberian ginseng helps the body cope with stress.

❑ Skullcap is good for nervous disorders. It also relieves headaches and aids sleep.

❑ Valerian keeps the nervous system from being overwhelmed. It also is a powerful sleep aid when taken at bedtime and helps to ease stress-related headaches.

❑ Wild oat is said to restore balance to the nervous system.

RECOMMENDATIONS

❑ Eat a diet composed of 50 to 75 percent raw foods. Fresh fruits and vegetables not only supply valuable vitamins and minerals, but are rich in compounds called flavonoids, many of which scavenge and neutralize dangerous free radicals.

❑ Avoid processed foods and all foods that create stress on the system, such as artificial sweeteners, carbonated soft drinks, chocolate, eggs, fried foods, junk foods, pork, red meat, sugar, white flour products, foods containing preservatives or heavy spices, and chips and similar snack foods.

❑ Eliminate dairy products from your diet for three weeks. Then reintroduce them slowly—and watch for returning symptoms of your "nervous" condition.

❑ Limit your intake of caffeine. Caffeine contributes to nervousness and can disrupt sleep patterns.

❑ Avoid alcohol, tobacco, and mood-altering drugs. While these substances may offer temporary relief from stress, they do nothing to really address the problem, and they are harmful to your health. The stress will still be there the next day.

❑ Follow a monthly fasting program. (*See* FASTING in Part Three.)

❑ Get regular exercise. Physical activity can clear your mind and keep stress under control. Some people like to run or walk by themselves, while others prefer team sports or group workouts. Any type of exercise will do the trick, as long as it is *regular*. Exercising only once a month will not do much to relieve stress.

❑ Learn to relax. Relaxation is often difficult for people suffering from the effects of stress, but it is necessary. A technique called *progressive relaxation* can be helpful. This involves tightening and relaxing the major muscle groups one at a time, being aware of each sensation. Start at your feet and work up to your head. Tense the muscles for a count of ten, concentrating on the tension, then let the muscles go lax and breathe deeply, enjoying the sensation of release.

❑ Get sufficient sleep each night. This may be difficult, because stress can keep you up at night (unless you are one of those people who welcomes sleep as an escape), but it is very important. The less sleep you get, the more stress will affect you, the more your immune system will weaken, and the greater your chance of becoming ill will be.

❑ Try meditation. Many people find that regular meditation helps them to relax and handle stress. Meditation does not have to have spiritual or religious connotations. For example, you can meditate on a word such as "peace," "calm," "relax," or "warm." Or you may find it helpful to meditate on a pleasant person, place, or event. It is good to have a store of pleasant thoughts to draw on during stressful times. While meditation can have some short-term benefits, it is more effective when practiced on a daily basis. Try meditating twice a day for ten to twenty minutes each time.

❑ Practice deep breathing. This can be done when facing a stressful situation—at home, at work, in your car, or elsewhere. Holding your breath is also good for relieving stress. Inhale deeply with your mouth closed, hold your breath for a few seconds (do not wait until you are uncomfortable), then exhale slowly through your mouth, with your tongue placed at the top of your teeth, next to the gum line. Do this four or five times, or until the tension passes. (*See* Breathing Exercises *under* PAIN CONTROL in Part Three.)

❑ Monitor your internal conversations. The way we talk to ourselves has a lot to do with how we feel about ourselves and our environments. Telling yourself things like "I should be able to handle this better," or "I shouldn't have let that idiot cut me off in traffic," or "I'll never get the hang of this computer" only adds to the stressfulness of situations and does nothing to resolve them. Learn to listen for—and then make yourself stop—these futile inner conversations. Some therapists recommend shouting "Get out!" (or any other phrase you choose) immediately when any intrusive and unpleasant worries enter your thoughts.

❑ Identify the sources of stress in your life. This can be an important first step in managing stress. Take a stress inventory periodically to help you understand what is causing you problems. You can use the following list of major stressors as a starting point:

• Death of a spouse or other close family member.
• Divorce.
• Death of a close friend.
• Financial problems.
• Legal separation from spouse.
• Job loss.
• Major injury.
• New marriage.
• Scheduled surgery.
• Change in family member's health.
• Serious trouble at work.
• Increased responsibility at work or at home.
• Sexual problems.
• Change of jobs.
• Child leaving home.
• Change in residence.
• Major change in diet.
• Vacation.
• Allergies.

Remember that this list is not exhaustive and that different people react to the same events differently. Also remember that children and young adults have different lists of stressful situations, which are just as serious for them as those above are for adults.

❏ Take a day off—that's what weekends are for. Take a drive, listen to music, go to the beach or lake, read—whatever you find rewarding and relaxing. Try to keep your thoughts in the present during this time so that you do not think about whatever it is that is causing the stress.

❏ Pursue a hobby. Hobbies are great for relieving stress. Take the time to do what you enjoy. Don't feel guilty about spending time doing something for yourself. Your health is worth it.

❏ Avoid hassles. Identify the things that are making you feel stressed out and either eliminate them from your life or prepare yourself to cope with them. If rush-hour traffic causes you stress, see if you can change your work hours slightly to avoid it. If that isn't possible, join a carpool or listen to a book on tape or a favorite piece of music while driving.

❏ Do not repress or deny your emotions. This only compounds stress. Admit your feelings and accept them. Keeping strong feelings bottled up only causes them to resurface later as illness. Don't be afraid to cry. Learning to cry can help you to manage stress. Crying can relieve anxiety and let loose bottled-up emotions.

❏ Work on creating a stress-free home environment. Keep the noise level down—noise contributes to stress. Turn down the radio, stereo, and television. Throw rugs and wall hangings absorb noise and are good additions to decor. Color is another important element of your environment to consider. Certain colors are much more calming and soothing than others (see COLOR THERAPY in Part Three). Also, use as much natural lighting in your home as possible. Unnatural fluorescent lighting can be especially aggravating.

❏ Investigate aromatherapy. This is the art of using highly concentrated distilled plant essences, called essential oils, for healing purposes. Essential oils affect both the mind and the body by means of olfactory stimulation of the brain. Essential oils that are particularly good for relieving stress include chamomile, bergamot, sandalwood, lavender, and sweet marjoram. Add 10 to 20 drops of one or more of these oils to a warm bath and relax in the tub, or simply dab a couple of drops of oil on a tissue or handkerchief and inhale the aroma periodically during the day. (See AROMATHERAPY AND ESSENTIAL OILS in Part Three.)

❏ Try not to take life too seriously. Learn to laugh.

❏ If stress-related symptoms become chronic or recurrent, consult your doctor to rule out an underlying illness.

❏ If you feel you simply cannot handle the stresses in your life, consider seeking outside help. It may be worth it to consult a qualified counselor or other practitioner who can help you to handle your problems and learn effective stress-reduction techniques. It is often enlightening and beneficial to talk with someone who can offer an objective response, whether a trusted friend or a professional counselor.

CONSIDERATIONS

❏ A study done at the University of Washington Medical School rated stressful situations according to their negative effects on physical and mental health. Rated highest was the death of a spouse. Divorce is next, followed by such circumstances as getting married, personal illness, and so on. The study found that the more stressful situations a person is experiencing, the greater the chance of illness.

❏ Stress in young people should never be underestimated. Problems at school, changing schools, peer pressures, personal image problems, sexual identity issues, the addition of a family member, or problems with boyfriends or girlfriends all lead to anxiety in young children and adolescents. Moreover, young people generally have fewer mechanisms or resources to cope with these situations than adults do. Often, adolescents or young children act out their feelings of stress in ways that are difficult for adults to understand.

❏ Research has shown that the hormone dehydroepiandrosterone (DHEA) can help people to cope with stress. (See DHEA THERAPY in Part Three.)

❏ Evidence shows that stress can trigger reactions to allergens and make allergic symptoms more severe.

❏ Stress can aggravate certain skin disorders, such as psoriasis and skin cancer, by damaging immune cells in the skin. The damage is done by a chemical released when nerve cells respond to stress.

❏ Dr. Hans Selye, stress expert and author of *Stress Without Distress* (J.B. Lippincott, 1974), said that it is not stress that is harmful—it is *dis*tress. Distress occurs when unresolved emotional stress is prolonged and not dealt with in a positive way.

❏ A group of Dutch researchers studied a group of eighty people for a period of six months. They found that individuals with high levels of stress had fewer than half the antibodies in their systems that subjects under less stress did.

❏ In a study done at the University of Pennsylvania, people who considered themselves chronic worriers found that they could reduce their anxiety levels by setting aside a specific time to worry each day. They reserved thirty minutes each day to worry and did not permit themselves to worry at other times.

❏ Heavy metal intoxication and food allergies can both cause symptoms that mimic those of stress. A hair analysis can reveal heavy metal poisoning. (See HAIR ANALYSIS in Part Three; see also ALLERGIES in Part Two.)

❏ The symptoms of hypoglycemia may mimic those of stress. (See HYPOGELYCEMIA in Part Two.)

❏ See also ANXIETY DISORDER and DEPRESSION in Part Two.

Stretch Marks

See under PREGNANCY-RELATED PROBLEMS.

Stroke

See under ARTERIOSCLEROSIS/ATHEROSCLEROSIS; CARDIOVASCULAR DISEASE.

Stye

See under EYE PROBLEMS.

Substance Abuse

See ALCOHOLISM; DRUG ADDICTION (SUBSTANCE ABUSE); SMOKING DEPENDENCY.

Sunburn

Sunburn is caused by excessive exposure to the sun's ultraviolet (UV) rays. The amount of exposure required to cause a burn depends on the individual, the geographical location, the time, and the atmospheric conditions. There are two types of ultraviolet rays, designated ultraviolet-A (UVA) and ultraviolet-B (UVB). Both are dangerous. UVB rays attack the skin's outer layers, while UVA rays attack the underlying layers.

Most sunburns are first-degree burns that cause the skin to become red, warm, and tender to the touch. Depending on the severity of the burn and the individual's skin type, the burn may subsequently "cool" into a suntan or thin layers of skin may peel off. A more serious sunburn can be a second-degree burn, causing extreme reddening, swelling, pain, and even blisters. This is a sign that the burn has gone deeper than just the surface layer of the skin and has caused damage and the release of fluids from cells in the lower layers of the skin. This results in eruptions and breaks in the skin where bacteria and other infectious organisms can enter. In the most severe cases, the burn may be accompanied by chills, fever, nausea, and/or delirium. Sunburn such as this is extremely painful and, for children, extremely dangerous. Dehydration often accompanies of sunburn.

Fair-skinned people are more prone to sunburn than darker skinned individuals, but no matter what your skin color, you will burn if you get enough exposure. Symptoms do not necessarily appear while you are in the sun; they may begin from one hour to twenty-four hours after sun exposure, and usually reach their peak in two to three days.

Today, the effects of sun exposure are becoming an increasing concern because of the decline in the earth's ozone layer. The ozone layer screens out the most harmful ultraviolet rays, but it is becoming steadily thinner all over the world, and holes that fluctuate in size have developed in various places. The incidence of skin cancer is growing at an alarming rate. Having two or more bad episodes of sunburn as a child makes you much more likely to develop skin cancer as an adult. (*See* SKIN CANCER in Part Two.)

Unless otherwise stated, the dosages recommended here are for adults. For a child between the ages of twelve and seventeen, reduce the dose to three-quarters of the recommended amount. For a child between the ages of six and twelve, use one-half the recommended dose, and for a child under six, use one-quarter of the recommended amount.

NUTRIENTS

SUPPLEMENT	SUGGESTED DOSAGE	COMMENTS
Important		
Cell Guard from Biotec Foods	As directed on label.	Provides high levels of antioxidants to protect and nourish the cells.
Coenzyme Q_{10}	60 mg daily.	Free radical scavenger that also increases the supply of oxygen to the cells.
Colloidal silver	Apply topically as directed on label.	Antiseptic to prevent infection. Subdues inflammation and promotes healing.
ConcenTrace from Trace Minerals Research	As directed on label.	Nourishes the skin by providing needed trace minerals.
Dimethylglycine (DMG) (Aangamik DMG from FoodScience of Vermont)	As directed on label.	Increases tissue oxygenation.
Free-form amino acid complex (Amino Balance from Anabol Naturals)	As directed on label.	To supply protein, needed for tissue repair.
Herpanacine from Diamond-Herpanacine Associates	As directed on label.	Promotes skin health, detoxifies the body, and enhances immunity.
L-Cysteine	500 mg daily, on an empty stomach. Take with water or juice. Do not take with milk. Take with 50 mg vitamin B_6 and 1,500 mg vitamin C.	Promotes healing of burns.
Multivitamin and mineral complex	As directed on label.	All nutrients are necessary in balance.
Potassium	99 mg daily.	Potassium lost through sunburn must be replaced.

Pycnogenol	As directed on label.	An antioxidant that has circulatory benefits and may reduce skin damage risks.
Vitamin A with mixed carotenoids including beta-carotene and vitamin E	25,000 IU daily for 2 weeks, then reduce to 10,000 IU daily until healed. If you are pregnant, do not exceed 10,000 IU daily. Start with 100 IU daily and increase slowly to 1,600 IU daily until healed.	To destroy free radicals released by sun exposure and aid in tissue repair and healing. Use d-alpha-tocopherol form.
or AE Mulsion Forte from American Biologics and natural carotenoid complex (Betatene)	As directed on label. As directed on label.	Contains vitamins A and E in emulsion form, which enters the system more rapidly. Allows for easier assimilation and greater safety at higher doses. Free radical scavengers and immune enhancers.
Vitamin C with bioflavonoids	10,000 mg daily and up.	Needed for tissue repair and healing. Also reduces scarring. Use calcium ascorbate form.
Helpful		
All-Purpose Bactericide Spray from Aerobic Life Industries	Apply topically as directed on label.	Destroys bacteria on the skin, reducing the possibility of infection.
Calcium and magnesium	2,000 mg daily. 1,000 mg daily.	Necessary for proper pH balance and potassium utilization. Also reduces stress on tissues.
Essential fatty acids (primrose oil and Ultimate Oil from Nature's Secret are good sources)	As directed on label.	Needed for tissue healing.
Silica or horsetail	As directed on label.	Supplies silicon, needed for repair of skin tissue. *See under* Herbs, below.
Vitamin B complex plus extra vitamin B₆ (pyridoxine) and para-aminobenzoic acid (PABA)	100 mg of each major B vitamin daily, with meals (amounts of individual vitamins in a complex will vary). 50 mg 3 times daily, with meals. 25 mg daily, with meals.	Important for tissue healing, especially for serious burns. A sublingual form is best. Needed for protein metabolism. Good for protecting the skin.
Vitamin E oil or ointment	Once the burn has cooled and healing has begun, apply topically to the affected area 3–4 times daily.	Promotes healing and helps prevent scarring. Purchase in oil or ointment form, or open a capsule to release the oil.
Zinc	100 mg daily for 1 month; then reduce to 50 mg daily. Do not exceed 100 mg daily.	Boosts the immune system and aids in tissue healing. Use zinc gluconate lozenges or OptiZinc for best absorption.

HERBS

❑ Aloe vera gel is a remarkably effective treatment for any kind of burn. It is even used in the burn units of some hospitals. Aloe relieves discomfort, speeds healing, and also helps to moisturize the skin and relieve dryness. Gen-

tly apply a thin layer of aloe vera gel to the sunburned area. Reapply it every hour until the pain is gone. Pulp taken directly from inside the fresh plant is best. If you use a commercial aloe product, make sure to choose one that contains no mineral oil, paraffin waxes, alcohol, or coloring.

❑ Apply a salve of calendula flowers and St. John's wort to badly burned areas. These two herbs have antiseptic properties, act as a painkiller for burns, and promote healing of skin wounds.

❑ An herbal bath can help minimize the stinging and pain of sunburn. Add 6 cups of chamomile tea or 6 drops of chamomile oil to a lukewarm tubful of water. Soak in the bath for thirty minutes or more. Lavender oil is also good and can be used in place of chamomile oil if you wish.

❑ Make a large pot of strong comfrey or gotu kola tea and let it cool. Soak sterile cotton gauze in the tea to make a compress and apply it to the affected area. Leave the compress in place for up to thirty minutes.

Note: Comfrey is recommended for external use only.

❑ Horsetail is a good source of silica, which is beneficial for tissue repair.

❑ A cream containing at least 5 percent tea tree oil helps to heal sunburn and other skin irritations.

RECOMMENDATIONS

❑ Eat high-protein foods for tissue repair, and raw fruits and vegetables to supply needed vitamins and minerals.

❑ Drink plenty of fluids; sunburn dehydrates the body.

❑ For immediate relief of sunburn pain, use cool-water compresses or cold clay poultices. (*See* USING A POULTICE in Part Three.) Or dissolve 1 pound of baking soda in a tubful of cool water, and soak in the bath for about thirty minutes. The herbal treatments described above are also excellent for relieving pain and stinging.

❑ Strictly avoid any further sun exposure until the burn is completely healed.

❑ When it comes to sunburn, prevention is better than cure. While most sunburns are minor burns that heal on their own, a history of sunburn is strongly linked to the development of skin cancer. Take precautions to prevent yourself from getting sunburned:

• Avoid spending time outdoors between the hours of 10:00 A.M. and 3:00 P.M.

• When you do spend time outdoors, wear a sun hat, protective clothing, and sunglasses that specify UV protection. The best type of clothing is made of light-colored, lightweight, tightly woven material.

• Always use a sunscreen with a sun protection factor (SPF) of 15 or higher. Apply the sunscreen to all exposed areas of skin. Reapply it frequently, at least every three to four hours, more often if you are swimming or perspiring. Make sure the sunscreen protects against both UVA and

UVB rays. Keep in mind that the SPF number refers only to the level of protection against UVB rays. Avobenezone appears to provide the best protection against UVA damage.

• Add to your sunscreen the contents of 1 capsule each of vitamin A, vitamin C, vitamin E, and selenium to help prevent free radical damage to the skin. After sunning, add these antioxidants to whatever skin cream you use for added protection and to aid in preventing wrinkles.

• Don't neglect your lips. The lips also are susceptible to sunburn. Use a sun protection product designed for the lips as well as a sunscreen for your face and body. Choose a formula containing natural ingredients such as aloe vera and vitamin E. Your health food store should carry such products in handy stick form.

• Do not rely on the weather to judge how strong the sun is. Cloudy or hazy days do not afford protection against sunburn; approximately 80 percent of the sun's ultraviolet rays pass through clouds. Reflections from water, metal, sand, or snow may increase—even double—the amount of ultraviolet rays you absorb. Take the same precautions on cloudy or hazy days that you do on bright, sunny days. Almost 90 percent of sunburn is caused by incidental sun exposure, not sunbathing. If you work outdoors, always wear sun screen and protect yourself by wearing a hat.

• To prevent dehydration, drink plenty of water while spending time in the sun.

❏ If you desire a tan, start with only fifteen-minute periods of sun exposure, and increase your exposure slowly, adding no more than fifteen more minutes every few days. This helps to prevent burning and results in a longer-lasting tan. Self-tanning lotions may be the safest way to get a tan.

❏ Always wear sunglasses to protect your eyes. Make sure your glasses protect your eyes from both UVA and UVB rays.

❏ For ordinary sunburn apply cool—not cold—compresses to the affected area(s) as often as needed. If the burn is severe, see a physician. If a child is sunburned, take special care. Do not apply any creams or anything to the burned area other than cool water or, *sparingly*, a bit of aloe vera gel twice a day. The burn will heal more readily if left exposed to the air.

❏ If you take any medications, ask your physician or pharmacist if they may increase your sensitivity to the sun.

CONSIDERATIONS

❏ Tretinoin (vitamin A acid), the active ingredient in the prescription medication Retin-A, is sometimes prescribed to help to repair skin that has been damaged by sun exposure. However, the use of tretinoin renders the skin significantly more vulnerable to additional sun damage. If you use this medication, you should *always* use a high-SPF sun block and avoid sun exposure as much as possible. This product should not be used during pregnancy, as it may cause birth defects.

❏ For a severe burn, a physician may prescribe silver sulfadiazine (Silvadene) cream and/or antibiotics to prevent infection, debridement to remove dead tissue, and/or hydrotherapy to loosen dead skin. Depending on the location and extent of the burn, physical therapy may be prescribed to keep muscles flexible. Muscle contracture can result from overlying skin damage and contraction.

❏ Your doctor may recommend taking an anti-inflammatory agent such as acetaminophen (Tylenol, Datril, and others) or ibuprofen (Advil, Nuprin, and others) to help relieve pain and inflammation. You should not give an aspirin-based product to a child with a sunburn.

❏ Berlock dermatitis is a heightened reaction to the sun caused by oil of bergamot, a common ingredient in perfumes, pomades, and colognes.

Sweating

See under PREGNANCY-RELATED PROBLEMS.

Swimmer's Ear

See under EAR INFECTION.

Temporomandibular Joint Syndrome

See TMJ SYNDROME.

Tendinitis

See under BURSITIS.

Thrombophlebitis

Phlebitis means inflammation of a vein. This problem usually occurs in the extremities, particularly the legs. If the inflammation is associated with the formation of a thrombus (a blood clot) in the vein, the condition is called *thrombophlebitis*.

Thrombophlebitis can be either superficial or deep. It is considered superficial if it affects a subcutaneous vein, one of the veins near the skin's surface. In superficial thrombophlebitis, the affected vein can be felt (it feels harder than normal), and may be seen as a reddish line under the skin, with localized swelling, pain, and tenderness to the touch. If there is widespread vein involvement, the lymphatic vessels (thin-walled vessels carrying fluid from the tissues to the bloodstream) may become inflamed. Superficial thrombophlebitis is a relatively common disorder. A superficial clot may be brought about by trauma, infection, standing for long periods of time, lack of exercise, and intravenous drug use. Pregnancy, varicose veins, obesity, and smoking increase the risk of superficial vein thrombophlebitis. Thrombophlebitis may also be associated with environmental sensitivities or allergies. Diagnosis of the condition is usually based on physical findings and/or a medical history indicating an increased risk.

Deep thrombophlebitis (known also as deep venous thrombosis, or DVT) affects the intermuscular or intramuscular veins further below the skin's surface. DVT is a much more serious condition than superficial thrombophlebitis because the veins affected are larger and located deep within the musculature of the leg. These are the veins responsible for the transport of 90 percent of the blood that flows back to the heart from the legs. Symptoms of DVT may include pain, warmth, swelling, and/or bluish discoloration of the skin of the affected limb. These symptoms are sometimes (but not often) accompanied by fever and chills. The pain is typically felt as a deep soreness that is worse when standing or walking and that gets better with rest, especially with the leg elevated. The veins directly under the skin may become dilated and more visible. Inflammation situated in a vein in the pelvis is called pelvic vein thrombophlebitis.

The primary risk associated with DVT is a sharp restriction in blood flow through the veins that can result in chronic venous insufficiency, a condition characterized by swelling, increased pigmentation, dermatitis, and ulceration of the affected leg. DVT can even be life-threatening if a blood clot breaks off from the venous lining and travels through the bloodstream to the heart, lung, or brain, where it may lodge in a blood vessel and cut off circulation to those vital organs. However, despite its potential seriousness, DVT can be completely without symptoms. Indeed, nearly half of all people who have it have no symptoms. In order to make a definitive diagnosis of DVT, a doctor must rule out a number of other disorders, including cellulitis and occlusive arterial disease. Doppler ultrasound, extremity arteriography (to rule out occlusive arterial disease), or blood coagulation tests may be carried out.

The reason or reasons for the formation of clots in the veins are often unknown. In most cases, clots are probably the result of a minor injury to the inside lining of a blood vessel. If the vessel lining receives a microscopic tear, for instance, this initiates clotting—a normal part of the body's repair processes. Platelets clump together to protect the injured area, and a series of biochemical events is initiated that results in the transformation of fibrinogen, a circulating blood protein, into strands of insoluble fibrin, which are deposited to form a net that traps blood cells, plasma, and yet more platelets. The result is a blood clot. Other possible causes of deep thrombus formation include abnormal clotting tendencies; poor circulation; certain types of cancer; and Behçet's syndrome, a condition affecting the small blood vessels that predisposes an individual to the formation of clots. Factors that increase the risk of DVT include recent childbirth, surgery, trauma, the use of birth control pills, and prolonged bed rest (some studies indicate that up to 35 percent of hospital patients develop DVT).

Anyone can get thrombophlebitis, but the disorder occurs more frequently in women than in men. The risk of developing DVT increases dramatically after the age of forty and triples with each additional twenty years.

NUTRIENTS

SUPPLEMENT	SUGGESTED DOSAGE	COMMENTS
Important		
Acetyl-L-carnitine	500 mg daily.	Protects the brain and blood vessels from fat accumulation.
Coenzyme Q10	100–200 mg daily.	Improves circulation and protects the heart.
Flaxseed oil or Ultimate Oil from Nature's Secret	2 tsp daily. As directed on label.	To supply essential fatty acids that minimize blood clot formation and keep veins and arteries soft and pliable, promoting cellular and cardiovascular health.
Garlic (Kyolic from Wakunaga)	2 capsules 3 times daily, with meals.	Improves circulation and thins the blood.
Heart Science from Source Naturals	As directed on label.	Contains powerful antioxidants and artery lining protectors.
L-Cysteine and L-methionine	500 mg each daily, on an empty stomach. Take with water or juice, not milk. Take with 50 mg vitamin B6 and 100 mg vitamin C for better absorption.	Protects and preserves cells; prevents accumulation of fat in the blood vessels. (See AMINO ACIDS in Part One.)
Lecithin granules or capsules	1 tbsp 3 times daily, before meals. 1,200 mg 3 times daily, before meals.	Fat emulsifier; to increase circulation.
L-Histidine	500 mg daily.	Important blood vessel dilator.
Magnesium plus calcium	1,000 mg daily. 1,500 mg daily.	A natural blood thinner that reduces abnormal clotting. Works with magnesium.
Methylsulfonyl-methane (MSM)	As directed on label.	Relieves pain and inflammation.
Pycnogenol or grape seed extract	50 mg 3 times daily. As directed on label.	Antioxidants that restore flexibility to arterial walls and reduce the risk of blood vessel disease and thrombophlebitis.

Vitamin C with bioflavonoids	4,000–8,000 mg daily.	Aids circulation and reduces clotting tendencies. Bioflavonoids prevent bruising and promote healing.
Vitamin E	Start with 400 IU daily and increase slowly to 1,600 IU daily. If you have a clotting disorder or high blood pressure, start with 100 IU daily and increase slowly to 400 IU daily.	Thins the blood and reduces platelet "stickiness." Use d-alpha-tocopherol form. Emulsion form is recommended for easier assimilation and greater safety at high doses.
Zinc	50 mg daily. Do not exceed a total of 100 mg daily from all supplements.	Aids in healing of ulcers and boosts immune function. Needed to maintain proper concentration of vitamin E in the body. Use zinc gluconate lozenges or OptiZinc for best absorption.
Helpful		
Advanced Carotenoid Complex from Solgar	As directed on label.	Contains antioxidants, immune enhancers, free radical scavengers, potential cancer fighters, and heart disease protectors.
Body Essential Silica Gel from Natureworks	As directed on label.	Good for healing of veins and skin tissues.
Body Language Super Antioxidant from OxyFresh	As directed on label.	Protects the body from free radical damage, environmental stresses, and pollutants.
Vitamin B complex	As directed on label.	Speeds healing time and and aids all bodily functions.

HERBS

❏ Alfalfa, pau d'arco, red raspberry, rosemary, and yarrow are antioxidant herbs that improve blood oxygenation.

❏ Butcher's broom improves circulation.

❏ Cayenne (capsicum) thins the blood, eases blood pressure, and improves circulation. It can also be combined with ginger, plantain, and witch hazel in a poultice and applied directly on the affected area.

❏ Ginger, skullcap, and valerian root dilate the blood vessels and aid circulation.

❏ Ginkgo biloba improves circulation and brain function, and is a powerful antioxidant.

❏ Leg ulcers can be treated with alcohol-free goldenseal extract. Moisten a sterile piece of gauze with a dropperful of extract and place it over the affected area.

❏ Hawthorn dilates the blood vessels, lowers cholesterol levels, and protects the heart.

❏ Olive leaf extract aids in preventing infection.

RECOMMENDATIONS

❏ Eat plenty of fresh fruits and vegetables; raw nuts and seeds; soybean products; and whole grains.

❏ Reduce your consumption of red meat. Better yet, eliminate it from your diet.

❏ Do not consume any dairy products, fried or salty foods, or processed or partially hydrogenated vegetable oils.

❏ Get regular moderate exercise. Walking, swimming, and other exercise improve circulation and prevent sluggishness in the veins, lessening the tendency to form clots.

❏ Take alternating hot and cold sitz baths, or apply alternating hot and cold compresses using the herbs recommended above. (*See* SITZ BATH in Part Three.)

❏ Lie on a padded slant board with your feet higher than your head for fifteen minutes a day. This is particularly helpful if you stand on your feet a lot.

❏ Ask your pharmacist about special elastic support stockings (antiembolism stockings) to improve circulation.

❏ If you smoke, *stop*. Smoking constricts the blood vessels, resulting in poor circulation and weakened blood flow. This is especially important if you are taking birth control pills. (*See* SMOKING DEPENDENCY in Part Two.)

❏ Avoid wearing tight-fitting clothing that cuts off circulation, such as knee socks with tight bands and girdles.

❏ If you experience a swollen, painful vein that does not get better within two weeks, talk to a health professional.

❏ If you are confined to bed, move your legs as much as possible to counteract pooling of the blood in the veins. Clean your legs daily to remove germs that can cause infection. Avoid using products that can dry your skin. Contact your health care provider if you notice any redness or swelling in the legs—these may be signs of infection.

❏ If you develop leg ulcers, keep the ulcers clean and germ-free to prevent infection. Follow your physician's recommendations concerning proper care for your ulcers, and be forewarned that leg ulcers may take three months to a year to heal. (*See* LEG ULCERS in Part Two.)

CONSIDERATIONS

❏ Superficial thrombophlebitis is usually treated by elevating the affected limb; applying warm moist compresses; and bed rest. A doctor may also prescribe anti-inflammatory drugs.

❏ Aspirin (less than one regular tablet per day) is an effective anticoagulant for treating DVT.

❏ DVT is a potentially serious health problem, and hospitalization may be recommended. An anticoagulant such as heparin or warfarin (Coumadin) is usually given, both intravenously and orally. Surgery may be needed to tie off the affected vein to prevent the clot from traveling to the lungs, a condition known as a pulmonary embolism. Recovery time varies, depending on the severity of the disease.

Note: Do not combine vitamin E and prescription blood-thinning drugs.

☐ Behçet's syndrome is a chronic multisystem disease distinguished by thrombophlebitis, plus arthritis, iritis, uveitis, and ulceration of the mouth and genitalia. This disease is found worldwide, but is most common in young men of eastern Mediterranean and eastern Asian descent. Persons with Behçet's syndrome should avoid needle punctures, as these can induce inflammatory skin lesions.

☐ *See also* CIRCULATORY PROBLEMS and LEG ULCERS, both in Part Two.

Thrush

See under FUNGAL INFECTION.

Thyroid Problems

See HYPERTHYROIDISM; HYPOTHYROIDISM.

Tic Douloureux

See under HEADACHE.

Tinnitus

See under HEARING LOSS.

TMJ Syndrome

An estimated 10 million Americans suffer from temporomandibular joint (TMJ) syndrome, a condition in which the temporomandibular joint does not function properly. This is the joint that connects the temporal bone (the bone that forms the sides of the skull) with the mandible (the jawbone). This painful affliction produces pain in the muscles and joints of the jaw that sometimes radiates to the face, neck, and shoulder. There may also be difficulty opening the mouth all the way, and clicking, grinding, and popping noises may occur during chewing and movement of the joint. Headaches, muscle spasms, toothaches, dizziness, feelings of pain and pressure behind the eyes, pain and ringing in the ears, and difficulty opening and closing the jaw normally are other possible symptoms.

The jaw joint is embedded in an intricate web of nerves and muscle. The force of chewing (something we do a lot of) and of clenching or gritting the teeth creates enormous tension and pressure in that region of the face. The cartilage disk that cushions the joint may become displaced or wear out. This causes the bones of the temporomandibular joint to rub against one another, rather than gliding smoothly past each other. In some instances, a misalignment of the jaw and teeth prevents smooth operation of the joint.

The most common underlying causes of TMJ syndrome are stress and a poor bite, together with clenching and grinding of the teeth (bruxism), especially at night. TMJ syndrome can also be caused by bad posture, habits such as cradling the telephone between the shoulder and jaw, repeated or hard blows to the jaw or chin, or whiplash. Poor dental work and orthodontia may aggravate the problem, as can habits such as gum chewing, thumb-sucking, and chewing exclusively on one side of the mouth. A common contributing factor is hypoglycemia; people tend to clench and grind their teeth more when their blood sugar is low.

To diagnose TMJ syndrome, a physician may use x-rays and a technique called arthrography, in which an opaque dye is injected into the joint and then viewed with fluoroscopy.

A correct diet and the proper supplements, possibly in conjunction with other treatments, are valuable for TMJ syndrome and often solve the problem. They are also helpful for bruxism (tooth-grinding).

TMJ SELF-TEST

Place your little fingers in your ears so that hearing is obstructed. Then slowly and steadily open and close your jaw. If at any point you hear a clicking, popping, and/or grinding noise, the jaw joints may be out of alignment, and examination by a professional experienced in diagnosing and treating TMJ syndrome is advisable.

NUTRIENTS

SUPPLEMENT	SUGGESTED DOSAGE	COMMENTS
Essential		
Calcium and	2,000 mg daily.	For proper muscular function and calming effect. Prevents
magnesium	1,500 mg daily, in divided doses, after meals and at bedtime.	bone softening and relieves stress. Use chelate forms.
Chondroitin sulfate plus	500–1,000 mg daily.	Nutritional support for strengthening joints, ligaments, and tendons.
glucosamine sulfate	As directed on label.	
Kyolic-EPA from Wakunaga		Increases activity of anti-inflammatory prostaglandins.
Methylsulfonyl-methane (MSM)	500–1,000 mg 3 times daily.	A sulfur compound that can reduce inflammation and aid in joint and tissue repair.

S-Adenosylmethio-nine (SAMe) (SAMe Rx-Mood from Nature's Plus)	400 mg 2 times daily.	Deficiency results in an inability to maintain cartilage properly. Aids in reducing pain and inflammation. *Caution:* Do not use if you have manic-depressive disorder or take prescription antidepressants.
Vitamin B complex plus extra pantothenic acid (vitamin B$_5$)	100 mg of each major B vitamin 3 times daily (amounts of individual vitamins in a complex will vary). 100 mg twice daily.	Anti-stress vitamins. Sublingual forms are recommended for best absorption.
Helpful		
Coenzyme Q$_{10}$ plus Coenzyme A from Coenzyme-A Technologies	60 mg daily. As directed on label.	Improves oxygenation of affected tissues. Works effectively with coenzyme Q$_{10}$ to support the immune system's detoxification of many dangerous substances.
L-Tyrosine	500 mg daily. Take at bedtime on an empty stomach with water or juice. Do not take with milk. Take with 50 mg vitamin B$_6$ and 500 mg vitamin C for better absorption.	Improves the quality of sleep and relieves anxiety and depression. (*See* AMINO ACIDS in Part One.) *Caution:* Do not take tyrosine if you are taking an MAO inhibitor drug.
Multivitamin and mineral complex	As directed on label.	For balanced nutrients. A hypoallergenic product is best.
Shark cartilage (BeneFin from Lane Labs)	Start with 1 gram per 15 lbs of body weight daily, divided into 3 doses. When relief is achieved, reduce the dosage to 1 gm per 40 lbs of body weight daily.	Treats pain and inflammation. Aids in repairing joints and bones.
Vitamin C with bioflavonoids	4,000–8,000 mg daily.	Combats stress and is necessary in adrenal gland function. Also necessary for healing and repair of connective tissue.

HERBS

❑ Blue violet, catnip, chamomile, hops, kava kava, lobelia, St. John's wort, skullcap, thyme, passionflower, red raspberry, valerian root, and wild lettuce have calming and anti-stress properties.

Caution: Do not use chamomile regularly, as ragweed allergy may result. Avoid it completely if you are allergic to ragweed. Do not take lobelia internally on an ongoing basis.

❑ Boswellia, an Ayurvedic herb, helps to restore blood vessels around inflamed connective tissue. It also reduces inflammation.

❑ Feverfew and ginger are good for pain and soreness. Ginger is also a powerful antioxidant that has anti-inflammatory effects.

Caution: Do not use feverfew during pregnancy.

❑ Nettle leaf has anti-inflammatory properties.

❑ SP-14 Valerian Blend from Solaray Products combats stress and is also beneficial.

❑ Turmeric and willow bark are good for pain and inflammation.

RECOMMENDATIONS

❑ Eat a diet including lightly steamed vegetables, fresh fruits, whole-grain products, white fish, skinless chicken and turkey, brown rice, and homemade soups and breads. Also eat more sulfur-containing foods, such as asparagus, eggs, garlic, and onions. Sulfur is needed for the repair and rebuilding of bone, cartilage, and connective tissue. It also aids in the absorption of calcium.

❑ Eat fresh pineapple frequently. Bromelain, an enzyme found in pineapple, is excellent for reducing inflammation. To be effective, the pineapple must be fresh. Freezing and canning destroy enzymes.

❑ Avoid high-stress foods: all forms of sugar, all white flour products, all junk foods, candy, colas, potato chips, pies, and fast foods.

❑ Do not consume any foods or beverages containing caffeine. As a stimulant, caffeine can increase tension, which often aggravates the problem. Also avoid taking over-the-counter medications containing decongestants, which can have a similar effect.

❑ Do not consume alcoholic beverages. These are a common contributing factor in bruxism (tooth-grinding), which can cause or aggravate TMJ syndrome.

❑ If you work at a desk, check your posture periodically throughout the day. Do not lean over the desk; keep your back comfortably straight, with your ears not too far in front of your shoulders. Try to keep your head aligned so that your cheekbones are over your collarbone.

❑ Sleep on your back to give your back, shoulder, and neck muscles plenty of rest. Do not sleep on your side or lie on your stomach with your head turned to the side. Avoid propping your head at a sharp angle to read or watch television in bed.

❑ Fast at least once a month to give the body and jaws a rest. (*See* FASTING in Part Three.)

❑ Do not chew gum. Avoid overly chewy foods such as red meat and bagels.

❑ Experiment with heat and cold therapy, and use hot or cold packs—whichever works best—for relief of pain, especially pain in the neck and shoulders.

❑ Be wary of any practitioner who rigidly adheres to one single approach in treating TMJ syndrome. A multidisciplinary team is a better choice. If possible, seek help from practitioners associated with a university dental or medical school.

CONSIDERATIONS

❑ TMJ syndrome is often treated with a special bite plate that is worn over the teeth to stabilize the bite and prevent tooth-clenching. To permanently correct the bite, you may have to have teeth reshaped, undergo orthodontia, or get crowns or a permanent oral appliance. Rarely, surgery is required to repair a damaged joint.

❏ Stress management, combined with heat and muscle relaxants, often relieves the symptoms of TMJ syndrome.

❏ Physical therapy is becoming a widely recognized, viable treatment for TMJ syndrome. This may involve jaw and tongue exercises to retrain stressed muscles and/or the use of a transcutaneous nerve stimulation (TENS) unit; ultrasound, which promotes tissue healing; and electrogalvanic stimulation, which helps relax muscles. These types of therapy should be prescribed in conjunction with an exercise and stress-reduction program.

❏ Some TMJ syndrome sufferers have been helped by biofeedback readings taken from the masseter muscle (the muscle that opens and closes the jaw). This treatment, combined with relaxation techniques such as controlled breathing, has proved effective.

❏ TMJ syndrome has become a much misdiagnosed and overtreated disorder. People with ambiguous pain in various parts of their bodies (such as menstrual cramps) have been misdiagnosed as having TMJ syndrome, for example. Some health care practitioners have voiced concern that TMJ syndrome may be providing inadequately trained or even disreputable practitioners with an opportunity to take advantage of patients. According to an article published in the February 1993 issue of the *New York State Journal of Medicine*, TMJ syndrome is an area in which "dental quackery" is quite common.

❏ Orthodontists, dentists, physical therapists, and many other "specialists" now offer various treatments for TMJ syndrome. However, it is estimated that 90 percent of all cases of TMJ syndrome respond to simple, inexpensive treatments, such as those recommended in this section. It therefore makes sense to try such measures *before* investing in expensive medical or dental treatment.

❏ TMJ syndrome is not the only disorder that can cause jaw pain. Another possible cause is rheumatoid arthritis. In this disorder, the symptoms are more severe in the morning and tend to ease somewhat as the day goes on (*see* ARTHRITIS in Part Two). This is not usually the case with TMJ syndrome. A displaced disk can also cause jaw pain. Treatment for this disorder involves realigning the ligaments with a plastic splint.

❏ *See also* BRUXISM and STRESS, both in Part Two.

Tonsillitis

Tonsillitis is an inflammation of the palatine tonsils, which are the accumulations of lymphatic tissue on the right and left sides of the upper throat. It can be caused by either viral or bacterial infection. Generally, younger children tend to get viral tonsillitis, while older children and adults tend to get bacterial tonsillitis—usually caused by *Streptococcus* bacteria. Symptoms include sore throat, difficulty swallowing, hoarseness, coughing, and redness, pain, and swelling of the tonsils. Other possible symptoms include headache, earache, fever and chills, nausea and vomiting, nasal obstruction and discharge, and enlarged lymph nodes throughout the body.

This disorder is most common in children, but it can occur at any age. In adults, it may be a sign that the body's resistance to disease is lower than it should be. An improper diet that is high in refined carbohydrates and low in protein and other nutrients may also predispose one to developing tonsillitis. Some people have repeated bouts of tonsillitis, and it can become a chronic condition. If untreated, tonsillitis can lead to a very severe condition called a *peritonsillar abscess*, in which the airways become obstructed, making breathing difficult. The infection can also spread into the neck and chest area. In general, the more repeated bouts of tonsillitis a person has, the more difficult it is to cure. Each time the tonsils become inflamed, scar tissue accumulates on the tonsils.

Unless otherwise specified, the dosages recommended here are for adults. For a child between the ages of twelve and seventeen, reduce the dose to three-quarters the recommended amount. For a child between six and twelve, use one-half the recommended dose, and for a child under the age of six, use one-quarter the recommended amount.

NUTRIENTS

SUPPLEMENT	SUGGESTED DOSAGE	COMMENTS
Important		
Vitamin C with bioflavonoids	5,000–20,000 mg daily. (*See* ASCORBIC ACID FLUSH in Part Three.)	To fight infection and boost the immune response.
Zinc lozenges	1 15-mg lozenge every 2–3 waking hours for 3 days, then reduce to 1 lozenge 4 times daily until healed.	An immunostimulant that aids healing.
Helpful		
Acidophilus (Kyo-Dophilus by Wakunaga is a good source)	As directed on label. Take on an empty stomach.	Necessary if antibiotics are prescribed. Use a nondairy formula.
Chlorophyll	Use as a gargle as directed on label.	Has an antibiotic effect and can heal irritations in the mouth and throat. Use a liquid form.
Cod liver oil	As directed on label.	Aids immune response and healing of tissue.
Colloidal silver	As directed on label.	An antibiotic that reduces inflammation and inhibits infection.
Maitake extract or shiitake extract or reishi extract	As directed on label. As directed on label. As directed on label.	Mushrooms with immune-boosting and antiviral properties.

Proteolytic enzymes	As directed on label. Take between meals.	Aids in reducing inflammation.
Pycnogenol or grape seed extract	As directed on label. As directed on label.	Antioxidants that protect the skin, reduce inflammation, and enhance immunity.
Vitamin A with mixed carotenoids including beta-carotene	10,000 IU daily for 3 days, then reduce to 5,000 IU daily.	Needed for repair of tissue. Aids healing. Emulsion form is recommended for easier assimilation.
Vitamin B complex	50 mg of each major B vitamin 3 times daily, with meals (amounts of individual vitamins in a complex will vary).	To help maintain a healthy mouth and throat.
plus extra pantothenic acid (vitamin B$_5$)	100 mg daily.	Plays a role in the production of the formation of antibodies and aids in the utilization of other vitamins.
and vitamin B$_6$ (pyridoxine)	50 mg daily.	Helps reduce swelling.
Vitamin E	400 IU daily.	Destroys free radicals and enhances the immune system Use d-alpha-tocopherol form.

HERBS

❑ Catnip tea enemas are good for reducing fever. (*See* EN-EMAS in Part Three.)

❑ Chamomile relieves fever, headaches, and pain.

Caution: Do not use this herb on an ongoing basis, as ragweed allergy may result. Avoid it completely if you are allergic to ragweed.

❑ ClearLungs from RidgeCrest Herbals is an herbal combination that helps to strengthen the immune system, enhances tissue repair, and controls inflammation.

❑ Echinacea fights infection and boosts the immune system. Make echinacea tea and drink as much of it as you can. Or take it in tincture form, ½ teaspoon every three to four hours until your symptoms improve.

❑ A hot infusion made from equal parts of dried elder flower, peppermint, and yarrow eases the pain of tonsillitis. Drink this throughout the day.

❑ Flaxseed oil reduces pain and inflammation, and aids recovery.

❑ Marshmallow tea coats inflamed mucous membranes. Steep 3 heaping teaspoons of marshmallow blossoms in 3 cups of cold water for twelve hours, then heat and strain. Drink 2 to 3 cups daily.

❑ Hot mullein poultices are soothing. (*See* USING A POULTICE in Part Three.)

❑ Pau d'arco is a natural antibiotic and potentiates immune function. It is also a powerful antioxidant.

❑ Sage tea, made with a bit of alum, can be used as a gargle. It can also be prepared with hot malt vinegar and taken orally in 2- to 3-ounce doses.

Caution: Do not use sage if you suffer from any type of seizure disorder.

❑ For sore throat, take alcohol-free extract of goldenseal or St. John's wort. Place 6 drops or ½ dropperful of extract under your tongue and leave it there for a few minutes before swallowing. Do this four times daily for three days.

Caution: Do not take goldenseal internally on a daily basis for more than one week, do not use it while pregnant or breastfeeding, and use it with caution if you are allergic to ragweed.

❑ Thyme reduces fever, headaches, and mucus. It is good for chronic respiratory problems and sore throat.

RECOMMENDATIONS

❑ Use a warm saltwater gargle. Dissolve ½ teaspoon of salt in 1 cup of warm water and gargle with the mixture three times a day to help reduce swelling, relieve pain, and remove mucus.

❑ Apply hot or cold compresses, whichever one provides more relief, to the throat area.

❑ Do not smoke, and avoid secondhand smoke. Tobacco smoke irritates the throat.

❑ Add humidity to the air at home with a humidifier, a pan of water placed on a radiator, or boiling a pot of water on the stove. Moistening steam stimulates the blood flow to the mucous membranes, promoting healing.

❑ For relief of tonsillitis pain, inhale essential oils of bergamot, lavender, tea tree, thyme, benzoin, and lemon.

❑ If you have a sore throat that does not improve within two weeks, consult your health care provider to determine what type of sore throat you have.

❑ If your physician prescribes antibiotics for bacterial tonsillitis, eat yogurt and take an acidophilus supplement to replace the "friendly" bacteria. Do not take the acidophilus at the same time as the antibiotic, however.

❑ Rest and drink plenty of fluids.

CONSIDERATIONS

❑ A cleansing juice fast for three days with vegetable broth can be helpful. (*See* FASTING in Part Three.)

❑ Bee propolis is good for treating tonsillitis.

❑ If an abscess develops, surgical drainage may be required.

❑ If tonsillitis becomes recurrent or chronic, tonsillectomy (removal of the tonsils) may be recommended. In the past, doctors removed tonsils on a very frequent basis. Today we know that the tonsils are important for the proper functioning of the immune system. Tonsils should not be removed unless absolutely necessary.

Tooth Decay

Tooth decay rivals the common cold as the most prevalent human disorder. It is not a natural process, as many people believe, but a bacterial disease. This bacteria can enter the bloodstream and cause other problems in the body. Bacteria in the mouth combine with mucus and food debris to create a sticky mass called plaque that sticks to the surfaces of the teeth. The bacteria in the plaque feed on ingested sugars and produce an acid that leaches calcium and phosphate from the teeth. Gradually, if the sticky deposits are not removed, the teeth erode—first the enamel (the outer layer) and then the dentin (the body of the tooth). If unchecked, decay can progress even further, into the pulp that contains the nerve in the center of the tooth, resulting in a toothache. Infection may result, leaving the tooth vulnerable to abscess.

Tooth decay depends on three factors: the presence of bacteria, the availability of sugars for the bacteria to feed on, and the vulnerability of tooth enamel. Poor nutrition and poor oral hygiene are probably the main factors behind most cavities. In particular, people who consume large quantities of refined carbohydrates—especially sticky-textured foods that cling to tooth surfaces—or who snack frequently without cleaning their teeth afterwards are much more likely to have a problem with tooth decay. There are also some people who, for reasons not yet understood, seem to have unusually acidic saliva and/or higher than normal levels of bacteria present in their mouths, and they too are more prone to tooth decay.

Tooth decay normally causes no symptoms until it is rather far advanced. Then the tooth may become sensitive to heat, cold, and the consumption of sugar. In later stages, a toothache may occur.

Unless otherwise specified, the dosages recommended here are for adults. For a child between the ages of twelve and seventeen, reduce the dose to three-quarters of the recommended amount. For a child between six and twelve, use one-half of the recommended dose, and for a child under the age of six, use one-quarter of the recommended amount.

NUTRIENTS

SUPPLEMENT	SUGGESTED DOSAGE	COMMENTS
Important		
Acidophilus (Kyo-Dophilus from Wakunaga is a good source)	As directed on label.	Important if taking antibiotics; protects "friendly" bacteria in the colon. Use a nondairy formula.
Calcium and magnesium	1,500 mg daily. 750 mg daily.	Necessary for strong, healthy teeth. Needed to balance with calcium.
Grape seed extract	As directed on label.	A powerful antioxidant and anti-inflammatory.
L-Tyrosine	As directed on label, on an empty stomach. Take with water or juice. Do not take with milk. Take with 50 mg vitamin B_6 and 500 mg vitamin C for better absorption.	Use for relief of pain and anxiety. (*See* AMINO ACIDS in Part One.) *Caution:* Do not take this supplement if you are taking an MAO inhibitor drug.
Vitamin A with mixed carotenoids including beta-carotene	10,000 IU daily.	Important for healing and for tooth formation.
Vitamin B complex	As directed on label.	Helps maintain healthy nerves and gums. A sublingual type is best.
Vitamin C with bioflavonoids	3,000 mg daily in divided doses.	Protects against infection and inflammation. Do not use a chewable form, as this may erode tooth enamel.
Vitamin D_3	400 mg daily.	Needed for absorption of calcium and healing of gum tissue.
Vitamin E	600 IU daily.	Promotes healing.
Vitamin K	As directed on label.	May aid in preventing tooth decay.
Helpful		
Coenzyme Q_{10} plus Coenzyme A from Coenzyme-A Technologies	As directed on label. As directed on label.	Provides energy needed for gum cell growth and healing of gum tissue. Works effectively with coenzyme Q_{10} to support the immune system's detoxification of many dangerous substances.
Multivitamin and mineral complex	As directed on label.	All nutrients are needed in balance.
S-Adenosylmethionine (SAMe) by (SAMe Rx-Mood from Nature's Plus)	400 mg twice daily.	Deficiency results in an inability to maintain cartilage properly. Aids in reducing pain and inflammation. *Caution:* Do not use if you have manic depressive-disorder or take prescription antidepressants.
Shark cartilage (BeneFin from Lane Labs)	Start with 1 gram per 15 lbs of body weight daily, divided into 3 doses. When relief is achieved, reduce the dosage to 1 gm per 40 lbs of body weight daily.	Treats pain and inflammation. Aids in repairing joints and bones.
Zinc	30 mg daily. Do not exceed a total of 100 mg daily from all supplements.	Boosts immune function. Use zinc gluconate or OptiZinc for best absorption.

HERBS

❑ Calendula, chamomile, peppermint, and yarrow are natural anti-inflammatories.

❑ Clove oil is helpful for toothache pain. Apply 1 or 2 drops to the affected tooth with a cotton swab as needed. If you find the clove oil too strong, dilute it with olive oil.

❑ Alcohol-free goldenseal extract can be used as an anti-bacterial mouthwash. If inflammation is present, put a few drops of goldenseal extract on a piece of sterile cotton and press against the gum by the affected tooth, pushing in place tightly, at bedtime. Leave the cotton in place overnight. Do this for three consecutive nights to destroy bacteria and reduce inflammation.

❑ Kava kava, St. John's wort, white willow bark, and wintergreen have analgesic properties. White willow bark is also an anti-inflammatory.

❑ Sage is good for its anti-inflammatory properties. Bring to a boil 2 tablespoons of dried, crushed sage leaves in 1 cup of water. Steep for 20 minutes and strain. Cool to a comfortable temperature and use the mixture to rinse your mouth several times daily.

❑ Thyme is a natural antiseptic that reduces the level of bacteria in the mouth.

RECOMMENDATIONS

❑ Eat plenty of raw fruits and vegetables. These contain minerals that help to keep the saliva from becoming too acidic.

❑ Avoid carbonated soft drinks. These are high in phosphates, which promote the loss of calcium from the tooth enamel.

❑ Avoid all refined sugars.

❑ Do not smoke.

❑ Practice good oral hygiene. Brush your teeth after eating and floss between the teeth daily. This is the only way to remove cavity-causing plaque. There are also mouth rinses available to enhance the plaque-removing power of brushing and flossing. Do not brush overzealously or more than two or, at most, three times a day. Too much brushing can cause the gums to recede, exposing the root areas of the teeth, which are more prone to decay than the rest of the tooth. Use a soft-bristle toothbrush and replace it with a new one every month.

❑ Do not use chewable vitamin C supplements, which can erode tooth enamel. Tablets or powders designed for swallowing do not pose this danger.

❑ To ease the pain of toothache or abscess until you can see your dentist, rinse the affected area with warm salt water (add ½ teaspoon of salt to 8 ounces of warm water).

CONSIDERATIONS

❑ Stim-U-Dent, found in drugstores, is beneficial for keeping the gums massaged and clean. It also aids in removing plaque. Before using one, to avoid damaging your gums, soak it in water or hold in your mouth until it softens. Massage between all your teeth.

❑ Regularly scheduled dental checkups are recommended at least once yearly.

❑ Researchers are looking into the possibility of adding cranberry extract to toothpaste and/or mouthwash. Evidence suggests that a compound present in cranberries may reduce plaque formation.

❑ Researchers in Britain believe that they have developed a vaccine that prevents tooth decay by eliminating bacteria from the mouth. The American Dental Association's (ADA) Division of Science is optimistic about the findings and looks forward to additional studies.

❑ At present, the only known way to stop tooth decay once it has started is to remove the decayed area and cover it with some type of filling. Many different materials are used to fill cavities. The most common is the "silver" amalgam filling. Amalgam formulas vary, but virtually all contain about 50 percent mercury, a toxic heavy metal. There are other filling choices, however, including gold and natural-looking ceramic-based materials called composites. You may wish to discuss concerns about filling materials with your dentist before treatment.

❑ It was once believed that having dental work done posed a risk of endocarditis, a heart infection, for some people. There is not sufficient evidence to prove a link between the two, however.

❑ Fluoride increases resistance to tooth decay. It is added to many toothpastes and community drinking water supplies. Many dentists recommend routine fluoride treatments to prevent cavities, especially for children. Fluoride is a substance derived from the element fluorine. Fluorine is a deadly chemical, but fluoride is not believed to be dangerous in small amounts. However, there is debate as to whether or not fluoride is a risk factor for cancer. Animal and human epidemiology studies conducted on fluoride so far have not been conclusive as to whether or not fluoride is a carcinogen.

❑ Seven out of ten Americans get medical or dental x-rays in an average year. These peeks inside the body can be valuable, even lifesaving, tools for diagnosing health problems. But x-rays are sometimes ordered when they are not needed. Other times, failure to follow precautions may expose people to more radiation than necessary.

❑ Air abrasive technology uses a targeted spray of powder to remove tooth decay with no drilling sound or vibrations. Laser technology may be used as an alternative to the conventional dental drill.

Toxicity

See ALUMINUM TOXICITY; ARSENIC POISONING; CADMIUM TOXICITY; CHEMICAL POISONING; COPPER TOXICITY; ENVIRONMENTAL TOXICITY; FOODBORNE/WATERBORNE DISEASE; LEAD POISONING; MERCURY TOXICITY; NICKEL TOXICITY.

Tuberculosis

Tuberculosis (TB) is a very old and highly contagious disease caused by the bacteria *Mycobacterium tuberculosis*. It is primarily a disease of the lungs, but it can affect any body organ, including the bones, kidneys, intestines, spleen, and liver. One of the most lethal among infectious diseases, TB is found throughout the world. It is especially devastating in places such as Asia and Africa, where HIV and AIDS are widespread and have compromised the immune systems of so many people that the tuberculosis bacteria often meet with little or no resistance. It is estimated that by the year 2020, there will be 200 million new cases of this disease, and 70 million people worldwide will die from it.

TB is usually spread by infected airborne droplets that are coughed up by individuals with the active disease and then inhaled by susceptible persons. Once inhaled, the bacteria normally lodge in the lungs. The body may successfully battle the infection at this point. If the immune system is not functioning optimally, however, or if another onslaught of the bacteria reaches the lungs, chances are the bacteria will multiply and proceed to liquefy and destroy lung tissue. Overcrowded, poorly ventilated housing and overpopulated prisons are fertile breeding grounds for the spread of TB. Tuberculosis may also be contracted from contaminated food or from milk that has not been pasteurized. In such cases, the primary focus of the infection usually is in the digestive tract. This type of tuberculosis is more common in developing countries. It is rare in the Western world.

Symptoms of TB may be slow in developing and initially resemble those of influenza—general malaise, coughing, loss of appetite, night sweats, chest pain, and low-grade fever. At first, the cough may be nonproductive, but as the disease progresses, increasing amounts of sputum are produced. As the condition worsens, fever, night sweats, chronic fatigue, weight loss, chest pain, and shortness of breath may occur, and the sputum may become bloody. In advanced cases, TB of the larynx can occur, making it impossible to speak above a whisper.

Antibiotic regimens that could successfully combat the disease have been developed, and living standards have risen so that the poor nutrition and inadequate hygienic standards that had once helped TB to spread and flourish are less prevalent in the United States. In spite of the fact that multi-drug-resistant strains of TB exist (if a strain of TB is resistant to both of the drugs most often widely prescribed for TB, it is considered multi-drug-resistant), rates of TB have declined in the United States since 1993. Just over 18,000 cases of the disease were reported in 1998.

But the global epidemic of tuberculosis, together with the migration of people from one country to another, probably means that, unless aggressive action is taken to eradicate TB everywhere in the world, America will see an upsurge of this disease in coming decades. The best defense against tuberculosis is a strong immune system and a healthy diet.

NUTRIENTS

SUPPLEMENT	SUGGESTED DOSAGE	COMMENTS
Very Important		
AE Mulsion Forte from American Biologics or vitamin A	As directed on label, to supply 200,000 IU vitamin A daily. If you are pregnant, do not exceed 10,000 IU daily. 25,000 IU daily. If you are pregnant, do not	To supply vitamins A and E, vital for healing of lung tissue and protection against free radicals. This emulsion form is easily assimilated and is safe at high doses.
plus natural carotenoid complex (Betatene) plus	exceed 10,000 IU daily. 25,000 IU daily.	
vitamin E	400–800 IU daily.	Use d-alpha-tocopherol form.
Coenzyme Q$_{10}$	75 mg daily.	Helps carry oxygen to tissues for healing.
Colloidal silver	As directed on label.	An antiseptic that subdues inflammation and heals lesions.
Free-form amino acid complex	As directed on label.	Needed for tissue repair. Free-form amino acids are rapidly absorbed and assimilated by the body.
Garlic (Kyolic from Wakunaga)	2 capsules 3 times daily, with meals.	Acts as a natural antibiotic; keeps infection in check and stimulates immune function.
Grape seed extract	As directed on label.	A powerful antioxidant that enhances immunity.
L-Cysteine and L-methionine	500 mg each twice daily, on an empty stomach. Take with water or juice. Do not take with milk. Take with 50 mg vitamin B$_6$ and 1,500 mg vitamin C for better absorption and prevention of cysteine kidney stones.	To protect the lungs and liver by detoxifying harmful toxins. (*See* AMINO ACIDS in Part One.)
Selenium	200 mcg daily. If you are pregnant, do not exceed 40 mcg daily.	Protects against free radicals and promotes a healthy immune system.
Vitamin B complex	100 mg of each major B vitamin 3 times daily. (amounts of individual vitamins in a complex will vary).	Needed for production of red blood cells and antibodies. Aids in utilization of oxygen. Use a high-stress formula. Injections (under a doctor's supervision) may be necessary. If injections are not available, use a sublingual form.
plus extra pantothenic acid (vitamin B$_5$) and	100 mg 3 times daily.	The anti-stress vitamin.
vitamin B$_6$ (pyridoxine)	50 mg 3 times daily.	Some drugs used to fight TB can cause a deficiency of this vitamin.
Vitamin C with bioflavonoids	5,000–20,000 mg daily, in divided doses. (*See* ASCORBIC ACID FLUSH in Part Three.)	Strengthens immune response and promotes healing.

Supplement	Suggested Dosage	Comments
Vitamin D₃	Start with 1,000 IU daily and decrease slowly to 400 IU daily over the course of 1 month.	Essential for utilization of calcium and phosphorus. People with TB need sunlight daily and/or vitamin D for healing.
Vitamin E	Start with 400 IU daily and increase slowly to 1,600 IU daily over the course of 1 month.	Powerful free radical scavenger. Protects the lung tissues and provides oxygen to the cells. Use d-alpha-tocopherol form. Emulsion form is recommended for easier assimilation and greater safety at high doses.
Important		
ACES + Zn from Carlson Labs	As directed on label. Do not exceed 100 mg zinc daily from all sources.	A formula that fights free radicals with enzymes and antioxidants.
CTR Support from PhysioLogics	As directed on label.	To diminish damage caused by inflammation.
Essential fatty acids (Ultimate Oil from Nature's Secret is a good source)	As directed on label.	Important in formation of all cells, including lung tissue.
Glutathione	500 mg daily, on an empty stomach.	Protects the lungs and cells from free radical damage.
Kelp	2,000–3,000 mg daily.	For a natural supply of minerals. Rich in iodine.
L-Serine	500 mg daily, on an empty stomach. Take with water or juice. Do not take with milk. Take with 50 mg vitamin B₆ and 100 mg vitamin C for better absorption.	Helps the body maintain immune function. (*See* AMINO ACIDS in Part One.)
Multienzyme complex plus proteolytic enzymes	As directed on label. Take with meals. As directed on label. Take between meals.	Needed to keep inflammation down, to digest essential nutrients, and to improve absorption.
Multimineral complex with boron and calcium and magnesium and silica	3 mg daily. Do not exceed this amount. 1,000 mg daily. 750 mg daily. 25–100 mg daily.	All nutrients are needed for strength and healing. Take with meals. Use a high-potency formula. Do not use a sustained-release formula.
Multivitamin complex	As directed on label.	To provide a balance of needed nutrients.
Oxy-5000 Forte from American Biologics	As directed on label.	An antioxidant with superoxide dismutase (SOD).
Zinc	50–80 mg daily. Do not exceed a total of 100 mg daily from all supplements.	Promotes immune function and healing. Use zinc gluconate lozenges or OptiZinc for best absorption.

HERBS

❏ Butcher's broom, calendula, cayenne (capsicum), chamomile, peppermint, and yarrow have anti-inflammatory properties.

❏ Elecampane, ephedra, goldenseal root, horehound, licorice, lobelia, marshmallow root, mullein, myrrh gum, and thyme have decongestant and expectorant properties.

❏ A combination echinacea and pau d'arco tea is beneficial. Echinacea is a powerful antioxidant and bolsters the immune system; pau d'arco benefits the body by cleansing the blood and acting as an antibacterial agent, as well as possessing anti-tumor agents. Drink 3 cups of this tea daily. Or combine echinacea tincture with equal parts of tinctures of elecampane and mullein, and take 1 teaspoon of this mixture three times daily.

❏ ClearLungs from RidgeCrest Herbals is a Chinese herbal formula that relieves bronchial and lung congestion.

❏ Lung Tonic from Herbs, Etc. supports lung function.

RECOMMENDATIONS

❏ If you suspect you may have tuberculosis, or that you may have been exposed to it, see your health care provider. Prompt, proper treatment is essential.

❏ Follow the prescribed treatment regimen exactly. If any medications cause side effects, contact your physician. *Do not* discontinue taking the medications on your own.

❏ To promote healing, eat a diet consisting of at least 50 percent raw vegetables and fruits. Also eat alfalfa sprouts, fish, fowl, pomegranates, raw cheeses, raw seeds and nuts, whole grains, and garlic.

❏ Drink fresh pineapple and carrot juice and a "green drink" daily. Drink fresh raw potato juice; potato juice contains compounds called protease inhibitors, which block carcinogens and prevent cell mutation. (*See* JUICING in Part Three.)

❏ Make purée of steamed asparagus in a blender. Refrigerate and take 4 tablespoons twice a day with meals. Asparagus stimulates immune function and is anticarcinogenic.

❏ Make kefir, buttermilk, and fresh sugar-free yogurt a part of your daily diet. Also take an acidophilus supplement for as long as you are taking antibiotics, to relieve stress on the gastrointestinal tract and enhance nutrient absorption. Do not take the acidophilus at the same time as the antibiotic, but do make sure you take it.

❏ Do not smoke or consume alcohol or use recreational drugs. All of these affect the ability of the immune system to fight infection. Smoking is even more dangerous than usual in the presence of a lung infection.

❏ Avoid stress. Rest, sunshine, and fresh air are most important. A dry climate is recommended.

CONSIDERATIONS

❏ People infected with TB should not use cortisone preparations. Cortisone suppresses immune function and makes the infection more difficult to treat.

❏ Vaccines and drugs cannot control TB if poor lifestyle practices are followed. Cleanliness and proper nutrition are vital in combating this disease.

❏ Experts estimate that up to 90 percent of the population may have encountered the tubercle bacillus sometime in their lives, but in the majority of cases, the immune system successfully keeps a full-blown infection from developing. People who do not defeat it outright often carry the germ in a dormant state, sometimes for decades, before immunity weakens and the bacteria begin replicating and infect the host.

❏ The Air Supply personal air purifier from Wein Products is a small unit worn around the neck. It sets up an invisible pure air shield against microorganisms (such as viruses, bacteria, and mold) and microparticles (including dust, pollen, and pollutants) in the air. It also eliminates vapors, smells, and harmful volatile compounds in the air. The Living Air XL-15 unit from Alpine Industries is an ionizing unit good for purifying the air in the home or workplace.

❏ The tubercle bacillus has an incredible capacity for reproduction. A single organism is capable of producing billions of descendants within one month.

❏ The American Lung Association estimates that tuberculosis affects approximately 6.8 of every 100,000 persons in the United States. The World Health Organization has singled out TB as a "global health emergency."

❏ People with AIDS are more likely than most to have tuberculosis at some point during their illness

❏ The Bacillus Calmette-Guerin vaccine (BCG), which consists of a weakened form of tubercle bacilli, can be used for vaccination against tuberculosis. Many medical authorities believe BCG is an effective preventive measure against TB, while others have serious doubts about its safety. A TB skin test may indicate if you are carrying TB bacteria even before you have symptoms of the disease.

❏ The World Health Organization has recommended a global strategy—directly observed treatment short course, or DOTS—as a method of conquering TB. The basis of this program is to both treat and then monitor the TB infected subjects very closely, making sure they complete their course of antibiotics. Cure rates in this type of program have reached as high as 95 percent, even in the poorest of conditions where TB used to thrive.

Tumor

A tumor, or neoplasm, is an abnormal new growth of tissue. It may be localized to one area or present on many sites in the body. Tumors can appear nearly anywhere in or on the body and can be cancerous (malignant) or benign (noncancerous). Polyps and papillomas are examples of benign tumors. Squamous cell and basal cell carcinomas are examples of malignant tumors.

Unlike benign tumors, malignant tumors are usually serious and are likely to grow, take over other organs, and metastasize (spread). They can be a life-threatening problem if they are not detected and treated at an early stage. The prognosis for a person who develops a malignant tumor depends on the location of that tumor. If it is difficult to detect and there are few discernable symptoms, then treatment may not begin soon enough to prevent the tumor from metastasizing.

Environmental factors and diet seem to play an important role in the development of tumors of all types. Tumors have been known to decrease in size and even disappear in response to dietary changes and supplementation with high-quality vitamins and minerals. The suggestions here are designed to enhance immune function and suppress the growth of tumors—both benign and malignant.

Unless otherwise specified, the dosages recommended here are for adults. For a child between the ages of twelve and seventeen, reduce the dose to three-quarters of the recommended amount. For a child between six and twelve, use one-half of the recommended dose, and for a child under the age of six, use one-quarter of the recommended amount.

NUTRIENTS

SUPPLEMENT	SUGGESTED DOSAGE	COMMENTS
Important		
Coenzyme Q$_{10}$ plus	100 mg daily.	Promotes immune function; carries oxygen to the cells.
Coenzyme A from Coenzyme-A Technologies	As directed on label.	Works with coenzyme Q$_{10}$.
Garlic (Kyolic from Wakunaga)	2 capsules 3 times daily, with meals.	May help to reduce the size of tumors.
Maitake extract or	As directed on label.	Mushroom extracts that strengthen the body and
reshii extract or	As directed on label.	improve overall health; have immunostimulant properties,
shiitake extract	As directed on label.	have anti-tumor action, and reverse T cell suppression caused by tumors.
Melatonin	5–10 mg daily, at bedtime.	People with brain tumors may have an increased survival rate if they take melatonin along with their radiation therapy.
Proteolytic enzymes or	As directed on label.	To help the immune system and aid in the breakdown
Inflazyme Forte from American Biologics or	As directed on label.	of undigested foods.
Wobenzym N from Marlyn Nutraceuticals	As directed on label.	
Shark cartilage (BeneFin from Lane Labs)	1 gm per 2 lbs of body weight daily, divided into 3 doses. If you cannot tolerate taking it orally, it can be administered in a retention enema.	Has been shown to inhibit and even reverse the growth of some types of tumors. Also stimulates the immune system.
or shark liver oil	100 mg 3 times daily for 20 days, then 10–15 days off. Maintain this schedule.	Immune system booster that can help protect the body from radiation damage.
Vitamin C with bioflavonoids	3,000–10,000 mg daily, in divided doses.	Promotes immune function.

Zinc	30–80 mg daily. Do not exceed a total of 100 mg daily from all supplements.	Promotes a healthy immune system and wound healing, and helps maintain the proper concentration of vitamin E in the blood. Use zinc gluconate lozenges or OptiZinc for best absorption.
Helpful		
Kelp	1,000–1,500 mg daily.	Promotes immune function. Supplies balanced minerals.
L-Arginine	500 mg daily, on an empty stomach. Take with water or juice. Do not take with milk. Take with 50 mg vitamin B₆ and 100 mg vitamin C for better absorption.	Retards tumor growth by enhancing immune function. (*See* AMINO ACIDS in Part One.)
and L-cysteine	500 mg daily, on an empty stomach. Take with 1,500 mg vitamin C to prevent cystine kidney stones.	Detoxifies harmful toxins, protects the body against radiation, and acts against carcinogens.
plus glutathione	500 mg daily, on an empty stomach.	Helps reduce side effects of chemotherapy and protect the liver.
plus taurine	500 mg daily, on an empty stomach.	Used in some clinics for treatment of breast cancer.
Lecithin granules or capsules	1 tbsp 3 times daily, with meals. 1,200 mg 3 times daily, with meals.	An important component of healthy cell membranes.
Multivitamin and mineral complex	As directed on label, with meals.	For necessary vitamins and minerals. Use a high-potency formula.
Primrose oil or flaxseed oil or salmon oil	1,000 mg 3 times daily, before meals. As directed on label. As directed on label.	To supply essential fatty acids, specifically useful for breast tumors. Both eicosapentaenoic acid (EPA) and docosahexaenoic acid (DHA) are helpful in protecting the body against toxic effects of some cancer treatments.
Raw thymus glandular	As directed on label.	Stimulates the thymus gland, which is important for immune function. (*See* GLANDULAR THERAPY in Part Three.)
Vitamin A plus natural carotenoid complex (Betatene) plus vitamin E or ACES from Carlson Labs	25,000 IU daily. If you are pregnant, do not exceed 10,000 IU daily. 25,000 IU daily. Start with 400 IU daily and increase slowly to 800 IU daily. As directed on label.	Powerful immunostimulants and antioxidants. Emulsion forms are recommended for easier assimilation and greater safety at higher doses. Use d-alpha-tocopherol form. Supplies vitamin C in addition to vitamins A and E and selenium.
Vitamin B complex plus extra vitamin B₆ (pyridoxine) plus pantothenic acid (vitamin B₅)	As directed on label. 50 mg 3 times daily. 100 mg daily.	Vital in intracellular metabolism and normal cell multiplication. A sublingual type is best. Required for normal cell growth and brain and nervous system function. Enhances immunity. Consider injections (under a doctor's supervision). An anti-stress vitamin that plays a role in hormone and antibody production, energy production, vitamin production, and in treating depression and anxiety.

HERBS

❑ Cat's claw boosts the immune system and has anti-tumor properties. Cat's Claw Defense Complex from Source Naturals is a combination of cat's claw and other herbs, plus antioxidant nutrients such as beta-carotene, N-acetyl-cysteine, vitamin C, and zinc.

Caution: Do not use cat's claw during pregnancy.

❑ Many people with external tumors have responded well to poultices made from comfrey, pau d'arco, ragwort, and wood sage. (*See* USING A POULTICE in Part Three.)

❑ For breast lumps, try using poultices made of poke root, which is effective in combating glandular swelling. (*See* USING A POULTICE in Part Three.)

Note: Poke root is recommended for external use only.

❑ Other beneficial herbs include barberry, burdock root, dandelion, milk thistle, pau d'arco, and red clover. These herbs purify the blood, stimulate liver activity, act as natural antibiotics, and generally help healing.

Caution: Do not use barberry during pregnancy.

RECOMMENDATIONS

❑ Eat a diet consisting of 50 percent raw fruits and vegetables. If possible, purchase produce from an organic source. Nuts, seeds, whole grains, and low-fat yogurt and yogurt products also should be included in the diet. Do not consume animal protein (eat soy protein instead), dairy products (except for yogurt), processed and packaged foods, salt (if you do use salt, use sea salt, which still retains its mineral content), sugar, white flour, or white flour products.

❑ *See* CANCER in Part Two and follow the recommended diet.

❑ *See* FASTING in Part Three and follow the program.

CONSIDERATIONS

❑ Although benign tumors are generally limited in growth, they usually should be removed; a small percentage may later become malignant.

❑ Malignant tumors must be treated as early as possible. Depending on the site and size of the tumor, there are many different methods of treatment. (*See* CANCER in Part Two.)

❑ Iron deficiency has been linked to the development of tumors. However, iron supplements should be taken only if tests show a deficiency. People with cancer should *not* take supplemental iron.

❑ Scientists of the University of California—Los Angeles School of Medicine have found that sodium linoleate, which contains linoleic acid (an essential fatty acid), has the ability to fight cancer cells in the laboratory.

❑ Studies done in Japan suggest that taking garlic supplements may help reduce the size of tumors.

❑ Regular physical checkups and tests for various cancers, such as breast, colon, cervical, prostate, and skin cancer, should be part of your routine, especially after the age of forty.

❑ *See also* BREAST CANCER; CANCER; FIBROCYSTIC BREASTS; FIBROIDS, UTERINE; POLYPS; PROSTATE CANCER; SKIN CANCER; and/or WARTS, all in Part Two.

Ulcer

See BEDSORES; CANKER SORES (APHTHOUS ULCERS); LEG ULCERS; PEPTIC ULCER. *See also under* EYE PROBLEMS.

Ulcerative Colitis

Ulcerative colitis is a chronic disorder in which the mucous membranes lining the colon become inflamed and develop ulcers, causing bloody diarrhea, pain, gas, bloating, and, at times, hard stools. The colon muscles then have to work harder to move these hardened stools through the colon. This can cause the mucous lining of the colon wall to bulge out into small pouchlike projections called diverticula. This usually occurs in the lower left section of the large intestine called the *sigmoid* ("S-shaped") colon, although it can occur in any part of the colon. *Enteritis* and *ileitis* are types of inflammation of the small intestine often associated with colitis.

Ulcerative colitis can range from relatively mild to severe. Common complications are diarrhea and bleeding, often causing the loss of vital nutrients and fluids. A rarer complication is toxic megacolon, in which the intestinal wall weakens and balloons out, threatening to rupture.

The cause or causes of most cases of colitis are unknown, but possible contributing factors include poor eating habits, stress, and food allergies. Colitis can also be caused by infectious agents such as bacteria. This type of colitis is often associated with the use of antibiotics, which alter the normal bowel flora and permit microorganisms that are normally held in check to proliferate. The symptoms can range from simple diarrhea to the more severe type of symptoms associated with ulcerative colitis.

Unless otherwise specified, the dosages recommended here are for adults. For a child between the ages of twelve and seventeen, reduce the dose to three-quarters of the recommended amount. For a child between six and twelve, use one-half of the recommended dose, and for a child under the age of six, use one-quarter of the recommended amount.

NUTRIENTS

SUPPLEMENT	SUGGESTED DOSAGE	COMMENTS
Essential		
Iron	As directed by physician.	Usually depleted in people with chronic inflammatory bowel disease. *Note:* Do not take supplemental iron unless anemia has been diagnosed.
Proteolytic enzymes	As directed on label. Take between meals.	Vital for proper digestion of proteins and helps to control inflammation.
plus multienzyme complex with pancreatin	As directed on label. Take after meals.	Anti-inflammatory enzymes. Use a formula that is high in pancreatin and low in hydrochloric acid (HCl).
Vitamin B complex	As directed on label.	Essential for the breakdown of fats, protein, and carbohydrates and for proper digestion. Use a hypoallergenic formula.
plus extra vitamin B_6 and	50 mg 2 times daily.	
vitamin B_{12} and	1,000 mcg twice daily.	A sublingual form is best.
folic acid	400 mcg twice daily.	Often depleted in people with this disorder. May protect against colon cancer.
Very Important		
Acidophilus (Kyo-Dophilus from Wakunaga is a good source) or Bio-Bifidus from American Biologics	As directed on label twice daily, on an empty stomach.	To normalize the intestinal bacteria. Very important if you are taking antibiotics. Use a nondairy formula.
Aerobic Bulk Cleanse from Aerobic Life Industries or psyllium husks	1 tbsp in water or juice on an empty stomach in the morning. Drink it down quickly, before it thickens. Take separately from other supplements and medications. As directed on label.	To keep the colon walls clean of toxic wastes.
Free-form amino acid complex	As directed on label twice daily, on an empty stomach.	To supply needed protein for tissue healing.
L-Glutamine	500 mg twice daily, on an empty stomach. Take with water or juice. Do not take with milk. Take with 50 mg vitamin B_6 and 100 mg vitamin C for better absorption.	A major metabolic fuel for the intestinal cells; maintains the villi, the absorption surfaces of the intestines. (*See* AMINO ACIDS in Part One.)
Vitamin A with mixed carotenoids including natural beta-carotene and	25,000 IU daily. If you are pregnant, do not exceed 10,000 IU daily.	An antioxidant that protects the mucous membranes and aids in healing. An antioxidant that promotes healing.
vitamin E	Up to 800 IU daily.	Deficiency has been associated with bowel cancer. Use d-alpha-tocopherol form.
Helpful		
Aerobic 07 from Aerobic Life Industries or	As directed on label twice daily.	Provides stabilized oxygen to the colon and destroys unwanted bacteria.
Dioxychlor from American Biologics	10–20 drops sublingually 1–2 times daily.	An important antibacterial, antifungal, and antiviral agent.

Colloidal silver	As directed on label.	A natural broad-spectrum antiseptic that fights infection, subdues inflammation, and promotes healing. Can be taken by mouth or applied topically.
Essential fatty acids (flaxseed oil and primrose oil are good sources)	As directed on label.	Important in cell formation. Protects the lining of the colon.
Garlic (Kyolic from Wakunaga)	2 capsules 3 times daily, with meals.	A natural antibiotic that has a healing effect on the colon.
Glucosamine sulfate or N-Acetylglucosamine (N-A-G from Source Naturals)	As directed on label. As directed on label.	An important component in the protective mucous secretions of the digestive tract.
Multimineral complex with calcium and chromium and magnesium and zinc	As directed on label.	Malabsorption of these essential minerals is a problem with colitis. Calcium also is needed for the prevention of cancer, which may occur due to constant irritation. Use a high-potency formula.
Raw thymus glandular	500 mg twice daily.	Important in immune function. (See GLANDULAR THERAPY in Part Three.)
VitaCarte from Phoenix BioLabs or shark cartilage	As directed on label. As directed on label.	Contains pure bovine cartilage, which can be effective in improving ulcerative colitis.
Vitamin C with bioflavonoids	3,000–5,000 mg daily, in divided doses.	Needed for immune function and healing of mucous membranes. Use a buffered form.

HERBS

❑ Aerobic Bulk Cleanse (ABC) from Aerobic Life Industries contains healing herbs that cleanse the colon. Take it mixed with half fruit or vegetable juice and half aloe vera juice, before meals.

Note: Always take this product separately from other supplements and medications.

❑ Alfalfa, taken in capsule or liquid form, supplies vitamin K and chlorophyll, needed for healing. Take it as directed on the product label three times daily.

❑ Aloe vera aids in healing the colon, thereby easing pain. Drink 1/2 cup of aloe vera juice in the morning and again at bedtime.

❑ Boswellia, bromelain, buchu leaves, and turmeric (curcumin) reduce inflammation.

❑ Burdock root, milk thistle, and red clover aid in cleansing the blood. Milk thistle also improves liver function.

❑ Chamomile, dandelion, feverfew, papaya, red clover, slippery elm, and yarrow extract or tea are beneficial for colitis, as is pau d'arco tea.

Caution: Do not use chamomile on an ongoing basis, and avoid it completely if you are allergic to ragweed. Do not use feverfew during pregnancy.

❑ Lobelia tea is good to drink. Also use it as an enema for inflammation of the colon; it gives quick relief. (*See* ENEMAS in Part Three.)

Caution: Do not take lobelia internally on an ongoing basis.

❑ Nettle and quercetin aid in inhibiting allergic reactions.

RECOMMENDATIONS

❑ Do not wear clothing that is tight around the waist.

❑ For acute pain, try drinking a large glass of water. This aids in flushing out particles caught in the crevices of the colon, relieving pain.

❑ During a flare-up, consume only soft foods until the pain has subsided. Put oat bran or steamed vegetables through a blender. Add 1 tablespoon of oat or rice bran daily to cereals and juice to add the bulk needed for cleansing the colon. Or add 1 tablespoon of Aerobic Bulk Cleanse to juice and drink it on an empty stomach upon arising.

❑ Eat plenty of dark green leafy vegetables. These are rich sources of vitamin K. Vitamin K deficiency has been linked to ulcerative colitis.

❑ Try eating junior baby foods for two weeks. Baby foods are easy to digest. Earth's Best baby foods are organic and are available in many health food stores and supermarkets. While on the baby food diet, take extra fiber such as glucomannan. Glucomannan should be taken one-half to one hour before meals with a large glass of water.

Note: Always take supplemental fiber separately from other supplements and medications.

❑ Do stretching exercises and take proteolytic enzymes to improve digestion.

❑ Use cleansing enemas made with 2 quarts of lukewarm water. This helps to rid the colon of undigested foods and relieve pain. Use wheatgrass juice as a retention enema. For severe gas and bloating, use an *L. bifidus* enema. See ENEMAS in Part Three.

❑ For long-term management of ulcerative colitis and to prevent flare-ups, *see* Diet for Colitis on page 668 and follow the suggestions there.

❑ *See* FASTING in Part Three, and follow the program once a month.

CONSIDERATIONS

❑ A food sensitivity test is advised for anyone who suffers from colitis. We have seen many people with colitis do well once they make changes in their diet and lifestyle.

❑ When magnesium is given intravenously with vitamin B6, it relaxes the muscles in the walls of the bowels and can control an attack of spastic colon.

❑ If serious complications arise and all other treatments have failed, surgery may be required.

Diet for Colitis

Ulcerative colitis can be an extremely painful and even temporarily disabling condition. Diet is probably the most significant factor in achieving and maintaining remission. Shari Lieberman, nutritionist and author, recommends the following dietary guidelines for people with colitis:

• The most important thing to do is keep a daily record of what you eat and what symptoms you experience. This way you can see which foods have aggravated or improved your condition. Some people are sensitive only to certain foods, such as yeast products, wheat products, or dairy products. By checking your daily record, you can see which food or foods have caused flare-ups or made you feel better.

• Eat a low-carbohydrate, high-vegetable-protein diet. Include alfalfa or barley in the diet. Baked or broiled fish, chicken, and turkey (without the skin) are acceptable sources of protein.

• Eat lots of vegetables. If you cannot tolerate raw vegetables, steam them.

• Eat a high-fiber diet. Oat bran, brown rice, barley and other whole grains, lentils, and related products such as rice cakes are good. Be sure grains are well cooked.

• Keep fats and oils out of your diet, and stay away from high-fat milk and cheeses. Fats and oils exacerbate the diarrhea that comes with colitis.

• Include garlic in the diet for its healing and antibiotic properties.

• Eat cooked foods that are broiled or baked, not fried or sautéed. Avoid sauces made with butter.

• Avoid carbonated soft drinks, spicy foods, and anything containing caffeine. These substances can irritate the colon. Also avoid red meat, sugar, and processed foods.

• Try soy-based cheese instead of dairy cheese; try soymilk or rice milk instead of cow's milk. If you do eat dairy foods, use nonfat types. If you have a lactose intolerance, try lactose-free milk. Many lactose-intolerant people can tolerate low-fat yogurt.

• Drink plenty of liquids—at least eight 8-ounce glasses of water daily to make up for the fluid lost with diarrhea. Carrot and cabbage juices and "green drinks" are also good. Or add chlorophyll liquid to juices.

• Do not eat fruit on an empty stomach. Eat it between meals instead. Avoid acidic fruits such as oranges and grapefruit. Fruit juices should be diluted with water and taken during or after meals.

❏ Vitamin K deficiency has been linked to ulcerative colitis. Sulfa drugs and mineral oil deplete vitamin K.

❏ Ulcerative colitis and Crohn's disease are both classified as inflammatory bowel diseases. Irritable bowel syndrome (IBS), although capable of causing some similar symptoms, is a condition that involves no inflammation. (See IRRITABLE BOWEL SYNDROME in Part Two.)

❏ The earliest signs of ulcerative colitis sometimes mimic the symptoms of arthritis—achiness and joint pain. These symptoms may or may not be accompanied by the abdominal discomfort typical of colitis. If you start experiencing arthritis-like symptoms, it may be beneficial to change your diet and see if improvement results. (See Diet for Colitis above.)

❏ Anyone who has had ulcerative colitis for at least five years—even if it is mild or inactive for a long time—should undergo regular colonoscopy, since people with this disease run a much greater risk of developing colon cancer than the general population. A colonoscopy is an examination performed with a long, flexible instrument that allows a physician to see inside the length of the colon.

❏ See also DIVERTICULITIS and MALABSORPTION SYNDROME, both in Part Two.

Underweight/Weight Loss

Some people are thinner than average all their lives and are perfectly healthy that way. For others, however, underweight may be associated with health problems. This is particularly true if the condition results from unintended, perhaps sudden, weight loss. Unintended weight loss can result from a malabsorption problem; intestinal parasites; certain types of cancer; a colon disorder such as Crohn's disease, ulcerative colitis, or diverticulitis; or a chronic illness such as diabetes, chronic diarrhea, or hyperthyroidism. Surgery, stress, or trauma, such as the loss of a loved one, can also contribute to loss of appetite and weight loss.

Underweight can also be caused by treatments such as cancer chemotherapy and radiation therapy, whose side effects include nausea, vomiting, and loss of appetite. An individual who is underweight but believes he or she weighs too much may be suffering from an eating disorder. People with AIDS often suffer from what is known as "wasting syndrome," in which they become more and more emaciated as the disease progresses.

Weight loss may in turn cause nutritional deficiencies that further impair health and complicate recovery. Two age groups for whom undernutrition is a special problem are the very young and the very old. Malnutrition in childhood, especially in infancy, can have permanent effects because it interferes with normal growth and development. Children also have less in the way of nutritional reserves in their bodies to draw upon if intake or absorption of nutrients is inadequate. At the other end of the lifespan, many elderly people find themselves less and less interested in eating as time goes by, and reduced financial resources may add to the incentive to skip meals. As a result, older people have an increased risk of becoming malnourished.

The suggestions in this section are intended for older people who require nutritional rehabilitation. They may also be useful for people who have higher than normal nutritional requirements, such as people who have hepatitis or are undergoing cancer treatment, those who are recovering from burns or trauma, and women who are pregnant or nursing. A child who is undernourished or stops gaining weight should be seen by a physician.

NUTRIENTS

SUPPLEMENT	SUGGESTED DOSAGE	COMMENTS
Essential		
Raw liver extract	As directed on label.	Excellent source of B vitamins and minerals. Use liver extract from organically raised beef. Use a liquid form for easy assimilation.
Vitamin A plus carotenoid complex with natural beta-carotene	10,000 IU daily. As directed on label.	Antioxidants that enhance immunity and aid in fat storage. Essential for protein utilization.
Vitamin B complex	100 mg of each major B vitamin daily, with meals. (amounts of individual vitamins in a complex will vary).	Increases the appetite and aids in digestion of fats, carbohydrates, and protein. Use a sublingual form for best absorption. Injections (under a doctor's supervision) may be necessary.
Vitamin C with bioflavonoids.	3,000 mg daily.	Helps prevent cancer, protects against infection, and enhances immunity.
Vitamin D$_3$	400 IU daily.	Necessary for healthy bone formation.
Vitamin E	600 IU daily.	A powerful antioxidant that helps prevent cancer and inhibits the formation of free radicals. Use d-alpha-tocopherol form.
Zinc	80 mg daily. Do not exceed this amount.	Improves the senses of taste and smell. Use zinc gluconate lozenges or OptiZinc for best absorption.
Important		
Essential fatty acids (Ultimate Oil from Nature's Secret is a good source)	As directed on label.	A most important element of the diet.

Free-form amino acid complex	As directed on label.	To supply needed protein in a form that is readily available and easily metabolized. Use a formula containing all the essential amino acids.
Garlic (Kyolic from Wakunaga)	2 capsules 3 times daily, with meals.	Provides protection against free radicals. Contains many essential nutrients.
Inflazyme Forte from American Biologics or Wobenzym N from Marlyn Nutraceuticals	4 tablets 3 times daily, with meals. 3–6 tablets 2–3 times daily, between meals.	Aids in the proper breakdown of proteins, fats, and carbohydrates for better absorption of foods. Destroys free radicals and aids in proper breakdown and absorption of foods.
Quercetin plus bromelain	As directed on label. As directed on label.	Aids in preventing reactions to certain foods, pollens, and other allergens. Increases immunity. Enhances effectiveness of quercetin.
Helpful		
Brewer's yeast	As directed on label.	Stimulates the appetite and supplies B vitamins.
Floradix Iron + Herbs from Salus Haus	As directed on label.	Increases appetite and helps digestion.
Multienzyme complex	As directed on label.	Aids digestion.
Multivitamin and mineral supplement	As directed on label.	To supply a balance of all needed vitamins and minerals. Use a high-potency formula.
Spiru-tein from Nature's Plus	As directed on label. Take between meals.	A safe protein supplement.

HERBS

❑ Alfalfa, blessed thistle, caraway, cayenne (capsicum), celery, dill, fennel, hyssop, and lady's mantle all work to stimulate the appetite.

❑ Astragalus protects the immune system, helps with digestion, and combats fatigue.

❑ Fenugreek and ginseng have long been used as appetite stimulants and digestive aids, especially for elderly people.

Caution: Do not use ginseng if you have high blood pressure.

RECOMMENDATIONS

❑ If you think you may be underweight, and particularly if you are experiencing unintended weight loss, have a complete medical examination to check for an underlying physical disorder. You may have a health problem that requires treatment. Be concerned about an infant or young child who suddenly seems to stop gaining weight normally.

❑ Eat a diet consisting of at least 300 grams of complex carbohydrates, 100 grams of protein, and 2,500 to 3,000 calories a day. Include starchy vegetables, such as potatoes and beans, as well as grains, turkey, chicken, fish, eggs, avocados, olive oil, safflower oil, raw cheeses, nuts, and seeds.

Eat only whole-grain breads, pasta, crackers, and hot and cold cereals.

❑ Eat nondairy soy-based cream soups. Soymilk can be used in the same ways as cow's milk. Cream soups are usually higher in protein and calories than broth soups.

❑ Drink herbal teas, fruit and vegetable juices, and mineral water.

❑ Eat frequent but small meals and snacks, and eat them slowly. If you are undernourished, you may lose your appetite if confronted with large amounts of food at one sitting. You can always have additional servings if you are still hungry after the first.

❑ Do not eat fried or junk foods for extra calories. Instead, eat high-calorie snacks such as the following between meals or before bedtime: raw cheese; banana soy pudding; turkey, chicken, or tuna sandwiches with cheese; raw nuts; rice crackers with nut butter; yogurt; yogurt fruit shakes; carob soymilk; almond milk; buttermilk; custard; nuts; and avocados.

❑ Eliminate from the diet coffee, tea, and anything else (such as soft drinks) that contains caffeine.

❑ If possible, get regular moderate exercise. Walking and similar activities are good. Moderate exercise helps in the assimilation of nutrients and in increasing the appetite. Avoid strenuous exercise.

❑ Eat in relaxed surroundings. Do not try to eat when you are upset or nervous.

❑ If you smoke, stop.

❑ Investigate the possibility of food allergies. (See ALLERGIES in Part Two.) Avoid any foods you think you may be allergic to.

❑ Consult your physician about any medications you may be taking. Some medications can cause a decrease in appetite and weight loss.

❑ If other people comment on your thinness but you feel you actually could stand to lose weight, consider professional evaluation for an eating disorder. (See ANOREXIA NERVOSA and/or BULIMIA in Part Two.)

CONSIDERATIONS

❑ Consideration of the appearance and smell of the food, as well as the eating environment, is important when trying to stimulate a poor appetite.

❑ The color red helps to stimulate taste buds. (See COLOR THERAPY in Part Three.)

❑ See also APPETITE, POOR.

Urinary Tract Infection

See BLADDER INFECTION (CYSTITIS); KIDNEY DISEASE (RENAL FAILURE); VAGINITIS.

Uterine Prolapse

See PROLAPSE OF THE UTERUS.

Uveitis

See under EYE PROBLEMS.

Vaginitis

The symptoms of vaginitis, or inflammation of the mucous membranes lining the vagina, include a burning and/or itching sensation and abnormal vaginal discharge. Vaginitis may be caused by bacterial or fungal infection, vitamin B deficiency, or irritation from excessive douching or the use of such products as deodorant sprays. Infectious vaginitis is often caused by trichomonas, gonococci, or other sexually transmitted organisms. Other factors, such as poor hygiene and tight, nonporous clothing, may contribute to the problem. Pregnancy, diabetes, and the use of antibiotics disturb the body's natural balance, creating an environment in which infectious organisms can thrive. Oral contraceptives also can produce vaginal inflammation.

Atrophic vaginitis is a condition primarily found in postmenopausal women and those whose ovaries have been surgically removed. This disorder can result in the formation of adhesions and a high susceptibility to infection. Common symptoms include itching or burning, painful intercourse, and a thin, watery discharge, occasionally tinged with blood.

Unless otherwise specified, the dosages recommended here are for adults. For a girl between the ages of twelve and seventeen, reduce the dose to three-quarters of the recommended amount.

NUTRIENTS

SUPPLEMENT	SUGGESTED DOSAGE	COMMENTS
Very Important		
Acidophilus (Kyo-Dophilus from Wakunaga is a good source)	As directed on label 3 times daily, with meals. Open 3 capsules and dissolve in 1 qt warm water with 6 drops tea tree oil added to use as a douche.	To replenish normal "friendly" bacteria. Use a nondairy formula.
Biotin	300 mcg 3 times daily.	Inhibits yeast.
Essential fatty acids	As directed on label.	Aids healing.
Garlic (Kyolic from Wakunaga)	1 capsule 3 times daily, with meals.	Has antifungal properties.

Vitamin B complex	50–100 mg 3 times daily, with meals.	Often deficient in people with vaginitis. Use a high-potency formula.
Yeast-Gard from Lake Consumer Products	As directed on label.	Excellent antifungal agent. Reduces pain.
Helpful		
Colloidal silver	As directed on label.	A broad-spectrum natural antibiotic that subdues inflammation and promotes healing.
N-Acetylglucosamine (N-A-G from Source Naturals)	As directed on label.	Amino acid compound. Forms the basis of complex molecular structures that are key parts of mucous membrane tissue.
Vitamin A with mixed carotenoids including beta-carotene	25,000 IU daily. If you are pregnant, do not exceed 10,000 IU daily.	Powerful antioxidants that aid healing.
and vitamin E	400 IU daily.	Use d-alpha-tocopherol form.
Vitamin B complex plus extra vitamin B₆ (pyridoxine)	As directed on label. 50 mg 3 times daily.	Regulates metabolism and promotes good health. Especially important if using estrogen cream for treatment of atrophic vaginitis.
Vitamin C with bioflavonoids	2,000–5,000 mg daily.	Important immune system stimulant. Necessary for tissue healing.
Vitamin D₃ with calcium and magnesium	1,000 mg daily. 1,500 mg daily. 1,000 mg daily.	To relieve stress. Women need extra supplements of these nutrients at this time.
Zinc	30 mg daily. Do not exceed a total of 100 mg daily from all supplements.	To increase immunity and promote proper utilization of vitamin A. Also reduces severity of herpes outbreaks. Use zinc gluconate lozenges or OptiZinc for best absorption.

HERBS

❏ Aloe vera is helpful for infections and is known for its healing effects. Aloe vera gel can be applied topically to relieve itching. It can also be taken internally or used in a douche.

❏ Barberry has remarkable infection-fighting properties.

❏ Douche with infusions made from antiseptic herbs such as calendula, garlic, goldenseal, fresh plantain, St. John's wort, or tea tree oil, along with herbs such as comfrey leaves, to soothe irritation. Echinacea and goldenseal can also be taken orally.

Note: Comfrey is recommended for external use only. Do not take goldenseal internally on a daily basis for more than one week at a time, do not use it during pregnancy, and use it with caution if you are allergic to ragweed.

❏ Calendula and vitamin A vaginal suppositories are soothing and healing to irritated tissues. Goldenseal suppositories are useful for all types of infection.

❏ Chamomile has antifungal properties.

❏ Cinnamon and dandelion inhibit the growth of *Candida albicans*. They can be used as a douche or taken internally.

❏ Echinacea has antifungal properties and enhances the immune system. It can be taken internally or used as a douche.

❏ Meno-Fem from Prevail Corporation is a combination of traditional herbs and nutrients designed to combat the symptoms of menopause. It is helpful for vaginitis related to hormonal imbalance.

❏ Pau d'arco contains natural antibiotic agents and has a healing effect. It can be taken in capsule form, made into a tea, or used as a douche.

❏ Tea tree oil is good for vaginitis. Topical tea tree oil cream is effective against fungal infection, herpes blisters, warts, and other types of infection. Tea tree oil suppositories have been used successfully for vaginal yeast infections.

RECOMMENDATIONS

❏ Eat plain yogurt that contains live yogurt cultures, or apply plain yogurt directly to the vagina. This can help fight infection and soothe inflammation. Also consume brown rice, millet, and acidophilus.

❏ Consume fiber daily. Oat bran is a good source.

❏ Eat a diet that is fruit-free, sugar-free, and yeast-free. Avoid aged cheeses, alcohol, chocolate, dried fruits, fermented foods, all grains containing gluten (wheat, oats, rye, and barley), ham, honey, nut butters, pickles, raw mushrooms, soy sauce, sprouts, sugar in any form, vinegar, and all yeast products. Also eliminate citrus and acidic fruits (grapefruits, lemons, limes, oranges, pineapple, and tomatoes) from your diet until the inflammation subsides. Then add them back slowly.

❏ Keep clean and dry. Wear cotton underwear, which absorbs moisture and allows air to circulate. Avoid tight clothing and synthetic fabrics. Change into dry clothing as soon as possible after swimming. Do not spend prolonged periods of time in a wet bathing suit.

❏ To relieve itching, open a vitamin E capsule and apply the oil to the inflamed area.

❏ Add 3 cups of pure apple cider vinegar to bath water to treat vaginitis. Soak in the tub for twenty minutes, allowing the water to flow into the vagina.

❏ Do not use corticosteroids or oral contraceptives until your condition improves. Oral contraceptives can upset the balance of microorganisms in the body.

❏ Do not use sweet-smelling douches. Try douching with 2 capsules of garlic or with 1 cup of fresh garlic juice added to a quart of warm water. Alternate this treatment with acidophilus douches: Open 2 acidophilus capsules and add them to either 1 quart of warm water or to 1 cup of plain yogurt. The garlic fights infection while the acidophilus helps to restore normal flora and acid balance.

❑ Avoid taking iron supplements until the inflammation subsides. Infectious bacteria require iron for growth. If a bacterial infection is present, the body naturally "hides" iron by storing it in the liver, spleen, and bone marrow to inhibit the growth of the bacteria.

❑ Drink steam-distilled water only.

CONSIDERATIONS

❑ Atrophic vaginitis is often treated with prescription estrogen ointments. The use of these products increases the body's need for vitamin B_6. Vaginal absorption of synthetic estrogen may be dangerous.

❑ Natural progesterone cream applied to the vagina is beneficial for atrophic vaginitis.

❑ *See also* BLADDER INFECTION (CYSTITIS); CANDIDIASIS; KIDNEY DISEASE (RENAL FAILURE); and SEXUALLY TRANSMITTED DISEASE (STD), all in Part Two.

Varicose Veins

Varicose veins are abnormally enlarged, bulging, bluish, and lumpy-looking veins, often associated with dull, nagging aches and pains. This is the result of malfunctioning valves inside the veins. When blood pulses through the arteries, powered by the beating of the heart, to provide nutrients and oxygen to the body tissues, it returns to the heart by means of the veins. Like the arteries, the veins are tube-shaped vessels in graduated sizes, but unlike the arteries, the veins have tiny valves on their inner walls to prevent the blood from flowing backward, toward the arteries. If the valves do not work properly, circulation is impaired and blood accumulates in the veins, stretching them. Swelling, restlessness, leg sores, itching, leg cramps, and a feeling of heaviness in the legs are characteristic of varicose veins.

Because poor circulation contributes to the formation of varicose veins, they are more common in people who sit or stand in one position for prolonged periods of time, people who habitually sit with their legs crossed, and those who lack proper regular exercise. Excess weight, heavy lifting, and pregnancy put increased pressure on the legs, increasing the likelihood of developing varicose veins. Constipation, heart failure, liver disease, and abdominal tumors can also play a role in the formation of varicose veins. A deficiency of vitamin C and bioflavonoids (mainly rutin) can weaken the collagen structure in the vein walls, which can lead to varicose veins. A tendency toward varicose veins may also run in families. Some experts believe that hormone replacement therapy (HRT) and birth control pills can contribute to the formation of varicose veins. It is esti-mated that approximately 50 percent of all middle-aged Americans have at least some varicosities. More women than men are affected.

Most cases of varicose veins do not pose a serious problem and can be managed with simple home measures. In some cases, however, if varicose veins are not treated properly, complications such as bleeding under the skin, deep-vein blood clots, an eczema-like condition near the affected veins, or ulcerated spots near the ankles may occur. Other possible, and more serious, complications that can arise include phlebitis (inflammation of a vein), thrombophlebitis (formation of a clot in an inflamed vein), postthrombotic syndrome (indicated by a number of symptoms including leg ulcers), hemorrhage from a ruptured vein, or pulmonary embolism (a blood clot that travels to the lung and lodges there).

NUTRIENTS

SUPPLEMENT	SUGGESTED DOSAGE	COMMENTS
Very Important		
Coenzyme Q_{10}	100 mg daily.	Improves tissue oxygenation, increases circulation, and enhances immunity.
plus Coenzyme A from Coenzyme-A Technologies	As directed on label.	Works with coenzyme Q_{10} to support the immune system's detoxification of many dangerous substances.
Dimethylglycine (DMG) (Aangamik DMG from FoodScience of Vermont)	50 mg 3 times daily.	Improves oxygen utilization in the tissues.
Essential fatty acids (Ultimate Oil from Nature's Secret is a good source)	As directed on label.	Reduces pain and helps to keep blood vessels soft and pliable.
Glutathione	As directed on label.	Protects the heart, veins, and arteries from oxidant damage.
Pycnogenol or grape seed extract	As directed on label. As directed on label.	Stimulate blood circulation, boost immunity, neutralize free radicals, and strengthen connective tissue, including that of the cardiovascular system.
Vitamin C plus bioflavonoid complex plus extra rutin	3,000–6,000 mg daily. 100 mg daily. 50 mg 3 times daily.	Aids circulation by reducing blood clotting tendencies. To promote healing and prevent bruising. A potent noncitrus bioflavonoid that helps maintain the strength of blood vessels.
Important		
Vitamin E	Start with 400 IU daily and slowly increase to 1,000 IU daily.	Improves circulation and aids in preventing heavy feeling in the legs. Use d-alpha-tocopherol form.
Helpful		
Aerobic Bulk Cleanse from Aerobic Life Industries	As directed on label. Take separately from other supplements and medications.	Keeping the colon clean is important.

Brewer's yeast	As directed on label.	Contains needed protein and B vitamins.
Lecithin granules or capsules	1 tbsp 3 times daily, with meals. 1,200 mg 3 times daily, with meals.	Fat emulsifier that aids circulation.
Multivitamin and mineral complex	As directed on label.	To maintain a balance of all necessary nutrients.
Vitamin A plus natural carotenoid complex (Betatene)	10,000 IU daily. As directed on label.	To enhance immunity, protect the cells, and slow the aging process.
Vitamin B complex plus extra vitamin B$_6$ (pyridoxine) and vitamin B$_{12}$	50–100 mg 3 times daily, with meals. 50 mg daily. 300–1,000 mcg daily.	B vitamins are needed to help in digestion of foods. Sublingual forms are best for all the B vitamins.
Vitamin D$_3$ plus calcium and magnesium	1,000 mg daily, at bedtime. 1,500 mg daily, at bedtime. 750 mg daily, at bedtime.	This combination helps to relieve leg cramps. Use calcium chelate form.
Zinc plus copper	80 mg daily. 3 mg daily.	Aids healing. Needed to balance with zinc.

HERBS

❏ Aloe vera gel is a cooling and soothing topical treatment for varicose veins.

❏ Bilberry supports the health of connective tissue, including that of the veins.

❏ Bromelain can reduce risk of clot formation in the blood vessels.

❏ Butchers broom, ginkgo biloba, gotu kola, and hawthorn berries improve circulation in the legs.

❏ Cayenne helps to relieve pain and inflammation, and also expands blood vessels, reducing stress on the capillaries. It is available in capsule and cream forms.

❏ Dandelion alleviates tissue swelling by reducing water retention.

❏ Horse chestnut makes a good treatment for the discomfort of varicose veins. Mix 1/2 teaspoon of horse chestnut powder with 2 cups of water, and moisten a sterile cotton gauze cloth with the mixture. Rub the cloth gently over the affected area. This is soothing to inflamed veins. Witch hazel can also be used this way to reduce discomfort.

❏ Horse Chestnut Cream from Planetary Formulas is a topical formula containing horse chestnut, butcher's broom, witch hazel, white oak, and myrrh. It can be used to reduce the appearance of varicose veins.

❏ Herbs used in traditional Chinese medicine that are helpful in alleviating symptoms include magnolia flower (*Magnolia liliflora*, also known as xho yi hua), scutellaria (*Scutellaria baicalensis*, or huang qin; also known as Baikal

skullcap), trichosanth (*Trichosanthes kirilowii*), and wild angelica (*Angelica dahurica*, or bai zhi).

❏ Bathing your legs or other affected area in white oak bark herb tea three times a day helps to stimulate blood flow. Simmer (but do not boil) a strong tea and use the tea to make compresses. Apply the compresses to affected areas.

RECOMMENDATIONS

❏ Eat a diet that is low in fat and refined carbohydrates and includes plenty of fish and fresh fruits and vegetables.

❏ Eat as many blackberries and cherries as you can. These may help prevent varicose veins, or ease the symptoms if you already have them.

❏ Include garlic, ginger, onions, and pineapple in your diet.

❏ Make sure that your diet contains plenty of fiber to prevent constipation and keep the bowels clean.

❏ Avoid animal protein, processed and refined foods, sugar, ice cream, fried foods, cheeses, peanuts, junk foods, tobacco, alcohol, and salt.

❏ Maintain a healthy weight and get regular moderate exercise. Walking, swimming, and bicycling all promote good circulation. Change your daily routine to allow more time for exercise and movement for your legs.

❏ Wear loose clothing that does not restrict blood flow. It is a good idea to wear supportive elastic stockings; these help to support the varicose veins and prevent swelling them increasing.

❏ Elevate your legs above heart level for twenty minutes at least once a day to alleviate symptoms.

❏ Avoid long periods of standing or sitting. Take rest periods several times during the day to elevate your legs above heart level. Avoid crossing your legs, doing heavy lifting, and putting any unnecessary pressure on your legs.

❏ If you sit at a desk all day at work, make sure to get up and walk around periodically. You can also flex your leg muscles and wiggle your toes to increase blood flow. If possible, try to rest your feet on an object that is elevated from the floor when seated.

❏ If you have to stand for long periods of time, shift your weight between your feet, stand on your toes, or take short walks to alleviate pressure.

❏ Elevate your feet in front of you while sitting down to read or watch television.

❏ After bathing, apply castor oil directly over the problem veins and massage the oil into your legs from the feet up.

❏ To help improve circulation and ease pain, fill a tub with cold water. Stand in the water and simulate walking.

❏ Try using homeopathic remedies to ease symptoms.

Homeopathic remedies that have been used to treat varicose veins include *Ferrum metallicum, Hamamelis virginiana,* and *Pulsatilla.*

❏ Avoid scratching the itchy skin above varicose veins. This can cause ulceration and bleeding.

CONSIDERATIONS

❏ Cellulose is an indigestible carbohydrate found on the outer layer of vegetables and fruits. Good for alleviating symptoms, it can be found in apples, beets, Brazil nuts, broccoli, carrots, celery, green beans, lima beans, pears, peas, and whole grains.

❏ Some physicians treat varicose veins by injecting a sodium tetradecyl sulfate (saline) solution into the affected vein and applying compression bandages for a period of time. The solution fuses the vein walls together permanently, closing the defective vein. The body compensates for lost vessels by finding an alternate route for blood flow.

❏ Spider veins are chronically dilated capillaries near the surface of the skin. They are harmless and rarely cause any problems, although they can be distressing for cosmetic reasons.

❏ Hemorrhoids are actually varicose veins of the anus or rectum. Symptoms of hemorrhoids include rectal itching, pain, and blood in the stool. (*See* HEMORRHOIDS in Part Two.)

❏ Massage therapy can aid in stimulating the legs. You should not massage the veins directly, but instead massage the area around them and upward toward the heart.

❏ Compression therapy, in which a compression garment of some type is used to exert pressure on the legs in an effort to help the venous valves close properly, may be helpful in alleviating symptoms.

❏ Dimethylsulfoxide (DMSO) has been used to relieve the swelling and pain of severe varicose veins. This liquid, a byproduct of wood processing, is applied topically to the affected area as needed. Only DMSO from a health food store should be used for therapeutic purposes.

❏ The symptoms of varicose veins are similar to those of thrombophlebitis. In addition, the chances of developing varicose veins increase greatly if you suffer from thrombophlebitis. (*See* THROMBOPHLEBITIS in Part Two.)

❏ Sclerotherapy is a treatment sometimes recommended for varicose veins. In this procedure, an irritant is injected into the vein, causing it to become nonfunctional, and subsequently shrink and fade. There are potential complications with this procedure, however.

❏ Surgical removal of varicose veins is a treatment option that may be recommended if the veins are causing a considerable amount of discomfort. The operation results in scarring.

❏ Vein stripping is a medical treatment in which a main superficial vein is removed and the veins connected to it tied off, forcing the blood to return to the heart through the deeper leg veins.

❏ Valve repair is another treatment option for varicose veins. In this procedure, a synthetic material is used to restore the valve.

❏ *See also* CIRCULATORY PROBLEMS in Part Two.

❏ *See also under* PREGNANCY-RELATED PROBLEMS in Part Two.

Venereal Disease

See SEXUALLY TRANSMITTED DISEASE (STD).

Vertigo

Vertigo is a sensation of dizziness, faintness, or lightheadedness that results from an impaired sense of balance and equilibrium. The term comes from *vertere,* the Latin verb meaning "to turn." A person suffering from vertigo may feel that he or she is sinking or falling and/or that the room and objects in it are spinning around. In some cases, the individual may feel that he or she is spinning, too. Vertigo is sometimes accompanied by nausea and hearing loss. Vertigo is not an illness in itself—it is a symptom of another condition.

Vertigo occurs when the central nervous system receives conflicting messages from the inner ear, eyes, muscles, and skin pressure receptors. This may result from a variety of causes, including brain tumors, high or low blood pressure, allergies, diabetes, head injuries, inadequate or interrupted supply of oxygen to the brain, anemia, viral infection, fever, the use of certain drugs, nutritional deficiencies, neurological disease, psychological stress, changes in atmospheric pressure, blockage of the ear canal or eustachian tube, middle ear infections, or excess wax in the ear. Poor cerebral circulation also can cause dizziness and the inability to maintain balance. Poor cerebral circulation may be due to either the narrowing of the blood vessels that supply the brain (arteriosclerosis), pinched blood vessels in the neck (cervical osteoarthritis), or a disorder such as diabetes or anemia.

There are at least 100 different syndromes that can include vertigo. There are also different types of vertigo. *Chronic vertigo* can occur as a result of hypertension or atherosclerosis. This type of vertigo either does not go away completely or recurs frequently. *Senile vertigo* can be caused by atherosclerosis, chronic eye disease, or a syndrome called benign paroxysmal positional vertigo. However, it is worth checking to see if side effects or interactions might be causing the problem. *Juvenile vertigo* is usually caused by anxiety or hyperventilation.

Positional vertigo is, as it states, an attack of vertigo that occurs when you assume a particular position. BPPV is an example of positional vertigo. It is thought to be caused by damage to the body's balance mechanisms in the inner ear. The crystals may be dislodged by injury, infection, or as a result of old age, causing all the symptoms of vertigo when you move your head.

Sudden onset vertigo is, as the name implies, vertigo that strikes suddenly and may last for minutes or hours. It can be caused by motion sickness, Ménière's disease, or insufficient oxygen supply to the brain. Low blood sugar can also cause dizziness similar to vertigo.

Because of the effects of aging on the body, older people are more prone to vertigo. The body maintains a sense of balance through a complex mechanism involving both the inner ears and visual input. Within the canals of the inner ears, there are structures called *otoliths,* which are minute calcium carbonate crystals that press upon the hairlike cells that line the inner membranes. Gravity acts on the otoliths so that they shift in response to head movements. This bends the fiber cells, which, in turn, transmit signals to the brain. The brain then uses these signals to calculate the positioning of the head. As people age, tiny bits of debris may accumulate in the inner ears and press against the hair cells, resulting in false signals being sent to the brain. This can interfere with the sense of balance and result in vertigo. In addition, with increasing age, nerve impulses require more time to travel from the eyes to the brain and spinal cord. This can cause dizziness and loss of balance upon sudden movement.

Dizziness is not synonymous with vertigo. Anyone may occasionally experience a feeling of lightheadedness, dizziness, unsteadiness, or the sensation of feeling faint. Those with low blood pressure may have this feeling upon rising quickly from a sitting or lying position. In some cases, dizziness can be a warning sign of a heart attack, stroke, concussion, or brain damage.

Unless otherwise specified, the dosages recommended here are for adults. For a child between the ages of twelve and seventeen, reduce the dose to three-quarters of the recommended amount. For a child between six and twelve, use one-half of the recommended dose, and for a child under the age of six, use one-quarter of the recommended amount.

NUTRIENTS

SUPPLEMENT	SUGGESTED DOSAGE	COMMENTS
Very Important		
Dimethylglycine (DMG) (Aangamik DMG from FoodScience of Vermont)	As directed on label.	Increases oxygen supply to the brain.
Vitamin B complex	100 mg of each major B vitamin 3 times daily, with meals (amounts of individual vitamins in a complex will vary).	B vitamins are necessary for normal brain and central nervous system function. Consider injections (under a doctor's supervision) for better absorption. If injections are not available, use sublingual forms. Improves cerebral circulation and lowers cholesterol. *Caution:* Do not take niacin if you have a liver disorder, gout, or high blood pressure.
plus extra vitamin B$_3$ (niacin)	100 mg 3 times daily. Do not exceed this amount.	
and vitamin B$_6$ (pyridoxine)	50 mg daily.	
and vitamin B$_{12}$	1,000–2,000 mcg daily.	A sublingual form is recommended.
Vitamin C with bioflavonoids	3,000–10,000 mg daily, in divided doses.	An antioxidant that also improves circulation.
Vitamin E	Start with 200 IU daily and increase slowly to 400–800 IU daily.	Improves circulation. Use d-alpha-tocopherol form.
Important		
Choline and inositol and/or lecithin	As directed on label 3 times daily.

As directed on label. | Necessary in nerve function. Helps to prevent hardening of the arteries and improve brain function. |
Coenzyme Q$_{10}$ plus Coenzyme A from Coenzyme-A Technologies	100–200 mg daily.	Improves circulation to the brain. Works well with coenzyme Q$_{10}$ to support the immune system's detoxification of many dangerous substances.
Vitamin A with mixed carotenoids including natural beta-carotene	10,000 IU daily.	Enhances immunity and acts as an antioxidant.
Zinc	30 mg daily. Do not exceed a total of 100 mg daily from all supplements.	Promotes a healthy immune system and helps maintain vitamin E levels. Use zinc gluconate lozenges or OptiZinc for best absorption.
Helpful		
Brewer's yeast	1/2 tsp daily for 3 days, then increase to 1 tbsp daily.	Contains balanced B vitamins.
Calcium and magnesium	1,500 mg daily.

750 mg daily. | Important in maintaining regular nerve impulses. To help prevent dizziness. |
Kelp	1,000–1,500 mg daily.	For necessary balanced minerals and vitamins.
Melatonin	1.5–5 mg daily, taken 2 hours or less before bedtime.	Helps to maintain equilibrium.
Multivitamin and mineral complex	As directed on label.	For necessary balance of vitamins and minerals.

HERBS

❏ Black cohosh lowers blood pressure.

Caution: Do not use this herb during pregnancy.

❑ Butcher's broom and cayenne (capsicum) help improve circulation.

❑ Dandelion tea or extract is very good for high blood pressure.

❑ Ginger relieves dizziness and nausea.

❑ Ginkgo biloba improves circulation and improves brain function by increasing the supply of oxygen to the brain. Take 120 mg of ginkgo biloba extract daily.

RECOMMENDATIONS

❑ Avoid making rapid or extreme movements and rapid changes in body position.

❑ Limit your total sodium intake to less than 2,000 milligrams per day. Too much sodium can disrupt the workings of the inner ear.

❑ Avoid alcohol, caffeine, nicotine, and all fried foods.

❑ To subdue dizziness, sit in a chair with your feet flat on the floor and stare at a fixed object for a few minutes.

❑ If you begin to experience dizziness soon after taking new medication, assume that the problem is drug related. Discuss the problem with your physician or pharmacist.

❑ If vertigo is a recurring problem, consult your health care provider. It may be a sign of an underlying problem that requires treatment.

CONSIDERATIONS

❑ People who have vertigo sometimes experience a phenomenon called nystagmus, involuntary rapid or jerky eye movements. It may occur spontaneously or as a result of changing positions. Nystagmus, or any other unusual eye movement, always requires the attention of a physician.

❑ Dizziness can be caused by many different things, some of them serious. If you feel dizzy and find it difficult to speak, swallow, or think clearly, seek medical attention. These may be the symptoms of a stroke. Numbness and tingling or loss of vision accompanied by dizziness also can be signs of a stroke.

❑ If dizziness is accompanied by nausea, sweating, and paleness of complexion with a racing heartbeat, seek medical attention. This can be a sign of a number of different health problems, including a heart attack, or, if you have diabetes, a hypoglycemic (low blood sugar) episode. Hypotension, or a sudden drop in blood pressure, also can cause sudden dizziness, especially after meals.

❑ Air contains less oxygen at altitudes high above sea level. Lower oxygen levels can cause mild, temporary dizziness or lightheadedness.

❑ Certain activities, such as taking amusement park rides, watching action movies, sailing, or playing video games, may bring on vertigo or dizziness. In such cases, symptoms diminish soon after the activity ceases.

❑ Treatment for benign paroxysmal positional vertigo usually entails special exercises and, sometimes, surgery.

❑ *See also* ARTERIOSCLEROSIS/ATHEROSCLEROSIS; CARDIO-VASCULAR DISEASE; and MENIÉRÈ'S DISEASE in Part Two.

Vitiligo

Vitiligo, also called leukoderma, is a skin condition characterized by chalky white patches of skin surrounded by a dark border. The spots can be few or many; they may be tiny or cover the body. They usually appear on both sides of the body in approximately the same place (for example, you may have exactly the same white patches on the top of your left and right foot), and they do not hurt or itch. These spots occur because, for some reason, the cells that normally produce the skin pigment melanin are absent. If the affected area is on the scalp, the hair that grows from it is likely to be white as well.

Vitiligo itself is not a threat to health. However, it has been linked with other diseases in some cases, including Addison's disease, pernicious anemia, and alopecia areata (patches of hair loss). The exact cause of vitiligo is not known, but it can run in families and may be related to an autoimmune problem. A thyroid gland malfunction may be involved as well. Vitiligo can also occur after physical trauma to the skin. Chemical agents such as catechol (used for tanning and dyeing) and phenol (often found in disinfectants) may be involved in the development of this condition. Physical and emotional stress may aggravate the condition. The unpigmented spots are a concern primarily for cosmetic reasons and are highly vulnerable to sunburn.

NUTRIENTS

SUPPLEMENT	SUGGESTED DOSAGE	COMMENTS
Very Important		
Vitamin B complex	50 mg of each major B vitamin and up, 3 times daily (amounts of individual vitamins in a complex will vary).	Needed for proper skin tone and texture. Helps to combat stress. A sublingual form is recommended.
plus extra pantothenic acid (vitamin B$_5$)	300 mg daily, in divided doses.	The anti-stress vitamin. Important in skin pigmentation. Sublingual form is best.
and para-aminobenzoic acid (PABA)	100 mg and up, 3 times daily.	Aids in stopping discoloration of the hair. Consider injections (under a doctor's supervision).
Important		
Essential fatty acids (primrose oil and Ultimate Oil from Nature's Secret are good sources)	As directed on label.	Stimulates hormone function and contains all the needed essential fatty acids.

Helpful		
Ageless Beauty from Biotec Foods	As directed on label.	Protects the skin from free radical damage.
Calcium and magnesium	1,000 mg daily. 500 mg daily.	Deficiency contributes to fragility of the skin. Needed to balance with calcium.
Methylsulfonyl-methane (MSM)	As directed on label.	Possesses remarkable therapeutic properties for the skin. Helps to detoxify the body on a cellular level.
Multivitamin and mineral complex	As directed on label.	To maintain a balance of all essential nutrients.
S-Adenosylmethio-nine (SAMe)	As directed on label.	Aids in relief of stress and depression, eases pain, and has antioxidant effects. *Caution:* Do not use if you have manic-depressive disorder or take prescription antidepressants.
Silica	As directed on label.	Important for developing skin's strength and elasticity; stimulates collagen formation.
Vitamin A plus carotenoid complex with beta-carotene	10,000 IU daily. As directed on label.	To promote healing and construction of new skin tissue.
Vitamin C with bioflavonoids	3,000–5,000 mg daily, in divided doses.	Necessary for the formation of collagen, a protein that gives skin its flexibility. Also fights free radicals and strengthens the capillaries that feed the skin.
Vitamin E	Start with 400 IU daily and increase slowly to 800 IU daily.	Protects against free radicals that can damage the skin. Use d-alpha-tocopherol form.
Zinc plus copper	50 mg daily. Do not exceed a total of 100 mg daily from all supplements. 3 mg daily.	For tissue strength and repair. Use zinc gluconate lozenges or OptiZinc for best absorption. Needed for collagen production and healthy skin. Also needed to balance with zinc.

HERBS

❑ The use of picrorrhiza (an Indian herb used in Ayurvedic medicine) has been shown to reduce the number and size of unpigmented skin patches.

❑ St. John's wort can help reduce stress and anxiety.

RECOMMENDATIONS

❑ Consult a nutritionally oriented physician for vitamin B complex plus PABA injections (*see under* Nutrients, above). This treatment is often effective.

❑ Treat the affected area gently—cleanse gently, apply moisturizers liberally, and protect exposed areas from cleansing agents or other chemicals by wearing protective gloves or clothing.

❑ Expose patches of affected skin to the sun—this may promote repigmentation—but don't overdo it. Use ade-quate sun protection on the affected area, and always apply a sunscreen with a sun protection factor (SPF) of 15 or higher to any unpigmented areas. They have no natural protection against the sun's ultraviolet rays.

CONSIDERATIONS

❑ Vitiligo sometimes responds to the use of PABA and magnesium. Small spots of pigment appear gradually, like freckles. The spots gradually merge until normal color is restored. Some people with vitiligo have prematurely gray or white hair. A small percentage of such people treated with PABA and magnesium have experienced a return of both skin and hair to the original color.

❑ Vitiligo lesions may be de-emphasized by the use of commercial cosmetics that cover the affected area with an opaque, waterproof layer. DermaBlend is one widely available product.

❑ Creams and lotions that contain antioxidants such as ginkgo biloga, green tea, vitamin C, and carotenes may be helpful.

❑ Creams containing fluorinated steroids may be prescribed to stimulate repigmentation of the skin.

❑ For persons with widespread vitiligo, bleaching of the unaffected skin with hydroquinone (a weak but safe depigmenting agent) may be recommended. This is done to minimize the difference in color between pigmented and depigmented areas. The process is irreversible, and it can take from several months to years to complete.

❑ Psoralen plus ultraviolet light A (PUVA) therapy is often used to treat vitiligo. This therapy combines ultraviolet light with an oral drug and has proven to be effective, even for those with advanced symptoms. However, this treatment has many potential side effects for some individuals, including eye problems, liver damage, nausea, and skin blistering.

❑ For mild forms of vitiligo, topical corticosteriods may be used to restore small patches of nonpigmented skin.

❑ An article in *Let's Live* magazine reported on a new treatment in which healthy pigment cells were transplanted into the affected area. These transplants were successful in all but one case and none of the recipients rejected the transplantation of healthy pigment cells.

❑ GH3 cream from Gero Vita International has given good results for many skin problems. This face cream is for adult use only.

Warts

Warts are small growths that are caused by human papillomaviruses (HPV). There are at least sixty known types of

HPV. Warts may appear singly or in clusters. This section addresses three types of warts: common warts, plantar warts, and genital warts.

Common warts can be found anywhere on the body, but are most common on the hands, fingers, elbows, forearms, knees, face, and the skin around the nails. Most often, they often occur on skin that is continually exposed to friction, trauma, or abrasion. They can also occur on the larynx (the voice box) and cause hoarseness. Common warts may be flat or raised, dry or moist, and have a rough and pitted surface that is either the same color as or slightly darker than the surrounding skin. They can be as small as a pinhead or as large as a small bean. Highly contagious, the virus that causes common warts is acquired through breaks in the skin. Common warts can spread if they are picked, trimmed, bitten, or touched. Warts on the face can spread as a result of shaving. Common warts typically do not cause pain or itching.

Plantar warts occur on the soles of the feet and the undersides of the toes. They are bumpy white growths that may resemble calluses, except that they can be tender to the touch and often bleed if the surface is trimmed. They also often have an identifiable hard center. Plantar warts do not tend to spread to other parts of the body.

Genital warts are soft, moist growths found in and around the vagina, anus, penis, groin, and/or scrotum. In men, they can grow in the urethra as well. They are usually pink or red in color and resemble tiny heads of cauliflower. Genital warts most often occur in clusters, but they can appear singly as well. They are transmitted through vaginal, oral, or anal sex, and are highly contagious. Because the warts do not usually appear until three months or more after an individual becomes infected with the HPV that causes them, the virus can be spread before the carrier is even aware that he or she has it. Although genital warts are not cancerous, they appear to cause changes in the cervix that may be a precursor to cervical cancer. An infant born to a mother with genital warts may contract the virus.

Unless otherwise specified, the dosages recommended here are for adults. For a child between the ages of twelve and seventeen, reduce the dose to three-quarters of the recommended amount. For a child between six and twelve, use one-half of the recommended dose, and for a child under the age of six, use one-quarter of the recommended amount.

NUTRIENTS

SUPPLEMENT	SUGGESTED DOSAGE	COMMENTS
Very Important		
Vitamin B complex	50 mg of each major B vitamin 3 times daily (amounts of individual vitamins in a complex will vary).	Important in normal cell multiplication.
Vitamin C with bioflavonoids	4,000–10,000 mg daily.	Has powerful antiviral capacity.
Important		
L-Cysteine	500 mg twice daily, on an empty stomach. Take with water or juice. Do not take with milk. Take with 50 mg vitamin B₆ and 100 mg vitamin C for better absorption.	Supplies sulfur, needed for prevention and treatment of warts. (*See* AMINO ACIDS in Part One.)
Methylsulfonyl-methane (MSM)	As directed on label.	MSM and vitamin C are used by the body to build healthy new cells.
Vitamin A with mixed carotenoids including natural beta-carotene	100,000 IU daily for 1 month, then 50,000 IU daily for 1 month, then reduce to 25,000 IU daily for 1 month or until warts disappear. If you are pregnant, do not exceed 10,000 IU daily.	Needed for normalizing skin and epithelial membranes. Use emulsion form for easier assimilation and greater safety at higher doses.
Vitamin E	400–800 IU daily. Can be applied topically; cut open capsule to release oil. Apply to warts daily.	Improves circulation and promotes tissue repair and healing. Use d-alpha-tocopherol form.
Zinc	50–80 mg daily. Do not exceed a total of 100 mg daily from all supplements.	Increases immunity against viruses. Use zinc gluconate lozenges or Zinc for best absorption.
Helpful		
Multivitamin and mineral complex	As directed on label.	Needed for normal cell division.
Reishi extract or shiitake extract	As directed on label. As directed on label.	Has antiviral properties.

HERBS

❑ Aloe vera gel; myrrh; oils of clove, lemongrass, peppermint, tea tree, or wintergreen; and tinctures of black walnut, chickweed, goldenseal, and pau d'arco have all been used externally to treat warts. Aloe vera gel has both antibacterial and antiviral properties. Place a small dab of one on the wart two or three times daily until the wart is gone. If irritation occurs, dilute the oil or extract with distilled water or cold-pressed vegetable oil.

❑ Astragalus protects the immune system, which is important in warding off warts.

❑ Black walnut has healing properties. It is particularly useful for warts in the mouth and throat.

RECOMMENDATIONS

❑ To remove common warts, try one or more of the following remedies:

• Crush a garlic clove and apply the garlic directly on the wart, avoiding the surrounding skin. Cover it with a bandage and leave it in place for twenty-four hours. Blisters should then form, and the wart should fall off in about a week.

- Apply a paste made from castor oil and baking soda to the wart. Put the mixture on each night and cover it with a bandage. This may remove the wart in three to six weeks.

❏ Increase the amount of sulfur-containing amino acids in your diet by eating more asparagus, citrus fruits, eggs, garlic, and onions. Desiccated liver tablets are also good.

❏ If you suspect you may have genital warts, see your health care provider promptly. This is especially important for women, because genital warts have been linked to cervical cancer. An immediate Pap test is advised.

❏ Keep genital warts dry. After bathing, use a hair dryer on a low setting to dry the area. Do not rub or irritate it. Wear only cotton underwear. Do not have sexual intercourse until the warts are completely healed.

❏ Do not cut or burn a wart off yourself. These are procedures that must be done by a qualified health care provider.

CONSIDERATIONS

❏ Plantar warts may not require treatment. However, if a wart is painful and interferes with walking, treatment is warranted. Several treatment sessions may be necessary to eliminate them, but doctors can usually eradicate even the most stubborn plantar warts.

❏ Adequate daily vitamin C intake is most important in maintaining effective immunity against the viruses that cause warts.

❏ People who take medications to suppress the immune system, such as those who have received organ transplants or who have certain autoimmune disorders, are more prone to develop warts.

❏ Most common warts disappear within a year or two, even without treatment. Unless a common wart becomes bothersome, there is no need to do anything about it. Commonly used medical treatments for common and plantar warts include fulguration (using electric current to destroy wart tissue); freezing with liquid nitrogen, and topical applications of some chemicals.

❏ Some physicians have achieved good results using the drug bleomycin (Blenoxane) to treat warts. It is injected or applied locally.

❏ Cantharidin is another chemical your physician may apply to get rid of warts.

❏ For larger genital warts, CO_2 laser surgery may be recommended. Interferon injections may be used for genital warts that do not go away with other treatment.

❏ Common warts can be treated with a mild acid solution such as salicylic acid. It is thought that the acid weakens the walls of the wart enough to allow some of the virus to enter the bloodstream, causing the production of antibodies that eventually attack and destroy the warts. Removal does not allow the body to build up immunity to the virus.

❏ There are a variety of treatments for genital warts, but none is a perfect cure and all have side effects. Treatment falls into three categories: prescription topical preparations that destroy wart tissue; surgical methods to remove wart tissue; and biological approaches that target the virus.

❏ A study on the injection of interferon alfa directly into genital warts found this treatment to be successful approximately 36 percent of the time. Interferon alfa is a powerful antiviral substance. However, using this treatment for large numbers of warts may be too uncomfortable and expensive.

❏ Women who have been diagnosed with genital warts should have a vaginal and uterine Pap smear every six months, as these warts are associated with an increased risk of cervical cancer.

Weakened Immune System

Modern conventional medicine battles disease directly by means of drugs, surgery, radiation, and other therapies, but true health can be attained only by maintaining a healthy, properly functioning immune system. It is the immune system that fights off disease-causing microorganisms and that engineers the healing process. The immune system is the key to fighting every kind of insult to the body, from that little shaving nick to the myriad of viruses that seem to abound these days. Even the aging process may be more closely related to the functioning of the immune system than to the passage of time.

Weakening of the immune system results in increased susceptibility to virtually every type of illness. Some common signs of impaired immune function include fatigue, listlessness, repeated infections, inflammation, allergic reactions, slow wound healing, chronic diarrhea, and infections that represent an overgrowth of some normally present organism, such as oral thrush, systemic candidiasis, or vaginal yeast infections. It is estimated that healthy adults in our society have an average of two colds a year. Persons who have significantly more colds and infectious illnesses than that are likely to have some problem with immune function. By understanding some of the basic elements of the immune system and how they work, plus the overall role the immune system plays in your health, you can take responsibility for your own health.

In its simplest terms, the task of the immune system is to identify those things that are "self" (that naturally belong in the body) and those that are "nonself" (foreign or otherwise harmful material), and then to neutralize or destroy that which is nonself. The immune system is unlike other bodily systems in that it is not a group of physical structures but a system of complex interactions involving many different organs, structures, and substances, among them white blood cells, bone marrow, the lymphatic vessels and organs, specialized cells found in various body tissues, and specialized substances, called serum factors, that are present in the blood. Ideally, all of these components work together to protect the body against infection and disease.

The human immune system is functional at birth, but it does not yet function well. This is termed *innate immunity*—the immunity you are born with. Immune function develops and becomes more sophisticated as the system matures and the body learns to defend itself against different foreign invaders called antigens. This is termed *adaptive immunity*. The immune system has the ability to learn to identify, and then to remember, specific antigens that have been encountered. It does this through two basic means, known as *cell-mediated immunity* and *humoral immunity*.

In cell-mediated immunity, white blood cells called T lymphocytes identify and then destroy cancerous cells, viruses, and microorganisms like bacteria and fungi. The T lymphocytes, or T cells, mature in the thymus gland (hence the "T" designation). This is where they learn to recognize what is "self," and therefore should be tolerated, and what is "nonself," and therefore should be destroyed. The thymus, a small gland located behind the top of the breastbone, is a major gland of the immune system. In the thymus, each T cell is programmed to identify one particular type of invading enemy. Not all prospective T cells make a successful passage through the thymus. Those whose programming is imperfect (for instance, those that mistakenly identify "self" as "nonself") are eliminated. The ones that do make it are released into the bloodstream to search out and destroy antigens that correspond to their programming. They attack the antigens in part through the secretion of proteins called cytokines. Interferon is one of the better known types of cytokines.

Humoral immunity involves the production of antibodies. These are not cells, but special proteins whose chemical structures are formed to match the surfaces of specific antigens. When they encounter their specific antigens, antibodies either damage the invasive cells or alert the white blood cells to attack. The antibodies are produced by another group of white blood cells, the B lymphocytes, which are manufactured by and mature in the bone marrow. When a B lymphocyte is presented with a particular antigen, it engineers an antibody to match it and stores a blueprint of the invader so that it can initiate the production of antibodies in case of subsequent exposure, even if a long period of time elapses in between. For this system to work, each B cell must come into existence prepared to produce an almost infinite variety of different antibodies, so that it can match whatever antigen it is presented with. This is made possible by a mechanism known as "jumping genes." Inside the B cells, the genes that determine the chemical structure of the protein to be produced can be shuffled around and linked up in an astronomical number of different combinations. As a result, any B cell is capable of producing an antibody molecule to match virtually any foreign invader. It is the phenomenon of humoral immunity that makes immunization possible.

Because of their crucial role in all aspects of immunity—both cell-mediated and humoral—white blood cells are considered the body's first line of defense. White blood cells are larger than red blood cells. In addition, they can move independently in the bloodstream and are able to pass through the cell walls. This enables them to travel quickly to the site of an injury or infection. There are different categories of white blood cells, each of which performs a specific function. These include the following:

- *Granulocytes.* There are three types of granulocytes:
  1. *Neutrophils,* the most abundant type of white blood cell, whose function is to ingest and destroy microorganisms such as bacteria.
  2. *Eosinophils,* which ingest and destroy antigen-antibody combinations (formed when antibodies intercept antigens) and also moderate hypersensitive (allergic) reactions by secreting an enzyme that breaks down histamine. High levels of eosinophils in the blood are often present in individuals with allergic disorders, presumably because the body is attempting to tame the allergic reaction.
  3. *Basophils,* which secrete compounds such as heparin or histamine in response to contact with antigens.

- *Lymphocytes.* The lymphocytes are responsible for the development of specific immunities. Three important types of lymphocytes are T cells, B cells, and NK cells:
  1. *T cells* undergo maturation in the thymus gland and play a major role in cell-mediated immunity.
  2. *B cells* mature in the bone marrow and are responsible for the production of antibodies.
  3. *NK (natural killer) cells* destroy body cells that have become infected or become cancerous.

- *Monocytes.* The largest cells in the blood, monocytes act as the "garbage collectors" of the body. They engulf and digest foreign particles as well as damaged or aging cells, including tumor cells. After spending about twenty-four hours circulating in the bloodstream, most monocytes enter the tissues and perform similar functions there. At this point, they are known as macrophages.

Another important component of immunity is the lymphatic system. This is a system of organs (including the spleen, the thymus, the tonsils, and the lymph nodes) and fluid, called lymph, that circulates through the lymphatic vessels in the body and also bathes the body's cells. The lymphatic system provides a kind of continuous cleansing that operates at the cellular level. It is through the lymphatic system that fluid from the spaces between cells is drained, taking with it waste products, toxins, and other debris from the tissues. The lymph flows through the lymph nodes, where the macrophages filter out the undesirables, and from it there returns to the venous circulation.

Other important components of the immune system are the spleen, the thymus, and the bone marrow. The spleen filters the blood and removes old red blood cells that need replacing. The spleen is populated by macrophages, dendritic cells (white blood cells that collect bits of antigens so that T cells can learn to recognize them), red blood cells, killer cells, and B and T cells. In the spleen, antigens are brought to the B cells, which use them to learn to manufacture the appropriate antigen response. People whose spleens have been removed tend to be more prone to illness because these important functions are no longer performed.

The thymus is the site where T cells mature. T cells play a role in immunity by secreting interleukin-1, interleukin-2, and interferon, as well as activating B cells so that they produce antibodies. The bone marrow produces new white blood cells, platelets, B cells, killer cells, granulocytes, and thymocytes. All white blood cells are made from stem cells. Stem cells are embryonic cells that have the capacity to mature into virtually any type of cells. Some of the white blood cells made in the bone marrow leave the bone marrow and mature elsewhere in the body, while others mature where they are and support the immune system. All the cells of the immune system come originally from the bone marrow.

Both the appendix and the tonsils also support the immune system.

Marvelous as it is, the immune system can work as it should only if it is cared for properly. This means getting all the right nutrients and providing the right environment, plus avoiding those things that tend to depress immunity. Many elements of the environment we live in today compromise our immune systems' defensive abilities. The chemicals in the household cleaners we use; the overuse of antibiotics and other drugs; the antibiotics, pesticides, and myriad additives present in the foods we eat; and exposure to environmental pollutants all place a strain on the immune system. Another factor that adversely affects the immune system is stress. Stress results in a sequence of biochemical events that ultimately suppresses the normal activity of white blood cells and places undue demands on the endocrine system, as well as depleting the body of needed nutrients. The result is impaired healing ability and lowered defense against infection.

Proper immune function is an intricate balancing act. While inadequate immunity predisposes one to infectious illness of every type, it is also possible to become ill as a result of an immune response that is too strong or directed at an inappropriate target. Many different disorders, including allergies, lupus, pernicious anemia, rheumatic heart disease, rheumatoid arthritis, and, possibly, diabetes, have been linked to inappropriate immune system activity. Consequently, they are known as autoimmune, or "self-attacking-self," disorders.

While much is known about the functioning of the immune system, much more remains to be learned; only in the past ten to fifteen years have many facets of immune function begun to be studied and understood by physicians and researchers. The field of immunology (the study of the immune system) is one of the fastest growing fields in medicine today.

The program of supplements outlined here is designed to strengthen the immune system, whether it is damaged as a result of disease, stress, inadequate nutrition, poor living habits, chemotherapy, or a combination of one or more of these factors. The dosages recommended here are for adults. For a child between the ages of twelve and seventeen, reduce the dose to three-quarters of the recommended amount. For a child between six and twelve, use one-half of the recommended dose, and for a child under the age of six, use one-quarter of the recommended amount.

NUTRIENTS

SUPPLEMENT	SUGGESTED DOSAGE	COMMENTS
Acetyl-L-carnitine	As directed on label.	An energy carrier, metabolic facilitator, and cell membrane protectant. Protects the heart.
Acidophilus (Kyo-Dophilus from Wakunaga is a good source)	As directed on label. Take on an empty stomach.	Restores important bacteria to the intestinal tract. Use a nondairy formula.
Aerobic 07 from Aerobic Life Industries	9 drops twice daily, taken in water.	For tissue oxygenation.
Béres Drops Plus from Nupharma Nutraceuticals	As directed on label.	Contains minerals and trace elements that boost and nourish the immune system.
Beta-1,3-glucan	As directed on label.	Stimulates macrophages to remove cellular debris and, possibly, to recognize and kill tumor cells.
Body Language Super Antioxidant from Oxyfresh	As directed on label.	To protect the body from free radical damage, environmental stresses, and pollutants.
Bovine colostrum	As directed on label.	Contains immunoglobulins and antibody-stimulating factors. Enhances immunity.
Coenzyme Q$_{10}$ plus	100 mg daily.	Supports the immune system. An oxygen enhancer to protect the cells and heart function.
Coenzyme A from Coenzyme-A Technologies	As directed on label.	Works well with coenzyme Q$_{10}$ to support the immune system and increase energy.
Essential fatty acids (Ultimate Oil from Nature's Secret is a good source)	As directed on label.	A most important element in the diet. Necessary for a healthy immune system.
Free-form amino acid complex (Amino Balance from Anabol Naturals)	As directed on label, on an empty stomach.	Protein that is broken down into a form the body can use. Use a formula containing all the essential amino acids.

Garlic (Kyolic from Wakunaga)	2 capsules 3 times daily.	Stimulates the immune system.
Glutathione	As directed on label.	Inhibits the formation of free radicals; aids in red blood cell integrity; reduces quantities of hydrogen peroxide; protects immune cells.
Kelp	2,000–3,000 mg daily.	Supplies a balance of minerals needed for immune system integrity.
Kyo-Green from Wakunaga	As directed on label.	Supplies nutrients and chlorophyll needed for tissue repair, and cleanses the blood. Important in immune response.
L-Arginine and L-ornithine	As directed on label, on an empty stomach. Take with water or juice. Do not take with milk. Take with 50 mg vitamin B$_6$ and 100 mg vitamin C for better absorption.	To enhance the immune system and retard the growth of tumors and cancer. Necessary for the immune system. (See AMINO ACIDS in Part One.)
L-Cysteine and L-methionine plus L-lysine	500 mg each twice daily, on an empty stomach.	To destroy free radicals and viruses and protect the glands, especially the liver. (See AMINO ACIDS in Part One.)
Lecithin granules or capsules	1 tbsp 3 times daily, with meals. 1,200 mg 3 times daily, with meals.	Aids in cellular protection.
Maitake extract or reishi extract or shiitake extract	As directed on label. As directed on label. As directed on label.	Mushrooms that build immunity and fight viral infections and cancer.
Manganese	2 mg daily.	Necessary for proper immune function. Works with the B vitamins to provide a general feeling of well-being.
Multivitamin and mineral complex	As directed on label.	All vitamins and minerals are necessary in balance. Use a high-potency formula.
Proteolytic enzymes or Inflazyme Forte from American Biologics or Wobenzym N from Marlyn Nutraceuticals	As directed on label. 4 tablets 3 times daily, with meals. 3–6 tablets 2–3 times daily, between meals.	To aid in proper breakdown of proteins, fats, and carbohydrates for better absorption of nutrients. Destroys free radicals and aids in proper breakdown and absorption of foods.
Pycnogenol and/or grape seed extract	As directed on label 3 times daily, with meals. As directed on label.	A unique bioflavonoid that is a potent antioxidant and immune enhancer. One of the most potent antioxidants; protects the cells.
Quercetin plus bromelain	As directed on label. As directed on label.	Helps to prevent reactions to certain foods, pollens, and other allergens. Increases immunity. Enhances effectiveness of quercetin.
Raw thymus glandular plus multiglandular complex with raw spleen glandular	As directed on label. As directed on label. As directed on label.	To enhance T cell production. Glandulars from lamb source are best.

Selenium	200 mcg daily. If you are pregnant, do not exceed 40 mcg daily.	Important free radical destroyer.
Squalene (shark liver oil)	As directed on label.	Aids in rebuilding and functioning of cells; has anticancer properties.
Superoxide dismutase (SOD) plus Dimethylglycine (DMG) (Aangamik DMG from FoodScience of Vermont)	As directed on label. As directed on label.	To improve oxygenation of tissues.
Taurine Plus from American Biologics	As directed on label.	An antioxidant and immune regulator necessary for white blood cell activation and neurological function.
Vitamin A plus natural carotenoid complex with beta-carotene	10,000 IU daily. As directed on label.	Needed for proper immune function. Powerful antioxidants, free radical scavengers, and immune enhancers. May protect against cancer and heart disease.
Vitamin B complex plus extra vitamin B$_6$ (pyridoxine) and vitamin B$_{12}$ plus raw liver extract	100 mg of each major B vitamin 3 times daily, with meals (amounts of individual vitamins in a complex will vary). 50 mg 3 times daily. 1,000–2,000 mcg daily. As directed on label.	Anti-stress vitamins, especially important for normal brain function. Consider injections (under a doctor's supervision). If injections are not available, use a sublingual form. Vitamins B$_6$ and B$_{12}$ potentiate amino acids and are necessary for best absorption of amino acids and for proper functioning of enzymes in the body. A good source of B vitamins and iron. Consider injections (under a doctor's supervision).
Vitamin C with bioflavonoids	5,000–20,000 mg daily, in divided doses. (See ASCORBIC ACID FLUSH in Part Three.)	An important antioxidant that decreases susceptibility to infection.
Vitamin E	400 IU daily.	An antioxidant that is an integral part of the body's defense system. Use d-alpha-tocopherol form. Use emulsion form for easier assimilation.
Zinc plus copper	50–80 mg daily. Do not exceed this amount. 3 mg daily.	Very important for the immune system. Use zinc chelate form. Needed to balance with zinc.

HERBS

❏ Astragalus boosts the immune system and generates anticancer cells in the body. It is also a powerful antioxidant and protects the liver from toxins.

Caution: Do not take this herb in the presence of a fever.

❏ Bayberry, fenugreek, hawthorn, horehound, licorice root, and red clover all enhance the immune response.

Caution: If overused, licorice can elevate blood pressure. Do not use this herb on a daily basis for more than seven days in a row. Avoid if you have high blood pressure.

❏ Black radish, dandelion, and milk thistle help to cleanse the liver and the bloodstream. The liver is *the* organ of detoxification and must function optimally.

❑ Boxthorn seed, ginseng, suma, and wisteria contain germanium, a trace element that aids immune function and has anticancer properties.

Caution: Do not use ginseng if you have high blood pressure.

❑ Echinacea boosts the immune system and enhances lymphatic function.

Note: Do not use this herb if you have an autoimmune disorder.

❑ Esberitox from Enzymatic Therapy is a combination of different herbs designed to promote a healthy immune system.

❑ Ginkgo biloba is good for the brain cells, aids circulation, and is a powerful antioxidant.

❑ Goldenseal strengthens the immune system, cleanses the body, and has antibacterial properties.

Caution: Do not take goldenseal internally on a daily basis for more than one week at a time, do not use it during pregnancy, and use it with caution if you are allergic to ragweed.

❑ ImmunoCare from Himalaya USA is a combination formula containing Ayurvedic herbs that may protect white blood cells.

❑ St. John's wort is a natural blood purifier and fights viruses such as HIV and Epstein-Barr virus.

❑ Ligustrum (known in Chinese herbology as *nu zhen zi*) increases bone marrow production of lymphocytes as well as their maturation into T cells. It is beneficial for thymus and spleen health and inhibits tumor growth.

❑ Picrorrhiza, an Indian herb used in Ayurvedic medicine, is a powerful immunostimulant that boosts all aspects of immune function.

RECOMMENDATIONS

❑ Take an inventory of the factors that may be compromising your immune system and take steps to correct them. Two of the most common immune suppressors include stress and an incorrect diet, especially a diet high in fat and refined processed foods.

❑ Supply your immune system with adequate amounts of nutrients that promote proper immune function. Some of the most valuable include:

• Vitamin A is the anti-infection vitamin. If used properly and in moderate doses, vitamin A is rarely toxic and is very important in the body's defense system.

• Vitamin C may be the single most important vitamin for the immune system. It is essential for the formation of adrenal hormones and the production of lymphocytes. It also has a direct effect on bacteria and viruses. Vitamin C should be taken with bioflavonoids, natural plant substances that enhance absorption and reinforce the action of this vitamin.

• Vitamin E interacts with vitamins A and C and the mineral selenium, acting as a primary antioxidant and scavenger of toxic free radicals. Vitamin E activity is an integral part of the body's defense system.

• Zinc boosts the immune response and promotes the healing of wounds when used in appropriate doses (100 milligrams or less daily). It also helps to protect the liver. Doses over 100 milligrams per day may actually depress immune function, however.

❑ Begin a diet of fresh fruits and vegetables (preferably raw) plus nuts, seeds, grains, and other foods that are high in fiber.

❑ Include in the diet chlorella, garlic, and pearl barley. These foods contain germanium, a trace element beneficial for the immune system. Also add kelp to the diet, in the form of giant red kelp or brown kelp. Kelp contains iodine, calcium, iron, carotene, protein, riboflavin, and vitamin C, which are necessary for the immune system's functional integrity.

❑ Consume "green drinks" daily.

❑ Avoid animal products, processed foods, sugar, and soda.

❑ Follow a fasting program once a month to rid your body of toxins that can weaken the immune system. (*See* FASTING in Part Three.)

❑ Use spirulina, especially while fasting. Spirulina is a naturally digestible food that aids in protecting the immune system. It supplies many nutrients needed for cleansing and healing.

❑ Be sure to get sufficient sleep. As much as possible, avoid stress.

❑ Get regular moderate exercise (but don't overdo it). Exercise reduces stress and elevates mood, which has a positive effect on immune response. In addition, T lymphocyte production is stimulated by exercise.

❑ Avoid overeating.

❑ Do not smoke or consume beverages containing alcohol or caffeine.

❑ Do not take any drugs except for those prescribed by your physician.

CONSIDERATIONS

❑ White blood cells are an indicator of health. Since the beginning of the AIDS epidemic, we have all become aware of white blood cell counts—and the implications of low numbers of white blood cells. The normal range of white blood cells in a person with a strong immune system is anywhere from 4,000 to 12,000 cells per microliter (µL, the equivalent of one-millionth liter) of blood.

❑ Marijuana use weakens the immune system. Delta-9 tetrahydrocannabinol (THC), the most active compound in marijuana, alters the normal immune response, making the white blood cells 35 to 40 percent less effective than normal.

❑ Mercury amalgam dental fillings have been linked to a weakened immune system. Toxic metals suppress the immune system. A hair analysis can be used to check for heavy metal intoxication. (*See* MERCURY TOXICITY in Part Two and HAIR ANALYSIS in Part Three.)

❑ A person's mental state can suppress his or her immune system. A positive frame of mind is important in building up the immune system. (*See* ANXIETY DISORDER; DEPRESSION; and/or STRESS in Part Two.)

❑ An underactive thyroid results in immune deficiency. (*See* HYPOTHYROIDISM in Part Two.)

❑ Food allergies and adverse food reactions can place stress on the immune system. (*See* ALLERGIES in Part Two.)

❑ Research has shown that dehydroepiandrosterone (DHEA), a hormone, may enhance the functioning of the immune system. (*See* DHEA THERAPY in Part Three.)

❑ Human growth hormone (HGH) is another naturally occurring hormone that strengthens the immune system. Treatment with HGH requires the supervision of a physician. (*See* GROWTH HORMONE THERAPY in Part Three.)

❑ *See also* AIDS in Part Two.

Weight Problems

See ANOREXIA NERVOSA; APPETITE, POOR; BULIMIA; OBESITY; UNDERWEIGHT/WEIGHT LOSS.

Wilson's Disease

Wilson's disease, also called *hepatolenticular degeneration* or *inherited copper toxicosis*, is a rare inherited disorder that affects approximately 1 in 30,000 persons worldwide. In persons with Wilson's disease, the body is unable to metabolize the trace element copper as it should, with the result that excess copper accumulates in the brain, kidneys, liver, and the corneas of the eyes. This causes organ damage and other complications, including neurological problems and psychotic behavior. Untreated, Wilson's disease leads to brain damage, cirrhosis of the liver, hepatitis, and, ultimately, death. Fortunately, early detection and treatment of the disease can minimize the symptoms and complications and possibly even prevent them altogether.

Symptoms of Wilson's disease may include bloody vomit; difficulty speaking, swallowing, and/or walking; drooling; an enlarged spleen; jaundice; loss of appetite; loss of coordination; progressive fatigue and/or weakness; progressive intellectual impairment; psychological deterioration manifested as personality changes and/or bizarre behavior; rigidity, spasms, or tremors of the muscles; swelling and/or fluid accumulation in the abdomen; and unex-

plained weight loss. Sometimes the first sign is the development of a pigmented ring, known as a Kayser-Fleischer ring, at the outer margin of the cornea, which may be detected during a routine eye examination. In the advanced stages of the disease, symptoms due to chronic active hepatitis or cirrhosis may appear, menstrual cycles may cease, and an individual may experience chest pains, heart palpitations, lightheadedness, pallor, and shortness of breath as a result of exertion.

Although persons with Wilson's disease are born with the disorder, symptoms are rarely seen before the age of six and most often do not appear until adolescence or even later. However, to prevent complications, treatment is required whether symptoms have appeared or not. Diagnosis is usually based on a study of individual and family medical history plus blood tests to determine levels of ceruloplasmin (a copper-carrying protein in the blood) and to check for anemia, plus a urine test to reveal elevated levels of copper in the urine. A liver biopsy to evaluate the amount of copper in liver tissue may be done to confirm the diagnosis.

The dosages recommended here are for adults. For a child between the ages of twelve and seventeen, reduce the dose to three-quarters of the recommended amount. For a child between six and twelve, use one-half of the recommended dose, and for a child under the age of six, use one-quarter of the recommended amount.

NUTRIENTS

SUPPLEMENT	SUGGESTED DOSAGE	COMMENTS
Very Important		
Garlic (Kyolic from Wakunaga)	As directed on label.	A powerful antioxidant that protects liver and heart function. Promotes normal healing and prevents cell damage.
Iron	As directed by physician. Take with 100 mg vitamin C for better absorption.	To correct and protect against anemia. *Caution:* Do not take iron unless anemia is diagnosed.
Multivitamin and mineral complex with	As directed on label.	A balance of all nutrients is essential for healing.
potassium and	99 mg daily.	Necessary for proper muscle contraction.
selenium	200 mcg daily. If you are pregnant, do not exceed 40 mcg daily.	Needed for proper adrenal gland function.
Vitamin A with mixed carotenoids including beta-carotene	10,000 IU daily.	Powerful antioxidants that also enhance immunity.
Vitamin B complex	75 mg of each major B vitamin 3 times daily. (amounts of individual vitamins in a complex will vary).	Protects the liver and is needed for proper brain function.
plus extra vitamin B₆ (pyridoxine)	50 mg 3 times daily.	Helps to prevent damage to the nervous system and guard against anemia. Also combats fluid retention.

684

Vitamin C with bioflavonoids	3,000–5,000 mg daily, in divided doses.	Protects against inflammation, anemia, and hepatitis, and reduces copper levels in the body. Use an esterified form.
Vitamin E	600 IU daily. Take separately from iron.	Promotes normal healing and prevents cell damage. Use d-alpha-tocopherol form.
Zinc	75 mg daily. Do not exceed this amount.	Decreases copper levels and enhances immunity. Zinc balances copper in the body.

Important

Acetyl-L-carnitine	As directed on label.	Protects liver and heart function.
Advanced Carotenoid Complex from Solgar	As directed on label.	Contains powerful free radical scavengers and immune enhancers.
Calcium and magnesium	1,500–2,000 mg daily. 750–1,000 mg daily.	Minerals that work together to prevent muscle spasms.
Coenzyme Q_{10} plus Coenzyme A from Coenzyme-A Technologies	As directed on label. As directed on label.	A powerful antioxidant that also increases circulation and energy. Works with coenzyme Q_{10}.
Flaxseed oil	As directed on label.	To supply essential fatty acids, which are vital for brain and nerve function and enhance immunity.
Free-form amino acid complex	As directed on label, on an empty stomach.	Necessary for protein synthesis. Use a formula containing all the essential amino acids.
Gamma-amino-butyric acid (GABA)	As directed on label, on an empty stomach.	Essential for proper brain function. Also has a tranquilizing effect. (*See* AMINO ACIDS in Part One.)
L-Arginine and L-ornithine plus L-cysteine	As directed on label, on an empty stomach. Take at bedtime with water or juice. Do not take with milk. Take with 50 mg vitamin B_6 and 100 mg vitamin C for better absorption. As directed on label, on an empty stomach.	To aid in liver and kidney detoxification. (*See* AMINO ACIDS in Part One.) Reduces the body's absorption of copper.
Methylsulfonyl-methane (MSM)	As directed on label.	Contains sulfur, which aids in removing copper from the body.
Pycnogenol and/or grape seed extract	As directed on label. As directed on label.	Powerful antioxidants that lessen mental deterioration.

HERBS

❑ Burdock, dandelion, milk thistle, and suma cleanse and support the liver and help to fight fatigue.

❑ Alfalfa, ginkgo biloba, gotu kola, kava, lobelia, parsley, oat straw, periwinkle, and skullcap are good for overall good health and the functioning of the brain and nervous system.

Caution: Do not take lobelia internally on an ongoing basis.

❑ Astragalus, echinacea, and pau d'arco are helpful for fatigue.

Caution: Do not use astragalus in the presence of a fever.

❑ Black radish and red clover strengthen the liver.

❑ Cat's claw is an anti-inflammatory, antioxidant, immune system enhancer, and internal cleanser. Cat's Claw Defense Complex from Source Naturals is a good source of this herb and also contains other beneficial ingredients.

Caution: Do not use cat's claw during pregnancy.

❑ Cayenne (capsicum) eases blood pressure, fights fatigue, and helps support the nervous system.

❑ Goldenseal is helpful if symptoms include difficulty swallowing, and it can ease fatigue as well. Licorice is also beneficial for swallowing difficulties, as is gargling with thyme tea.

Caution: Do not take goldenseal internally on a daily basis for more than one week at a time, do not use it during pregnancy, and use it with caution if you are allergic to ragweed. Do not use licorice on a daily basis for more than seven days in a row, and avoid it if you have high blood pressure.

❑ St. John's wort is beneficial for the nervous system and also helps to overcome fatigue and difficulty swallowing.

❑ Siberian ginseng is a tonic herb that helps reduce fatigue and supports brain and nervous system function.

Caution: Do not use this herb if you have hypoglycemia, high blood pressure, or a heart disorder.

❑ Valerian root is calming and is good for the brain and nervous system. It can also be beneficial for swallowing difficulties.

RECOMMENDATIONS

❑ Increase your consumption of onions. They contain sulfur, which helps to rid the body of copper.

❑ Eat fresh (not canned) pineapple frequently. It contains bromelain, an enzyme that helps to keep down swelling and inflammation.

❑ Have the copper level of your drinking water tested. Look in the yellow pages of your local telephone directory or consult your state's environmental agency for laboratories that can do this type of testing. If your tap water contains more than 1 part per million of copper, drink quality bottled water instead (steam-distilled is best) or check the pipes in your home; if you can determine that all or most of the copper in your water is coming from the pipes, it may be worthwhile to replace them with copper-free ones.

❑ If you take a multivitamin and/or mineral supplement, be sure to choose a formula that does *not* contain copper.

❑ Eliminate from the diet foods high in copper. These include barley, beets, blackstrap molasses, broccoli, chocolate, enriched cereals, garlic, lentils, liver, mushrooms, nuts, organ meats, salmon, and shellfish, as well as avocados, beans and other legumes, egg yolks, oats, oranges, pecans, raisins, soybeans, whole grains, and green leafy vegetables.

❏ If you suffer from tremors, avoid caffeine.

❏ Avoid alcohol consumption. Wilson's disease increases the risk of cirrhosis of the liver.

❏ Do not use copper cookware or utensils.

CONSIDERATIONS

❏ Wilson's disease can be neither prevented nor cured. With appropriate management, however, the prognosis is excellent.

❏ Anyone with a family history of Wilson's disease should undergo diagnostic testing—the sooner the better, and whether or not symptoms are present—so that treatment, if necessary, may begin as soon as possible.

❏ Treatment of Wilson's disease is a lifelong proposition. Most often, it involves taking penicillamine (Cuprimine, Depen), a drug that removes copper from the body by increasing its excretion in the urine. Possible side effects of this drug include deficiencies of vitamin B_6 (pyridoxine) and iron, and many people experience an allergic reaction to the drug within ten days of taking it. The most serious potential side effects of this medication include kidney disease, blood cell problems, and Goodpasture's syndrome (a potentially life-threatening syndrome characterized by bleeding of the lungs and kidney failure). Penicillamine has also been suspected of being linked to leukemia development in at least two cases. A person with a sensitivity to penicillamine may also be given a steroid such as prednisone (Deltasone and others) to decrease the reaction to the penicillamine, or the drug trientine (Syprine) may be prescribed instead. This medication also chelates copper so that it can be eliminated from the body.

❏ Some doctors prescribe high doses of zinc in place of, or in conjunction with, conventional drugs to keep copper levels under control. Zinc naturally balances with copper in the body. Zinc acetate (Galzin) is another medication that may be prescribed. It should be taken exactly as the doctor has prescribed.

❏ Regardless of the treatment regimen, regular checkups are required to monitor possible side effects from medication and to check the level of copper in the urine.

❏ If you develop any personality changes or problems linked to Wilson's disease, consulting a psychologist or other mental health professional may be helpful for both and your family.

❏ Elevated copper levels in the body result in the depletion of vitamin C and zinc. Persons with Wilson's disease therefore always require a higher than normal intake of these nutrients.

❏ Wilson's disease is not the only cause of elevated levels of copper in the body. Toxic levels of copper can also accumulate in the body as a result of excessive exposure to the metal. If a person with elevated copper levels has normal liver function and no corneal abnormalities, it is likely that the toxicity is due to something other than Wilson's disease. In addition, copper toxicity as a result of excessive copper ingestion can be demonstrated by hair analysis, whereas persons with Wilson's disease do not exhibit elevated levels of copper in the hair.

❏ *See also* COPPER TOXICITY in Part Two.

❏ The Wilson's Disease Association offers aid and support to people with Wilson's and related diseases (*see* HEALTH AND MEDICAL ORGANIZATIONS in the Appendix).

Wilson's Syndrome

See under HYPOTHYROIDISM.

Worms (Parasites)

Worms are parasites that live in the gastrointestinal tract. The most common types of worms are roundworms (including ascarids, hookworms, pinworms, and threadworms) and tapeworms. Roundworms are contagious intestinal parasites that are shaped like earthworms but smaller in size. They can easily be seen with the naked eye. Pinworms are white, threadlike worms about one-third inch long. Tapeworms vary in length from an inch up to thirty feet and can survive for up to twenty-five years in the body. In the United States, pinworm infestation in young children is by far the most prevalent parasitic worm problem.

Depending on the type of worm involved and the severity of the infestation, there may be a variety of symptoms. In some cases, there may be no perceptible symptoms at all. In some cases, worms may be seen in the stool.

Pinworms can cause severe anal itching (especially at night, as the worms tend to migrate outside the anus to lay their eggs), insomnia, and restlessness. Hookworms can cause itching on the soles of the feet, and in some cases, bloody sputum, fever, rash, and loss of appetite. Threadworms can cause coughing or bronchitis, abdominal pain, diarrhea, and gas, preceded by tiny red abrasions that sometimes itch. Small tapeworms can cause weight and appetite loss, abdominal pain, vomiting, and diarrhea. Large tapeworms can cause similar symptoms, but usually without weight loss. Ascariasis, caused by ascarids, is characterized by bloating, stomach pain, vomiting, and difficulty breathing. Trichinosis is a disease caused by a microscopic roundworm that, if left untreated, can lead to muscle damage and cardiac or neurologic complications.

Worm infestations can range from mild to severe, even life threatening, particularly in children. They result in poor absorption of essential nutrients, and in some cases, loss of blood from the gastrointestinal tract. They can therefore lead to such deficiency-related disorders as anemia and growth problems. Malabsorption resulting from parasitic infection makes one susceptible to many diseases because it results in diminished immune function.

Worms can be contracted through a variety of mechanisms, including improper disposal of human or animal waste, walking barefoot on contaminated soil, and ingestion of eggs or larvae from uncooked or partially cooked meat. In some cases, eggs may become airborne and be inhaled.

Parasites are more common than most people suppose, and they can be behind many illnesses, including colon disorders. They are more common in children than in adults. They are also common in people with AIDS, chronic fatigue syndrome, candidiasis, and many other disorders. Unfortunately, physicians often do not check for worm infestation.

The dosages recommended here are for adults. For a child between the ages of twelve and seventeen, reduce the dose to three-quarters of the recommended amount. For a child between six and twelve, use one-half of the recommended dose, and for a child under the age of six, use one-quarter of the recommended amount.

NUTRIENTS

SUPPLEMENT	SUGGESTED DOSAGE	COMMENTS
Important		
Acidophilus (Kyo-Dophilus from Wakunaga is a good source)	As directed on label.	Restores normal intestinal flora. Use a nondairy formula.
Beta-carotene	50,000 IU daily until you are healed.	Acts as an anti-infective.
Essential fatty acids (Ultimate Oil from Nature's Secret is a good source)	As directed on label.	Helps to protect the gastrointestinal tract.
Garlic (Kyolic)	2 capsules 3 times daily, with meals. A fresh clove of garlic can also be put in the shoes to be absorbed through the skin.	Has antiparasitic properties.
Kyolic-EPA from Wakunaga	As directed on label.	Restores proper fatty acid balance. Repairs tissues and aids in healing.
Liquid Kyolic with B_1 and B_{12}	As directed on label.	An excellent blood builder.
Multivitamin and mineral complex	As directed on label.	To promote overall health and proper nutrition. All nutrients are needed by persons with these disorders.
Parasitin+ from Växa International	As directed on label.	To cleanse and detoxify the body of parasites and worms.
Vitamin B complex plus extra vitamin B_{12}	50 mg of each major B vitamin 3 times daily, with meals (amounts of individual vitamins in a complex will vary). 1,000–2,000 mcg twice daily.	To prevent anemia associated with parasitic infestation. Use sublingual forms to assure absorption.
Vitamin C with bioflavonoids	3,000 mg daily.	Protects against infection and enhances immune function.
Zinc	50 mg daily. Do not exceed a total of 100 mg daily from all supplements.	Promotes a healthy immune system and proper wound healing.

HERBS

❑ Aloe vera juice, taken twice daily as directed on the product label, has an alkalinizing and anti-inflammatory effect.

❑ Black walnut extract destroys many types of worms. Take black walnut extract on an empty stomach three times per day.

❑ Butternut bark, fennel seed, flaxseed, licorice root, and senna leaf are good for bowel and colon cleansing.

Caution: If overused, licorice can elevate blood pressure. Do not use this herb on a daily basis for more than seven days in a row. Avoid if you have high blood pressure.

❑ Calendula ointment or witch hazel can be used to help relieve anal itching and irritation.

❑ Cascara sagrada, chamomile, chaparral, echinacea root, ficus, gentian root, mugwort, mullein oil, parsley, pau d'arco, rhubarb root, slippery elm, thyme, valerian, and wormwood are effective against many types of worms.

Caution: Do not use wormwood during pregnancy. It is not recommended for long-term use. It can be habit-forming.

❑ Cayenne (capsicum), garlic, and turmeric help to strengthen the immune system and destroy many types of worms.

❑ Grapefruit seed extract is very effective for destroying parasites. It can be taken internally and is also good for washing vegetables before eating (mix 10 drops of extract in 2 quarts of water) to remove any bacteria or parasites.

❑ Pinkroot works well against roundworms.

❑ Pumpkin extract contains zinc and aids in expelling worms.

RECOMMENDATIONS

❑ Eat a high-fiber diet consisting primarily of raw vegetables and whole grains.

❑ Eat pumpkin seeds, sesame seeds, and figs (or drink fig juice) on an empty stomach three times per day. This can be combined with the black walnut extract mentioned under Herbs, above.

❑ Drink only filtered or bottled steam-distilled water.

❏ Monitor your intake and output of fluids, and replace fluids as needed.

❏ Eliminate *all* sugar, refined carbohydrates, fruits (except figs and pineapples), and pork and pork products from the diet until the worms have been completely eradicated. Pork can harbor parasites. Worms thrive on sugar.

❏ For tapeworms, fast for three days on raw pineapple. (*See* FASTING in Part Three.) The bromelain in pineapple destroys tapeworms.

❏ Drink plenty of papaya juice.

❏ For pinworms, eat bitter melon, a cucumber-shaped vegetable found in Asian markets. This is effective against pinworms and is a good immune system strengthener. Eat one or two melons a day for seven to ten days. Do this again after two months to ensure that the infestation has not returned.

❏ *Never* eat meat, fish, or poultry that is not fully cooked or that has been left out at room temperature for too long. (*See* FOODBORNE/WATERBORNE DISEASE in Part Two.)

❏ Take a warm bath using ½ cup of Epsom salts per gallon of water. Before getting into the water, apply zinc oxide to the opening of the anus. Repeat for three days in a row.

❏ Have pet cats and dogs checked and, if appropriate, treated for parasites when you first get them, and in the spring and fall of each year thereafter.

❏ Always wear shoes in soiled areas.

❏ Maintain meticulous personal hygiene. Avoid scratching the anal area, and wash your hands frequently, preferably with antibacterial soap, scrubbing well under the fingernails. If children are affected, teach them proper hygiene as well.

❏ Wash all utensils and surfaces that come in contact with raw meat, pork, or fish with antibacterial soap.

❏ Wash underwear, bed linens, and towels after each use in very hot water with chlorine bleach added, if possible. Change linens and towels daily.

❏ For a severe infestation, use high colonics (also known as colonic irrigation). This procedure is usually performed in a professional office. If this treatment is not available, follow the procedure for colon cleansing described in this book. (*See* COLON CLEANSING and ENEMAS, both in Part Three.) A product called 10-Day Colon Cleanse from Aerobic Life Industries is also recommended.

CONSIDERATIONS

❏ Worm infestations can be persistent and stubborn. It may be necessary to treat all members of the household to finally eradicate the parasites. All family members should be examined for possible infection. In addition, it is a good idea to compile a list of people who have been in close contact with the affected individual and advise them to seek the evaluation and advice of a health care provider.

❏ The following are the routes through which different types of worms can enter the body:

• Ascarids: Through the soil; or in contaminated raw or undercooked food.

• Hookworms and threadworms: Through the feet or drinking water.

• Pinworms: Eggs can be transferred by touch from an infected individual that has eggs on the fingers from scratching the affected area.

• Tapeworms: In raw or undercooked beef, fish, or pork, or through inadvertently swallowing infested fleas or lice that live on pets.

❏ Doctors treat most types of worms with prescription medications such as mebendazole (Vermox) or thiabendazole (Mintezol), or with pyrantel pamoate (Antiminth), which is available over the counter. Creams or ointments may be prescribed to relieve anal itching and irritation.

❏ Some sushi has been found to be contaminated with a wormlike parasite called anisakis, which can cause illness similar to Crohn's disease if ingested. This parasite is a tightly coiled, clear worm, about one-half to three-quarters inch in length. It commonly embeds itself in herring and other fish. Fortunately, an experienced sushi chef can spot this parasite easily, so its presence in sushi is relatively rare.

❏ The risk of parasitic infection is increased by travel to places with inadequate public sanitation, personal hygiene levels, and/or food handling practices.

❏ Because of the generalized nutritional deficiency associated with this disorder, good nutrition is vital. Foods high in protein and iron are particularly important.

Wrinkles

Wrinkles form when the skin thins and loses its elasticity. As long as the skin is supple, any creasing of the skin disappears as soon as you stop making the expression that caused it. But skin that has lost its suppleness retains the lines formed by smiling or frowning, for instance, even after you have assumed a more neutral expression. Over time, these lines deepen into wrinkles.

Some amount of wrinkling is a result of aging and is probably inevitable; no matter what you do, you will develop some lines if you simply live long enough. The first signs of wrinkles usually appear in the delicate tissue around the eyes—smile lines or "crow's feet." The cheeks and lips show damage next. As we age, our skin becomes thinner and dryer, both of which contribute to the formation of wrinkles. But other factors help to determine the rate and the extent of wrinkling, including diet and nutrition, muscle tone, habitual facial expressions, stress, proper skin care (or lack thereof), exposure to environmental pollutants, and lifestyle habits such as smoking. Heredity probably also plays a role.

The most important factor of all is sun exposure, which not only dries out the skin but also leads to the generation of free radicals that can damage skin cells. The sun is your skin's worst enemy. It is estimated that 90 percent of what we think of as signs of age are actually signs of overexposure to sunlight. Furthermore, overexposure does not necessarily mean sunbathing or sunburn; approximately 70 percent of sun damage is incurred during such everyday activities as driving and walking to and from your car. The ultraviolet-A (UVA) rays that do this damage are present all day long and in all seasons. These rays erode the elastic tissues in the skin, causing wrinkling. Worse, the effects of the sun are cumulative, although they may not be obvious for many years.

NUTRIENTS

SUPPLEMENT	SUGGESTED DOSAGE	COMMENTS
Very Important		
Methylsulfonyl-methane (MSM)	As directed on label.	Has been shown to help prevent wrinkling of the skin.
Primrose oil or black currant seed oil	1,000 mg 3 times daily. As directed on label.	Good healers for dermatitis, acne, and most other skin disorders. These oils contain linoleic acid, which is needed by the skin.
Vitamin A	25,000 IU daily for 3 months, then reduce to 15,000 IU daily. If you are pregnant, do not exceed 10,000 IU daily.	Necessary for healing and construction of new skin tissue.
plus natural carotenoid complex (Betatene)	As directed on label.	Antioxidants and vitamin A precursors.
Vitamin B complex plus extra vitamin B$_{12}$	As directed on label. 1,000–2,000 mcg daily.	Anti-stress and anti-aging vitamins. Sublingual forms are best.
Important		
Kelp	1,000–1,500 mg daily.	Supplies balanced minerals needed for good skin tone.
Selenium	200 mcg daily. If you are pregnant, do not exceed 40 mcg daily.	An antioxidant that works are synergistically with vitamin E.
Silica	As directed on label.	Important for skin strength and elasticity. Stimulates collagen formation.
Topical vitamin C (Hyper-C Serum from Jason Natural Cosmetics)	As directed on label. Apply topically to the face after washing and before applying moisturizer for best absorption.	Studies have shown that applying vitamin C topically promotes collagen production, improving skin tone and can slightly reduce the appearance of fine wrinkles.
Vitamin C with bioflavonoids	3,000–5,000 mg daily, in divided doses.	Necessary for the formation of collagen, a protein that gives the skin its flexibility. Also fights free radicals and strengthens the capillaries that feed the skin.
Vitamin E	Start with 400 IU daily and increase slowly to 800 IU daily.	Protects against free radicals that can damage the skin and contribute to aging. Use d-alpha-tocopherol form.
Zinc plus copper	50 mg daily. Do not exceed a total of 100 mg daily from all supplements. 3 mg daily.	For tissue strength and repair. Use zinc gluconate lozenges or OptiZinc for best absorption. Needed for collagen production and healthy skin. Also needed to balance with zinc.
Helpful		
Ageless Beauty from Biotec Foods	As directed on label.	Protects the skin from free radical damage.
Calcium and magnesium	1,500 mg daily. 750 mg daily.	Deficiency contributes to fragility of the skin. Needed to balance with calcium.
Collagen cream	Apply topically as directed on label.	Good for very dry skin. A nourishing cream.
Elastin cream	Apply topically as directed on label.	Helps smooth existing wrinkles. Prevents formation of new ones.
Flaxseed oil capsules or liquid or Ultimate Oil from Nature's Secret	1,000 mg daily. 1 tsp daily. As directed on label.	To supply needed essential fatty acids.
GH3 cream from Gero Vita	Apply topically as directed on label.	Excellent for the prevention of wrinkles. Also good for any discoloration of the skin.
Glucosamine sulfate or N-Acetylglucosamine (N-A-G from Source Naturals)	As directed on label. As directed on label.	Important for the formation of healthy skin and connective tissue.
Grape seed extract	As directed on label.	An antioxidant that protects the skin from damage.
Herpanacine from Diamond-Herpanacine Associates	As directed on label.	Contains antioxidants, amino acids, and herbs that promote skin health.
Pycnogenol	As directed on label.	A free radical scavenger that also strengthens collagen.
Superoxide dismutase (SOD)	As directed on label.	A free radical destroyer. Also good for brown age spots.
Tretinoin (Retin-A)	As prescribed by physician.	Removes fine lines and smoothes out wrinkles; also excellent for age spots, precancerous lesions, and sun-damaged skin. Available by prescription only. Takes around 6 months to show results.
Vitamin D$_3$	400 IU daily.	Deficiency can contribute to aging of the skin.

HERBS

❑ Acerola hydrates the skin.

❑ Alfalfa, borage, burdock root, chamomile, horsetail, oat straw, red raspberry, and thyme are all good for general nourishment of the hair, skin, and nails.

❑ Aloe vera has soothing, healing, and moisturizing properties. Apply pure aloe vera gel to dry skin as directed on the product label.

❑ Comfrey is good for alleviating dry skin.

Caution: This herb is recommended for external use only. Do not take it internally.

❑ Witch hazel is very useful in skin care.

❑ Other herbs that are beneficial for skin tone include borage seed, cranberry, flaxseed, ginger root, lavender, lemongrass, parsley, and pumpkin seed.

RECOMMENDATIONS

❑ Eat a well-balanced diet that includes many and varied fruits and vegetables, preferably raw, to provide your skin with the nutrients it needs. Also eat whole grains, seeds, nuts, and legumes.

❑ Drink at least 2 quarts of water every day, even if you do not feel thirsty. This helps to keep the skin hydrated and to flush away toxins, discouraging the formation of wrinkles.

❑ Obtain fatty acids from cold-pressed vegetable oils. Avoid saturated and animal fats.

❑ Do not smoke, and avoid alcohol and caffeine. All of these substances dry out the skin, making it more vulnerable to wrinkling. In addition, the smoking habit means pursing one's lips hundreds of times each day. The creases that form when you inhale from a cigarette often develop into wrinkles at a comparatively early age.

❑ No matter what your age or skin type, protect yourself from the sun. Always apply a sunscreen with a sun protection factor (SPF) of at least 15 to all exposed areas of skin, especially your face, regardless of the season or the weather. Sun exposure is the single greatest source of skin damage.

❑ Get regular exercise. Like other organs of the body, skin gets its nourishment from the bloodstream. Exercise increases the circulation of blood to the skin.

❑ Exercise your face. Sit in a chair and extend your jaw in an exaggerated chewing motion. Stretch the muscles under your chin and the front of your neck. Lying on a slant board for fifteen minutes a day is also good.

❑ Avoid alcohol-based toning products. Use witch hazel or an herbal/floral water instead.

❑ Pay attention to your facial expressions. If you find yourself squinting, raising your eyebrows, or making some other potentially wrinkle-inducing expression over and over again, you can make a conscious effort to stop.

❑ Practice good skin care and keep your skin well lubricated, especially if it is dry. (See DRY SKIN in Part Two.)

❑ Avoid using harsh soaps or solid cleansing creams such as cold cream on your face. Use natural oils such as avocado oil instead to remove dirt and old makeup. Apply it gently to your face and rinse it off with warm water. E-Gem Skin Care Soap from Carlson Laboratories is also good. Use a facial sponge or loofah several times a week to remove dead, dry skin cells and stimulate circulation.

❑ After cleansing your skin, apply a moisturizing lotion, preferably while the skin is still damp. Vitamin A Moisturizing Gel from Derma-E Products is a good nongreasy moisturizer that is quickly absorbed and diminishes the appearance of fine lines. It is available in health food stores.

❑ Open a capsule of ACES + Zn from Carlson Labs and add the contents to your moisturizing cream before applying. This will help protect the skin from free radical damage. Do the same with your sunscreen.

❑ Do not apply heavy oils around the eye area before going to bed. This may cause eyes to be puffy in the morning.

❑ Limit your use of cosmetics, and choose the ones you do use carefully. Do not share your cosmetics, and replace them every three months.

CONSIDERATIONS

❑ Selecting good skin care products can be confusing. We recommend that you seek out products containing natural ingredients, and avoid those that contain petrolatum, mineral oil, or any hydrogenated oils. Some good ingredients to look for in skin care products include the following:

• *Allantoin,* a soothing agent derived from comfrey.

• *Alpha-hydroxy acids,* natural fruit acids that encourage the shedding of dead surface skin cells and the formation of fresh, new skin cells.

• *Aloe vera,* which is rich in nutrients and softens the skin.

• *Arnica,* an herb with astringent and skin-soothing properties.

• *Burdock,* an herb that helps the body eliminate poisons from the skin.

• *Calendula,* an herb that promotes skin cell formation and stimulates tissue growth, and also soothes and softens sensitive skin.

• *Chamomile,* an anti-inflammatory, antibacterial herb that is good for sensitive skin.

• *Collagen,* a protein found in healthy young skin tissue.

• *Comfrey,* an herb that aids healing and soothes chapped, irritated, or blemished skin.

• *Cucumber,* which contains amino and organic acids that cool and refresh the skin and tighten the pores.

• *Essential fatty acids* (including linoleic, linolenic, and arachidonic acids), which smooth rough skin, protect against moisture loss, and prevent invasion by free radicals.

• *Ginkgo biloba,* an antioxidant that helps skin stay younger looking.

• *Glycerine,* a soap byproduct that attracts and holds moisture in the skin.

• *Ivy,* an herb that stimulates circulation and aids other ingredients in penetrating the skin.

• *Liposomes,* microscopic bubbles that deliver active ingredients deep into the skin.

• *Panthenol (provitamin B$_5$)*, a nutrient that builds moisture and soothes irritation.

• *Retinoic acid*, a form of vitamin A that smoothes skin, promotes cell renewal, and improves circulation to the skin.

• *Sage*, an herb with astringent properties that can help relieve dry, itchy skin.

• *Witch hazel*, a natural astringent that tones the skin.

• *Yarrow*, an astringent herb that acts as an anti-inflammatory and tightens and firms saggy skin.

❏ There are many excellent home facial treatments that can help with specific skin problems. Some of the best include:

• *To add color to sallow skin*, mash $\frac{1}{2}$ cup or so of strawberries in a blender and apply them to your face. Leave them on for ten minutes, then rinse with tepid water.

• *To alleviate puffiness in the eye area*, place cool cucumber slices over your eyes for ten minutes or more, as needed.

• *To cleanse the pores*, rub mashed tomato over your face.

• *To help protect your skin from free radical damage*, add a few drops of green tea extract to your lotions, astringents, and other beauty products.

• *To moisturize your skin*, mash together grapes (a natural source of collagen and alpha-hydroxy acids) with enough honey to make a paste, and apply the mixture to your face as a mask. Leave it in place for twenty to thirty minutes while you relax, then rinse it off.

• *To remove dead surface skin cells and improve skin texture*, gently rub a small handful of dry short-grain rice against your face for a few minutes. This technique has been used by Japanese women for centuries.

• *To soften and nourish the skin*, mash half of an avocado and apply it to your face. Leave it on until it dries, then rinse off with warm water. Avocado contains essential fatty acids and other nutrients that help prevent premature wrinkling.

• *To tighten and refine pores*, whip up the white of an egg with a pinch of alum and apply it to your face as a mask. After fifteen to twenty minutes, rinse it off with lukewarm water.

❏ Wrinkle lines from the lips toward the nose may be due to a deficiency of vitamin B$_2$ (riboflavin).

❏ Researchers studying premature aging have found that vitamin E may help prevent wrinkling.

❏ Chemical peels, used by many dermatologists and skin care professionals, trigger collagen production deep underneath the skin by destroying the upper layer of skin cells. The new collagen produced helps to improve elasticity and give the skin a more youthful look. Chemical peels can irritate the skin, and they can also cause sun sensitivity. Alpha-hydroxy acids (AHAs) are acids derived from various fruits that act in much the same way, but they are natural, less irritating to the skin, and do not produce sun sensitivity. Glycolic acid (the best for exfoliation), tartaric acid, citric acid, and malic acid are all AHAs. While these are gentler than chemical peels, they still can irritate sensitive or fair skin.

❏ Ester-C Gel with E Skin Recovery Complex from Derma-E Products is a good product that combines esterified vitamin C, vitamin E, borage oil, green tea extract, and herbs that help repair dull, aging, sun-damaged skin.

❏ Dermatologists are constantly searching for ways to prevent or treat wrinkles. Doctors perform a wide range of treatments for wrinkles, including facial peels, cosmetic skin surgery, laser resurfacing, local BoTox (purified botulinum toxin) or collagen injections, and fat transfers, to name a few. All of these treatments can cause unpleasant side effects. If you are considering medical treatment for this condition, do plenty of research and discuss your options with a qualified dermatologist.

Xerophthalmia

See under EYE PROBLEMS.

Yeast Infection (Yeast Vaginitis)

See under CANDIDIASIS; FUNGAL INFECTION; VAGINITIS.

Part Three

Remedies
and Therapies

INTRODUCTION

In Part Two, various treatment programs were recommended for each of the health problems discussed. Part Three explains how to implement these remedies and therapies. It describes when each treatment can be beneficial, and, when appropriate, offers instructions for effective use. You can choose from among the more traditional remedies, such as fasting, juicing, and poultices, or from more alternative treatments, such as aromatherapy, Ayurvedic remedies, homeopathy, hyperbaric oxygen therapy, magnetic field therapy, and many others. These remedies can be used in conjunction with a healthy diet and supplementation program. After learning about the available treatments, you will be able to choose the options that are most suitable for you.

Acupressure

See under PAIN CONTROL.

Acupuncture

See under PAIN CONTROL.

Aromatherapy and Essential Oils

Aromatherapy is the use of pure essential oils to enhance physical and mental well-being. Essential oils are aromatic, highly concentrated distilled essences of plants. These oils can have many different applications in our lives. They can sometimes be used as a natural adjunct to, or substitute for, prescription or over-the-counter drugs. We can also use them simply to make ourselves feel better.

Aromatherapy uses the sense of smell to enrich our experience of the world. Smell plays a significant role in our daily perceptions and how we react physically, emotionally, and mentally to what is going on around us. Various scents help us orient ourselves to the season of the year, our location, and situations of danger. Essential oils not only affect the physical but also the mental and emotional aspects of our lives. The inhalation of certain essential oils has been associated with the release of brain chemicals that simulate various emotions. For example, lavender oil has the ability to evoke and increase the release of serotonin, thus producing a calming effect on the body. Some essential oils also have healing properties when applied topically to the skin.

When purchasing essential oils, make sure they are 100-percent pure botanical extracts, not chemical reproductions of different fragrances. Chemical reproductions are not effective in aromatherapy because they do not evoke the same biochemical response as natural, pure essential oils. Pure essential oils are extracted directly from various parts of different plants. The oils can be obtained by a variety of methods, including distillation, solvent extraction, carbon dioxide extraction, expression (pressing), and enfleurage (a process in which some type of odorless oil is used to extract essential oil from flower petals). The type and part of the plant being used determines which type of extraction process is appropriate.

The following are some helpful hints to keep in mind when shopping for essential oils:

- Buy in small quantities (the oxygen in partially filled bottles deteriorates the oil).
- Read the label carefully and make sure it says "pure essential oil."
- Be aware that the availability of different plants and the extraction methods used affect prices, so there can be great variations in the costs of different oils. This is normal.
- Certain plant oils, such as apple blossom and peach blossom, cannot be extracted. If you find oils with such scents, they are not true essential oils.

Using essential oils is really very simple. Basically, you dilute a small amount of essential oil in a base of some kind (either water or another oil, termed a carrier oil, depending on the intended use), and apply or inhale it. For inhalation therapy, there are special devices available, including diffusers, simmer pots, aromatherapy lamps, and light bulb rings. When using one of these devices, follow the manufacturer's instructions. Or you can inhale an essential oil directly from the bottle. For topical applications, you can use any of the following to dilute essential oils:

- Almond oil.
- Apricot oil.
- Grapeseed oil.
- Jojoba oil.
- Olive oil.
- Water.

The following are some suggested dilution ratios for topical applications:

- Baths. Add 8 drops essential oil to 1 cup water and add to the bath.
- Body lotion. Add 25 drops essential oil to 8 ounces of unscented lotion.
- Carpet freshener. Add 25 drops essential oil to 16 ounces of water.
- Cleaning. Add 25 drops essential oil to 2 gallons of water.
- Facial oil. Add 6 drops essential oil to 1 ounce of jojoba oil.
- Hair conditioner. Add 1 drop essential oil to 4 to 6 ounces of unscented conditioner.
- Hair rinse. Add 10 drops essential oil to 16 ounces water.
- Massage oil. Add 25 drops essential oil to 2 ounces almond, apricot, grape seed, jojoba, or olive oil.
- Perfume. Add 12 drops essential oil to $\frac{1}{2}$ ounce water or jojoba oil.
- Room deodorizer. Add 25 drops essential oil to 16 ounces water.

Common Essential Oils

There are many different essential oils available, each with its own special properties. The table below lists some of the more commonly used oils and their qualities. Use it to determine which essential oil or oils you might like to try.

Essential Oil	Uses
Bergamot	A balancing oil. Lifts melancholy and depression.
Cedarwood	An antiseptic, astringent, expectorant, and sedative. Normalizes sweat gland function. Good for bronchial problems and useful for controlling mold and mildew.
Chamomile	An analgesic, anti-inflammatory, and antispasmodic. Excellent for headaches (apply as a compress to head). Good in baths, hair rinse, and massage oil.
Cinnamon bark	Useful for scent enhancement in the home or office. Makes a good air freshener and is also antifungal.
Clary Sage	A very aromatic oil that is enjoyed by both men and women. An antidepressant, anxiety-reducer, anti-inflammatory, antispasmodic, and aphrodisiac. Helps to counteract insomnia. Good used in skin and hair care products. *Caution:* Should not be used in the first months of pregnancy.
Cypress	An astringent, antiseptic, antispasmodic, and deodorant. Constricts the blood vessels. Repels fleas. Reduces coughing and excessive perspiration.
Eucalyptus	An antiseptic, antiviral, chest rub, decongestant, disinfectant, and expectorant. Reduces fever. Used as an ointment for muscular aches and pains. Good for repelling insects, and for use on insect bites or stings. Has a normalizing, balancing effect.
Frankincense	An anti-inflammatory, antiseptic, sedative, and expectorant. Promotes cellular regeneration. Good for cleansing and purifying the home. Helpful for bronchitis.
Geranium	An antidepressant, antidiabetic, antiseptic, hormone balancer, and insect repellent. A normalizing and balancing, mildly sedating oil good for PMS, nervous tension, skin concerns, and neuralgia. Good as a bath additive.
Grapefruit	Reduces appetite; useful in treating obesity. Balances moods, relieves depression, cleanses the body of toxins, reduces water retention, and cleanses and detoxifies the skin. Useful in baths, skin care products, and colognes.
Hyssop	An antiseptic and tonic. Useful for cleansing and detoxifying. Stimulates the respiratory system. Good for bronchitis as it helps clear the lungs of congestion. *Caution:* Do not use if you have epilepsy or other seizure disorder.
Jasmine	An antidepressant, antiseptic, and sedative. Useful for anxiety, emotional imbalances, frigidity, and impotence. Benefits scalp and skin.
Juniper	An antiseptic, detoxifier, diuretic, and internal cleanser. Helps rid the body of toxins and parasites, reduces spasms, improves arthritis, and reduces cellulite. *Caution:* Do not use during pregnancy. Do not use if you have kidney problems.
Lavender	Useful as an antiseptic and for improving immune system function, calming and normalizing the body, fighting bacterial and fungal infection, easing depression, and reducing inflammation. Good for acne, burns, eczema, skin healing, sleep disorders, and stress.
Lemon	An antiseptic, astringent, and bacteriostat. Helps to increase the body's defense against infections. Good for varicose veins, stomach ulcers, anxiety, depression, and digestive disorders. Emulsifies and disperses grease and oil. Helpful in cleaning products and hair rinses and for wound cleansing.
Linden	A calming, sedating, and soothing tonic. Moisturizing for the skin.
Orange	Balances and uplifts emotions. Has antispasmodic and regenerative properties. Useful in skin care products. *Caution:* This oil increases sensitivity to the sun. Do not use it if you will be spending considerable time outdoors.

Patchouli	An earthy scent used in personal fragrances, baths, and hair care products. Good for dry skin. Has antidepressant, anti-inflammatory, antiseptic, aphrodisiac, and fungicidal properties.
Peppermint	Helpful for headaches, congestion, fatigue, fever, indigestion, muscle soreness, sinus problems, and stomach problems. An antiseptic, antispasmodic, mental stimulant, and regenerative. Good for use in baths and oral care products.
Pine	An antiseptic, antiviral, expectorant, restorative, and stimulant. Helps to clear the mind.
Rose	An antidepressant, antiseptic, and tonic astringent. Also a mild sedative. Good for female complaints, impotence, insomnia, and nervousness. Used in skin care products.
Rosemary	An analgesic, antiseptic, antispasmodic, astringent, and mental stimulant. Enhances circulation. Helpful for cellulite, dandruff, hair loss, memory problems, headache, and sore muscles. Used in hair care products as a conditioner and shine enhancer. *Caution:* If irritation occurs, discontinue use. Do not use directly on the skin without diluting. Use caution inhaling it if you have asthma or bronchitis. Do not use if you have epilepsy.
Rosewood	An antiseptic and regenerative. Calms and helps restore emotional balance. Good for anxiety, cellular regeneration, depression, headaches, nausea, PMS, and tension. Good in facial or massage oils.
Sandalwood	An antidepressant, antiseptic, expectorant, aphrodisiac, and skin moisturizer. Good for bronchitis and nervousness; it is soothing for both mind and body. Good in skin care blends.
Tea tree	A potent anti-infective, anti-inflammatory, antiseptic, antiviral, expectorant, fungicide, and parasiticide. Good for athlete's foot, bronchial congestion, dandruff, insect bites, ringworm, and yeast infections.
Thyme	An antiseptic, antispasmodic, and expectorant. Calming.
Vanilla	Mainly used as a fragrant scent for the bath and body. Used in skin care products.
Yarrow	An anti-inflammatory and antispasmodic. Improves digestion and lowers blood pressure. Similar in function to chamomile.
Ylang ylang	An antidepressant, antiseptic, aphrodisiac, and calming sedative. Lifts mood, eases anxiety, reduces stress, normalizes the heartbeat, and lowers blood pressure. Good for frigidity, high blood pressure, and impotence.

• Shampoo. Add 12 drops essential oil to 16 ounces unscented shampoo.

To help you determine which essential oil or oils may be suited to your particular needs, see Common Essential Oils on page 696.

When using essential oils, be aware that they are highly concentrated and very potent. Keep the following commonsense precautions in mind:

• Do not use oils full strength. Always dilute them first.

• Do not use oils near the eyes.

• Do not touch your face, mucous membranes, or genitals if your hands have been in direct contact with the oils.

• Keep essential oils out of the reach of children.

• Be cautious about using essential oils for children, especially young children. If you do use essential oils on a child, reduce the concentration of the essential oil by half or more.

• Be cautious using essential oils during pregnancy.

• Avoid sun exposure when using bergamot and other citrus oils.

Ascorbic Acid Flush

Because vitamin C (ascorbic acid) promotes the healing of wounds and protects the body from bacterial infection, allergens, and other pollutants, it is often beneficial to flush the body with ascorbic acid. This therapy can help treat chemical allergies and chemical poisoning, arsenic and radiation poisoning, influenza, and sprains, and it can help prevent other illnesses, including cancer and AIDS.

PROCEDURE FOR ADULTS

Place 1,000 milligrams of ascorbic acid in a cup of water or juice. To make this drink, use ascorbic acid in the form of either esterified vitamin C, such as Ester-C, or a buffered product, such as calcium ascorbate. Take every half hour, keeping track of how much has been taken, until diarrhea results. Count the number of teaspoons needed to produce diarrhea. Subtract 1 from this amount, and take the resulting ascorbic acid drink every four hours for one to two days. During therapy, make sure the stool retains a tapioca-like consistency. If it again becomes watery, decrease dosage as necessary. Repeat therapy once a month.

PROCEDURE FOR INFANTS AND CHILDREN

Place 250 milligrams of ascorbic acid in a cup of water or juice, using an esterified vitamin C product, such as Ester-C, or a buffered product, such as calcium ascorbate. Give to the child every hour until a stool of tapioca-like consistency is produced. If the child or infant does not produce this stool within 24 hours, increase dose to 500 milligrams every hour, and keep the child on this schedule for one or two days. *Do not exceed 500 milligrams per hour.* Children should be given treatment only under medical supervision.

NUTRIENTS

SUPPLEMENT	SUGGESTED DOSAGE	COMMENTS
Very Important		
Multivitamin and mineral complex	As directed on label.	To replace any lost vitamins and minerals during therapy.

Ayurvedic Remedies

Ayurvedic medicine is one of the oldest forms of medicine in the world. It incorporates tools such as diet, exercise, breathing exercises, meditation (yoga), mental visualization, therapeutic massage, and herbs to treat illness and maintain health. This ancient healing method also uses color therapy, sound therapy, and aromatherapy to help create balance within the body.

In Ayurveda, the fundamental healing philosophy is the concept of the three *doshas*, or basic types of energy or functional principles. These are vata (from ether and air), pitta (from fire and water), and kapha (from water and earth), and according to the principles of Ayurveda, they are present in everyone and everything. Vata is the energy of movement. Pitta is the energy of digestion or metabolism. Kapha is the energy of lubrication and structure. All three doshas are present in everyone, but one is usually predominant in any given individual. Ayurvedic medicine sees disease as a result of an excess or deficiency in vata, pitta, or kapha, and also the presence of toxins. Good health indicates a balance of these three energies in a body that is relatively toxin-free. Ayurvedic herbs are used to treat illness by restoring this balance. Herbs that deal with energy or movement are used to increase vata. Herbs that treat digestion, assimilation, absorption, and metabolism are pitta, and those involved with structure and the musculoskeletal system—the "glue" that holds the body together—are kapha.

Ayurvedic medicine regards the human body as a manifestation of cosmic energy that is transferred to all levels, both mental and physical. This can be difficult for people from Western cultures to grasp, but practitioners believe the two systems of energy are closer than we can conceive. At Ayurveda's core is the belief that we are a totality of body and soul within the universe, and if we can live in harmony with nature and our inner beings, we will stay healthy.

Biofeedback

See under PAIN CONTROL.

Blood Purification

Blood is composed of four components: plasma, the watery, colorless liquid in which the other components float; red blood cells; white blood cells; and platelets. Through these components, the blood performs several life-sustaining functions. The red blood cells transport oxygen to the cells. The platelets are needed for the blood-clotting process. The white blood cells destroy bacteria and other disease-producing organisms. In addition, blood transports nutrients to the cells and carries away wastes; transports hormones from the endocrine glands to other parts of the body; helps regulate the amounts of acids, bases, salts, and water in the cells; and helps regulate body temperature. If any of these functions is impaired, the consequences can have a direct bearing on your health.

There are several ways in which the functions carried out by the blood may be hampered. First, hundreds of chemicals—ranging from gases such as carbon monoxide to toxic metals such as lead to natural substances such as fat—can find their way into the blood and impair its function. These foreign substances enter the body through the air we breathe, the water we drink, the food we eat, and the surfaces with which we come in contact through our skin. Because these substances act on the blood in different ways, the adverse effects they produce may vary widely.

Second, the performance of the blood may be hampered by a lack of specific nutrients. A classic example is an iron deficiency that results in anemia. However, there are many nutrients that the blood requires on a daily basis if it is to perform normally.

Finally, genetics can play a role in creating blood disorders. Sickle cell anemia and hemophilia are two common examples of such disorders.

Blood purification techniques can act in two ways. Some help draw foreign substances out of the body, while others provide important nutrients to help restore the blood's normal structure and maximize its performance.

PROCEDURE

Blood purification is achieved through the use of a special

fast. Once you have decided to follow a blood purification program, it is vital to choose an appropriate time for the fast. Consider that fasting requires the conservation of energy. Therefore, avoid fasting on a week when, for instance, you are moving your office or participating in a sports event. Also keep in mind that the cold-weather months are not an ideal time for a fast, as some of the heat you need to withstand the cold is created during the digestive process. Most important is the need to be mentally prepared. If you are "psyched up" for the fast, it is the right time to fast.

Once you have chosen the time for the fast and have prepared yourself mentally, you can begin to prepare yourself physically. For one week prior to the fast, follow a raw vegetable diet, including lots of "green drinks." Chlorophyll, obtained from tablets or fresh juice, "pre-cleanses" the body, making the fast less of a shock to your system.

While on the fast, consume only steam-distilled water; juices; and dandelion, milk thistle, licorice root, yellow dock root, burdock root, or red clover tea or extract. Drink at least 8 to 10 cups of distilled water daily to aid in cleansing and to help carry toxins out of the body. The best juices for blood purification are lemon juice, beet juice and its tops, carrot juice, and the juices of all leafy greens. Leafy green juices are particularly important because they supply chlorophyll, an essential part of any blood purification therapy. Chlorophyll not only cleanses the blood of impurities, but also builds up the blood with important nutrients, promotes regularity, and inhibits cellular damage from radiation. This makes chlorophyll helpful in the treatment of many disorders. Wheatgrass, barley, and alfalfa juices are all rich in chlorophyll.

Stay on the fast for three days, or as directed by your health-care provider. Once you have completed the fast, avoid white flour and all sugars—substances that are highly refined and hard to digest. The stress placed on your body by such foods can "undo" all of the good accomplished by the fast. Ideally, these foods should be avoided all of the time. At the very least, eliminate them—as well as heated fats and oils—for at least one month after your fast.

NUTRIENTS

SUPPLEMENT	SUGGESTED DOSAGE	COMMENTS
Very Important		
Chlorophyll tablets or	As directed on label.	Cleanses and refurbishes red blood cells. Aids immune system function.
liquid chlorophyll (fresh wheatgrass juice is a good source)	As directed on label. Take with juice.	
Important		
Cell Guard from Biotec Foods	As directed on label.	A good antioxidant formula.
Helpful		
Kyo-Green from Wakunaga	As directed on label.	Good for the liver and the colon. Contains wheatgrass and barley grass.

| Ultimate Cleanse from Nature's Secret | As directed on label. | A 2-part system that helps stimulate and detoxify the organs, blood, and channels of elimination. |

HERBS

❏ Barberry, black radish, eyebright, lobelia, milk thistle, Oregon grape, pau d'arco, wild yam, and yellow dock cleanse and detoxify the liver and the endocrine system. You can use these herbs independently or in any combination.

Caution: Do not take lobelia internally on an ongoing basis. Do not use Oregon grape during pregnancy.

❏ Borage seed, chamomile, dandelion, ginkgo biloba, and sarsaparilla help to restore the acid/alkaline balance to the bloodstream. Ginkgo biloba is also a powerful antioxidant and improves circulation.

Caution: Do not use chamomile on an ongoing basis, as ragweed allergy may result. Avoid it completely if you are allergic to ragweed.

❏ Burdock, dandelion, hawthorn, licorice, pau d'arco, red clover, rhubarb, sage, shiitake mushroom, and Siberian and other ginsengs detoxify and cleanse the blood. These herbs can be used independently or in any combination.

Caution: Do not use licorice on a daily basis for more than seven days in a row, and avoid it completely if you have high blood pressure. Do not use sage if you have any kind of seizure disorder. Do not use Siberian ginseng if you have hypoglycemia or a heart disorder. Do not use any type of ginseng if you have high blood pressure.

❏ Echinacea cleanses the lymphatic glands.

Caution: Do not use this herb if you have any kind of autoimmune disease.

❏ Goldenseal cleanses the mucous membranes.

Caution: Do not take this herb internally on a daily basis for more than one week at a time, as it may disturb normal intestinal flora. Do not use it during pregnancy, and use it with caution if you are allergic to ragweed.

❏ Green tea is a powerful antioxidant. Drink two or three cups daily.

CONSIDERATIONS

❏ *See also* ENEMAS and FASTING in Part Three.

Chelation Therapy

Chelation (pronounced *key-LAY-shun*) therapy is a safe, nonsurgical treatment used to rid the body of excess toxins, particularly metals. Chelating agents used in this therapy are available in over-the-counter formulas that can be taken orally at home, and in intravenous solutions that must be administered under the supervision of a physician. These chelators draw out toxic metals and other harmful substances that impair body function, and help the body eliminate these toxins via the kidneys. Oral chelating agents can often prevent problems from occurring by restoring circulation to the body's tissues. If serious health problems already exist, intravenous therapy is usually necessary.

Chelation therapy is used to treat a variety of health problems. First, chelating agents are used to bind with heavy toxic metals such as cadmium, lead, and mercury—substances that enter the body through food, water, and other means—and excrete these metals from the body. As certain minerals accumulate in the body, they interact with other minerals, promoting the actions of some and inhibiting the actions of others. Lead, for instance, has been shown to inhibit the actions of calcium, iron, and potassium, all of which are important nutrients. When chelating agents are used to eliminate toxic metals such as lead from the body, essential nutrients are better able to do their job.

Chelation therapy is also used in the treatment of atherosclerosis and other circulatory disorders, as well as in the treatment of gangrene, which often is the result of poor circulation. In atherosclerosis, deposits of cholesterol, fats, and other substances collect on the walls of large and medium-sized arteries in the form of hard plaque. It has been found that calcium acts as the "glue" that holds the atherosclerotic plaque together. Chelating agents bind with this calcium and carry it out of the body, breaking up the plaque deposits, unclogging the arteries, and permitting more normal blood flow.

ORAL CHELATION THERAPY

Oral chelating agents offer a safe, convenient alternative for persons who are at risk for circulatory problems or problems caused by toxic metal accumulation. Among the many disorders that may be helped by chelation therapy are multiple sclerosis, Parkinson's disease, Alzheimer's disease, and arthritis. Despite reservations voiced by many in the medical establishment, many severely disabled, high-risk individuals have reported dramatic improvement in arterial circulation after chelation treatment.

Procedure

The following chelating agents can be used to prevent many degenerative illnesses and can often alleviate the symptoms of existing conditions. These agents can be purchased in the combinations shown below in health food stores and drugstores. Follow package directions regarding dosage.

- Alfalfa, fiber, rutin, and selenium.
- Calcium and magnesium chelate with potassium.
- Chromium, garlic, pectin, and potassium.
- Coenzyme A.
- Coenzyme Q_{10}.
- Copper chelate, iron, sea kelp, and zinc chelate.

In addition, the following supplements can act as oral chelating agents to rid the body of excess toxic metals and minerals. Mineral supplements can be used with intravenous chelation to replace lost minerals and to control free radical damage, which has been linked to heart disease.

NUTRIENTS

SUPPLEMENT	SUGGESTED DOSAGE	COMMENTS
Aangamik DMG from FoodScience of Vermont	200 mg daily.	Increases available oxygen and prevents cellular and tissue oxidation.
Alfalfa liquid or tablets	Double the amount directed on the label.	Detoxifies the liver and alkalizes the body. Chelates toxic substances from the body.
Apple pectin and rutin	As directed on label. As directed on label.	To bind with unwanted toxic metals and remove them from body through the intestinal tract.
Calcium plus magnesium	1,500 mg daily. 700–1,000 mg daily.	Replaces calcium lost by using chelating substances. Use calcium citrate form. Displaces calcium within the cells of the artery walls.
Coenzyme Q_{10}	60–90 mg daily.	Improves circulation, lowers blood pressure, and acts as a chelating agent.
Garlic (Kyolic from Wakunaga)	2 capsules twice daily, with meals.	A good chelating agent and detoxifier.
L-Cysteine and L-methionine	500 mg each twice daily, on an empty stomach. Take with water or juice. Do not take with milk. Take with 50 mg vitamin B_6 and 100 mg vitamin C for better absorption.	Two of the most important natural dietary chelators. Cysteine is effective for nickel toxicity.
L-Lysine plus glutathione	500 mg each daily.	Aids in detoxifying harmful toxins and metals. Powerful free radical scavengers and antioxidants that remove unwanted substances from the body. Caution: Do not take lysine longer than 6 months at a time.
Selenium	200 mcg daily. If you are pregnant, do not exceed 40 mcg daily.	A powerful free radical scavenger.
Vitamin A with mixed carotenoids including natural beta-carotene or carotenoid complex	25,000 IU daily. If you are pregnant, do not exceed 10,000 IU daily. As directed on label.	To aid in excreting toxic substances. Use emulsion forms for easier assimilation.
Vitamin B complex plus extra vitamin B_3 (niacin) and pantothenic acid (vitamin B_5) and vitamin B_{12} and folic acid	100 mg of each major B vitamin 3 times daily (amounts of individual vitamins in a complex will vary). 50 mg 3 times daily. 50 mg 3 times daily. 1,000 mcg 3 times daily. As directed on label.	B vitamins aid in protecting the body from harmful substances and are needed for all cellular functions. Caution: Do not take niacin if you have a liver disorder, gout, or high blood pressure.

Vitamin C with bioflavonoids	5,000–15,000 mg daily, in divided doses.	Powerful chelating agents and immunostimulants.
Vitamin E	Start with 600 IU daily and increase slowly to 1,000 IU daily.	Removes toxic substances and destroys free radicals. Use d-alpha-tocopherol form. Emulsion form is recommended for easier assimilation and greater safety at higher doses.

Recommendations

❑ Follow a diet designed to treat heart disease and/or high cholesterol. Avoid fried foods; dairy products; mayonnaise, oils, and other fats; red meat; processed and fast foods; salt; and gravies. Drink only steam-distilled water. Eat as many fiber-rich foods as possible. Oats, brown rice, and wheat bran are all good sources of fiber. See CARDIO-VASCULAR DISEASE and HIGH CHOLESTEROL in Part Two for more information.

❑ Add a high-protein drink to your diet, or take the essential amino acids in supplement form. A deficiency of any one essential amino acid will reduce the effectiveness of all the others.

❑ Increase your intake of manganese by eating Brazil nuts, pecans, barley, buckwheat, whole wheat, and dried split peas. Manganese is an important chelating agent when consumed in manganese-rich foods. It is a major factor in blocking calcium from entering the cells of the arterial lining.

❑ Incorporate onions into your daily meals. Onions produce a natural chelating effect in the body and tend to decrease the "clotting power" of blood.

❑ When using chelation therapy, make sure to replace any essential minerals that might be displaced by chelating agents. Alfalfa, iron, kelp, and zinc supplements are recommended. Use a natural source of iron, such as blackstrap molasses or Floradix Iron + Herbs from Salus Haus.

❑ If taking zinc supplements, eat sulfur-rich foods, like garlic, onions, and legumes. Zinc inhibits the action of sulfur.

INTRAVENOUS CHELATION THERAPY

Intravenous chelation therapy is often used to remove calcified, hardened plaque from the arterial walls, improving circulation. When used under the care of a physician, this procedure can be a safe alternative to vascular surgery. This therapy is also used to remove heavy metals, such as lead, from the body. Most serious illnesses require repeated injections of the chelating agents.

The most common chelating agent now used in intravenous therapy is ethylenediaminetetraacetic acid (EDTA). A strong substance, EDTA attracts lead, strontium, and many other metals, as well as calcium. Although there is controversy surrounding the use of this agent, it has not been found to be toxic when used correctly.

Prior to beginning a course of EDTA chelation therapy, you must undergo a thorough physical examination. This includes a series of laboratory tests, including evaluations of cholesterol, blood, kidney function, liver function, glucose, and electrolytes. In addition, an electrocardiogram and chest x-ray are routinely performed. Other studies often assess vitamin B_{12} and mineral status. Typically, kidney function studies are repeated several times during the course of chelation therapy. Blood studies may have to be repeated, too, depending on the initial laboratory results.

The course of chelation therapy varies from person to person, but a typical course includes two treatments per week, each of three hours' duration. In addition to EDTA, physicians frequently administer supplements—including vitamin C, magnesium, and trace minerals—with the intravenous infusion, depending on the individual's particular illness and the results of the laboratory studies.

Recommendations

❑ While undergoing EDTA chelation therapy, be sure to take supplemental vitamins and minerals, particularly zinc, chromium, and the B-complex vitamins. This is important, as chelation agents are known to bind with and remove certain vitamins and minerals from the body. During therapy, take these supplements as directed in NUTRITION, DIET, AND WELLNESS in Part One.

Considerations

❑ When supervised by a qualified physician, EDTA intravenous chelation therapy is safe and causes few side effects.

❑ A 1989 study, published in the *Journal of Advancement in Medicine*, used EDTA to treat 3,000 people with coronary artery disease and other vascular problems. Nearly 90 percent experienced significant improvement.

❑ Hair analysis is an excellent means of determining the concentration of minerals in the body. (*See* HAIR ANALYSIS in Part Three.)

❑ There are over 150 doctors in the United States who are certified by the American Board of Chelation Therapy as approved chelation therapists. For information on the approved physicians in your area, you can contact the American College for Advancement in Medicine (*see* HEALTH AND MEDICAL ORGANIZATIONS in the Appendix).

Chinese Medicine

Traditional Chinese medicine (TCM) is an ancient form of medicine. It is based mainly on the prevention of illness, although it has helped many people to find a cure for a wide variety of health problems.

Chinese medicine uses herbs, acupuncture, acupressure,

massage, and diet to promote health. It especially emphasizes changing lifestyle habits. The key to understanding Chinese medicine is to understand the idea of *balance*. The goal in using any of the tools of Chinese medicine is to supply the body with what it requires to retain balance. Once balance is attained, the person regains health.

For centuries the Chinese have taught how to achieve balance in life using the concept of yin and yang, which are present in human beings and in all of nature. Yang is characterized as heat and light; yin as shadow and cold. Dryness and summer are yang; wetness and winter are yin. Chinese philosophy also classifies energy as yang and blood as yin. A person with an excess of yang might be overweight, have an angry temperament, and high blood pressure. Such an individual would benefit from such foods as asparagus, bananas, cucumbers, soy products (tofu), and watermelon. A person with a quiet personality, who is listless or tires easily, may have an excess of cooling yin. Foods recommended for this type of person include beef, garlic, ginger, lamb, and pepper. Yin foods are cooling and have a cooling effect, whereas yang foods are warming. Neutral foods include black beans, cabbage, carrots, lemons, and rice and other whole grain foods. These foods provide balance. To maintain health, one must consume the proper balance of yin, yang, and neutral foods.

Like foods, medicinal herbs are seen in terms of yin and yang. Chinese herbs are very powerful and should be used under the advice of a healer trained in traditional Chinese medicine. Traditional Chinese remedies that have recently become more widely available in the United States include cordyceps and velvet antler. Cordyceps is a plant that is found only in certain isolated places in southwest China, more than 12,000 feet above sea level. Chinese researchers have found more than 200 species of wild cordyceps. Studies on this herb suggest that it can reduce the ill effects of radiation treatment, lower blood pressure, reduce symptoms of asthma and other respiratory problems, increase energy levels, improve memory, and improve male sexual ability. Velvet antler has been reported to increase energy, mental alertness, and sex drive; decrease blood pressure and cholesterol levels; and reduce PMS symptoms. Velvet antler may also be effective as an anti-inflammatory.

Chiropractic

See under PAIN CONTROL.

Colon Cleansing

Retained debris in the colon leads to the absorption of toxins, resulting in systemic intoxication (poisoning). Symptoms of this condition can include mental confusion, depression, irritability, fatigue, gastrointestinal irregularities, and even allergic reactions such as hives, sneezing, and coughing. Many nutritionists and researchers believe that this toxicity can eventually lead to more serious disorders. Colon cleansing can rid the colon of debris, and help prevent and treat a variety of health problems.

PROCEDURE

The best means of removing toxins and wastes from the body is a fast. This should be the first step in any colon cleansing program. (*See* BLOOD PURIFICATION and FASTING in Part Three.) In addition to following a fast, use a wheatgrass, fresh lemon juice, garlic, or coffee enema. (*See* ENEMAS in Part Three.) If bowel problems or related symptoms are chronic, repeat this program once monthly.

The following supplements aid in cleansing the colon.

NUTRIENTS

SUPPLEMENT	SUGGESTED DOSAGE	COMMENTS
Very Important		
Fiber (ground flaxseeds, oat bran, and psyllium seed husks are good sources)	1 capsule or 1 teaspoon 4 times daily. Take separately from other supplements and medications.	Essential for a clean colon. Not habit forming.
Important		
Acidophilus or Kyo-Dophilus from Wakunaga	As directed on label. Take on an empty stomach. As directed on label. Take on an empty stomach.	Restores the normal "friendly" bacteria in the colon. If you are allergic to dairy products, use a nondairy formula.
Aloe vera juice	$1/2$ cup 3 times daily.	Heals colon inflammation. Use a pure form.
Bio-Bifidus from American Biologics	As directed on label. For fast results, also use as an enema (do this only once).	Replaces the bowel flora.
Helpful		
Apple pectin	As directed on label.	Source of quality fiber. Helps to detoxify heavy metals.
Kyo-Green from Wakunaga or ProGreens from Nutricology or wheatgrass juice or capsules	As directed on label. As directed on label. As directed on label. As directed on label.	To assist in keeping the colon clear of toxic debris and aid in healing of an inflamed colon.
Sonne's #7 from Sonne Organic Foods	As directed on label.	An intestinal cleanser. Contains liquid bentonite, which absorbs and eliminates toxins.
Ultimate Cleanse from Nature's Secret	As directed on label.	An excellent detoxification program.
Vitamin C with bioflavonoids	6,000–10,000 mg daily, in divided doses. (*See* ASCORBIC ACID FLUSH in Part Three.)	Protects the body from pollutants. Use a buffered or esterified form.

HERBS

❏ Aloe vera, calendula, and peppermint help to restore the acid/alkaline balance of the colon and promote healing.

❏ Burdock, echinacea, horsetail, and licorice have detoxifying properties. Licorice also supports the organs.

Caution: If overused, licorice can elevate blood pressure. Do not use this herb on a daily basis for more than seven days in a row. Avoid it completely if you have high blood pressure.

❏ Barberry, butternut bark, cascara sagrada, flaxseed, red raspberry, rhubarb, and senna can be used to flush the colon and release waste.

Caution: Do not use barberry during pregnancy.

❏ Boneset, elecampane, fenugreek, lobelia, and yarrow loosen and flush mucus from the intestines.

Caution: Do not use lobelia on an ongoing basis.

❏ Burdock root, milk thistle, and red clover cleanse the blood and support the liver.

❏ Fennel restores the acid/alkaline balance of the colon, promotes healing, flushes the colon, and releases waste.

❏ Garlic eliminates certain parasites.

❏ Marshmallow restores the acid/alkaline balance of the colon, promotes healing, and loosens and flushes mucus from the intestines.

❏ Pau d'arco restores the acid/alkaline balance of the colon, promotes healing, and has detoxifying properties.

❏ Slippery elm soothes inflammation and cleanses excess waste from the colon. For quick relief, use slippery elm tea as an enema.

RECOMMENDATIONS

❏ Eat only raw foods for two weeks, and then maintain a diet of 50 percent raw foods, including plenty of raw vegetables and noncitrus fruits such as apples, bananas, berries, grapes, and pears.

❏ Drink at least eight 8-ounce glasses of water each day, even if you are not thirsty. Insufficient liquid intake promotes hard stools, which can stay in the colon for weeks or even months, causing symptoms such as headache, fatigue, and depression, and resulting in a toxic bloodstream.

❏ Avoid saturated fats, sugar, and highly processed foods. Avoid oils and fried foods until the colon returns to normal and the stools are normal. Use olive oil, canola oil, or essential fatty acids sparingly during this cleansing period. Dairy products should be avoided because they create excess mucus in the colon. This diet helps to maintain a clean colon.

❏ If you have a blood sugar problem, avoid sweet fruits.

❏ Upon arising and at bedtime, drink the juice of a fresh lemon squeezed into a cup of warm water to cleanse the bloodstream and detoxify and neutralize the system.

❏ Each morning, take a brisk walk and drink fresh carrot and apple juice, "green drinks," or fresh pineapple and papaya juice.

❏ Make a colon-cleansing drink by mixing 1 tablespoon of bentonite with 1 teaspoon of psyllium seed, 1/2 cup of apple juice, 1/2 cup of aloe vera juice, and 1/2 cup of steam-distilled water. Drink this mixture once daily until the colon is clean and not foul smelling.

❏ Use a fiber supplement such as psyllium seed on a daily basis. Mix the supplement with water or juice, and drink it immediately, as the mixture thickens quickly. Avoid fiber supplements in capsule and pill form.

Color Therapy (Chromotherapy)

The effects of color on our moods, health, and way of thinking have been studied by scientists for years. Even an individual's preference for one color over another may be related to the way that color makes the individual feel.

Color can be described as light—visible radiant energy—of certain wavelengths. Photoreceptors in the retina, called cones, translate this energy into colors. The retina contains three kinds of cones: one for blue, one for green, and one for red. We perceive other colors by combining these colors.

According to Dr. Alexander Schauss, director of the American Institute for Biosocial Research in Tacoma, Washington, when the energy of color enters our bodies, it stimulates the pituitary and pineal glands. This in turn affects the production of certain hormones, which in turn affect a variety of physiological processes. This explains why color has been found to have such a direct influence on our thoughts, moods, and behavior—an influence that many experts believe is distinctly separate from psychological and cultural factors. Remarkably, color seems to have an effect even on blind people, who are thought to sense color as a result of energy vibrations created within the body.

Clearly, the colors you choose for your clothes and for your home, office, car, and other surroundings can have a profound effect on you. Colors have been known to ease stress, to fill you with energy, and even to alleviate pain and other physical problems. This idea, it should be noted, is far from new. In fact, the "color your world" concept is part of the ancient Chinese design technique *feng shui.*

When selecting a color to effect a change in mood or to relieve discomfort, it is vital to choose the color suited to your particular objective. For instance, blue has a relaxing, peaceful, and calming effect. Blue lowers the blood pressure, the heart rate, and respiration. In one study, children prone to aggressive behavior became calmer when placed in a blue classroom. Blue has also been found to make people feel cooler in hot and humid environments. To help relieve the pain of ulcers, back problems, insomnia, pain, rheumatism, and inflammatory disorders, surround yourself with blue, and focus your mind on the body part you want to heal while looking at the color. One good place to do this is in the countryside, where the blue of the sky and the water can impart a feeling of calming "oneness" with the universe.

As another of nature's most abundant colors, green, like blue, has a soothing and relaxing effect on the body as well as on the mind. People who are depressed or anxious can benefit from green surroundings. Green also helps nervous disorders, exhaustion, heart problems, and cancer. When you are ill, try sitting on a hillside or by a green pasture, and focus on the body part you want to heal. Green may also be a good environmental color for the dieter.

Like blue and green, violet creates a peaceful environment. Violet also suppresses the appetite and is good for scalp and kidney problems and for migraine headaches.

The color red stimulates, excites, and warms the body. Red increases the heart rate, brain wave activity, and respiration. The color of passion and energy, red is also good for impotence and frigidity, as well as for anemia, bladder infections, and skin problems. Those who have poor coordination should avoid wearing the color red. In addition, people suffering from hypertension (high blood pressure) should avoid rooms with a red decor, as this can cause their blood pressure to rise. Conversely, red has a good effect on those with hypotension (low blood pressure).

Pink has a soothing effect on the body, relaxing the muscles. Because it has been found to have a tranquilizing effect on aggressive and violent people, pink is often used in prisons, hospitals, and juvenile and drug centers. Those suffering from anxiety or withdrawal symptoms can benefit from pink surroundings. Pink is also a good color for the bedroom, where it can help evoke feelings of romance.

Orange is the color of choice for stimulating the appetite and reducing fatigue. Use this color in place mats and tablecloths, for instance—to encourage a finicky eater or to pique the appetite of a person who is ill. This color should be avoided by those who are trying to lose weight. If you are feeling tired or run down, try wearing an orange garment to lift your energy level. General weakness, allergies, and constipation may also improve.

Yellow is the most memorable of all the colors. Whenever you want to remember something, jot it down on yellow paper. This color also raises the blood pressure and increases the pulse rate, but to a lesser degree than red does. As the color of sunshine, yellow has an energizing effect; it can help relieve depression. A chromotherapist may use this color to treat muscle cramps, hypoglycemia, overactive thyroid, and gallstones.

Black is a "power" color. Try wearing black clothes for a feeling of strength and self-confidence. Black also suppresses the appetite. If you want to lose weight, cover your dining table with a black tablecloth.

Crystal and Gemstone Therapy

Some people believe colorful crystals hold incredible powers. For example, Thomas Edison is said to have believed that his success was due in part to a pocketful of quartz crystals he always carried with him. He felt that the stones allowed him the opportunity to take notice of his inner self and his creativity. Gemstone therapists believe that gems possess a specific healing energy that can be transferred to the body.

Certain gemstones are used for healing specific organs by contact with the body's related energy centers, called *chakras*. Certain stones also direct energies towards emotional states. Quartz crystals are probably the most popular. Quartz can be a beautiful white, such as milk quartz, or colorless and shiny like rock crystal. The rock crystal's therapeutic properties are aimed at soothing resentment and envy. It is also used to calm weak kidneys, cardiac pain, and upset stomachs.

In some cases, the healing properties of gems are used to stimulate energy flow to certain areas of the body. Amber (yellow to brown) is believed to aid in kidney and bladder function. Agate (gray, blue, and beige) promotes self-confidence and energy. Amethyst (purple) is used to unlock blocked energy, bring calm in times of grief, and promote positive thinking. Diamonds (many colors) protect energy fields and cleanse the blood. Emerald (green) improves memory and intellect. Jade (green or white) attracts loyal friends, brings good fortune, composure, peacefulness, and wisdom. Onyx (black) improves devotion and concentration. Ruby (red) increases energy, improves circulation, and promotes intuitive thinking. Sapphire (blue) gives the wearer self-esteem, purity of mind, and contentment. Turquoise is used to protect against harmful energy. Black onyx aids in changing bad habits. These are only a few examples of the powers ascribed to gemstones.

All crystals and gemstones should be "cleansed" periodically in running water to wash away the negative energies they may have picked up, particularly if they have been used for healing.

DHEA Therapy

The most abundant hormone found in the bloodstream, dehydroepiandrosterone (DHEA) is produced by the adrenal glands, which sit atop the kidneys. Much like human growth hormone (HGH) and melatonin—two other hormones now known to have anti-aging properties—DHEA is produced abundantly during youth, with production peaking around age twenty-five. After this, though, production wanes. By the age of eighty, people are thought to have only 10 to 20 percent of the DHEA they had at twenty.

Research has shown that DHEA has many functions in the body pertaining to health and longevity. Among other things, it helps to generate the sex hormones estrogen and testosterone; increases the percentage of muscle mass; decreases the percentage of body fat; and stimulates bone deposition, thereby helping to prevent osteoporosis. As the production of DHEA declines with age, the structures and systems of the body appear to decline with it. This leaves the body vulnerable to various cancers, including cancer of the breast, prostate, and bladder, as well as to atherosclerosis, high blood pressure, Parkinson's disease, diabetes, nerve degeneration, and other age-related conditions.

Research suggests that DHEA replacement therapy can have a number of highly beneficial effects. In a 1986 study based on twelve years of research involving 242 middle-aged and elderly men, small doses of DHEA appeared to be linked with a 48-percent reduction in death from heart disease, and a 36-percent reduction in death from other causes. In a twenty-eight-day study, DHEA therapy enabled men to lose 31 percent of mean body fat without changing body weight. DHEA is thought to have caused this loss of fat by blocking an enzyme that is known to produce fat tissue and promote cancer cell growth. In another study, middle-aged and elderly men taking DHEA for one year experienced a markedly greater sense of well-being, including a better ability to cope with stress, increased mobility, decreased pain, and higher quality sleep. Research also indicates that DHEA supplements can help prevent cancer, arterial disease, multiple sclerosis, and Alzheimer's disease; treat lupus and osteoporosis; enhance the activity of the immune system; and improve memory. Laboratory studies in animals have indicated that DHEA can increase lifespan by as much as 50 percent.

DHEA comes both in nonprescription-strength pills and capsules, and in higher-dosage prescription-strength pills and capsules. Most of the DHEA that you can buy is made in laboratories from substances extracted from wild yams, the most common substance being *diosgenin.* Also available are extracts of the wild yams that have *not* been processed into DHEA, but which the body may convert into DHEA.

DHEA therapy should be undertaken with caution. Some physicians believe that high doses of DHEA suppress the body's natural ability to synthesize the hormone. Women should take no more than 10 milligrams daily. Animal studies have indicated that high doses can also lead to liver damage. For this reason, while undergoing DHEA replacement therapy, it is important to take supplements of the antioxidants vitamin C, vitamin E, and selenium to prevent oxidative damage to the liver. 7–Keto DHEA may be a better source of DHEA than ordinary DHEA. 7–Keto DHEA plays the same role as DHEA in the body, such as strengthening the immune system and enhancing memory, but, unlike ordinary DHEA, it is not converted into estrogens or testosterone.

Enemas

Over time, toxic wastes can accumulate in the colon and liver, and then circulate throughout the body via the bloodstream. A clean and healthy colon and liver, then, are essential for the health of all the organs and tissues of the body.

There are two types of enemas—the retention enema and the cleansing enema. Retention enemas, also known as suppositories or implants, are held in the body for about fifteen minutes. Their primary action is to help rid the liver of impurities. Cleansing enemas, which are retained for only a few minutes, are used to flush and cleanse the colon.

When using any enema, keep in mind that enemas should never be used if there is rectal bleeding. In such a case, contact a physician immediately.

If you experience tension or spasms in the bowel while using an enema, try using warmer water—99°F is a good temperature—to help relax the bowel. If the bowel is weak or flaccid, try using colder water—75°F to 80°F—to help strengthen it.

After using any enema, be sure to wash and sterilize the tip of the enema bag.

THE CATNIP TEA ENEMA

Catnip tea enemas are a good way to bring a high fever down quickly and keep it down. These also relieve constipation and congestion, which keep fever up. When body temperature goes above 102°F (103°F in children over two), take a cleansing catnip tea enema. Repeat the procedure every four to six hours, and continue taking the enemas twice daily as long as fever persists. Catnip tea enemas should *not* be used by children under two years of age.

Procedure

To make the solution for the catnip tea enema, place about 8 tablespoons of fresh or dried catnip leaves in a glass or enameled pot. (If you are using bagged catnip tea, use the amount recommended on the package to make 1 quart of tea.) In a separate pot, bring 1 quart of steam-distilled water to a boil. Remove the water from the heat and pour it over the herbs. Cover the pot and let the tea steep for five to ten minutes. Then strain out the catnip and allow the tea to cool to a comfortable, slightly warm temperature.

Place all of the solution in an enema bag. Do not use petroleum jelly to lubricate the tip of the enema bag. Instead, use vitamin E oil (buy it in oil form or pierce the end of a vitamin E capsule and squeeze the liquid onto the tip). The liquid will both ease insertion and have a healing effect on the anus and the lining of the colon, if these areas are inflamed. Aloe vera may also be used for this purpose.

The best position to assume when receiving the enema is

"head down and rear up." If you experience any pain during insertion, stop the flow of the enema bag and, remaining in the same position, take deep breaths until the pain subsides. Then resume the enema flow. If you expel the liquid before all of it has been inserted, simply begin the process over again. If pain persists, discontinue the enema procedure.

After the liquid has been inserted, roll onto your back, and finally roll over and lie on your left side. As you are doing this, massage your colon to help loosen any fecal matter. Start on your right side and gradually move your fingers up toward the bottom of your rib cage, then across your abdomen and down the left side. Hold the solution in your body for three or four minutes before expelling it.

THE COFFEE OR WHEATGRASS RETENTION ENEMA

This type of enema is not hard to retain, since it is only a cup of liquid. When used as a retention enema—an enema that is held in the body for a specified period of time—coffee does not go through the digestive system and does not affect the body as a coffee beverage does. Instead, the coffee solution stimulates both the liver and the gallbladder to release toxins, which are then flushed from the body.

A coffee retention enema is quite helpful during a serious illness, after hospitalization, and after exposure to toxic chemicals. This enema can also be used while fasting to relieve the headaches sometimes caused by a fast-induced release of toxins.

Some alternative clinics use fresh wheatgrass retention enemas for the treatment of cancer and other chronic illnesses. Use 1 ounce of fresh wheatgrass juice in one cup of warm water. Wheatgrass contains nearly all the nutrients and enzymes the body needs for healing. If you cannot obtain fresh wheatgrass, Sweet Wheat from Sweet Wheat, Inc., a freeze-dried product, is a good alternative. Try using coffee and wheatgrass enemas on alternating days.

Procedure

To make the coffee enema solution, place 2 quarts of steam-distilled water in a pan, and add 6 heaping tablespoons of ground coffee (do not use instant or decaffeinated). Boil the mixture for fifteen minutes, cool to a comfortable temperature, and strain. Use only 1 pint of the strained coffee at a time, and refrigerate the remainder in a closed jar.

Place 1 pint of the enema solution in an enema bag. Do not use petroleum jelly to lubricate the tip of the enema bag. Instead, use vitamin E oil (buy it in oil form or pierce the end of a vitamin E capsule and squeeze the liquid onto the tip). The liquid will both ease insertion and have a healing effect on the anus and the lining of the colon, if these areas are inflamed. Aloe vera gel may also be used for this purpose.

The best position to assume when receiving the enema is "head down and rear up." After the liquid has been in-

serted, roll onto your right side and hold the solution in your body for fifteen minutes before allowing the fluid to be expelled. Do not roll from side to side.

Do not be concerned if the liquid is not expelled after fifteen minutes. Simply stand up and move around as usual until you feel the urge to expel the liquid.

Recommendations

❑ Use steam-distilled water, not tap water. This is especially important for retention enemas—you do not want to absorb any chemicals from the tap water.

❑ To maximize the benefits of this or any other retention enema, use a cleansing enema first.

❑ Do not abuse coffee enemas by using them too often. Use them only once daily while following a program for a specific disorder, unless you are being treated for cancer. People with cancer may need up to three enemas a day. You may also use coffee and wheatgrass enemas occasionally as needed.

❑ Remember that excessive use of coffee enemas over six months or more may deplete the body's stores of iron, as well as other minerals and vitamins, causing anemia. Do not use coffee enemas for longer than four to six weeks at a time. If you develop anemia during treatment—or whenever you use this enema daily for a long period of time—be sure to take desiccated liver tablets as directed on the label.

❑ If you have cancer, AIDS, or another serious illness, or if you have a malabsorption problem, add 1 cc of B-complex vitamins or 2 cc of injectable liver extract, plus a dropperful of liquid kelp or sea water concentrate (found in health food stores) to the enema solution. If you are unable to locate injectable forms of these supplements, open 2 capsules of a B-complex supplement and add the contents to the enema solution, making sure it dissolves before use. You can open up a capsule of probiotics and add the contents to the solution. Used daily, these supplements replace any lost B vitamins, help rebuild the liver, and provide an extra boost of energy. You can also add burdock root and milk thistle extract to the enema. Use only alcohol-free liquid extract and 5 drops of each to the enema solution. This will help to cleanse the blood and the liver.

❑ To kill unwanted bacteria in the colon—or for any type of colon disorder, including diarrhea and constipation—add 5 drops of either Aerobic 07 from Aerobic Life Industries or Dioxychlor from American Biologics to the enema solution.

THE LEMON JUICE CLEANSING ENEMA

The lemon juice enema is an excellent means of cleansing the colon of fecal matter and other impurities and of detoxifying the system. This enema also balances the pH of the colon and is useful whenever cleansing of the colon is desired, as well as for colon disorders, such as constipation.

Procedure

To make the solution for the lemon enema, add the juice of 3 lemons to 2 quarts of lukewarm steam-distilled water. (Be sure to avoid using either very cold or very warm water.) If desired, add 2 droppersful of liquid kelp to boost the mineral content of the solution.

Place all of the solution in an enema bag. Do not use petroleum jelly to lubricate the tip of the enema bag. Instead, use vitamin E oil (buy it in oil form or pierce the end of a vitamin E capsule and squeeze the liquid onto the tip). The liquid will both ease insertion and have a healing effect on the anus and the lining of the colon, if these areas are inflamed. Aloe vera gel may also be used for this purpose.

The best position to assume when receiving the enema is "head down and rear up." After the liquid has been inserted, roll onto your back, and finally roll over and lie on your left side. As you are doing this, massage your colon to help loosen any fecal matter. Start on your right side and gradually move your fingers up toward the bottom of your rib cage, then across your abdomen and down the left side.

Note that 2 quarts is a lot of liquid. If you experience any pain during insertion, stop the flow of the enema bag and, remaining in the same position, take deep breaths until the pain subsides. Then resume the enema flow. If you expel the liquid before all of it has been inserted, simply begin the process over again. If pain persists, discontinue the enema procedure.

Hold the solution in your body for three or four minutes before allowing it to be expelled. After two or three such sessions, you will find it easier to insert and hold the liquid.

Recommendations

❏ If you have trouble with constipation, use the lemon juice enema once a week, and the coffee retention enema once a week. The bowels will shortly move on their own, the colon will be clean, and the stool will not be foul-smelling.

❏ If you suffer from colitis, use the lemon juice enema once a week. Any time pain from colitis is experienced, this enema will quickly relieve the discomfort.

❏ If you are allergic to lemons, prepare the enema solution with 1 to 2 ounces of wheatgrass juice or 1 ounce of liquid aged garlic extract (Kyolic) in 2 quarts of steam-distilled water. Or fill the enema bag with plain steam-distilled water.

THE PROFLORA WHEY ENEMA

This remedy may be beneficial if you have used high colonics or taken antibiotics over a long period of time—practices that can kill the body's "friendly" bacteria. The whey enema helps the body fight yeast infections and improves digestion and the assimilation of nutrients.

Procedure

To make the enema solution, mix 2 quarts of lukewarm steam-distilled water and 5 tablespoons of ProFlora whey. Pour the mixture into the enema bag. Release any air from the enema tube before insertion, and lubricate the tip with vitamin E oil (buy it in oil form or pierce the end of a vitamin E capsule and squeeze the liquid onto the tip). Do not use petroleum jelly to lubricate the tip of the bag.

For best results, use a plain water enema before using the ProFlora whey enema, as this makes it easier to retain the solution for the necessary period of time. Do not use this type of enema on a daily basis. Limit it to three times a year.

To replace the friendly bacteria in the colon, do a probiotic retention enema after the ProFlora whey enema. Open up 8 capsules of Kyo-Dophilus from Wakunaga and add the contents to 1 cup of lukewarm (body-temperature) water. The best position to assume when receiving the enema is "head down and rear up." This implant will normalize the pH of the colon and restore healthy bacteria so that constipation will be eliminated. After the liquid has been inserted, roll onto your right side and hold the solution in your body for fifteen minutes before allowing the fluid to be expelled. Do not roll from side to side.

Do not be concerned if the liquid is not expelled after fifteen minutes. Simply stand up and move around as usual until you feel the urge to expel the liquid. Do not use this type of enema on a daily basis. Limit it to three times a year.

Exercise

The closest thing to a "magic bullet" for maintaining youth and optimal health is a well-balanced combination of exercise and proper nutrition. The entire body benefits from this formula, both physically and psychologically.

Regular exercise improves digestion and elimination, increases endurance and energy levels, promotes lean body mass while burning fat, and lowers overall blood cholesterol while increasing the proportion of "good" cholesterol (HDL) to "bad" cholesterol (LDL). Exercise also reduces stress and anxiety, which are contributing factors to many illnesses and conditions. In addition to the physical benefits, studies have shown that regular exercise elevates mood, increases feelings of well-being, and reduces anxiety and depression.

The power of exercise in maintaining health was underscored by the continuing Aerobics Center Longitudinal Study, which was designed to examine the effects of different fitness levels. According to its 1996 report, published in the *Journal of the American Medical Association*, low fitness may pose as great a risk to health as smoking, and a greater risk than high cholesterol, high blood pressure, or obesity. It was reported that smokers who are moderately physically fit, but have high blood pressure and high cholesterol, live longer than nonsmokers who are healthy but sedentary. Moderate fitness, it was stated, can be achieved in ten weeks through many different forms of exercise, including daily sessions of walking, bicycling, or even gardening.

Exercise includes a variety of movements and different activities. *Recreational* exercise is meant for enjoyment and relaxation, while *therapeutic* exercise is intended to alleviate or prevent a particular problem. Sometimes an exercise can be both recreational and therapeutic. Take swimming, for example. With careful attention to arm and shoulder movements, swimming can meet both the recreational and therapeutic needs of someone who has arthritis of the shoulder.

There are a number of exercise types, each of which has a specific purpose:

• *Aerobic or endurance exercise* improves the body's capacity to use fuel and oxygen. Swimming, bicycle riding, jogging, and power walking are examples of this type of exercise. The body's cardiovascular system benefits through increased blood supply to the muscles and enhanced oxygen delivery throughout the body. Just twenty minutes a day of sustained aerobic activity can lower blood pressure and strengthen heart function.

• *Range-of-motion exercise* helps maintain a joint's complete movement by putting a body part through its maximum available range of motion. Extending and moving one's arms in wide circular motions is an example of this. Some degree of flexibility is required to perform range-of-motion exercises, so stretching is recommended beforehand.

• *Strengthening exercise* helps a muscle's ability to contract and do work. Doing sit-ups, for example, is a way of strengthening abdominal muscles.

One exercise rarely achieves two goals. For instance, a strengthening exercise will not significantly affect endurance, and range-of-motion exercises will not necessarily improve strength. A total exercise program must consider the individual's goals and include activities designed to achieve those goals. (*See* PAIN CONTROL in Part Three for other types of exercises that can be used for relaxation, meditation, and healing.)

Exercise should not be looked at as a chore. Try to select activities that you enjoy and look forward to doing. Whatever you choose, start out slowly, listen to your body, and gradually increase the intensity and duration of your workout.

A word of caution: If you are over thirty-five and/or have been sedentary for some time, consult with your health care provider before beginning any new exercise program.

Fasting

Over time, toxins build up in the body as the result of the pollutants in the air we breathe, the chemicals in the food and water we consume, and other means. Periodically, the body seeks to rid itself of these toxins and releases them from the tissues. The toxins then enter the bloodstream, causing the body to experience a "low" or "down" cycle. During such a cycle, you may suffer from headaches, diarrhea, or depression. Fasting is an effective and safe method of helping the body detoxify itself and move through this low cycle with greater speed and fewer symptoms. In fact, fasting is recommended for any illness, as it gives the body the rest it needs to recover. Acute illnesses, colon disorders, allergies, and respiratory diseases are most responsive to fasting, while chronic degenerative diseases are the least responsive. By relieving the body of the work of digesting foods, fasting permits the system to rid itself of toxins while facilitating healing.

But fasting is helpful not just in times of poor health or during the body's low cycles. By fasting regularly, you give all of your organs a rest, and thus help reverse the aging process and live a longer and healthier life. During a fast, the following happens:

• The natural process of toxin excretion continues, while the influx of new toxins is reduced. This results in a reduction of total body toxicity.

• The energy usually used for digestion is redirected to immune function, cell growth, and eliminatory processes.

• The immune system's workload is greatly reduced, and the digestive tract is spared any inflammation due to allergic reactions to food.

• Due to a lowering of serum fats that thins the blood, tissue oxygenation is increased and white blood cells are moved more efficiently.

• Fat-stored chemicals, such as pesticides and drugs, are released.

• Physical awareness and sensitivity to diet and surroundings are increased.

Due to these effects of fasting, a fast can help you heal with greater speed; cleanse your liver, kidneys, and colon; purify your blood; help you lose excess weight and water; flush out toxins; clear the eyes and tongue; and cleanse the breath. It is recommended that you fast at least three days a month, and follow a ten-day fast at least twice a year.

Depending on the length of the fast, it accomplishes different things. A three-day fast helps the body rid itself of toxins and cleanses the blood. A five-day fast begins the process of healing and rebuilding the immune system. A ten-day fast can take care of many problems before they arise and help to fight off illness, including the degenerative diseases that have become so common in our chemically polluted environment.

Certain precautions should be taken during fasts. First, *do not* fast on water alone. An all-water fast releases toxins too quickly, causing headaches and worse. Instead, follow the live-juice diet detailed below, as this both removes toxins and promotes healing by supplying the body with vitamins, minerals, and enzymes. Such a fast is also more likely to lead to a continued healthy diet once the fast is over, as it will accustom you to the taste of raw vegetables and the vitality that this diet promotes. Second, whenever you fast for more than three days, do so only under the supervision of a qualified health care professional. If you have diabetes, hypoglycemia, or another chronic health problem, even short fasts should be supervised by a doctor. Pregnant and lactating women should *never* fast.

A final word of advice: It took years to wear your body down, and it will take time to build it back up to its peak condition. But believe that it can be done. Then, whenever you start to feel unwell, fast and feel better.

PROCEDURE

To prepare for the fast, eat only raw vegetables and fruits for two days. This will make the fast less of a shock to the system.

While on the fast, consume at least eight 8-ounce glasses of steam-distilled water a day, plus pure juices and up to 2 cups of herbal tea a day. Dilute all juices with the water, adding about 1 part water to 3 parts juice. Do not drink orange or tomato juice, and avoid all juices made with sweeteners or other additives.

The best juice to use during your fast is fresh lemon juice. Add the juice of one lemon to a cup of warm water. Fresh apple, beet, cabbage, carrot, celery, and grape juices are also good, as are "green drinks," which are made from green leafy vegetables. These green drinks are excellent detoxifiers. Raw cabbage juice is particularly good for ulcers, cancer, and all colon problems. Just be sure to drink the cabbage juice as soon as it is prepared. As this juice sits, it loses its vitamin content.

As a general rule, you should not combine fruit and vegetable juices. Apples are the only fruit that should be added to vegetable juices.

Follow the juice-water-and-tea fast with a two-day diet of raw fruits and vegetables. The desired effects of the fast can be ruined by eating cooked foods immediately afterward. Because both the size of the stomach and the amount of secreted digestive juices may decrease during fasting, the first meals after a fast should be frequent and small.

HERBS

❏ Herbal teas may be consumed throughout the fast, once or twice per day or more if you wish. Try the following teas:

• Use alfalfa, burdock, chamomile, dandelion, milk thistle, red clover, and rose hips tea to rejuvenate the liver and cleanse the bloodstream.

Caution: Do not use chamomile on an ongoing basis, as ragweed allergy may result. Avoid it completely if you are allergic to ragweed.

• Drink 2 parts echinacea and pau d'arco tea mixed with 1 part unsweetened cranberry juice. Used four times a day,

this will rebuild the immune system, aid in bladder function, and rid the colon of unwanted bacteria.

Note: Do not use echinacea herb if you have any kind of autoimmune disorder.

• Use peppermint tea for its calming and strengthening effect on the nerves, and for indigestion, nausea, and flatulence.

• Use slippery elm tea for inflammation of the colon. This tea also is beneficial when used as an enema solution.

❏ Take 2 capsules of garlic twice a day. If you prefer a liquid supplement, add 1 tablespoon of liquid aged garlic extract (Kyolic) to a cup of water. Garlic supplements may be taken on a daily basis before, during, and after a fast to promote overall health, aid in the healing process, and rid the colon of many types of parasites.

RECOMMENDATIONS

❏ If you must have something to eat during the fast, eat a piece of watermelon. Always eat watermelon by itself, with no additional foods. You can also try applesauce—fresh, not canned—made in a blender or food processor. Leave the skin on the apples, and do not cook them.

❏ Take a fiber supplement on a daily basis before and after your fast, but not during the fast. To promote cleansing of the colon before and after your fast, be sure to make extra fiber a part of your daily diet. Bran, especially oat bran, is an excellent source of fiber. Try to avoid supplements containing wheat bran, as they may be irritating to the colon wall. Another good fiber source is Aerobic Bulk Cleanse (ABC) from Aerobic Life Industries. To use this colon cleanser, mix it with half aloe vera juice and half natural cranberry juice. This mixture adds fiber and has a healing and cleansing effect also. Psyllium seed husks and ground flaxseed are other good-quality fiber products. Be certain to accompany any fiber capsule with a large glass of water, because the capsules expand and soak up a good deal of water.

❏ Do not chew gum while on the fast. The digestive process starts when chewing prompts the body to secrete enzymes into the gastrointestinal tract. If there is no food in the stomach for the enzymes to digest, trouble occurs.

❏ If desired, take spirulina during the fast. Spirulina is high in protein and contains a wide range of vitamins and minerals, plus chlorophyll for cleansing. If you are using tablets, take 5 tablets three times daily. If you are using powder, take 1 teaspoon three times daily, mixing the powder with a cup of unsweetened juice.

❏ If you have hypoglycemia, never fast without also using a protein supplement. Spirulina, described above, is a good choice. Make sure the spirulina is of good quality, has been laboratory tested, and has been cleaned before processing. Kyo-Green from Wakunaga is also valuable. Before starting any fast, consult a qualified health care professional.

❑ If you are over sixty-five, or if you need daily supplements for another reason, continue taking your vitamin and mineral supplements during the fast. Older people need certain vitamins and minerals daily. When you are drinking fresh juices, reduce the dosage of supplements that you take.

❑ If desired, before, during, and after your fast, use Kyo-Green from Wakunaga of America and ProGreens from Nutricology. These products contain all the nutrients needed to aid in the healing process. If used during the fast, these products should replace a cup of "green drink."

❑ During a fast, as toxins are released from your body, you may experience fatigue; body odor; dry, scaly skin; skin eruptions; headaches; dizziness; irritability; anxiety; confusion; nausea; coughing; diarrhea; dark urine; dark, foul-smelling stools; body aches; insomnia; sinus and bronchial mucus discharge; and/or visual or hearing problems. These symptoms are not serious and will quickly pass. To alleviate any of these symptoms, use a daily lemon juice enema to cleanse the colon, and a daily coffee enema to rid the liver of impurities. (See ENEMAS in Part Three.)

❑ During your fast, be sure to get adequate rest. If necessary, try napping during the day to recharge your batteries.

❑ If desired, before, during, and after your fast, use Desert Delight from Aerobic Life Industries. This product, which contains cranapple, papaya, and aloe vera juice, helps keep the colon clean, and also supports kidney and bladder function, aids digestion, and has a healing effect on ulcers. If used during the fast, substitute this product for a cup of juice.

❑ To make an excellent juice for healing many illnesses, juice together 3 carrots, 3 kale leaves, 2 stalks celery, 2 beets, 1 turnip, ¼ pound spinach, ½ head of cabbage, ¼ bunch of parsley, ¼ of an onion, and ½ clove of garlic. If you don't have a juicer, place the vegetables in pure water and gently boil them, adding no seasonings. A cup of this juice may be substituted for any other juice while fasting. Save the vegetables from the broth to eat after your fast. Remember that no solid food is allowed during the fast.

❑ During a fast, as toxins are released from your body, you will probably experience a coated tongue and an unpleasant taste in your mouth. To relieve this problem, try rinsing your mouth with fresh lemon juice.

❑ If desired, before, during, and after your fast, use Daily Detox Tea from Houston International to help the bloodstream and organs eliminate toxins. If used during the fast, this product should replace a cup of herbal tea.

❑ If you are a denture wearer, keep your dentures in your mouth throughout the fast to prevent shrinkage of the gums.

❑ While fasting, continue your normal daily routine, including moderate exercise. Avoid any strenuous exercise.

❑ Be aware that when you fast during a low phase, you help your body experience the "up" phase of the cycle—a period during which you feel great. This occurs because the body has been cleansed of impurities. However, when you start to pollute your body again, the toxins once again begin to build up, and, in time, you will again have a low phase. When this occurs, the fast should be repeated.

❑ Before, during, and after your fast, use dry-brush massages to help rid the skin of toxins and dead cells. Perform the massage with a *natural* bristle brush that has a long handle, so that you can reach your back. Always brush toward the heart—from wrist to elbow, elbow to shoulder, ankles to knees, knees to hips, and so on. This massage will flake away large amounts of dead skin, freeing the pores of impediments, and, in turn, helping the skin to excrete poisons. It will also greatly improve circulation. *Do not* use this technique on areas of the body affected by acne, eczema, or psoriasis. Also avoid brushing areas that are broken or recently scarred, or that have protruding varicose veins.

Glandular Therapy

The glandular system is both important and complex. Virtually all body functions—from digestion to reproduction to growth—depend on a healthy glandular system.

To a large degree, the health of the glands, like the health of any organ of the body, can be greatly improved by adequate vitamin and mineral supplementation. Glandular therapy, the use of concentrated forms of various raw animal glands, can also improve the health of specific glands.

Early endocrinologists hypothesized that glandulars worked by providing nutrients the body lacked. Once supplied with the missing nutrients, the malfunctioning organ was able to repair itself and function properly.

In the 1930s, Dr. Royal Lee, a pioneering biochemical researcher, began his own work with glandulars, and developed a different explanation for the substances' effectiveness—an explanation that has been supported by more recent research. Dr. Lee hypothesized that the organs were malfunctioning not because of missing nutrients, but because the body was attacking its own organs. This attack—which may be compared to the immune system's attack of a transplanted organ, although it is milder in nature—impairs organ function, causing chronic health problems. According to Dr. Lee, glandulars neutralize such attacks, allowing the organs to heal themselves.

Some of the most important glandulars are the following:

- Raw adrenal gland.
- Raw brain.
- Raw heart.
- Raw kidney.
- Raw liver.

Maintaining a Healthy Glandular System

A gland is an organ that manufactures and releases fluids and other substances into the body for the body's use. The function of these fluids is so wide-ranging that virtually all body processes depend on a healthy glandular system. An imbalance or malfunction of any one glandular substance or gland can create tremendous problems throughout the body.

Glands fall into two categories: the exocrine glands and the endocrine glands. The exocrine glands, each of which secretes a specialized substance, open onto a surface of an organ or other structure through a duct. Examples of such glands are the salivary glands of the mouth, and the sweat and oil glands of the skin. Other exocrine glands can be found in the kidneys, the mammary glands, and the digestive tract. These glands perform a variety of functions. The salivary glands, for instance, secrete saliva, which aids in the digestion of food, while the sweat glands help rid the body of waste products.

Unlike the exocrine glands, the endocrine glands are ductless, and thus secrete the substances they produce—specifically, hormones—directly into the bloodstream. Examples of these glands include the adrenal glands, found atop the kidneys; the gonads, found in the reproductive organs; the pancreas, found behind the stomach; the pituitary gland, found at the base of the brain; the thyroid and parathyroid glands, found in the neck; and the thymus gland, found below the thyroid. The pineal gland, which is attached to the brain, is also thought to be an endocrine gland.

By secreting hormones—chemicals that start or control the activity of an organ or group of cells—the endocrine glands help regulate practically all body functions. For instance, the pancreas secretes insulin, an important regulator of sugar metabolism. The female gonads, called the ovaries, produce hormones like estrogen, which aids the development of secondary sex characteristics, prepares the walls of the uterus to receive a fertilized egg, and performs many other important functions. The thymus secretes thymosin, a hormone that is critical to proper immune system function. The pituitary gland, which is often called the "master gland," regulates the functions of the other glands, and also produces a hormone that stimulates body growth. It should be noted that the pituitary gland, like many of the other endocrine glands, produces more than one hormone. Similarly, some hormones, such as estrogen, are secreted by more than one gland.

Like all organs, the glands need nutritional support, especially when stress depletes the body's stores of nutrients. Glandulars—concentrated forms of various organic animal glands—are one means of improving the health of the glands. In addition, nutritional supplements can help maintain the health of these glands, and thereby ensure proper functioning of the glandular system.

NUTRIENTS

SUPPLEMENT	SUGGESTED DOSAGE	COMMENTS
Very Important		
Kelp	Up to 200 mg daily.	Rich in minerals and the element iodine, which are necessary for thyroid function.
L-Arginine plus	500 mg daily.	Increases the size and activity of the thymus gland.
L-lysine	500 mg daily.	Add this supplement if you are prone to herpes outbreaks.
L-Glycine	500 mg daily.	Essential for the health of the thymus gland, spleen, and bone marrow.
L-Tyrosine	500 mg daily.	Important to the health and function of the adrenal, thyroid, and pituitary glands.
Manganese	As directed on label. Take separately from calcium.	Crucial to the production of thyroxine, the hormone that regulates the metabolic process. This nutrient is stored and used by the liver, kidneys, pancreas, lungs, prostate gland, and brain.
Vitamin A plus natural beta-carotene and other carotenoids	As directed on label. As directed on label.	Nutrients that nourish the thymus gland and increase antibody production. All organs with duct systems require these nutrients.
Vitamin B complex plus extra vitamin B$_2$ (riboflavin) and pantothenic acid (vitamin B$_5$)	100 mg of each major B vitamin twice daily (amounts of individual vitamins in a complex will vary). 50 mg 3 times daily. 50 mg 3 times daily.	B vitamins work best when all are taken together. Especially important if you are under stress. Vital to the health of the entire glandular system, especially the adrenal glands. The anti-stress vitamin.
Vitamin C with bioflavonoids	1,500 mg daily.	Important for adrenal function, and should be taken when using L-cysteine to prevent formation of cystine kidney stones.
Zinc plus copper	50 mg daily. Do not exceed 100 mg daily from all supplements. 3 mg daily.	Needed by the immune system, and for thymus and pancreas health. Especially important for the sex glands (gonads). Needed to balance with zinc.
Important		
Lecithin granules or capsules	1 tsp 3 times daily, before meals. 1,200 3 times daily, before meals.	All cells and organs have lecithin surrounding them for protection. Also helps cleanse the liver.
Raw thymus glandular plus multiglandular complex	As directed on label. As directed on label.	To stimulate immune function and aid glandular function. A sublingual form is best.

Helpful		
Essential fatty acids (flaxseed oil, primrose oil, and salmon oil are good sources)	As directed on label.	Needed to nourish the glands.
L-Cysteine and L-methionine plus glutathione	500 mg each daily, on an empty stomach. Take with water or juice. Do not take with milk. Take with 50 mg vitamin B$_6$ and 100 mg vitamin C for better absorption.	Aid in detoxifying glands of harmful pollutants. Also necessary for insulin production, and act as powerful antioxidants.
Selenium	As directed on label. If you are pregnant, do not exceed 40 mcg daily.	Nourishes the liver and pancreas.
Silica or horsetail or oat straw	500 mg twice daily.	To supply silicon, a trace mineral that aids in healing the glands and tissues. *See under* Herbs, below. *See under* Herbs, below.
Superoxide dismutase (SOD) or Cell Guard from Biotec Foods	As directed on label, on an empty stomach. Take with a large glass of water. As directed on label.	A potent detoxifier that also transports oxygen for healing in the glandular system. An antioxidant complex that contains SOD.
Vitamin E	400–800 IU daily.	Rids the body of toxic substances when combined with vitamin C and selenium. Use d-alpha-tocopherol form.

HERBS

❑ Black cohosh, black radish extract, goldenseal, licorice, lobelia, mullein, and red clover, taken in tea form, help strengthen and rebuild the liver, and restore glandular balance.

Caution: Do not take goldenseal internally on a daily basis for more than one week at a time, do not use it during pregnancy, and use it with caution if you are allergic to ragweed. Do not use licorice on a daily basis for more than seven days in a row, and avoid it completely if you have high blood pressure. Do not take lobelia on an ongoing basis, and do not take it in capsule form.

❑ Burdock root and red clover aid in cleansing the lymphatic glands and ridding the body of toxins.

❑ Cedar stimulates pancreatic function.

❑ Celery seed and hydrangea are diuretics that can be used to stimulate the kidneys.

❑ Chicory, milk thistle, and stillingia root stimulate and cleanse the liver.

❑ Cordyceps exerts its primary effects on the kidneys and increases lung capacity.

❑ Dandelion stimulates and cleanses the liver. It also stimulates bile production, thereby benefiting the spleen and improving the health of the pancreas.

❑ Echinacea cleanses and strengthens the kidneys, liver, pancreas, and spleen.

❑ Horsetail and oat straw are good sources of silicon, which aids in healing, and are also high in calcium. They can be taken in tea or capsule form.

❑ Parsley is a diuretic that stimulates kidney function. It also helps strengthen and rebuild the liver, and maintain glandular balance.

❑ Safflower flowers encourage the pancreas to manufacture insulin.

❑ Uva ursi is a diuretic that stimulates kidney function. It also has a germicidal effect, and thereby destroys any bacteria that may be present. It is a tonic for a weakened liver, kidneys, and other glands.

❑ Gentian contains elements that are known to normalize the functions of the thyroid gland.

RECOMMENDATIONS

❑ *See* BLOOD PURIFICATION in Part Three and follow the instructions.

❑ Use alfalfa, beet, black radish, and dandelion juice for cleansing the liver, which is the largest gland in the body. (*See* JUICING in Part Three.)

❑ Use olive oil and lemon juice (3 tablespoons of olive oil mixed with the juice of a fresh lemon), plus plenty of pure apple juice, to stimulate the gallbladder and help excrete bile and even small gallstones. (*See* GALLBLADDER DISORDERS in Part Two.)

❑ *See* FASTING in Part Three and follow the program once monthly to allow glands time to heal and rest.

❑ *See* HYPOTHYROIDISM in Part Two and follow the temperature self-test to determine how well your thyroid gland is functioning.

CONSIDERATIONS

❑ When toxic substances circulate through the bloodstream due to poor eating habits, the use of drugs, or other factors, the presence of these substances is reflected in the lymphatic system. The lymph glands act as a filter, removing poisons from the body.

❑ *See also* GLANDULAR THERAPY in Part Three.

- Raw lung.
- Raw mammary gland.
- Raw ovary.
- Raw pancreas.

- Raw pituitary gland.
- Raw spleen.
- Raw thymus.
- Raw thyroid gland.

Care should be taken in the purchase of glandulars. Many glandular products are byproducts of the meat-processing industry and are taken from adult animals that show the effects of aging and exposure to toxins. This impairs the quality of the glandular. For best results, make sure that the glandulars you buy come from young, organically raised free-range animals that have not received hormones.

Growth Hormone Therapy

Human growth hormone (HGH) is secreted by the pituitary gland in the brain. Like all hormones, HGH works to regulate the activities of vital organs, and thus helps maintain health throughout the body. HGH was originally called a growth hormone because it is produced in greatest amounts during adolescence, when growth is most rapid. HGH does indeed help control growth. Because of the link between this hormone and the growth process, HGH therapy was first used to treat children who were failing to grow normally because of a deficiency of this hormone. Without HGH therapy, these children would have become dwarfs; with it, their growth was normal.

However, it has been found that HGH regulates more than just growth. Tissue repair, healing, cell replacement, organ health, bone strength, brain function, enzyme production, and the health of nails, hair, and skin all require adequate amounts of HGH. In addition, this hormone strengthens the immune system and helps the body resist oxidative damage.

Unfortunately, after adolescence, levels of HGH begin to decline at a rate of about 14 percent per decade. As production of the hormone decreases, so does the function of all vital organs. Because of this correlation between declining HGH production and aging, another application of HGH therapy has developed: the use of the hormone to reverse or retard age-related symptoms of physical and mental decline, and to treat some non-age-related disorders as well. It is this newer use of HGH therapy that we are concerned with in this discussion.

According to reports in scientific literature, benefits from HGH replacement therapy include a reversal of declining pulmonary function, decreased body fat, increased capacity to exercise, increased bone mass in people with osteoporosis, and the improvement or reversal of many other age-related symptoms and disorders. HGH has also been shown to strengthen the immune system and to improve the quality of life for people with AIDS by treating "wasting syndrome"—severe weight and muscle loss. People receiving HGH have reported a general enhancement of health and well-being, including a more positive outlook.

Although HGH injections may be self-administered, therapy must be prescribed and supervised by a physician. This is particularly important in light of the fact that as the therapy promotes tissue repair and other processes, the need for many nutrients increases. Therefore, treatment should include the supplementation of various vitamins, minerals, and, in some cases, other hormones.

As long as the dosage remains low—4 to 8 international units of the hormone per week—HGH therapy appears to be free of significant side effects. Those side effects that do occur usually pass as the body adjusts to the therapy.

RECOMMENDATIONS

❏ Avoid the consumption of excessively sweet foods, as it results in a blood sugar level that is counterproductive to the release and utilization of HGH. High-sugar foods should especially be avoided before going to bed, as the primary supply of HGH is released during sleep.

❏ Avoid eating immediately before exercising. Although vigorous exercise usually stimulates the production of HGH, blood sugar levels must be stable during exercise for HGH release to take place.

❏ To stimulate the body's production of HGH, take the amino acid arginine, which has been shown to encourage HGH production. This amino acid is best taken in supplement form (500 milligrams daily), as foods that are high in arginine also contain amino acids that inhibit its ability to reach the pituitary gland, the site of HGH release.

CONSIDERATIONS

❏ Triple Strength Growth Hormone from Fountain of Youth Technologies is an Ayurvedic herbal formula whose ingredients include naturally occurring levodopa (L-dopa) and Ayurvedic herbs to stimulate the pituitary gland to release human growth hormone (HGH).

❏ The use of some brands of HGH has resulted in the production of antibodies to growth hormone.

❏ For information about other anti-aging hormones, *see* Melatonin *under* NATURAL FOOD SUPPLEMENTS in Part One, and DHEA THERAPY in Part Three.

Guided Imagery

See under PAIN CONTROL.

Hair Analysis

Hair analysis offers an accurate assessment of the concentration of minerals in the body—those that are toxic in any amount, those that are essential, and those that are needed in small amounts, but toxic in larger amounts. By allowing early detection of toxic substances such as mercury, lead, cadmium, and aluminum, hair analysis makes it possible to identify and treat toxicity before overt symptoms appear; and by showing levels of minerals such as calcium, it makes it possible to identify and treat a range of nutritional deficiencies well before health problems become serious.

Before the technique of hair analysis was developed, medical practitioners who were interested in the concentration of trace elements in the body had to rely on urine and serum sampling. Unfortunately, these tests have been shown to be inaccurate. They simply do not reflect the concentration of minerals in the cells and organs, but instead show the level of *circulating minerals.* The correlation between mineral concentrations in the internal organs of the body and concentrations in hair has been found to be much more reliable. In fact, hair analysis has been found to be such an accurate measure of substance exposure that it is often used to detect drug use.

Hair analysis begins with the removal of a small amount of hair, usually from the nape of the neck. Because harsh chemical treatment of the hair through coloring, bleaching, and permanent-waving can result in inaccuracies, a pubic hair specimen may be used instead. The hair sample is chemically washed and stripped of all substances found on it. A specific amount (by weight) of the resulting sample is then dissolved in a known volume of acid. Finally, using a method of chemical analysis called atomic absorption photospectrometry, each mineral is isolated and measured on a parts-per-million (ppm) basis.

Hair analysis also provides a relatively permanent record of mineral concentrations, which can be analyzed by computer to determine the correlation between various elements in the hair. Treatment of any identified problems, using chelation therapy and/or other programs, can then be designed and implemented before the condition becomes irreversible. (*See* CHELATION THERAPY in Part Three.) Later, follow-up hair analyses can be compared with the initial results to learn the effectiveness of the treatment.

The table that follows lists the minerals that can be measured through hair analysis. Next to each element is its symbol. In addition, the table shows the way in which each mineral interacts with other elements. In the case of lead, for instance, note that the presence of lead does not promote the action of any other mineral (second column). On the other hand, lead does inhibit the action of calcium, iron, and potassium (third column)—all important nutrients. Finally, the action of lead itself is inhibited by the presence of selenium and zinc (fourth column).

Your health care professional should be able to help you obtain an analysis of your hair. Do be sure that the laboratory you are dealing with is a reputable one. Questions you might ask about the lab include the following:

- Does the laboratory conform to the standards set by the American Society of Elemental Testing Laboratories, or the Hair Analysis Standardization Board?
- How long has this laboratory been in business?
- How old is the equipment being used?

- How experienced is the staff?

Two organizations that can provide a complete hair analysis are The Legacy Corporation and Doctor's Data Inc. (*see* MANUFACTURER AND DISTRIBUTOR INFORMATION in the Appendix).

INTERACTION OF MINERALS

Mineral Name	Elements Promoted by Mineral	Elements Inhibited by Mineral	Inhibitors of the Mineral
Aluminum (Al)	P	F	
Arsenic (As)	Co, I	Se	
Beryllium (Be)		Mg	
Cadmium (Cd)		Cu	
Calcium (Ca)	Fe, Mg, P	Cu, F, Li, Mn, Zn	Cr, Pb, S
Chlorine (Cl)*			
Chromium (Cr)		Ca	
Cobalt (Co)	As, F	Fe, I	
Copper (Cu)	Fe, Mo, Zn	P	Ag, Ca, Cd, Mn, S
Fluorine (F)		Mg	Al, Ca
Iodine (I)	As, Co		
Iron (Fe)	Ca, Cu, K, Mn, P		Co, Mg, Pb, Zn
Lead (Pb)		Ca, Fe, K	Se, Zn
Lithium (Li)		Na	Ca
Magnesium (Mg)	Ca, K, P	Fe	Mn
Manganese (Mn)	Cu, Fe, K, P	Mg	Ca
Mercury (Hg)*			
Molybdenum (Mo)	Cu, S	P	N
Nickel (Ni)*			
Nitrogen (N)		Mo	
Phosphorus (P)	Al, Be, Ca, Fe, Mg, Mn, Zn	Na	Cu, Mo
Potassium (K)	Fe, Mg, Mn, Na		Pb
Selenium (Se)		Cd, Pb	As, S
Silver (Ag)		Cu	
Sodium (Na)	K		Li, P
Sulfur (S)	Mo	Ca, Cu, Se	Zn
Zinc (Zn)	Cu, P	Cd, Fe, Pb, S	Ca

Mineral interactions have not been documented.

Heat and Cold Therapy

See under PAIN CONTROL.

Homeopathy

The practice of homeopathic medicine was started 200 years ago by Samuel Hahnemann, a German physician. The basic principles of homeopathy are that the natural state of the human body is one of health and that we possess the natural ability to heal ourselves. What we describe as symptoms are actually the body's efforts to protect itself against disease. Therefore, to effect a cure, we should not suppress the symptoms, but seek to stimulate the body's own natural healing processes.

Conventional Western medicine often seeks a cure by administering large doses of suppressant drugs. This can be a harmful approach for three reasons. First, suppressing symptoms can hamper the body's ability to cure itself. Second, the use of some drugs can have serious side effects. Third, this can rob the body of the opportunity to develop its own natural immunity.

It is possible to increase the healing power of a medicine and reduce its toxicity while at the same time proportionately and progressively diluting the medicine. In homeopathy, the more a remedy is diluted, the greater its potency. This allows homeopathic physicians to administer extremely powerful but minute therapeutic doses with no unpleasant side effects and no danger of toxic reactions. The reverse is often true in conventional medicine.

The patient and not the illness is the focal point in homeopathic medicine. Homeopathy considers the state of the whole individual—physical, mental, and emotional—whereas conventional physicians are often concerned only with the physical aspects of illness. Of course, no system of healing can cure all diseases. A good guideline to follow is homeopathy as the general rule, conventional medicine as a last resort.

Homeopathic medicines are among the safest preparations known to medical science. Most of them (about 80 percent) are derived from plants. Some examples of plant-derived homeopathic remedies are *Bryonia* (wild hops), *Calendula* (marigold), and *Rhus toxicodendron* (poison ivy). Other remedies are derived from animals or animal products. These include *Apis mellifica* (honeybee) and *Sepia* (inky fluid from the cuttlefish). Still other remedies are prepared from minerals or mineral ores. Examples include *Natrum muriaticum* (sodium chloride), *Silicea* (flint), and *Sulfur*.

Homeopathic remedies are prepared by grinding the active ingredient and mixing it with alcohol and water, then allowing it to soften and steep. Finally, the liquid is filtered to produce a tincture. The medicines are then potentized by progressive dilutions, which increase the healing power while decreasing the concentration. There are various potency ranges. The base, or mother tincture, has a potency of 1x. To make a 2x potency, one part of the base tincture is attenuated (mixed) with 9 parts of alcohol and shaken ten times. To make a 3x potency, one part of the 2x potency is mixed with 9 parts of alcohol and shaken again. This process is continued until the desired potency is attained. Other mixing agents that can be used in addition to alcohol are glycerin, water, and lactose. In addition to x potencies, there are c potencies. These are prepared in the

same way as the x potencies, except they are mixed at a ratio of 99 to 1, instead of 9 to 1. There are also k potencies. The 1,000k potency is labeled as 1m, a 10,000k potency as 10m, and so on.

Homeopathic remedies come in pellets, tablets, and dilutions (liquids). The potenizing (mixing) affects the way a homeopathic medicine works. Generally speaking, the lower potencies, such as 3x or 6x, have a greater effect on the organs and are suited to acute illness. Medium potencies, such as 12x and 30x, affect the senses and nervous system. High potencies, 60x and above, affect mental condition. The following is a rough guide to the various potencies, their effects, and uses:

Potency	What It Affects	Frequency of Dosage
6x, 12x, 6c, 12c	Body organs. Used for symptoms of acute conditions.	One dose every $1/4$ hour to every 4 hours.
30x, 30c	Body organs plus the senses and nervous system. Used for symptoms of chronic conditions.	Once a day to 3 times a day.
200x, 1m, 10m, LM	Body organs, senses, nervous system, mind, and emotions.	Once a month to once a year.

A typical dose of a homeopathic remedy is 3 tablets or 10 pellets for adults, 2 tablets or 5 pellets for children. Remedies should be taken on an empty stomach. The tablets should be placed under the tongue and held there for as long as possible while they dissolve. If possible, you should not swallow the tablets.

Hydrotherapy

Hydrotherapy—the therapeutic use of water, steam, and ice—has been used for centuries to effectively treat injuries and a wide range of illnesses. Treatment techniques include baths (full body and specific body parts), compresses, showers, sitz baths, steam baths, and whirlpools. Hospitals, clinics, and spas worldwide use forms of hydrotherapy as safe and effective methods for treating such conditions as AIDS, back pain, bronchitis and other respiratory problems, cancer, hypertension, muscle pain and inflammation, and rheumatoid arthritis. Hydrotherapy is also useful in treating the discomfort caused by spinal trauma.

There are three categories of external hydrotherapy: hot water, cold water, and alternating hot and cold water. *Hot water* stimulates the immune system and increases circulation, helping to relieve the body of toxins. By soothing nerves, hot water calms and relaxes the body. *Cold water,* which constricts blood vessels, is effective in reducing inflammation. Cold-water treatments are also used to reduce fever. *Alternating hot- and cold-water treatments* have been found to alleviate upper respiratory congestion and stimulate organ function through improved circulation.

Many hydrotherapy techniques for a range of conditions can be effectively performed at home. For instance, muscular pain and swelling caused by a sprain or strain respond favorably to an immediate application of cold. An ice pack, applied continually (up to twenty minutes on, followed by twenty minutes off) during the initial twenty-four hours following a trauma, can reduce swelling and provide relief.

Sitz baths, in which the pelvis is immersed in water, increase blood flow in the pelvic region and help to relieve problems in that area. Hot-water sitz baths are commonly used for the treatment of inflamed hemorrhoids, painful ovaries and testicles, muscular disorders, prostate disorders, and uterine cramps. Cold-water sitz baths are used to treat constipation, impotence, inflammation, sore muscles, and vaginal discharge. Alternating hot- and cold-water sitz baths are helpful in relieving abdominal disorders, blood poisoning, congestion, foot infection, headaches, muscle disorders, neuralgia, and swollen ankles. (*See* SITZ BATH in Part Three.)

Other effective hydrotherapy methods include simple, soothing baths and showers, body wraps, foot and hand baths, steam inhalation, and hot and/or cold compresses.

Although many hydrotherapy methods can be performed at home, certain treatments such as hyperthermia, neutral baths, and whirlpool baths, are available only in clinics or hospitals. These treatments must be performed under the careful supervision of a licensed therapist or other health care provider:

• *Hyperthermia.* Fever stimulates the body's immune system to produce the antibodies necessary for fighting certain illnesses. Hyperthermia is a hot-immersion bath used to induce fever in those who cannot achieve one naturally. This hydrotherapy method has been used effectively in the treatment of AIDS, cancer, and upper respiratory infections.

• *Neutral bath.* This therapy, in which the body is submerged to the neck in warm water (92°F to 98°F), helps to soothe the body. Neutral baths are effective in calming nervousness and emotional upsets, reducing joint swelling, and helping the body rid itself of toxins.

• *Whirlpool bath.* Used effectively in treating muscle and joint injuries, whirlpool baths are also used to soothe burns and to stimulate circulation in those with paralysis.

If you are interested in locating a hydrotherapy facility in your area, check with your local hospital. You can also look in the yellow pages of your local telephone directory under "Health Resorts" or "Physical Therapists."

A word of caution: If you have any health-related problems or conditions, be sure to consult with your health care provider before beginning *any* hydrotherapy treatment. All of the treatments presented in this section are recommended for those who are in generally good health.

Hyperbaric Oxygen Therapy

All human tissues and organs need oxygen in order to function. Hyperbaric oxygen therapy (HBOT) is the administration of oxygen at high atmospheric pressure. This saturates the body with oxygen, increasing the total available amount. HBOT is useful in the treatment of a variety of conditions that are associated with an insufficient amount of oxygen in part or all of the body.

HBOT is administered by placing the individual being treated in a special chamber that delivers pure oxygen at three times the normal atmospheric pressure. In most cases, the entire chamber is pressurized for treatment, and then depressurized before the person is removed. In some cases, oxygen is delivered by mask, making pressurization and depressurization unnecessary.

In the United States, HBOT is most commonly used in cases of trauma, including burns, wounds, injuries from motor vehicle accidents, carbon monoxide poisoning, acute cyanide poisoning, smoke inhalation, and the death of tissues from radiation therapy. HBOT is also used to treat skin grafts that are failing to take, gangrene, decompression sickness, and certain cases of blood loss and anemia. When used after surgery, HBOT has been shown to greatly improve early healing in a majority of cases. It has also been used to bring near-drowning victims out of comas, and it has proved to be a valuable adjunctive treatment for people who have opportunistic infections resulting from immunosuppression, as occurs in people with HIV and AIDS.

In other countries, HBOT has been widely used to treat people who have had strokes and those afflicted with alcoholism, drug addiction, arterial and vascular disorders, and multiple sclerosis. While the therapy has occasionally been used to treat such problems in the United States, at this time many of these applications are still controversial among American practitioners. Nevertheless, HBOT is now being used by both conventional and alternative physicians, and continues to gain acceptance for new applications.

Although HBOT is strictly controlled for safety, it may not be appropriate for all individuals. People with a history of emphysema, middle ear infection, or spontaneous pneumothorax (accumulation of air in the chest cavity) may encounter problems with this therapy.

Hypnotherapy

See under PAIN CONTROL.

Juicing

Fruits and vegetables are excellent sources of a wide range of vitamins, minerals, enzymes, and other nutrients, including phytochemicals—compounds that have been shown to combat cancer. Since more of the healthful substances found in fruits and vegetables are being discovered all the time, no supplement pill can contain all of these compounds. Also, because each plant appears to produce particular phytochemicals that work against cancer in particular ways, it is suggested that a rich assortment of fruits and vegetables be included in the diet. It is also recommended that you consume two glasses of live juices a day for health maintenance. Four glasses a day is recommended if you want to speed healing and recovery from illness.

Juicing is an excellent means of adding fruits and vegetables to your diet. Since juice contains the whole fruit or vegetable—except for the fiber, which is the indigestible part of the plant—it contains virtually all of the plants' health-promoting components. Because fresh juices are made from *raw* fruits and vegetables, all of the components remain intact. Vitamin C and other water-soluble vitamins can be damaged by overprocessing or overcooking. Enzymes, which are proteins needed for digestion and other important functions, can also be damaged by cooking. Fresh juice, however, provides all of the plants' healthful ingredients in a form that is easy to digest and absorb. In fact,

it has been estimated that fruit and vegetable juices can be assimilated in twenty to thirty minutes.

Ideally, the juices recommended in this book should be made fresh in your kitchen and consumed immediately. Many commercial juices are heat-treated to lengthen shelf life. As just discussed, this process can destroy important nutrients. In addition, preservatives may have been added. Even pure, freshly made juices can lose some of their nutrients by being allowed to sit for long periods of time. By buying the best produce available, properly preparing it for juicing, and processing it in your own juicer, you will produce the most healthful, nutrient-rich drinks possible.

The individual entries in Parts Two and Three recommend the use of specific juices for the treatment of specific disorders. It is helpful, though, to be familiar with the three categories into which juices generally fall: green juices, vegetable juices, and fruit juices.

GREEN JUICES OR "GREEN DRINKS"

Green juices cleanse the body of pollutants and have a rejuvenating effect. Made from a variety of green vegetables, green juices are rich in chlorophyll, which helps to purify the blood, build red blood cells, detoxify and heal the body, and provide the body with fast energy.

Green juices can be made with alfalfa sprouts, barley grass, cabbage, kale, dandelion greens, spinach, and other green vegetables, including wheat grass. Wheat grass juice is particularly important in any cancer treatment, especially when radiation therapy is involved.

Preparing Produce for Juicing

Juicing is an easy way to make delicious drinks that can boost your health and help you treat a number of disorders. By following these guidelines, you will ensure that your juices are as pure, nutrient-rich, and appetizing as possible:

• Whenever possible, buy and use organically grown produce—produce that is grown without the use of pesticides and other harmful chemicals. This prevents chemical residues from ending up in your juice.

• If you are unable to obtain organically grown fruits and vegetables, peel or thoroughly wash the produce, using a vegetable brush to remove chemical residues and waxes. Most health food stores carry vegetable washes that will help remove any residues.

• When purchasing potatoes for juicing, avoid those with a green tint, and be sure to remove any sprouts or eyes. The chemical solanine, which gives the potato its green cast, can cause diarrhea, vomiting, and abdominal pain.

• When using organically grown produce, feel free to leave the skin on in most cases. Do remove the skin, though, before juicing apricots, grapefruits, kiwis, oranges, papayas, peaches, and pineapples. The skins of oranges and

grapefruits are quite bitter, and also contain a toxic substance that should not be consumed in large amounts. Because kiwis and papayas are tropical fruits, their skins are likely to contain residues of the harmful sprays often used in foreign countries, where some chemicals outlawed in the United States may still be legal. The skins of pineapples are too thick to be processed by most juicers.

• When juicing fruits, leave in small seeds, except when using apples. Apple seeds actually contain cyanide, a toxic substance. Because of their size and hardness, all pits *must* be removed.

• Juice most produce with stems and leaves intact. However, remove carrot and rhubarb greens, as they contain toxic substances.

• When using soft fruits that contain very little water—avocados, bananas, and papayas, for instance—purée the fruits in a blender rather than using a juicer. Then stir the purée into other juices.

• Remember to rotate vegetables and fruits so you get a variety of nutrients.

To sweeten and dilute your green juices, try adding fresh carrot and apple juice. (No other fruit juices should be added.) Steam-distilled water is another good addition.

Although green juices have great health benefits, they should be consumed in moderation. Try drinking about 8 to 10 ounces a day. The following is an excellent "green drink":

Ageless Cocktail

4–5 carrots
3 sprigs fresh parsley
1 large handful spinach
1 large handful kale
1 beet, including tops
1 clove garlic, peeled
1/4 head cabbage

1. Thoroughly wash all vegetables, peeling the carrots and beet if they were not grown organically. Cut the vegetables into pieces small enough to fit into the juicer.
2. Process the vegetables in the juicer, and drink immediately.

VEGETABLE JUICES

Fresh vegetable juices are restorers and builders. They boost the immune system, remove acid wastes, and balance the metabolism. They also aid in the control of obesity by removing excess body fat.

Among the most healthful and delicious of the vegetable juices are beet, cabbage, carrot, celery, cucumber, kale, parsley, turnip, spinach, watercress, and wheat grass juice. Carrot juice is probably the most popular of the juices and is packed with carotenoids, including beta-carotene, the vitamin A precursor that helps fight cancer. Because carrots are the sweetest of the vegetables, their juice is not just delicious on its own, but is also great for mixing with other vegetables to increase their appeal. On the other hand, strong-flavored vegetables—broccoli, celery, onions, parsley, radishes, rutabaga, and turnips, for instance—should be used in small amounts only.

Garlic is a great addition to vegetable drinks. Before juicing, drop the garlic into vinegar for 1 minute to destroy any bacteria and mold on its surface. To avoid irritating the lining of the intestinal tract, use only 1 fresh garlic clove in 2 glasses of juice.

For the greatest health benefits, use many different vegetables when making your juices. That way, you will provide your body with a variety of important nutrients. The recipes that follow are just two of the many healthful vegetable juice drinks that you might want to try.

Potassium/Raw Potato Juice

1 pound potatoes (3 medium potatoes)
1 carrot or 1 stalk celery (optional)
6–8 ounces steam-distilled water

1. Scrub the potatoes well, and cut out any eyes. Do not use potatoes that are part green.
2. Cut each potato in half. Cut the peel from the potato, making sure to keep about 1/2 inch of potato on the peel. Set aside the potato center for another use.
3. Cut the potato skins into small enough pieces to fit into the juicer. If desired, wash the carrot or celery, peeling the carrot if it was not grown organically. Cut into pieces.
4. Process the vegetables in the juicer. Add the water, and drink immediately. Do not allow to stand.

Cabbage Juice for Ulcers

1/4–1/2 head cabbage
1 apple or 2 carrots
1/4 cup steam-distilled water

1. Thoroughly wash the vegetables and fruit, peeling the apple or carrots if they were not grown organically. Cut the produce into small enough pieces to fit into the juicer.
2. Process the vegetables and fruit in the juicer. Add the water, and drink immediately. Do not allow it to stand, so as not to lose its benefits.

FRUIT JUICES

Fruit juices help cleanse the body and nourish it with important nutrients, including cancer-fighting antioxidants.

Although any fruit can be juiced, certain juices are particularly healthful and delicious. One favorite cleansing juice is watermelon. To make this refreshing drink, place a whole piece of watermelon—with the rind intact—in the juicer. Other delicious juices can be made with apples, apricots, bananas, berries, citrus fruits, kiwi, melons, pears—with just about any fruit that you want to use.

You can enjoy fruit juices at any time of the day. About 10 to 12 ounces per day is recommended. The following is just one of the delicious fruit juice drinks you can make at home.

Kiwi Deluxe

1 firm kiwi, peeled
1 small bunch red grapes
1 green apple
1/2 cup berries (blueberries, blackberries,
and raspberries are good choices)

1. Wash all of the fruit thoroughly, peeling the apple if it was not grown organically. Cut the fruit into small enough pieces to fit into the juicer.
2. Process the fruit in the juicer. Pour over ice, and drink.

Variation: Frozen fruit mixes can take the place of ice. This will make the drink taste like a shake. Add a cup of frozen fruit mix to the recipe above. You can also add rice milk or soymilk and a banana if desired.

Light Therapy

The body's circadian rhythm—its inner clock—is regulated by the pineal gland. Affected by the absence or presence of light, the pineal gland is responsible for controlling such bodily functions as hormone production, body temperature, and the timing of sleep. Disturbances in the circadian rhythm can lead to depression as well as insomnia and other sleep disorders. The use of natural sunlight and various forms of light therapy has been effective in reestablishing the body's natural rhythm.

Natural sunlight contains the full-wavelength spectrum needed for maintaining health. It triggers the impulses that regulate most bodily functions. Artificial lighting—incandescent and fluorescent—lacks the complete balanced spectrum found in sunlight. Without certain wavelengths, the body cannot absorb some nutrients. Inadequate exposure to proper light can contribute to or worsen such illnesses and conditions as fatigue, depression, stroke, hair loss, suppressed immune function, cancer, hyperactivity, osteoporosis, and Alzheimer's disease.

A variety of light therapies has been used effectively in the treatment of a number of disorders. Some of the most common therapies are:

• *Bright Light Therapy.* This therapy involves the use of bright white light that ranges in intensity from 2,000 to 5,000 lux. (A lux is equal to the light of one candle: the average indoor light ranges from 50 to 500 lux.) Bright light therapy has proven helpful in treating cases of bulimia, sleep phase syndrome (a condition in which the person cannot fall asleep until the middle of the night), and irregular menstrual cycles.

• *Cold Laser Therapy.* Utilizing a low-intensity beam of laser light that stimulates the natural healing process at a cellular level, cold laser therapy has proven effective in the treatment of pain, trauma, and orthopedic myofascial syndrome. It has also been used in dentistry, dermatology, and neurology.

• *Full-Spectrum Light Therapy.* Exposure to natural sunlight and other forms of full-spectrum light is effective in relieving a number of disorders, including depression, hyperactivity, hypertension, insomnia, migraines, and premenstrual syndrome. Sunlight has long been used to treat babies with jaundice. Full-spectrum light, as well as bright white light, is effective in the treatment of seasonal affective disorder (SAD). Common symptoms of SAD, which is also called the "winter blues," are depression, fatigue, overeating, and lowered libido.

• *Photodynamic Light Therapy.* This therapy involves injecting light-absorbing dye into specific types of malignant tumors, then exposing the tumors to certain light. The dye absorbs the light, causing a chemical reaction that, in turn, kills the cancer cells.

• *Syntonic Optometry.* In this treatment, colored light is applied directly into the eyes to intensify the control centers of the brain that regulate various body functions. Syntonic optometry has been useful in treating pain, inflammation, headaches, and traumatic brain injuries.

• *Ultraviolet Light Therapy.* Ultraviolet light therapies are used to treat illnesses such as asthma and cancer, as well as conditions like high cholesterol and premenstrual syndrome. The sun's UVA rays, which have longer wavelengths than UVB and UVC rays, are considered the least harmful. There are a variety of ultraviolet light therapies. *UVA-1 therapy* isolates a portion of the UVA wavelength. It is used in the treatment of systemic lupus erythematosus. *Hemoirradiation therapy* involves removing an amount of blood (up to a pint) from the body, irradiating it with ultraviolet light, then reinjecting it. This therapy has been used successfully in treating asthma, blood poisoning, cancer, infections, rheumatoid arthritis, and symptoms stemming from AIDS. Patients with vitiligo and psoriasis can benefit from the treatment of *PUVA light therapy* (psoralen UV-A). First, patients are injected with psoralen, a light-sensitive drug; then they are exposed to UV light.

Magnet Therapy

See under PAIN CONTROL.

Massage

See under PAIN CONTROL.

Meditation

See under PAIN CONTROL.

Music and Sound Therapy

Music therapy is the controlled use of music in the treatment of physical, mental, or emotional disorders. A variety of problems—including depression, high blood pressure, asthma, migraines, ulcers, and a range of physical disabilities—are currently treated with music. In general, the nature of the problem dictates the precise form of the therapy. For some problems, specific musical pieces are played for the person being treated. In other instances, individuals actively participate in rhythm bands, group singing, individual or group music lessons, or music-accompanied physical activities.

Music has been shown to have various therapeutic capabilities. When played for individuals or groups with mental or emotional problems or with stress-related ailments, music can reduce anxiety and lessen irritability. In work with blind people, music has facilitated the development of better auditory perception. As a part of physical therapy, music has been used to stimulate or regulate movement. Also as a means of physical therapy, the playing of instruments has been employed both for its psychological benefits, such as greater self-confidence, and for its physical benefits, such as the strengthening of weak mouth and lip muscles.

Music is not the only type of sound that has been found to have therapeutic value. For many years, environmental sounds—the sound of a running stream, a waterfall, or bird songs, for instance—have been used by therapists and psychologists as a means of treatment. These sounds, it appears, can do much to relieve stress and lift depression.

Anyone can take advantage of the ability of music and other sounds to induce relaxation, with or without professional guidance. Soft music and soothing sounds, used alone or with relaxation techniques, can effectively alleviate stress, relax muscles, and evoke a positive mood. Researchers suggest that these sounds promote the production of endorphins, the body's own painkillers, and can thereby also help in the control of pain. In some cases, of course—when music is to be applied to physical therapy, for instance—an experienced practitioner should be consulted.

Pain Control

Pain is a message sent by the body to the brain, signaling that disease, injury, or strenuous activity has caused trouble in some area. Without pain, you would remain unaware of many problems—from torn ligaments to appendicitis—until the disorders became serious. At low levels, pain can motivate you to rest the injured area so that tissues can be repaired and additional damage can be prevented. When severe, pain can motivate you to seek treatment as well.

Not all pain, though, appears to serve a useful function. While *acute pain*, the pain described above, can alert us to a problem that needs immediate attention, in some cases pain lasts long after an injured area has healed. In other instances, pain may be caused by recurring backache, migraines and other headaches, arthritis, and other disorders. Referred to as *chronic pain*—which may be defined as pain that occurs, continually or intermittently, for more than six

months—this pain may signal an ongoing problem that cannot be eliminated through treatment. In such a case, pain management often becomes the treatment goal.

For some people, pain is cyclical—pain produces anxiety, and this anxiety intensifies the pain. Fear and anticipation of the physical problem can also heighten the pain, leading to feelings of depression and helplessness. When experiencing such pain, it is natural to limit one's activities. This can lead to a "chronic pain cycle," which can adversely affect one's confidence and self-esteem.

Being aware of the chronic pain cycle as well as understanding its psychological effects can help you avoid being drawn into it:

1. The cycle generally begins with prolonged periods of rest and inactivity, causing a loss in physical strength, endurance, and flexibility. As a result, you may begin to lose confidence in your ability to do things, causing a lowering of personal goals.

2. Inability to perform usual activities at home or work is likely to promote feelings of frustration, and you may begin perceiving yourself as unproductive. This sense of lowered self-esteem may further lead to depression.

3. During times when the pain subsides or is more tolerable than usual, you may overexert yourself in an effort to prove to yourself and others that you can still do the things you did before the chronic pain began.

4. As a result of the overexertion, the pain often returns and may be more severe than before. You may find yourself unable to finish tasks or accomplish goals. Discouraged and in pain, you begin limiting your activities, and the cycle begins again.

One way to keep from getting caught up in the chronic pain cycle is through pain management. Often, the reduction of physical pain can prevent the cycle from starting.

There are a variety of treatments that can help alleviate pain. Some do so on a purely physical level, perhaps by interrupting the pain process or desensitizing nerve endings. Others approach pain control on a psychological level, by affecting the mind's perception of the pain. In the treatment of pain, however, there often is no clear-cut separation of the physical and the psychological. Just as a physical reduction of pain may decrease anxiety and improve outlook, so can the mind be used to relax muscles and effect other physical changes that then reduce symptoms.

The following sections are meant to introduce you to some of the many pain-control techniques now available. Depending on the cause of your pain, the level of your pain, and your own treatment preferences, you may want to try one or more of these techniques. While some of these approaches, like the use of hot and cold packs, can easily be used on your own; other techniques, like biofeedback, require at least initial training by a qualified practitioner; and some, like chiropractic, must be performed by a professional. When possible, get referrals from your health care provider or from friends. If a reputable pain clinic is available to you, this can be a wonderful resource—one that offers a range of practitioners experienced in using a variety of pain-control techniques. Make sure that the professional you consult has successfully treated a condition such as yours. Try to obtain the names of others who have used this practitioner and speak to them about their therapies.

ACUPRESSURE

Based on the same beliefs that are the foundation of acupuncture (see the above discussion), acupressure—also known as "contact healing"—is actually the older of the two methods. Acupressure and the healing art of shiatsu (a massage technique) are commonly referred to as "acupuncture without needles." Like acupuncture, acupressure seeks to restore health by restoring the normal flow of *chi*, the life energy that flows through the body along pathways called meridians. While acupuncture uses the insertion of needles to promote energy flow, acupressure uses finger and hand pressure. During pressure stimulation, neurotransmitters, which help to inhibit the reception and transmission of pain, are released.

Acupressure is a safe, simple, and inexpensive treatment. Although it may be performed by a skilled practitioner, because of the treatment's noninvasive nature, acupressure may also be performed by the individual for the immediate relief of pain. In fact, a number of self-acupressure techniques, including Acu-Yoga, *Do-In*, and *Tui Na*, can help you control pain through finger pressure, massage, body positioning, and a variety of other means.

More information on acupressure is available from the Acupressure Institute (see HEALTH AND MEDICAL ORGANIZATIONS in the Appendix).

ACUPUNCTURE

This ancient Chinese practice is based on the belief that health is determined by *chi*, the vital life energy that flows through every living thing. This energy is thought to move through the body along pathways called meridians, each of which is linked to a specific organ. If the flow of energy is balanced, the individual enjoys good health. If something interrupts this flow, however, various problems, including pain, can result. Acupuncture is used to restore proper energy flow, and, as a result, good health.

In acupuncture treatment, the acupuncturist inserts thin needles at specific points in the body. Although slight discomfort may occasionally be felt upon insertion of the needle, the treatment is virtually painless. The needles may be left in place for anywhere from a few minutes to a half-hour. To support the acupuncture therapy, the practitioner may recommend taking herbs in the form of teas and capsules, and may also suggest specific lifestyle changes and exercises. Relief may be experienced after only one treatment or after a series of treatments.

Although used for a variety of health problems, including addictions and mental disorders, in the United States, acupuncture is perhaps most commonly used to relieve pain, including backache and migraine headaches. Studies have indicated that acupuncture may stimulate the production of endorphins, the body's own painkillers. Completely safe, acupuncture has no known side effects.

For more information on acupuncture and a list of practitioners in your area, you can contact the American Association of Oriental Medicine (*see* HEALTH AND MEDICAL ORGANIZATIONS in the Appendix).

BIOFEEDBACK

Biofeedback combines a variety of relaxation methods such as guided imagery and meditation with the use of instruments that monitor the individual's responses. Over time, this teaches you to consciously regulate a number of your own *autonomic functions*—heart rate, blood pressure, and other processes previously believed to be involuntary. By consciously regulating these functions, you can control a number of problems, including pain.

During a biofeedback session, electrodes connected to a monitoring unit are taped or otherwise painlessly attached to the skin. The machine may measure any one of a number of things, including skin temperature, pulse, blood pressure, muscle tension, and brain wave activity. As you use various techniques, such as relaxation, to create the desired response—lower blood pressure, for instance—the machine, through sound or images, provides moment-by-moment feedback on your progress. Eventually, with the practitioner's help, you should become able to effect the desired response without the use of the machine.

Although biofeedback has been successfully used to help control a wide range of health problems, it is perhaps best known for its use in the treatment of headaches and migraines. In a large number of cases, biofeedback has been successfully used to avert the onset of migraines. It has also been used to treat injuries, as well as to relieve the pain of TMJ syndrome.

It should be noted that biofeedback only measures stress; it does not cure it. Sessions should be conducted in conjunction with other therapies under the watchful eye of a qualified health care practitioner.

If you are considering biofeedback training, you can contact the Association for Applied Psychophysiology and Biofeedback (*see* HEALTH AND MEDICAL ORGANIZATIONS in the Appendix).

BREATHING EXERCISES

Shallow or poor breathing can contribute to many disorders. We need to learn to breathe deeply, and from the abdomen rather than from the chest, which produces short and shallow breathing. Learning this technique helps one to breathe in more oxygen, which then passes through the lungs and is absorbed into the bloodstream and into our bodies. Oxygen is needed for cellular respiration, cell metabolism, and proper brain function. If you breathe too shallowly, the body cannot eliminate sufficient carbon dioxide for good health. Proper breathing technique increases lung capacity, increases energy levels, speeds the healing process of many disorders, and helps to relieve anxiety, asthma symptoms, insomnia, and stress.

To practice deep breathing, do the following:

• Slowly breathe in through your nose and from your abdomen as deeply as you can and hold the breath for a count of 10.

• Place your tongue between your front teeth and the roof of your mouth. Slowly breathe out through your mouth.

Do this for five minutes three times daily. Choose an environment with fresh air when doing this exercise, not a place with a lot of traffic or pollution.

If you want to relax quickly—say, if you are under tension or stress, or are having an anxiety attack—place your arms down along the sides of your body. As you are inhaling deeply, stretch your arms up and out as if to form a V shape. Then exhale slowly through your mouth and bring your arms back down to your side. This is a stretching and breathing exercise at the same time. Repeat this as many times as is comfortable every hour until you find relief.

CHIROPRACTIC

Chiropractic is a form of treatment that seeks to eliminate pain—and, in some cases, other problems—through the manipulation of the spinal column. Chiropractors believe that if the spinal vertebrae are properly aligned, impulses from the brain are able to travel freely along the spinal cord to the various organs, maintaining healthy function throughout the body. If a misalignment of the spine occurs, however, the normal flow of impulses is disrupted, resulting in pain as well as other physical disorders. Chiropractors seek to return the spine's alignment to its normal, healthy state. This permits the nervous system to regain normal function, allowing the body to heal itself and eliminate the pain.

After the chiropractor locates any spinal misalignments, chiropractic adjustment is used to reestablish normal function. This adjustment may involve touch; active motion, in which the patient bends and stretches in specific ways; and passive movement, in which the doctor assists the patient's movements. A hand-held rubber-tipped instrument may be used to gently manipulate the vertebrae. Some chiropractors support adjustment therapy with applications of heat and cold, electrical stimulation, nutrition, and other natural therapies. Chiropractic does not use drugs or surgery.

After physicians and dentists, chiropractors are the third largest group of health care professionals in our nation. They are licensed in all fifty states and most health insurance plans cover the treatment they provide. Chiropractors are the most widely used practitioners in the alternative health care field. The U.S. Department of Health and Human Services lists spinal manipulation as a "proven treatment" for low back pain. Chiropractic therapy is also used to treat arthritis, bursitis, and a variety of other disorders, including many nonpainful ailments.

GUIDED IMAGERY

Much research has indicated that bodily functions previously thought to be totally beyond conscious control can be modified using psychological techniques. Guided imagery, a technique that has grown in popularity in the last several years, uses this mind-body connection to help people cope with a variety of disorders, including pain.

Researchers have established a link between negative emotions and lowered immune function. Conversely, they have found a connection between positive emotions and a healthy immune response. Guided imagery—the mind thinking in pictures—is an effective tool for eliminating negative thoughts and replacing them with positive ones.

Through guided imagery, the mind conjures up mental pictures or scenes in order to better direct the body's energy. You can, for instance, close your eyes and visualize the pain as a sharp knife in the affected body area. Then you can imagine that the knife is being withdrawn, and that a cooling, soothing cream is being applied to the area. Through imagery, people with cancer commonly visualize the cancer cells in their bodies as weak and their white "fighter" cells as strong and destructive. In other instances, people have found that, rather than visualizing the pain, focusing on a pleasant scene, such as a beautiful day at the beach, promotes relaxation and substantially controls pain.

Used successfully in the treatment of rheumatoid arthritis, cancer, and other illnesses, guided imagery has also been shown to reduce stress, slow the heart rate, and stimulate the immune system. Taught properly, guided imagery can be an effective form of self-care; however, it is not meant to replace your doctor's care or prescribed medication. Rather, it can be used to enhance your prescribed course of treatment.

HEAT AND COLD THERAPY

Hot and cold packs are simple-to-use pain-control tools that have been widely employed for many years. When applied singly or in combination, these techniques often provide relief not only from the pain itself, but, in some cases, from any accompanying swelling.

Heat

Pain from backaches, arthritis, and similar disorders often responds well to heat therapy. By increasing the temperature in selected areas of the body, this treatment enhances blood circulation and helps muscles to relax, reducing stiffness and increasing mobility.

Heat can be applied to the affected area through a number of means, including hot water bottles and electric heating pads. Often, moist heat works better than dry heat. Some electric heating pads are capable of producing moist heat, as are some gel packs. Hot showers and wet towels are other means of concentrating moist heat on a painful area. Poultices can also be effective and, for certain disorders, sitz baths are helpful. (*See* USING A POULTICE and SITZ BATH in Part Three.)

Use all forms of heat therapy with caution. Monitor the intensity of the heat and the duration and frequency of the treatment. Do not allow yourself to fall asleep while using an electric heating pad. Regardless of the heat source, a good rule of thumb is twenty minutes on, twenty minutes off. After removing the heat, firmly rub or massage the affected area. This will both dissipate the heat and help relieve tension. Do not massage the area if it is inflamed or has just sustained a serious injury. And never massage the area if you have phlebitis or other vascular problems.

Cold

Because of its ability to prevent swelling, cold packs are often the treatment of choice directly following a strain, sprain, or other injury. In such cases, cold packs alone should be used during the first twenty-four to thirty-six hours. Cold packs can also help relieve certain types of chronic pain.

Ice packs are probably the most common means of applying cold. These packs can simply be applied to the painful area, or they can be rubbed on the area using a circular motion for five to seven minutes. Lower back pain seems to be particularly responsive to ice rubs. Cold gel packs, which are kept in the freezer between uses, are also effective, and, because of their pliable consistency, are often more comfortable than ice packs. If none are available, a pack of frozen peas works just as well and can mold to the area. When you are done with it, mark the bag so it can be used over again for this purpose (do not eat them) and place it back in the freezer.

Like heat therapy, cold therapy should be used with caution. Wrap ice packs, gel packs, or frozen peas in a towel before applying them to the affected area. Then apply the packs for no more than twenty minutes at a time.

Heat and Cold

In some cases, alternating hot and cold treatments work best. For a painful and stiff neck, for instance, try using a warm shower to relieve tension. After the shower, use a five- to seven-minute ice massage to reduce swelling and further relieve pain.

Experimentation is the best way to discover whether heat, cold, or alternating heat and cold best relieves your discomfort. If several applications of one type of treatment—say, heat—do not provide any relief, try the opposite treatment. If your pain persists, and especially if you are not sure of its cause, consult your health care provider.

Counterirritants

A variety of over-the-counter topical products, such as capsaicin cream, Ben-Gay, and Icy Hot, can be used in lieu of a heat pack to treat localized pain. As counterirritants, these products stimulate blood flow to the affected area, acting much like heat. Boswellin Cream from Nature's Herbs, Glucosamine/Chondroitin MSM Ultra Rx-Joint Cream from Nature's Plus, Traumeel from Heel Inc., and many others natural products found in health food stores are good for arthritis, inflammation, bruising, and sprains. While such products may be relatively convenient and easy to use, they should be used with discretion. Do not apply anything but ordinary clothing to an area that has been treated with a counterirritant. Heating pads placed over treated areas can increase the medication's rate of absorption into the skin, thus causing serious damage.

HERBS

Many herbs have been used for centuries for their pain-relieving properties. Some of the best include:

- Angelica, black haw, cramp bark, kava kava, rosemary, and valerian root are good for pain related to cramps and muscle spasms.

- A tea made of blue violet, catnip, chamomile, gotu kola, licorice, rosemary, white willow, or wood betony is effective in relieving tension and nerve pain. DLPA complex by Nature's Plus, containing white willow bark plus DL-phenylalanine and bromelain, is a good natural pain reliever.

Caution: Do not use chamomile on an ongoing basis, and avoid it completely if you are allergic to ragweed. Do not use licorice on a daily basis for more than seven days in a row, and avoid it completely if you have high blood pressure. Do not take a product containing phenylalanine if you are pregnant or nursing a baby; if you take an MAO inhibitor drug; or if you suffer from panic attacks, diabetes, or phenylketonuria (PKU). If you have high blood pressure, start with the lowest dosage and monitor your blood pressure before increasing the dose.

- Capsaicin, an ingredient in cayenne (capsicum), can provide pain relief when regularly applied to the affected area. Now available in Zostrix, an over-the-counter topical cream, capsaicin is thought to relieve pain by limiting the production of a neural pain transmitter called substance P. Although the application of capsaicin may cause a burning sensation at first, repeated use keeps nerves from replenishing their supply of substance P, so that pain is not transmitted to the brain. In studies, capsaicin has been used to control the pain of postherpetic neuralgia, diabetic neuropathy, rheumatoid arthritis, osteoarthritis, and cluster headaches. Cayenne may also help to alleviate pain if taken orally in capsule form.

- Hops, kava kava, passion flower, valerian root, wild lettuce, and wood betony have muscle-relaxing properties and may help to relieve lower back pain.

• Essential oils of jasmine, juniper, lavender, peppermint, rose, rosemary, and thyme have been effective in the treatment of a variety of types of pain.

• Migraine Pain Reliever from Natural Care is an herbal blend that has been effective in relieving migraines.

• Fresh papaya juice and/or fresh pineapple is highly recommended for the treatment of inflammation, heartburn, ulcers, back pain, and digestive disorders.

• Saffron has been found to be effective in treating abdominal pain after childbirth.

HYPNOTHERAPY

Like meditation and visualization, hypnotherapy is a method by which a qualified physician or therapist can induce a positive mental state in an individual. The therapist attempts to quiet the person's conscious mind to make the unconscious mind more accessible. Hypnosis is designed to generate a state of deep relaxation in which there is a heightened receptivity to suggestion through the calm repetition of words and statements. Once an individual is in this state, the practitioner provides simple verbal suggestions that help the mind block the awareness of pain and replace it with a more positive feeling, such as a feeling of warmth. If the pain is the result of an earlier injury, the practitioner may also help the individual more clearly remember the incident—a practice that often helps alleviate anxiety and thus reduce pain.

Hypnotherapy enhances positive imagery, helps to reduce anxiety, and induces a deep level of relaxation. During a hypnotic state, the mind is highly focused and fully aware of the situation, enabling the person to concentrate without being distracted. During hypnosis, breathing and pulse rate slow down and blood pressure may drop.

No one can be forced into hypnosis. You must be a willing participant in the process. Good rapport between therapist and client is important.

Hypnosis has been used successfully to control back pain, joint pain, burn pain, and the pain of migraines and other headaches. This technique can be a valuable self-help tool, as you can learn to hypnotize yourself whenever you need it. However, self-hypnosis must first be learned from a licensed psychologist, a certified hypnotherapist, or another professional with experience in hypnotherapy.

MAGNET THERAPY

Magnet therapy has been used in the Far East and Europe for some time and is becoming popular in the United States. Magnets can be used to provide relief from pain and to hasten healing. Research on the effectiveness of magnet therapy is in its preliminary stage here in the United States. However, many experts claim that this therapy has many benefits. In a report published in the January issue of the *American Journal of Pain Management,* researchers noted that magnets sewn into socks alleviated the chronic pain of dia-

betic peripheral neuropathy (nerve deterioration and chronic pain in the feet due to diabetes). A double-blind study conducted at the Technion-Israel Institute of Technology demonstrated that magnetic stimulation of the brain can ease severe depression, a disorder that affects some 10 million Americans. At the Baylor College of Medicine in Houston, researcher Carlos Valbona found that magnets could provide signficant relief for the pain of postpolio syndrome.

Magnets are believed to work by increasing circulation and blood flow to affected areas, which in turn reduces swelling and inflammation. Arthritis, asthma, carpal tunnel syndrome, fibromyalgia, infections, migraines, osteoporosis, ruptured disks, sports injuries, and tennis elbow are a few of the conditions that may be helped by magnet therapy.

Negative or north field (designated "−") magnets are effective. Positive or south field (designated "+") magnets are not. Usually, magnets in the range of 400 to 2,500 gauss strength are used. (To give you an idea of the relative strength of these magnets, the average refrigerator magnet is about 200 gauss.) You should never use magnets that are not designed for bodily use. Purchase magnets from a reputable company that offers a money-back guarantee, and follow the directions on how to use them.

There are magnets made especially for different disorders. They are available as small chips and on pillows, mattress pads, knee pads, chair pads, bracelets, wraps for the back, neck, and other body parts. If you sleep on a magnetized mattress pad and the person next to you is not sleeping on one, he or she will be subjected to a positive (+) field rather than a negative (−) one. You should not wear a single magnet while resting on a magnetized mattress pad, as this will result in conflicting fields.

Caution: Magnets should not be used during pregnancy or in the presence of pacemakers, insulin pumps, and automatic defibrillators. People who take anticoagulants or use drug patches also should not use magnets. Keep your magnets away from your computer's hard drive and storage disks.

MASSAGE

Massage, which falls under the category of bodywork, involves the manipulation of muscles and other soft tissues. It is beneficial in treating a wide range of conditions, including muscle spasms and pain, soreness from injury, and headaches. Massage works to relieve pain in a number of ways: by promoting muscle relaxation; by increasing lymphatic circulation and thereby reducing inflammation; by breaking up scar tissue and adhesions; by promoting blood flow through the muscles; and by promoting drainage of the sinus fluids.

Massage is not advisable for everyone. Those with a history of phlebitis, high blood pressure, or any other vascular disorder should not receive any type of deep muscle massage performed with strong pressure. Always check with a physician before receiving deep muscle massage. Massage should not be performed on inflamed areas or on individuals with malignant or infectious conditions.

A variety of massage therapies are currently in use. Each is based on a different theory and utilizes specific techniques. The following bodywork systems represent some of those most widely used:

- *Deep Tissue Massage.* Used to release chronic muscular tension, deep tissue massage is applied with greater pressure and on deeper muscles than classic Swedish massage. It generally focuses on a specific problem area.

- *Esalen Massage.* This massage technique attempts to bring about a sense of well-being through deep and beneficial states of consciousness. Esalen massage focuses on the mind and body as a whole. It is a hypnotic method that uses slow, rhythmic movements to bring about a general state of relaxation.

- *The Feldenkrais Method.* The idea of "self-image" is central to the theory and technique of this method. Through exercise and "touch," the therapist helps eliminate negative muscle patterns and the feelings and thoughts associated with them. This method uses two approaches: *Awareness through Movement* and *Functional Integration.* Awareness through Movement employs a group approach in which the participants are guided through a slow, gentle sequence designed to replace old movement patterns with new ones. Functional Integration is an individualized approach that uses hands-on touch and movement. The Feldenkrais Method differs from most other types of massage in that there is no attempt to alter the body's structure. Rather, it is through touch that the practitioner attempts to communicate a sense of improved self-image and movement.

- *Neuromuscular Massage.* This form of deep tissue massage concentrates on a specific muscle. Through the use of concentrated finger pressure, sensitive "trigger points" are released and blood flow is increased.

- *Reflexology.* Reflexology originated thousands of years ago in China. It was taken up in the United States in the 1950s. Reflexologists apply pressure to different spots on the feet, hands, and ears that correlate with the body's organs. This opens a channel for energy to flow to the affected part of the body. There may be pain when pressure is applied to some spots, and in some cases it is necessary to use prolonged pressure. The reflexologist should inform you about which body part any pressure point represents so that if you feel pain, you can apply pressure and massage the spot yourself to reduce the pain.

- *Reiki.* In Japanese, *reiki* (ray-key) means "universal life energy." The practice of reiki promotes a return to health through "wholeness." The treatment consists of the health professional gently placing his or her hands on a relaxed body. You keep your clothes on for a reiki session. The practitioner's hands touch a variety of places, such as the head, chest, abdomen, and back, to promote energy to flow through the body. For some people, this treatment promotes deep relaxation, while to others it may be invigorating. Reiki originated many thousands of years ago and is easy to learn, but powerful. It is used to relieve stress, empower goals, overcome obstacles, and heal illness. It can also be a tool for spiritual growth.

- *Rolfing or Structural Integration.* This method is based on the belief that function is improved when body parts are properly aligned. Through manipulation of connective tissue linking muscles to bones, the therapist attempts to restore fuller movement, resulting in a more balanced body. The Rolfer applies deep tissue pressure to the muscles of the neck, head, back, pelvis, legs, and arms. This pressure stretches and guides the connective tissues, allowing for more flexible movement. Rolfing is also effective for muscle pain, neck tension, back pain, headaches, and increasing the range of motion. Before treating you, a Rolfer will evaluate your motion as you walk, bend, and turn.

- *Shiatsu.* Literally meaning "finger pressure" in Japanese, this Oriental massage technique focuses on acupressure points to restore and maintain health. Through firm, rhythmic pressures applied to specific points for three to ten seconds each, the shiatsu therapist attempts to unblock the energy that flows through the acupuncture meridians. The pressure used depends on the person's needs. Other techniques used include kneading, stroking, tapping, and stretching done by a shiatsu instructor.

- *Sports Massage.* A combination of kneading, passive stretching, and range of deep-tissue motions, sports massage is designed to ease muscle strain and promote flexibility. It is most effective when applied before or after exercising.

- *Swedish Massage.* This technique, developed by Peter Hendricks Ling in the early 1800s, uses kneading, stroking, tapping, and shaking to induce the body to relax. Swedish massage can also relieve soreness and swelling, as well as promote rehabilitation after an injury.

So numerous are your massage choices that before making a decision, you might wish to visit your local library. There, resources will familiarize you with what is available and will help to you either learn techniques of self-massage or choose the type of massage therapist who can best provide the help you need.

For organizations that can provide further information about massage therapy, *see* HEALTH AND MEDICAL ORGANIZATIONS in the Appendix.

MEDICATION

Several over-the-counter medications are available to help you control your pain. Two of the simplest nonnarcotic pain relievers are acetylsalicylic acid (aspirin) and acetaminophen (found in Tylenol, Datril, and many other products). Both of these medications can help relieve mild to moderate pain. Aspirin can also reduce swelling and inflammation. If you take aspirin for pain relief, you should also take supplements of vitamin C, as this nutrient has been shown to make the effects of the analgesic last longer.

Nonsteroidal anti-inflammatory drugs, another type of nonnarcotic analgesic, may also be helpful in the relief of aches and pains. These products include ibuprofen (Advil, Nuprin, and others), ketoprofen (Orudis), and naproxen sodium (Aleve).

Although over-the-counter analgesics are generally regarded as safe, discretion should be exercised in their use. If you take acetaminophen, be sure to avoid the consumption of alcohol, as this can both decrease the effectiveness of the drug and cause damage to the liver. If you take aspirin, be aware that it may affect the stomach. More important, you should *never* give aspirin to a child, especially a child with a cold or flulike symptoms. Regardless of the pain reliever being used, you should never take more than the dosage directed on the label without first consulting your health care provider. Virtually any medication can cause problems when used inappropriately.

MEDITATION

Meditation, which has been practiced for thousands of years, is an effective means of treating stress and managing pain. Broadly defined, meditation is an activity that calms the mind and keeps it focused on the present. In the meditative state, the mind is not cluttered with thoughts or memories of the past, nor is it concerned with future events.

There are hundreds of meditation techniques, most of which fall into one of two categories: *concentrative* and *mindfulness*. During concentrative meditation, attention is focused on a single sound, an object, or one's breath, to bring about a calm, tranquil mind. One simple, common technique involves sitting or lying comfortably in a quiet environment, closing your eyes, and focusing attention on your breath as you inhale through your nose for a count of three, then exhale through your mouth for a count of five. This focus on your breathing rhythm—slow, deep, regular breaths—allows your mind to become tranquil and aware.

During mindfulness meditation, the mind becomes aware of but does not react to the wide variety of sensations, feelings, and images tied in with a current activity. By sitting quietly and allowing the images of your surroundings to pass through your mind without reacting to or becoming involved with them, you can attain a calm state of mind.

Much research has been done on transcendental meditation (TM). TM brings about a state of deep relaxation in which the body is totally at rest, but the mind is highly alert. Studies show that meditation, especially TM, is effective in controlling anxiety, enhancing the immune system,

and reducing conditions such as high blood pressure. Meditation has also been used successfully to treat chronic pain and to control substance abuse.

Meditation is an effective self-care technique that can be a useful part of your health care program. However, it is not an alternative to recommended medical treatment.

QI GONG

Qi gong (pronounced chie-gong) is a slow-motion exercise that is older than tai chi. Both concentrate on movement and breath meditation. *Qi* means "life force, energy," and *gong* means "work, a skill of practice." Qi gong increases vital energy for emotional and physical health.

According to traditional Chinese medicine, this type of exercise wards off illness. It has been linked to reduced blood pressure and increased levels of endorphins, natural body chemicals that relieve pain and maintain mental health. Work with a trained professional to begin with, and in a half-hour you will be able to practice qi gong on your own. You will not find the exercises too strenuous. They are done as if in slow motion.

This particular discipline not only improves your mind, but also tones the muscles and joints and improves your balance. Remember to move your body slowly, with concentration, and remove all other thoughts from your mind. Proper breathing is also a part of qi gong. You want to enable your physical and mental processes to operate in balance for healing, relaxation, and internal energy.

RELAXATION TECHNIQUES

Once pain occurs—whether from injury or another source—your psychological reaction to it can have a profound effect on the duration and intensity of the pain. In some people, pain is cyclical; pain produces anxiety and tension, and tension intensifies pain. In the case of disorders such as migraines, tension can be a significant cause of the initial pain. By releasing tension, relaxation techniques can greatly reduce certain types of pain and actually prevent some pain from occurring.

A variety of relaxation techniques are available, including biofeedback, deep breathing, guided imagery, meditation, progressive relaxation, and yoga. These techniques facilitate deep relaxation and reduce stress. The advantage of relaxation therapy is that you can easily master these methods, either on your own or with the help of a professional, and then use them whenever they are needed.

TAI CHI

Tai chi, known as "meditation in motion," is similar to qi gong. It is used for meditation and complete relaxation. Both techniques are characterized by slow, soft, flowing movements that emphasize energy forces. These arts are very unlike the "strong" martial arts, such as karate and kung fu (wushu). Tai chi releases the flow of energy throughout the body. When this energy becomes blocked, one becomes ill.

TENS UNIT THERAPY

Transcutaneous electric nerve stimulation (TENS) units can be helpful in dealing with localized pain and are widely used both in doctors' offices and physiotherapy clinics. TENS therapy can also be performed at home.

With this technique, electrodes are placed on the skin and joined to the TENS unit with wires. Electric signals are then sent to the nerve endings, blocking pain signals before they reach the brain. It is believed that these signals may also stimulate the production of endorphins, the body's natural painkillers. TENS therapy is not considered painful, although some people report feelings of mild discomfort.

Pain relief from TENS therapy can be long- or short-term in nature. Because the treatments are safe and have no known side effects, they can be repeated as necessary.

Using a Poultice

A poultice is made of a soft, moist substance that is mixed to the consistency of a paste, and then spread on or between layers of cloth. The cloth is then placed on a body surface. Poultices act by increasing blood flow, relaxing tense muscles, soothing inflamed tissues, or drawing toxins from an infected area. Thus, they can be used to relieve the pain and inflammation associated with abscesses; boils; bruises; carbuncles; fibrocystic disease; fractures; enlarged glands in the neck, breast, or prostate; leg ulcers; sprains; sunburn; tumors; and ulcerated eyelids. They are also used to break up congestion, draw out pus, and remove embedded particles from the skin.

PROCEDURE

An herbal poultice may be made with dried or fresh herbs. The two types of poultices are prepared in slightly different ways. (For information on choosing the best herbal poultice for your condition, as well as cautions regarding the use of specific herbs, *see* Types of Poultices in this section.)

Preparing a Dried Herb Poultice

If you are using dried herbs, use a mortar and pestle to grind the herbs to a powder. Place the herbs in a bowl, and add enough warm water to make a thick paste that can be easily applied. Make a quantity sufficient to cover the affected area. The ratio of ground herbs to water will vary according to the herb being used. Add the water in small increments, just until the mixture is thick but not stiff.

Arrange a clean piece of gauze, muslin, linen, or white cotton sheeting on a clean, flat surface. The material should be large enough to cover the affected area completely. Spread the herbal paste over the cloth. Cleanse the affected area with hydrogen peroxide, and place the poultice over the area. Wrap a towel or plastic wrap around the poultice to prevent the soiling of clothes or sheets. Use a pin or other fastener to secure the poultice in place.

Preparing a Fresh Herb Poultice

If using fresh herbs for your poultice, place 2 ounces of the whole herb—about ½ cup—and 1 cup of water in a small saucepan. Simmer for 2 minutes. Do not drain.

Arrange a clean piece of gauze, muslin, linen, or white cotton sheeting on a clean, flat surface. The material should be large enough to cover the affected area completely. Pour the herbal solution over the cloth. Cleanse the affected body part with hydrogen peroxide, and place the poultice over the area. Wrap a towel or plastic wrap around the poultice to prevent the soiling of clothes or sheets. Use a pin or other fastener to secure the poultice in place.

Treatment Duration

Herbal poultices should be kept in place for one to twenty-four hours, as needed. During this period, you may experience a throbbing pain as the poultice draws out infection and neutralizes toxins. When the pain subsides, you will know that the poultice has accomplished its task and should be removed. Apply fresh poultices as needed until the desired level of healing has been reached. Wash the skin thoroughly after each poultice is removed.

TYPES OF POULTICES

By making your poultice with the appropriate herbs or other substances, you will help ensure that the treatment is effective. Herbs commonly used in poultices are listed below, along with the conditions for which they are appropriate. Note that when the mixture used to make the poultice contains an irritant, such as mustard, it should not come into direct contact with the skin, but should be placed between pieces of cloth.

• Chaparral, dandelion, and yellow dock can be used to treat skin disorders such as acne, eczema, itchy or dry skin, psoriasis, and rashes. You can use one herb or combine two or three. The greatest benefit will be obtained from using all three. Use chaparral only if you grow it yourself or purchase it from a reputable organic grower.

• Elderberry can relieve pain associated with hemorrhoids.

• Fenugreek, flaxseed, and slippery elm can be combined to treat inflammation. Slippery elm can also be used alone for the inflamed gangrenous sores often associated with diabetes, and for leg ulcers. The use of a slippery elm poultice upon the appearance of sores and ulcers can help prevent gangrene. Slippery elm can also be combined with lobelia to treat abscesses, blood poisoning, and rheumatism.

- Goldenseal is good for inflammations of all kinds.

- Lobelia and charcoal (available in health food stores) can be combined and used to treat insect bites, bee stings, and almost all wounds. Lobelia can be combined with slippery elm to treat abscesses, blood poisoning, and rheumatism.

- Mullein is used for inflamed hemorrhoids, lung disorders, mumps, tonsillitis, and sore throat. To make the poultice, mix 4 parts mullein with 1 part hot vinegar and 1 part water.

- Mustard is beneficial for inflammation, lung congestion, and swelling, and can help relax tense muscles. Because mustard is an irritant, place the mixture between two pieces of cloth, rather than placing it in direct contact with the skin.

- Onion is good for ear infections and for boils and sores that have difficulty healing. To make this poultice, place finely chopped onion between two pieces of cloth, rather than placing it in direct contact with the skin.

- Pau d'arco, ragwort, and wood sage can be combined and used to treat tumors and external cancers.

- Poke root is good for an inflamed or sore breast.

- Sage, like poke root, can help relieve breast inflammation and soreness.

Sitz Bath

As a form of hydrotherapy—the use of hot and cold water, steam, and ice to restore and maintain health—the sitz bath increases blood flow to the pelvic and abdominal areas, and thus can help reduce inflammation and otherwise alleviate a variety of problems. Sitz baths can use hot or cold water only, or can alternate heat and cold. Hot sitz baths are particularly helpful for such disorders as hemorrhoids, muscular disorders, painful ovaries and testicles, prostate problems, and uterine cramps. Cold sitz baths are helpful in the treatment of constipation, impotence, inflammation, muscle disorders, and vaginal discharge. Alternating hot and cold sitz baths can help relieve abdominal disorders, blood poisoning, congestion, foot infection, headaches, muscle disorders, neuralgia, and swollen ankles.

PROCEDURE

To prepare a sitz bath, fill a tub or basin so that the water covers the hips and reaches the middle of the abdomen. If possible, place the water in a basin that will allow you to immerse just the pelvic and abdominal regions. In this case, you can fill another basin with water that is a few degrees warmer, and immerse your feet in it while sitting in the sitz bath. If no suitable basins are available, place the sitz bath water in a bathtub. You may wish to cover your body with a sheet or blanket to increase your comfort.

As discussed above, the temperature of the water should vary according to the type of illness you are treating. When using a hot sitz bath, the bathtub or basin should be filled with water of about 110°F. (Make sure that the temperature of the water does not exceed 120°F.) You might want to make the water 90°F to 100°F at the beginning of the bath and then gradually increase the temperature to 110°F. As already mentioned, your feet can be immersed in slightly hotter water. You might wish also to apply a cold compress to your forehead, as the compress will make it easier for you to withstand the heat of the bath. (Make sure that the sitz bath, foot bath, and cold compress are all prepared ahead of time.)

Stay in the bath for twenty to forty minutes. After the moist heat of the bath has soothed the area being treated, you can further stimulate the body by taking a quick cold shower or simply splashing your body with cool water. Then towel yourself dry.

When using a cold sitz bath, fill the bathtub or basin with ice water. Stay in the cold bath for thirty to sixty seconds only. By no means should you stay in the water for more than sixty seconds, as this added time will provide no additional benefits, and may even be harmful. Then towel yourself dry.

When using alternating hot and cold baths, fill one basin with water of about 110°F, and a second basin with ice water. Immerse yourself first in the hot sitz bath, and remain there for three to four minutes. Then move to the cold sitz bath, and remain there for thirty to sixty seconds. Repeat this two to four times, and towel yourself dry.

A word of caution: If you have any health related problems or conditions, be sure to consult with your health care provider before using any type of sitz bath.

Steam Inhalation

Steam inhalation therapy is helpful for relieving the congestion of bronchitis, the common cold, and a variety of other respiratory and sinus conditions. Steam inhalation opens up congested sinuses and lung passages, allowing you to discharge mucus, breathe more easily, and heal faster. To make the steam, you may use water only, or you may add dried or fresh herbs or herbal oils to enhance the effects of the treatment.

PROCEDURE

To provide the steam for the inhalation treatment, you may place the hot water in either a sink or a pot. In most cases, you can choose whichever method you find most convenient and comfortable. But if you are using fresh or dried herbs, you should use a glass or enameled pot, rather than the sink, to hold the water.

Using a Sink

If using your bathroom sink to hold the water, fill the sink with very hot water. If desired, add 2 to 5 drops of herbal oil. Keep the water hot and steaming during the treatment by allowing a small, continuous trickle of hot water to flow into the basin. (The overflow outlet of your sink should prevent the water from spilling over.) As the water becomes diluted, add a few more drops of the herbal oil as needed.

Hold your head over the sink, and breathe in the steam. Usually, five to ten minutes of steam should be sufficient to clear your congestion. In some cases, you may choose to extend the session. Keep your face far enough from the water so that the steam does not irritate or burn your skin. This is particularly important when a child is being treated, as a child's skin is more sensitive to heat.

Using a Pot

If you choose to use a pot to hold the water, and you are using fresh or dried herbs, be sure to select glass or enameled cookware only. This is important, as a metal pot can cause herbs to lose some of their medicinal properties. If you are using water only, any type of pot is appropriate.

Fill a wide pot with water, and bring it to a boil. Then remove the pot from the heat source, and place it on a heat-proof pad or cutting board at a convenient height for the inhalation treatment.

Once the water stops bubbling, if desired, add fresh or dried herbs or several drops of essential oil to the water. Allow the water to cool slightly. Then hold your head over the pot, and breathe in the steam. Capture the steam by draping a towel over your head and the pot, creating a "tent." Usually, five to ten minutes of steam should be sufficient to clear your congestion. In some cases, you may choose to extend the session. Keep your face far enough from the water so that the steam does not irritate or burn your skin. This is particularly important when a child is being treated, as a child's skin is more sensitive to heat.

Whichever method you use, after each steam inhalation treatment, take several deep, full breaths to clear lung congestion. Repeat the therapy as needed.

HERBS

❏ Coltsfoot, comfrey, elecampane, ephedra, eucalyptus, fennel, fenugreek, horseradish, licorice, lobelia, lungwort, mullein, pleurisy root, thyme, vervain, and yerba santa are expectorants that facilitate the excretion of mucus from the throat, lungs, and sinuses. These herbs may be used singly, in combination with one another, or in combination with the demulcent herbs listed below.

❏ Burdock, chickweed, coltsfoot, Irish moss, lungwort, marshmallow, mullein, peach bark, and slippery elm are demulcents—substances that soften and relieve irritation of the mucous membranes. These herbs may be used singly, in

combination with one another, or in combination with the expectorant herbs listed above.

Preparing for and Recovering from Surgery

Although few people enjoy the prospect of surgery, sometimes surgery is the best available means of improving the quality of life or extending life. Thousands of Americans face surgery each year, often with fear and doubt. Not knowing what is involved can mean putting yourself through far more discomfort than is necessary. Whether you are undergoing surgery for the first time or the tenth, understanding why you need it and knowing about the risks involved, available alternative treatments, and the aftereffects will help you make the right decision. Being educated about your illness will enable you to deal more effectively with the outcome.

After you have been informed of all your options and have decided that surgery is the only viable alternative, use the nutritional guidelines provided in the table below to prepare for the surgery. (For more information on making the decision to have surgery, see the inset on that subject in this section.) By taking these nutrients both before and after surgery, you will support the healing process and lessen postsurgical discomfort and pain. Make sure that your diet is well balanced and healthy. Remember that your general health *after* surgery partly depends on your general health *before* surgery. Do not take any supplements that thin the blood before surgery. Eicosapentaenoic acid (EPA), feverfew, garlic, ginger, gingko biloba, kava kava, and vitamin E are among the supplements that should not be used prior to surgery.

Unless otherwise stated, the dosages recommended here are for adults. For a child between the ages of twelve and seventeen, reduce the dose to three-quarters of the recommended amount. For a child between the ages of six and twelve, use one-half the recommended dose, and for a child under six, use one-quarter of the recommended amount.

NUTRIENTS

SUPPLEMENT	SUGGESTED DOSAGE	COMMENTS
Acidophilus (Kyo-Dophilus from Wakunaga is a good source)	As directed on label 3 times daily.	To stabilize the intestinal bacterial flora if antibiotics are used. Use a high-potency powdered form.
Coenzyme Q10	60 mg daily.	A free radical destroyer that improves tissue oxygenation.
Essential fatty acids (salmon oil and Ultimate Oil from Nature's Secret are good sources)	As directed on label.	Important for proper cell growth and healing of all tissues. *Caution:* Do not take for one week prior to surgery. Take this supplement after the surgery.

Free-form amino acid complex	As directed on label.	Aids in collagen synthesis and wound healing. Is a readily available form of protein, easily absorbed by the body.
Garlic (Kyolic from Wakunaga)	2 capsules 3 times daily.	A natural antibiotic that enhances immune function.
L-Cystine	500 mg twice daily.	Speeds healing of wounds.
L-Glutamine	500 mg 3 times daily and at bedtime.	Speeds healing of wounds.
L-Lysine	500 mg daily.	Speeds healing of wounds and aids collagen formation. Caution: Do not take lysine for longer than 6 months at a time.
Methylsulfonyl-methane (MSM)	As directed on label.	Good for pain and healing of tissues.
Multivitamin complex with vitamin A and mixed carotenoids including natural beta-carotene	As directed on label.	Provides necessary vitamins and minerals. Vitamin A is needed for protein utilization in tissue repair and is a free radical scavenger.
Pcynogenol or grape seed extract	As directed on label.	Surgery depletes the body of antioxidants. These are powerful antioxidants.
Vitamin C with bioflavonoids	6,000–10,000 mg daily, in divided doses.	Aids in tissue repair and healing of wounds. Vital in immune function. Use a buffered form.
Vitamin E	Beginning the day after surgery, take 600 IU daily. Do not take any vitamin E during the 2 weeks before surgery, as it thins the blood.	Improves circulation and repairs tissues. Use d-alpha-tocopherol form.
Vitamin E oil	After the stitches are removed and healing has begun, apply topically to the area of the incision 3 times daily.	Promotes healing and reduces scar formation. Purchase in oil form or cut open a capsule to release the oil.
Vitamin K	As directed on label.	This important vitamin is needed for blood clotting.
Zinc plus calcium and magnesium and silica and vitamin D	50 mg daily. 1,500 mg daily. As directed on label. As directed on label. 400 IU daily.	Important for tissue repair. Look for a supplement that contains all of these nutrients.

HERBS

❏ Herbal teas are highly recommended before and after surgery. Try the following teas:

• Alfalfa, dandelion, and nettle are high in vitamins, minerals, and can also increase the appetite. Alfalfa is also a good source of iron.

• Bromelain and turmeric (curcumin) have potent anti-inflammatory properties.

• Burdock root and red clover aid in cleansing the blood and the liver.

• Echinacea enhances immune system function.

• Goldenseal is a natural antibiotic and helps to prevent infection.

Caution: Do not take this herb internally on a daily basis for more than one week at a time, as it may disturb normal intestinal flora. Do not use it during pregnancy, and use it with caution if you are allergic to ragweed.

• Green tea contains powerful antioxidants that aid in the healing process.

• Kelp, reishi, and St. John's wort may help protect against the adverse effects of x-ray radiation.

• Milk thistle protects the liver from the toxic buildup of drugs and chemicals resulting from surgical procedures.

• Pau d'arco is a natural antibacterial herb. It enhances healing, cleanses the blood, and aids in the prevention of candidiasis.

• Rose hips are a good source of vitamin C and enhance healing.

RECOMMENDATIONS

❏ Consult with your physician about minimally invasive surgery, also called laparoscopic, "keyhole," and "band-aid" surgery. This type of procedure—involving one or more small incisions rather than a large one—does less damage to the skin, muscles, and nerves than does conventional "open" surgery. It also involves a shorter hospital stay and less recovery time. Be aware that such procedures can be used for certain surgeries only.

❏ If you are overweight and have sufficient time to diet before surgery, try to gradually lose the extra weight. Studies show that excess weight can increase both the difficulty of performing surgery and the length of the recovery time. It has also been linked to an increased likelihood of postoperative infection.

❏ If you smoke, stop. Smoking delays healing and interferes with the actions of certain drugs.

❏ Make sure your doctor and those who will care for you are aware of any allergies you have to drugs, chemicals, or foods.

❏ Ask your surgeon if there is anything that you can do to prepare for the surgery. In addition to the surgeon's recommendations, avoid taking vitamin E supplements, aspirin, and all compounds containing aspirin for two weeks prior to surgery. These substances thin the blood.

❏ Make sure your doctor and those who will care for you are aware of any supplements and medications—including natural medicines—you take regularly.

❏ Because blood transfusions are sometimes required during surgery, speak to your doctor about the possibility of storing your own blood for use during the operation. By using your own blood, you will avoid the risk of contracting hepatitis or the AIDS virus. Remember that even disease-free blood can cause reactions such as rashes if not perfectly matched. Your doctor will tell you if you need to take iron supplements a week before the first blood collection. Arrange the appointments so that the last time you give blood is at least four days before the surgery. (Whole blood can be stored for thirty-five days.)

❏ Many operations require that the patient be shaved. If this is necessary, tell the surgeon that you prefer to be shaved the day of surgery. Studies show that the infection rate is lower for patients who are shaved the day of surgery when compared with those who are shaved the night before.

❏ Add fiber to your diet. It ensures better intestinal tract function.

❏ Check with your surgeon before using any treatments at home prior to surgery. If the surgeon concurs, take two cleansing enemas using the juice of a fresh lemon before entering the hospital. It is important to have a clean colon prior to surgery. Taking a half glass of aloe vera juice in the morning and before bedtime will help to keep your colon clean. Take a bottle of this remedy with you to the hospital. It tastes like spring water and needs no refrigeration.

❏ Many hospitals employ massage with therapeutic essential oils to promote relaxation and relieve the inevitable stress of the presurgical period. If your hospital does not practice this therapy, make arrangements for a qualified massage therapist who is knowledgeable about aromatherapy to give you a massage prior to surgery.

❏ Keep a positive attitude about your surgery, and look forward to getting out of bed and back to normal as soon as possible. The sooner you get out of bed, the better your chances of avoiding postoperative infection.

❏ The practice of ordering routine laboratory tests before admission for surgery is commonplace in most hospitals. Many doctors believe that urinalysis, chest x-rays, or complete blood counts, for example, can identify potential problems that might complicate the surgery if not detected and treated early. Tests that are commonly performed before surgery, and the symptoms that prompt doctors to order them, include the following:

• Blood glucose: Alcoholism, altered mental status, cystic fibrosis, diabetes, excessive sweating with tremor or anxiety, muscle weakness, or pancreatitis.

• Blood potassium: Congestive heart failure, diabetes, diarrhea, high blood pressure, kidney failure, muscle weakness, tissue damage, use of drugs known to affect potassium levels, or vomiting.

• Blood sodium: Central nervous system disease, cirrhosis, congestive heart failure, diarrhea, excessive sweating, pulmonary disease, thirst or fluid intake, or vomiting.

• Chest x-ray: Abnormal sounds when breathing, chest pain, cough, fever with no known source, or shortness of breath.

• Electrocardiogram (EKG): Chest pain, distant heart sound, heart murmur, irregular heartbeat, or palpitations.

• Platelet count: Alcoholism, blood loss, easy bruising, or use of drugs known to affect platelet count.

• Urinalysis: Diabetes, discharge, kidney disease, side pain, urinary frequency or hesitancy, or use of drugs known to cause kidney disease.

• White blood count: Fever, suspicion of infection, or use of drugs known to affect white blood cell count.

Discuss with your doctor the necessity of having certain tests performed prior to surgery.

❏ Before deciding to have surgery, ask your physician the following types of questions:

• Why do I need the operation?

• Are there alternatives to surgery?

• What are the benefits of having the operation?

• What are the risks of having the operation?

• What if I do not have this operation?

• What is your experience in performing this surgery?

• What kind of anesthesia will I need?

• How will the surgery improve my quality of life and/or my chances for survival?

• Are there other forms of treatment that might be used instead of surgery?

• What percentage of the operations performed of this type are successful?

• What physical changes will result from this operation, and what improvements can you expect?

• How long is the recovery period?

• What is the cost of the operation?

❏ Ask about the potential risks and side effects of having anesthesia. Be sure to mention any medical problems you have, including allergies, and any medications you have been taking, since they may affect your response to the anesthesia.

❏ After surgery, don't overwork your body by eating highly processed foods. Try to consume at least 8 cups of liquids each day, including distilled water, herbal teas, juices, and protein drinks. The appetite is often poor after surgery, and large meals can be overwhelming. Try eating five to seven small, light, nutritious meals a day.

❏ After surgery, exercise caution when engaging in strenuous activity such as lifting. Most doctors advise patients to avoid lifting anything in excess of 10 pounds for two weeks after surgery. Ask your doctor when you can begin light exercise, which has been shown to aid circulation and speed physical recovery. Also ask if there are any specific exercises that can aid your recovery.

❏ After surgery, the homeopathic remedy *Arnica montana* is good for reducing swelling and promoting healing.

CONSIDERATIONS

❏ After major surgery, people generally experience a rapid breakdown of skeletal muscle, which increases any feelings of weakness. In studies in which the amino acid glutamine was added to postsurgical intravenous solutions, muscle breakdown rates were greatly diminished.

❏ Nicholas Cavarocchi, M.D., of Temple University recommends that patients be given 2,000 international units of vitamin E twelve hours prior to heart surgery. This amount of vitamin E lowers free radical levels in the blood. This is recommended only under a physician's supervision.

❏ Some foods interfere with the actions of certain medications. Milk, dairy products, and iron supplements may interfere with some forms of antibiotics. Acidic fruits, such as oranges, pineapples, and grapefruits, can inhibit the action of penicillin and aspirin. *See* Substances That Rob the Body of Nutrients on page 336 for a list of the nutrients that are lost with the use of different drugs.

❏ Postsurgical depression is not uncommon. A healthy dietary program can help fight depression.

❏ An article in the May 1999 issue of *American Health* reported that research from the University of Chicago Medical Center found that patients who ate potatoes, tomatoes, and eggplants prior to surgery reacted unpredictably to anesthesia. These foods contain natural chemicals that affect metabolism and may alter the effect of anesthesia.

❏ Remember: It takes the body a few weeks to recover from the trauma of surgery. During this period, hormonal imbalances are corrected, and the rate of metabolism is adjusted. Most incisions close within two days and heal within a week to the point that the skin will hold together under normal stress and body movement. However, you should obtain your doctor's approval before engaging in any exercise or lifting anything over 10 pounds in weight.

Therapeutic Liquids

The benefits of vegetables and grains are discussed throughout this book. This section offers two recipes that provide these benefits in broths that have healing properties.

The first of the broths derives its healthful properties—including its high potassium content—from potatoes and other vegetables. When purchasing potatoes, choose ones that do not have a green tint. The chemical solanine, which gives the potato its green cast, can interfere with nerve impulses and cause diarrhea, vomiting, and abdominal pain. Use Potato Peeling Broth as a nutritious drink when fasting. This broth is also good for heart disorders.

The second broth—Barley Water—has healing and fortifying properties and is useful during convalescence from many different illnesses. You can also add powdered slip-pery elm to the water to make a drink that is not only nourishing, but also soothing to the throat and digestive tract.

Many other therapeutic liquids can also be made from vegetables and grains, as well as from fruits. To learn about nutritious juices, *see* JUICING in Part Three.

Potato Peeling Broth

---

3 potatoes
1 carrot, sliced
1 celery stalk, sliced
2 quarts steam-distilled water
1 onion, sliced and/or 3 cloves garlic, peeled

1. Scrub the potatoes well, and cut out any eyes.
2. Cut the potatoes in half. Cut the peel from the potatoes, making sure to keep about $1/2$ inch of potato with the peel. Set aside the potato centers for another use.
3. Place the potato peelings, carrot, and celery in a large pot. Cover with the water. Add the onion and/or garlic to taste, and boil for about 30 minutes.
4. Cool the broth. Strain out and discard the vegetables, and serve the broth as desired.

Barley Water

---

1 cup barley
3 quarts steam-distilled water

1. Place the barley and the water in a large pot, and boil for about 3 hours.
2. Cool the broth. Strain out and discard the barley, and serve the broth as desired.

TENS Unit Therapy

See under PAIN CONTROL.

Yoga

Yoga is not new; it was developed in India over 5,000 years ago, and was used to unite the body, mind, and spirit. Often, people think of yoga as physical exercise. However, the progress of learning to still the mind and unify consciousness is also important in yoga exercises. It can be difficult to turn off the voices in your head, especially when your body is motionless.

Hatha is a Sanskrit word meaning "willful" and *yoga* is translated as "union" or "communion." This is understood as meditation in action. *Hatha yoga* is a term familiar to many who practice yoga, but it is not actually a particular style of yoga.

There are many different styles of yoga to choose from. Some are softer and easier to do and some are strenuous and hard to do. If you are a beginner, it is probably best to try the easier forms, and it is necessary to work with a teacher. The following are a few approaches to choose from:

• *Ananda yoga* will appeal to the beginner who desires to cultivate spirituality and learn how to meditate. Ananda is a slower-paced style.

• *Ashtanga yoga* becomes more strenuous as the student progresses. The postures are linked together in a continuous flow, performed while practicing ujjayi breathing. This builds stamina, strength, and flexibility. It is challenging, and not for the beginner.

• *Bikram yoga* is not for the beginner. It requires a great deal of work. It is a sequential series of twenty-six postures done in a continuous flow. The room this practice is done in is heated to 100 degrees or more to promote sweating that helps cleanse the body of toxins.

• *Kundalini* and *tantra yoga* focus on activating the energy centers in the body called *chakras*. The chakras are seven cores of energy in the body. This type of yoga involves exploring the core of the body rather than the limbs—moving to the center and seeing the body as rivers of energy.

• *Raja yoga* concentrates more on meditation and less on strength and is good for the beginner.

• *Sevananda yoga* is a holistic approach. There are five basic principles that unite the body, mind (intellect), spirit, and heart. They include proper breathing (pranayama), a vegetarian diet, proper relaxation (savasana), study of the Vedic scriptures, and meditation.

• *Tivamukti yoga* focuses on spiritual teachings, postures, chanting, meditation, music, readings, and are all incorporated into the class.

There are many other types of yoga including kripalu yoga, integral yoga, and phoenix rising yoga therapy. There are many unique techniques and teaching methods. The goals, however, are the same: to teach a greater understanding and awareness of the body; to free oneself from negative thoughts that drain one's energies; and to strengthen mental and spiritual balance. Yoga postures remove obstructions from the body to enhance energy and well-being and achieve inner peace.

APPENDIX

Glossary

absorption. Nutritionally, the process by which nutrients are absorbed through the intestinal tract into the bloodstream to be used by the body. If nutrients are not properly absorbed, nutritional deficiencies can result.

acetic acid. A weak inorganic acid that is the active ingredient in vinegar; a 4- to 5-percent solution of acetic acid in water makes vinegar.

acid. Any of a class of compounds that share certain basic chemical characteristics. Acids have low pH, are usually sour to the taste, and, in their pure form, are often corrosive. They can be either organic or inorganic compounds. Acids found in plant tissues (especially fruits) tend to prevent the secretion of fluids and shrink tissues.

acidosis. A condition characterized by excessive acidity of bodily fluids.

acute illness. An illness that comes on quickly and may cause relatively severe symptoms, but is of limited duration.

adaptogen. A term for a substance, usually an herb, that produces suitable adjustments in the body. Adaptogens tend to normalize body functions, and when the job is completed, they are eliminated or incorporated into the body without side effects. Some beneficial adaptogens include garlic, ginseng, echinacea, ginkgo, goldenseal, and pau d'arco.

adrenal gland. One of a pair of glands situated atop the kidneys. The adrenal glands are the source of the stress hormones epinephrine (adrenaline) and cortisol, among others.

allergen. A substance that provokes an allergic response.

allergy. An inappropriate response by the immune system to a normally harmless substance. Allergies can affect any of the body's tissues. Hay fever is a common type of allergy.

allyl sulfides. Phytochemicals found in leeks, onions, garlic, and chives that act to detoxify the body.

alternative therapy. The treatment of disease by means other than conventional medical, pharmacological, and surgical techniques.

amino acid. Any of twenty-two nitrogen-containing organic acids from which proteins are made.

anabolic compound. A substance that allows the conversion of simple nutritive materials into complex materials that are part of living tissue during the constructive phase of metabolism.

analgesic. Tending to relieve pain, or a substance that relieves pain.

anemia. A deficiency in the blood's ability to carry oxygen to the body tissues.

anesthetic. Causing loss of sensation, or a substance that causes the loss of sensation, especially the ability to feel pain.

angina pectoris. A syndrome of chest pain with sensations of suffocation, typically brought on by exertion and relieved by rest.

antacid. A substance that neutralizes acid in the stomach, esophagus, or the first part of the duodenum.

antibiotic. Tending to destroy or inhibit the growth of microorganisms, especially bacteria and/or fungi; or a substance that has this property.

antibody. A protein molecule made by the immune system that is designed to intercept and neutralize a specific invading organism or other foreign substance.

antigen. A substance that can elicit the formation of an antibody when introduced into the body.

antihistamine. A substance that interferes with the action of histamines by binding to histamine receptors in various body tissues (*see* histamine).

antioxidant. A substance that blocks or inhibits destructive oxidation reactions. Examples include vitamins C and E, the minerals selenium and germanium, the enzymes catalase and superoxide dismutase (SOD), coenzyme Q_{10}, and some amino acids.

arrhythmia. *See* cardiac arrhythmia.

arteriosclerosis. A circulatory disorder characterized by a thickening and stiffening of the walls of large and medium-sized arteries, which impedes circulation.

artery. A blood vessel through which blood is pumped from the heart to all the organs, glands, and other tissues of the body.

ascorbate. A mineral salt of vitamin C. Taken as nutritional supplements, ascorbates are less acidic (and therefore less irritating) than pure ascorbic acid and also provide for better absorption of both the vitamin C and the mineral.

ascorbic acid. The organic acid more commonly known as vitamin C.

atherosclerosis. The most common type of arteriosclerosis, caused by the accumulation of fatty deposits in the inner linings of the arteries.

autoimmune disorder. Any condition in which the immune system reacts inappropriately to the body's own tissues and attacks them, causing damage and/or interfering with normal functioning. Examples include Bright's disease, diabetes, multiple sclerosis, rheumatoid arthritis, and systemic lupus erythematosus.

autologous transfusion. A transfusion of one's own blood that has been collected and kept for later use.

bacteria. Single-celled microorganisms. Some bacteria can cause disease; other ("friendly") bacteria are normally present in the body and perform such useful functions as aiding digestion and protecting the body from harmful invading organisms.

benign. Literally, "harmless." Used to refer to cells, especially cells growing in inappropriate locations, that are not malignant (cancerous).

beta-carotene. A substance the body uses to make vitamin A.

bile. A bitter, yellowish substance that is released by the liver into the intestines for the digestion of fats.

biofeedback. A technique for helping an individual to become conscious of usually unconscious body processes, such as heartbeat or body temperature, so that he or she can gain some measure of control over them, and thereby learn to manage the effects of various disorders, including acute back pain, migraines, and Raynaud's disease.

bioflavonoid. Any of a group of biologically active flavonoids. They are essential for the stability and absorption of vitamin C. Although they are not technically vitamins, they are sometimes referred to as vitamin P.

biopsy. Excision of tissue from a living being for diagnosis.

blood count. A basic diagnostic test in which a sample of blood is examined and the number of red blood cells, white blood cells, and platelets determined; or the results of such a test.

blood sugar. The glucose (a form of sugar) present in the blood.

blood-brain barrier. A mechanism involving the capillaries and certain other cells of the brain that keeps many substances, especially water-based substances, from passing out of the blood vessels to be absorbed by the brain tissue.

bowel tolerance. The amount of any substance the body can tolerate before it results in diarrhea.

bronchi. The two main branches of the trachea (windpipe) that lead to the lungs.

Candida albicans. A type of fungus normally present at some level in the body. If it is present in overabundance, it causes yeast infection. Known as candida.

capillaries. Tiny blood vessels (their walls are about one cell thick) that allow the exchange of nutrients and wastes between the bloodstream and the body's cells.

carbohydrate. Any one of many organic substances, almost all of them of plant origin, that are composed of carbon, hydrogen, and oxygen, and serve as the major source of energy in the diet.

carcinogen. An agent that is capable of inducing cancerous changes in cells and/or tissues.

cardiac. Pertaining to the heart.

cardiac arrhythmia. An abnormal heart rate or rhythm.

carotene. A yellow to orange pigment that is converted into vitamin A in the body. There are several different forms, including alpha-, beta-, and gamma-carotene.

carotenoids. A group of phytochemicals that act as antioxidants and includes the carotenes as well as some other substances.

CAT scan. Computerized axial tomography scan. A computerized x-ray scanning procedure used to create a three-dimensional picture of the body, or part of the body, for the purpose of detecting abnormalities.

cauterization. A technique used to stop bleeding that involves applying electrical current, a laser beam, or a chemical such as silver nitrate directly to a broken blood vessel.

cell. A very small but complex organic unit consisting of a nucleus, cytoplasm, and a cell membrane. All living tissues are composed of cells.

cellulose. An indigestible carbohydrate found in the outer layers of fruits and vegetables.

cerebral. Pertaining to the brain.

chelation. A chemical process by which a larger molecule or group of molecules surround or enclose a mineral atom.

chelation therapy. The introduction of certain substances into the body so that they will chelate, and then remove, foreign substances such as lead, cadmium, arsenic, and other heavy metals. Chelation therapy can also be used to reduce or remove calcium-based plaque from the linings of the blood vessels, easing the flow of blood to vital organs and tissues.

chemotherapy. Treatment of disease by the use of chemicals (such as drugs), especially the use of chemical treatments to combat cancer.

chiropractic. A system of healing based on the belief that many disorders result from misalignments (called subluxations) of the spinal vertebrae and other joints. Chiropractors primarily treat illness by using physical manipulation techniques to bring the body into proper alignment and thus restore normal health and functioning.

chlorophyll. The pigment responsible for the green color of plant tissues. It can be taken in supplement form as a source of magnesium and trace elements.

cholesterol. A crystalline substance that is soluble in fats and that is produced by all vertebrates. It is a necessary constituent of cell membranes and facilitates the transport and absorption of fatty acids. Excess cholesterol, however, is a potential threat to health.

chromosome. Any of the threadlike strands of DNA in the nuclei of all living cells that carry genetic information. There are normally forty-six chromosomes (twenty-three pairs) in all human cells, with the exception of egg and sperm cells.

chronic illness. A disorder that persists or recurs over an extended period, often for life. Chronic illnesses can be as relatively benign as hay fever or as serious as multiple sclerosis.

citric acid. An organic acid found in citrus fruits. Often used to lower the pH of cosmetic products to bring them closer to the natural pH of the skin.

clotting factor. One of several substances, especially vitamin K, that are present in the bloodstream and are important in the process of blood clotting.

co-carcinogen. An agent that acts with another to cause cancer.

coenzyme. A molecule that works with an enzyme to enable the enzyme to perform its function in the body. Coenzymes are necessary in the utilization of vitamins and minerals.

cold-pressed. A term used to describe food oils that are extracted without the use of heat in order to preserve nutrients and flavor.

colic. Sharp abdominal pains that result from spasm or obstruction of certain organs or structures, especially the intestines, uterus, or bile ducts.

colonoscope. An instrument for examining the colon.

complete protein. A source of dietary protein that contains a full complement of the eight essential amino acids.

complex carbohydrate. A type of carbohydrate that, owing to its chemical structure, releases its sugar into the body relatively slowly and also provides fiber. The carbohydrates in starches and fiber are complex carbohydrates. Also called *polysaccharides*.

complication. A secondary infection, reaction, or other negative event that makes recovery from illness more difficult and/or longer.

congenital. Present from birth, but not necessarily inherited.

contraceptive. Tending to prevent conception, or a device, substance, or method used to prevent pregnancy.

contusion. A bruise; an injury in which the skin is not broken.

convulsion. A seizure characterized by intense, uncontrollable contraction of the voluntary muscles that results from abnormal cerebral stimulation.

coryza. The nasal symptoms of the common cold.

cruciferous. Literally, "cross-shaped." A term used to refer to a group of vegetables—including broccoli, Brussels sprouts, cabbage, cauliflower, turnips, and rutabagas—that have characteristic cross-shaped blossoms and that contain substances that may help to prevent colon cancer.

cystoscope. Instrument used to examine the urinary bladder.

dementia. A permanent acquired impairment of intellectual function that results in a marked decline in memory, language ability, personality, visuospatial skills, and/or cognition (orientation, perception, reasoning, abstract thinking, and calculation). Dementia can be either static or permanent, and can result from many different causes.

demulcent. Soothing, especially to mucous membranes.

dermis. The layer of skin that lies underneath the epidermis. Blood and lymphatic vessels and the glands that secrete perspiration and sebum are all found in the dermis.

detoxification. The process of reducing the buildup of various poisonous substances in the body.

disorientation. The loss of a normal relationship to one's surroundings; the inability to comprehend time, people, and place.

dithiolthiones. Phytochemicals found in broccoli that increase levels of enzymes that help protect against certain types of cancer.

diuretic. Tending to increase urine flow, or a substance that promotes the excretion of fluids.

dosha. Any of the three types of vital energy in Ayurvedic medicine. It is the balance between the doshas that determines health.

DNA. Deoxyribonucleic acid. Substance in the cell nucleus that genetically contains the cell's genetic blueprint and determines the type of life form into which a cell will develop.

echocardiogram. A diagnostic test that uses ultrasound to detect structural and functional abnormalities of the heart.

edema. Retention of fluid in the tissues that results in swelling.

EDTA. Ethylenediaminetetraacetic acid. An organic molecule used in chelation therapy.

EEG. Electroencephalogram. A test used to measure brain wave activity.

EKC (or ECG). Electrocardiogram. A test that monitors heart function by tracing the conduction of electrical impulses associated with heart activity.

elastin. A protein that gives tissue its elasticity.

electrolyte. Soluble salts dissolved in the body's fluids. Electrolytes are the form in which most minerals circulate in the body. They are so named because they are capable of conducting electrical impulses.

ELISA. Enzyme-linked immunoadsorbent assay. A test that determines the presence of a particular protein, such as an antibody, by detecting the presence of an enzyme that is linked to that protein.

ellagic acid. A phytochemical found in strawberries and grapes that helps rid the body of free radicals.

embolus. A loose particle of tissue, a bloot clot, or a tiny air bubble that travels through the bloodstream and, if it lodges in a narrowed portion of a blood vessel, can block blood flow.

emulsion. A combination of two liquids that do not mix with each other, such as oil and water; one substance is broken into tiny droplets and is suspended within the other. Emulsification is the first step in the digestion of fats.

endemic. Native to or prevalent in a particular geographic region. Often used to describe diseases.

endocrine system. The system of glands that secrete hormones into the bloodstream. Endocrine glands include the pituitary, thyroid, thymus, and adrenal glands, as well as the pancreas, ovaries, and testes.

endorphin. One of a number of natural hormonelike substances found primarily in the brain. One function of endorphins is to suppress the sensation of pain, which they do by binding to opiate receptors in the brain.

endoscope. Instrument for examining the interior of a hollow organ.

enteric. Pertaining to the small intestines.

enzyme. One of many specific protein catalysts that initiate or speed chemical reactions in the body without being consumed.

epidemic. An extensive outbreak of a disease, or a disease occurring with an unusually high incidence at certain times and places.

epidermis. The outer layer of the skin.

Epstein-Barr virus (EBV). A virus that causes infectious mononucleosis and that may cause other health problems as well, especially in people with compromised immune systems.

erythema. Reddening, especially of the skin.

essential. A term for nutrients needed for building and repair that cannot be manufactured by the body, and that therefore must be supplied in the diet. At present, there are some forty-two known essential nutrients.

essential fatty acids (EFAs). Three unsaturated fatty acids—arachidonic acid, linoleic acid, and linolenic acid—that are essential for health and cannot be manufactured by the body.

excision. Surgical cutting away and/or removal of tissue.

fat-soluble. Capable of dissolving in the same organic solvents as fats and oils.

fatty acid. Any one of many organic acids from which fats and oils are made.

FBS. Fasting blood sugar. The level of glucose present in a blood sample drawn at least eight hours after the last meal.

fiber. The indigestible portion of plant matter. Fiber is an important component of a healthy diet because it is capable of binding to toxins and escorting them out of the body.

flatulence. Excessive amounts of gas in the stomach or other parts of the digestive tract.

flavonoid. Any of a large group of crystalline compounds found in plants. Also called bioflavonoid.

free radical. An atom or group of atoms that is highly chemically reactive because it has at least one unpaired electron. Because they join so readily with other compounds, free radicals can attack cells and can cause a lot of damage in the body. Free radicals form in heated fats and oils, and as a result of exposure to atmospheric radiation and environmental pollutants, among other things.

free radical scavenger. A substance that removes or destroys free radicals.

fungus. One of a class of organisms that includes yeasts, mold, and mushrooms. A number of fungal species, such as *Candida albicans*, are capable of causing severe disease in immunocompromised hosts.

gastritis. Inflammation of the stomach lining.

gastroenteritis. Inflammation of the mucous lining of the stomach and the intestines.

gastrointestinal. Pertaining to the stomach, small and large intestines, colon, rectum, liver, pancreas, and gallbladder.

genetic. Inherited.

genistein. An isoflavone (a type of phytochemical) found in alfalfa sprouts, broccoli, cabbage, collard greens, kale, and soybeans. It aids with symptoms of perimenopause and may prevent some cancers.

GERD. Gastroesophageal reflux disease. Medical term for a syndrome characterized by frequent indigestion or heartburn.

gingivitis. Inflammation of the gums surrounding the teeth.

gland. An organ or tissue that secretes a substance(s) for use elsewhere in the body rather than for its own functioning.

globulin. A type of protein found in the blood. Certain globulins contain disease-fighting antibodies.

glucose. A simple sugar that is the principal source of energy for the body's cells.

gluten. A protein found in many grains, including wheat, rye, barley, and oats.

glycogen. A polysaccharide (complex carbohydrate) that is the main form in which glucose is stored in the body, primarily in the liver and muscles. It is converted back into glucose as needed to supply energy.

hair analysis. A method of determining the levels of minerals, including both toxic metals and essential minerals, in the body by measuring the concentrations of those minerals in the hair. Unlike mineral levels in the blood, those in the hair reflect the person's status over several preceding months.

HDL cholesterol. A type of lipoprotein (a protein molecule that transports cholesterol in the bloodstream) that is commonly referred to as "good cholesterol" because high levels normally indicate a low risk for heart disease.

heavy metal. A metallic element whose specific gravity (a measurement of mass as compared with the mass of water or hydrogen) is greater than 5.0. Some heavy metals, such as arsenic, cadmium, lead, and mercury, are extremely toxic.

hematocrit. The percentage of blood (by volume) that is composed of red blood cells.

hematoma. A bulge or swelling that is filled with blood. Hematomas are usually the result of a blunt injury or other trauma that causes a blood vessel under the skin to break.

hemicellulose. An indigestible carbohydrate resembling cellulose, found in plant cell walls, that absorbs water.

hemoglobin. The iron-containing red pigment in the blood that is responsible for the transport of oxygen.

hemorrhage. Profuse or abnormal bleeding.

hepatic. Pertaining to the liver.

hepatitis. A general term for inflammation of the liver. It can result from infection or exposure to toxins.

herbal therapy. The use of herbal combinations for healing or cleansing purposes. Herbs can be used in tablet, capsule, tincture, or extract form, as well as in baths and poultices.

hernia. A condition in which part of an internal organ protrudes, inappropriately, through an opening in the tissues that are supposed to contain it.

histamine. A chemical released by the immune system that acts on various body tissues. It has the effect of constricting the smooth bronchial tube muscles, dilating small blood vessels, allowing fluid to leak from various tissues, and increasing the secretion of stomach acid.

HIV. Human immunodeficiency virus. The virus that causes AIDS.

Hodgkin's disease. A type of lymphoma (cancer of the lymphatic system).

homeopathy. A medical system based on the belief that "like cures like"—that is, that illness can be cured by taking a *minute* dose of a substance that, if taken by a healthy person, would produce symptoms like those being treated. Homeopathy employs a variety of plant, animal, and mineral substances in very small doses to stimulate the body's natural healing powers and to bring the body back into balance.

hormone. One of numerous essential substances produced by the endocrine glands that regulate many bodily functions.

host. An organism in or on which another organism lives and from which the invading organism obtains nourishment.

hyaluronic acid. An organic acid known as the most effective natural skin moisturizer. It is present in human skin and is able to hold 500 times its own weight in water.

hydrochloric acid. A strong, corrosive inorganic acid that is produced in the stomach to aid in digestion.

hydrogenation. A chemical process used to turn liquid oils into more solid form by bombarding the oil molecules with hydrogen atoms. Hydrogenation destroys the nutritional value of the oil and also results in the formation of potentially cis- and trans-fatty acids, strangely altered fatty acid molecules that do not occur in nature.

hypercalcemia. The presence of abnormally high amounts of calcium in the blood.

hypertension. High blood pressure. Generally, hypertension is defined as a regular resting pressure over 140/90.

hypoallergenic. Having a low capacity for inducing hypersensitive (allergic) reactions.

hypocalcemia. The presence of abnormally low amounts of calcium in the blood.

hypotension. Low blood pressure.

hypothalamus. A portion of the brain that regulates many aspects of metabolism, including body temperature and the hunger response.

idiopathic. Term describing a disease of unknown cause.

immune globulin. A protein that functions as an antibody in the body's immune response. Immune globulins are manufactured by certain white blood cells and found in body fluids and on mucous membranes.

immune system. A complex system that depends on the interaction of many different organs, cells, and proteins. Its chief function is to identify and eliminate foreign substances such as harmful bacteria that have invaded the body. The liver, spleen, thymus, bone marrow, and lymphatic system all play vital roles in the proper functioning of the immune system.

immunity. The condition of being able to resist and overcome disease or infection.

immunodeficiency. A defect in the functioning of the immune system. It can be inherited or acquired, reversible or permanent. Immunodeficiency renders the body more susceptible to illness of every type, especially infectious illnesses.

immunology. The branch of medical science that deals with the functioning of the immune system.

immunotherapy. Treatment of disease by using techniques to stimulate or strengthen the immune system.

incubation period. The period of time between exposure to an infectious disease and the appearance of symptoms, during which the infection is developing.

infection. Invasion of body tissues by disease-causing organisms such as viruses, protozoa, fungi, or bacteria.

infestation. An invasion of the body by parasites such as insects, worms, or protozoa.

inflammation. A reaction to illness or injury characterized by swelling, warmth, and redness.

inguinal. Pertaining to the groin.

insomnia. The inability to sleep.

insulin. A hormone produced by the pancreas that regulates the metabolism of glucose (sugar) in the body.

interaction. A phenomenon that occurs when two or more substances affect one another's activity or combine to create a different effect than any of them would have on its own. Any substance introduced into the body can potentially interact with another substance or substances already present. Drugs, foods, herbs, minerals, and vitamins can all interact with one another.

interferon. A protein produced by the cells in response to viral infection that prevents viral reproduction and is capable of protecting uninfected cells from viral infection. There are different types of interferon, designated alpha, beta, and gamma.

interleukin. Any of a number of immune system chemicals manufactured by the body to aid in fighting infection.

intestinal flora. The "friendly" bacteria present in the intestines that are essential for the digestion and metabolism of certain nutrients.

intolerance. Nutritionally, the inability to digest a particular food, usually due to a lack or deficiency of certain enzymes.

intravenous (IV) infusion. The use of a needle inserted in a vein to assist in fluid replacement or the giving of medication.

ischemia. The condition of being starved for blood. Ischemia affecting the heart or brain can cause a heart attack or stroke.

isoflavones. A class of phytochemical that inhibits the uptake of estrogen, which may help prevent estrogen based cancers such as breast cancer.

IU. International unit. A measure of potency based on an accepted international standard. Dosages of vitamin A and E supplements, among others, are usually measured in international units. Because this is a measurement of potency, not weight or volume, the number of milligrams in an international unit varies, depending on the substance being measured.

lactase. An enzyme that converts lactose into glucose and galactose. It is necessary for the digestion of milk and milk products.

lactic acid. An acid that results from anaerobic glucose metabolism. It is present in certain foods, including certain fruits and sour milk (when milk becomes sour, this means that some of the lactose, or milk sugar, it contained has been converted into lactic acid). Lactic acid is also produced in the muscles during anaerobic exercise. It is the buildup of lactic acid that causes muscle fatigue during strenuous activity. Synthetic lactic acid is used in food products as a flavoring and preservative.

lactobacilli. Any of a number of species of bacteria that are capable of transforming lactose (milk sugar) into lactic acid through fermentation. Lactobacilli are naturally present in the colon and are sometimes referred to as "friendly" bacteria because they aid in digestion and fight certain disease-causing microorganisms. The two species of lactobacilli most commonly available in supplement form are *L. acidophilus* and *L. bifidus*.

laser. Light amplification by stimulated emission of radiation. An instrument that focuses highly amplified light waves. Lasers are used in surgical procedures, especially eye surgery.

LDL cholesterol. A type of lipoprotein (a protein molecule that transports cholesterol in the bloodstream) that is commonly referred to as "bad cholesterol" because high levels normally indicate a high risk of heart disease.

lecithin. A mixture of phospholipids that is composed of fatty acids, glycerol, phosphorus, and choline or inositol. All living cell membranes are largely composed of lecithin.

leukemia. Cancer of the blood-producing tissues, especially the bone marrow and lymph nodes, resulting in an overabundance of white blood cells. It can be either acute (most common in children) or chronic (most common in adults). It is similar in certain respects to Hodgkin's disease.

limbic system. A group of deep brain structures that, among other things, transmit the perception of pain to the brain and generate an emotional reaction to it.

limonoids. Phytochemicals found in citrus fruits that may inhibit the production of cancerous tumors.

lipid. Substances found in nature that are soluble in the same organic solvents as fats and oils are. Important nutritional lipids include choline, gamma linolenic acid, inositol, lecithin, and linoleic acid.

lipoprotein. A type of protein molecule that incorporates a lipid. Lipoproteins act as agents of lipid transport in the lymph and blood.

lipotropic. Any of a number of substances that help to prevent the accumulation of abnormal or excessive amounts of fat in the liver, control blood sugar levels, and enhance fat and carbohydrate metabolism. Commonly used lipotropics include choline, inositol, and methionine.

lutein. A phytochemical (one of the carotenoids) found in kale, spinach, and other dark green leafy vegetables that is beneficial for the eyes. It may help protect against macular degeneration.

lycopene. A phytochemical found in tomatoes that appears to afford protection against prostate cancer and to protect the skin against harm from ultraviolet rays.

lymph. A clear fluid derived from blood plasma that circulates throughout the body, is collected from the tissues, and flows through the lymphatic vessels, eventually returning to the bloodstream. Its function is to nourish tissue cells and return waste matter to the bloodstream.

lymph nodes. Organs located in the lymphatic vessels that act as filters, trapping and removing foreign material. They also form lymphocytes, immune cells that develop the capacity to seek out and destroy specific foreign agents.

lymphadenopathy. Enlargement of a lymph node or nodes as a result of the presence of a foreign substance or disease. This condition is often referred to as "swollen glands."

lymphocyte. A type of white blood cell found in lymph, blood, and other specialized tissues, such as the bone marrow and tonsils. There are several different categories of lymphocytes, designated B-lymphocytes, T-lymphocytes, and null (or non-B, non-T) lymphocytes. These cells are crucial components of the immune system. B-lymphocytes are primarily responsible for antibody production, whereas the T-lymphocytes are involved in the direct attack against invading organisms. It is the T-helper cell, a subtype of T-lymphocyte, that is the primary cell infected and destroyed by human immunodeficiency virus (HIV), the virus that causes AIDS.

lymphokine. Any of a group of substances produced by the cells of the immune system when exposed to antigens. They are not antibodies, but rather perform such functions as stimulating the production of additional lymphocytes and activating other immune cells.

lymphoma. Cancer of the lymphatic tissues.

macrobiotics. A dietary approach adapted from Far Eastern philosophy whose basic principle consists of balancing the yin and yang energies of foods. Yin foods, such as water, are expansive; yang foods, such as salt or meat, are contractile. For the most part, the macrobiotic diet consists of whole grain cereals, millet, rice, soups, and vegetables, with beans and supplementary foods depending on the individual and the condition. Different conditions are considered either yin or yang, so the macrobiotic program must be adapted to each individual.

macrophage. A type of immune cell that surrounds and digests foreign materials and cellular debris in the body.

malabsorption. Nutritionally, a defect in the absorption of nutrients from the intestinal tract into the bloodstream.

malignant. Literally, "evil." Used to refer to cells or groups of cells that are cancerous and likely to spread.

mammography. An x-ray examination of the breast.

melanoma. A malignant tumor originating from pigment cells in the deep layers of the skin.

menopause. The cessation of menstruation, caused by a sharp decrease in the production of the sex hormones estrogen and progesterone. Menopause usually occurs after the age of forty-five or following the removal of the female reproductive organs.

metabolism. The physical and chemical processes necessary to sustain life, including the production of cellular energy, the synthesis of important biological substances, and degradation of various compounds.

metabolite. A substance produced as a result of a metabolic process.

metastasis. The spread of cancer to a site or sites away from the original tumor.

microgram. A measurement of weight equivalent to $1/1,000$ milligram.

milligram. A measurement of weight equivalent to $1/1,000$ gram (a gram is equal to approximately $1/28$ ounce).

mineral. An inorganic substance required by the body in small quantities.

monoterpenes. Phytochemicals found in citrus fruits, eggplant, green vegetables, tomatoes, and yams that act as antioxidants and help protect the immune system.

MRI. Magnetic resonance imaging. A technique used in diagnosis that combines the use of radio waves and a strong magnetic field to produce detailed images of the internal structures of the body.

mucous membranes. Membranes that line the cavities and canals of the body that communicate with the air. Examples include the membranes lining the inside of the mouth, nose, anus, and vagina.

myelin sheath. A fatty covering that protects nerve cells. Myelin sheaths are noticeably damaged or missing in people with multiple sclerosis.

naturopathy. A form of health care that uses diet, herbs, and other natural methods and substances to cure illness. The goal is to produce a healthy body state without the use of drugs by stimulating innate defenses.

neuropathy. A complex of symptoms caused by abnormalities in motor or sensory nerves. Symptoms may include tingling or numbness, especially in the hands or feet, followed by gradual, progressive muscular weakness.

neurotransmitter. A chemical that transmits nerve impulses from one nerve cell to another. Major neurotransmitters include acetylcholine, dopamine, gamma-aminobutyric acid, norepinephrine, and serotonin.

nucleic acid. Any of a class of chemical compounds found in all viruses and plant and animal cells. Ribonucleic acid (RNA) and deoxyribonucleic acid (DNA), which contain the genetic instructions for every living cell, are two principal types.

nutraceutical. A food- or nutrient-based product or supplement designed and/or used for a specific clinical and/or therapeutic purpose.

nutrient. A substance that is needed by the body to maintain life and health.

occult blood test. A test that detects the presence of blood in bodily excretions such as stool, sputum, or urine. It is most often used in screening for cancer.

oncologist. A cancer specialist.

oncology. The medical specialty dealing with cancer.

organic. A term used to describe foods that are grown without the use of synthetic chemicals, such as pesticides, herbicides, and hormones.

osteopathy. A system of medicine based on the belief that the body is a vital mechanical organism whose structural and functional integrity are coordinated and interdependent, and that disturbances in the musculoskeletal system can therefore cause disorders elsewhere in the body. Because of this philosophy, although osteopaths can prescribe drugs and perform surgery, they are more likely to recommend physical therapy or musculoskeletal manipulation as the treatment of first choice.

osteoporosis. A disorder in which minerals leach out of the bones, rendering them progressively more porous and fragile.

oxidation. A chemical reaction in which oxygen reacts with another substance, resulting in a chemical transformation. Many oxidation reactions result in some type of deterioration or spoilage.

Pap test. Microscopic examination of cells collected from the vagina and cervix to test for signs of cancer.

parasite. An organism that lives on or in another organism and obtains nourishment from it.

pathogen. A toxin or small organisms that can cause disease.

peptide. A substance composed of two or more amino acids.

perimenopause. The period before menopause—possibly starting as much as ten years before—during which women may experience uncomfortable symptoms because of fluctuating hormones.

peristalsis. The rhythmic contractions of the muscles of the digestive tract that move matter into the stomach, through the intestines, and, ultimately, out of the body.

pH. Potential of hydrogen. A scale used to measure the relative acidity or alkalinity of substances. The scale runs from 0 to 14. A pH of 7 is considered neutral; numbers below 7 denote increasing acidity and numbers above 7 denote increasing alkalinity.

pharyngitis. Sore throat.

phenylketonuria (PKU). An inherited disorder caused by a lack of an enzyme necessary to convert the amino acid phenylalanine into another amino acid, tyrosine, so that excesses can be eliminated from the body. A buildup of excess phenylalanine in the blood can lead to neurological disturbances and mental retardation.

phytochemical. Any one of many substances present in fruits and vegetables (*phyto* means "plant" in Greek). There are hundreds of phytochemicals, and more are being identified every day. Some appear to help protect the body against illness, including such serious diseases as cancer and heart disease.

pituitary. A gland located at the base of the brain that secretes a number of different hormones. Pituitary hormones regulate growth and metabolism by coordinating the actions of other endocrine glands.

placebo. A pharmacologically inactive substance, primarily used in experiments to provide a basis for comparison with pharmacologically active substances.

plaque. An unwanted deposit of a certain substance on tissues, often with the potential to cause some type of health problem. The buildup of plaque in the arteries is a leading cause of cardiovascular disease; plaque deposits on the teeth can lead to gum disease; Alzheimer's disease is associated with the accumulation of characteristic plaques in brain tissue.

precancerous lesion. Abnormal tissue that is not malignant, but that may be in the process of becoming so.

probiotics. Elements that encourage the growth of beneficial bacteria in the body.

prognosis. A forecast as to the likely course and/or outcome of a disorder or condition.

progesterone. A hormone whose functions include preparing a woman's body for pregnancy in the second half of the menstrual cycle. Progesterone cream is used in hormone replacement therapy to prevent vaginal atrophy.

prostaglandin. Any of a number of hormonelike chemicals that are made in the body from essential fatty acids and that have important effects on target organs. They influence the secretion of hormones and enzymes, and are important in regulating the inflammatory response, blood pressure, and blood-clotting time.

protein. Any of many complex nitrogen-based organic compounds made up of different combinations of amino acids. Proteins are basic elements of all animal and vegetable tissues. Biological substances such as hormones and enzymes also are composed of protein. The body makes the specific proteins it needs for growth, repair, and other functions from amino acids that are either extracted from dietary protein or manufactured from other amino acids.

proteolytic enzymes. Enzymes that break down dietary proteins, yet do not attack the proteins that make up the normal cells of the body. Proteolytic enzymes may have value in fighting cancer and other diseases. Cancer cells have a type of protein coating; theoretically, if this coating is destroyed by proteolytic enzymes, the white blood cells would be able to attack the cancer cells and destroy them.

pruritus. Itching.

pulmonary. Pertaining to the lungs.

purulent. Containing or causing the production of pus.

radiation. Energy that is emitted or transmitted in the form of waves. The term is often used to refer to radioactivity; however, radioactivity is a specific type of radiation that comes from the decay of unstable atoms.

radiation therapy. A type of treatment, most often used for cancer, that involves the use of ionizing radiation, including Roentgen rays, radium, or other radioactive substances to destroy specific areas of tissue. Also called *radiotherapy.*

RAST. Radioallergosorbent test. A blood test that measures levels of specific antibodies produced by the body's immune system, used to test for allergic reactions.

RDA. Recommended daily allowance. The amount of a vitamin or other nutrient that should be consumed daily in order to prevent nutritional deficiency. RDAs are determined by the U.S. Food and Drug Administration.

red blood cell. A blood cell that contains the red pigment hemoglobin and transports oxygen and carbon dioxide in the bloodstream.

remission. Lessening or reversal of the signs and symptoms of disease. This term is used particularly of serious and/or chronic illnesses such as cancer and multiple sclerosis.

renal. Pertaining to the kidneys.

retinoic acid. Vitamin A acid. A form of retinoic acid is the active ingredient in the medication Retin-A.

retrovirus. A type of virus that has RNA as its core nucleic acid and contains an enzyme called *reverse transcriptase* that permits the virus to copy its RNA into the DNA of infected cells, in effect taking over the cells' genetic machinery. Human immunodeficiency virus (HIV), the virus that causes AIDS, is a retrovirus. Retroviruses are also known to cause certain types of cancer in animals and are suspected of causing forms of leukemia and lymphoma in humans.

RNA. Ribonucleic acid. A complex protein found in plant and animal cells. RNA carries coded genetic information from DNA, in the cell nucleus, to protein-producing cell structures called ribosomes, where these instructions are translated into the form of protein molecules—the basic component of all living tissue.

saturated fat. A fat that is solid at room temperature. Most saturated fats are of animal origin, although a few, such as coconut oil and palm oil, come from plants.

saturation. With regard to fats, the term "saturation" refers to the chemical structure of the fatty acid molecules, specifically the number of hydrogen atoms present. Fat molecules that cannot incorporate any additional hydrogen atoms are said to be *saturated;* those that could incorporate one additional hydrogen atom are referred to as *monounsaturated;* and those that could incorporate two or more additional hydrogen atoms are referred to as *polyunsaturated.*

scratch test. A procedure in which a small amount of a suspected allergen is applied to a lightly scratched area of skin to test for an allergic reaction.

sebum. The oily secretion produced by glands in the skin.

secondary infection. An infection that develops after and is made possible by the presence or effect of a previous infection, inflammation, or other condition, but that is not necessarily directly caused by it.

seizure. A sudden, brief episode characterized by changes in consciousness, perception, muscular motion, and/or behavior. A convulsion is a type of seizure.

serotonin. A neurotransmitter found principally in the brain that is considered essential for relaxation, sleep, and concentration.

serum. The fluid portion of the blood.

simple carbohydrate. A type of carbohydrate that, owing to its chemical structure, is rapidly digested and absorbed into the bloodstream. Glucose, lactose, and fructose are examples of simple carbohydrates.

sorbic acid. An organic acid used as a food preservative.

steroid. One of a group of fat-soluble organic compounds with a characteristic chemical composition. A number of different hormones, drugs, and other substances—including cholesterol—are classified as steroids.

stroke. An attack in which the brain is suddenly deprived of oxygen as a result of interrupted blood flow. If it continues for more than a few minutes, brain damage and even death may result.

sublingual. Literally, "under the tongue." Sublingual medications and supplements often look like tablets or liquids meant for swallowing, but they are designed to be held in the mouth while the active ingredient is absorbed into the bloodstream through the mucous membranes.

symptom. An alteration in normal feeling or functioning experienced as a result of a bodily disorder.

syncope. Temporary loss of consciousness; fainting.

syndrome. A group of signs and symptoms that together are known or presumed to characterize a disorder.

synergy. An interaction between two or more substances in which their action is greater when they are together than the sum of their individual actions would be.

systemic. Pertaining to the entire body.

T cell. A type of lymphocyte that is a crucial part of the immune system.

teratogen. An agent that causes malformation of a developing embryo or fetus.

thrombus. An obstruction in a blood vessel.

thrush. A fungal infection caused by *Candida albicans* that is characterized by small whitish spots on the tongue and the insides of the cheeks. It occurs most often in infants and in persons with compromised immune systems.

topical. Pertaining to the surface of the body.

toxicity. The quality of being poisonous. Toxicity reactions in the body impair bodily functions and/or damage cells.

toxin. A poison that impairs the health and functioning of the body.

trace element. A mineral required by the body in extremely small quantities.

tremor. Involuntary trembling.

triglyceride. A compound consisting of three fatty acids plus glycerol. Triglycerides are the form in which fat is stored in the body and are the primary type of lipid in the diet.

tumor. An abnormal mass of tissue that serves no function. Tumors are usually categorized as either benign or malignant (cancerous).

type A personality. A personality that tends to be impatient and aggressive. Persons with type A personalities tend to have stronger stress reactions and may be more susceptible to cardiovascular disease.

type B personality. A personality that tends to be relaxed and patient, and less reactive to stress. Those with type B personalities may be less prone to develop stress-related illnesses such as high blood pressure and heart disease.

ultrasound. Ultra-high-frequency sound waves. Ultrasound technology is used in a number of different medical diagnostic and treatment tools.

unsaturated fat. Any of a number of dietary fats that are liquid at room temperature. Unsaturated fats come from vegetable sources and are good sources of essential fatty acids. Examples include flaxseed oil, sunflower oil, safflower oil, and primrose oil.

urticaria. Hives.

vaccine. A preparation administered to achieve immunity against a specific agent by inducing the body to make antibodies to that agent. A vaccine may be a suspension of living or dead microorganisms, or a solution of an allergen or viral or bacterial antigens.

vascular. Pertaining to the circulatory system.

vein. One of the blood vessels that returns the blood from the body tissues to the heart.

venom. A poisonous substance produced by an animal, such as certain snakes and insects.

virus. Any of a vast group of minute, often disease-causing, structures composed of a protein coat and a core of DNA and/or RNA. Because they are incapable of reproducing on their own (they must reproduce inside the cells of an infected host), viruses are not technically considered living organisms. Unlike bacteria, viruses are not affected by antibiotics.

visualization. A technique that involves consciously using the mind to influence the health and functioning of the body. Also called creative visualization.

vital signs. Basic indicators of an individual's health status, including pulse, breathing, blood pressure, and body temperature.

vitamin. One of approximately fifteen organic substances that are essential in small quantities for life and health. Most vitamins cannot be manufactured by the body and so need to be supplied in the diet.

water-soluble. Capable of dissolving in water.

white blood cell. A blood cell that functions in fighting infection and in wound repair.

withdrawal. The process of adjustment that occurs when the use of a habit-forming substance to which the body has become accustomed is discontinued.

yang. In Chinese medicine, one of the two vital principles that must be in balance to create harmony and balance in the body. Yang is heat, light, and dryness. Yang organs include the spleen, gallbladder, intestines, and the skin.

yeast. A type of single-celled fungus. Certain types of yeast can cause infection, most commonly in the mouth, vagina, or gastrointestinal tract. Common yeast infections include vaginitis and thrush.

yin. In Chinese medicine, one of the two vital principles that must be in balance to create harmony and balance in the body. Yin is cold, shadow, and moisture. Yin organs include the heart, liver, kidneys, lungs, and bones.

Manufacturer and Distributor Information

Below are the manufacturers and distributors of some of the brand-name products mentioned in this book, plus their addresses and phone numbers. This information is provided to enable you to contact these companies to order or to obtain further information about their products. None of the manufacturers or distributors mentioned has had any connection with the production of this book. Rather, we list these companies because we believe their products to be effective and of high quality. Be aware that addresses and telephone numbers are subject to change.

A. Vogel Homeopathic
See Bioforce USA.

Ab Diagnostics
1383 Carriage Hill Drive SE
Grand Rapids, MI 49508-6232
800–211–6636 616–455–1945
http://www.abdiagnostics.com
Home testing kits for Hepatitis C and HIV.

Abkit, Inc.
207 East 94th Street, 2nd Floor
New York, NY 10128
800–226–6227 212–860–8358
CamoCare cream.

ABRA, Inc.
10365 Highway 116
Forestville, CA 95436
707–869–0761
http://www.abratherapeutics.com
VitaSerum.

Advanced Health Solutions
P.O. Box 937
Cardiff, CA 92007
800–943–0054
Acidophilus; colon health books; ProFlora Whey; Webster Witt Implant Kit.

Aerobic Life Industries
2916 North 35th Avenue, Suite 8
Phoenix, AZ 85017
800–798–0707 602–455–6380
http://www.aerobiclife.com
Aerobic Bulk Cleanse; Aerobic Heart; Aerobic 07; All-Purpose Bactericide Spray; Bee Venom Balm; Burn Gel; China Gold; Colon Formula; 45-Day MAX Colon Cleanse Kit; Homozon; Mag 0₇; MSM Capsules; MSM Lotion; 10-Day Colon Cleanse Kit.

AIM International
3904 East Flamingo Avenue
Nampa, ID 83687
800–456–2462 208–465–5116
http://www.theaimcompanies.com
Barleygreen.

AkPharma, Inc.
P.O. Box 111
Pleasantville, NJ 08232
800–732–6441 609–645–5100
Beano.

Alacer Corporation
19631 Pauling
Foothill Ranch, CA 92610
800–854–0249 949–951–9660
Emergen-C.

Aller//Guard Corporation
40 Cindy Lane
Ocean, NJ 07712–7248
800–234–0816 908–988–6868
X-MITE powder.

Allergy Control Products
96 Danbury Road
Ridgefield, CT 06877
800–422–3878
http://www.allergycontrol.com

Allergy Research Group
30806 Santana Street
P.O. Box 55907
Hayward, CA 94544
800–545–9960 510–487–8526
http://www.nutricology.com
ChronoSet.

Allovedic Remedies
American Formulary, Inc.
140 Ethel Road, Suites S–T
Piscataway, NJ 08854
732–985–9899
E-mail: info@americanformulary.com
http://www.americanformulary.com
Antioxidant Formula; Blood Sugar Balance Formula; Cardiotonic Support Formula; Energy Formula; Joint Support Formula; Liver Support Formula; Memory Support Formula; Probiotic with B-Complex Formula; Rejuvenator Support Formula; Respiratory Support Formula.

Alpine Industries
220 Reservoir
Needham Heights, MA 02194
800–628–2209
http://www.alpineindustries.com
Living Air XL-15.

American Biologics
1180 Walnut Avenue
Chula Vista, CA 91911
800–227–4473 619–429–8200
http://www.americanbiologics.com
AE Mulsion Forte; Bio-Bifidus; Bio-Dophilus; Bio-Rizin; Brain Power; Dioxychlor DC-3; Dioxychlor Oxy C-2 Gel; GE-132; Inflazyme Forte; Liquid Chlorophyll; Micellized Vitamin A emulsion; Multi-Glandular; Oxy-5000 Forte; Panoderm I; Selenium Forte; Sharkilage; Sub-Adrene; Taurine Plus; Ultra Brain Power; Ultra Connexin; Ultra Osteo Synergy.

America's Finest, Inc.
140 Ethel Road West, Suites S–T
Piscataway, NJ 08854
800–350–3305 732–985–9899
http://www.afisupplements.com
Bacopin & Ginkgo Complex.

Amerifit Nutrition
166 Highland Park Drive
Bloomfield, CT 06002
800–990–3476 860–242–3476
http://www.amerifit.com
Glucosamine & Chondroitin chewable wafers; Estroven.

Anabol Naturals
1550 Mansfield Street
Santa Cruz, CA 95062
800–426–2265 408–479–1403
Amino Balance; crystalline free-form amino acids; Muscle Octane.

Anurex Labs
P.O. Box 414760
Miami, FL 33141
305–757–7733
http://www.anurex.com
Anurex cryotherapy device for hemorrhoids.

Apollo Light Systems, Inc.
352 West 1060 South
Orem, UT 84058
800–545–9667 801–226–2370
http://www.apollolight.com
Brite Lite IV.

ASN, Inc.
P.O. Box 1277
Hood River, OR 97031
800–800–9119 541–387–4500
http://www.a-s-n.com
Humagro; Testatropinol.

Astrological Health
P.O. Box 19319
Boulder, CO 80308
877–700–9890 303–444–9890
Holistic herbal supplements; Zodiac Sign Wellness Formulas.

Ayurvedic Concepts
See Himalaya USA.

Bay to Bay Distribution, Inc.
453 Ravendale Drive, Suite A
Mountain View, CA 94043
800–647–5749 650–691–0108
http://www.baytobay.com
Maximum Living supplements, including Maximum Living Ginkgo Biloba with DHA.

Bayer Diagnostics
511 Benedict Avenue
Tarrytown, NY 10591
914–631–8000
http://bayerus.com/diagnostics
Glucometer Elite; Glucometer Encore.

BDP America, Inc.
See Nupharma Nutracueticals.

Bio-Nutritional Formulas
41 Bergen Line Avenue
Westwood, NJ 07675
201–666–2300
Eugalan Forte.

bioAllers
See NatraBio Homeopathic.

Bioforce USA
437 Route 295
Chatham, NY12037
800–641–7555 518–392–8787
http://www.bioforceUSA.com
Distributor of Bioforce AG and A. Vogel herbal and homeopathic products, including Calcium Absorption Formula; Cardiaforce; Echinaforce; Geriaforce; Menopause Relief; Molkosan Whey of Life; Prostasan.

Biomax Laboratories
P.O. Box 130803
Carlsbad, CA 92013-0803
800–541–3550 760–599–1142
http://www.tennis-elbow.net
CT Cream.

Biotec Foods
Division, AgriGenic Food Corporation
5152 Bolsa Avenue, Suite 101
Huntington Beach, CA 92649
800–788–1084 714–899–3477
http://www.biotec-foods.com
Ageless Beauty; Anti-Stress Enzymes; Bio-Gestin; Cell Guard.

Biotech Corporation
107 Oakwood Drive
Glastonbury, CT 06033
860–633–8111
Cellu-Rid; CholestaMax; Prostate R_x; Shen Min Hair Nutrient; Shen Min Topical Solution.

Biotics Research
8122 East Fulton
Ada, MI 49301
800–437–1298 616–676–3380
http://www.bioticsresearch.com
A.D.P.; Bio-Cardiozyme Forte; Cytozyme-F; Cytozyme-M; Intenzyme Forte; Neonatal Multi-Gland; Osteo-B-Plus.

Bluebonnet Nutrition Corporation
12915 Dairy Ashford
Sugar Land, TX 77478
800–580–8866 281–240–3332
http://www/bluebonnetnutrition.com
Diet Chrome-Care.

Bodyonics
140 Lauman Lane
Hicksville, NY 11801
800–588–9898 516–822–1230
Age Erasers; BotanImmune; CellaFree; Cold Immune; EstroGentle.

Boiron
6 Campus Boulevard, Building A
Newtown Square, PA 19073
800–BLU–TUBE 610–325–7464
Homeopathic remedies.

BotanicLab
2900-B Saturn Street
Brea, CA 92821
714–524–5533
http://www.botaniclab.com
Spes.

CamoCare
See Abkit Inc.

Cardinal Nutrition
1000 West 8th Street
Vancouver, WA 98660
888–733–5676 360–693–1883
http://www.cardinalmsm.com
OptiMSM.

Cardiovascular Research, Ltd.
1061 Shary Circle
Concord, CA 94518
800–888–4585 510–827–2636
Elastase; Essential Fatty Acid Complex; Lipothiamine; Serraflazyme.

Carlson Laboratories, Inc.
15 College Drive
Arlington Heights, IL 60004-1985
888–234–5656 847–255–1600
http://www.carlsonlabs.com
ACES; ACES + Zn; Amino Blend; Amino-VIL; D.A. #34; Co-Q-10; E-Gem Skin-Care Soap; E-Sel; Glutathione Booster; Key-E suppositories; salmon oil.

CC Pollen Company
3627 East Indian School Road, Suite 209
Phoenix, AZ 85018
800–875–0096 602–957–0096
http://www.ccpollen.com
Aller Bee-Gone.

Century Systems, Inc
P.O. Box 43725
120 Selig Drive
Atlanta, GA 30336
800–843–9662
http://www.1800thewoman.com
Miracle 2000.

CircAid Medical Products, Inc.
9323 Chesapeake Drive, Suite B-2
San Diego, CA 92123
800–247–2243 858–576–3550
http://www.circaid.com
Compression garments and bandages for treating lymphedema, venous insufficiency, and venous ulcers.

Coenzyme-A Technologies
12512 Beverly Park Road, B1
Lynnwood, WA 98037
425–438–8586
http://www.coenzyme-a.com
Body Image; Clear Skin Image; Coenzyme A; Healthy Cholesterol Image; Healthy Joint Image.

Continental Vitamin Company
4510 South Boyle Avenue
Los Angeles, CA 90058
800–421–6175 323–581–0176
http://www.cvc4health.com
Superior Source sublingual nutritional supplements, including Allergy Helper; Chromium Picolinate; Instant Enerjetz; No Shot B-6/B-12/Folic; Slumber Helper.

Country Life
101 Corporate Drive
Hauppauge, NY 11788
516–231–1031
http://www.country-life.com
Biochem Sports & Fitness products; Desert Essence tea tree oil products; Herbal Mood Boost; Long Life Teas; Saw Palmetto & Pygeum Capsules; Soy-Licious.

Custom Probiotics
3000 Honolulu Avenue, #4
Glendale, CA 91214
818–248–3529
High potency acidophilus and bifidus dietary supplements.

CWR Environmental Products Inc.
100 Carney Street
Glen Cove, NY 11542
800–444–3563 516–674–2441
http://www.cwrenviro.com
Ceramic water-filtration systems.

CX Research Inc.
275 Lotus Circle
Austin, TX 78737
512–288–2700
OmegaBrite.

Cytodyne Technologies
1920 Swarthmore Avenue
Lakewood, NJ 08701
732–363–3032
http://www.cytodyne.com
CytoPro.

DaVinci Laboratories
20 New England Drive, C-1504
Essex Junction, VT 05453-1504
800–325–1776 800–510–3676 (Canada)
http://www.davincilabs.com
*Flora; Olivir. Products available through
health professionals only.*

Derma-E Products Inc.
975 Independence Avenue
Chatsworth, CA 91311
800–521–3342
http://www.derma-e.com
*Ester-C Gel; Itch Relief Lotion; Pycnogenol
Crème (or Gel) with Vitamins E, C, & A;
Scar Gel; Vitamin A Moisturizing Gel;
Vitamin A Wrinkle Treatment; Vitamin E
Moisturizing Gel; Wrinkle Treatment Oil.*

Diamond-Herpanacine Associates
P.O. Box 544
Ambler, PA 19002
215–542–2981
http://www.diamondformulas.com
*Diamond Mind; Diamond Trim; Healthy
Horizons; Herpanacine.*

Doctor's Data, Inc.
P.O. Box 111
West Chicago, IL 60186
800–323–2784 630–377–8139
http://www.doctorsdata.com
Hair analysis services.

Earth Science
350 West Rincon Street
Corona, CA 92880
909–371–7565
*Skin care, hair care, and nutrition products,
including Micellized Multiple Vitamin and
Minerals.*

Earth's Bounty
See Matrix Health Products.

Eclectic Institute
14385 SE Lusted Road
Sandy, Oregon 97055
800–332–4372
*Organic herbs, herbal extracts, nutritional
supplements.*

Ecological Formulas
1061 Shary Circle
Concord, CA 94518
800–888–4585 510–827–2636
*B Cell Formula; Buffered Vitamin C Powder;
Caprystatin; Essential Fatty Acid Complex;
Free-Form Amino Acid Crystals;
Hypomultiple Vitamin-Mineral Formula;
Inflazyme; Novagest Cream; Orithrush;
Quercitin-C; Tri-Salts.*

Eden Foods, Inc.
701 Tecumseh Road
Clinton, MI 49236
888–424–3336 517–456–7424
http://www.edenfoods.com
Bifa-15.

Efamol Nutraceuticals, Inc.
23 Dry Dock Avenue
Boston, MA 02210
888–332–6651
http://www.efamol.com
*Essential fatty acid supplements, including
Efalex Focus.*

Emu Country, Inc.
1900 George Washington Boulevard
Wichita, KS 67218-3950
316–685–5666
http://www.emucountryusa.com
Emu Oil; Emu Plus.

En Garde Health Products
7702 Balboa Boulevard, Building #10
Van Nuys, CA 91406
800–955–4633 818–901–8505
http://www.engardehealth.com
DynamO2.

Enhanced Fitness
P.O. Box 189
Toronto, OH 43964
888–820–4675
http://www.enhancedfitness.com
Calorad.

Enzymatic Therapy
825 Challenger Drive
Green Bay, WI 54311
800–783–2286 414–469–1313
http://www.enzy.com
*Arthogesic; Asparagus Extract; Cell Forté
with IP-6; Cell Forté with IP-6 and Inositol;
Derma-Klear; Enada NADH; Esberitox;
GastroSoothe; GS-500; Grape Seed (PCO)
Phytosome; HyperiCalm; IP_6; Ivy Extract;
Kava-30; Liquid Liver Extract; Mega-Zyme;
Phytodolor; Remifemin; Remifemin Plus;
7-Keto; SinuCheck; ThymuPlex; Vira-Plex.*

Enzyme Process International
2035 East Cedar Street
Tempe, AZ 85281
602–731–9290
SAMe.

E'Ola International
3879 South River Road
St. George, UT 84790
435–634–9780
http://www.eola.com
Smart Longevity.

Esteem Products Ltd.
15015 Main Street, Suite 204
Bellevue, WA 98007
800–954–5515 425–562–1281
http://www.esteemproducts.com
Diet Esteem Plus.

Ethical Nutrients
100 Avenida La Pata
San Clemente, CA 92673
800–668–8743 949–366–0818
http://www.ethicalnutrients.com
*Bone Builder; Bone Builder With Boron;
Mycel Baby Vites.*

Flora Manufacturing & Distributing, Ltd.
805 East Badger Road
Lynden, WA 98264
800–446–2110 360–354–2110
*U.S. distributor of Salus Haus products,
including Floradix Iron + Herbs.*

FoodScience Laboratories
20 New England Drive
Essex Junction, VT 05453
800–874–9444 802–878–5508
http://www.fslabs.com
*Aangamik DMG; Coenzyme Q_{10}; Energy
Now; Glucosamine Plus; Multi-Zyme; Olive
Leaf Extract.*

Forest Pharmaceuticals, Inc.
2510 Metro Boulevard
St. Louis, MO 63043
314–569–3610
Armour Thyroid Tablets.

Freeda Vitamins and Pharmacy
36 East 41st Street
New York, NY 10017
800–777–3737 212–685–4980
AntiAllergy; FemCal; ferrous fumarate.

Futurebiotics
145 Rice Field Lane
Hauppauge, NY 11788
800–367–5433
http://www.futurebiotics.com
*Colloidal mineral supplements; Cholestatin;
Megavital Forte.*

Gaia Herbs, Inc.
108 Island Ford Road
Brevard, NC 28712
828–884–4242
http://www.gaiaherbs.com
Saw Palmetto Supreme.

Gero Vita International
4936 Yonge Street
Toronto, Ontario M2N 6S3
Canada
http://www.gvi.com
*GH3; GH3 cream; Lung Support Formula;
Prostata.*

Global Health Services Inc.
P.O. Box 4746
Fort Lauderdale, FL 33338-4746
http://www.herpes.com/vir-immune.shtml
VIR-L-Lysine.

Global Marketing Associates, Inc.
3536 Arden Road
Hayward, CA 94545-3908
800–869–0763
Garlitech.

Good Things Naturally
610 West Main Street
Greenfield, IN 45140
317–462–2004.
Retail supplier of a wide variety of supplement products.

Green Foods Corporation
320 Graves Avenue
Oxnard, CA 93030
800–777–4430   805–983–7470
http://www.greenfoods.com
Carrot Essence; Green Magma; Green Tea Barley Essence; Veggie Magma; Wheat Germ Essence.

Health From The Sun
P.O. Box 179
22 North Main Street
Newport, NH 03773
800–447–2229
http://www.healthfromthesun.com
Borage oil; EFA Attention Formula; EFA Derma-Skin Formula; EFA Heart Formula; EFA Joint Formula; evening primrose oil; flaxseed oil; Intestamend; pumpkin seed oil; Total EFA; Ultra DHA; Ultra Omega-3 Fish Oil.

Heart Foods Company
2235 East 38th Street
Minneapolis, MN 55407
800–229–3663   612–724–5266
Cayenne products including Heart Food Caps; Power Caps; Power Plus.

Heel Inc.
11600 Cochiti Road Southeast
Albuquerque, NM 87123
505–293–3843
http://www.heelbhi.com
Traumeel; Vertigoheel.

Henkel Corporation
5325 South Ninth Avenue
LaGrange, IL 60525
708–579–6150
Betatene; Pycnogenol.

HerbaSway Therapeutic Formulas
342 Quinnipiac Street, Building 8A
Wallingord, CT 06492-4048
800–672–7322   203–269–6991
http://www.herbasway.com
Cholestra; Diabetica Tea; HerbaGreen Tea; Kudja; Liver-Enhancer; Premenstra; Soy Futura; Stamina.

Herbs, Etc.
1345 Cerrillos Road
Santa Fe, NM 87505
800–634–3727   505–982–1265
Alcohol-free herbal extracts, including Deep Chi Builder; Deep Sleep; Lung Tonic; Singer's Saving Grace.

Herbs for Kids
151 Evergreen Drive, Suite D
Bozeman, MT 59715
406–587–0180
Alcohol-free organic herbal extracts.

Himalaya USA (formerly Ayurvedic Concepts)
6950 Portwest Drive, Suite 170
Houston, TX 77024
800–869–4640   713–863–1622
http://www.himalayausa.com
GastriCare; GlucoCare; HeartCare; ImmunoCare; JointCare; LaxaCare; LeanCare; LiverCare; MindCare; ProstaCare; StressCare; UriCare; VeinCare; VigorCare.

Home Health Access Corporation
2401 West Hassell Road, Suite 1510
Hoffman Estates, IL 60195-5200
847–781–2500
http://www.homeaccess.com
Home Access Express HIV-1 Test System.

Hybrivet Systems
17 Erie Drive
Natick, MA 01760
800–262–5323   508–651–7881
LeadCheck Aqua; LeadCheck Swabs.

Hyland's
See P&S Laboratories.

Immune-Tree
1177 South 1680 West
Orem, UT 84058
801–434–8129
http://www.immunetree.com
Colostrum 6 Maximum Strength.

Integrated Health
12832 Chardron Avenue
Hawthorne, CA 90250
800–799–3232
ATP.

Jarrow Formulas Inc.
1824 South Robertson Boulevard
Los Angeles, CA 90035
800–726–0886   310–204–6936
http://www.jarrow.com
BioSil; Colostrum Specific; IP$_6$; Jarro-Dophilus; Methylcobalamin.

Jason Natural Cosmetics
8468 Warner Drive
Culver City, CA 90232
800–527–6605   310–838–7543
http://www.jason-natural.com
Bosom Buddies breast self-examination kit; Hyper-C Serum; Woman Wise Wild Yam products.

Johnson & Johnson
1001 US Highway 202
Raritan, NJ 08869–0610
800–421–6736
Advanced Care Cholesterol Kit.

Kelco
See Natural Alternatives International.

KAL Dietary Supplements
Division, Nutraceutical Corporation
1400 Kearns Boulevard
Park City, UT 84060
800–669–8877   800–579–4665
products@nutraceutical.com
http://www.nutraceutical.com/kal.cfm
Bone Defense; Enada NADH; Virility Two.

Kingchem Inc. Nutritional Products
296 Kinderkamack Road
Oradell, NJ 07649
201–261–6002
http://www.kingchem.com
Huperzine A.

LactAid, Inc.
McNeil Consumer Products Compapny
7050 Camp Hill Road
Fort Washington, PA 19034–2299
800–522–8243   215–233–7000
http://www.lactaid.com
LactAid.

Lake Consumer Products
625 Forest Edge Drive
Vernon Hills, IL 60061
800–635–3696   847–793–0230
Yeast-Gard.

Lane Labs-USA, Inc.
172 Broadway
Woodcliff Lake, NJ 07675
800–526–3001   201–391–8600
BeneFin shark cartilage.

Legacy Corporation
2261 East Somerset Drive
Salt Lake City, UT 84121
800–375–0339
Hair analysis services.

Liddell Laboratories
1036 Country Club Road
Moraga, CA 94556
800–460–7733
Brain Energy; Female Energy; Male Energy; Vital HGH.

Life Extension Foundation
P.O. Box 229120
Hollywood, FL 33022
800–544–4440   954–766–8433
http://www.lef.org
Prolongevity supplements, including Cognitex with Pregnenolone; Gamma E Tocopherol Formula; Pro Fem progesterone cream; Super Green Tea Extract.

Lifestar Millennium, Inc.
2175 Francisco Boulevard East, #A2
San Rafael, CA 94901
800–858–7477 415–457–1400
http://www.lifestar.com
Micronic Silver; Protec Probiotic; Salute Santé Grapeseed Oil.

Liverite Products, Inc.
15405 Redhill Avenue, Suite C
Tustin, CA 92780
888–425–5483
http://www.liveriteproducts.com
Liverite.

Maharishi Ayurveda Products
1068 Elkton Drive
Colorado Springs, CO 80907
800–255–8332 719-260-5500
http://www.mapi.com
Amrit Ambrosia and Amrit Nectar Ayurvedic formulas.

Maitake Products, Inc.
222 Bergen Turnpike
Ridgefield Park, NJ 07660
800–747–7418 201–229–0101
http://www.maitake.com
Grifron Maitake caplets; Grifron Maitake D-fraction; Mai Green Tea; Mai Tonic Tea; Prost-Mate.

Marlyn Nutraceuticals
14851 North Scottsdale Road
Scottsdale, AZ 85254
800–462–7596 480–991–0200
Wobenzym N.

Matrix Health Products, Inc.
8400 Magnolia Avenue, Suite N
9316 Wheatlands Road
Santee, CA 92071
800–736–5609 619–448–7550
http://www.earthsbounty.com
http://www.matrixhealth.com
Earth's Bounty supplements, including Earth's Bounty Noni, O_2 Spray; Oxy-Caps; Oxy Cleanse; Oxy Max; Oxy Mist.

MegaFood
8 Bowery Road
Derry, NH 03038
800–848–2542 603–432–5022
http://www.megafood.com
MegaZymes.

Menuco Corporation
350 Fifth Avenue, Suite 7509
New York, NY 10118
800–636–8261 212–736–1039
http://www.menuco.com
Enada NADH.

Metabolic Maintenance Products
68994 North Pine Street
P.O. Box 3600
Sisters, OR 97759
800–772–7873 541-549-7800
http://www.metabolicmaintenance.com

SAMe. Products available through health care professionals only.

Metabolic Response Modifiers
2633 West Coast Highway, Suite B
Newport Beach, CA 92663-4708
800–948–6296
http://www.metabolicresponse.com
Bone Maximizer; CM+TM; Colon Clear; Liver-X; Neuro-Max; Osteo-Max.

Metagenics, Inc.
100 Avenida La Pata
San Clemente, CA 92673
800–692–9400 949–366–0818
http://www.metagenics.com
Essentials, Ethical Nutrients, MetaBotanica, Metadocs, Metagenics, MetaPharma, and Unipro brand nutritional supplements, including Bio-Zyme; Cal Apatite; Calcitite Hi-Strength; Collagenics; Endurabolic; Fibroplex; Hepatagen; HP 2 Influenza; Metazyme; Omega EFA; Ultra Clear Sustain; Ultrabalance Protein. Available through health care professionals only.

Miller Pharmacal Group, Inc.
350 Randy Road, Suite 2
Carol Stream, IL 60188-1831
800–323–2935 630–871–9557
http://www.millerpharmacal.com
A/G-Pro; Carozyme; Karbozyme; LipoComplex; Mg-Taurine Forte; Milco-Zyme; MM-Zyme; Proteolytic Enzymes; Theramill Forte. Available through health care professionals only.

Montana Naturals International, Inc.
19994 Highway 93
Arlee, MT 59821
800–872–7218 406–726–3214
Royal jelly.

Muscle-Link
1701 Ives Avenue
Oxnard, CA 93033
800–667–4626 805–385–3510
http://www.muscle-link.com
GH Stak.

MuscleTech
1785 South Park Avenue
Buffalo, NY 14220
716–822–4974
http://www.muscletech.com
Cell-Tech.

National Allergy Supply, Inc.
1620 Satellite Boulevard, Suite D
Duluth, GA 30097
800–522–1448
http://www.natlallergy.com/
Drug-free allergy-relief products.

National Enzyme Company
15366 US Highway 160
Forsyth, MO 65653
800–825–8545 417–546–4796
http://www.nationalenzymecompany.com
Plant-derived digestive enzyme products.

Natra-Bio Homeopathic
1441 West Smith Road
Ferndale, WA 98248
800–232–4005 360–384–5656
http://www.natrabio.com
Homeopathic remedies: bioAllers Allergy Relief formulas, including Animal Hair/ Dander; Grain/Dairy; Grass Pollen; Mold/ Yeast/Dust; Pollen/Hayfever; Sinus & Allergy Nasal Spray; and Tree Pollen.

Natren, Inc.
3105 Willow Lake
Westlake Village, CA 91361
800–992–3323
http://www.natren.com
Bifido Factor; Digesta-Lac; Gy-na-tren; Healthy Trinity; LifeStart; Megadophilus.

Natrol Inc.
21411 Prairie Street
Chatsworth, CA 91311
800–326–1520
http://www.natrol.com
Cravex; DHEA; Digest Support; Ester C Plus Bioflavonoids; PreNatal Care; Tonalin 1000-CLA; Tonalin 750-CLA.

Natural Alternatives
See RidgeCrest Herbals.

Natural Alternatives International
1185 Linda Vista Drive
San Marcos, CA 92069
1–800–455–1740
760–744–7340
http://www.nai-online.com
Juice Plus.

Natural Balance
3155 North Commerce Court
Castle Rock, CO 80104
800–833–8737
http://www.naturalbalance.com
AndroMax; Brain Pep; Cobra; Colon Clenz; Diet Pep; 5-HTP; HTP.Calm; Iprical Plus; Moducare; MSM Cream; Pyruvate; SeroThin; Turbo Charge.

Natural Organics
548 Broadhollow Road
Melville, NY 11747-3708
800–645–9500 800–525–0200
631–293–0030
http://www.naturesplus.com
Nature's Plus supplements, including Bioperine 10; Bromelain; Candida Forte; Coenzyme Q_{10}; Detoxygen; Fuel for Thought; Glucosamine/Chondroitin MSM Ultra Rx-Joint Cream; Herbal Actives, including Artichoke; ImmunActinZinc lozenges; Liv-R-Actin; Ocu-Care; Prost-Actin; SAMe Rx-Mood; Spiru-tein; Ultra Bromelain; Ultra Hair; Ultra Juice Green; Ultra Nails.

NaturalMax
Division, Nutraceutical Corporation
1400 Kearns Boulevard
Park City, UT 84060
800–669–8877 800–579–4665
http://www.nutraceutical.com/naturalmax.cfm
Breast Health.

Nature's Answer
85 Commerce Dr.
Hauppauge, NY 11788
800–439–2324 631–231–7492
http://www.naturesanswer.com
Bio-Strath; FOR KIDS herbal supplements, including Bubble B-Gone; E-KID-nacea; E-KID-nacea Plus; Ginger KID; KID B-Well Tonic; KID Catnip; KID Chamomile; NAT-Choo; Tummie Tonic; Slumber.

Nature's Best Inc.
195 Engineers Road
Hauppauge, NY 11788
631–232–3355
http://www.naturesbest.com
Perfect IsoPure.

Nature's Herbs
A Twinlab Company
701 South 600 East
American Fork, UT 84003
800–437–2257
http://www.naturesherbs.com
Boswellin Cream; Bronc-Ease.

Nature's Life
7180 Lampson Avenue
Garden Grove, CA 92841
800–854–6837 714–379–6500
Bromelain Joint Ease, Ginger & Curcumin Joint Ease.

Nature's Path, Inc.
P.O. Box 7862
Venice, FL 34287
877–723–6248 941–426–3375
Flora-Lyte; herbal pet products; liquid trace minerals.

Nature's Plus
See Natural Organics.

Nature's Products
2525 Davie Road
Davie, FL 33317
800–752–7873 305–474–9049
EPA Pure/300; EPA Pure/1200.

Nature's ScienCeuticals
See Neways, Inc.

Nature's Secret
Division, Omni Nutraceuticals
5310 Beethoven Street
Los Angeles, CA 90066
800–841–8448
http://www.naturessecret.com
Ultimate Cleanse; Ultimate Fiber; Ultimate Oil.

Nature's Sources, LLC
5653 West Howard Street
Niles, IL 60714
800–827–7656 847–647–8484
http://www.naturessources.com
AbsorbAid; Kolorex; Kolorex cream.

Nature's Way Products
10 Mountain Springs Parkway
Springville, UT 84663
800–962–8873 801–489–1500
http://www.naturesway.com
Attention Focus; Fenu-Thyme; Kidney Bladder Formula; Naturalax 2; Primadophilus; Silent Night Formula.

NatureWorks
c/o Abkit, Inc.
207 East 94th Street
New York, NY 10128
800–226–6227
http://www.NatureWorks.com
Betatene; Body Essential Silica gel; Calendula Ointment.

New Chapter, Inc.
22 High Street
Brattleboro, VT 05301
800–543–7279 802–257–0018
http://www.newchapterinc.com
Flora; Tum-Ease.

Neways, Inc.
150 East 400 North
Salem, UT 84653
801–423–2800
http://www.neways.com
Nature's ScienCeuticals products, including Cell Pill; Orbitol; Osteo Solutions.

Nonu International
50 East 100 South, Suite 205
St. George, Utah 84770
877–438–6668 435–628–3013
http://www.nonuinc.com
Nonu Juice.

Nordic Naturals
3040 Valencia Avenue, Suite 2
Aptos, CA 95003-4126
800–662–2544 831–662–2852
http://www.nordicnaturals.com
ProDHA; ProOmega. Products available through health care professionals only.

North American Herb & Spice
P.O. Box 4885
Buffalo Grove, IL 60089
847–229–1701
Oil of rosemary.

Nupharma Nutraceuticals, Inc.
4045 Sheridan Avenue PMB # 363
Miami Beach, Florida 33140
305-861-3355
http://www.dldewey.com
Béres Drops Plus.

Nutramax Laboratories, Inc.
2208 Lakeside Boulevard
Edgewood, MD 21040
800–925–5187 410–776–4000
http://www.nutramaxlabs.com
Cosamin.

Nutramedix
212 North US Highway One, Suite 17
Tequesta, FL 33469
800–288–2844 561–745–2917
http://www.nutramedix.com
Cat's claw; maca.

NutriCology Inc.
30806 Santana Street
Hayward, CA 94544
800–545–9960 510–639–4572
http://www.nutricology.com
ProGreens.

Nutri-Health
218 Justin Drive
Cottonwood, AZ 86326
800–991–9286
Flora Source.

Nutrition Now, Inc.
6350 NE Campus Drive
Vancouver, WA 98661
800–929–0418 360–737–6800
http://www.nutritionnow.com
Quercetin Plus.

Nutrition 21
4 Manhattanville Road
Purchase, NY 10577-2197
800–343–3082
http://www.nutrition21.com
Mineral supplements.

Nx Generation Ltd.
175 L Commerce Drive
Hauppauge, NY 11788
800–623–3727 516–231–2900
http://www.nxgeneration.com
Anti-Alcohol Reviver; Cholesterol Buster; Fat Burners; Joint Guard; Serenity.

Olympian Labs
P.O. Box 12461
Scottsdale, AZ 85267
800–756–1072 800–473–5883
602–483–2302
http://www.olympian-labs.com
Anxiety-X; Asthma-X$_5$; Biogra; Cold-X10, Fibro-X, Gastro-Calm; Glucosalage S04 (regular and extra strength); Herp-Eeze; Lycopene; Menoflash; Pedia-Calm; Quercetin Plus.

Omega-Life, Inc.
15355 Woodbridge Road
Brookfield, WI 53005
800–328–3529 414–786–2070
Fortified Flax.

Omega Nutrition
1924 Franklin Street
Vancouver, BC Z5L IR2
Canada
800–661–3529
Organic oil products.

Omni Nutraceuticals, Inc.
5310 Beethoven Street
Los Angeles, CA 90066
800–841–8448 310–845–3154
http://www.irwinnaturals.com
Cholestaid; Diet System 6 Cellulite Removal Program; Inholtra Joint Pain Formula; Inholtra Sulfamax MSM Formula.

Only Natural Inc.
31 Saratoga Boulevard
Island Park, NY 11558
516–897–7001
Glucosamine chondroitin sulfate.

Optimal Nutrients
1163 Chess Drive, Suite F
Foster City, CA 94404
800–966–8874
Coenzyme Q_{10}.

Optimum Nutrition
600 North Commerce Street
Aurora, IL 60504
800–705–5226
http://wwew.optimumnutr.com
Pro Complex.

Oxyfresh USA, Inc.
P.O. Box 3723
Spokane, WA 99220
800–999–9551 509–924–4999
Body Language Essential Green Foods; Body Language Super Antioxidant.

Padma Health Products, Inc.
River Vale, NJ 07675
877–723–6250 201–664–2100
Padma Basic herbal supplements. Products available only through health care professionals.

P&S Laboratories
Division, Standard Homeopathic
  Company
210 West 131 Street
Los Angeles, CA 90061
800–624–9659 213–321–4284
http://www.hylands.com
Hyland's homeopathic remedies, including *Earache Tablets; Poison Ivy/Oak Tablets.*

Papaya John's
P.O. Box 441
Paia, HI 96779
888–972–7292
http://www.papayajohn.com
Mature Green Papaya Powder; Papaya Almond papaya bars; Papaya Ginger & NONI Turmeric Milk Thistle & Flax papaya bars; Papaya Honey concentrate; Papaya Macadamia Nut papaya bars.

Parametric Associates, Inc.
10934 Lin-Valle Drive
St. Louis, MO 63123
800–747–1601 314–892–0988
Brain Alert; Calcium-Collagen Complex; Cardio-Power; Cold & Sinus; Digest-All; D-Yeast; Fat Metabolizer; Fatigue Free; Female Harmony; G.O.U.T.; Male Formula; Mobility; Multiple "Plus"; Nutra-Mune; Para-Cleans; Pure & Regular; Stress Free; Super Antioxidant; Sweet Dreams.

Pep Products, Inc.
3130 North Commerce Court
P.O. Box 8002
Castle Rock, CO 80104
800–833–8737 303–688–6633
PEP Formula.

Pharmaceutical Purveyors of Oklahoma
1709 North Portland
Oklahoma City, OK 73107
800–234–1091 405–943–1091
Perfect B.

Pharmanex, Inc.
75 West Center
Provo, UT 84601
888–742–7626
http://www.pharmanex.com
Cholestin.

Phoenix BioLabs
2794 Loker Avenue West, Suite 104
Carlsbad, CA 92008
800–947–8482
http://www.vitacarte.com
VitaCarte.

PhysioLogics
6565 Odell Place
Boulder, CO 80301
800–765–6775
Coloklysis; CTR Support. Products available through health care professionals only.

PhytoPharmica
825 Challenger Drive
Green Bay, WI 54311
800–553–2370 920–469–9099
http://www.phytopharmica.com
Cellular Forte with IP-6; Esberitox; Glucosamine Sulfate; Glucosamine Sulfate Complex; Phytodolor; Remifemin.

Planetary Formulas
23 Janis Way
Scotts Valley, CA 95066
800–606–6226 800–777–5677
408–438–1700
http://www.planetaryformulas.com
http://www.planetherbs.com
Horse Chestnut Cream; Triphala Internal Cleanser.

Plantes & Medecines, Inc.
3014 Rigel Avenue
Las Vegas, NV 89102
877–723–6248 702–871–7153
Elusan Digest; Elusan Elimin; Elusan Garlic; Elusan Natural Sleep; Elusan Relax; Elusan St. John's Wort; Elusan Tranquil; Elusan Veins.

Prevail Corporation
2204-8 NW Birdsdale
Gresham, OR 97030
800–248–0885
http://www.prevail.com
Acid-Ease; Cardio Enzyme Formula; Cholesterol Enzyme Formula; Maxi-Calm; Meno-Fem; Osteo Formula; Prostate Enzyme Formula; Sinease.

Primary Source
1150 Post Road
Fairfield, CT 06430
800–667–1538
OPC-85.

Priorities
1451 Concord Street
Framington, MA 01701
800–553–5398
Allergy and asthma relief catalog.

Probiologic Inc.
8711 148th Avenue NE
Redmond, WA 98052
253–881–8218
Capricin.

Products of Nature
211 Greenwood Avenue 2-2 PMB116
Bethel, CT 06801
800–527–0762
http://theproductsofnature.com
Natural Woman Essential Body Cream.

Professional Health Products, Ltd.
211 Overlook Drive, Suite 5
Sewickley, PA 15143
800–929–4133
Osseoapatite Plus. Products available through health care professionals only.

Progressive Research Labs, Inc.
9219 Katy Freeway
Houston, TX 77024
800–877–0966 713–365–9334
http://www.prlabs.com
Cardio Nutrition Rx; Depression Nutrition Rx; Diabetic Nutrition Phase II; Diabetic Nutrition Rx; Hypoglycemic Nutrition Rx; Vision Nutrition Rx.

Prolongevity
See Life Extension Foundation.

Pure-Gar, Inc.
P.O. Box 98813
Tacoma, WA 98498
800–537–7695 206–582–6421
Nutritional supplements.

Pure n Natural Industries
12402 Nordesta Drive
Norwalk, CA 90650
888–848–2932
Portable air purification unit.

Quantum
P.O. Box 2791
Eugene, OR 97402
800–448–1448
SuperLysine Plus Cream.

Queen Helene Products
Para Laboratories, Inc.
100 Rose Avenue
Hempstead, NY 11550
800–645–3752 516–538–4600
http://www.queenhelene.com
Batherapy; Footherapy.

Regenesis Network LLC
5835 South Eastern Avenue
Los Angeles, CA 90040
323–890–4820
http://www.regenesis1.com
Regenesis Pro.

Rene M. Caisse Research Institute
P.O. Box 23155
Ottawa, Ontario, Canada K2A 4E2
613–729–9111
Essiac Herbal Tea. Products available through health care professionals only.

Rexall Sundown
851 Broken Sound Parkway Northwest
Boca Raton, FL 33487
561–241–9400
http://www.rexallsundown.com
Cellasene.

R-Garden Internationale
3881 Enzyme Lane
P.O. Box 417
Kettle Falls, WA 99141
800–800–1927 509–738–2345
http://www.rgarden.com
Cordyceps.

Ridgecrest Herbals, Inc.
1151 South Redwood Road, Suite 106
Salt Lake City, UT 84104
800–242–4649 801–978–9633
http://www.ridgecrestherbals.com
ClearLungs.

RX Vitamins
200 Myrtle Boulevard
Larchmont, NY 10538
800–326–5772 914–834–1804
ARTH-9; CDA-21; CV-10; DB-7; Menopause Formula; Ocular Formula.

Sabinsa Corporation
121 Ethel Road West, #6
Piscataway, NJ 08854
732–777–1111
http://www.sabinsa.com
Ayurvedic extracts and nutraceuticals, including ashwagandha; Bacopin; Bioperine; Boswellin; Citrin; Coleus forskohlii; C^3

Complex; Ginger Dry Extract; Ginger Soft Extract; Gymnema Sylvestre GS_4.

Safe Home Products Inc.
P. O. Box 5319
1708 Brown Deer Trace
Coralville, IA 52241-5319
319–354–7301
http://www.safehomeproducts.com
EarCheck otitis media detector.

Salus Haus
See Flora Manufacturing & Distributing, Ltd.

Samra Health & Beauty, Inc.
3000 South Robertson Boulevard, Room 420
Los Angeles, CA 90034
888–417–2672
Anti-Aging; Brain Power; Calm Colon; Children's Vita Herb; Digest Ease; Healthy Hair; Immune Booster; Ultra Circulation; Traditional Chinese Medicine.

Sawyer Products of Safety Harbor, Florida
P.O. Box 188
Safety Harbor, FL 34695
800–940–4464 727–725–1177
http://www.sawyerproducts.com
The Extractor.

Scandinavian Naturals Health & Beauty Products, Inc.
13 North Seventh Street
Perkasie, PA 18944
800–288–2845 215–453–2505
Glucosamine/Chrondroitin Sulfate Complex. Products available through health care professionals only.

Schiff Products
P.O. Box 26708
Salt Lake City, UT 84126
801–975–1166
Phytocharged nutritional supplements.

Silver Sage
949 Pioneer Road
Draper, UT 84020
800–898–5153 801–571–6500
http://www.silversage.com
ThyroStart.

Similasan
108 North Ridge Street
P.O. Box 7429
Breckenridge, CO 80424
800–426–1644 970–547–5060
http://www.similasan.ch/deutsch.htm
Similasan Eye Drops #1; Similasan Eye Drops #2.

Skin-Lyte Nature's Path, Inc.
5621 Reistertown Road
North Port, FL 34287
800–326–5772 941–426–3375
Electrolyte products for the hair and skin.

Solaray Products
Division, Nutraceutical Corporation
1400 Kearns Boulevard
Park City, UT 84060
800–669–8877 800–579–4665
http://www.nutraceutical.com/
   solaray.cfm
5-HTP; Gastroveda; Intestiveda; ParasiVeda; SP-6 Cornsilk Blend; SP-8 Hawthorn Motherwort Blend; SP-14 Valerian Blend; SP-6 Cornsilk Blend.

Solgar Vitamin and Herb Company, Inc.
500 Willow Tree Road
Leonia, NJ 07605
877–765–4274 201–944–2311
Advanced Carotenoid Complex; EarthSource Greens & More; MaxEPA; Whey to Go.

Sonne Organic Foods
P.O. Box 2160
Cottonwood, CA 96022
916–347–5868
Sonne's #7.

Source Naturals
23 Janis Way
Scotts Valley, CA 95066
831–438–1144
http://www.sourcenaturals.com
Activated Quercetin; Calcium Night; Cat's Claw Defense Complex; Coenzymate B Complex; Daily Essential Enzymes; GlucosaMend; Heart Science; N-A-G; Proangenol 100; Proanthodyn; Urban Air Defense; Visual Eyes; Wellness Formula.

Soy Biotics
3 Pearl Court
Allendale, NJ 07401
800–769–1288
Soyfood supplements.

Spectrum Naturals
133A Copeland
Petaluma, CA 94952
707–778–8900
Flaxseed oil.

Sun Precautions
2815 Wetmore Avenue
Everett, WA 98201
800–882–7860
Solumbra sun-protective clothing.

The SunBox Company
19217 Orbit Drive
Gaithersburg, MD 20879
800–548–3968 301–869–5980
Dawn Simulator.

Superior Source
See Continental Vitamin Company.

Sweet Wheat, Inc.
P.O. Box 187
Clearwater, FL 33757
888–227–9338
http://www.sweetwheat.com
Sweet Wheat.

Symbiotics, Inc.
2301 West Highway 89A, Suite 107
Sedona, AZ 86336
800–784–4355 520–203–0277
http://www.symbiotics.com
New Life Colostrum (original and high-Ig formulas).

The Synergy Company
HC 64 Box 2901
Castle Valley, UT 84532-9613
800–723–0277 435–259–5366
http://www.synergy-co.com
Vita Synergy for Men; Vita Synergy for Women.

Synergy Plus/International Vitamins
500 Halls Mill Road
Freehold, NJ 07728–8811
800–375–8482
http://www.synergyplus.net
Bone Support; Capralin.

Terra Maxa, Inc.
3301 West Central Avenue
Toledo, OH 43606
800–783–7817 419–385–3001
E-mail: terramaxa@solarstop.net
P.S.I.

Terra Tech Inc.
International Reforestation Suppliers
P.O. Box 5547
Eugene, OR 97405
800–321–1037
http://www.terratech.net
Lil Sucker venom extractor.

Thompson Nutritional Products
Division, Rexall Sundown
851 Broken Sound Parkway, NW
Boca Raton, FL 33487
800–421–1192 561–241–9400
http://www.rexallsundown.com
Life Guard.

Threshold Enterprises
23 Janis Way
Scotts Valley, CA 95066
800–777–5677
Vitamin and mineral supplements.

Thursday Plantation
P.O. Box 5613
Montecito, CA 93150
800–848–8966 805–963–2297
Tea tree oil.

Tom's of Maine
P.O. Box 710
Kennebunk, ME 04043
207–985–2944
Tom's of Maine Natural Toothpaste and other natural body care products.

Trace Minerals Research
1990 West 3300 South
Ogden, UT 84401
800–624–7145 801–731–6051
Arth-X; Complete Calcium; ConcenTrace; Electrolyte; MSM; PowerHouse Sports Recovery.

TriMedica International
1895 South Los Feliz Drive
Tempe, AZ 85282
800–800-8849 480–998–1041
http://www.trimedica.com
Acid/Alkaline Placemat; All Complete Enzymes; Colloidal liquid silver; Cold Combat!; Grobust; MSM Liquid; pH Papers; PREG; ProG+; Vitamin O2.

Twinlab
2120 Smithtown Avenue
Ronkonkoma, NY 11779
800–645–5626 631–467–3140
http://www.twinlab.com
Bone Support with Ostivone; GABA Plus; Mega Bromelain; OcuGuard; Phos Fuel.

UniTea Herbs
828 Pearl Street
Boulder, CO 80302
800–864–8327 303–443–1248
SensualiTea.

Växa International, Inc.
7835 Tern Drive
Orlando, FL 32822
800–248–8292 813–870–2904
407–273–9999
http://www.vaxa.com
Anti-Oxin+; Attend; Buffer-pH+; Cell-U-Lite; Clearin; Medical pH-Test Strips; Parasitin+; PMS-Ease; Prostatin+.

Wakunaga of America Company, Ltd.
23501 Madero
Mission Viejo, CA 92691–2764
800–421–2998 949–855–2776
http://www.kyolic.com
Arthritic Pain Relief Cream; Be Sure; Bifido Factor; Cardio Logic; Ginkgo Biloba Plus; Kyo-Chlorella; Kyo-Dophilus; Kyo-Green; Kyolic aged garlic extract; Kyolic-EPA; Kyolic Super Formula 102; Kyolic Super Formula 105; Liquid Kyolic with B_1 and B_{12}; Neuro Logic; Probiata; ProFlora whey.

Waterwise
P.O. Box 494000
Leesburg, FL 34749-4000
800–874–9028
Showerwise filter with showerhead.

Wein Products Inc.
115 West 25th Street
Los Angeles, CA 90007
213–749–6049
http://www.weinproducts.com
Air Supply personal air purifier.

Windmill Health Products
21 Dwight Place
Fairfield, NJ 07004
800–822–4320
http://www.windmillvitamins.com
Menocom.

ZAND Herbal Formulas
1722 14th Street, Suite 230
Boulder, CO 80302
800–371–8420 303–786-8558
http://www.zand.com
Allergy Season; Decongest Herbal; HerbalMist throat spray; Herbs for Kids; Insure Herbal; Quick Cleanse Program.

Health and Medical Organizations

The following is a list of organizations that can provide assistance for specific disorders and situations. The services offered by these organizations vary. Some provide information only; others offer various types of referrals, support groups, and even access to medical or social services. In most cases, the organizations' areas of interest are obvious from their names. Where this is not the case, a brief description of the organization's focus is offered. Be aware that addresses and telephone numbers are subject to change.

RESOURCE ORGANIZATIONS

Academy of Chinese Healing Arts
505 South Orange Avenue
Sarasota, FL 34236
941–955–4456
Program includes acupuncture, Chinese herbology, homeopathy, and German electro-acpuncture.

Acupressure Institute
1533 Shattuck Avenue
Berkeley, CA 94709
800–442–2232 510–845–1059
http://www.acupressure.com

AIDS Action Committee of Massachusetts
131 Clarendon Street
Boston, MA 02116
617–437–6200 617–450–1423 (TTY)
Hotline: 800–235–2331 617–450–1427
http://www.aac.org

Alcoholics Anonymous
P.O. Box 459
New York, NY 10163
212–870–3400
http://www.aa.org

Alexander Graham Bell Association for the Deaf
3417 Volta Place NW
Washington, DC 20007–2778
202–337–5220 (voice and TTY)
http://www.agbell.org

ALS Association
27001 Agoura Road, Suite 150
Calabasas Hills, CA 91301–5104
800–782–4747 818–880–9007
http://www.alsa.org

Alzheimer's Association
919 North Michigan Avenue, Suite 1100
Chicago, IL 60611–1676
800–272–3900 312–335–8700
http://www.alz.org

American Academy of Allergy, Asthma, and Immunology
611 East Wells Street
Milwaukee, WI 53202
800–822–2762 414–272–6071
http://www.aaaai.org

American Academy of Child and Adolescent Psychology
3615 Wisconsin Avenue NW
Washington, DC 20016–3007
202–966–7300
http://www.aacap.org

American Academy of Dermatology
930 North Meacham Road
Schaumburg, IL 60173
888–462–3376 847–330–0238
http://www.aad.org

American Academy of Otolaryngology—Head and Neck Surgery
One Prince Street
Alexandria, VA 22314
703–836–4444
http://www.entnet.org
Services include providing information about Ménière's disease.

American Academy of Sleep Medicine
6301 Bandel Road NW, Suite 101
Rochester, MN 55901
507–287–6006
http://www.asda.org

American Anorexia Bulimia Association (AABA)
165 West 46th Street, Suite 1108
New York, NY 10036
212–575–6200
http://www.aabainc.org

American Apitherapy Society
5390 Grande Road
Hillsboro, OH 45133
937–364–1108
http://www.apitherapy.org/aas/default.htm

American Association of Clinical Endocrinologists
1000 Riverside Avenue, Suite 205
Jacksonville, FL 32204
904–353–7878
http://www.aace.com
Provides information about thyroid and other glandular disorders.

American Association of Nutritional Consultants
302 East Winona Avenue
Warsaw, IN 46580
888–828–2262
http://www.aanc.net
Offers certified nutritional counseling (CNC) certification.

American Association of Oriental Medicine (AAOM)
433 Front Street
Catasauqua, PA 18032
888–500–7999 610–266–1433
http://www.aaom.org
Specializes in Oriental healing and exercise.

American Association of Sex Educators, Counselors, and Therapists
P.O. Box 238
Mount Vernon, IA 52314
http://www.aasect.org

American Association on Mental Retardation (AAMR)
444 North Capitol Street NW, Suite 846
Washington, DC 20001–1512
800–424–3688 202–387–1968
http://www.aamr.org

American Board of Chelation Therapy
1407-B North Wells
Chicago, IL 60601
800–356–2228 312–787–2228

American Brain Tumor Research Association
2720 River Road, Suite 146
Des Plains, IL 60018
800–886–2282 847–827–9910
http://www.abta.org

American Cancer Society
1599 Clifton Road
Atlanta, GA 30329
800–ACS–2345
http://www.cancer.org

American Chronic Pain Association, Inc.
P.O. Box 850
Rocklin, CA 95677
916–632–0922
www.theacpa.org
Services include providing information about shingles and postherpetic neuralgia.

American College for Advancement in Medicine (ACAM)
23121 Verdugo Drive, Suite 204
Laguna Hills, CA 92653
800–532–3688 714–583–7666
http://www.acam.org
Provides a list of chelation therapists.

American Council for Headache Education (ACHE)
819 Mantua Road
Mount Royal, NJ 08061
856–423–0258
http://www.achenet.org

American Council of the Blind
1155 15th Street NW, Suite 1004
Washington DC 20005
800–424–8666 202–467–5081
http://www.acb.org

American Dental Association
211 East Chicago Avenue
Chicago, IL 60611
312–440–2500
http://www.ada.org

American Diabetes Association
1660 Duke Street
Alexandria, VA 22314
800–232–3472 703–549–1500

American Foundation for AIDS Research (AMFAR)
120 Wall Street, 13th Floor
New York, NY 10005-3902
800–392–6327 212–806–1600
http://www.amfar.org

American Foundation for the Blind
11 Penn Plaza, Suite 300
New York, NY 10001
800–232–5463 212–502–7600
http://www.afb.org

American Genetic Association
Frederick, MD 21701
301–695–9292

American Heart Association
7272 Greenville Avenue
Dallas, TX 75231
800–242–8721 214–373–6300
http://www.aha.org

American Industrial Hygiene Association
2700 Prosperity Avenue, Suite 250
Fairfax, VA 22031
703–849–8888
http://www.aiha.org
Provides information on occupational and environmental health and safety issues.

American Institute of Holistic Theology
5600 Market Street, Suite 10
Youngstown, OH 44512
800–650–4325
http://www.aiht.edu
Provides instruction in a variety of natural approaches to health care and maintenance.

American Kidney Fund (AKF)
6110 Executive Boulevard, Suite 1010
Rockville, MD 20852
800–638–8299 301–881–3052
http://www.akfinc.org

American Liver Foundation
75 Maiden Lane, Suite 603
New York, NY 10038
800–465–4837
http://www.liverfoundation.org

American Lung Association
1740 Broadway
New York, NY 10019
800–5864–872 212-315-8700
http://www.lungusa.org

American Medical Association (AMA)
515 North State Street
Chicago, IL 60610
312–464–5000
http://www.ama-assn.org

American Mental Health Foundation
1049 Fifth Avenue
New York, NY 10028
212–737–9027

American Pain Society
4700 West Lake Avenue
Glenview, IL 60025
847–375–4715
http://www.ampainsoc.org

American Parkinson Disease Association
1250 Hylan Boulevard, Suite 4B
Staten Island, NY 10305–1946
800–223–2732 718–981–8001
http://www.apdaparkinson.org

American Preventive Medical Association
9912 Georgetown Pike, Suite D-2
P.O. Box 458
Great Falls, Virginia 22066
800–230–2762 703–759–0662
http://www.apma.net

American Reflexology Certification Board
11129 West Tulane Avenue
Littleton, CO 80127
303–933–6921
Can provide information on programs for learning this technique.

American Society for Reproductive Medicine
1209 Montgomery Highway
Birmingham, AL 35216
205–978–5000
http://www.asrm.org

American Society of Cataract and Refractive Surgery
3702 Pender Drive, Suite 250
Fairfax, VA 22030
703–591–2220
http://www.ascrs.org

American Speech-Language-Hearing Association
10801 Rockville Pike
Rockville, MD 20852
800–638–8255 301–897–5700
http://www.asha.org

American Tinnitus Association
P.O. Box 5
Portland, OR 97207
503–248–9985
http://www.ata.org

Anorexia Nervosa and Related Eating Disorders (ANRED)
P.O. Box 5102
Eugene, OR 97405
503–344–1144
http://www.anred.com

Anxiety Disorders Association of America
11900 Parklawn Drive, Suite 100
Rockville, MD 20852
301–231–9350
http://www.adaa.org

Arthritis Foundation
1330 West Peachtree Street
Atlanta, GA 30309
800–283–7800
http://www.arthritis.org

Asbestos Victims of America
P.O. Box 66594
Scotts Valley, CA95067
408–438–5864

Association for Applied Psychophysiology and Biofeedback
10200 W. 44th Avenue, Suite 304
Wheat Ridge, CO 80033-2840
303–422–8436

Association for the Education and Rehabilitation of the Blind and Visually Impaired
4600 Duke Street, Suite 430
P.O. Box 22397
Alexandria, VA 22314
703–823–9690
http://www.aerbvi.org

Asthma and Allergy Foundation of America (AAFA)
1233 20th Street NW, Suite 402
Washington, DC 20036
800–727–8462
Website:http://www.aafa.org

Autism Society of America
7910 Woodmont Avenue, Suite 300
Bethesda, MD 20814–3015
800–328–8476 extension 150
301–657–0881
http://www.autism-society.org

Bradford Research Institute
1180 Walnut Avenue
Chula Vista, CA 91911
800–227–4473 619–429–8200
http://www.bradfordresearchinst.org
Provides a variety of alternative and integrative therapies.

Brain Injury Association
105 North Alfred Street
Alexandria, VA 22314
703–236–6000
http://www.biausa.org

Brain Research Foundation
120 South LaSalle Street, Suite 1300
Chicago, IL60603
312–759–5150

Cancer Information Service
National Cancer Institute
Building 31, Room 10A24
9000 Rockville Pike
Bethesda, MD 20892
800–422–6237
http://cis.nci.nih.gov

Cancer Research Foundation of America
1600 Duke Street, Suite 110
Alexandria, VA 22314
800–227–2732 703–836–4412
http://www.preventcancer.org

Cancer Treatment Centers of America
Midwestern Regional Medical Center
2501 Emmaus Avenue
Zion, IL 60099
800–615–3055 888–624–9143
http://www.cancercenter.com
Offers information on alternatives for the diagnosis and effective treatment of cancer.

Celiac Disease Foundation
13251 Ventura Boulevard, Suite 1
Studio City, CA 91604–1838
818–990–2354
http://www.celiac.org

Center for the Study of Anorexia and Bulimia
1841 Broadway, 4th Floor
New York, NY 10023
212–333–3444

Centers for Disease Control and Prevention (CDC)
1600 Clifton Road
Atlanta, GA 30333
800–311–3435 404–639–3534
STD Hotline: 800–227–8922
http://www.cdc.gov

Childhelp USA
15757 North 78th Street
Scottsdale, AZ 85260
480–922–8212
Hotline: 800–422–4453
800–222–4453 (TDD)
http://www.childhelpusa.org
Provides help for abused children.

Children and Adults with Attention-Deficit/Hyperactivity Disorder
8181 Professional Place, Suite 201
Landover, MD 20785
800–233–4050 301–306–7070
http://www.chadd.org

Children of Aging Parents (CAPS)
1609 Woodburne Road, Suite 302A
Levittown, PA 19057
800–227–7294 215–945–6900

Choice in Dying
475 Riverside Drive, Room 1852
New York, NY 10115
212–870–2003
http://www.choices.org

CFIDS Association of America
P.O. Box 220398
Charlotte, NC 28222–0398
800–442–3437 704–365–2343
http://www.cfids.org
Provides information and services related to chronic fatigue and immune dysfunction syndrome.

Clayton College of Natural Health
2140 11th Avenue South, Suite 305
Birmingham, AL 35205-2841
800–995–4590 205-323-8236
Provides degree programs in nutrition, naturopathy, and other holistic disciplines.

Crohn's and Colitis Foundation of America
386 Park Avenue South, 17th floor
New York, NY 10016–8804
800–932–2423 212–685–3440
http://www.ccfa.org

Cystic Fibrosis Foundation (CFF)
6931 Arlington Road, Suite 2000
Bethesda, MD 20814
800–344–4823 301–951–4422
http://www.cff.org

Designs for Health Institute
1750 30th Street, Suite 319
Boulder, CO 80301
303–415–0229
Website://http://www.dfhi.com
Offers advanced training in clinical nutrition.

Do It Now Foundation
P.O. Box 27568
Tempe, AZ 85285–7568
480–491–0393
Publishes substance abuse and behavioral health information.

Dogs for the Deaf
10175 Wheeler Road
Central Point, OR 97502
541–826–9220 (voice and TDD)
http://www.dogsforthedeaf.org

Endometriosis Association
8585 North 76th Place
Milwaukee, WI 53223
800–992–3636 414–355–2200
http://www.endometriosisassn.org

Epilepsy Foundation of America
4351 Garden City Drive
Landover, MD 20785–2267
800–332–1000 301–459–3700
http://www.efa.org

Esalen Institute
Highway 1
Big Sur, CA 93920-9616
831-667-3000
http://www.esalen.org
Provides information on Esalen massage therapy.

The FDA Cancer Liaison Program
Office of Special Health Issues
Food and Drug Administration
5600 Fishers Lane HF-12 Room 9-49
Rockville, MD 20857
888–463–6332 301–827–4460
http://www.fda.gov/oashi/cancer/
   cancer.html

Feingold Association of the United States
127 East Main Street, #106
Riverhead, NY 11901
800–321–3287 631–369–9340
http://www.feingold.org
Provides information on the effects of food and food additives on health, behavior, and learning.

Feldenkrais Guild of North America
3611 SW Hood Avenue, Suite 100
Portland, OR 97201
800–775–2118 503–221–6612
http://www.feldenkrais.com
Provides information on the Feldenkrais method of therapeutic touch.

Fibromyalgia Network
P.O. Box 31750
Tucson, AZ 85751
800–853–2929
http://www.fmnetnews.com

Food Allergy Network
10400 Eaton Place, Suite 107
Fairfax, VA 22030
800–929–4040 703–691–3179
http://www.foodallergy.org

Foundation Fighting Blindness
Executive Plaza I, Suite 800
11350 McCormick Road
Hunt Valley, MD 21031-1014
888–394–3937 410–785–1414
TDD: 800–683–5551 410–785–9687
http://www.blindness.org
*Provides information on retinal disorders,
including macular degeneration, retinitis
pigmentosa, and Usher syndrome.*

Gay Men's Health Crisis (GMHC)
119 West 24th Street
New York, NY 10011
800–243–7692 212–807–6655
212–645–7470 (TTY)
http://www.gmhc.org
*Provides information and services relating to
HIV and AIDS.*

The Genetic Alliance
4301 Connecticut Avenue NW, Suite 404
Washington, DC 20008-2304
800–336–4363 202–966–5557
http://www/geneticalliance.org
*Works to enhance the lives of people with
genetic health conditions.*

Gerontology Research Group
P.O. Box 905
661–775–3995 extension 2511
Santa Clarita, CA 91380-9005
http://www.grg.org
*Physicians, scientists, and engineers
dedicated to the quest to slow and ultimately
reverse human aging.*

Glaucoma Research Foundation
200 Pine Street, Suite 200
San Francisco, CA 94104
800–826–6693 415–986–3162
http://www.glaucoma.org

Guiding Eyes for the Blind
611 Granite Springs Road
Yorktown Heights, NY 10598
800–942–0149 914–245–4024
http://www.guiding-eyes.org

Harvard Medical School
Harvard University
25 Shattuck Street
Boston, MA 02115
617–495–1000
http://www.hms.harvard.edu
*Provides a variety of health-related
publications and information.*

Herpes Resource Center
American Social Health Association
P.O. Box 13827
Research Triangle Park, NC 27709
919–361–8400
http.//www.ashastd.org

Human Growth Foundation
997 Glen Cove Avenue
Glen Head, NY 11545
800–451–6434
http://www.hgfound.org

Immune Deficiency Foundation
40 West Chesapeake Avenue, Suite 308
Towson, MD 21204
800–296–4433
http://www.primaryimmune.org
*Specializes in primary immunodeficiency
diseases.*

**Institute for the Psychology of
Air Travel**
551 Boylston Street, Suite 202
Boston, MA 02116
617–437–1811
http://www.techadvisers.com/psyair/

**International Academy of Classical
Homeopathy**
P.O. Box 242
Gardiner, NY 12525
877–973–6339
http://www.classicalhomeopathy.com

**International Association for Medical
Assistance to Travelers**
736 Center Street
Lewiston, NY 20402
716–754–4883
http://www.sentex.net/~iamat/ci.html

International Diabetes Center
3800 Park Nicollet Boulevard
Minneapolis, MN 55416
612–927–3393
http://www.idcdiabetes.org

International Tremor Foundation
7046 West 105th Street
Overland Park, KS 66212–1803
913–341–3880
http://www.essentialtremor.org

Interstitial Cystitis Association
51 Monroe Street, Suite 1402
Rockville, MD 20850
800–435–7422 301–610–5300
http://www.ichelp.org

Juvenile Diabetes Foundation
120 Wall Street
New York, NY 10005–4001
800–533–2873 212–785–9500
http://jdf.org

La Leche League International
1400 N. Meacham Road
Schaumberg, IL 60173-4048
847–519–7730

**Learning Disabilities Association of
America (LDA)**
4156 Library Road
Pittsburgh, PA 15234
412–341–1515
http://www.ldfnatl.org

The Leukemia and Lymphoma Society
600 Third Avenue
New York, NY 10011
800–955-4572 212–573–8484
http://www.leukemia.org

The Living Bank
P.O. Box 6725
Houston, TX 77265
800–528–2971 713–961–9431
http://www.livingbank.org
*Provides information and maintains registry
of donated organs, tissues, bones, and bodies
for transplants or research.*

Lung Line Information Service
National Jewish Hospital
1400 Jackson Street
Denver, CO 80226
800–222–5864 303–355–5864
http://www.http://www.nationaljewish.
  org/ll1.html

Lupus Foundation of America
1300 Piccard Drive, Suite 200
Rockville, MD 20850–3226
800–558–0121 301–670–9292
http://www.lupus.org

March of Dimes National Foundation
1275 Mamaroneck Avenue
White Plains, NY 10605
888–663–4637
Website://www.modimes.org

Medic Alert Foundation
2323 Colorado Avenue
Turlock, CA 95382
800–432–5378 800–344–3226
209–668–3333
http://www.medicalert.org
*Maintains files on individuals who wear a
medical bracelet to provide information in
case of an emergency.*

**Mothers Against Drunk Driving
(MADD)**
P.O. Box 541688
Dallas, TX 75354–1688
800–438–6233
http://www.madd.org

Multiple Sclerosis Foundation
6350 North Andrews Avenue
Fort Lauderdale, FL 33309
800–441–7055
http://www.msfacts.org

Muscular Dystrophy Association–USA
3561 East Sunrise Drive
Tucson, AZ 85718
800–572–1717
http://www.mdausa.org

Myasthenia Gravis Foundation of America
123 West Madison Street, Suite 800
Chicago, IL 60602
800–541–5454 312–853–0522
http://www.myasthenia.org

National Aging Information Center
330 Independence Avenue SW,
Room 4656
Washington, DC 20201
202–619–7501
http://www.aoa.dhhs.gov/naic/

National Alliance of Breast Cancer Organizations
9 East 37th Street, 10th Floor
New York, NY 10016
888–806–2226 212–889–0606
http://www.nabco.org

National Alopecia Areata Foundation
710 C Street, Suite 11
San Rafael, CA 94901
415–456–4644
http://www.naaf.org

National Association for Continence
P.O. Box 8310
Spartanburg, SC 29305
800–252–3337 864–579–7900
http://www.nafc.org

National Association for the Visually Handicapped
3201 Balboa Street
San Francisco, CA 94121
415–221–3201
22 West 21st Street
New York, NY 10010
212–889–3141
http://www.navh.org

National Association of the Deaf
814 Thayer Avenue
Silver Spring, MD 20910
301–587–1788
http://www.nad.org

National Association of People With AIDS (NAPWA)
1413 K Street NW, Suite 700
Washington, DC 20005
202–898–0414
http://www.napwa.org

National Attention Deficit Disorder Association (ADDA)
1788 Second Street, Suite 200
Highland Park, IL 60035
847–432–2332
http://www.add.org

National Autism Hotline
Autism Services Center
P.O. Box 507
Huntington, WV 25710
304–525–8014

National Burn Victim Foundation
246-A Madisonville Road
P.O. Box 409
Basking Ridge, NJ 07920
908–953–9091
http://www.nbvf.org

National Cancer Institute
Building 31, Room 10A03
31 Center Drive, MSC 2580
Bethesda, MD 20892-2580
800–422–6237 301–435–3848
http://www.nci.nih.gov

National Center for Injury Prevention and Control
Mailstop K65
4770 Buford Highway NE
Atlanta, GA 30341-3724
770–488–1506
http://www.cdc.gov/ncipc/
Services include providing information about fracture prevention and treatment and advice on making homes safer for elderly or frail individuals.

National Chronic Pain Outreach Association
7979 Old Georgetown Road, Suite 100
Bethesda, MD 20814
301–652–4948

National Clearinghouse for Alcohol and Drug Information
11426–28 Rockville Pike, Suite 200
Rockville, MD 20847–2345
800–729–6686 301–443–6500

National Council on Aging
409 Third Street SW, 2nd Floor
Washington, DC 20024
202–479–1200
http://www.ncoa.org

National Council on Alcoholism and Drug Dependence
12 West 21st Street
New York, NY 10010
800–622–2255 212–206–6770
http://www.ncadd.org

National Diabetes Information Clearinghouse (NDIC)
1 Information Way
Bethesda, MD 20892–3560
301–654–3327
http://www.niddk.nih.gov/health/
diabetes/ndic.htm

National Digestive Diseases Information Clearinghouse
2 Information Way
Bethesda, MD 20892–3570
301–654–3810
http://www.niddk.nih.gov/health/
digest/nddic.htm

National Down Syndrome Congress
7000 Peachtree-Dunwoody Road, NE
Lake Ridge 400 Office Park Building #5,
Suite 100
Atlanta, GA 30328
800–232–6372 770–604–9500
http://www.ndsccenter.org

National Down Syndrome Society (NDSS)
666 Broadway
New York, NY 10012
800–221–4602 212–460–9330
http://www.ndss.org

National Eating Disorders Organization
6655 South Yale Avenue
Tulsa, OK 74136
918–481–4044

National Eye Institute (NEI)
2020 Vision Place
Bethesda, MD 20892-3655
301–496–5248
http://www.nei.nih.gov

National Foundation for Depressive Illness
P.O. Box 2257
New York, NY 10116
800–239–1265
http://www.depression.org

National Headache Foundation
428 West Saint James Place
Chicago, IL 60614
800–643–5552 773–388–6399
http://www/headaches.org

National Health Information Center
P.O. Box 1133
Washington, DC 20013–1133
800–336–4797 301–565–4167
http://nhic-nt.health.org

National Heart, Lung, and Blood Institute
Information Center
P.O. Box 30105
Bethesda, MD 20824–0105
301–251–1222
http://www.nhlbi.nih.gov

National Hemophilia Foundation (NHF)
116 West 32nd Street, 11th Floor
New York, NY 10001
800–424–2634· 212–328–3700
http://www.hemopohilia.org

National Hospice and Palliative Care Organization
1700 Diagonal Road, Suite 300
Alexandria, VA 22314
703–243–5900
http://www.nho.org

National Institute for Occupational Safety and Health
200 Independence Avenue, SW
Washington, DC 20201
800–356–4674

National Institute of Allergies and Infectious Diseases
Building 31, Room 7A-50
31 Center Drive MSC 2520
Bethesda, MD 20892–2520
301–496–5717
http://www.niaid.nih.gov

National Institute of Arthritis, Musculoskeletal, and Skin Diseases
National Institutes of Health
Box AMS
Bethseda, MD 20892
301–496–8188
http://www.nih.gov/niams/
Services include providing information about fibromyalgia syndrome.

National Institute of Diabetes and Digestive and Kidney Diseases (NIDDK)
National Institutes of Health
31 Center Drive, MSC 2560
Bethesda, MD 20892–2560
301–496–3583
http://www.niddk.nih.gov

National Institute of Mental Health (NIMH)
6001 Executive Boulevard Room 8184
 MSC 9663
Bethesda, MD 20892–9663
301–443–4513
http://www.nimh.nih.gov

National Institute on Aging
Building 31, Room 5C27
31 Center Drive, MSC 2292
Bethesda, MD 20892
301–496–1752
http://www.nih.gov/nia/

National Institute on Alcohol Abuse and Alcoholism
6000 Executive Boulevard, Willco
 Building
Rockville, MD 20892–7003
301–443–3860
http://www.niaaa.nih.gov

National Institute on Drug Abuse
6001 Executive Boulevard
Bethesda, MD 20892–9561
301–443–1124
http://www.nida.nih.gov

National Kidney and Urologic Diseases Information Clearinghouse
3 Information Way
Bethesda, MD 20892–3580
301–654–4415
Internet: http://www.niddk.nih.gov

National Kidney Foundation
30 East 33rd Street, Suite 1100
New York, NY 10016
800–622–9010 212–889–2210
http://www.kidney.org

National Lead Information Center
1019 19th Street NW Suite 401
Washington, DC 20036
800–424–5323 800–532–3394
http://www.healthy.net/pan/cso/cioi/
 nlic.htm

National Library Service for the Blind and Physically Handicapped
Library of Congress
Washington, DC 20542
202–707–5100 202–707–0744 (TDD)
http://lcweb.loc.gov/nls/

National Mental Health Association
1021 Prince Street
Alexandria, VA 22314
800–969–6642 703–684–7722
800–433–5959 (TTY)
http://www.nmha.org

National Multiple Sclerosis Society
733 Third Avenue
New York, NY 10017
800–344–4867 212–986–3240
http://www.nmss.org

National Neurofibromatosis Foundation
95 Pine Street, 16th Floor
New York, NY 10005
800–323–7938 212–344–6633
http://www.nf.org

National Organization for Rare Disorders
P.O. Box 8923
New Fairfield, CT 06812-8923
800–999–6673
http://www.rarediseases.org

National Osteoporosis Foundation
1232 22nd Street NW
Washington, DC 20037–1292
202–223–2226
http://www.nof.org

National Parkinson Foundation (NPF)
1501 NW 9th Avenue
Miami, FL 33136–1494
800–327–4545 305–547–6666
http://www.parkinson.org

National Pediculosis Association
P.O. Box 610189
Newton, MA 02461
781–449–6487
http://www.headlice.org

National Pesticide Telecommunications Network (NPTN)
Oregon State University
333 Weiniger
Corvallis, OR 97331–6502
800–858–7378
http://www.ace.orst.edu/info/nptn/
Provides information on health hazards of and safety precautions against pesticides.

National Psoriasis Foundation
6600 SW 92nd Avenue, Suite 300
Portland, OR 97223
800–723–9166 503–244–7404
http://www.psoriasis.org

National Reye's Syndrome Foundation
P.O. Box 829
Bryan, OH 43506
800–233–7393
http://www.bright.net/~reyessyn/

National Rosacea Society
800 South Northwest Highway, Suite 200
Barrington, IL 60010
888–662–5874 708–382–8971
http://www.rosacea.org

National Safety Council
1121 Spring Lake Drive
Itasca, IL 60143–3201
630–285–1121
http://www.nsc.org

National Sudden Infant Death Syndrome Resource Center
2070 Chain Bridge Road, Suite 450
Vienna, VA 22182
703–821–8955
http://www.circsol.com/SIDS/

National Stroke Association
96 Inverness Drive East
Englewood, CO 80112
800–787–6537 303–649–9299
http://www.stroke.org

Natural Healing Institute
P.O. Box 230294
Encinitas, CA 92023-0294
Offers license and certificate programs in naturopathic medicine, holistic health, nutrition, herbology, and massage.

NSF International, Inc.
P.O. Box 130140
789 N. Dixboro Road
Ann Arbor, MI 48113-0140
800–673–6275 734–769–8010
http://www.nsf.com

Nursing Home Information Service
National Senior Citizens Education
 and Research Council
8403 Colesville Road
Silver Spring, MD 20910
301–578–8938
http://www.nscerc.org/nursing.htm

Obsessive-Compulsive Anonymous
P.O. Box 215
New Hyde Park, NY 10041
516–739–0662
http://hometown.aol.com/west24th/
 index.html

**Osteoporosis and Related Bone
Diseases—National Resource Center**
National Institutes of Health
1232 22nd Street NW
Washington, DC 20037-1292
800–624–2663 202–223–0344
    202–466–4315 (TTY)
http://www.osteo.org

Paget Foundation
120 Wall Street, Suite 1602
New York, NY 10005
800–237–2438 212–509–5335
http://www.paget.org

**Planned Parenthood Federation
of America**
810 Seventh Avenue
New York, NY 10019
212–541–7800
http://www.plannedparenthood.org

PMS Access
429 Gammon Place
P.O. Box 259690
Madison, WI 53725
800–222–4767
http://www.womenshealth.com/
    hotline.html

Prevent Blindness America
500 East Remington Road
Schaumburg, IL 60173
800–331–2020 847–843–2020
http://www.prevent-blindness.org

Project Inform
205 13th Street, #2001
San Francisco, CA 94103
800–822–7422 415–558–9051
http://www.projectinform.org
*Provides information to help educate people
with HIV and their health care providers
about treatment.*

Rational Recovery
Box 800
Lotus CA 95651
800–303–2873 530–621–2667
http://www/rational.org/recovery/
Abstinence-based recovery.

Rolf Institute of Structural Integration
205 Canyon Boulevard
Boulder, CO 80302
800–530–8875 303–449–5903
http://www.rolf.org
*Provides information on the Rolfing method
of massage.*

**School of Shiatsu and Massage at
Harbin Hot Springs**
P.O. Box 889
Middletown, CA 95461
707–987–3801
http://aspen.forest.net/waba/school/
    school.htm

Scleroderma Federation
89 Newbury Street, Suite 201
Danvers, MA 01923
800–722–4673 978–750–4499
http://www.scleroderma.org

Scoliosis Association
P.O. Box 811705
Boca Raton, FL 33481–1705
800–800–0669 561–994–0669
http://www.spine-surgery.com/Assoc/
    scoliosis.htm

**Self Management and Recovery
Training (SMART)**
24000 Mercantile Road, Suite 11
Beachwood, OH 44122
216–292–0220
http://smartrecovery.org
*Abstinence-based recovery using cognitive-
behavioral techniques.*

Self-Help for Hard of Hearing People
7910 Woodmont Avenue, Suite 1200
Bethesda, MD 20814
301–657–2248 301–657–2249 (TTY)
http://www.shhh.org

Simon Foundation
P.O. Box 835-F
Wilmette, IL 60091
800–237–4666
http://www.simonfoundation.org
*Provides information on dealing with
incontinence.*

Sjögren's Syndrome Foundation
333 North Broadway, Suite 2000
Jericho, NY 11753
800–475–6473 516–933–6365
http://www.sjogrens.com

Skin Cancer Foundation
P.O. Box 561
New York, NY 10156
800–754–6490 212–725–5176
http://www.skincancer.org

Somerset School of Massage Therapy
7 Cedar Grove Lane
Somerset, NJ 08873
732–356–0787
http://www.ssmt.org

**Spina Bifida Association of America
(SBAA)**
4590 MacArthur Boulevard NW, Suite 250
Washington, DC 20007–4226
800–621–3141 202–944–3285
http://www.sbaa.org

**Sudden Infant Death Syndrome
Alliance**
1314 Bedford Avenue, Suite 210
Baltimore, MD 21208
800–221–7437 410–653–8226
http://www.sidsalliance.org

Thyroid Foundation of America
Ruth Sleeper Hall—RSL 350
40 Parkman Street
Boston, MA 12114–2698
800–832–8321 617–726–8500
http://www.tsh.org

Unicorn Children's Foundation
100 Greenwood Avenue
Evanston, IL 60201
888–782–8321
http://www.eunicorn.com
*Can provide a list of physicians who treat
autistic disorders and learning disabilities.*

United Cerebral Palsy Association
1660 L Street NW, Suite 700
Washington, DC 20036
800–872–5827
http://www.ucpa.org

United Ostomy Association
19772 MacArthur Boulevard, Suite 200
Irvine, CA 92612–2405
800–826–0826 714–660–8624
http://www.uoa.org

United Parkinson Foundation
833 West Washington Boulevard
Chicago, IL 60607
312–733–1893

Utah College of Massage Therapy
25 South 300 East
Salt Lake City, Utah 84111
800–617–3302
http://www.ucmt.com

VZV Research Foundation
40 East 72nd Street
New York, NY 10021
212–472–7148
http://vzvfoundation.org
*Information aabout chickenpox, shingles,
and postherpetic neuralgia.*

Water Quality Association
4151 Naperville Road
Lisle, IL 60532
708–505–0160
http://www/wqa.org
*Provides information on types of water and
methods of water treatment.*

Wilson's Disease Association
4 Navaho Drive
Brookfield, CT 06810
800–399–0266 203–775–9666
http://www.wilsonsdisease.org

Wilson's Syndrome Foundation
P.O. Box 539
Summerfield, FL 34492
800–621–7006
http://www.wilsonssyndrome.org

Women for Sobriety
P.O. Box 618
Quakerstown, PA 18951-0618
800–333–1606 215–536–8026
http://www/womenforsobriety.com

Abstinence-based recovery for women only.

Y-ME National Breast Cancer Organization
212 West Van Buren Street
Chicago, IL 60607
800–221–2141   312–986–8338
http://www.y-me.org

HEALTH TREATMENT AND RETREAT CENTERS

The following are centers that can provide assistance in maintaining or improving upon your health. The services offered by these organizations vary.

American Metabolic Institute
555 Saturn Building B
M/S 432
San Diego, CA 92154
800–388–1083   619–267–1107
http://www.ami-health.org
Provides alternative treatment for cancer and other diseases.

BioPulse Clinics
10421 South Jordan Gateway, Suite 500
South Jordan, Utah 80499
888–552–2855
Provides alternative treatment for cancer and other diseases.

Cenegenics Medical Institute
851 South Rampart Boulevard
Las Vegas, Nevada 89128
888–968–6437
http://www.cenegenics.com
Specializes in anti-aging medicine, including nutritional, exercise, and hormone management programs.

The Douglass Center for Nutrition and Preventative Medicine
101 Timberlachen Circle, Suite 101
Lake Mary, FL 32746
888–324–0888
Provides treatments focusing on restoring health without serious side effects.

Dr. Dean Ornish
Preventative Medicine Research Institute
900 Bridgeway, Suite 1
Sausalito, CA 94965
415–332–2525 extension 230
http://www.pmri.org
Offers health retreats for those interested in achieving a healthier lifestyle. The main sites are in California and Georgia, but Dr. Ornish has set up a site network at the following hospitals:

Alegent Bergan Mercy Medical Center
7500 Mercy Road
Omaha, NE 68124
402–398–6778

Alegent Immanuel Medical Center
6901 North 72nd Street
Omaha, NE 68122
402–572–2015

BroMenn Healthcare
Department of Cardiology
P.O. Box 2850
Bloomington, IL 61702
309–827–4321 extension 2522

Broward General Medical Center
Wellness Center
1625 SE Third Avenue
Fort Lauderdale, FL 33316
800–528–4888   954–355–4386
954–355–5463,

Highmark Blue Cross Blue Shield HEALTHPLACE
Health Education Center, Suite 1721
120 Fifth Avenue
Pittsburgh, PA 15222
800–447–1352
http://www.highmark.com

Highmark Blue Cross Blue Shield at Windber Medical Center
600 Somerset Avenue
Windber, PA 15963
814–467–3634

The Hippocrates Health Institute
1443 Palmdale Court
West Palm Beach, FL 33411
561–471–8876
http://www.hippocratesinst.org
Practices a holistic approach to the treatment of cancer and other illnesses.

Mercy Health Partners of Southwestern Ohio
Mercy Franciscan Hospital
Holistic Health Center
2366 Kipling Avenue
Cincinnati, OH 45239
513–853–5097

Midwest Center for Health and Healing
Swedish American Health System
4230 Newburg Road
Rockford, IL 61108
815–484–8710

St. Francis Hospital & Health Center
Cardiac Services
12935 South Gregory Street
Blue Island, IL 60406
800–721–8000   708–597–2000
extension 5560

Scripps Center for Integrative Medicine
Scripps Heart Shiley Sports & Health Center
10820 North Torrey Pines Road
La Jolla, CA CA 92037
858–554–3300

Swedish Medical Center
1101 Madison, 10th floor
Seattle, WA 98104
206–215–3500

Walter Reed Medical Center
6900 Georgia Avenue
NW Building 2 Room 4A34
Washington, DC 20307–5001
202–782–1555
Services only for military health care beneficiaries on active duty or retired military beneficiaries and their spouses and children.

Fertility Research Foundation
875 Park Avenue
New York, NY 10021
888–373–2229   212–744–5500
http://www.frfbaby.com
A treatment and research facility specializing in diagnosing and treating infertility problems.

Gillette Centers for Women's Cancers
Brigham and Women's Hospital
75 Francis Street
Boston, MA 02115
Dana-Farber Cancer Institute
44 Binney Street
Boston, MA 02115
Massachusetts General Hospital
Fruit Street
Boston, MA 02108
800–320–0022
http://cancercare.harvard.edu/cancer care/breast_gyn/breast_gyn.html

International Bio Care Hospital
U.S. Office
111 Elm Street
San Diego, CA 92101
800–785–0490   800–701–7345
http://www.ibchospital
Specializes in the treatment of cancer, arthritis, diabetes, lupus, hepatitis C, lyme disease, multiple sclerosis, degenerative diseases, and chronic fatigue syndrome. Therapies used include ultraviolet blood irradiation therapy (UBIT), chelation therapy, and other alternative treatments. Treatment facility located in Mexico.

The Johns Hopkins Breast Center
550 North Broadway
Baltimore, MD 21205
410–614–2853
http://ww2.med.jhu.edu/breastcenter/

The Johns Hopkins Hospital
600 North Wolfe Street
Baltimore, Maryland 21287
410–955–5000
http://hopkins.med.jhu.edu/ johnshopkinshospital/

Mayo Clinic
200 First Street SW
Rochester, MN 55905
507–284–2511   507–284–9786 (TDD)
http://www.mayo.edu

Mayo Clinic Hospital
5777 East Mayo Boulevard
Scottsdale, AZ 85054
480–515–6296 480–342–0169 (TDD)

Mayo Clinic Jacksonville
4500 San Pablo Road
Jacksonville, FL 32224
904–953–2000 904–953–2300 (TDD)
http://www.mayo.edu/mcj/

Mayo Clinic Scottsdale
13400 East Shea Boulevard
Scottsdale, AZ 85259
480–301–8000 480–301–7683 (TDD)
http://www.mayo.edu/mcs/

The McDougall Program at St. Helena Health Center
St. Helena Hospital
Deer Park, CA 94576
800–358–9195 707–963–6207
http://www.drmcdougall.com/
sthelena.html
Offers a twelve-day health-improvement program focusing on diet and lifestyle modifications.

Memorial Sloan-Kettering Cancer Center
1275 York Avenue
New York, NY 10021
800–525–2225
http://www.mskcc.org

New York Presbyterian Hospital
Complementary Care Center
177 Fort Washington Avenue
MHB-9GN-425
New York, NY 10032
212–305–9622
http://www.nyp.org
Offers massage, hypnosis, acupressure, reflexology, and many other treatments.

Pritikin Longevity Center
1700 Ocean Avenue
Santa Monica, CA 90401
310–458–6700
http://www.pritikinca.com

The St. John's Breast Center
St. John's Regional Health Center
1235 East Cherokee
Springfield, Missouri 65804
800–364–6120

Strang Cancer Prevention Center
428 East 72nd Street
New York, NY 10021
212–794–4900
http://www.strang.org

Weimar Institute
P.O. Box 486
Weimar, CA 95736
800–525–9192
Offers an eighteen-day health-improvement program including hydrotherapy, massage, exercise, and lifestyle counseling.

Wildwood Lifestyle Center and Hospital
P.O. Box 129
Wildwood, GA 30757
800–634–9355
http://www.tagnet.org/wildwood/

HEALTH SPAS

Doral Saturnia International Spa Resort
8755 NW 36th Street
Miami, FL 33178
305–593–6030

Fit For Life Spa
1460 South Ocean Blvd.
Pompano Beach, FL 33062
954–941–6688

Foxhollow by the River Wellness Spa
609 West Main Street, 2nd Floor
Louisville, KY 40202
502–584–3692

The Golden Door
P.O. Box 463077
Escondido, CA 92046-3077
800–424–0777

Lake Austin Resort
1705 South Quinlan Park Road
Austin, Texas 78732
800–847–5637

L'Auberge Del Mar Resort and Spa
1540 Camino Del Mar
Del Mar, CA 92014
619–259–1515

The Raj
Maharishi Ayur Veda Health Center
1734 Jasmine Avenue
Fairfield, IA 52556
800–248–9050

The Wetlands Wellness Spa at Foxhollow
9601 Covered Bridge Road
Prospect, KY 40059
502–241–7005

The Wiesbaden Hot Springs Spa and Lodgings
P.O. Box 349
Ouray, CO 81427
970–325–4347

Suggested Reading

The following list of books is provided for those who wish to explore a particular topic further. The books mentioned here are good sources of further information.

Airola, Paavo. *Cancer Causes, Prevention, and Treatment: The Total Approach.* Phoenix, AZ: Health Plus Publishers, 1972.

Airola, Paavo. *How to Get Well.* Phoenix, AZ: Health Plus Publishers, 1974.

Airola, Paavo. *How to Keep Slim, Healthy, and Young With Juice Fasting.* Phoenix, AZ: Health Plus Publishers, 1971.

Aladjem, Henrietta. *Understanding Lupus.* New York: Scribner, 1986.

Antol, Marie Nadine. *Healing Teas.* Garden City Park, NY: Avery Publishing Group, 1996.

Appleton, Nancy. *Lick the Sugar Habit.* Garden City Park, NY: Avery Publishing Group, 1996.

Astor, Stephen. *Hidden Food Allergies.* Garden City Park, NY: Avery Publishing Group, 1989.

Balch, Phyllis A. *Prescription for Dietary Wellness.* Garden City Park, NY: Avery Publishing Group, 1995.

Barnes, Broda O., and Lawrence Galton. *Hypothyroidism: The Unsuspected Illness.* New York: Cromwell, 1976.

Becker, Robert O., and Gary Selden. *Body Electric: Electromagnetism and the Foundation of Life.* New York: William Morrow & Co., 1987.

Bland, Jeffrey. *Medical Applications of Clinical Nutrition.* New Canaan, CT: Keats Pub., 1983.

Bliznakov, Emile, and Gerry Hunt. *The Miracle Nutrient: Coenzyme Q$_{10}$.* New York: Bantam Books, 1987.

Bradford, Robert W., and Michael Culbert. *Now That You Have Cancer.* Chula Vista, CA: The Bradford Foundation, 1992.

Brighthope, Ian. *The AIDS Fighters.* New Canaan, CT: Keats Publishing, 1988.

Brinkley, Ginny, Linda Goldberg, and Janice Kukar. *Your Child's First Journey.* Garden City Park, NY: Avery Publishing Group, 1989.

Buist, Robert. *Food Chemical Sensitivity.* Garden City Park, NY: Avery Publishing Group, 1988.

Cabot, Sandra. *Smart Medicine for Menopause.* Garden City Park, NY: Avery Publishing Group, 1995.

Carter, Mildred, and Tammy Weber. *Body Reflexology: Healing At Your Fingertips.* West Nyack, NY: Parker Publishing Company, 1994.

Cass, Hyla, and Terrence McNally. *KAVA: Nature's Answer to Stress, Anxiety, and Insomnia.* Rocklin, CA: Prima Publishing, 1998.

Cawood, Frank. *Super Life, Super Health.* Peachtree, GA: FC & A, 1999.

Check, William A., and Ann G. Fettner. *The Truth About AIDS: Evolution of an Epidemic.* New York: Holt, Rinehart & Winston, 1985.

Clare, Sally, and David Clare. *Creative Vegetarian Cookery.* Dorset, England: Prism Press, 1988.

Clark, Daniel and Kaye Wyatt. *Colostrum: Life's First Food The Ultimate Anti-Aging Weight Loss And Immune Supplement.* Salt Lake City, UT: CNR Publications.1998.

Crook, William. *Help For The Hyperactive Child.* Jackson, TN: Professional Books. 1991.

Crook, William G. *The Yeast Connection,* rev. ed. New York: Vintage Books, 1986.

Davidson, Paul. *Are You Sure It's Arthritis?* New York: Macmillan Publishing Co., 1985.

de Haas, Cherie. *Natural Skin Care.* Garden City Park, NY: Avery Publishing Group, 1989.

Editors of East West Journal. *Shopper's Guide to Natural Foods.* Garden City Park, NY: Avery Publishing Group, 1988.

Edwards, Linda. *Baking for Health.* Garden City Park, NY: Avery Publishing Group, 1988.

Erasmus, Udo. *Fats That Heal Fats That Kill.* Burnaby, British Columbia, Canada: Alive Books, 1993.

Evans, Gary. *Chromium Picolinate: Everything You Need to Know.* Garden City Park, NY: Avery Publishing Group, 1996.

Evans, Richard A. *Making the Right Choice: Treatment Options in Cancer Surgery.* Garden City Park, NY: Avery Publishing Group, 1995.

Feingold, Ben F. *Why Your Child Is Hyperactive.* New York: Random House, 1985.

Feingold, Helene, and Ben Feingold. *The Feingold Cookbook for Hyperactive Children and Others With Problems Associated With Food Additives and Salicylates.* New York: Random House, 1979.

Fink, John. *Third Opinion: An International Directory to Alternative Therapy Centers for the Treatment and Prevention of Cancer.* Garden City Park, NY: Avery Publishing Group, 1997.

Foster, Cynthia. *Stop the Medicine.* Scottsdale, AZ: Break On Through Press, LLC., 1999.

Frankel, Paul. *The Methylation Miracle.* New York, NY: St. Martin's Press, 1999.

Fujita, Takuo. *Calcium and Your Health.* Tokyo: Japan Publications, 1987.

Fulder, Stephen. *The Ginger Book.* Garden City Park, NY: Avery Publishing Group, 1996.

Fulder, Stephen. *The Ginseng Book.* Garden City Park, NY: Avery Publishing Group, 1996.

Germann, Donald R. *The Anti-Cancer Diet.* New York: Wyden Books, 1977.

Gittleman, Ann Louise. *Guess What Came to Dinner: Parasites and Your Health.* Garden City Park, NY: Avery Publishing Group, 1993.

Graedon, Joe, and Teresa Graedon. *The People's Guide To Deadly Drug Interactions.* New York: St. Martin's Press.

Gregory, Scott J., and Bianca Leonardo. *They Conquered AIDS!* True Life Publications, 1989.

Griffith, H. Winter. *Complete Guide to Symptoms, Illness and Surgery for People Over 50.* Los Angeles: The Body Press, 1992.

Grogan, Bryanna Clark. *Soyfoods: Cooking For A Positive Menopause*. Summertown, TN: Book Publishing Company. 1999.

Gutman, Jimmy, and Stephen Schettini. *The Ultimate GSH Handbook*. Montreal, Canada: Gutman & Schettini Enr. 1998.

Halpern, Georges. *Cordyceps: China's Healing Mushroom*. Garden City Park, NY: Avery Publishing Group, 1999.

Heidenry, Carolyn. *Making the Transition to a Macrobiotic Diet*. Garden City Park, NY: Avery Publishing Group, 1988.

Heinerman, John. *Aloe Vera, Jojoba & Yucca*. New Canaan, CT: Keats, 1982.

Heinerman, John. *Heinerman's Encyclopedia Of Nature's Vitamins And Minerals*. Paramus, NJ: Prentice Hall, 1998.

Hobbs, Christopher. *The Ginsengs: A User's Guide*. Santa Barbara, CA: Botanica Press, 1996.

Howard, Mary Ann. *Blueprint for Health*. Grand Rapids, MI: Zondervan Publishing House, 1985.

Howell, Edward. *Enzyme Nutrition*. Garden City Park, NY: Avery Publishing Group, 1987.

Huggins, Hal A. *It's All in Your Head*. Garden City Park, NY: Avery Publishing Group, 1993.

Jacobson, Michael. *Safe Food: Eating Wisely in a Risky World*. Washington, DC: Living Planet Press, 1991.

Krumholz, Harlan M., and Robert H. Phillips. *No If's, And's or Butts, The Smoker's Guide to Quitting*. Garden City Park, NY: Avery Publishing Group, 1993.

Kushi, Aveline, and Wendy Esko. *The Macrobiotic Cancer Prevention Cookbook*. Garden City Park, NY: Avery Publishing Group, 1987.

Kushi, Michio, with Edward Esko. *The Macrobiotic Approach to Cancer*. Garden City Park, NY: Avery Publishing Group, 1991.

Kushi, Michio. *The Macrobiotic Way*. Garden City Park, NY: Avery Publishing Group, 1993.

Lance, James W. *Migraine and Other Headaches*. New York: Scribner, 1986.

Lane, I. William, and Linda Comac. *Sharks Don't Get Cancer: How Shark Cartilage Could Save Your Life*. Garden City Park, NY: Avery Publishing Group, 1992.

Lane, I. William, and Linda Comac. *Sharks Still Don't Get Cancer*. Garden City Park, NY: Avery Publishing Group, 1996.

Lau, Benjamin. *Garlic For Health*. Wilmot, WI: Lotus Light Publications, 1988.

Lerman, Andrea. *The Macrobiotic Community Cookbook*. Garden City Park, NY: Avery Publishing Group, 1989.

Levenstein, Mary Kerney. *Everyday Cancer Risks and How to Avoid Them*. Garden City Park, NY: Avery Publishing Group, 1992.

Levitt, Paul, and Elissa Guralnick. *The Cancer Reference Book*. New York: Paddington Press, 1979.

Lundberg, Paul. *The Book Of Shiatsu*. New York, NY: Fireside, 1992.

Majeed, Muhammed and Lakshmi Prakash. *Lactospore: The Effective Probiotic*. Piscataway, NJ: NutriScience Publishers, Inc., 1998.

Margolis, Simeon. *The Johns Hopkins Encyclopedia Of Drugs*. New York, NY: Medletter Associates, Inc., 1998.

Marks, Edith. *Coping With Glaucoma*. Garden City Park, NY: Avery Publishing Group, 1997.

McFarland, Judy Lindberg. *Aging Without Growing Old*. Palos Verdes, CA: Western Front, LTD, 2000.

Messina, Mark, and Virginia Messina, with Ken Setchell. *The Simple Soybean and Your Health*. Garden City Park, NY: Avery Publishing Group, 1994.

Meyerowitz, Steve. *Power Juices—Super Drinks*. New York, NY: Kensington Publishing Corp., 2000.

Mindell, Earl. *Unsafe at Any Meal*. New York, NY: Warner Books, 1986.

Moss, Ralph. *Cancer Therapy: The Independent Consumer's Guide to Non-Toxic Treatment & Prevention*. Brooklyn, NY: Equinox Press, 1995.

Murray, Michael. *Encyclopedia Of Nutritional Supplements*. Rocklin, CA: Prima Publishing, 1996.

Olkin, Sylvia Klein. *Positive Pregnancy Fitness*. Garden City Park, NY: Avery Publishing Group, 1987.

Ott, John N. *Light, Radiation, and You: How to Stay Healthy*. Old Greenwich, CT: Devin-Adair Publishers, 1982.

Papon, R. Donald. *Homeopathy Made Simple*. Charlottesville, VA: Hampton Roads Publishing Company, Inc., 1999.

Passwater, Richard A., and Elmer Cranton. *Trace Elements, Hair Analysis and Nutrition*. New Canaan, CT: Keats Publishing, 1983.

Pearsall, Paul. *Superimmunity: Master Your Emotions and Improve Your Health*. New York: McGraw-Hill, 1987.

Phillips, Robert H. *Coping With Osteoarthritis*. Garden City Park, NY: Avery Publishing Group, 1989.

Phillips, Robert H. *Coping With Prostate Cancer*. Garden City Park, NY: Avery Publishing Group, 1994.

Podell, Ronald M. *Contagious Emotions: Staying Well When Your Loved One Is Depressed*. New York: Pocket Books, 1993.

Randolph, Theron G. *Human Ecology and Susceptibility to the Chemical Environment*. Springfield, IL: Charles C. Thomas, 1981.

Rapp, Doris J. *Allergies and the Hyperactive Child*. New York: Sovereign Books, 1979.

Sahelian, Ray. *DHEA: A Practical Guide*. Garden City Park, NY: Avery Publishing Group, 1996.

Sahelian, Ray. *5-HTP: Nature's Serotonin Solution*. Garden City Park, NY: Avery Publishing Group, 1998.

Selye, Hans. *Stress Without Distress*. Philadelphia: J.B. Lippincott Co., 1974.

Shelton, Herbert M. *Fasting Can Save Your Life*, rev. ed. Natural Hygiene, 1981.

Shute, Wilfrid. *Dr. Wilfrid E. Shute's Complete Updated Vitamin E Book*. New Canaan, CT: Keats Publishing, 1975.

Smith, Lendon. *Feed Your Kids Right: Dr. Smith's Program for Your Child's Total Health*. New York: McGraw-Hill, 1979.

Svoboda, Robert. *Prakruti: Your Ayurvedic Constitution*. Albuquerque, NM: Geocom Limited, 1989.

Swanson, David. *Mayo Clinic On Chronic Pain*. New York, NY: Kensington Publishing Corporation, 1999.

Steinman, David, and Samuel S. Epstein. *The Safe Shoppers Bible*. New York: Macmillan, 1995.

Teitelbaum, Jacob. *From Fatigued to Fantastic*. Garden City Park, NY: Avery Publishing Group, 1996.

Treben, Maria. *Health from God's Garden: Herbal Remedies for Glowing Health and Glorious Well-Being*. Rochester, VT: Thorsons Publishers, 1987.

Ulene, Art. *Complete Guide To Vitamins, Minerals, And Herbs*. New York, NY: Avery Books (an imprint of Penguin Putnam), 2000.

University of California, Berkeley. *Wellness Letter: The Newsletter Of Nutrition, Fitness, And Stress Management*. Berkeley, CA.

Wade, Carlson. *Carlson Wade's Amino Acids Book*. New Canaan, CT: Keats Publishing, 1985.

Walker, Lynne. *Nature's Pharmacy*. Paramus, NJ: Reward Books, 1998.

Walker, Morton. *The Chelation Way*. Garden City Park, NY: Avery Publishing Group, 1990.

Walters, Richard. *Options: The Alternative Cancer Therapy Book.* Garden City Park, NY: Avery Publishing Group, 1993.

Warren, Tom. *Beating Alzheimer's.* Garden City Park, NY: Avery Publishing Group, 1991.

Weber, Marcea. *Macrobiotics and Beyond.* Garden City Park, NY: Avery Publishing Group, 1989.

Weber, Marcea. *Whole Meals.* Dorset, England: Prism Press, 1983.

Webster, David. *Acidophilus And Colon Health.* New York, NY: Kensington Publishing, 1999.

Weiner, Michael A. *Maximum Immunity.* Boston: Houghton Mifflin Co., 1986.

Wigmore, Ann. *Recipes for Longer Life.* Garden City Park, NY: Avery Publishing Group, 1982.

Wigmore, Ann. *The Wheatgrass Book.* Garden City Park, NY: Avery Publishing Group, 1985.

Williams, Xandria. *What's in My Food?* Dorset, England: Prism Press, 1988.

Wilson, Roberta. *Aromatherapy for Vibrant Health and Beauty.* Garden City Park, NY: Avery Publishing Group, 1995.

Wlodyga, Ronald R. *Health Secrets From the Bible.* Triumph Publishers, 1979.

Woessner, Candace, Judith Lauwers, and Barbara Bernard. *Breastfeeding Today.* Garden City Park, NY: Avery Publishing Group, 1988.

Wolfe, Sidney and Rose-Ellen Hope. *Worst Pills Best Pills II.* Washington, D.C.: Public Citizen's Health Research Group, 1993.

Ziff, Sam. *Silver Dental Fillings: The Toxic Timebomb.* Santa Fe, NM: Aurora Press, 1984.

Index

Abscess, 120–21
AbsorbAid, 61
ACE inhibitors, 275, 326
Acerola (*Malpighia glabra*), 88
Acetaminophen, 195, 726
Achondroplasia, 400
Acid/alkali imbalance, 122–25
Acid-Ease, 61
Acidophilus. *See Lactobacillus acidophilus*
Acidosis, 122–23
Acne, 125–28
Acquired immunodeficiency syndrome. *See* AIDS
Actinic keratoses, 628, 631
Acupressure, 721
Acupuncture, 211, 721
Acute mastitis, 229
Acute seasonal allergic rhinitis, 154
Acyclovir (Zovirax), 285, 624
Adaptive immunity, 680
Addison's disease, 129
Additives, 8
Adenomyosis, 349
Adenosine triphosphate (ATP), 63, 66–67, 73
Adrenal disorders, 129–31
Adrenal hormones, 647
Adrenaline, 129
Adrenocorticotropic hormone (ACTH), 131, 239, 647
Aerobic Bulk Cleanse, 70
Aerobic Colon Care, 70
Aged garlic extract, 55
Age spots, 131–32
Aging, 132–38
AIDS (acquired immunodeficiency syndrome), 138–47, 499, 629, 668
Alanine, 44
Alcoholism, 147–53
Aldosterone, 129
Alendronate (Fosamax), 553
Alexander, Dale, 68
Alfalfa (*Medicago sativa*), 63, 88
Alkalosis, 123–25
All Complete Enzymes, 61
Allergens, 153
Allergic dermatitis, 319
Allergies, 153–67
Allergy Relief, 81
Allopathy, 85
Allopurinol (Zyloprim), 399
Aloe (*Aloe vera*), 63–64, 89
Alopecia, 401
Alpha-hydroxy acids, 339, 549, 691
Alpha-lipoic acid, 152
Alprazolam (Xanax), 182

Alternative cancer therapies, 248–49
Alternative Medicine, Office of, 86
Aluminum, 169
   cookware, 10, 219
   toxicity, 167–68, 355
Alzheimer's disease, 168–74, 506
American diet, 26
American Health, 732
American Journal of Cardiology, 45
American Journal of Clinical Nutrition, 136
American Journal of Epidemiology, 262
American Journal of Pain Management, 724
American Journal of Public Health, 135
Amiloride (Midamor, Moduretic), 313
Amino acids, 4, 42–43, 546
   branched-chain, 42
   daily dosages, 6
   D- and L- forms, 44
   essential, 43
   free-form, 43
   functions in body, 44
   list of, 44–52
   over-the-counter, 43–44
Amino sugar, 72
Amniocentesis, 584
A.M./P.M. Ultimate Cleanse, 70
Analgesics, 299, 725–26
Anasarca, 342
Androstenedione, 129
Anemia, 174–77, 576
Angelman syndrome, 353
Angiogenesis inhibitor, 79
Animal protein, 483–85, 559
Anisakis, 688
Anise (*Pimpinella anisum*), 89
Annals of Internal Medicine, 195, 390, 422
Annals of Neurology, 528
Annatto (*Bixa orellana*), 89
Anorexia nervosa, 177–79
Antacids, 423, 462, 563
Antibiotics, 8, 219, 286, 300, 627
Antidepressants, 318
Antihistamines, 299
Antioxidants, 15, 309, 417, 560
   combination supplements, 58
   and free radicals, 53–54
   list of, 53–58
Anti-sense compounds, 146
Anxiety disorder, 179–82
Apis mellifica, 216
APO-E4, 173
Appendicitis, 183–84
Appetite, poor, 184–85
Arachidonic acid (AA), 313
Archives of General Psychiatry, 51
Archives of Internal Medicine, 638

Archives of Opthalmology, 367
Arginine, 44–45
Ariboflavinosis, 16
Aromatherapy, 650, 695–97
Arrhythmias, 269
Arsenic poisoning, 185
Arterial ulcers, 491
Arteriosclerosis/Atherosclerosis, 186–88
Arteriosclerosis obliterans, 186
Artesian water, 40
Arthogesic, 81
Arthritis, 188–95
Artichoke, 81
Artificial ingredients, 8
Asai, Kazuhiko, 28
Ascarids, 686, 688
Ascorbic acid, 13, 20–21
Ascorbic acid flush, 697–98
Ashwagandha (*Withania somnifera*), 89
Asparagine, 45
Aspartame, 10, 355
Aspartic acid, 45
Aspirin, 8, 604, 726
Astemizole (Hismanal), 407
Asthma, 195–200, 576
Astragalus (*Astragalus membranaceus*), 89
Atherosclerosis. *See* Arteriosclerosis/Atherosclerosis
Athlete's foot, 200–201, 387
Atopic dermatitis, 319
Atrophic vaginitis, 670
Attention deficit disorder (ADD)/ Attention deficit hyperactivity disorder (ADHD), 201–5
Autism, 205–8
Autistic savants, 206
Autoimmune disorders, 681
Ayurvedic remedies, 156, 197, 698
Azoles, 201

Backache, 208–12, 576–77
Bacterial pneumonia, 568
Bad breath. *See* Halitosis
Bags under the eyes, 358
Balch, Phyllis, 547
Baldness. *See* Hair loss
Barberry (*Berberis vulgaris*), 89
Barium enema, 328
Barley grass, 64
Barley Green, 72
Barrett's esophagus, 422, 424
Basal cell carcinoma, 627
Basophils, 680
Bayberry (*Myrica cerifera*), 90
B cells, 680

Beans, 4
Beating Alzheimer's (Warren), 173
Bedsores, 212–14
Bed-wetting, 214–15
Bee pollen, 64
Bee propolis, 64, 261
Bee sting, 215–16
Behçet's syndrome, 654, 656
Belladonna, 238
Benign prostatic hyperplasia (BPH), 591
Berson, Eliot, Dr., 368
Beta-amyloid, 172
Beta-blockers, 275, 397
Beta-carotene, 15
Beta-1,3–D-glucan, 64, 467
Betatene, 81
Bifidobacterium bifidum, 64–65
Bilberry (*Vaccinium myrtillus*), 53–54, 90
Bile, 389
Bilirubin, 479
Biofeedback, 721
Bioflavonoids, 13, 23, 397
Bio-Gestin, 61
Bioperine 10, 62
Biotin, 18, 616
Bio-Zyme, 61
Bipolar disorders, 315
Birch (*Betula alba*), 90
Birth plan, 586
Bites. *See* Bee sting; Dog bite; Insect
    allergy; Snakebite; Spider bite
Bitot's spots, 358–59
Black cohosh (*Cimicifuga racemosa*), 90
Black walnut (*Juglans nigra*), 90
Black widow spider, 641–42
Bladder cancer, 254
Bladder discomfort/infection, 577
Bladder infection (cystitis), 216–19
Bladder polyps, 574
Bleeding gums, 577
Blepharitis, 359
Blessed thistle (*Cnicus benedictus*), 90
Blood-brain barrier, 42
Blood clot, 654
Blood pressure problems. *See* High
    blood pressure
Blood purification, 698–99
Bloodshot eyes, 359
Blood sugar problems. *See* Diabetes;
    Hypoglycemia
Blue cohosh (*Caulophyllum
    thalictroides*), 90
Blurred vision, 359–60
B lymphocytes, 680
Body Language Essential Green
    Foods, 81
Body mass index, 545–46
Boil, 120, 219–21
Boldo (*Peumus boldus*), 91
Bone density measurement, 550
Bone marrow, 681
    transplant, 228
Bone Maximizer, 81
Boneset (*Eupatorium perfoliatum*), 91
Bone spur, 424–25
Bone Support with Ostivone, 81
Books on nutritional healing, 764–66

Borage (*Borago officinalis*), 91
Boron, 25–26
Borrelia burgdorferi, 496
Boswellia (*Boswellia serrata*), 91
BotanImmune, 82
Bottled water, 40
Bovine cartilage, 65
Breast cancer, 221–29
Breastfeeding-related problems, 229–32
Breast Health, 82, 226
Breast self-examination, 222–23
Breathing exercises, 721–22
Brewer's yeast. *See* Yeast
Bright's disease, 481
British Medical Journal, 157, 318
Bronchitis, 232–35. *See also* Asthma;
    Emphysema; Hay fever;
    Pneumonia; Sinusitis
Brown recluse spider, 641–42
Brown rice, 4
Bruising, 235–37
Bruxism, 237–38
Buchu (*Barosma betulina*), 91
Bulimarexia, 177
Bulimia, 177, 238–41
Bupropion (Zyban), 319, 638
Burdock (Arctium lappa), 54, 91
Burns, 241–43
Butcher's broom (*Ruscus aculeatus*), 91
B vitamins, 13, 15–20, 587

Cadmium toxicity, 245–46, 361
Caffeine, 8, 552
Calcified bursitis, 244
Calcitonin, 554, 556
Calcium, 26–27, 29, 253, 440, 485
    forms of, 553
    and osteoporosis, 550
Calcium channel blockers, 275
Calendula (*Calendula officinalis*), 92
CamoCare, 82
Campylobacter jejuni, 380
Cancer, 246–62. *See also* Individual
    cancers
Cancer (journal), 222
Candida albicans, 263
Candida infection of the nipples, 387
Candida septicemia, 263
Candidiasis, 263–66, 319
Canker sores (aphthous ulcers), 266–67
Capecitabine (Xeloda), 227
Capsaicin, 624, 723
Carbamazepine (Tegretol), 172
Carbohydrate addicts, 545
Carbohydrates, 3–4
    complex, 3, 204, 590
    simple, 3, 204, 544
Carbonic anhydrase inhibitors, 397
Carbozyme, 62
Carbuncle, 219–20
Cardiac asthma, 196
Cardiaforce, 82
Cardio Enzyme Formula, 61
Cardiovascular disease, 267–75
Carnitine, 45–46
Carotenoids, 15, 57–58
Carpal tunnel syndrome, 275–79

Cascara sagrada (*Frangula purshiana*), 92
Catalase, 59
Cataracts, 360–62
Catnip (*Nepeta cataria*), 92
Catnip tea enema, 705–6
Cat's claw (*Uncaria tomentosa*), 92
Cavarocchi, Nicholas, Dr., 732
Cavities. *See* Tooth decay
Cayenne (*Capsicum frutescens*), 92
Cedar (*Cedrus libani*), 92
Celecoxib (Celebrex), 193
Celery (*Apium graveolens*), 93
Celiac disease, 279–81
Cell-mediated immunity, 680
Cellular targets, 146–47
Cellulose, 70
Cerasomal-cis-9–cetylmyristoleate, 65
Cerebral allergies, 157
Cervical cancer, 254–55
Cervical polyps, 574
Chamomile (*Matricaria recutita*), 93
Chanca piedra (*Phyllanthus niruri*), 93
Chaparral (*Larrea tridentata*), 93
Chaste tree (*Vitex agnus-castus*), 93
Chelation therapy, 699–701
Chemical allergies, 281–82
Chemical peels, 691
Chemical poisoning, 283
Chickenpox, 283–85
Chickweed (*Stellaria media*), 93
Chinese medicine, 86, 156, 701–2
Chiropractic, 722
Chiropractors, 211
Chlamydia, 285–86, 463
Chlamydia pneumoniae, 418, 528
Chlamydia trachomatis, 568
Chlorella, 65
Chlorine, 36
Chlorophyll, 699. *See also* Chlorella;
    Green drinks
Cholecystokinin-pancreozymin
    (CCK), 241
Cholesterol, 5, 440–43
Cholesterol Enzyme Formula, 61
Cholesterol problems. *See* High
    cholesterol
Choline, 18–19
Chondroitin sulfate, 65–66
Chorionic villus sampling, 584
Chromium, 27–28
Chromium Picolinate, 27, 82
Chromosome 21, 331
Chronic fatigue syndrome, 286–90
Chronic Fatigue Syndrome (Stoff), 287
Chronic obstructive pulmonary
    disease (COPD), 343
Chronic vertigo, 674
Chuchuhuasi (*Maytenus krukovit*), 94
Cinnamon (*Cinnamomum verum*), 94
Circulatory problems, 290–92
Cirrhosis of the liver, 292–95
Citrin, 66
Citrulline, 46
Clostridium
    botulinum, 379–80
    difficile, 229
    perfringens, 380

tetani, 330
Clove *(Syzygium aromaticum),* 94
Coenzyme A, 66
Coenzyme Q$_{10}$, 23–24, 54, 66, 136–37
Coffee retention enema, 706
Colchicine, 399
Cold. *See* Common cold
Cold sores (fever blisters), 295–96
Cold therapy, 723
Cold water therapy, 715–16
Colitis. *See* Ulcerative colitis
Colloidal silver, 66, 219, 266
Colon cleansing, 702–3
Colonoscopy, 328
Colorblindness, 362
Colorectal cancer, 255, 303
Color therapy (chromotherapy), 703–4
Colostrum, 66, 137
Comfrey *(Symphytum officinale),* 94
Common cold, 297–300, 577
Common warts, 678–79
Complementary Medicine for the
    Physician, 197
Complete Guide to Symptoms, Illness
    and Surgery for People Over 50
    (Griffith), 172
Complexion problems. *See* Acne; Dry
    skin; Oily skin; Psoriasis; Rosacea;
    Wrinkles
Compresses, 87
Compression therapy, 674
Conjunctivitis (pinkeye), 362–63
Constipation, 300–303, 577
Cooking, 2
Coping with Prostate Cancer (Phillips), 596
Copper, 28, 208
    deficiency, 303–4
    toxicity, 304–5, 612, 684–86
Corneal stroma, 342
Corneal ulcer, 363
Corn germ, 66–67
Corns and calluses, 305–6
Corn silk *(Zea mays),* 94
Coronary arteries, 268
Cortisol, 129
Cough medicines, 299
Coughs, 577
Cow's milk, 177
Cradle cap, 616
Cramer, Daniel W., 349
Cramp bark *(Viburnum opulus),* 94
Cramps. *See* Muscle cramps;
    Premenstrual syndrome
Cranberry *(Vaccinium macrocarpon),* 95
C-reactive protein, 418
Creams, 87
Creatine, 67
Crohn's disease, 306–10
Crook, William, Dr., 81
Croup, 310
Cryosurgery, 595, 631
Crystal therapy, 704
Cushing's syndrome, 129
Cu/Zn SOD, 57
Cyanocobalamin, 18
Cyclophilin inhibitors, 147
Cysteine, 46

Cystic fibrosis, 311–13
Cystine, 46
Cystitis, 217
Cytomegalovirus, 521

D.A. #34 Food Enzymes, 61
Daily Essential Enzymes, 61
Daily Value (DV), 13
Dairy products, 204
Damiana *(Turnera diffusa),* 95
Danazol (Danocrine), 349, 372
Dandelion *(Taraxacum officinale),* 95
Dandruff, 313–14
Deafness. *See* Hearing loss
Decoctions, 87
Decongestants, 299
Deep breathing, 649
Deep venous thrombosis (DVT), 654–55
DEET, 473, 498
Dehydroepiandrosterone (DHEA), 67,
    129, 137, 261, 554, 684
    therapy, 704–5
Deionized water, 40
Delayed-onset muscle soreness, 208
Dementia, 168, 617–19
Demodex folliculorum, 610
Dependent edema, 342
Depression, 314–19, 577–78
Dermatitis, 319–21
Dermatitis herpetiformis, 279, 319
Desiccated liver, 67
Developmental Pharmacology and
    Therapy, 304
Devil's claw *(Harpagophytum*
    procumbens), 95
Deyo, Richard, Dr., 211
D-glucaric acid, 253
Diabetes, 321–26
Diabetic nephropathy, 325
Diabetic neuropathy, 325
Diabetic retinopathy, 325, 363
Diabetic ulcers, 491
Diadzein, 253
Diagnostic and Statistical Manual of
    Mental Disorders (DSM-IV), 201
Diamond Mind, 82
Diamond Trim, 82
Diarrhea, 326–28
Diclofenac sodium (Voltaren), 195
Digest Support, 61
Dimethylaminoethanol (DMAE), 67, 138
Dimethylglycine (DMG), 67, 138
Dimethylsulfoxide (DMSO), 67–68, 194,
    214, 245, 261, 399, 492, 674
Dimness of vision, 363–64
Dinarello, Charles, Dr., 193
Dioxins, 349
Diphosphates, 556
Discoid lupus erythematosus, 493–94
Disorders, 116. *See also* under individual
    disorders
    troubleshooting for, 117–19
Disulfiram (Antabuse), 152
Diverticulitis, 328–30
Diverticulosis, 328
Dizziness, 578, 675. *See also* Ménière's
    disease; Vertigo

DL-phenylalanine (DLPA), 182
DNA, 45, 48, 65, 246, 601, 636, 638
DNAase (Dornase), 313
Docosahexaenoic acid (DHA), 229, 313
Dog bite, 330–31
Donepezil (Aricept), 173
Dong quai *(Angelica sinensis),* 95
Dopamine, 315, 558
Doq, Tieraona Low, Dr., 144
Double depression, 315
Down syndrome, 331–33
Doxepin (Sinequan), 290
Drug addiction (substance abuse), 334–37
Dry eyes, 364
Dry mouth, 566–67
Dry skin, 337–39
Ductal carcinoma in situ, 221
Dwarfism, 400
Dyspepsia. *See* Indigestion
Dysplastic nevi, 628
Dysthymia, 315

Ear infection, 340–41
Earth's Bounty NONI, 82
Earthsource Greens & More, 72
Eating disorders. *See* Anorexia nervosa;
    Appetite, poor; Bulimia; Obesity;
    Underweight
Ebersole, Jeffrey, Dr., 566
Echinacea *(Echinacea species),* 95, 300
Echinaforce, 82
Eclampsia, 578–79
Ectopic pregnancy, 579
Eczema, 319
Edema, 342–43, 579
Edison, Thomas, 704
Edwards, Nancy, Dr., 174
Elastase, 61
Elder *(Sambucus nigra),* 96
Electromyography (EMG), 276
Emphysema, 343–46
Emu oil, 68
Endometriosis, 346–49
Endoscopic technique, 278
Enemas, 705–7
Engorgement (breast), 229
Enlarged prostate. *See* Prostatitis/
    Enlarged prostate
Enteritis, 666
Enuresis. *See* Bed-wetting
Environmental Protection Agency (EPA),
    36, 38, 350
Environmental toxicity, 350–52
Enzymes, 13, 59
    commercially available, 60–61
    digestive, 59
    food, 60
    functions in body, 59
    metabolic, 59
    over-the-counter, 61–62
Eosinophils, 680
Ephedra *(Ephedra sinica),* 96
Epicondylitis, 244
Epilepsy, 352–55
Epinephrine, 216, 397, 471
Epirubicin (Ellence), 227
Epistaxis, 538

Epstein-Barr virus, 521
Escherichia coli, 217, 380
Esophageal cancer, 255–56
Essential fatty acids (EFAs), 68–69
Essential oils, 86, 623, 695–97
Estriol excretion studies, 585
Estrogen, 221–22, 511, 514
Estrogen replacement therapy, 222, 455
EstroGentle, 82
Eucalyptus (*Eucalyptus globulus*), 96
European Journal of Cancer, 261
Evening primrose oil. *See* Primrose oil
Everyday Cancer Risks and How to Avoid Them (Levenstein), 253
Exercise, 649, 707–8
External otitis, 340
Extracts, 86
Eyebright (*Euphrasia officinalis*), 96
Eye problems, 355–69
Eyestrain, 364–65

Fad diets, 544
False unicorn root (*Chamaelirium luteum*), 96
Familial polyposis, 574
Fasting, 708–10
Fatigue. *See* Chronic fatigue syndrome
Fats, 4–5, 442–43, 501
Fennel (*Foeniculum vulgare*), 69, 96
Fentanyl (Actiq), 227
Fenugreek (*Trigonella foenum-graecum*), 97
Fertility tests, 465
Fever, 369–71
Feverfew (*Chrysanthemum parthenium*), 97
Fiber, 3, 69–70, 300–301
Fibrocystic breasts, 371–72
Fibroids, uterine, 372–74
Fibromyalgia syndrome, 374–78
Fibroplex, 82
Fibrositis, 208
Filtration, water, 39–40
Finasteride (Proscar), 598
Firshein, Richard, 199
Fish oil, 68, 309
5–alpha-reductase, 594
5–hydroxy L-tryptophan (5–HTP), 70–71, 241
Flavonoids, 55
Flax (*Linum usitatissimum*), 68–69, 97
Floaters, 365
Flu. *See* Influenza
Fluoridation, 37–38
Fluoride, 556, 567
Fluoxetine (Prozac), 290
Folate, 19
Folic acid, 355, 587
Follicle-stimulating hormone (FSH), 516
Food allergies, 154
Food and Drug Administration (FDA), 5, 40, 51
Foodborne/Waterborne disease, 378–84
Foods
  acceptable, 11
  additives and artificial ingredients in, 8

to avoid, 11
  cookware for, 10
  overcooking, 9–10
  phytochemicals in, 9
  raw, 8
Fracture, 384–86
Frankt, Robert, Dr., 458
Free radicals, 53–54, 247
Free radical scavengers, 53
Free radical theory of aging, 132
Frigidity, 386–87
Fruits, 8
Fungal infection, 387–89
Fungal pneumonia, 568
Furuncle, 219

Gallbladder disorders, 389–91
Gamma-aminobutyric acid (GABA), 46–47, 205
Gamma-globulin, 290, 394
Gamma-linolenic acid (GLA), 193, 545
Gangrene, 391–92
Garlic (*Allium sativa*), 55, 71, 97, 231, 383
Gas, 579–80. *See also* Heartburn/Gastroesophageal reflux disease; Indigestion
Gastroenteritis. *See* Foodborne/Waterborne disease
Gastroesophageal reflux disease. *See* Heartburn/Gastroesophageal reflux disease
GastroSoothe, 82
Gemstone therapy, 704
Genistein, 253
Genital herpes, 433
Genital warts, 678–79
Gentian (*Gentiana lutea*), 97
Germanium, 28
German measles (rubella), 392–94
Gestational diabetes, 321, 578
Giardia lamblia, 380
Gigantism, 400
Ginger (*Zingiber officinale*), 98
Gingivitis, 564
Ginkgo (*Ginkgo biloba*), 55, 71, 98
Ginseng (*Panax quinquefolius; Panax ginseng*), 71–72, 98
Glandular therapy, 710–13
Glaucoma, 365–66, 394–97
Gleason score, 592
Glomerulonephritis, 481
Glossary, 737–45
Glucaric acid, 226
Glucomannan, 69–70
Glucosamine, 72
Glucose tolerance factor, 27
Glucose tolerance test (GTT), 448
Glucosidase inhibitors, 147
Glutamate, 173
Glutamic acid, 47
Glutamine, 47
Glutathione, 48, 55–56, 138
Gluten, 279, 321, 616
Glycine, 48
Glycolic acid, 691
Glycosaminoglycans, 65
Glycosylation, 325

Goldenseal (*Hydrastis canadensis*), 98, 565, 626
Gonorrhea, 619–20
Gonzalez, Nicholas, Dr., 253
Gotu kola (*Centella asiatica*), 99
Gout, 189–90, 397–400
Grape seed extract, 57, 138, 261
Grape seed oil, 69
Gravel root (*Eupatorium purpureum*), 99
Graves' disease, 447
Green drinks, 72, 717–18
Green Magma, 72
Green papaya, 72–73
Green tea (*Camellia sinensis*), 56, 99
Griffith, H. Winter, Dr., 172
Groin spasm, stitch, or pressure, 580
Ground water, 40
Growth hormone therapy, 713
Growth problems, 400–401
Guarana (*Paullinia cupana*), 99
Guar gum, 70
Guided imagery, 722
Gum disease. *See* Periodontal disease

Hahnemann, Samuel, 714
Hair analysis, 713–14
Hair loss, 401–4
Halitosis (bad breath), 404–5
Halsted radical mastectomy, 227
Hand tremors, 560
Harman, Denham, Dr., 132
Harvard Mental Health Letter, 241
Hashimoto's disease, 451
Hawthorn (*Crataegus laevigata*), 99
Hay fever, 154, 405–7
Headache, 408–13
Health and medical organizations, 755–63
Hearing aids, 416
Hearing loss, 413–17
Heart attack, 268, 417–22
Heartburn/Gastroesophageal reflux disease (GERD), 422–24, 580
Heart disease. *See* Cardiovascular disease; Heart attack
Heart failure, 269
Heat therapy, 722–23
Heel spur, 424–25
Helicobacter pylori, 418, 561, 563
Hemicellulose, 70
Hemophilia, 425–26
Hemorrhoids, 426–29, 580, 674
Hepatitis, 292, 429–32
Hepatolenticular degeneration, 684
Herbal Mood Boost, 82
Herbs, 85
  actions and targets in body, 113–14
  alternative healing systems, 86
  buying, 88
  essential oils, 86
  extracts, 86
  guidelines for taking, 88
  list of, 88–112
  pain relieving, 723–24
  phytomedicines, 85–86
  plasters, compresses, and poultices, 87
  powders, 87

salves, ointments, and creams, 87
steam inhalation, 729
stimulating, 85
syrups, 87
teas, infusions, and decoctions, 87
tinctures, 87
tonics, 85
vinegars, 87
wines, 87
Herniated disk, 208
Herpesvirus infection, 433–35
Herpes zoster. *See* Shingles
Hiatal hernia, 422
High blood pressure (hypertension), 268, 290, 436–40
High cholesterol, 440–43
High-density lipoproteins (HDL) cholesterol, 417, 440–41, 707
Hill, David, 383
Hirschsprung's disease, 301
Histidine, 48
Hives, 443–46
HIV (human immunodeficiency virus), 138–41, 426. *See also* AIDS
Hoffer, Abram, Dr., 14
Homeopathy, 157, 204–5, 714–15
Homocysteine, 48–49, 172, 417
Honey, 73
Honeybee venom, 195, 399
Hookworms, 686, 688
Hops (*Humulus lupulus*), 100
Horehound (*Marrubium vulgare*), 100
Hormone replacement therapy, 514–15, 554, 567
Horse chestnut (*Aesculus hippocastanum*), 100
Horsetail (*Equisetum arvense*), 100
Hot water therapy, 715
Howell, Edward, Dr., 59
Huggins, Hal, Dr., 518
Human body, 2
Human growth hormone (HGH), 138, 546, 554, 684
therapy, 713
Human papilloma viruses (HPV), 677–78
Humoral immunity, 680
Hydrangea (*Hydrangea arborescens*), 100
Hydrazine sulfate, 261
Hydrochloric acid, 60, 460, 532
Hydrolysis, 42
Hydronephrosis, 481
Hydrotherapy, 715–16
Hydroxycitric acid, 545
Hyperbaric oxygen therapy, 716
Hypercalciuria, 483
Hyper-C Serum, 82
Hyperemesis gravidarum, 581
Hyperglycemia, 321–22
HyperiCalm, 82
Hyperkeratosis, 305
Hyperosmolar syndrome, 322
Hypertension. *See* High blood pressure
Hyperthermia, 261
Hyperthyroidism, 446–48
Hypnotherapy, 724
Hypochlorhydria, 319
Hypoglycemia (low blood sugar), 448–50

Hypokalemia, 177
Hypothyroidism, 450–53
Hyssop (*Hyssopus officinalis*), 100
Hysterectomy-related problems, 453–55

Idiopathic epilepsy, 353
IgE, 157
Ileitis, 666
Imipramine hydrochloride (Janimine; Tofranil), 182
Immune system, weakened. *See* Weakened immune system
Impaired glucose tolerance, 321
Impotence, 455–59
Incontinence, 459–60
Indigestion (dyspepsia), 460–62
Infertility, 463–66
Infiltrating ductal carcinoma, 221
Inflammation, 466–68
Inflammatory carcinoma, 221
Inflazyme, 62
Infla-Zyme Forte, 61–62
Infliximab (Remicade), 309
Influenza, 468–70
Infusions, 87
Inherited copper toxicosis, 684
Injuries of the muscles and joints, 643–46
Innate immunity, 680
Inosine, 73
Inositol, 19, 231
Inositol hexaphosphate (IP$_6$), 73, 253
Insect allergy, 470–71
Insect bite, 471–73
Insomnia, 473–76, 580–81
Instant Enerjetz, 82
Insulin, 324–25
Interferon alfa, 679
Interferons, 300
Interleukin-2, 261
Intermittent claudication, 186
Intracellular adhesion molecule (ICAM-1), 418
Intraductal carcinoma in situ, 221
Intravenous chelation therapy, 701
Intrinsic asthma, 196
Intrinsic factor, 18, 133
Iodine, 29
Ionizing radiation, 601
Irish moss (*Chondrus crispus*), 101
Iron, 29–30, 672
deficiency, 665
Irritable bowel syndrome, 303, 476–79
Isoleucine, 49
Itchy eyes, 366
It's All in Your Head (Huggins), 518

Jaborandi (*Pilocarpus jaborandi*), 101
Jatoba (*Hymenaea courbaril*), 101
Jaundice, 479–80
Jaw pain. *See* Bruxism; Stress; TMJ syndrome
Jerusalem artichoke tablets, 82–83
Jock itch, 387
Johns Hopkins Medical Letter, 424, 462
Journal of Advancement in Medicine, 701
Journal of Allergy and Clinical Immunology, 199

Journal of Burn Care and Rehabilitation, 243
Journal of Clinical Nutrition, 552
Journal of Family Practice, 554
Journal of Neurology, Neurosurgery, & Psychiatry, 173
Journal of Pineal Research, 361
Journal of the American Academy of Dermatology, 632
Journal of the American Medical Association, 30, 55, 171, 274, 347, 349, 361, 390, 552, 707
Journal of the National Cancer Institute, 144, 594
Juicing, 717–18
Juniper (*Juniperus communis*), 101
Juvenile vertigo, 675

Kagnoff, Martin F., Dr., 281
Kamen, Betty, Dr., 455
Kaposi's sarcoma, 628–29
Karbozyme, 62
Kava kava (*Piper methysticum*), 101, 316–17
Kava-30, 83
Kayser-Fleischer ring, 684
Kelp, 73–74
Ketogenic diet, 355
Ketosis, 544
Kidney disease (renal failure), 480–83
Kidney stones, 481, 483–85
Kinesiology, 211
Klevay, Leslie, 304
Kolorex, 83
Kombucha tea, 74
Kragballe, Knud, Dr., 600
Krumholz, Harlan, 638
Kudzu (*Pueraria lobata*), 101
Kyo-Green, 72
Kyolic Neuro Logic, 83

Lactobacillus acidophilus, 4, 74, 461
Lactoferrin, 74
Lactose intolerance (lactase deficiency), 485–87
Lady's mantle (*Achillea millefolium*), 101–2
The Lancet, 171, 177, 281, 513, 521, 613
Langer, Stephen, Dr., 325
Laryngeal cancer, 256
Lavender (*Lavandula angustifolia*), 102
Lawrence, Ruth, Dr., 231
Laxatives, 302–3
Lead poisoning, 487–90
Leaky gut syndrome, 60, 309
Lecithin, 74–75, 173
Ledum palustre, 216
Lee, Royal, Dr., 710
Leg cramps, 581. *See also* Muscle cramps
Legionella pneumophila, 492
Legionnaire's disease, 492–93
Leg ulcers, 490–92
Lemongrass (*Cymbopogon citratus*), 102
Lemon juice cleansing enema, 706–7
Lennox-Gastaut syndrome, 353
Let's Live, 677
Leucine, 49
Leukemia, 256–57

Leuprolide (Lupron), 598
Levodopa, 560
Licorice (*Glycyrrhiza glabra*), 102, 562
Lifestyle Heart Trial study, 188
Light therapy, 719
Lignin, 70
Lin, Robert I-San, Dr., 55
Lin Yutang, 86
Lipofuscin accumulation, 131
Lipoic acid, 138
Lipothiamine, 62
Lithium, 504
Liver, 148–49, 294
Liver disease. *See* Cirrhosis of the liver;
    Hepatitis
Lobular carcinoma, 221
Loss of vision, 363–64
Low-density lipoproteins (LDLs), 5, 48,
    188, 326, 417, 440–41, 707
Lumbago, 209
Lumpectomy, 227
Lung cancer, 257–58
Lupus, 493–96
Lutein, 253, 361
Lycopene, 144
Lyme disease, 496–99
Lymphatic system, 680–81
Lymphocytes, 680
Lymphoma (non-Hodgkin's), 258
Lysine, 26, 49

Maca (*Lepidium meyenii*), 103
Macela (*Achyrocline satureoides*), 103
Macrosomia, 578
Macular degeneration, 366–67
Magnesium, 30, 215, 440, 677
    deficiency, 612
Magnet therapy, 211, 724
Maitake (*Grifola frondosa*), 75, 138
Malabsorption syndrome, 499–502
Male menopause, 516
Malnutrition. *See* Malabsorption
    syndrome; Underweight
Manganese, 30–31, 552
Manic-depressive disorder/Bipolar
    mood disorder, 315, 502–4
Manufacturer and distributor
    information, 746–54
Maple syrup urine disease, 42
Marfan's syndrome, 290
Marijuana, 683
Marshmallow (*Althaea officinalis*), 103
Massage, 674, 724–25
Massage therapists, 211
Mastitis (breast infection), 229–30
Maxi-Calm, 83
Meadowsweet (*Filipendula ulmaria*), 103
Measles, 504–5
Meditation, 726
Mega-Zyme, 62
MegaZymes, 62
Melatonin, 56, 75–76, 138, 262
Memory problems, 505–8
Ménière's disease, 508–10
Meningitis, 510–11
Menopausal problems, 511–16
Menopause, 453–54

Mercury, 169, 266
    toxicity, 516–18
Mercury amalgam dental fillings, 517,
    661, 684
Metabolic acidosis, 122
Metastasis, 246
Metazyme, 62
Methionine, 49–50, 56
Methylation, 79
Methyl donors, 79
Methylphenidate (Ritalin), 204
Methylsulfonylmethane (MSM), 76
Methyl tertiary butyl ether (MTBE), 37
Micellized Multiple Vitamin and
    Mineral, 83
Micronutrients, 5–8
Middle ear infections, 340
Migraine, 518–21
Milcozyme, 62
Milk thistle (*Silybum marianum*), 103
Minerals, 5
    bulk, 25
    daily dosages, 6
    deficiency in, 7
    list of, 25–34
    over-the-counter, 25
    supplements needed for
        assimilation, 7
    trace, 25
Mineral water, 40
Minton, John Peter, Dr., 372
Miotics, 397
Miracle 2000, 83
Miscarriage (spontaneous abortion), 581
Misoprostol (Cytotec), 195
Mitral valve prolapse, 269
MM-Zyme, 62
Mn SOD, 57
Molds, 153–54
Molybdenum, 31
Monoamine oxidase (MAO) inhibitors,
    318, 438
Monocytes, 680
Mononucleosis, 521–23
Monounsaturated fatty acids, 5
Morning sickness, 581–82
Motherwort (*Leonurus cardiaca*), 104
Motion sickness, 523–25
Mouth (oral) cancer, 258–59
Mouth disease. *See* Halitosis;
    Periodontal disease
Mucopolysaccharides, 65
Mucus in the eyes, 367
Muira puama (*Ptychopetalum
    olacoides*), 104
Mullein (*Verbascum thapsus*), 104
Multiple sclerosis, 525–28
Multi-Zyme, 62
Mumps, 529–30
Muscle cramps, 530–32
Muscle injuries. *See* Sprains; Strains
Music and sound therapy, 719–20
Mustard (*Brassica nigra*), 104
Mutual supplementation, 4
Myasthenia gravis, 357
Mycobacterium tuberculosis, 662
Mycoplasma pneumonia, 568

Mycosis fungoides, 628
Myocardial infarction, 268, 417
Myrrh (*Commiphora myrrha*), 104
Myxedema coma, 451

N-acetylcysteine (NAC), 56
Nader, Ralph, 36
Nail problems, 532–35
Naltrexone (ReVia), 151–52
Naproxen (Naprosyn), 300
Narcolepsy, 535–37
Nasal congestion, 582
Nasal polyps, 574
Native American medicine, 86
Natural food supplements, 63
    list of, 63–81
    over-the-counter, 63
    special use, 81–84
Natural spring water, 41
Nature's Answer FOR KIDS, 83
Needle biopsy, 592
Neisseria
    gonorrhoeae, 619
    meningitis, 510
Nephrotic syndrome, 481
Nervousness. *See* Anxiety disorder;
    Stress
Neti pot, 626
Nettle (*Urtica dioica*), 104
Neurology, 173
Neurotransmitters, 334, 506, 612
Neutrophils, 680
New England Journal of Medicine, 21, 172,
    225–26, 442, 490, 495, 560, 578, 595
New York State Journal of Medicine, 658
Niacin, 16–17, 253
Niacinamide, 16–17
Nickel toxicity, 537–38
Nicotinamide adenine dinucleotide
    (NADH), 56, 76, 173
Nicotinic acid, 16–17
Nieper, Hans, Dr., 253, 595
NK (natural killer) cells, 680
*No If's, And's or Butts, The Smoker's
    Guide to Quitting* (Krumholz
    & Phillips), 638
Non-rapid-eye-movement (REM)
    sleep, 535
Nonsteroidal, anti-inflammatory drugs
    (NSAIDs), 173, 195, 726
Nonstress test, 585
Norepinephrine, 129, 315
Nosebleed, 538–40, 582
Nucleoside analogues, 146
Nummular dermatitis, 319
Nutraceuticals, 2
Nutrition
    acceptable foods, 11
    deficiencies in, 132–33
    foods to avoid, 11
    four basic nutrients, 3–5
    micronutrients, 5–8
    during pregnancy, 583
Nutrition Health Review, 199
Nystatin, 266

Oat bran, 70

Oat straw (*Avena sativa*), 105
Obesity, 540–47
Octacosanol, 77
Oily skin, 547–49
Ointments, 87
Oligomeric proanthocyanidins, 56–57, 138
Olive leaf (*Olea europaea*), 77, 105
Omega-3 EFAs, 68, 188, 193, 225
Omega-6 EFAs, 68, 188
Oncogene AC, 602
Optimum daily intakes, 13
Oral chelation therapy, 700–701
Oral contraceptives, 590
Orchiectomy, 595
Oregon grape (*Mahonia aquifolia*), 105
Organic produce, 8
Ornithine, 50
Orthopedic surgeons, 211
Osmotic agents, 396
Osteoarthritis, 189
Osteomalacia. *See* Rickets/Osteomalacia
Osteo-Max, 83
Osteopaths, 211
Osteoporosis, 549–54
Otitis media, 340, 413
Otoliths, 675
Ototoxic drugs, 413
Ovarian cancer, 259
Oxalic acid, 483
Oxytocin challenge test, 585
Ozone layer, 651

Packer, Lester, Dr., 53
Paget's disease of bone, 554–56
Paget's disease of the nipple, 221
Pain control, 720–27
Pallidotomy, 560
Pancreatitis, 556–58
Pancrelipase, 313
Panic attacks, 179–80
Pantothenic acid, 17
Papaya (*Carica papaya*), 105
Pap tests, 262–63
Para-aminobenzoic acid (PABA), 20, 138, 677
Parkinson's disease, 558–61
Paronychia, 387
Parotid glands, 529
Parsley (*Petroselinum crispum*), 105
Partial mastectomy, 227
Passionflower (*Passiflora incarnata*), 105
Patent ductus arteriosus, 304
Pau d'arco (*Tabebuia heptaphylla*), 105
Pectin, 70
Penicillamine (Cuprimine, Depen), 686
Penland, James, Dr., 475
Peppermint (*Mentha piperita*), 106
Peptic ulcer, 561–64
Peptide bonds, 42
Perilla, 77
Perimenopausal problems, 511–16
Periodontal disease, 564–67
Periorbital edema, 342
Peritonsillar abscess, 658
Pernicious anemia, 175
Pesticides, 36

Peyronie's disease, 459
Phenylalanine, 50, 317, 409
Phenylpropanolamine, 547
Phillips, Robert, Dr., 596, 638
Phlebitis, 653
Phosphates, 204
Phosphatidyl choline, 77
Phosphatidyl serine, 77
Phosphorus, 31
Photophobia, 367
Physiatrists, 211
Physical therapists, 211
Physical therapy, 658
Phytochemicals, 2, 9
Phytodolor, 83
Phytomedicines, 85–86
Pinworms, 686, 688
Pityrosporum ovale, 313, 615
Plantain (*Plantago major*), 106
Plantar warts, 678–79
Plasters, 87
Pleurisy root (*Asclepias tuberosa*), 106
Pliamycin (Mithracin), 556
PMS. *See* Premenstrual syndrome
Pneumocystis carinii, 568
Pneumonia, 567–69
Poison control centers, list, 572–73
Poisoning, 571–74
Poison ivy/Poison oak/Poison sumac, 570–71
Polycystic kidney disease, 481
Polyols, 326
Polyps, 574–75
Polyunsaturated fatty acids, 5
Polyunsaturates, 68
Positional vertigo, 675
Potassium, 31–32, 440
Poultices, 87, 727–28
Powders, 87
Preeclampsia, 342, 578–79
Pregnancy-related problems, 575–87
Pregnenolone, 77–78
Premenstrual syndrome (PMS), 516, 587–90
PreNatal Care from Natrol, 83
Prescription for Dietary Wellness (Balch), 547
Primrose (*Oenothera biennis*), 69, 106
Probiotics, 78
Pro Fem progesterone cream, 226
ProFlora whey enema, 707
Progesterone, 78, 511, 514
ProGreens, 72
Progressive relaxation, 649
Prolactin, 594
Prolapsed disk, 208
Prolapse of the uterus, 590–91
Proline, 50
Prostaglandin analogs, 397
Prostate cancer, 591–96
Prostate specific antigen (PSA), 592
Prostatitis/Benign prostatic hypertrophy (BPH), 596–98
Protease inhibitors, 146
Protein, 4
    complementary, 4
    complete, 4

deficiency, 42
incomplete, 4
Proteoglycans, 65
Proteolytic Enzymes, 62
Pseudodementia, 617
Pseudomonas aeruginosa, 311
Psoralen plus ultraviolet A (PUVA) therapy, 677
Psoriasis, 599–600
Psyllium seed, 70
Pulmonary embolism, 290
Pumpkin (*Curcurbita pepo*), 106
Puncture vine (*Tribulus terrestris*), 106
Purines, 399
Pycnogenol. *See* Oligomeric proanthocyanidins
Pyelonephritis, 217, 481
Pygeum (*Pygeum africanum*), 107
Pyorrhea, 564
Pyridoxine, 17–18

Qi gong, 726
Quercetin, 23
Quick Cleanse Program, 83

Radiation exposure, 601–3
Radioallergosorbent (RAST) test, 405
Radon, 603
Rainforests, 86
Raloxifene (Evista), 227, 349, 554
Ranitidine (Zantac), 195
Rapid-eye-movement (REM) sleep, 535
Rash. *See* Skin rash
Raw foods, 2, 8
Raynaud's disease/Raynaud's phenomenon, 290, 603–4
Recommended Dietary Allowances (RDAs), 5, 13
Red clover (*Trifolium pratense*), 107
Red raspberry (*Rubus idaeus*), 107
Red yeast rice, 78
Reflux menstruation theory, 346
Reishi (*Ganoderma lucidum*), 80, 138
Relaxation techniques, 726
Remifemin, 83
Remifemin Plus, 83
Rems (radiation), 601
Renal tubular acidosis, 481
Repetitive motion injury. *See* Carpal tunnel syndrome
Resistance, 147
Respiratory acidosis, 122
Restless leg syndrome, 473, 475
Retinitis pigmentosa, 367–68
Reverse osmosis filter, 39
Reverse transcriptase inhibitors, 147
Reye's syndrome, 604–6
Rheumatic fever, 606–7
Rheumatoid arthritis, 189
Rhubarb (*Rheum rhabarbarum*), 107
Rhus toxicodendron, 278
Riboflavin, 16
Rice bran, 70
Rickets/Osteomalacia, 607–8
Ringworm, 387
RNA, 45, 48, 65
Rosacea, 608–10

Rose (*Rosa canina*), 107
Rosemary (*Rosmarinus officinalis*), 107
Rosiglitazone (Avandia), 326
Rotation diet, 165–67
Roundworms, 686
Royal jelly, 78–79

S-adenosylmethionine (SAMe), 79
The Safe Shopper's Bible (Steinman & Epstein), 252–53
Sage (*Salvia officinalis*), 108
St. John's wort (*Hypericum perforatum*), 108, 319
S-allyl-mercaptocysteine (SAMC), 596
Salmonella, 379
Saltman, Paul, 552
Salves, 87
Sampson, John, Dr., 346
Sangre de grado (*Croton lechleri*), 108
Sarsaparilla (*Smilax species*), 108
Saturated fatty acids, 5
Saw palmetto (*Serenoa repens*), 108
Scabies, 610–11
Schauss, Alexander, Dr., 703
Schizophrenia, 611–14
Schmidt's syndrome, 129
Sciatica, 208, 582
Science, 361
Sclerotherapy, 674
Scombroid poisoning, 380
Scotoma, 368
Sea cucumber, 79
Sea mussel (*Perna canaliculus*), 79
Seasonal affective disorder (SAD), 315
Sebaceous cyst, 614–15
Seborrhea, 319, 615–17
Seborrheic keratoses, 631
Secretin, 207–8
Seddon, Johanna, Dr., 367
Segmental mastectomy, 227
Seizures, 352–53
Selegiline (Eldepryl), 136, 560
Selenium, 32, 57, 253, 313
Selye, Hans, Dr., 650
Senile vertigo, 674
Senility (dementia), 168, 617–19
Serotonin, 315
Serraflazyme, 62
7-keto DHEA, 595
Sexually transmitted diseases (STDs), 619–21
Shark cartilage, 79–80, 262
Shiitake (*Lentinus edodes*), 80, 138
Shingles (herpes zoster), 621–24
Sigmoid colon, 666
Sigmoidoscopy, 328
Sildenafil (Viagra), 275, 325, 458
Silicon, 32
Silymarin, 57
Sinusitis, 624–27
Sitz bath, 728
Skin cancer, 627–32
Skin care products, 690–91
Skin problems, 582
Skin rash, 632–35
Skullcap (*Scutellaria laterfolia*), 109
Sleep apnea, 473–76

Sleeping pills, 476
Sleep problems. *See* Insomnia; Narcolepsy
Slipped disk, 208
Slippery elm (*Ulmus rubra*), 109
Smart Longevity, 83
Smoking dependency, 262, 319, 326, 343, 635–38
Snakebite, 638–40
Sodium, 12, 33
Sodium fluoride, 552
Soft drinks, 552
Solar keratoses, 628
Sore nipples, 230
Sore ribs, 582
Sore throat, 640–41
Soy, 552, 594
Soy-Licious, 83
Sparkling water, 41
Spider bite, 641–43
Spider veins, 674
Spirulina, 80
Spleen, 681
Spondyloarthropathies, 189
Sprains, 643–46
Squamous cell carcinoma, 627–28
Squawvine (*Mitchella repens*), 109
Staphyloccus aureus, 219, 379
Steam-distilled water, 41
Steam inhalation, 626, 728–29
Stoff, Jesse, Dr., 287
Stomach cancer, 259–60
Stomatitis, 564
Stone root (*Collinsonia canadensis*), 109
Strains, 643–46
Streptococcus pneumoniae, 510, 568
Stress, 646–50
Stress hormones, 129
Stress Without Distress (Selye), 650
Stretch marks, 583
Stroke. *See* Arteriosclerosis/ Atherosclerosis; Cardiovascular disease
Stye, 368–69
Sub-Adrene, 83
Substance abuse. *See* Alcoholism; Drug addiction (substance abuse); Smoking dependency
Substantia nigra, 558
Substrate, 59
Sucralfate (Carafate), 195
Sudden onset vertigo, 675
Sugar, 263–64, 325
Sulfite allergies, 158, 199
Sulfur, 33
Suma (*Pfaffia paniculata*), 109
Sumatriptan (Imitrex), 521
Sunburn, 651–53
Sun exposure, excessive, 131
Sunscreen, 631–32
Superficial thrombophlebitis, 654–55
Super Green Tea Extract, 83–84
Superoxide dismutase (SOD), 30, 33, 57, 59–60, 138
Surgery, 729–32
Sweating, 583
Swimmer's ear. *See* Ear infection

Synergy, 13
Synovial joints, 188–89
Syphilis, 620
Syrup of ipecac, 573–74
Syrups, 87
Systemic candidiasis, 263
Systemic lupus erythematosus, 493–94

Tacrine (Cognex), 173
Tai chi, 726–27
Tanning salons, 630
Tapeworms, 686, 688
Tap water, 35
    analysis of, 38
    fluoridation, 37–38
    hard versus soft, 37
    safety of, 36–37
    treatment methods, 38–40
Taurine, 50–51
T cells, 680–81
Teas, 87
Tea tree (*Melaleuca alternifolia*), 109
Temporomandibular joint syndrome. *See* TMJ syndrome
Tendinitis, 244
TENS unit therapy, 727
Teratogens, 587
Testicular cancer, 260
Testosterone, 512, 514
Tetracyclic antidepressants, 318
Theo-Dur Sprinkle, 199
Therapeutic liquids, 732
Thermogenesis, 545
They conquered AIDS! True Life Adventures (Gregory & Leonardo), 146
Thiamine, 16
Thinning eyelashes, 369
Threadworms, 686, 688
Threonine, 51
Thromboangiitis obliterans, 290
Thrombolytic agents, 274
Thrombophlebitis, 653–56
Thrush, 263
Thyme (*Thymus vulgaris*), 109
Thymus, 681
Thyroid problems. *See* Hyperthyroidism; Hypothyroidism
Tic douloureux, 411
Tick bites, 496–99
Time, 141
Tinctures, 87
Tinea capitis, 387
Tinnitus. *See* under Hearing loss
Tired eyes, 366
TMJ syndrome, 237, 374, 656–58
TNM system, 628
Tobramycin (Nebcin), 313
Tocotrienols, 226
Tomatoes, 144
Tonsillectomy, 659
Tonsillitis, 658–59
Tooth decay, 660–61
Total mastectomy, 227
Tranquilizers, 476
Trans-fatty acids, 5
Transurethral incision of the prostate (TUIP), 598

Transurethral resection of the prostate (TURP), 598
Transurethral vaporization of the prostate (TVP), 598
Treponema pallidum, 620
Trichinella spiralis, 380
Trichinosis, 686
Tricyclic antidepressants, 318, 578
Trochanteric bursitis, 244
Troubled Waters on Tap, 36
Tryptophan, 51, 315
Tuberculosis, 662–64
Tumor, 664–66
Turmeric (*Curcuma longa*), 55, 110
Tyler, Varro, Dr., 87
Tyramine, 409
Tyrosine, 51–52, 317–18

Ulcer. *See* Bedsores; Canker sores; Leg ulcers; Peptic ulcer
Ulcerated eyelid, 369
Ulcerative colitis, 666–68
Ultimate Oil, 69
Ultra High Performance Dietary Supplement, 84
Ultra Juice Green, 84
Ultrasound, 584–85
Ultraviolet light (UVL) therapy, 600
Ultraviolet (UV) rays, 628, 651, 689
Underweight/Weight loss, 668–70
Unipolar disorders, 315
Uremia, 481
Urethritis, 217
Uric acid, 397
Urinary tract infection. *See* Bladder infection (cystitis); Kidney disease (renal failure); Vaginitis
USA Today, 86
Uterine prolapse. *See* Prolapse of the uterus
Uva ursi (*Arctostaphylos uva-ursi*), 110
Uveitis, 363
UV radiation, 632

Vaginitis, 670–72
Valerian (*Valeriana officinalis*), 110
Valine, 52
Valvular disease, 269
Vanadium, 33
Varicella zoster, 283–84, 621
Varicose veins, 583, 672–74
Vegetables, 8
Vegetarian Enzyme Complex, 62
Vein stripping, 674
Venereal disease. *See* Sexually transmitted diseases (STDs)

Venous ulcers, 491
Vertebroplasty, 211
Vertigo, 674–76
Vervain (*Verbena officinalis*), 110
Vinegars, 87
Viral pneumonia, 568
Vitamin A, 14–15, 57–58
toxicity, 587
Vitamin B$_5$ (pantothenic acid), 17, 138
deficiency, 399
Vitamin B$_1$ (thiamine), 16
Vitamin B$_6$ (pyridoxine), 17–18
Vitamin B$_3$ (niacin, nicotinic acid, niacinamide), 16–17
Vitamin B$_{12}$ (cyanocobalamin), 18, 172
deficiency, 133, 136, 175–76
Vitamin B$_2$ (riboflavin), 16
Vitamin C (ascorbic acid), 13, 20–21, 58, 396, 636, 679
deficiency, 237
Vitamin D, 21, 550, 552
deficiency, 607–8
Vitamin E, 21–22, 29, 32, 58, 172, 313, 631
deficiency, 399
Vitamin F, 68
Vitamin K, 22–23
deficiency, 265, 281
Vitamins, 5
balance and synergy of, 13
cautions when taking, 8
daily dosages, 6
deficiency in, 7
list of, 14–24
oil-soluble, 13
over-the-counter, 14
protein-bonded, 14
RDA versus RDI versus ODA, 13
supplements needed for assimilation, 7
synthetic versus natural, 13–14
water-soluble, 13
VitaSerum, 84
Vita Synergy, 84
Vitiligo, 676–77
Vocal cord polyps, 574
Volatile oils, 86

Warfarin (Coumadin), 275
Warren, Tom, 173
Warts, 677–79
Water, 3
artesian, 40
bottled, 40
deionized, 40
ground, 40

mineral, 40
natural spring, 41
sparkling, 41
steam-distilled, 41
tap, 35–40
Weakened immune system, 679–84
Weight problems. *See* Anorexia nervosa; Appetite, poor; Bulimia; Obesity; Underweight/Weight loss
Wellness Formula, 84
Wheat germ, 80
Wheatgrass, 80
Wheatgrass retention enema, 706
Whey protein, 80–81
White blood cell counts, 683
White blood cells, 680
White oak (*Quercus alba*), 110
White willow (*Salix alba*), 110
Wigmore, Ann, Dr., 80
Wild cherry (*Prunus serotina*), 111
Wild oregano (*Origanum vulgare*), 111
Wild yam (*Discorea villosa*), 111
Wilkinson, Richard S., Dr., 504
Wilson's disease, 684–86
Wilson's syndrome, 453
Wines, 87
Wintergreen (*Gaultheria procumbens*), 111
Witch hazel (*Hamamelis virginiana*), 111
Wobenzym N, 62
Women's Health Advisor, 475
Wood betony (*Stachys officinalis*), 111
World Health Organization, 86
Worms (parasites), 686–88
Wormwood (*Artemisia absinthium*), 112
Wright, Jonathan, Dr., 199
Wrinkles, 688–91

Xerophthalmia, 369

The Yeast Connection (Crook), 81
Yeast infection, 81, 205, 263–66, 387
Yellow dock (*Rumex crispus*), 112
Yerba maté (*Ilex paraguariensis*), 112
Yin and yang, 702
Yoga, 732–33
Yogurt, 4
Yohimbe (*Pausinystalia yohimbe*), 112
Yucca (*Yucca baccata*), 112

Zanamivir (Relenza), 199, 470
ZAND cold, flu, and allergy formulas, 82
Zeaxanthin, 361
Zinc, 13, 33–34, 58, 300, 686
deficiency, 151, 304–5, 598, 612
Zyban, 319

Acknowledgments

There are many people who have come and gone in my life and have contributed to my books in many different ways, but I want to dedicate this to three loyal and true friends who are no longer with me:

Judge Wendell W. Mayer
Charles R. Cripe
Skeeners Balch

I also wish to acknowledge the following people, who both advised and supported me as I prepared and wrote the third edition of this book: my daughters, Ruby Hines and Cheryl Keene; my grandchildren, Lisa, Ryan, and Rachel; my brother, Al Henning; my research and editing staff, Suzanne Kaminiski and Avery editor Amy Tecklenberg; Theresa Auman, who manages Good Things Naturally; Tom Witman, who researched the section on sports nutrition for bodybuilders; and the manufacturers and suppliers who allowed me to evaluate their products before recommending them to my readers. Finally, I would like to thank all the readers who have remained loyal throughout the years.

Phyllis A. Balch

About the Author

Phyllis Balch is a certified nutritional consultant who received her certification from the American Association of Nutritional Consultants, and has been a leading nutritional counselor for over two decades. She came to the field as a result of experiencing firsthand the benefits of using diet and nutrition as remedies for sickness.

In the 1970s, she and her children suffered from a number of undiagnosed (or misdiagnosed) illnesses and, although they had expert medical knowledge very close at hand, these maladies continued to disrupt their lives. Ms. Balch felt that there was something missing in the typical approach that treated the symptoms rather than the cause of illness. Her first introduction to the relationship between nutrition and well-being was through the late Paavo Airola, a well-known naturopath and writer. Ms. Balch then pursued her own intensive research into the science of nutrition and, by making radical changes in diet, was able to transform her own health and the health of her children.

Convinced that nutrition was, in many cases, the answer to regaining and maintaining health, Ms. Balch opened a health food store called Good Things Naturally. In 1983, she published *Nutritional Outline for the Professional and the Wise Man*—now known as *Prescription for Nutritional Healing*—to share her knowledge with a broader audience. Through its first two editions, this book has had millions of readers in many different countries, and it has been translated into seven foreign languages. This is its third edition.

Ms. Balch continues to share her knowledge with others, and has convinced many traditionally schooled medical practitioners to incorporate nutritional methods of restoring health into their practice. She is highly sought after as a visiting lecturer and also appears on television and radio programs throughout Canada and North America. Ms. Balch currently resides in Fort Myers, Florida, and Greenfield, Indiana.

Some Physical Constants

Avogadro's number	N_A		$6.022\ 136\ 7 \times 10^{23}$ particles/mol
Boltzmann's constant	k		$1.380\ 658 \times 10^{-23}$ J/K
Bohr magneton	$m_B = e\hbar/2m_e$		$9.274\ 015\ 4 \times 10^{-24}$ J/T
Coulomb constant	$k = 1/4\pi\epsilon_0$		$8.987\ 551\ 788 \times 10^{9}$ N·m²/C²
Compton wavelength	$\lambda_C = h/2e$		$2.426\ 310\ 58 \times 10^{-12}$ m
Fundamental charge	e		$1.602\ 177\ 33 \times 10^{-19}$ C
Gas constant	$R = N_A k$		$8.314\ 51$ J/mol·K $= 1.987\ 22$ cal/mol·K
			$= 8.205\ 78 \times 10^{-2}$ L·atm/mol·K
Gravitational constant	G		$6.672\ 6 \times 10^{-11}$ N·m²/kg²
Mass, of electron	m_e		$9.109\ 389\ 7 \times 10^{-31}$ kg
			$= 510.999\ 1$ keV/c^2
of proton	m_p		$1.672\ 623\ 1 \times 10^{-27}$ kg
			$= 938.272\ 3$ MeV/c^2
of neutron	m_n		$1.674\ 929 \times 10^{-27}$ kg
			$= 939.565\ 6$ MeV/c^2
Permeability of free space	μ_0		$4\pi \times 10^{-7}$ N/A²
Planck's constant	h		$6.626\ 075\ 5 \times 10^{-34}$ J·s
			$= 4.135\ 669\ 2 \times 10^{-15}$ eV·s
	$\hbar$		$1.054\ 572\ 66 \times 10^{-34}$ J·s
			$6.582\ 122\ 0 \times 10^{-16}$ eV·s
Speed of light	c		$2.997\ 924\ 58 \times 10^{8}$ m/s
Unified mass unit	u		$1.660\ 540 \times 10^{-27}$ kg
			$= 931.494\ 32$ MeV/c^2

Mathematical Symbols

$=$	is equal to		Δx	change in x
$\neq$	is not equal to		$\lvert x \rvert$	absolute value of x
$\approx$	is approximately equal to		$n!$	$n(n-1)(n-2)\cdots 1$
$\sim$	is of the order of		Σ	sum
$\propto$	is proportional to		$\lim$	limit
$>$	is greater than		$\Delta t \rightarrow 0$	Δt approaches zero
$\geq$	is greater than or equal to		$\dfrac{dx}{dt}$	derivative of x with respect to t
$\gg$	is much greater than			
$<$	is less than		$\dfrac{\partial x}{\partial t}$	partial derivative of x with respect to t
$\leq$	is less than or equal to			
$\ll$	is much less than		$\int$	integral

Some Conversion Factors

1 m = 39.37 in = 3.281 ft = 1.094 yd

$1 \text{ m} = 10^{15} \text{ fm} = 10^{10} \text{ Å} = 10^9 \text{ nm}$

1 km = 0.6215 mi

1 mi = 5280 ft = 1.609 km

$1 \text{ lightyear} = 1 \, c{\cdot}y = 9.461 \times 10^{15} \text{ m}$

1 in = 2.540 cm

$1 \text{ L} = 10^3 \text{ cm}^3 = 10^{-3} \text{ m}^3 = 1.057 \text{ qt}$

1 h = 3.6 ks

$1 \text{ y} = 365.24 \text{ d} = 3.156 \times 10^7 \text{ s}$

1 km/h = 0.278 m/s = 0.6215 mi/h

1 ft/s = 0.3048 m/s = 0.6818 mi/h

$1 \text{ rev} = 2\pi \text{ rad} = 360°$

1 rad = 57.30°

1 rev/min = 0.1047 rad/s

1 slug = 14.59 kg

$1 \text{ tonne} = 10^3 \text{ kg} = 1 \text{ Mg}$

$1 \text{ atm} = 101.3 \text{ kPa} = 1.013 \text{ bar} = 76.00 \text{ cmHg} = 14.70 \text{ lb/in}^2$

$1 \text{ N} = 10^5 \text{ dyn} = 0.2248 \text{ lb}$

1 lb = 4.448 N

1 Pa·s = 10 poise

$1 \text{ J} = 10^7 \text{ erg} = 0.7373 \text{ ft·lb} = 9.869 \times 10^{-3} \text{ L·atm}$

1 kW·h = 3.6 MJ

$1 \text{ cal} = 4.184 \text{ J} = 4.129 \times 10^{-2} \text{ L·atm}$

1 L·atm = 101.3 J = 24.22 cal

$1 \text{ eV} = 1.602 \times 10^{-19} \text{ J}$

1 Btu = 778 ft·lb = 252 cal = 1054 J

1 horsepower = 550 ft·lb/s = 746 W

$1 \text{ W/m·K} = 6.938 \text{ Btu·in/h·ft}^2{\cdot}°\text{F}$

$1 \text{ T} = 10^4 \text{ G}$

1 kg weighs about 2.205 lb

Atomic Numbers and Atomic Masses

Name	Symbol	Atomic Number	Mass	Name	Symbol	Atomic Number	Mass
Actinium	Ac	89	227.03	Mercury	Hg	80	200.59
Aluminum	Al	13	26.98	Molybdenum	Mo	42	95.94
Americium	Am	95	(243)	Neodymium	Nd	60	144.24
Antimony	Sb	51	121.75	Neon	Ne	10	20.179
Argon	Ar	18	39.948	Neptunium	Np	93	237.05
Arsenic	As	33	74.92	Nickel	Ni	28	58.69
Astatine	At	85	(210)	Niobium	Nb	41	92.91
Barium	Ba	56	137.3	Nitrogen	N	7	14.007
Berkelium	Bk	97	(247)	Nobelium	No	102	(259)
Beryllium	Be	4	9.012	Osmium	Os	76	190.2
Bismuth	Bi	83	208.98	Oxygen	O	8	15.9994
Boron	B	5	10.81	Palladium	Pd	46	106.4
Bromine	Br	35	79.90	Phosphorus	P	15	30.974
Cadmium	Cd	48	112.41	Platinum	Pt	78	195.09
Calcium	Ca	20	40.08	Plutonium	Pu	94	(244)
Californium	Cf	98	(251)	Polonium	Po	84	(210)
Carbon	C	6	12.011	Potassium	K	19	39.102
Cerium	Ce	58	140.12	Praseodymium	Pr	59	140.91
Cesium	Cs	55	132.905	Promethium	Pm	61	(147)
Chlorine	Cl	17	35.453	Protactinium	Pa	91	231.04
Chromium	Cr	24	52.00	Radium	Ra	88	(226)
Cobalt	Co	27	58.93	Radon	Rn	86	(222)
Copper	Cu	29	63.55	Rhenium	Re	75	186.2
Curium	Cm	96	(247)	Rhodium	Rh	45	102.905
Dysprosium	Dy	66	162.50	Rubidium	Rb	37	85.47
Einsteinium	Es	99	(252)	Ruthenium	Ru	44	101.1
Erbium	Er	68	167.26	Rutherfordium	Rf	104	(261)
Europium	Eu	63	152.0	Samarium	Sm	62	150.36
Fermium	Fm	100	(257)	Scandium	Sc	21	44.96
Fluorine	F	9	19.00	Selenium	Se	34	78.96
Francium	Fr	87	(223)	Silicon	Si	14	28.09
Gadolinium	Gd	64	157.25	Silver	Ag	47	107.870
Gallium	Ga	31	69.72	Sodium	Na	11	22.990
Germanium	Ge	32	72.59	Strontium	Sr	38	87.62
Gold	Au	79	196.97	Sulfur	S	16	32.064
Hafnium	Hf	72	178.49	Tantalum	Ta	73	180.95
Hahnium	Ha	105	(260)	Technetium	Tc	43	(98)
Helium	He	2	4.003	Tellurium	Te	52	127.60
Holmium	Ho	67	164.93	Terbium	Tb	65	158.92
Hydrogen	H	1	1.00797	Thallium	Tl	81	204.37
Indium	In	49	114.82	Thorium	Th	90	232.04
Iodine	I	53	126.90	Thulium	Tm	69	168.93
Iridium	Ir	77	192.2	Tin	Sn	50	118.69
Iron	Fe	26	55.85	Titanium	Ti	22	47.88
Krypton	Kr	36	83.80	Tungsten	W	74	183.85
Lanthanum	La	57	138.91	Uranium	U	92	238.03
Lawrencium	Lr	103	(260)	Vanadium	V	23	50.94
Lead	Pb	82	207.19	Xenon	Xe	54	131.29
Lithium	Li	3	6.941	Ytterbium	Yb	70	173.04
Lutetium	Lu	71	174.97	Yttrium	Y	39	88.906
Magnesium	Mg	12	24.31	Zinc	Zn	30	65.38
Manganese	Mn	25	54.94	Zirconium	Zr	40	91.22
Mendelevium	Md	101	(258)				

Review of Mathematics

In this appendix, we will review some of the basic results of algebra, geometry, trigonometry, and calculus. In many cases, we will merely state results without proof. Table D-1 lists some mathematical symbols.

Equations

The following operations can be performed on mathematical equations to facilitate their solution:

1. The same quantity can be added to or subtracted from each side of the equation.

2. Each side of the equation can be multiplied or divided by the same quantity.

3. Each side of the equation can be raised to the same power.

It is important to understand that the preceding rules apply to each *side* of the equation and not to each *term* in the equation.

Table D-1

Mathematical Symbols

$=$	is equal to
$\neq$	is not equal to
$\approx$	is approximately equal to
$\sim$	is of the order of
$\propto$	is proportional to
$>$	is greater than
$\geq$	is greater than or equal to
$\gg$	is much greater than
$<$	is less than
$\leq$	is less than or equal to
$\ll$	is much less than
Δx	change in x
$|x|$	absolute value of x
$n!$	$n(n-1)(n-2)\cdots 1$
Σ	sum
lim	limit
$\Delta t \to 0$	Δt approaches zero
$\dfrac{dx}{dt}$	derivative of x with respect to t
$\dfrac{\partial x}{\partial t}$	partial derivative of x with respect to t
$\int$	integral

Example D-1

Solve the following equation for x: $(x - 3)^2 + 7 = 23$.

1. Subtract 7 from each side: $(x - 3)^2 = 16$

2. Take the square root of each side: $x - 3 = \pm 4$

3. Add 3 to each side: $x = 4 + 3 = 7$ or $x = -4 + 3 = -1$

Remark Note that in step 2 we do not need to write $\pm(x - 3) = \pm 4$ because all possibilities are included in $x - 3 = \pm 4$.

Check the Result We check our result by substituting each value into the original equation: $(7 - 3)^2 + 7 = 16 + 7 = 23$ and $(-1-3)^2 + 7 = 16 + 7 = 23$.

Example D-2

Solve the following equation for x:

$$\frac{1}{x} + \frac{1}{4} = \frac{1}{3}$$

1. Subtract $\frac{1}{4}$ from each side: $\dfrac{1}{x} = \dfrac{1}{3} - \dfrac{1}{4} = \dfrac{4}{12} - \dfrac{3}{12} = \dfrac{1}{12}$

2. Multiply each side by $12x$: $x = 12$

Remark This type of equation occurs both in geometric optics and in analyses of electric circuits. Although it is easy to solve, errors are often made. A typical mistake is to take the reciprocal of each *term*, obtaining $x + 4 = 3$. Taking the reciprocal of each term is not allowed; taking the reciprocal of each *side* of an equation is allowed. Note that multiplying each side by $12x$ in step 2 is equivalent to taking the reciprocal of each side of the equation.

Direct and Inverse Proportion

The relationships of direct proportion and inverse proportion are so important in physics that they deserve special consideration. Often much algebraic manipulation can be avoided through a simple knowledge of these relationships. Suppose, for example, that you work for 5 days at a certain pay rate and earn $400. How much would you earn at the same pay rate if you worked 8 days? In this problem, the money earned is *directly proportional* to the time worked. We can write an equation relating the money earned M to the time worked t using a constant of proportionality R:

$$M = Rt$$

The constant of proportionality in this case is the pay rate. We can express R in dollars per day. Since $400 was earned in 5 d, the value of R is $400/(5\ \text{d}) = $80/\text{d}$. In 8 d, the amount earned is therefore

$$M = (\$80/\text{d})(8\ \text{d}) = \$640$$

However, we do not have to find the pay rate explicitly to work the problem. Since the amount earned in 8 d is $\frac{8}{5}$ times that earned in 5 d, this amount is

$$M = \tfrac{8}{5}(\$400) = \$640$$

We can use a similar example to illustrate inverse proportion. If you get a 25% raise, how long would you need to work to earn \$400? Here we consider R to be a variable and we wish to solve for t:

$$t = \frac{M}{R}$$

In this equation, the time t is *inversely proportional* to the pay rate R. Thus, if the new rate is $\frac{5}{4}$ times the old rate, the new time will be $\frac{4}{5}$ times the old time or 4 d.

There are some situations in which one quantity varies as the square or some other power of another quantity where the ideas of proportionality are also very useful. Suppose, for example, that a 10-in diameter pizza costs \$8.50. How much would you expect a 12-in diameter pizza to cost? We expect the cost of a pizza to be approximately proportional to the amount of its contents, which is proportional to the area of the pizza. Since the area is in turn proportional to the square of the diameter, the cost should be proportional to the square of the diameter. If we increase the diameter by a factor of 12/10, the area increases by a factor of $(12/10)^2 = 1.44$, so we should expect the cost to be $(1.44)(\$8.50) = \$12.24$.

Example D-3

The intensity of light from a point source varies inversely with the square of the distance from the source. If the intensity is 3.20 W/m² at 5 m from a source, what is it at 6 m from the source?

1. Write an equation expressing the fact that the intensity varies inversely with the square of the distance:

$$I = \frac{C}{r^2}$$

where C is some constant.

2. Let I_1 be the intensity at $r_1 = 5$ m and I_2 be the intensity at $r_2 = 6$ m, and express the ratio I_2/I_1 in terms of r_1 and r_2:

$$\frac{I_2}{I_1} = \frac{C/r_2^2}{C/r_1^2} = \frac{r_1^2}{r_2^2} = \left(\frac{r_1}{r_2}\right)^2 = \left(\frac{5}{6}\right)^2 = 0.694$$

3. Solve for I_2:

$$I_2 = 0.694I_1 = (0.694)(3.20 \text{ W/m}^2) = 2.22 \text{ W/m}^2$$

Linear Equations

An equation in which the variables occur only to the first power is said to be linear. A linear equation relating y and x can always be put into the standard form

$$y = mx + b \qquad \text{D-1}$$

where m and b are constants that may be either positive or negative. Figure D-1 shows a graph of the values of x and y that satisfy Equation D-1. The constant b, called the **intercept**, is the value of y at $x = 0$. The constant m is the **slope** of the line, which equals the ratio of the change in y to the correspond-

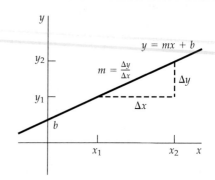

Figure D-1 Graph of the linear equation $y = mx + b$, where b is the intercept and $m = \Delta y/\Delta x$ is the slope.

ing change in x. In the figure, we have indicated two points on the line, x_1, y_1 and x_2, y_2, and the changes $\Delta x = x_2 - x_1$ and $\Delta y = y_2 - y_1$. The slope m is then

$$m = \frac{y_2 - y_1}{x_2 - x_1} = \frac{\Delta y}{\Delta x}$$

If x and y are both unknown, there is no unique solution for their values. Any pair of values x_1, y_1 on the line in Figure D-1 will satisfy the equation. If we have two equations, each with the same two unknowns x and y, the equations can be solved simultaneously for the unknowns.

Example D-4

Find the values of x and y that satisfy

$$3x - 2y = 8 \qquad \text{D-2}$$

and

$$y - x = 2 \qquad \text{D-3}$$

Picture the Problem Figure D-2 shows a graph of each of these equations. At the point where the lines intersect, the values of x and y satisfy both equations. We can solve two simultaneous equations by first solving either equation for one variable in terms of the other variable and then substituting the result into the other equation. An alternative method is to multiply one equation by a constant such that one of the unknown terms is eliminated when the equations are added or subtracted.

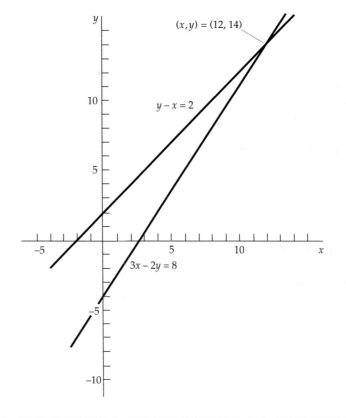

Figure D-2 Graph of Equations D-2 and D-3. At the point where the lines intersect, the values of x and y satisfy both equations.

1. Solve Equation D-3 for y:	$y = x + 2$
2. Substitute this value for y into Equation D-2:	$3x - 2(x + 2) = 8$
3. Simplify and solve for x:	$3x - 2x - 4 = 8$
	$x = 12$
4. To solve these equations using the alternative method, we first multiply Equation D-3 by 2:	$2y - 2x = 4$
5. Add this equation to Equation D-2:	$2y - 2x = 4$
	$\underline{3x - 2y = 8}$
	$3x - 2x = 12$
	$x = 12$

Factoring

Equations can often be simplified by factoring. Three important examples are

1. Common factor: $2ax + 3ay = a(2x + 3y)$
2. Perfect square: $x^2 \pm 2xy + y^2 = (x \pm y)^2$
3. Difference of squares: $x^2 - y^2 = (x + y)(x - y)$

The Quadratic Formula

An equation that contains a variable to the second power is called a *quadratic equation*. The standard form for a quadratic equation is

$$ax^2 + bx + c = 0 \qquad \text{D-4}$$

where a, b, and c are constants. The general solution of this equation is

$$x = -\frac{b}{2a} \pm \frac{1}{2a}\sqrt{b^2 - 4ac} \qquad \text{D-5}$$

When b^2 is greater than $4ac$, there are two solutions corresponding to the $+$ and $-$ signs. Figure D-3 shows a graph of y versus x where $y = ax^2 + bx + c$. The curve, called a **parabola**, crosses the x axis twice. The values of x for which $y = 0$ are the solutions to Equation D-4. When $b^2 < 4ac$, the graph of y versus x does not intersect the x axis, as is shown in Figure D-4, and there are no real solutions to Equation D-4. When $b^2 = 4ac$, the graph of y versus x is tangent to the x axis at the point $x = -b/2a$.

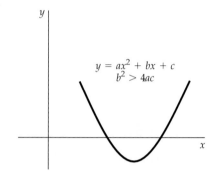

Figure D-3 Graph of y versus x when $y = ax^2 + bx + c$ for the case $b^2 > 4ac$. The two values of x for which $y = 0$ satisfy the quadratic equation (Equation D-4).

Exponents

The notation x^n stands for the quantity obtained by multiplying x times itself n times. For example, $x^2 = x \cdot x$ and $x^3 = x \cdot x \cdot x$. The quantity n is called the **power,** or the **exponent,** of x. When two powers of x are multiplied, the exponents are added:

$$(x^m)(x^n) = x^{m+n} \qquad \text{D-6}$$

This can be readily seen from an example:

$$x^2 x^3 = (x \cdot x)(x \cdot x \cdot x) = x^5$$

Any number raised to the 0 power is defined to be 1:

$$x^0 = 1 \qquad \text{D-7}$$

Then

$$x^n x^{-n} = x^0 = 1$$

$$x^{-n} = \frac{1}{x^n} \qquad \text{D-8}$$

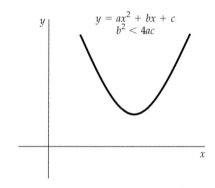

Figure D-4 Graph of y versus x when $y = ax^2 + bx + c$ for the case $b^2 < 4ac$. In this case, there are no (real) values of x for which $y = 0$.

When two powers are divided, the exponents are subtracted:

$$\frac{x^n}{x^m} = x^n x^{-m} = n^{n-m} \qquad \text{D-9}$$

Using these rules, we have

$$x^{1/2} \cdot x^{1/2} = x$$

so

$$x^{1/2} = \sqrt{x}$$

When a power is raised to another power, the exponents are multiplied:

$$(x^n)m = x^{nm} \qquad \text{D-10}$$

Logarithms

When y is related to x by $y = a^x$, the number x is said to be the logarithm of y to the base a and is written

$$x = \log_a y$$

If $y_1 = a^n$ and $y_2 = a^m$, then

$$y_1 y_2 = a^n a^m = a^{n+m}$$

and

$$\log_a y_1 y_2 = n + m = \log_a y_2 + \log_a y_1 \qquad \text{D-11}$$

It then follows that

$$\log_a y^n = n \log_a y \qquad \text{D-12}$$

Since $a^1 = a$ and $a^0 = 1$,

$$\log_a a = 1 \qquad \text{D-13}$$

and

$$\log_a 1 = 0 \qquad \text{D-14}$$

There are two bases in common use: base 10, called **common logarithms,** and base e ($e = 2.728...$), called **natural logarithms.** When no base is specified, the base is understood to be 10. Thus, $\log 100 = \log_{10} 100 = 2$ since $100 = 10^2$.

The symbol ln is used for natural logarithms. Thus,

$$y = \ln x \qquad \text{D-15}$$

implies

$$x = e^y \qquad \text{D-16}$$

Logarithms can be changed from one base to another. Suppose that

$$z = \log x \qquad \text{D-17}$$

Then

$$10^z = x \qquad \text{D-18}$$

Taking the natural logarithm of both sides of Equation D-18, we obtain

$$z \ln 10 = \ln x$$

or

$$\ln x = (\ln 10)\log x \qquad \text{D-19}$$

The Exponential Function

When the rate of change of a quantity is proportional to the quantity itself, the quantity increases or decreases exponentially. An example of *exponential decrease* is nuclear decay. If N is the number of radioactive nuclei at some time, then the change dN in some very small time interval dt will be proportional to N and to dt:

$$dN = -\lambda N \, dt$$

where the constant of proportionality λ is the decay rate. The function N satisfying this equation is

$$N = N_0 e^{-\lambda t} \qquad \text{D-20}$$

where N_0 is the number at time $t = 0$. Figure D-5 shows N versus t. A characteristic of exponential decay is that N decreases by a constant factor in a given time interval. The time interval for N to decrease to half its original value is its half-life $t_{1/2}$, which is related to the decay rate by

$$t_{1/2} = \frac{\ln 2}{\lambda} = \frac{0.693}{\lambda} \qquad \text{D-21}$$

An example of *exponential increase* is population growth. If the number of organisms is N, the change in N after a small time interval dt is given by

$$dN = +\lambda N \, dt$$

where λ is a constant that characterizes the rate of increase. The function N satisfying this equation is

$$N = N_0 e^{\lambda t} \qquad \text{D-22}$$

A graph of this function is shown in Figure D-6. An exponential increase is characterized by a doubling time T_2, which is related to λ by

$$T_2 = \frac{\ln 2}{\lambda} = \frac{0.693}{\lambda} \qquad \text{D-23}$$

If the rate of increase λ is expressed as a percentage, $r = \lambda/100\%$, the doubling time is

$$T_2 = \frac{69.3}{r} \qquad \text{D-24}$$

For example, if the population increases by 2% per year, the population will double every $69.3/2 \approx 35$ years. Table D-2 lists some useful relations for exponential and logarithmic functions.

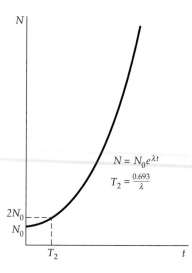

Figure D-6 Graph of N versus t when N increases exponentially. The time T_2 is the time it takes for N to double.

Graph labels: $N = N_0 e^{\lambda t}$, $T_2 = \frac{0.693}{\lambda}$, $2N_0$, N_0, T_2, t

Figure D-5 Graph of N versus t when N decreases exponentially. The time $t_{1/2}$ is the time it takes for N to decrease by one-half.

Graph labels: N, N_0, $\frac{1}{2}N_0$, $N = N_0 e^{-\lambda t}$, $t_{1/2} = \frac{0.693}{\lambda}$, $t_{1/2}$, t

Table D-2

Exponential and Logarithmic Functions

$e = 2.71828; \qquad e^0 = 1$

If $y = e^x$, then $x = \ln y$.

$e^{\ln x} = x$

$e^x e^y = e^{(x+y)}$

$(e^x)^y = e^{xy} = (e^y)^x$

$\ln e = 1; \qquad \ln 1 = 0$

$\ln xy = \ln x + \ln y$

$\ln \dfrac{x}{y} = \ln x - \ln y$

$\ln e^x = x; \qquad \ln a^x = x \ln a$

$\ln x = (\ln 10) \log x$

$\qquad = 2.3026 \log x$

$\log x = \log e \ln x = 0.43429 \ln x$

$e^x = 1 + x + \dfrac{x^2}{2!} + \dfrac{x^3}{3!} + \cdots$

$\ln(1 + x) = x - \dfrac{x^2}{2} + \dfrac{x^3}{3} - \dfrac{x^4}{4} + \cdots$

Geometry

The ratio of the circumference of a circle to its diameter is a natural number π, which has the approximate value

$$\pi = 3.141592$$

The circumference C of a circle is thus related to its diameter d and its radius r by

$$C = \pi d = 2\pi r \qquad \text{circumference of circle} \qquad \text{D-25}$$

The area of a circle is

$$A = \pi r^2 \qquad \text{area of circle} \qquad \text{D-26}$$

The area of a parallelogram is the base b times the height h (Figure D-7) and that of a triangle is one-half the base times the height (Figure D-8). A sphere of radius r (Figure D-9) has a surface area given by

$$A = 4\pi r^2 \qquad \text{spherical surface area} \qquad \text{D-27}$$

and a volume given by

$$V = \tfrac{4}{3}\pi r^3 \qquad \text{spherical volume} \qquad \text{D-28}$$

A cylinder of radius r and length L (Figure D-10) has surface area (not including the end faces) of

$$A = 2\pi r L \qquad \text{cylindrical surface} \qquad \text{D-29}$$

and volume of

$$V = \pi r^2 L \qquad \text{cylindrical volume} \qquad \text{D-30}$$

Area of parallelogram
$A = bh$

Figure D-7 Area of a parallelogram.

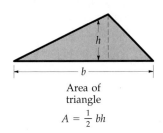

Area of
triangle

$A = \tfrac{1}{2}\, bh$

Figure D-8 Area of a triangle.

Spherical surface area
$A = 4\pi r^2$
Spherical volume
$V = \tfrac{4}{3}\pi r^3$

Figure D-9 Surface area and volume of a sphere.

Cylindrical surface area
$A = 2\pi r L$
Cylindrical volume
$V = \pi r^2 L$

Figure D-10 Surface area (not including the end faces) and volume of a cylinder.

Trigonometry

The angle between two intersecting straight lines is measured as follows. A circle is drawn with its center at the intersection of the lines, and the circular arc is divided into 360 parts called **degrees.** The number of degrees in the arc between the lines is the measure of angle between the lines. For very small angles, the degree is divided into minutes (') and seconds (") with $1' = 1°/60$ and $1'' = 1'/60 = 1°/3600$. For scientific work, a more useful measure of an angle is the radian (rad), which is defined as the length of the circular arc between the lines divided by the radius of the circle (Figure D-11). If s is the arc length and r is the radius of the circle, the angle θ measured in radians is

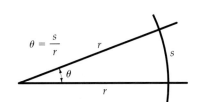

Figure D-11 The angle θ in radians is defined to be the ratio s/r, where s is the arc length intercepted on a circle of radius r.

$$\theta = \frac{s}{r} \qquad \text{D-31}$$

Since the angle measured in radians is the ratio of two lengths, it is dimensionless. The relation between radians and degrees is

$$360° = 2\pi \text{ rad}$$

or

$$1 \text{ rad} = \frac{360°}{2\pi} = 57.3°$$
D-32

Figure D-12 shows some useful relations for angles.

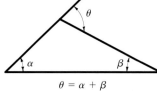

Figure D-12 Some useful relations for angles.

Figure D-13 shows a right triangle formed by drawing the line BC perpendicular to AC. The lengths of the sides are labeled a, b, and c. The trigonometric functions $\sin\theta$, $\cos\theta$, and $\tan\theta$ for an acute angle θ are defined as

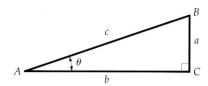

Figure D-13 A right triangle with sides of length a and b and a hypotenuse of length c.

$$\sin\theta = \frac{a}{c} = \frac{\text{opposite side}}{\text{hypotenuse}}$$
D-33

$$\cos\theta = \frac{b}{c} = \frac{\text{adjacent side}}{\text{hypotenuse}}$$
D-34

$$\tan\theta = \frac{a}{b} = \frac{\text{opposite side}}{\text{adjacent side}} = \frac{\sin\theta}{\cos\theta}$$
D-35

Three other trigonometric functions are the reciprocals of these functions and are defined as

$$\sec\theta = \frac{c}{b} = \frac{1}{\cos\theta}$$
D-36

$$\csc\theta = \frac{c}{a} = \frac{1}{\sin\theta}$$
D-37

$$\cot\theta = \frac{b}{a} = \frac{1}{\tan\theta} = \frac{\cos\theta}{\sin\theta}$$
D-38

The angle θ whose sine is x is called the arcsine of x, and is written $\sin^{-1} x$. That is, if

$$\sin\theta = x$$

then

$$\theta = \arcsin x = \sin^{-1} x \qquad \text{D-39}$$

The arcsine is the inverse of the sine. The inverse of the cosine and tangent are defined similarly. The angle whose cosine is y is the arccosine of y. That is, if

$$\cos \theta = y$$

then

$$\theta = \arccos y = \cos^{-1} y \qquad \text{D-40}$$

The angle whose tangent is z is the arctangent of z. That is, if

$$\tan \theta = z$$

$$\theta = \arctan z = \tan^{-1} z \qquad \text{D-41}$$

The Pythagorean theorem

$$a^2 + b^2 = c^2 \qquad \text{D-42}$$

gives some useful identities. If we divide each term in this equation by c^2, we obtain

$$\frac{a^2}{c^2} + \frac{b^2}{c^2} = 1$$

or, from the definitions of $\sin \theta$ and $\cos \theta$,

$$\sin^2 \theta + \cos^2 \theta = 1 \qquad \text{D-43}$$

Similarly, we can divide each term in Equation D-42 by a^2 or b^2 and obtain

$$1 + \cot^2 \theta = \csc^2 \theta \qquad \text{D-44}$$

and

$$1 + \tan^2 \theta = \sec^2 \theta \qquad \text{D-45}$$

These and other useful trigonometric formulas are listed in Table D-3.

Table D-3

Trigonometric Formulas

$\sin^2 \theta + \cos^2 \theta = 1; \qquad \sec^2 \theta - \tan^2 \theta = 1; \qquad \csc^2 \theta - \cot^2 \theta = 1$

$\sin 2\theta = 2 \sin \theta \cos \theta$

$\cos 2\theta = \cos^2 \theta - \sin^2 \theta = 2 \cos^2 \theta - 1 = 1 - 2 \sin^2 \theta$

$\tan 2\theta = \dfrac{2 \tan \theta}{1 - \tan^2 \theta}$

$\sin \dfrac{1}{2}\theta = \sqrt{\dfrac{1 - \cos \theta}{2}}; \qquad \cos \dfrac{1}{2}\theta = \sqrt{\dfrac{1 + \cos \theta}{2}}; \qquad \tan \dfrac{1}{2}\theta = \sqrt{\dfrac{1 - \cos \theta}{1 + \cos \theta}}$

$\sin(A \pm B) = \sin A \cos B \pm \cos A \sin B$

$\cos(A \pm B) = \cos A \cos B \mp \sin A \sin B$

$\tan(A \pm B) = \dfrac{\tan A \pm \tan B}{1 \mp \tan A \tan B}$

$\sin A \pm \sin B = 2 \sin[\tfrac{1}{2}(A \pm B)] \cos[\tfrac{1}{2}(A \mp B)]$

$\cos A + \cos B = 2 \cos[\tfrac{1}{2}(A + B)] \cos[\tfrac{1}{2}(A - B)]$

$\cos A - \cos B = 2 \sin[\tfrac{1}{2}(A + B)] \sin[\tfrac{1}{2}(B - A)]$

$\tan A \pm \tan B = \dfrac{\sin(A \pm B)}{\cos A \cos B}$

Example D-5

Use the isosceles right triangle shown in Figure D-14 to find the sine, cosine, and tangent of 45°.

Picture the Problem It is clear from the figure that the two acute angles of this triangle are equal. Since the sum of the three angles in a triangle must equal 180°, and the right angle is 90°, each acute angle must be 45°. If we multiply each side of any triangle by a common factor, we obtain a similar triangle with the same angles as the first. We can therefore choose any convenient length for one side. We choose the equal sides to have a length of 1 unit.

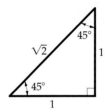

Figure D-14 An isosceles right triangle.

1. Find the length of the hypotenuse from the Pythagorean theorem:

$$c = \sqrt{a^2 + b^2} = \sqrt{1^2 + 1^2} = \sqrt{2} \text{ units}$$

2. Calculate sin 45° from its definition:

$$\sin 45° = \frac{a}{c} = \frac{1}{\sqrt{2}} = 0.707$$

3. Calculate cos 45° from its definition:

$$\cos 45° = \frac{b}{c} = \frac{1}{\sqrt{2}} = 0.707$$

4. Calculate tan 45° from its definition:

$$\tan 45° = \frac{a}{b} = \frac{1}{1} = 1$$

Example D-6

The sine of 30° is exactly 0.5. Find the ratios of the sides of a 30–60° right triangle.

Picture the Problem This common triangle is shown in Figure D-15. We choose a length of 1 unit for the side opposite the 30° angle.

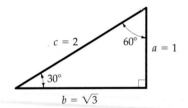

Figure D-15 A 30–60° right triangle.

1. Calculate the hypotenuse from the definition of the sine and the choice of 1 unit for the opposite side:

$$\sin 30° = \frac{a}{c} = \frac{1}{c} = 0.5$$

$$c = \frac{1}{0.5} = 2$$

2. Use the Pythagorean theorem to find the length b of the side opposite the 60° angle:

$$b = \sqrt{c^2 - a^2} = \sqrt{2^2 - 1^2} = \sqrt{3}$$

3. Use these results to calculate cos 30°, tan 30°, sin 60°, cos 60°, and tan 60°:

$$\cos 30° = \frac{b}{c} = \frac{\sqrt{3}}{2} = 0.866$$

$$\tan 30° = \frac{a}{b} = \frac{1}{\sqrt{3}} = 0.577$$

$$\sin 60° = \frac{b}{c} = \cos 30° = 0.866$$

$$\cos 60° = \frac{a}{c} = \sin 30° = 0.500$$

$$\tan 60° = \frac{b}{a} = \frac{\sqrt{3}}{1} = 1.732$$

For small angles, the length a is nearly equal to the arc length s, as can be seen in Figure D-16. The angle $\theta = s/c$ is therefore nearly equal to $\sin\theta = a/c$:

$$\sin\theta \approx \theta \qquad \text{for small values of } \theta \qquad\qquad \text{D-46}$$

Similarly, the lengths c and b are nearly equal, so $\tan\theta = a/b$ is nearly equal to both θ and $\sin\theta$ for small values of θ:

$$\tan\theta \approx \theta \sin\theta \approx \theta \qquad \text{for small values of } \theta \qquad\qquad \text{D-47}$$

Figure D-16 For small angles, $\sin\theta = a/c$, $\tan\theta = a/b$, and the angle $\theta = s/c$ are all approximately equal.

Equations D-46 and D-47 hold only if θ is measured in radians. Since $\cos\theta = b/c$ and these lengths are nearly equal for small values of θ, we have

$$\cos\theta \approx 1 \qquad \text{for small values of } \theta \qquad\qquad \text{D-48}$$

Example D-7

By how much do sin θ, tan θ, and θ differ when $\theta = 15°$?

1. Convert 15° to radians:

$$\theta = 15° \frac{2\pi \text{ rad}}{360°} = 0.262 \text{ rad}$$

2. Find sin 15° and tan 15° using a calculator:

$$\sin 15° = 0.259$$
$$\tan 15° = 0.268$$

3. Compute the percentage difference between θ and sin θ:

$$\frac{|\sin\theta - \theta|}{\theta} = \frac{|0.259 - 0.262|}{0.262} = \frac{0.003}{0.262} = 0.011 \approx 1\%$$

4. Compute the percentage difference between θ and tan θ:

$$\frac{|\tan\theta - \theta|}{\theta} = \frac{|0.268 - 0.262|}{0.262} = \frac{0.006}{0.262} = 0.023 \approx 2\%$$

Remark For smaller angles, the approximation $\theta \approx \sin\theta \approx \tan\theta$ is even more accurate.

Example D-7 shows that if accuracy of a few percent is needed, small angle approximations can be used only for angles of about 15° or less. Figure D-17 shows graphs of θ, sin θ, and tan θ versus θ, for small values of θ.

Figure D-18 shows an obtuse angle with its vertex at the origin and one side along the x axis. The trigonometric functions for a general angle such as this are defined by

$$\sin \theta = \frac{y}{c} \qquad \text{D-49}$$

$$\cos \theta = \frac{x}{c} \qquad \text{D-50}$$

$$\tan \theta = \frac{y}{x} \qquad \text{D-51}$$

Figure D-17 Graphs of tan θ, θ, and sin θ versus θ for small values of θ.

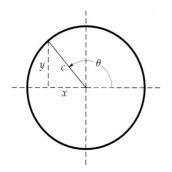

Figure D-18 Diagram for defining the trigonometric functions for an obtuse angle.

Figure D-19 shows plots of these functions versus θ. All trigonometric functions have a period of 2π. That is, when an angle changes by 2π rad, the function returns to its original value. Thus, $\sin(\theta + 2\pi) = \sin \theta$ and so forth. Some other useful relations are

$$\sin(\pi - \theta) = \sin \theta \qquad \text{D-52}$$

$$\cos(\pi - \theta) = -\cos \theta \qquad \text{D-53}$$

$$\sin(\pi/2 - \theta) = \cos \theta \qquad \text{D-54}$$

$$\cos(\pi/2 - \theta) = \sin \theta \qquad \text{D-55}$$

The trigonometric functions can be expressed as power series in θ. The series for sin θ and cos θ are

$$\sin \theta = \theta - \frac{\theta^3}{3!} + \frac{\theta^5}{5!} - \frac{\theta^7}{7!} + \cdots \qquad \text{D-56}$$

$$\cos \theta = 1 - \frac{\theta^2}{2!} + \frac{\theta^4}{4!} - \frac{\theta^6}{6!} + \cdots \qquad \text{D-57}$$

When θ is small, good approximations are obtained using only the first few terms in the series.

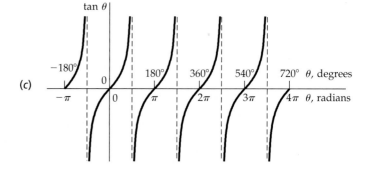

Figure D-19 The trigonometric functions sin θ, cos θ, and tan θ versus θ.

The Binomial Expansion

The binomial theorem is very useful for making approximations. One form of this theorem is

$$(1 + x)^n = 1 + nx + \frac{n(n - 1)}{2!}x^2 + \frac{n(n - 1)(n - 2)}{3!}x^3$$

$$+ \frac{n(n - 1)(n - 2)(n - 3)}{4!}x^4 + \cdots \qquad \text{D-58}$$

If n is a positive integer, there are $n + 1$ terms in this series. If n is a real number other than a positive integer, there are an infinite number of terms. The series is valid for any value of n if x^2 is less than 1. It is also valid for $x^2 = 1$ if n is positive. The series is particularly useful if $|x|$ is much less than 1. Then each term is much smaller than the previous term and we can drop all but the first two or three terms in the equation. If $|x|$ is much less than 1, we have

$$(1 + x)^n \approx 1 + nx, \qquad |x| \ll 1 \qquad \text{D-59}$$

Example D-8

Use Equation D-59 to find an approximate value for the square root of 101.

1. Write $(101)^{1/2}$ so it is in the form $(1 + x)^n$ with x much less than 1:

   $(101)^{1/2} = (100 + 1)^{1/2} = (100)^{1/2}(1 + 0.01)^{1/2}$

   $= 10(1 + 0.01)^{1/2}$

2. Use Equation D-59 with $n = \frac{1}{2}$ and $x = 0.1$ to expand $(1 + 0.01)^{1/2}$:

   $(1 + 0.01)^{1/2} \approx 1 + \frac{1}{2}(0.01) = 1.005$

3. Substitute this result into the equation in step 1:

   $(101)^{1/2} = 10(1 + 0.01)^{1/2} \approx 10.05$

Remarks We can assess the accuracy of this result by computing the first term in Equation D-58 that was neglected. This term is

$$\frac{n(n - 1)}{2}x^2 = \frac{\frac{1}{2}(-\frac{1}{2})}{2}(0.01)^2 = -\frac{0.0001}{8} \approx -0.00001 = -0.001\%$$

We therefore expect our answer to be correct to within about 0.001%. The value of $(101)^{1/2}$ to eight significant figures is 10.049875, which differs from 10.05 by 0.000124 or about 0.001% of 10.05.

Complex Numbers

A general complex number z can be written

$$z = a + bi \qquad \text{D-60}$$

where a and b are real numbers and $i = \sqrt{-1}$. The quantity a is called the real part and the quantity ib is called the imaginary part of z. We can represent a complex number in a plane as shown in Figure D-20, where the x axis is the real axis and the y axis is the imaginary axis. We can use the relations $a = r \cos \theta$ and $b = r \sin \theta$ from Figure D-20 to write the complex number z in polar coordinates:

$$z = r \cos \theta + (r \sin \theta)i \qquad \text{D-61}$$

where $r = \sqrt{a^2 + b^2}$ is called the magnitude of z.

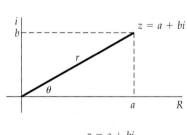

$z = a + bi$
$= r \cos \theta + (r \sin \theta)i$
$= r(\cos \theta + i \sin \theta)$

Figure D-20 Representation of a complex number in a plane. The real part of the complex number is plotted along the horizontal axis, and the imaginary part is plotted along the vertical axis.

When complex numbers are added or subtracted, the real and imaginary parts are added or subtracted separately:

$$z_1 + z_2 = (a_1 + b_1i) + (a_2 + b_2i) = (a_1 + a_2) + (b_1 + b_2)i \qquad \text{D-62}$$

However, when two complex numbers are multiplied, each part of one number is multiplied by each part of the other number:

$$z_1 z_2 = (a_1 + b_1i)(a_2 + b_2i) = a_1a_2 + b_1b_2i^2 + (a_1b_2 + a_2b_1)i \qquad \text{D-63}$$
$$= a_1a_2 - b_1b_2 + (a_1b_2 + a_2b_1)i$$

where we have used $i^2 = -1$.

The complex conjugate of a complex number, z^*, is that number obtained by replacing i with $-i$:

$$z^* = (a + bi)^* = a - bi \qquad \text{D-64}$$

The product of a complex number and its complex conjugate equals the square of the magnitude of the number:

$$zz^* = (a + bi)(a - bi) = a^2 + b^2 \qquad \text{D-65}$$

A particularly useful function of a complex number is the exponential $e^{i\theta}$. Using the expansion for e^x given in Table D-2, we have

$$e^{i\theta} = 1 + i\theta + \frac{(i\theta)^2}{2!} + \frac{(i\theta)^3}{3!} + \frac{(i\theta)^4}{4!} + \cdots$$

Using $i^2 = -1$, $i^3 = -i$, $i^4 = +1$, and so forth and separating the real parts from the imaginary parts, this expansion can be written

$$e^{i\theta} = 1 - \frac{\theta^2}{2!} + \frac{\theta^4}{4!} + \cdots + i\left(\theta - \frac{\theta^3}{3!} + \cdots\right)$$

Comparing this result with Equations D-56 and D-57, we can see that

$$e^{i\theta} = \cos\theta + i\sin\theta \qquad \text{D-66}$$

Using this result, we can express a general complex number as an exponential:

$$z = a + bi = r\cos\theta + (r\sin\theta)i = re^{i\theta} \qquad \text{D-67}$$

where $r = \sqrt{a^2 + b^2}$.

Differential Calculus

When we say that x is a function of t, we mean that for each value of t there is a corresponding value of x. An example is $x = At^2$, where A is a constant. To indicate that x is a function of t, we sometimes write $x(t)$ for x. Figure D-21 is a graph of x versus t for a typical function $x(t)$. At a particular value $t = t_1$, x has the value of x_1 as indicated. At another value t_2, x has the value x_2. The change in t, $t_2 - t_1$, is written $\Delta t = t_2 - t_1$ and the corresponding change in x is written $\Delta x = x_2 - x_1$. The ratio

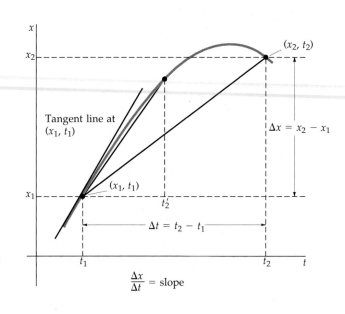

Figure D-21 Graph of a typical function $x(t)$. The points (x_1, t_1) and (x_2, t_2) are connected by a straight line. The slope of this line is $\Delta x / \Delta t$. As the time interval beginning at t_1 is decreased, the slope for that interval approaches the slope of the line tangent to the curve at time t_1, which is the derivative of x with respect to t.

$\Delta x / \Delta t$ is the slope of the straight line connecting (x_1, t_1) and (x_2, t_2). If we make Δt smaller and smaller, the line connecting (x_1, t_1) and (x_2, t_2) approaches the line that is tangent to the curve at the point (x_1, t_1). The slope of this tangent line is called the derivative of x with respect to t and is written dx/dt:

$$\frac{dx}{dt} = \lim_{\Delta t \to 0} \frac{\Delta x}{\Delta t} \qquad \text{D-68}$$

The derivative of a function of t is another function of t. If x is a constant, the graph of x versus t is a horizontal line with zero slope. The derivative of a constant is thus zero. In Figure D-22, x is proportional to t:

$$x = Ct$$

This function has a constant slope equal to C. Thus the derivative of Ct is C. Table D-4 lists some properties of derivatives and the derivatives of some particular functions that occur often in physics. It is followed by comments aimed at making these properties and rules clearer. More detailed discussion can be found in most calculus books.

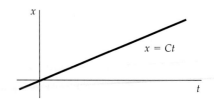

Figure D-22 Graph of the linear function $x = Ct$. This function has a constant slope C.

Table D-4

Properties of Derivatives and Derivatives of Particular Functions

Linearity

1. The derivative of a constant times a function equals the constant times the derivative of the function:

$$\frac{d}{dt}[Cf(t)] = C\frac{df(t)}{dt}$$

2. The derivative of a sum of functions equals the sum of the derivatives of the functions:

$$\frac{d}{dt}[f(t) + g(t)] = \frac{df(t)}{dt} + \frac{dg(t)}{dt}$$

Chain rule

3. If f is a function of x and x is in turn a function of t, the derivative of f with respect to t equals the product of the derivative of f with respect to x and the derivative of x with respect to t:

$$\frac{d}{dt}f(x) = \frac{df}{dx}\frac{dx}{dt}$$

Derivative of a product

4. The derivative of a product of functions $f(t)g(t)$ equals the first function times the derivative of the second plus the second function times the derivative of the first:

$$\frac{d}{dt}[f(t)g(t)] = f(t)\frac{dg(t)}{dt} + \frac{df(t)}{dt}g(t)$$

Reciprocal derivative

5. The derivative of t with respect to x is the reciprocal of the derivative of x with respect to t, assuming that neither derivative is zero:

$$\frac{dx}{dt} = \left(\frac{dt}{dx}\right)^{-1} \quad \text{if} \quad \frac{dt}{dx} \neq 0$$

Derivatives of particular functions

6. $\dfrac{dC}{dt} = 0$ where C is a constant

7. $\dfrac{d(t^n)}{dt} = nt^{n-1}$

8. $\dfrac{d}{dt}\sin \omega t = \omega \cos \omega t$

9. $\dfrac{d}{dt}\cos \omega t = -\omega \sin \omega t$

10. $\dfrac{d}{dt}\tan \omega t = \omega \sec^2 \omega t$

11. $\dfrac{d}{dt}e^{bt} = be^{bt}$

12. $\dfrac{d}{dt}\ln bt = \dfrac{1}{t}$

Example D-9

Find the derivative of $x = at^2 + bt + c$, where a, b, and c are constants.

Picture the Problem From rule 2, we can differentiate each term separately and add the results.

1. Use rules 1 and 7 to find the derivative of the first term:

$$\frac{d(at^2)}{dt} = 2at^1 = 2at$$

2. Compute the derivatives of the second and third terms:

$$\frac{d(bt)}{dt} = b, \qquad \frac{d(c)}{dt} = 0$$

3. Add these results:

$$\frac{dx}{dt} = 2at + b$$

Comments on Rules 1 Through 5

Rules 1 and 2 follow from the fact that the limiting process is linear. We can understand rule 3, the chain rule, by multiplying $\Delta f / \Delta t$ by $\Delta x / \Delta x$ and noting that, since x is a function of t, both Δx and Δf approach zero as Δt approaches zero. Since the limit of a product of two functions equals the product of their limits, we have

$$\lim_{\Delta t \to 0} \frac{\Delta f}{\Delta t} = \lim_{\Delta t \to 0} \frac{\Delta f}{\Delta x} \frac{\Delta x}{\Delta t} = \left(\lim_{\Delta x \to 0} \frac{\Delta f}{\Delta x} \right) \left(\lim_{\Delta t \to 0} \frac{\Delta x}{\Delta t} \right) = \frac{df}{dx} \frac{dx}{dt}$$

Rule 4 is not immediately apparent. The derivative of a product of functions is the limit of the ratio

$$\frac{f(t + \Delta t)g(t + \Delta t) - f(t)g(t)}{\Delta t}$$

If we add and subtract the quantity $f(t + \Delta t)g(t)$ in the numerator, we can write this ratio as

$$\frac{f(t + \Delta t)g(t + \Delta t) - f(t + \Delta t)g(t) + f(t + \Delta t)g(t) - f(t)g(t)}{\Delta t}$$

$$= f(t + \Delta t)\left[\frac{g(t + \Delta t) - g(t)}{\Delta t} \right] + g(t)\left[\frac{f(t + \Delta t) - f(t)}{\Delta t} \right]$$

As Δt approaches zero, the terms in brackets become $dg(t)/dt$ and $df(t)/dt$, respectively, and the limit of the expression is

$$f(t)\frac{dg(t)}{dt} + g(t)\frac{df(t)}{dt}$$

Rule 5 follows directly from the definition:

$$\frac{dx}{dt} = \lim_{\Delta t \to 0} \frac{\Delta x}{\Delta t} = \lim_{\Delta t \to 0} \left(\frac{\Delta t}{\Delta x} \right)^{-1} = \lim_{\Delta x \to 0} \left(\frac{\Delta t}{\Delta x} \right)^{-1} = \left(\lim_{\Delta t \to 0} \frac{\Delta t}{\Delta x} \right)^{-1}$$

Chapter 13

Opener p. 374 Michael Dunn/The Stock Market; **p. 381** Chuck O'Rear/Woodfin Camp and Assoc.; **p. 382 (a)** PAR/NYC, Inc. Archives; **(b)** David Burnett/Woodfin Camp and Assoc.; **p. 384 (a)** Estate of Harold E. Edgerton/Palm Press, Inc.; **(b)** Richard Megna/Fundamental Photographs; **p. 388 (a) and (b)** Office National d'Etudes et de Recherches Areospatiales; **p. 392 (top)** Picker International; **(bottom)** Dr. Owen M. Griffin, Naval Research Laboratory.

Chapter 14

Opener p. 403 Citibank; **p. 405** N.A.S.A. (73-HC-787); **p. 409** Institute for Marine Dynamics; **p. 417** Berenice Abbott/Commerce Graphics Ltd, Inc.; **p. 422** Estate of Harold E. Edgerton/Palm Press Inc.; **p. 423** Monroe Auto Equipment; **p. 426** Royal Swedish Academy of Music.

Chapter 15

Opener p. 442 (top) Four by Five Inc.; **(bottom)** Berenice Abbott/Photo Researchers; **p. 443** Berenice Abbott/Photo Researchers; **p. 454 (Figure 15-11)** *PSSC Physics*, 2nd ed., 1965. D.C. Heath & Co., and Education Development Center Inc., Newton, MA; **(Figure 15-12)** From Winston E. Kock, *Lasers and Holography*, Dover Publications, New York, 1981; **p. 459 (a) and (b)** *PSSC Physics*, 2nd ed., 1965. D.C. Heath & Co., and Education Development Center Inc., Newton, MA; **p. 461 (Figure 15-22)** *PSSC Physics*, 2nd ed., 1965. D.C. Heath & Co., and Education Development Center Inc., Newton, MA; **p. 462 (left)** Naval Research Laboratory; **(right)** Courtesy San Francisco Symphony; **(Figures 15-23 and 15-25)** *PSSC Physics*, 2nd ed., 1965. D.C. Heath & Co., and Education Development Center Inc., Newton, MA; **p. 463** Courtesy of the author; **p. 464** *PSSC Physics*, 2nd ed., 1965. D.C. Heath & Co., and Education Development Center Inc., Newton, MA; **p. 467 (left)** Sandia National Laboratory; **(right)** Robert de Gast/Photo Researchers; **(bottom)** Estate of Harold E. Edgerton/Palm Press Inc.; **p. 468 (Figure 15-28)** *PSSC Physics*, 2nd ed., 1965. D.C. Heath & Co., and Education Development Center Inc., Newton, MA; **(right)** Department of Energy.

Chapter 16

Opener p. 480 Dr. John S. Shelton; **p. 486** Berenice Abbott(8J 1328)/Photo Researchers; **p. 489** David Yost/Steinway & Sons; **p. 490 (bottom)** University of Washington; **p. 492** *PSSC Physics*, 2nd ed., 1965. D.C. Heath & Co., and Education Development Center Inc., Newton, MA; **p. 496 (top)** David Hathaway/N.A.S.A.; **(bottom)** Professor Thomas D. Rossing, Northern Illinois University, DeKalb.

Chapter 17

Opener p. 509 (a–d) Courtesy of Akira Tonomura, Advanced Research Laboratory, Hitachi, Ltd.; **p. 519 (a, b)** *PSSC Physics*, 2nd ed., 1965. D.C. Heath & Co., and Education Development Center Inc., Newton, MA; **(c)** C.G. Shull; **(d)** Claus Jönsson; **(bottom)** Jack Griffith/University of North Carolina.

Chapter 18

Opener p. 541 Lockheed Corporation; **p. 544** Courtesy Honeywell, Inc.; **p. 545** Dr. William Magnum/National Bureau of Standards; **p. 559 (top)** N.A.S.A.; **(bottom)** Jet Propulsion Laboratory/N.A.S.A.

Chapter 19

Opener p. 566 Phoenix Pipe and Tube/Lana Berkovich; **p. 572 (b)** Science Museum, London; **p. 588** Will and Deni McIntyre/Photo Researchers.

Chapter 20

Opener p. 600 Sandia National Laboratory; **p. 603** J.M. Mejuto/FPG International; **p. 610** Michael Collier/Stock, Boston; **p. 611 (b)** Jean-Pierre Horlin/The ImageBank; **(c)** Sandia National Laboratories; **(d)** Peter Miller/The Image Bank; **(e)** Sandia National Laboratories.

Chapter 21

Opener p. 633 Michael Melford/The Image Bank.

ILLUSTRATION CREDITS

Part Openers

Part I p. 18 James Sugar/Black Star
Part II p. 402 Michael Freeman
Part III p. 540 Sandia National Laboratory

Chapter 1

Opener **p. 1** The Granger Collection; **p. 4 (a)** The Granger Collection; **(b)** Frequency Electronics, Inc.; **p. 5 (a)** McDonald Observatory; **(b)** Bruce Coleman; **p. 7** Owen Franken/Stock, Boston; **p. 12 (a)** IBM Almaden Research Center; **(b)** from *The Body Victorius,* The Delacourt Press/Lennart Nilsson; **(c)** Kent and Donnan Dannen/Photo Researchers; **(d)** N.A.S.A. (68-HC-74); **(e)** Smithsonian Institution.

Chapter 2

Opener **p. 19** Barry O'Rourke/The Stock Market; **p. 26** George Hall/Woodfin Camp and Assoc.; **p. 27 (top)** Estate of Harold E. Edgerton/Palm Press, Inc.; **(bottom)** Gunter Ziesler/Peter Arnold Inc.; **p. 29** Sidney Harris; **p. 32** Courtesy General Motors Corporation; **p. 34 (a)** Stanford Linear Accelerator, U.S. Department of Energy; **(b)** John Seeman/Stanford Linear Accelerator Center.

Chapter 3

Opener **p. 54** Lewis Portnoy/Spectra-Action, Inc.

Chapter 4

Opener **p. 83** The Granger Collection; **p. 84** Arthur Tilley/FPG International; **p. 86** N.A.S.A./Science Source/Photo Researchers; **p. 88** Berenice Abbott/Commerce Graphics, Ltd., Inc.; **p. 90** Culver Pictures; **p. 91 (a)** Cotton Coulson/Woodfin Camp and Assoc.; **(b)** Gary Ladd; **(c)** Los Alamos Scientific Laboratory; **(d)** Science Photo Library/Photo Researchers; **p. 93 (b)** Fundamental Photographs; **Figure 4-6** David J. Phillip/AP Wide World; **p. 110** Bruce Hayes/Photo Researchers.

Chapter 5

Opener **p. 114** Courtesy Center for Engineering Design, University of Utah, Salt Lake City; **p. 115 (left)** F.P. Bowden and D. Tabor, *Friction and Lubrication of Solids,* Oxford University Press; **(right)** Uzi Landman, David W. Luedtke/Georgia Institute of Technology; **p. 118** Jean-Claude LeJeune/Stock, Boston; **p. 129** N.A.S.A. (85-HC-345); **p. 130** Malraux Photography/The Image Bank; **p. 131** Sandia National Laboratories; **p. 136** Richard Megna/Fundamental Photographs; **p. 143** David de Lossy/The Image Bank.

Chapter 6

Opener **p. 148** Estate of Harold E. Edgerton/Palm Press Inc.; **p. 152** Courtesy of Dr. Roger Craig; **p. 165** David J. Phillip/AP Wide World.

Chapter 7

Opener **p. 178** M.C. Escher Heirs/Cordon Art, De Baarn, Holland; **p. 180** Berenice Abbott/Photo Researchers; **p. 188 (a)** Visual Horizons/FPG International; **(b)** New York State Commerce Dept.; **(c)** L. Grant/FPG International; **p. 193** Stan Sholik/FPG International; **p. 195 (top left)** Courtesy of Omega Engineering, Inc.; **(top right)** Lennart Nilsson; **(bottom left)** Bruce Iverson; **(bottom right)** Lennart Nilsson; **p. 196** Leicester University/Science Photo Library/Photo Researchers.

Chapter 8

Opener **p. 212** Daniel Wray/The Image Works; **p. 218** Estate of Harold E. Edgerton/Palm Press Inc.; **p. 223** N.A.S.A.; **p. 227** Robert R. Edwards/ BOB-E Photography; **p. 228** Romilly Lockyer/The Image Bank; **p. 230** Courtesy of Mercedes-Benz of North America, Montvale, NJ; **p. 233** Estate of Harold E. Edgerton/Palm Press Inc.; **p. 236 (left and right)** Estate of Harold E. Edgerton/Palm Press Inc.; **p. 238 (left)** Berenice Abbot/Photo Researchers; **(right)** Brookhaven National Laboratory; **p. 239 (top left)** Courtesy Central Scientific Company; **(top right)** David Parker/Science Photo Library/Photo Researchers; **(bottom left)** Alar and Juri Toomre, from *Cambridge Atlas of Astronomy,* Cambridge University Press, 1985; **(bottom right)** Kitt Peak National Observatory, from *Cambridge Atlas of Astronomy,* Cambridge University Press, 1985; **p. 243** N.A.S.A./Shostal Superstock.

Chapter 9

Opener **p. 257** David Malin/Anglo-Australian Telescope Board; **p. 258** University of Utah/Center for Engineering Design; **p. 262** Culver Pictures; **p. 267** Michael Furman/The Stock Market; **p. 271** David Malin/Anglo-Australian Telescope Board; **p. 274** PAR/NYC, Inc. Archives; **p. 285** © Treë.

Chapter 10

Opener **p. 295** National Oceanographic and Atmospheric Administration; **p. 301** Dick Luria/Science Source/Photo Researchers; **p. 303** Richard Minnix; **p. 304 (Figure 10-19)** Estate of Harold E. Edgerton/Palm Press Inc.; **(Figure 10-20)** Focus on Sports; **p. 305** Dick Luria/FPG International; **p. 307 (left and right)** N.A.S.A./Goddard Space Flight Center; **p. 318** Chris Sorenson/The Stock Market.

Chapter 11

Opener **p. 321 (top)** Collection of Historical Scientific Instruments, Harvard University; **(bottom)** Erich Lessing/Magnum; **p. 325** Courtesy Central Scientific Company; **p. 331** N.A.S.A. (69-HC-905); **p. 341** N.A.S.A.

Chapter 12

Opener **p. 351** Thomas Zimmerman/FPG International.

The function y is the area under the f-versus-t curve from t_1 to a general value t. For a small interval Δt, the change in the area Δy is approximately $f\,\Delta t$.

$$\Delta y \approx f\,\Delta t$$

$$f \approx \frac{\Delta y}{\Delta t}$$

If we take the limit as Δt approaches 0, we can see that f is the derivative of y:

$$f = \frac{dy}{dt}$$

The relation between y and f is often written

$$y = \int f\,dt$$

where $\int f\,dt$ is called an **indefinite integral**. To evaluate an indefinite integral, we find the function y whose derivative is f. The definite integral of f from t_1 to t_2 is $y(t_1) - y(t_2)$, where $df/dt = y$:

$$\int_{t_1}^{t_2} f\,dt = y(t_2) - y(t_1)$$

Example D-10

Find the indefinite integral of $f(t) = t$.

1. The function whose derivative is t is $\frac{1}{2}t^2$ plus any constant:

$$\int t\,dt = \tfrac{1}{2}t^2 + C$$

where C is any constant

Table D-5 lists some important integration formulas. More extensive lists of differentiation and integration formulas can be found in handbooks such as Herbert Dwight's *Tables of Integrals and Other Mathematical Data*, fourth edition, Macmillan Publishing Company, Inc., New York, 1961.

Table D-5

Integration Formulas†

1. $\int A\,dt = At$	5. $\int e^{bt}\,dt = \dfrac{1}{b}e^{bt}$
2. $\int At\,dt = \frac{1}{2}At^2$	6. $\int \cos \omega t\,dt = \dfrac{1}{\omega}\sin \omega t$
3. $\int At^n\,dt = A\dfrac{t^{n+1}}{n+1}$, $n \neq -1$	7. $\int \sin \omega t\,dt = -\dfrac{1}{\omega}\cos \omega t$
4. $\int At^{-1}\,dt = A\ln t$	

†In these formulas, A, b, and ω are constants. An arbitrary constant C can be added to the right side of each equation.

Comments on Rule 11

Again we use the chain rule

$$\frac{de^{\theta}}{dt} = b\frac{de^{\theta}}{d\theta} \qquad \text{with} \qquad \theta = bt$$

and the series expansion for the exponential function:

$$e^{\theta+\Delta\theta} = e^{\theta}e^{\Delta\theta} = e^{\theta}\left[1 + \Delta\theta + \frac{(\Delta\theta)^2}{2!} + \frac{(\Delta\theta)^3}{3!} + \cdots\right]$$

Then

$$\frac{e^{\theta+\Delta\theta} - e^{\theta}}{\Delta\theta} = e^{\theta} + e^{\theta}\frac{\Delta\theta}{2!} + e^{\theta}\frac{(\Delta\theta)^2}{3!} + \cdots$$

As $\Delta\theta$ approaches zero, the right side of the equation above approaches e^{θ}.

Comments on Rule 12

Let

$$y = \ln bt$$

Then

$$e^y = bt \qquad \text{and} \qquad \frac{dt}{dy} = \frac{1}{b}e^y = t$$

Then using rule 5, we obtain

$$\frac{dy}{dt} = \left(\frac{dt}{dy}\right)^{-1} = \frac{1}{t}$$

Integral Calculus

Integration is related to the problem of finding the area under a curve. It is also the inverse of differentiation. Figure D-23 shows a function $f(t)$. The area of the shaded element is approximately $f_i\,\Delta t_i$, where f_i is evaluated anywhere in the interval Δt_i. This approximation improves if Δt_i is very small. The total area from t_1 to t_2 is found by summing all the area elements from t_1 to t_2 and taking the limit as each Δt_i approaches zero. This limit is called the integral of f over t and is written

$$\int_{t_1}^{t_2} f\,dt = \text{Area} = \lim_{\Delta t_i \to 0} \sum_i f_i\,\Delta t_i$$

If we integrate some function $f(t)$ from t_1 to some general value of t, we obtain another function of t. Let us call this function y:

$$y = \int_{t_1}^{t} f\,dt$$

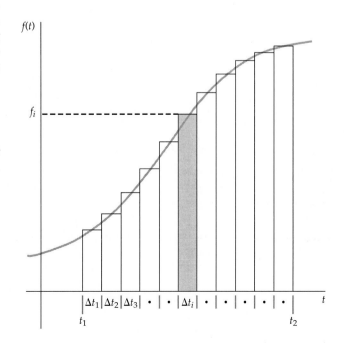

Figure D-23 A general function $f(t)$. The area of the shaded element is approximately $f_i\,\Delta t_i$, where f_i is evaluated anywhere in the interval.

Comments on Rule 7

We can obtain this important result using the binomial expansion. We have

$$f(t) = t^n$$

$$f(t + \Delta t) = (t + \Delta t)^n = t^n\left(1 + \frac{\Delta t}{t}\right)^n$$

$$= t^n\left[1 + n\frac{\Delta t}{t} + \frac{n(n-1)}{2!}\left(\frac{\Delta t}{t}\right)^2 + \frac{n(n-1)(n-2)}{3!}\left(\frac{\Delta t}{t}\right)^3 + \cdots\right]$$

Then

$$f(t - \Delta t) - f(t) = t^n\left[n\frac{\Delta t}{t} + \frac{n(n-1)}{2!}\left(\frac{\Delta t}{t}\right)^2 + \cdots\right]$$

and

$$\frac{f(t - \Delta t) - f(t)}{\Delta t} = nt^{n-1} + \frac{n(n-1)}{2!}t^{n-2}\,\Delta t + \cdots$$

The next term omitted from the last sum is proportional to $(\Delta t)^2$, the following to $(\Delta t)^3$, and so on. Each term except the first approaches zero as Δt approaches zero. Thus

$$\frac{df}{dt} = \lim_{\Delta x \to 0} \frac{f(t + \Delta t) + f(t)}{\Delta t} = nt^{n-1}$$

Comments on Rules 8 to 10

We first write $\sin \omega t = \sin \theta$ with $\theta = \omega t$ and use the chain rule,

$$\frac{d\sin\theta}{dt} = \frac{d\sin\theta}{d\theta}\frac{d\theta}{dt} = \omega\frac{d\sin\theta}{d\theta}$$

We then use the trigonometric formula for the sine of the sum of two angles θ and $\Delta\theta$:

$$\sin(\theta + \Delta\theta) = \sin\Delta\theta\cos\theta + \cos\Delta\theta\sin\theta$$

Since $\Delta\theta$ is to approach zero, we can use the small-angle approximations

$$\sin\Delta\theta \approx \Delta\theta \qquad \text{and} \qquad \cos\Delta\theta \approx 1$$

Then

$$\sin(\theta + \Delta\theta) \approx \Delta\theta\cos\theta + \sin\theta$$

and

$$\frac{\sin(\theta + \Delta\theta) - \sin\theta}{\Delta\theta} \approx \cos\theta$$

Similar reasoning can be applied to the cosine function to obtain rule 9.

Rule 10 is obtained by writing $\tan\theta = \sin\theta/\cos\theta$ and applying Rule 4 along with Rules 8 and 9.

$$\frac{d}{dt}(\tan\theta) = \frac{d}{dt}(\sin\theta)(\cos\theta)^{-1} = \sin\theta\frac{d}{dt}(\cos\theta)^{-1} + \frac{d(\sin\theta)}{dt}(\cos\theta)^{-1}$$

$$= \sin\theta(-1)(\cos\theta)^{-2}(-\sin\theta) + (\cos\theta)(\cos\theta)^{-1}$$

$$= \frac{\sin^2\theta}{\cos^2\theta} + 1 = \tan^2\theta + 1 = \sec^2\theta$$

ANSWERS

Problem answers are calculated using $g = 9.81$ m/s^2 unless otherwise specified in the Problem. Differences in the last figure can easily result from differences in rounding the input data and are not important.

To help you master the techniques in Examples and to solve the intermediate-level problems at the end of each chapter, the problem maps preceding the answers for the chapters indicate which Examples and odd-numbered intermediate-level Problems deal with similar material.

Chapter 1

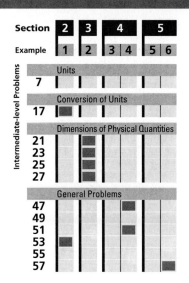

1. (c)

3. (a) 1 MW; (b) 2 mg; (c) 3 μm; (d) 30 ks

5. (a) 1 picoboo; (b) 1 gigalow; (c) 1 microphone; (d) 1 attoboy; (e) 1 megaphone; (f) 1 nanogoat; (g) 1 terabull

7. (a) C_1: ft, C_2: ft/s; (b) C_1: ft/s^2; (c) C_1: m/s^2; (d) C_1: ft, C_2: s^{-1}; (e) C_1: ft/s, C_2: s^{-1}

9. 2450 km/h, 1520 mi/h

11. (a) 62.1 mi/h; (b) 23.6 in; (c) 91.4 m

13. 1.61 km/mi

15. (a) 3.784 L; (b) 0.1589 m^3

17. (a) 0.505 ft^3; (b) 0.0143 m^3; (c) 14.3 L

19. (a) C_1: L, C_2: L/T; (b) C_1: L/T^2; (c) C_1: L/T^2; (d) C_1: L, C_2: 1/T; (e) C_1: L/T, C_2: 1/T

21. $L^3/(MT^2)$, m^3/kg·s^2

23. $M(L/T^2)(L/T) = ML^2/T^3$

25. $(ML/T^2)(L/T)$

27. $T = Cr^{3/2}/\sqrt{M_s G}$

29. (d)

31. (c)

33. (a) 30,000; (b) 0.0062; (c) 0.000004; (d) 217,000

35. (a) 1.14×10^5; (b) 2.24×10^{-8}; (c) 8.27×10^3; (d) 6.27×10^2

37. 4×10^6 membranes

39. (a) 1.69×10^3; (b) 4.8; (c) 5.6; (d) 10

41. One advantage of using your arm is that a measure of standard length is always available. The disadvantage is that arm lengths are not uniform. For example, if you wish to purchase a board of "two arm lengths," it may be shorter or longer than you expected, depending on the owner's arm length.

43. (a) True; (b) False; (c) True

45. 31.7 yr

47. 2.0×10^{23}

49. 3.51 Mm

51. 3.86×10^2 mi^2

53. (a) 1.8×10^2; (b) 3.4; (c) 2.9×10^8; (d) 0.45

55. (a) 6.6×10^3 electrons/m^3; (b) 3.6 protons/m^3

57. (a) 1×10^{11} cans/yr; (b) 2×10^9 kg/yr; (c) $2 billion

59. (a) In a plot of T versus m^n, $n = 1/2$ provides the best fit to a straight line.

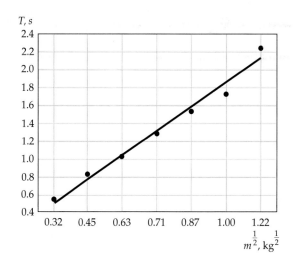

The slope of the line $C \approx 1.77$ s/kg$^{1/2}$. (b) The points with the greatest deviation are $T = 1.75$ s and $T = 2.22$ s.

61. (a) $C\sqrt{L/g}$; (b) Check by using pendulums of lengths 1 m and 0.5 m; the periods should be about 2 s and 1.4 s.

63. (a) 1.6×10^{10} bits; (b) 350 books

Chapter 2

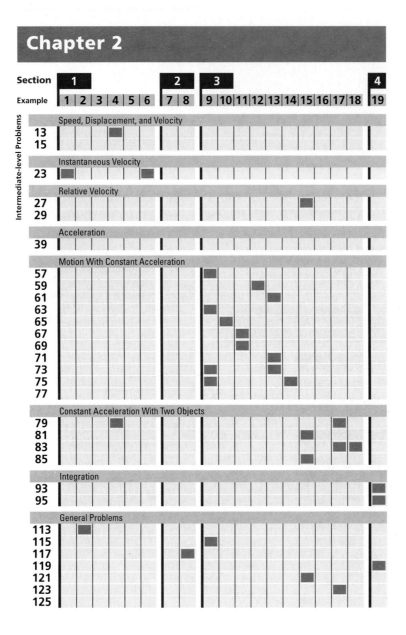

1. Since the cars go round a closed circuit and return nearly to the starting point, the displacement is nearly zero, and the average velocity is zero.

3. Yes. In a round trip, A to B and back to A, the average velocity is zero; the average velocity between A and B is not zero.

5. (a) 4 ns; (b) 4 ks

7. (a) 260 km; (b) 65 km/h

9. (a) 73.3 mi/h; (b) 44.3

11. (a) 434 yr; (b) 4.34×10^6 yr; he need not pay for pizza.

13. (a) 13 m; (b) 2.2 s

15. (a) 7.9×10^4 m/s; (b) 3.16×10^7 m/s; (c) 2×10^{10} yr

17. No, because for constant velocity, the instantaneous velocity and average velocities are equal.

19. (b)

21. (a) 1 m/s; (b) 2 m/s

23. (a) 2 m, 2 m/s; (b) $\Delta x = [(2t - 5) \Delta t + \Delta t^2]$ m; (c) $(2t - 5)$ m/s

25. (a)

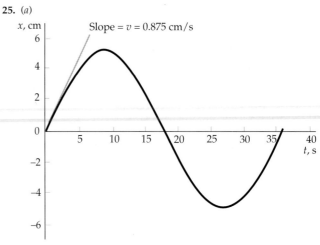

(b) 0.875 cm/s; (c) 0.723, 0.835, 0.857, 0.871, 0.874, 0.875; (d) 0.875 cm/s

27. 120 km

29. 6 h

31. (*a*) After getting started, walk in the opposite (negative) direction. Gradually slow the speed of walking, until the other end of the room is reached.

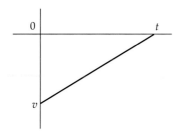

33. Yes. An object tossed up has a constant downward acceleration; at the top its instantaneous velocity is zero.

35. (*a*) $a = 0$; (*b*) $a > 0$; (*c*) $a < 0$; (*d*) $a = 0$

37. (*a*) 2.42 m/s², (*b*) 89.2 km/h

39. (*a*) 8 m/s², 8 m/s²; (*b*) 8 m/s²

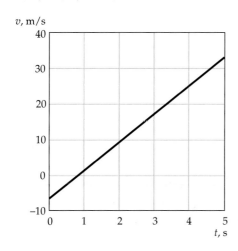

41. The initial downward velocities of the two rocks are not the same.

43. (*b*)

45. (*a*)

47. (*d*)

49. (*c*)

51. (*a*) 80 m/s; (*b*) 400 m; (*c*) 40 m/s

53. 15.6 m/s²

55. 4.59×10^3 m

57. (*a*) 4.08 s; (*b*) 20.4 m; (*c*) 0.99 s or 3.09 s are both acceptable.

59. (*a*) -5.1×10^5 m/s²; (*b*) 0.686 ms

61. 1467 m

63. (*a*)

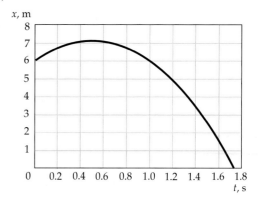

(*b*) 7.27 m; (*c*) 1.73 s; (*d*) 11.9 m/s

65. 1.62 m

67. 43.6 m

69. ±68 m/s; the stone may be thrown either up or down.

71. (*a*) 666 m; (*b*) 13.6 m/s

73. (*a*) 19.0 km; (*b*) 2 min 18 s; (*c*) 610 m/s

75. (*a*) 2.24 s; (*b*) 6.17 m

77. 145.7 m

79. 15.6 m

81. 100.4 km/h

83. Deceleration ≥ 0.754 m/s², $v_{rel} = 3.77$ m/s, distance = 518 m

85. 4.8 m/s

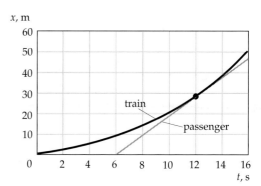

87. $2h/3$

89. 32.4 km

91. (*a*)

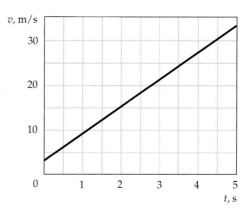

(*b*) 90 m

93. $x(t) = \int (7t^2 - 5)\, dt = (7/3)\, t^3 - 5t + C$

95. (a) 0.25 m/s; (b) 0.9 m/s, 3 m/s, 6 m/s; (c) 6.5 m

97.

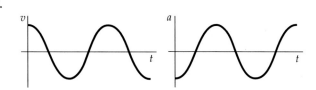

99. (c)

101. (a)

103. (d)

105. (d)

107. (a) t_0, t_1; (b) t_3, t_1, t_6, t_7; (c) t_2, t_5; (d) t_4; (e) t_2, t_6; (f) t_0, t_1, t_3, t_5, t_7

109. (a) a, f, i; (b) c, d; (c) a, d, e, f, h, i; (d) b, c, g. The graphs d and h and the graphs f and i are mutually consistent.

111. (a) 36 m; (b) −36 m; (c) −9 m/s

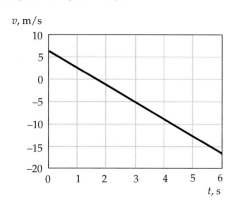

113. 134 m/s

115. 24 m, 1.4 s

117. $v(t) = (50 - 10t)$ m/s, $a = -10$ m/s^2, $x(t) = 50t - 5t^2$

119. (a) $x(t) = Ct^3/6 + At + B$; (b) 37.5 m/s, 62.5 m

121. (a) 6.67 s; (b) 6.67 s

123. (a) $\Delta x_s = 100.3$ m; $\Delta x_p = 232.3$ m; Note that $\Delta x_s + 100$ m $< x_p$, so the cars collide. (b) 5.52 s. (c) With added reaction time, the collision will occur sooner and be more severe.

125. The running time of the ball player is 2.42 s and the flight time of the ball is 2.19 s. A good umpire will call him out!

127. (a) Initially, $v = 0$ and increases as gt, but as v becomes finite, the acceleration diminishes to $g - bv$. Ultimately, the acceleration approaches zero and v remains constant, $v_{\text{term}} = g/b$.

(b)

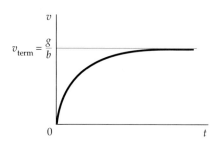

129. $x(t) = x_0\, e^{t - t_0}$.

131. (a)

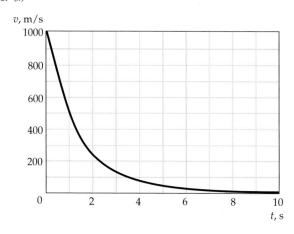

(b) 144.1 m/s

Chapter 3

1. The magnitude of the displacement can be less than but never more than the distance traveled.

3. (e)

5. $D = (-5\hat{i} + 5\hat{j})$ m

7.

(a)

(b)

(c)

(d)

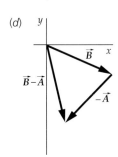

(e)

9. No, the magnitudes can be equal if the vector is along the component direction.

11. No, if $\vec{B} = -\vec{A}$, then $\vec{C} = 0$.

13. (b)

15. (a) $A_x = 8.66$ m, $A_y = 5$ m; (b) $A_x = 3.54$ m, $A_y = 3.54$ m; (c) $A_x = 3.5$ km, $A_y = 6.06$ km; (d) $A_x = 0$ km, $A_y = 5$ km; (e) $A_x = -13$ km/s, $A_y = 7.5$ km/s; (f) $A_x = -5$ m/s, $A_y = -8.66$ m/s; (g) $A_x = 0$, $A_y = -8$ m/s^2

17. (a) $A = 5.83$, $\theta = 31°$; (b) $B = 12.2$, $\theta = -35°$; (c) $C = 5.39$, $\theta = 42°$, $\phi = 236°$

19. (a) 5 m/s $\hat{i} + 8.66$ m/s $\hat{j}$; (b) -3.54 m $\hat{i} - 3.54$ m $\hat{j}$; (c) 14 m $\hat{i} - 6$ m $\hat{j}$

21. $\vec{B} = -1.5\vec{A}$

23. No

25. A particle moving at constant speed in a circular path is accelerating (the direction of the velocity vector is changing). If a particle is moving at constant velocity, it is not accelerating.

27. (a) The velocity vector is always tangent to the path.

(b)

29.

31. 14.1 km/h $\hat{i} - 4.1$ km/h $\hat{j}$

33. (b)

35. (a) -10 m/s; (b) $90°$; (c) 40 m/s $\hat{i} + 30$ m/s $\hat{j}$; (d) 10 m/s^2 at $37°$ with x axis

37. (a) 10 m/s $\hat{i} - 3$ m/s $\hat{j}$; (b) 44 m $\hat{i} - 9$ m $\hat{j}$; $r = 44.9$ m, $\theta = -11.6°$

39. (a) $\vec{v} = [6t\,\hat{i} + 4t\,\hat{j}]$ m/s, $\vec{r} = [(10 + 3t^2)\,\hat{i} + 2t^2\,\hat{j}]$ m

(b)

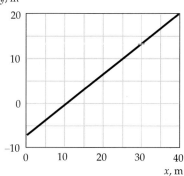

41. (d)

43. (a) 0.8 m/s; (b) 1.79 m/s; (c) $30°$ upstream

45. 5.18 km/h

47. (a) -120 m $\hat{i} + 4$ m $\hat{j}$; (b) -20 m/s $\hat{i} - 12$ m/s $\hat{j}$; (c) -2 m/s^2 $\hat{j}$

49. 261.7 km/h, $6.58°$ west of north

51. True

53. (e)

55. (a) A and E; (b) C; (c) A and E have the same speed, but not the same velocities.

57. 1.1 m

59. 15 m/s, 9.81 m/s^2 downward

61. 33.8 m/s

63. 20.3 m/s, $36.2°$

65. $69.3°$

67. (a) 49.5 s; (b) 12.4 km; (c) 12.0 km

69. (a) 8.14 m/s; (b) 23.2 m/s

71. $-63.4°$

73. $d[(v_0^2 \sin 2\theta)/g]/d\theta = (v_0^2/g)\,d(\sin 2\theta)/d\theta = (2v_0^2/g)\cos 2\theta$; set equal to 0; $2\theta = 90°$, $\theta = 45°$

75. $2v^2 \tan\phi/(g\cos\phi)$

77. 18.2 m from wall

79. $-1.93°$

81. 3.19 m/s

83. (a) 44.3 m/s, $9.33°$ above horizontal; (b) 0.733 s; (c) 3.23 m

85. 0.785 m

87. (a) 11.0 m; (b) $v_{0x} = 10$ m/s; $v_{0y} = 14.7$ m/s; (c) 17.8 m/s; (d) $55.8°$

89. (*a*) False; (*b*) False; (*c*) True

91.

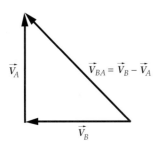

93. (*a*) north, northeast, east, southeast, south; (*b*) AB north, BC southeast, CD $\vec{a} = 0$, DE southwest, EF north; (*c*) equal

95. $4.9 \text{ m/s}^2\,\hat{i} + 8.5 \text{ m/s}^2\,\hat{j}$

97. (*a*)

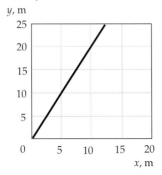

(*b*) $(5\hat{i} + 10\hat{j})$ m/s, 11.2 m/s

99. 4.29 m

101. Assuming an initial height of 1.5 m and an initial speed of 25 min/s: (*a*) 14 m; (*b*) 64 m; (*c*) 41 m; (*d*) 75 m

103. 14.8 m/s

105. (*a*) $(\hat{i} + \hat{j})$ m/s; (*b*) $(2\hat{i} - 3.5\hat{j})$ m/s^2;
(*c*) $[\hat{i} + \hat{j} + (2\hat{i} - 3.5\hat{j})t]$ m/s;
(*d*) $[4\hat{i} + 3\hat{j} + (\hat{i} + \hat{j})t + \frac{1}{2}(2\hat{i} - 3.5\hat{j})t^2]$ m

107. (*a*) $(25\hat{i} + 7.07\hat{j} + 7.07\hat{k})$ m/s; (*b*) $(39.9\hat{i} + 11.3\hat{j})$ m

109. Yes, if it is a high fly.

111. (*a*) 0.98 km/h; (*b*) 39.6 west of north; (*c*) 3 h 19 min

113. $v_y^2 = v_{0y}^2 + 2gh$, regardless of direction (up or down).
$v^2 = v_x^2 + v_y^2$, and since $v_x = v_{0x}$, $v^2 = v_{0x}^2 + v_{0y}^2 + 2gH = v_0^2 + 2gH$,
for any angle. $v = (v_0^2 + 2gh)^{1/2}$

1. If Newton's first law is obeyed, the reference frame is an inertial reference frame.

3. No

5. No

7. (*d*)

9. (*b*)

11. $F_2 = 3F_1$

13. 4.46 m/s^2

15. (*a*) 250 N; (*b*) 400 N

17. (*a*) $(1.5\hat{i} - 3.5\hat{j})$ m/s^2; (*b*) $(4.5\hat{i} - 10.5\hat{j})$ m/s;
(*c*) $(6.75\hat{i} - 15.75\hat{j})$ m

19. To accelerate, she must exert a force proportional to her mass.

21. (*c*)

23. 74.8 kg

25. (*a*) 395 N; (*b*) No

27. (*b*)

29. (*c*)

31.

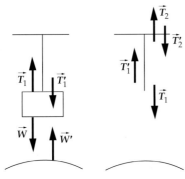

33. (*a*) 60 N; (*b*) 57.7 N

35. (*a*)

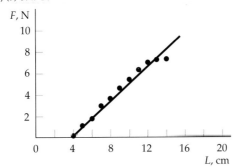

(*b*) 7.15 N; (*c*) 5.3 cm

37. No, the tension in the line must have a vertical component to support the weight of the towel.

39. (*b*)

41. (*c*)

43. (*a*) -8.81 m/s^2; (*b*) -7.81 m/s^2; (*c*) 10.19 m/s^2

45. (*a*) $v = -10.8$ m/s; (*b*) $v = -7.7$ m/s

47. (*a*) $T = w/2 \, (\sin \theta)$; $\theta = 90°$, T least; $\theta \to 0°$, T greatest; (*b*) 19.6 N

49. (*a*) 11,810 N; (*b*) 9810 N; (*c*) 7810 N

51. (*a*) $T_1 = 60$ N, $T_2 = 52$ N, $M = 5.3$ kg; (*b*) $T_1 = 46.2$ N, $T_2 = 46.2$ N, $M = 4.71$ kg; (*c*) $T_1 = T_3 = 34$ N, $T_2 = 58.9$ N, $M = 3.46$ kg

53.

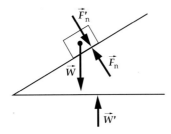

55. (*a*) and (*b*) = 98.1 N; (*c*) 49 N; (*d*) 49 N

57. (*a*) 149 N; (*b*) 3.41 m/s^2

59. (*a*)

61. high

63. 5.19 m/s^2

65. (*a*) 19.6 N; (*b*) 19.6 N; (*c*) 39.6 N; for $0 \le t \le 2$ s, $F = 19.6$ N; for 2 s $\le t \le 4$ s, $F = 9.62$ N

67. (*d*)

69. (*a*) $a = F/(m_1 + m_2)$; $F_c = F [m_2/(m_1 + m_2)]$; (*b*) $a = 0.4$ m/s^2; $F_c = 2.4$ N

71. $F_A = 160$ N, $F_B = 161.2$ N, $F_C = 321.6$ N

73. (*a*) 492 N, 3.71 m/s; (*b*) 20.7 m/s

75. (*a*) $m_1 = m_2(g - a)/(a + g \sin \theta) = 48$ kg; (*b*) 424 N

77. (*a*) 10 m/s^2; (*b*) $60 + 8x$ N

79. $a_{10} = 1.12$ m/s^2, $a_{20} = -1.12$ m/s^2, $T = 44.8$ N

81. $\Sigma F_x = m_1 a = T - m_1 g \sin \theta$, $\Sigma F_y = m_2 a = m_2 g - T$. Add the two equations and solve for a, using $\theta = 90°$. Use the expression for a to solve for T.

83. $2 m_1 m g/(m_1 + m_2)$

85. (*a*) $(2L/t^2) [(m_1 + m_2)/(m_1 - m_2)]$; (*b*) Differentiate with respect to t; $dg/dt = -2g/t$ or $dg/g = -2dt/t$; $m_2 = 0.926$ kg or 1.08 kg

87. (*a*)

89. 3 kg

91. 14.3 m/s^2

93. 20.8 lb

95. (*a*) The object will swing backward; (*b*) $T_x = ma$, $T_y = mg$, $\tan \theta = T_x/T_y = ma/mg$, $a = g \tan \theta$; (*c*) 1.6 m/s^2, 9.3°

97. (*a*) $a = F/(m_1 + m_2)$; (*b*) $F_{net} = Fm_2/(m_1 + m_2)$; (*c*) $Fm_1/(m_1 + m_2)$

99. 4000 N

101. (*a*) 55 g; (*b*) 2.45 m/s^2

103. (*a*) $T = (F_2 + 2F_1)/3$; (*b*) $3T_0/4C$

105. $a_1 = \dfrac{m_2 - m_1}{m_1 + m_2} g + \dfrac{2m_2}{m_1 + m_2} a$

$a_2 = \dfrac{m_1 - m_2}{m_1 + m_2} g + \dfrac{2m_1}{m_1 + m_2} a$

$T = \dfrac{2m_1 m_2}{m_1 + m_2} (g + a)$

Chapter 5

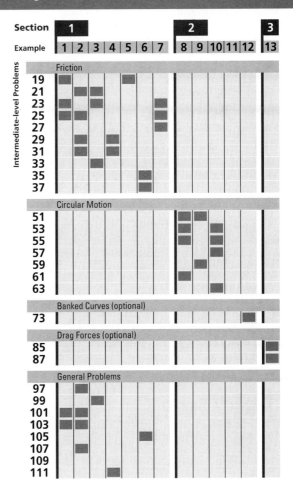

1. The force of friction between the objects and the floor of the truck

3. (a) False; (b) True; (c) True; (d) True

5. (d)

7. (e)

9. (b)

11. 0.417

13. (a) $\mu_s > \mu_k$; therefore f is greater if wheels do not spin; (b) $\mu_s = 0.425$

15. (a) 49.05 N; (b) 123 N

17. (a) $\theta > 0$ is preferable; it reduces F_n and therefore f_s; (b) 294 N

19. (b)

21. (a) 0.614 kg, 3.39 kg; (b) 9.81 N

23. 83.9 m

25. (a) 49.1 m; (b) 110 m

27. (a) 2.75 m/s^2; (b) 10.1 s

29. (a) -0.809 m/s^2; (b) $T = 0.176$ N

31. (a) -0.944 m/s^2; (b) -0.425 N

33. (a) One expects that F will increase with increasing magnitude of the angle since the normal component increases and the tangential component decreases.

(b) A force applied at a 0° angle will be most efficient.

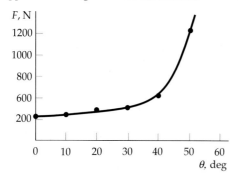

35. (a) 0.238; (b) 1.4 m/s^2

37. (a) 17.7 N; (b) 2.95 m/s^2, 5.9 N; (c) $a_1 = 1.96$ m/s^2, $a_2 = 7.87$ m/s^2

39. (a) $F = \mu_s mg/(\cos \theta + \mu_s \sin \theta)$; (b) F is a minimum when the denominator is a maximum. Differentiate $(\cos \theta + \mu_s \sin \theta)$ and set to 0. Solve for θ: $\theta = \tan^{-1} \mu_s$. For $\mu_s = 0.6$, $\theta = 31°$

41. $a_{min} = g(\sin \theta - \mu_s \cos \theta)/(\cos \theta + \mu_s \sin \theta)$, $a_{max} = g(\sin \theta + \mu_s \cos \theta)/(\cos \theta - \mu_s \sin \theta)$

43. True, it requires centripetal force.

45. (e)

47. 33.4 rpm

49. (a) 1.41 m/s; (b) 8.5 N

51. (a) 4660 N; (b) 110 m

53. $R = m_1 v^2/m_2 g$

55. $T_1 = [m_1 L_1 + m_2(L_1 + L_2)](2\pi/T)^2$; $T_2 = m_2(L_1 + L_2)(2\pi/T)^2$

57. 410 N, 53.3°

59. 640 N to 1000 N

61. (a) 2.61 N; (b) 1.21 m/s

63. 51.6°

65. (a) $a_c = \dfrac{v_0^2}{r}\left[\dfrac{1}{1 + (\mu_k v_0/r)t}\right]^2$; (b) $-\mu_k a_c$; (c) $a = a_c(1 + \mu_k^2)^{1/2}$

67. (d)

69. Bonita

71. (a) 7.25 m/s; (b) 0.536

73. (a) 8245 N; (b) 1565 N; (c) 0.19

75. 176 m

77. The constant b should increase with density as more air molecules collide with the object as it falls.

79. (d)

81. 3.27×10^{-9} kg/s

83. (a) 589 N; (b) 0.942 kg/m

85. 88.2 km/h

87. (a) 21.8 kg/m; (b) 78.48 kN. This initial acceleration would cause internal damage.

89. (a) 2.42 cm/s; (b) 1.15 h

91. (d)

93. (b)

95. (a) 10.7 m/s; (b) 8.0 N

97. (a) 0.289; (b) 600 N

99. 1486 N

101. (d)

103. $\mu_s = 0.577$, $\mu_k = 0.342$

105. $(m_1 + m_2)g\mu_s \cos \theta$

107. 0.433

109. 23.6 rpm

111. 1.22 kg, 0.672

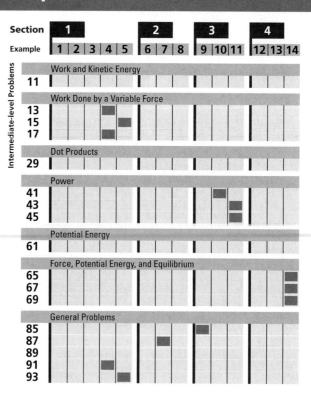

1. (*a*) False; (*b*) True; (*c*) True

3. Yes, if your center of mass is higher when standing than when lying in bed. Otherwise, no.

5. No, $dW = \vec{F} \cdot d\vec{r}$ and here $\vec{F}$ is perpendicular to $d\vec{r}$.

7. (*a*) 10.8 kJ; (*b*) 2.7 kJ; (*c*) 43.2 kJ

9. (*a*) 240 J; (*b*) −177 J; (*c*) 63 J

11. 54.4 kg

13. (*a*) 6 J; (*b*) 12 J; (*c*) 3.46 m/s

15. 19*C* J

17. (*a*) 2.75 J; (*b*) 11.4 J; (*c*) 2.76 m/s; (*d*) 3.5 J; (*e*) 2.84 m/s

19. No. Since the force is perpendicular to the motion, it will cause the particle to depart from straight-line motion.

21. (*a*) $F_{3m} = 417$ N, $F_{4m} = 313$ N, $F_{5m} = 250$ N; (*b*) 1.25 kJ for each *L*; (*c*) Choosing a longer length means one can exert a smaller force.

23. 180°

25. (*a*) −24; (*b*) −10; (*c*) 0

27. (*a*) 1 J; (*b*) 0.213 N

29. (*a*) $(d/dt)(\vec{r} \cdot \vec{r}) = \vec{r} \cdot (d\vec{r}/dt) + (d\vec{r}/dt) \cdot \vec{r} = 2\vec{v} \cdot \vec{r} = 0$. Therefore $\vec{v} \perp \vec{r}$. (*b*) $(d/dt)(\vec{v} \cdot \vec{v}) = 2\vec{a} \cdot \vec{v} = 0$. Therefore $\vec{a} \perp \vec{v}$. The above implies that the component of $\vec{a}$ in the plane formed by $\vec{r}$ and $\vec{v}$ is colinear with $\vec{r}$. (*c*) $(d/dt)(\vec{v} \cdot \vec{r}) = \vec{v} \cdot (d\vec{r}/dt) + \vec{r} \cdot (d\vec{v}/dt)$ $= v^2 + \vec{r} \cdot \vec{a} = 0$. Therefore, $a_r = -v^2/r$.

31. (*d*)

33. (*a*)

35. F_B

37. (*a*) 2 m/s; (*b*) 24 J

39. (*a*) 24 W; (*b*) −50 W; (*c*) 24 W

41. 26.7 kW

43. From Example 6-11, $x = (8P/9m)^{1/2}t^{3/2}$. From $v = (2P/m)^{1/2}t^{1/2}$, solve for $t^{3/2}$ and substitute this into the expression for *x*. Simplifying, one obtains $x = (m/3P)v^3$.

45. 4.9 m/s, 19.6 m

47. (*c*)

49. (*a*)

51. (*c*)

53. No. The steeper trail requires fewer steps, but more effort per step.

55. 4.71 kJ

57. 879 MW

59. (*a*) $U(x) = -6(x - x_0)$; (*b*) $U(x) = 24 - 6x$; (*c*) $U(x) = 50 - 6x$

61. $m_1 = 5.68$ kg, $m_2 = 4.32$ kg

63. (*a*) A, E: $F_x < 0$; B, D, E: $F_x = 0$; C: $F_x > 0$; (*b*) A; (*c*) B: unstable equilibrium; D: stable equilibrium

65. (*a*) $F_x = C/x^2$; (*b*) directed away from the origin; (*c*) $U(x)$ decreases as *x* increases; (*d*) If *C* is a negative constant, F_x is directed toward the origin and $U(x)$ increases as *x* increases.

67. $U(x) = a/x + U_0$

69. (*a*) $U(y) = 2Mg[(d^2 + y^2)^{1/2} - d] - mgy$; (*b*) $y = d(m/2M)/\sqrt{1 - (m/2M)^2}$; (*c*) $y_0 = d(m/2M)/\sqrt{1 - (m/2M)^2}$

71. Stable equilibrium at $x = 0$, unstable equilibrium at $x = \pm 2$. $U(x)$ is local minimum at $x = 0$, local maximum at $x = \pm 2$.

73. (*a*) $U(x)$ decreases; (*b*) $U(x) = 4/x^2$ J;
(*c*)

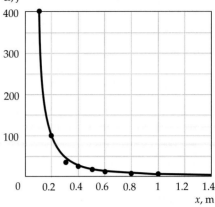

75. (*d*)

77. (*a*) $2h$; (*b*) wh; (*c*) $F \times 2h = wh$

79. (*a*) 706 MJ; (*b*) 11.8 MW

81. 0.5 m

83. 39.3 m

85. (*a*) 12 MW; (*b*) 1261 citizens

87. (*a*) 0; (*b*) 78 J

89. (*a*) 9 J; (*b*) −22 W

91. (*a*)

x, m	−4	−3	−2	−1	0	1	2	3	4
W, J	−11	−10	−7	−3	0	1	0	−2	−3

(*b*)

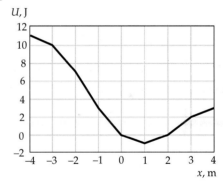

93. (*a*) μyg; (*b*) $\mu g(l^2/2)$

95. (*a*) Answer given in the problem. (*b*) $W = 10\pi F_0$ for clockwise rotation, $W = -10\pi F_0$ for counterclockwise rotation. The force is not conservative.
(*c*) $P = T\sqrt{2[(T/M) - g\sin\theta]x}$

Chapter 7

Section	1					2							3	
Example	1	2	3	4	5	6	7	8	9	10	11	12	13	14

Intermediate-level Problems

The Conservation of Mechanical Energy
17 19 21 23 25 27 29 31 33

The Conservation of Energy
43

Kinetic Friction
51 53 55

Mass and Energy
65

General Problems
73 75 77 79 81 83 85 87 89 91 93 95

1. Using conservation of mechanical energy is generally simpler, involving only scalars; however, some details can't be obtained (e.g., trajectories).

3. (c)

5. (c)

7. (a) 1.215 J; (b) 3.49 m/s; (c) 2.34 m

9. (a) 0.858 m; (b) The spring will accelerate the mass and it will then retrace the path, rising to a height of 5 m.

11. (a)

13. 26.7 m/s

15. 25.6°

17. 1.40 m/s

19. $[mg(\sin \theta + \mu_s \cos \theta)]^2/2k$

21. 8.0 m/s

23. $6mg$

25. 27.2 m/s

27. (a) 60°; (b) 51.3°

29. (a) 3.52 m/s; (b) 7.89 J; (c) 25.3 N; (d) 49°

31. (a) $(5/2) mgL$; (b) $6 mg$

33. Assuming your weight is 650 N: (a) 20.2°; (b) 6.4 m/s

35. $v = L\theta\sqrt{g/L + (k/m)\theta^2}$

37. The kinetic energy of the man increases at the expense of metabolic (chemical) energy.

39. (b)

41. (a) 0; (b) 560 J; (c) The increase in kinetic energy is at the expense of a loss in metabolic (chemical) energy.

43. (a) 94.2 kJ; (b) The energy comes from metabolic energy. (c) 471 kJ

45. Metabolic (chemical) energy converted to thermal energy is released through friction.

47. (a) 104 J; (b) 70.2 J; (c) 33.8 J; (d) 2.91 m/s

49. (a) 7.67 m/s; (b) 58.9 J; (c) 1/3

51. (a) 13.73y J; (b) −13.73y J; (c) 1.98 m/s

53. (a) $(3/8)\, mv_0^2$; (b) $(3v_0^2)/(16\pi gr)$; (c) 1/3 revolution

55. (a) 2.15 m; (b) 0.63 m/s; (c) 133 J

57. (a) $d = (mg/k)(\sin \theta + \mu_s \cos \theta)$; (b) $\mu_k = \tan \theta - \frac{1}{2}(1 + \mu_s \cot \theta)$

59. (a) 9×10^{13} J; (b) $\$2.5 \times 10^6$; (c) 9×10^{11} s = 28,400 yr

61. 3.56×10^{14} reactions

63. 0.782 MeV

65. 1.05 kg; (b) 3.06×10^9 kg

67. (b)

69. (a) 8.64 MJ; (b) 2065 kcal

71. 57.6 MJ

73. 350 kW

75. 45.1 kW

77. $\Delta E_{therm} = 0.602$ J; $v = 17.3$ m/s

79. (a) 1600 J; (b) 619 J; (c) 16 m/s

81. 18 kW

83. (a) $y = y_0 = 0$; (b) $F = mg - ky$; (c) $y = y_{max} = 2mg/k$; (d) $y_{eq} = mg/k$; (e) $W_f = \frac{1}{2}(m^2g^2/k)$

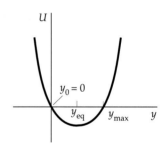

85. (a) 17.34 m; (b) 4905 N; (c) 4.905 m/s²; (d) 13.41 kN; (e) 5461 N; (f) 1440 N

87. (a) $F_{20} = 491$ N; $F_{30} = 981$ N; (b) $P_{20} = 9.82$ kW; $P_{30} = 29.4$ kW; (c) 8.85°; (d) 6.36 km/L

89. (a) 0.989 m; (b) 0.783 m; (c) 1.54 m

91. (a) 115.7 kJ; (b) 90 kJ; (c) 1.58

93. 10.96 m/s, 9.12 s. The pole vaulter uses additional metabolic energy to raise himself on the pole.

95. $\theta_2 = \cos^{-1}\left[1 - \dfrac{L}{L - x}(1 - \cos \theta_1)\right]$

97. (a) $F_{tan} = -mg \sin \theta$; therefore $a = dv/dt = -g \sin \theta$;
(b) For circular motion, $v = r\omega = L\, d\theta/dt$; $d\theta/dt = v/L$;
(c) $dv/dt = (dv/d\theta)(d\theta/dt) = (v/L)(dv/d\theta)$;
(d) $dv/d\theta = (L/v)(dv/dt) = -(L/v) g \sin \theta$; $v\, dv = -gL \sin \theta\, d\theta$;

(e) $\displaystyle\int_0^v v\, dv = \int_{\theta_0}^0 - gL \sin \theta\, d\theta$; $\frac{1}{2}v^2 = gL(1 - \cos \theta_0)$;

Note that $L(1 - \cos \theta_0) = h$; consequently, $v = \sqrt{2gh}$.

Chapter 8

1. hollow sphere

3. 15.6 m

5. 3.36 m

7. (2 m, 1.4 m)

9. (1.5 m, 1.36 m)

11. $(9/16)L$

13. $(0, 0, R/2)$

15. The external force is the force of the static friction between the tires and the road.

17. (b)

19. 4 m/s east

21. (a) Yes. Initially the scale reads $(M + m)g$. After m drops, the scale reads Mg. (b) $mg/(M + m)$ directed downward; (c) $F_{net} = (M + m)g - (M + m) a_{cm} = Mg$.

23. (a) $[(m_1 - m_2)^2 g]/[(m_1 + m_2)(m_1 + m_2 + m_c)]$; (b) $4gm_1m_2/(m_1 + m_2) + m_cg$; (c) Since $T = 2gm_1m_2/(m_1 + m_2)$, then $F = 2T + m_cg$

25. (a) True; (b) True; (c) True

27. If the man throws something forward, he will move backward.

29. Because of the conservation of momentum, the rocket can move without having something to push against. By expelling fuel, the rocket increases in velocity in the opposite direction.

31. 1.83 m/s to the left

33. (c)

35. 40 m

37. $\sqrt{gh/2}$

39. rolling ball

41. (a) 60 J; (b) 3.75 m/s to the right; (c) v of 3-kg block = 1.25 m/s to the right, v of 5-kg block = 0.75 m/s to the left; (d) 3.75 J; (e) 56.25 J

43. Assume that the ball travels 80 mi/h = 35 m/s and that the ball stops in a distance of 1 cm. The collision time is the distance for which the ball and bat are in contact divided by the average speed. Thus the collision time ≈ 0.02 m/18 m/s = 1 ms.

45. (a) 10.75 N·s; (b) 1344 N

47. $I = 1.81 \times 10^6$ MN·s; $F_{av} = 0.602$ MN

49. 1.15 kN

51. (a) If $d = 0.7$ m, then $F_{av} = 84$ N. (b) Yes, the weight of the ball is much less than the average force.

53. (a) 4.95×10^{-5} N; (b) The weight of the water droplet is about six times the average force due to 10 drops.

55. (a) False; (b) True; (c) True

57. (a) The energy losses are the same. (b) The percentage loss is greater for the two objects with oppositely directed velocities of $v/2$.

59. 0.56 m/s

61. 3.13 m/s

63. $3v$

65. (a) 1.5 m/s to the right; (b) v of 0.3-kg muffin = 2.5 m/s, v of 0.5-kg muffin = 4.5 m/s

67. v of 2-kg mass = 4.8 m/s, v of 3-kg mass = 0.8 m/s

69. (a) 5 m/s; (b) 25 cm; (c) $v_1 = 0$ m/s, $v_2 = 7$ m/s

71. (a) $0.2v_0$; (b) $0.4\,v_0$

73. $[2(m_1 + m_2)/m_1]\,\sqrt{gL}$

75. (a) 9 m/s $\hat{i}$ − 2 m/s $\hat{j}$; (b) 6 m/s $\hat{i}$

77. $v_p = 1.74 \times 10^7$ m/s, $v_\alpha = 4.34 \times 10^6$ m/s

79. (a) $v_x = 312$ m/s, $v_y = 66.6$ m/s; (b) 5610 m; (c) 35.8 kJ

81. 0.913

83. 0.894

85. (a) 1.7 m/s; (b) 0.83

87. (a) $\frac{1}{2}v_0\hat{i} + v_0\hat{j}$; (b) $mv_0^2/16$

89. (a) $v_2 = \sqrt{2}v$, $\theta_2 = 45°$; (b) $K_i = \frac{1}{2}m(3v_c)^2 = 4.5\,mv_0^2$, $K_f = \frac{1}{2}m(\sqrt{5}v_0)^2 + \frac{1}{2}(2m)(\sqrt{2}v_0)^2 = 4.5mv_0^2$

91. (a) Let m_1 and m_2 be the incoming and struck particles; assume $\vec{v}_0$ is in the x direction. From $\vec{p}_i = \vec{p}_f$ one obtains $m_1v_0 = m_1v\cos\phi + m_2v_2\cos\theta$ (1) and $m_1v\sin\phi = m_2v_2\sin\theta$ (2). Rearrange the first equation to $m_1(v_0 - v\cos\phi) = m_2v_2\cos\phi$ (1a). Divide (2) by (1a) to obtain $\tan\theta = (v\sin\phi)/(v_0 - v\cos\phi)$. (b) Did not use energy conservation; therefore, the result is valid for elastic and inelastic collisions.

93. $K_i = p_1^2/2m_1 + p_1^2/2m_2$; $K_f = p_1'^2/2m_1 + p_1'^2/2m_2$. In an elastic collision, $K_f = K_i$, thus $p_1'^2 = p_1^2$ and $p_1' = \pm p_1$. If $p_1' = +p_1$, the particles do not collide.

95. (a) 3.75 m/s; (b) $u_{3kg} = 1.25$ m/s, $u_{5kg} = -0.75$ m/s; (c) $u'_{3kg} = -1.25$ m/s, $u'_{5kg} = 0.75$ m/s; (d) $v'_{3kg} = 2.5$ m/s, $v'_{5kg} = 4.5$ m/s; (e) $K_i = K_f = 60$ J

97. 15 km/s

99. (a) 3.6×10^5 N; (b) 120 s; (c) 1.72 km/s

101. (e)

103. $v_f = 0.192$ m/s, $K_i = 31.25$ mJ, $K_f = 12.0$ mJ

105. 0.46 m/s

107. (a) -1.1×10^5 kg·km/h $\hat{i}$ + 1.05×10^5 kg·km/h $\hat{j}$; (b) $v_f = 43.4$ km/h, $\theta = 43°$ north of west

109. (a) 81 J; (b) 0 m/s; (c) $K_{cm} = 0$; (d) $K_{rel} = 81$ J

111. (a) 2.5 m from the pier; (b) $K_{total} = 330$ J, $K_{on\ land} = 270$ J; (c) 60 J derives from the chemical energy of the woman. (d) Shot will land in the water.

113. (a) Momentum of the system is not conserved because the rails will exert a vertical reaction force. (b) 4.33 m/s in direction opposite to shell; (c) 346 kJ

115. (a) 2.3 s; (b) The pumpers hit the ground at 24 km/h.

117. $0.75v\hat{i} - v\hat{j}$

119. (a) 29.6 km/s away from planet; (b) 8.1: This energy comes from the slowing of Saturn.

121. (a) -0.6 m/s; (b) 960 N

123. No

125. 8.85 kg

127. $r/14\hat{k}$

129. (a) From Problem 128, the fraction of energy retained after collision is $-\Delta K/K = 4(m/M)/(1 + m/M)^2 = 0.284$. The fraction of energy retained $= 1 - 0.284 = 0.716$. After N collisions, $K_f = K_i \times 0.716^N$. (b) 55

131. (a) $v^2 l^2/2L$; (b) v^2/L; (c) $Mv^3 t/L^2 + Mvtg/L$

133. (a) $(m_p + m_b)g$; (b) $F = g[m_p + m_b\sqrt{(2kh)/g(m_c + m_b)}]$

135. (a) 4670 km; (b) gravitational force of sun and other planets; (c) acceleration is toward the sun; (d) 9330 km

137. -1.5×10^{-22} kg·m/s $\hat{j}$

139. $1.2\sqrt{L}$

Chapter 9

1. The point on the rim moves the greater distance. Both turn through the same angle. The point on the rim has the greater speed. Both have the same angular velocity. Both have zero tangential acceleration. Both have zero angular acceleration. The point on the rim has the greater centripetal acceleration.

3. (c)

5. (a) 15.6 rad/s; (b) 46.8 rad; (c) 7.45 rev; (d) 4.68 m/s, 73 m/s^2

7. (a) 40 rad/s; (b) 0.96 m/s^2; 192 m/s^2

9. (a) 0.233 rad/s; (b) 2.8 m/s; 0.65 m/s^2

11. 7.27×10^{-5} rad/s

13. (a)

15. 1.04 rad/s, 9.93 rev/min

17. (d)

19. No, it may cause a rotating object to come to rest.

21. (b)

23. (a) 1.87 N·m; (b) 124 rad/s^2; (c) 620 rad/s

25. (a) $g \sin \theta$; (b) $mgL \sin \theta$; (c) $g \sin \theta$

27. (a) $2(M/R^2) \mu_k g r^2 \, dr$; (b) $(2/3) MR\mu_k g$; (c) $3Rw/4\mu_k g$

29. 4.66×10^{-5} kg·m^2

31. 28 kg·m^2

33. $(7/5)MR^2$

35. (a) $m_1 x^2 + m_2 (L - x)^2$; (b) $2 (m_1 x + m_2 x - m_2 L)$, $dI/dx = 0$ when $x = m_2 L/(m_1 + m_2)$

37. (a) 0.04 kg·m^2/0.04145 kg·m^2 = 0.965; (b) The moment of inertia would increase because I_{cm} of the hollow sphere $> I_{cm}$ of the solid sphere.

39. Let the element of mass be $dm = \rho \, dV = 2\pi \rho h r \, dr$, where h is the height of the cylinder. The mass m of the hollow cylinder is $m = \pi \rho h(R_2^2 - R_1^2)$, so $\rho = m/[\pi h(R_2^2 - R_1^2)]$. The element $dI = r^2 \, dm = 2\pi \rho h r^3 \, dr$. Integrate dI from R_1 to R_2 and obtain $I = \frac{1}{2}\pi \rho h(R_2^4 - R_1^4) = \frac{1}{2}\pi \rho h(R_2^2 + R_1^2)(R_2^2 - R_1^2) = \frac{1}{2}m(R_2^2 + R_1^2)$.

41. (a) $0.509 \, M/R^3$; (b) $0.329 \, MR^2$

43. $(\frac{1}{2})MR^2$

45. $(\frac{1}{2})MR^2$

47. (b)

49. (a) 52 kg·m^2; (b) 20.9 rev/min

51. 155 kW

53. $K_{tot} = 2.6 \times 10^{29}$ J, $K_{orb} = 2.7 \times 10^{33}$ J; $K_{orb} \simeq 10^4 \, K_{rot}$

55. (a) $\sqrt{(8mg/R)/2m + M}$; (b) $mg \, [1 + 8m/(2m + M)]$

57. 1.95 m

59. $\sqrt{(1 + M/2m)/(1 + M/3m)}$

61. 3.11 m/s^2; $T_1 = 12.4$ N, $T_2 = 13.4$ N

63. 1.56 m/s^2; $T_1 = 16.0$ N, $T_2 = 16.5$ N

65. 8.2 m/s

67. (a) $g/[1 + (2M/5m)]$; (b) $2mMg/(5m + 2M)$

69. (a) 72 kg; (b) 1.37 rad/s^2, $T_1 = 294$ N, $T_2 = 745$ N

71. (a) mg; (b) $2g/R$; (c) $2g$

73. (a) $(g \sin \theta)/(1 + m_1/2m_2)$; (b) $(\frac{1}{2}m_1 g \sin \theta)/(1 + m_1/2m_2)$; (c) $m_2 gh$; (d) $m_2 gh$; (e) $\sqrt{(2gh)/(1 + m_1/2m_2)}$; (f) For $\theta = 0$: $a = T = 0$; for $\theta = 90°$: $a = g/(1 + m_1/2m_2)$, $T = \frac{1}{2}m_1 a$, $v = \sqrt{(2gh)/(1 + m_1/2m_2)}$; for $m_1 = 0$: $a = g \sin \theta$, $T = 0$, $v = \sqrt{2gh}$

75. True

77. (b)

79. (c)

81. Assume the ball is rolling to the right. If f acts to the right along the direction of motion, the center of mass will then accelerate to the right and its linear speed will increase. But the torque produced by f about the center of mass will be counterclockwise tending to decrease the angular speed. But $v = R\omega$, so ω cannot decrease while v is increasing. If f acts to the left so that v decreases, it produces a clockwise torque that tends to increase ω. The only possibility consistent with $v = R\omega$ is $f = 0$.

83. 1125 J

85. 45.9 m

87. 3/2

89. 1.09L

91. 0.325°

93. 233 J

95. (a) From the figure it is evident that $x = r_0 \cos \theta$ and $y = r_0 \sin \theta$ relative to the center of the wheel. Therefore, if the coordinates of the center are X and R, those of point P are as stated.
(b) $v_{Px} = d(X + r_0 \cos \theta)/dt = dX/dt - r_0 \sin \theta \, d\theta/dt$. Note that $dX/dt = V$ and $d\theta/dt = -\omega = -V/R$; therefore, $v_{Px} = V + (r_0 V \sin \theta)/R$. $v_{Py} = d(R + r_0 \sin \theta)/dt = r_0 \cos \theta \, d\theta/dt$ ($dR/dt = 0$). Again, $d\theta/dt = -\omega$, so $v_{Py} = -(r_0 V \cos \theta)/R$.

(c) $\vec{v} \cdot \vec{r} = v_{Px}r_x + v_{Py}r_y = (V + r_0V \sin \theta/R)(r_0 \cos \theta) - (r_0V \cos \theta/R)(R + r_0 \sin \theta) = 0$

(d) $v^2 = v_x^2 + v_y^2 = V^2[1 + (2r_0/R) \sin \theta + r_0^2/R^2]; r^2 = r_x^2 + r_y^2 = R^2[1 + (2r_0/R) \sin \theta + r_0^2/R^2];$ so $v/r = V/R = \omega.$

97. $2F/R(M + 3m)$, counterclockwise; (b) $F/(M + 3m)$; (c) $-2F/(M + 3m)$.

99. $54°$

101. (a)

103. With $I = (2/5)mr^2$ one then obtains $\omega_0 = 5v_0(h - r)/2r^2.$ The translational impulse $P_t = F_0 \Delta t = mv_0$. The rotational impulse about the center of mass is $P_\tau = P_t(h - r) = I\omega_0.$

105. (a) 200 m/s; (b) 8000 rad/s; (c) 257 m/s; (d) 11.6 s

107. (a) $5v_0/3R$; (b) $(5/21)v_0$; (c) $1.056\ mv_0^2$; (d) $-1.016\ mv_0^2$

109. (a) $(2/3)\ v_0$; (b) $5v_0^2/18\mu_k g$; (c) $1/3$

111. 2.7×10^{-6} rad/s

113. (a) 0.0873 rad/s²; (b) 572 N·m; (c) 6550 kg·m²

115. (a) 7.36 m/s²; (b) 14.7 m/s²; (c) 2.43 m/s

117. $(6gL/7)^{1/2}$

119. (a) 780 kJ; (b) 211 N·m, 151 N; (c) 1375 rev

121. (a) 15 m; (b) 15.4 rad/s

123. (a), (b) $I_z = \int r^2\ dm = \int(x^2 + y^2)\ dm = \int x^2\ dm + \int y^2\ dm = I_y + I_x;$ (c) Let the z axis be the axis of rotation of the disk. By symmetry, $I_x = I_y$. So $I_x = \frac{1}{2}I_z = (1/4)MR^2.$ See Table 9-1.

125. (a) The spool will move down the plane at a constant acceleration, spinning in a counterclockwise direction as the string unwinds. $v = \sqrt{(2MgD \sin \theta)/(M + I/r^2)}$; (b) The direction of the friction force is up along the plane. $f_s = (Mg \sin\theta)/(1 + R/r)$

127. $0.75mg, 0.5mg, 0.25mg, 0, 0, 0$

129. (a) 230.4 N/m; (b) 122.7 J

131. (a) The only force is F; therefore, $a_{cm} = F/M.$ The torque about the center of mass is $\tau = FR$ and $I = MR^2/2$. Thus $\alpha = \tau/I = 2F/MR.$ If the cylinder rolls without slipping, $a_{cm} = \alpha R.$ Here, $\alpha = 2a_{cm}/R.$ (b) $f = F/3$, same direction as F; $a_{cm} = 4F/3M$

133. (a) $T(2r/R - 1)/3$; (b) $(2T/3m)(1 + r/R)$; (c) $r > R/2$ (d) Same direction as T.

Chapter 10

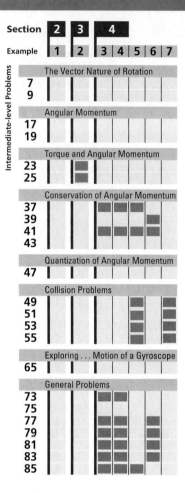

1. (a) True; (b) True; (c) True

3. $\vec{F} = -F\hat{i}, \vec{r} = R\hat{j}, \tau = +FR\hat{k}$

5. (a) $24\hat{k}$; (b) $-24\hat{j}$; (c) $13\hat{k}$

7. (a) Let $\vec{r}$ be in the x-y plane. If $\vec{\omega}$ points in the positive z direction, i.e., $\vec{\omega} = \omega\hat{k}$, the particle's velocity is in the $\hat{j}$ direction when $\vec{r} = r\hat{i}$ (see Figure) and has the magnitude $r\omega$. Thus, $\vec{v} = \vec{\omega} \times \vec{r} = r\omega\hat{j}$.

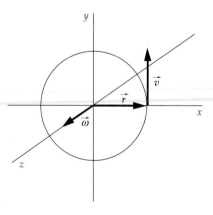

(b) $\vec{a} = d\vec{v}/t = (d\vec{\omega}/dt) \times \vec{r} + \vec{\omega} \times (d\vec{r}/dt) = (d\vec{\omega}/dt) \times \vec{r} + \vec{\omega} \times \vec{v} = \vec{a}_t + \vec{\omega} \times (\vec{\omega} \times \vec{r}) = \vec{a}_t + \vec{a}_c,$ where $\vec{a}_t$ and $\vec{a}_c$ are the tangential and centripetal accelerations, respectively.

9. $4\hat{j} + 3\hat{k}$

11. (b)

13. constant

15. (a) 28 kg·m²/s; (b) 32 kg·m²; (c) 0.875 rad/s²

17. The area at $t = t_1$ is $A_1 = \frac{1}{2}br_1\cos\theta_1 = \frac{1}{2}bx_1$, where θ_1 is the angle between $\vec{r}_1$ and $\vec{v}$ and x_1 is the component of $\vec{r}_1$ in the direction of $\vec{v}$. At $t = t_1 + dt$, $A = A_1 + dA = \frac{1}{2}b(x + dx) = \frac{1}{2}b(x + v\,dt)$. Thus, $dA/dt = \frac{1}{2}bv = $ constant. Note that $r\sin\theta = b$; consequently, $\frac{1}{2}bv = \frac{1}{2}L/m$.

19. $\vec{\tau} = \vec{r}_1 \times \vec{F}_1 + \vec{r}_2 \times \vec{F}_2 = (\vec{r}_1 - \vec{r}_2) \times \vec{F}_1$ since $\vec{F}_2 = -\vec{F}_1$. But $\vec{r}_1 - \vec{r}_2$ points along $-\vec{F}_1$ so $(\vec{r}_1 - \vec{r}_2) \times \vec{F}_1 = 0$.

21. (a) 4 N·m; (b) 0.192t rad/s

23. (a) $Rg(m_2\sin\theta - m_1)$ into the page; (b) $vR(I/R^2 + m_1 + m_2)$; (c) $(m_2\sin\theta - m_1)g/(I^2/R + m_1 + m_2)$

25. (a) 0.785 N·m; (b) 2.75 kg·m²/s; (c) 0.131 kg·m²; (d) 0.317, 0.634, 0.048

27. False

29. (e)

31. No

33. (b)

35. (c)

37. (a) $\omega_i/(1 + mR^2/I_0)$; (b) ω_f

39. (a) r_0mv_0; (b) $\frac{1}{2}mv_0^2$; (c) mv_0^2/r_0, $(3/2)\,mv_0^2$

41. 0.11 ms or 1.31×10^{-9} days

43. (a) 4 m/s; (b) 3.2 N/m

45. 54.7°

47. (a) 3.46×10^{-47} kg·m²; (b) 2.0 meV, 6.0 meV, 12 meV

49. 14 J·s

51. $L[(M - m)/12m]^{1/2}$

53. 7.75 m/s

55. 0.88

57. 7.36 rad/s; 11.1 J

59. (a) False; (b) True; (c) False

61. (d)

63. First, imagine that $\vec{L}$ points vertically upward and the car is moving directly away from you, rounding the top of a hill. The original $\vec{L}$ is now altered by the addition of a ΔL pointing to the left, hence $\vec{L}$ is rotated counterclockwise and the car rolls to its left. If the original $\vec{L}$ had pointed downward, the same ΔL would have been added, but now it causes a clockwise rotation of $\vec{L}$, and hence the car rolls to the right. Similarly, imagine $\vec{L}$ points forward, the car is moving away from you, and is turning to the left. The torque exerted by the road on the car in this case points upward. This means an upward component of angular momentum is added to $\vec{L}$, thus tending to lift the front of the car. If $\vec{L}$ had pointed backward, the same left turn would add the same angular momentum increment, this time raising the rear of the car.

65. (a) 3.27 rad/s; (b) 0.163 m/s; (c) 0.535 m/s²; (d) 24.5 N, 1.34 N

67. To prevent body of helicopter from rotating. If rear rotor fails, body of helicopter will tend to rotate on its main axis.

69. (e) The ball rotates counterclockwise. The torque about the center of the pole is clockwise and of magnitude RT, where R is the pole's radius and T is the tension. So L must decrease.

71. (a) $-47.7\hat{k}$; (b) $15.9\hat{k}$ N·m

73. 4.2 rev/s with $m_{arm} = 4$ kg

75. (a) 1. Use Newton's laws to determine v; $T\cos\theta = mg$; $T\sin\theta = mv^2/(r\sin\theta)$; $v = (rg\sin\theta\tan\theta)^{1/2} = 2.06$ m/s;

$\vec{v} = d\vec{r}/dt = -2.06\sin\omega t\,\hat{i} + 2.06\cos\omega t\,\hat{j}$

2. Find $\vec{L} = m\vec{r} \times \vec{v} = 6.18[\sin 30°(\cos\omega t\,\hat{i} + \sin\omega t\,\hat{j}) - \cos 30°\,\hat{k}] \times (-\sin\omega t\,\hat{i} + \cos\omega t\,\hat{j}) = [(3.09\hat{k} + 5.35(\sin\omega t\,\hat{j} + \cos\omega t\,\hat{i})]$ J·s

(b) $dL/dt = 14.7$ N·m, $\tau = mgr\sin 30° = 14.7$ N·m

77. $\omega_f = [(M + 5\,m\ell^2/L^2)/(M + 5m)]\omega$; $K_i = (ML^2 + 5m\ell^2)\omega^2/20$; $K_f = [(ML^2 + 5m\ell^2)^2/(ML^2 + 5mL^2)]\omega^2/20$

79. 30 rad/s; 10.5 rad/s; 176 J, 61.7 J

81. $\omega_i = 30$ rad/s, $\omega_f = 14.13$ rad/s; 93.3 J

83. 6.32 rad/s; 1.54 J

85. 0.55 s

87. $\omega = 12.5$ rad/s in both instances

89. (a) 21.4 rad/s; (b) $0.378\,e^{1.14t}$ J·s

Chapter 11

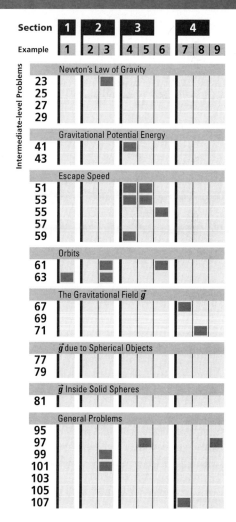

1. (a) False; (b) True

3. 4.39×10^{11} m

5. 3.91×10^{13} m

7. 11.7 y

9. The mass of the building is negligible compared to the mass of the earth.

11. (d)

13. (a) 1.88×10^9 m; (b) 1.9×10^{27} kg

15. 6.02×10^{24} kg

17. 2.45 m/s^2

19. 39.2 m/s^2

21. 2.63×10^6 m/s

23. (a) 37.6 N; (b) 2.66 km/s; (c) 1.33×10^5 s

25. $F \propto 1/R^3$

27. (a) 0.0027 N; (b) 0.48 N; (c) -0.061%

29. 0.605

31. Because gravity is weak compared to other forces of nature, either an extremely massive object or an extremely accurate instrument is needed to see its effects.

33. (a) 2.45×10^{-9} N; (b) $\tau = 4.41 \times 10^{-10}$ N·m

35. (a) His effectiveness would depend on his mass rather than his weight. (b) The power requirement would not be determined by the car's weight, but by its mass. (c) No significant effect.

37. (a) 5.77 kg; (b) gravitational mass

39. GMm_0/R

41. 6.95 km/s

43. (a) Outside: $\vec{F} = -(GMm_0/r^2)\hat{r}$. Inside: $\vec{F} = 0$. (b) $U(r) = -GMm_0/r$; $U(R) = -GMm_0/R$. (c) Since $F = 0$ for $r < R$, $dU/dr = 0$ and $U = $ constant. (d) Since U is continuous, then for $r < R$, $U(r) = U(R) = -GMm_0/R$.

(e)

45. (a) $M/2\pi R$; (b) $-\dfrac{GM}{R} \ln\left(\dfrac{R + \sqrt{x^2 + R^2}}{x}\right)$

(c) $GM/(x\sqrt{x^2 + R^2})$

47. Yes, if a large enough amount of momentum was imparted to the earth, say through a collision with a huge comet.

49. 35.5 km/s

51. 19.4 km/s

53. 61.0 km/s

55. From Example 11-6, the kinetic energy of a mass m in a circular orbit is $K = \frac{1}{2}|U|$. Note that this result is true for any circular orbit of a mass m about a massive center. But $|U|$ is the escape energy of $\frac{1}{2}mv_e^2$. Consequently, $K = \frac{1}{2}mv_c^2 = \frac{1}{2}(\frac{1}{2}mv_e^2)$ and $v_c = v_e/\sqrt{2}$.

57. $v_{eS} = 42.2$ km/s, $v_{e,\,solar} = 43.7$ km/s

59. To determine H use energy conservation: $\frac{1}{2}mv^2 = -\Delta U = GMm[1/R_E - 1/(R_E + H)]$ or $v^2 = 2gR_E^2[1/R_E - 1/(R_E + H)]$. So $H' = R_E H/(R_E + H)$ and, solving for H, $H = R_E H'/(R_E - H')$.

61. (a) 7.3 h; (b) 1.04×10^9 J; (c) 8.73×10^{10} J·s

63. $v = \sqrt{GM_S/r - GM_E r/(D-r)^2}$

65. 1×10^{-8} N $\hat{j}$

67. (a) 9.66×10^{-8} N $\hat{j}$; (b) 4.83×10^{-8} N/kg $\hat{j}$

69. (a) g of opposite elements of mass $R\lambda\, d\theta$ cancel. By symmetry, $g = 0$ at center. (b) 1. $m_1/m_2 = r_1/r_2$; 2. $g_1 > g_2$; 3. toward m_1; (c) toward m_1; (d) $g = 0$; (e) 1. $m_1/m_2 = r_1^2/r_2^2$; 2. $g_1 = g_2$; 3. $g = 0$; $g = 0$

71. (a) $CL^2/2$; (b) $-GC\displaystyle\int_0^L \dfrac{x\,dx}{(x_0 - x)^2} = \dfrac{2GM}{L^2}\left[\ln\left(\dfrac{x_0}{x_0 - L}\right) - \left(\dfrac{L}{x_0 - L}\right)\right]\hat{i}$

73. g is proportional to the mass within the sphere and inversely proportional to the radius, i.e., proportional to $r^3/r^2 = r$.

75. Zero. The gravitational field inside the 2-m shell is zero; therefore, it exerts no force on the 1-m shell, and, by Newton's third law, that shell exerts no force on the larger shell.

77. $g_1 (R_1^2/R_2^2)$

79. (a) $(Gm/a^2)(M_1/4.84 + M_2/9)$; (b) $GmM_1/1.21\, a^2$; (c) 0

81. $G\left(\dfrac{4\pi\rho_0 R_3}{3}\right)\left[\dfrac{1}{x^2} - \dfrac{1}{8(x - \frac{1}{2}R)^2}\right]$

83. $\sqrt{4\pi\rho_0 G/3}$

85. 1.04×10^{-5} m/s

87. (a) $-(GMm/d^2)[1 - (d^3/4)/(d^2 + R^2/4)^{3/2}]\hat{i}$; (b) $-0.821(GMm/R^2)\hat{i}$

89. (d)

91. 1.9×10^{27} kg

93. (a) 1.16×10^6 s; (b) 8.79×10^{25} kg

95. (a) $GM_E m\left(\dfrac{1}{r_1} - \dfrac{1}{r_2}\right)$; (b) In the above expression, replace $GM_E m$ by mgR_E^2, r_1 by R_E, and r_2 by $R_E + h$ to obtain the result given. (c) $[(1/R_E) - 1/(R_E + h)] = h/[R_E(R_E + h)]$; if $h \ll R_E$, the denominator $\approx R_E^2$ and $W = mgh$.

97. (a) $-0.56/r^2$; (b) $-(5.6 \times 10^{-7})r$

99. 8.94×10^7 m

101. 1700 m

103. Take the coordinate origin at the center of mass. Then $r_1 m_1 = r_2 m_2$ and $r = r_1 + r_2$. The force holding m_2 in orbit is $Gm_1 m_2/(r_1 + r_2)^2 = m_2 r_2 \omega^2$. $\omega^2 = Gm_1/r_2(r_1 + r_2)^2$. Now $r_2 = rm_1/(m_1 + m_2)$, so $\omega^2 = 4\pi^2/T^2 = G(m_1 + m_2)/r^3$ and $T^2 = 4\pi^2 r^3/G(m_1 + m_2)$.

105. (a) $gmR_E/2$; (b) $\sqrt{gR_E}$; (c) $\sqrt{3gR_E}$

107. (a)

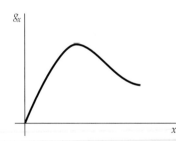

(b) $x = R/\sqrt{2}$

109. $Gm^2/[a(a + L)]$

111. (a) Since force on a mass m is $F = GMm/r^2$, then $F_s/F_m = M_s r_m^2/M_m r_s^2 = 179$. (b) $dF/dr = -2Gm_1 m_2/r^3 = -2F/r$; $dF/F = -2dr/r$. (c) Since $\Delta F = -2(F/r)\,\Delta r$, then $\Delta F_s/\Delta F_m = (F_s/F_m)(r_m/r_s) = (M_s r_m^3)/(M_m r_s^3) = 0.46$.

Chapter 12

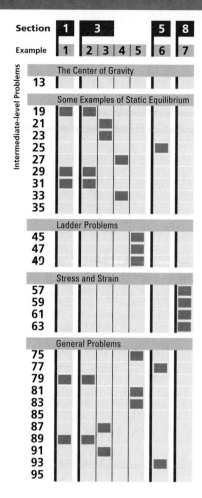

1. (a) False; (b) True; (c) True; (d) False

3. 318 N

5. 101 N

7. False. Location depends on mass distribution.

9. center of gravity

11. 3.4 m

13. $(0.94a, a)$

15. Left support, $F = 245$ N; right support, $F = 736$ N

17. $T_B = 692$ N, $F_{horizontal} = 0$, $F_{vertical} = 2540$ N, No, so no block is needed

19. 4.17 m

21. (a) 182 N; (b) 456 N; (c) $\vec{F} = 157$ N, $\vec{F}_{hinge} = 508$ N

23. (a) $\vec{T}_1, \vec{T}_2, \vec{F}_H$ (the force exerted on the strut by the hinge); (b) $\Sigma\tau$ about hinge = 0, so $T_{2y} = T_1 = 80$ N; (c) 139 N

25. 27°

27. $\dfrac{Mg\sqrt{2Rh - h^2}}{h - R}\,\hat{i} + Mg\hat{j}$

29. Force on middle support = 2920 N, compression. Force on end support = 1940 N, tension.

31. If her boss is 1 m from the left end, Julie must stand 2.33 m or less from the right end.

33. (a) $Mg - F\sqrt{(2R - h)/h}$; (b) $-F$; (c) $F\sqrt{(2R - h)/h}$

35. (a) 49 N; (b) 73.6 N·m; (c) 736 N, acting upward; (d) 687 N, acting downward

37. 636 N, 21.5°

39. $F_{2m} = 49.1$ N, $F_{6m} = 147$ N; both forces act in a direction 60° above the x axis.

41. (a) Cube is stationary, thus $f_s = -F$. $\tau = Fa$. (b) $x = a/3$ from center of cube. (c) $Mg/2$

43. No. The wall exerts a horizontal force on the ladder, so there must be friction between the floor and the ladder to balance that horizontal force on the ladder.

45. $\mu_s L \sin\theta \tan\theta$

47. $2h/L \sin\theta \tan\theta$

49. 59°

51. (a) $0.361mg$; (b) $0.313mg$; (c) $0.820mg$

53. 0.98 mm

55. 0.83 mm

57. 3.00181 m

59. (a) 34.7 cm; (b) 0.0776 J

61. 0.515 mm

63. 0.686

65. $A = A_0 - T/Y$

67. (c)

69. The body's center of gravity must be above the feet.

71. 99 cm

73. (a) 392 N; (b) 3

75. 0.577

77. 0.5

79. 304 kg

81. $(\cot\theta - 1)/2$

83. (a) 147 N; (b) 72.4% of total length

85. 0.207

87. (a) $T = 10,260$ N, $F_x = 5130$ N, $F_y = -4520$ N; (b) $T = 5924$ N, $F_x = 5130$ N, $F_y = 1403$ N

89. $2g$

91. (a) Since the center of gravity of the picture is in front of the wall, the torque due to mg about the nail must be balanced by an opposing torque due to the force of the wall on the picture, acting horizontally. So that $\Sigma F_x = 0$, the tension in the wire must have a horizontal component, and the picture must therefore tilt forward. (b) 3.43 N

93. (a) 83 km/h; (b) 105 km/h

95. 1.5 m

97. (a) 7.9 N; (b) 29.4 N; (c) 7.9 N

99. (a) Forces that act on the beam: weight = 49.1 N; force of the cylinder on the beam, $F_c = 28.3$ N; normal force of the ground, $F_{nb} = 24.5$ N; and friction force, $f_{sb} = 14.2$ N. Forces that act on the cylinder: weight = 78.5 N; force of the beam on the cylinder, $F_b = 28.3$ N; normal force of the ground, $F_{nc} = 103$ N; and friction force, $f_{sc} = 14.2$ N. (b) μ_s(beam–floor) = 0.58; μ_s(cylinder–floor) = 0.14.

101. $d/a = 1$

Chapter 13

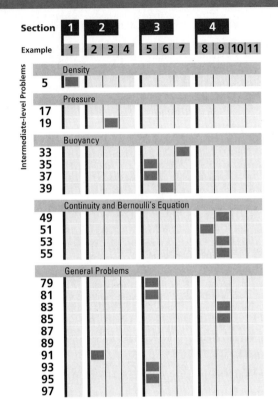

1. 0.673 kg

3. 103 kg

5. 13,621 kg/m^3

7. 29.8 inHg

9. (a) 1.5 atm; (b) 0.5 atm

11. 230 N

13. 200 atm

15. (a) 14,800 N; (b) 340 g

17. 45 cm

19. $W = Fh$; $F_1 = F_2 (A_1/A_2)$; $h_1A_1 = h_2A_2$; $h_1 = h_2 (A_2/A_1)$; $W_1 = F_1h_1 = F_2 (A_1/A_2)h_2 (A_2/A_1) = F_2h_2 = W_2$

21. (a) $V = 5.89 \times 10^{-3}$ m^3; $w = 57.8$ N; (b) $F = 173$ N; the water exerts a force that has an upward component on the slanting walls of the cone, so the walls exert a downward force on the water. This downward force plus the weight of the water must be balanced by the upward force exerted by the base on the water, which equals the downward force of the water on the base.

23. (c)

25. Nothing. The fish is in neutral buoyancy, so the upward acceleration of the fish is balanced by the downward acceleration of the displaced water.

27. (b) Volume of copper > volume of lead.

29. 4.36 N

31. (a) 11.1×10^3 kg/m^3; (b) lead

33. $\rho = 800$ kg/m^3; sp. gr. = 1.11

35. 250 kg/m^3

37. 183 m^3

39. 3.89 kg in freshwater

41. 2.06×10^7 kg

43. It blows over the ball, reducing the pressure above the ball below atmospheric pressure.

45. As the water falls, its velocity increases, causing the internal pressure to decrease; the pressure of air pushes it into a smaller stream.

47. (a) 12 m/s; (b) 132.5 kPa; (c) The volume flows are equal.

49. (a) 4.58 L/min; (b) 763 cm^2

51. $2\sqrt{h(H - h)}$

53. 1.85 m/s

55. 241 kPa

57. 1.47 kPa

59. 3.98 mPa·s

61. The water level remains constant.

63. The density of humid air is less than that of dry air.

65. The force acting is the difference in pressure between the wide and narrow parts times the area of the narrow part.

67. (a) Water spills over because the amount displaced is now greater than the volume of the lead block.

69. $F = 6.48 \times 10^4$ N. The table doesn't collapse because the atmosphere also exerts an upward force on the bottom surface of the table.

71. 1061 kg/m^3

73. 5000 kg/m^3

75. 72% of the block will be submerged.

77. 0.06 m^3 if mass = 60 kg

79. 40.2 g

81. The additional weight on the beaker side equals the weight of the displaced water, i.e., 64 g. That is the mass that must be placed on the other cup to maintain balance.

83. $h_A = 12.6$ m; $h_B = 5.3$ m

85. 6.5 mm

87. Since the object floats, the volume of displaced liquid is $m/\rho_0 = 4A \, \Delta h$; $\Delta h = m/4\rho_0 A$

89. (a) $dF = \rho gyL \, dy$; (b) 9.20×10^7 N; (c) Atmospheric pressure is exerted on each side of the dam and can therefore be neglected.

91. 1.37

93. (a) 70 m^3; (b) 6.61 m/s^2

95. 150 N (mass ≈ 15 kg)

97. (a) 2.4%; (b) 59 m^3

99. (a) 5.3 g; (b) 8 cm; (c) 1.17

Chapter 14

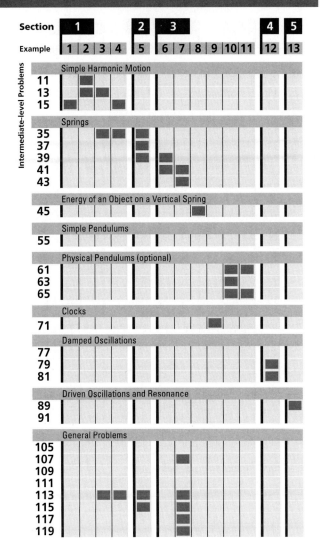

1. $4A, 0$

3. $0, A(2\pi f)^2$

5. (a) False; (b) True; (c) True

7. (a) 1.3 m/s; (b) 25 m/s

9. (a) $x(t) = (0.25 \text{ m}) \cos(4\pi/3)t$;
(b) $v(t) = dx/dt = -(\pi/3 \text{ m/s}) \sin(4\pi/3)t$;
(c) $a(t) = dv/dt = -(4\pi^2/9 \text{ m/s}^2) \cos(4\pi/3)t$

11. (a) $x(t) = (0.277 \text{ m}) \cos(4\pi t/3 - 0.445)$; (b) $v(t) = dx/dt = -(1.16 \text{ m/s}) \sin(4\pi t/3 - 0.445)$; (c) $a(t) = dv/dt = -(4.86 \text{ m/s}^2) \cos(4\pi t/3 - 0.445)$

13. (a) $x(t) = 10 \cos(\pi t/4)$

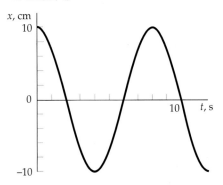

(b) 2.9 cm, 7.1 cm, 7.1 cm, 2.9 cm

15. (a) $v_{max} = 7.85$ m/s, $a_{max} = 24.7$ m/s^2; (b) $|v| = 6.28$ m/s, $a = -14.8$ m/s^2

17. (a) $f = 0.32$ Hz, $\omega = 2$ rad/s; (b) 3.1 s; (c) $x(t) = (40 \text{ cm}) \cos(2t)$

19. 9

21. 23 J

23. (a) 0.37 J; (b) 3.8 cm

25. 1.4×10^3 N/m

27. (a) True; (b) True

29. (a) 6.89 Hz; (b) 0.145 s; (c) 0.1 m; (d) 4.33 m/s; (e) 187 m/s^2; (f) $t = T/4 = 36.3$ ms; $a = 0$

31. (a) 680 N/m; (b) 0.42 s; (c) 1.5 m/s; (d) 23 m/s^2

33. (a) 3.1 kN/m; (b) 4.2 Hz; (c) 0.24 s

35. (a) 0.44 m/s; (b) 0.38 m/s, 1.2 m/s^2; (c) 0.095 s

37. 0.26 s

39. 10 kJ

41. 25 cm

43. (a) yes; (b) $A_{max} = 0.25$ m

45. (a) 0.13 J; (b) -0.32 J; (c) 0.45 J; (d) 0.13 J

47. False, the amplitude must be small.

49. The clock would run too slowly.

51. 12 s

53. 11.7 s

55. $T = 2\pi\sqrt{L/g}(1 - \sin\theta)$

57. 1.1 s

59. 0.5 kg·m^2

61. $0.0918L$

63. 2.4 s

65. (a) 0.25 m; (b) 0.57 m, 2.1 s

67. (a) $T = 2\pi\sqrt{I/mgL}$. Since $I = \frac{2}{5}mr^2 + mL^2$,
$T = 2\pi\sqrt{L/g + 2r^2/5gL} = 2\pi\sqrt{L/g}(\sqrt{1 + 2r^2/5L^2}) = T_0\sqrt{1 + 2r^2/5L^2}$; (b) $\sqrt{1 + x} \approx 1 + x/2$ for small x. When $r \ll L$, $T = T_0\sqrt{1 + 2r^25L^2} \approx T_0(1 + r^2/5L^2)$; (c) 0.008%, 22 cm

69. (a)

71. 6.43°

73. True

75. 3.1%

77. $A(t + T)/A(t) = e^{-T/2\tau}$

79. (a) 31%; (b) 0.031%

81. (a) 3.6 cm, 2.2 cm; (b) 38 J, 14 J

83. (a) 2.6 s; (b) 3.6 s; (c) 6.0 J

85. Pendulum of a clock, violin string when bowed

87. (a) $f_0 = 1.01$ Hz; (b) $f_0 = 2.01$ Hz; (c) $f_0 = 0.352$ Hz

89. (a) 0.498 m; (b) 14.1 rad/s; (c) 0.354 m; (d) 1 rad/s

91. 180 J; (b) 57 J; (c) 19 W

93. (a) 0; (b) 4 m/s

95. (a) 0.14 m, 0.44 s; (b) 0.23 m, 0.36 s; (c) For inelastic collisions, $x(t) = (0.14 \text{ m}) \sin[(14 \text{ rad/s})t]$; for elastic collisions, $x(t) = (0.231 \text{ m}) \sin[(17 \text{ rad/s})t]$

97. 1. B; 2. D; 3. A, C

99. (d)

101. (c)

103. (a) $v(t) = -(1.2 \text{ m/s}) \sin(3t + \pi/4)$; (b) -0.85 m/s; (c) 1.2 m/s; (d) 0.26 s or 1.3 s

105. (*a*) Since there is no friction, the only forces acting on the particle are mg and the normal force acting radially inward; the normal force is identical to the tension in the string that keeps the particle moving in a circular path if attached to a string of length r. (*b*) The particles meet at the bottom of the bowl because in simple harmonic motion, the period is independent of amplitude.

107. (*a*) 2.3 kg; (*b*) 0.65

109. $T = (2\pi/a)\sqrt{m/\rho g}$

111. The error is greater when the clock is elevated.

113. (*a*) $\mu_s = kA/(m_1 + m_2)g$; (*b*) A and E are unchanged, $\omega_f = \sqrt{m_1/(m_1 + m_2)}\,\omega_i$, $T_f = \sqrt{(m_1 + m_2)m_1}\,T_i$

115. (*a*) 2.3 Hz, 43 J; (*b*) maximum compression: 3.2 Hz, 0.60 m, 22 J; maximum extension: 3.2 Hz, 0.60 m, 43 J.

117. (*a*) If $\omega^2 A > g$, then the piston's acceleration is greater than the maximum acceleration of the block. (*b*) 2.4×10^{-2} s

119. (*a*) 2.5; (*b*) 6.4 cm

121. (*a*)

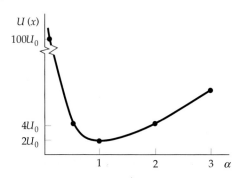

(*b*) $x_0 = 1$; (*c*) $U(x) = (1 - \epsilon)^2 + \dfrac{1}{(1 - \epsilon)^2}$; (*d*) $U(x) = $ constant $+ 4\epsilon^2$;

(*e*) $f = (1/\pi)\sqrt{2/m}$

123. $T = 8.59\sqrt{R/g}$

125. (*a*) $F = -(Gm\,M_E/R_E^3)r$; $F_x = (\sin\theta)F = (x/r)F = -(Gm\,M_E/R_E^3)x$; (*b*) $T = 2\pi\sqrt{m/k}$; $k = GmM_E/R_E^3 = gm/R_E$. Substituting k, $T = 2\pi\sqrt{R_E/g}$; $T = 84.4$ min.

127. Answer given in the problem.

129. Answer given in the problem.

Chapter 15

1. They move faster as they move up because the tension increases due to the weight of the rope below.

3. 1.32 km/s

5. 19.6 g

7. (*a*) 265 m/s; (*b*) 15 g

9. (*a*) 0.340 km/s; (*b*) 98% accurate; (*c*) No, because the speed of light is much greater than the speed of sound.

11. (*a*) 78 m; (*b*) 0.23 s, 70 m; (*c*) 70 m

13. (*a*) $v = \sqrt{\gamma RT/M}$; $dv/dt = \frac{1}{2}\sqrt{\gamma R/MT} = \sqrt{\gamma RT/M/2T} = v/2T$. Thus $dv/v = dT/2T$; (*b*) 4.95%; (*c*) $v_{\text{approximate}} = 347.4$ m/s, $v_{\text{exact}} = 347$ m/s

15. The lightning struck 680 m from the ballpark, 58.4° W or E of North.

17. (*a*) $d^2y/dx^2 = 6k(x + vt)$, $d^2y/dt^2 = 6kv^2(x + vt)$; thus $d^2y/dx^2 = (1/v^2)(d^2y/dt^2)$; (*b*) $d^2y/dx^2 = A(ik)^2 e^{ik(x-vt)} = -Ak^2 e^{ik(x-vt)}$, $d^2y/dt^2 = A(ikv)^2 e^{ik(x-vt)} = -Ak^2v^2 e^{ik(x-vt)}$; thus $d^2y/dx^2 = (1/v^2)(d^2y/dt^2)$; (*c*) $d^2y/dx^2 = -k^2/[k(x - vt)]^2 = -1/(x - vt)^2$, $d^2y/dt^2 = -(-kv)^2/[k(x - vt)]^2 = -v^2/(x - vt)^2$; thus $d^2y/dx^2 = (1/v^2)(d^2y/dt^2)$

19. For $y(x,t) = A\sin(kx - \omega t)$: $d^2y/dx^2 + i\,dy/dt = -Ak^2\sin(kx - \omega t) - Ai\omega\cos(kx - \omega t) \neq 0$. For $y(x,t) = Ae^{i(kx - \omega t)}$: $d^2y/dx^2 + i\,dy/dt = -k^2y + \omega y = 0$ if $k^2 = \alpha\omega$.

21. True

23. 20 cm

25. (a) 7.5×10^{14} to 4.3×10^{14} Hz; (b) 10 GHz

27. 171 Hz

29. (a) $y(x,t) = (0.025 \text{ m}) \sin(42x - 500t)$; (b) 13 m/s; (c) 6.3 km/s

31. (a) $P_0 = \frac{1}{2}\mu\omega^2 A_0^2 v$; (b) $P(x) = \frac{1}{2}\mu\omega^2 A_0^2 v e^{-2bx}$

33. (a) 0.75 Pa; (b) 4 m; (c) 85 Hz; (d) 340 m/s

35. (a) 36.7×10^{-5} m; (b) 8.27×10^{-2} Pa

37. (a) 0; (b) 3.67×10^{-7} m

39. (a) 138 Pa; (b) 21.7 W/m²; (c) 0.217 W

41. (a) 50 W; (b) 2 m; (c) 4.4×10^{-3} W/m²

43. False

45. (a) 10^{-11} W/m²; (b) 2×10^{-12} W/m²; (c) for (a) 9.4×10^{-5} Pa, for (b) 4.2×10^{-5} Pa

47. (a)

49. 99%

51. (a) 100 m; (b) 0.13 W

53. (a) 100 dB; (b) 50 W; (c) 20 m; (d) 96 dB

55. (a) 81 dB; (b) Eliminating the two least intense sources will not help much in reducing the intensity level of the noise. Most of the intensity comes from the 80-dB source.

57. 88 dB

59. 57 dB

61. (a)

63. (a) 15 m, 20 pies/min; (b) 13.5 m, 22.2 pies/min; (c) 15 m, 22 pies/min

65. (a) 1.3 m; (b) 262 Hz

67. (a) 2.1 m; (b) 162 Hz

69. (a) 80 m/s toward listener; (b) 420 m/s; (c) 1.7 m; (d) 247 Hz

71. (a) 24°; (b) 50 km high and 11.5 km over

73. 22 m/s = 79.2 km/h

75. $\Delta f = 9.2 \times 10^4$ Hz, $f = 30.00092$ GHz

77. 4.45 kHz

79. (a) 8.1×10^{-2} J; (b) 29 cm, 0.14 s

81. Both students must walk 0.75 m/s away from each other.

83. $f' = 1000 + 9.4 \sin 4t$ Hz

85. (a) 823.5 Hz; (b) 848.5 Hz

87. 183 m, 713 Hz.

89. 6.73×10^{10} m, 4.3×10^{34} kg

91. No; the frequencies are the same, but since the propagation speeds differ, so do the wavelengths.

93. (a) True; (b) False; (c) False

95. Segments 2 cm $< x \le 3$ cm are moving up. Segments 1 cm $\le x <$ 2 cm are moving down. $x = 2$ cm is instantaneously at rest.

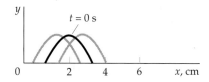

97. Cars behind slow down and then speed up in turn, as each reacts to the reduced distance between them and the car in front of them. This gives rise to a longitudinal wave pulse propagating backwards along the line of cars. No energy is transported. The speed of propagation is proportional to the length of a car and inversely proportional to the average driver's reaction time.

99. 21 cm

101. (a) 34 m/s to the left; (b) 20 m/s to the right; (c) 10 m/s to the right

103. (a) 110 Hz; (b) 1.1×10^4 Hz; (c) 570 Hz, 5.7×10^4 Hz

105. (a) 0.59 Hz; (b) 1.59 Hz

107. 8.0 m from the left end

109. 65 km/h

111. 1.07 kHz

113. (a) $A_r = A/2$, $A_t = 3A/2$; (b) $P_r = P_{in}/4$, $P_t = 3P_{in}/4$; (c) $A_1 = A + A_r = A_t$ so the amplitudes of displacement are the same.

115. (a) 4.5 m/s; (b) 887 Hz; (c) 842 Hz

117. (a) $T = 2.5 \times 10^{-3}$ s, $f = 400$ Hz; (b) 316 m/s; (c) $\lambda = 79$ cm, $k = 7.9$ m^{-1} (d) $y(x,t) = [5 \times 10^{-4} \sin(7.9x - 2.5 \times 10^3 t)]$ m; (e) $v_{max} = 1.26$ m/s, $a_{max} = 3.16$ km/s²; (f) 2.5 W

119. (a) $F = \mu v_0^2$; (b) $v_0 = \sqrt{F/\mu}$; (c) With respect to a fixed point on the chain, the pulse travels through 360°.

121. (a) The speed is given by $v = \sqrt{F/\mu}$. At a distance y from the bottom, $F = \mu gy$. Thus, $v = \sqrt{gy}$. (b) 2.2 s

123. (a) For $\Delta y/\Delta x \ll 1$, $\Delta \ell = \Delta x[1 + \frac{1}{2}(\Delta y/\Delta x)^2]$; so, $\Delta \ell - \Delta x = \frac{1}{2}(\Delta y/\Delta x)^2 \Delta x$ and $\Delta U = \frac{1}{2}F(\Delta y/\Delta x)^2 \Delta x$. (b) $(dy/dx)^2 = A^2 k^2 \cos^2(kx - \omega t)$. So $\Delta U = \frac{1}{2}FA^2 k^2 \Delta x \cos^2(kx - \omega t)$. (c) Replace F by $\mu v^2 = \mu \omega^2/k^2$. This gives Eq. 15-16b.

Chapter 16

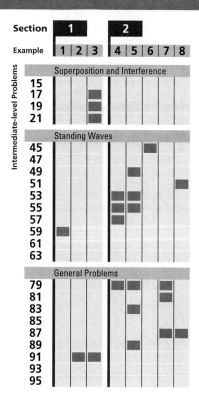

1. (*a*) False; (*b*) False; (*c*) True

3.

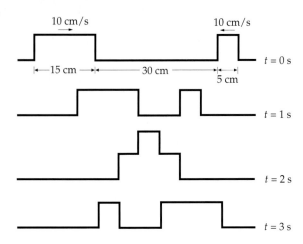

5. (*a*) 3.86 cm; (*b*) 3.46 cm

7. 0.071 m

9. (*a*) $\pi/2$ rad; (*b*) $\sqrt{2}A$

11. (*a*) 85 Hz, 255 Hz; (*b*) Some sound will reflect off walls, thus giving a variety of path differences.

13. (*a*) $4I_0$; (*b*) $2I_0$; (*c*) 0

15. For destructive interference, $\delta = \pi = 2\pi\Delta x/\lambda$. $\Delta x = d\sin\theta \le d$, where d is the source separation. So if $\Delta x < \lambda/2$, $\delta < \pi$ and there is no complete destructive interference in any direction.

17. 0.8π rad

19. 2361 Hz, 7083 Hz

21. 1.81 m; $\theta = 51°$

23. (*a*) 0.279 m; (*b*) 1220 Hz; (*c*) $\theta_3 = 0.432$ rad, $\theta_4 = 0.592$ rad, $\theta_5 = 0.772$ rad, $\theta_6 = 0.992$ rad, $\theta_7 = 1.354$ rad; (*d*) 0.07 rad

25. 1.98 rad

27. True

29. 4 Hz

31. (*a*) 496 Hz, 504 Hz; (*b*) If the beat frequency is diminished, the second fork has a frequency of 496 Hz, whereas if the beat frequency is increased, the frequency of the second fork is 504 Hz.

33. (*b*)

35. (*c*)

37. 180 m/s

39. (*a*) 17 Hz; (*b*) 8.5 Hz

41. (*a*) 1.25 Hz; (*b*) No second harmonic is excited. (*c*) 3.75 Hz

43. (*a*) 4.25 m; (*b*) 8.5 m

45. (*a*) $\lambda = 31$ cm, $f = 48$ Hz; (*b*) 15 m/s; (*c*) 63 cm

47. (*a*)

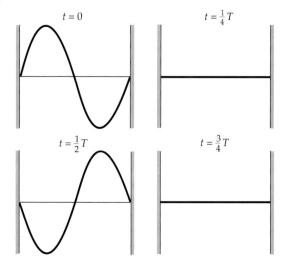

(*b*) 0.0126 s; (*c*) All the energy is kinetic.

49. (*a*) 75 Hz/125 Hz = 3/5, 125 Hz/175 Hz = 5/7; (*b*) The even harmonics are missing. (*c*) 25 Hz; (*d*) 3rd, 5th, 7th harmonics; (*e*) 4 m

51. (*a*) 345 m/s; (*b*) 0.45 cm

53. (*a*) 0.8 m; (*b*) 480 N; (*c*) 9.2 cm from the end

55. (*a*) 75 Hz; (*b*) 5th, 6th; (*c*) 2 m

57. 16.2 Hz

59. (*a*) The two sounds produce a beat because the third harmonic of 440 Hz equals the second harmonic of 660 Hz, and the original frequency of the E string is slightly greater than 660 Hz. If $f_E = (660 + \Delta f)$ Hz, a beat of $2\Delta f$ will be heard. (*b*) 661.5 Hz; (*c*) 79.6 N

61. 12.5 cm

63. (*a*) $y = 0.03\sin(3\pi/4)x\cos 200\pi t$;
(*b*) $dK = \frac{1}{2}\mu\,[6\pi\sin(3\pi/4)x\sin 200\pi t]^2\,dx$, $t = 2.5\times 10^{-3}$ s, straight;
(*c*) 89*m* J

65. (*a*) $N \simeq f_0\,\Delta t$; (*b*) $\lambda \simeq \Delta x/N$; (*c*) $k \simeq 2\pi N/\Delta x$; (*d*) N is uncertain because the waveform dies out gradually, rather than stopping abruptly at some time; hence, where the pulse starts and stops is not well defined. (*e*) $\Delta k \approx 2\pi\,\Delta N/\Delta x$. Since $\Delta N = 1$, $\Delta k \approx 2\pi/\Delta x$.

67. No

69. When the edges of the glass vibrate, sound waves are produced in the air in the glass. The resonance frequency of the air columns depends on the length of the air column, which depends on how much water is in the glass.

71. (*b*)

73. The pitch is determined in large part by the resonant cavity of the mouth. Since $v_{He} > v_{air}$, the resonance frequency is higher if helium is the gas in the cavity.

75. (*a*) 3400*n* Hz, $n = 1, 3, 5\ldots$; (*b*) Frequencies near 3400 Hz will be the most readily perceived.

77. (*a*) 2270 Hz; (*b*) 8th harmonic ($f_8 = 18.1$ kHz) or 9th harmonic ($f_9 = 20.4$ kHz)

79. (*a*) $f_n = n(0.66)$ Hz, $n = 1, 2, 3\ldots$; (*b*) $f_n = n(0.33)$ Hz, $n = 1, 3, 5\ldots$

81. (*a*) 4 m; (*b*) $\pi/2$ m^{-1}; (*c*) 800π rad/s;
(*d*) $y = 0.03[\sin(\pi/2)x][\cos 800\pi t]$

83. (*a*) $n = 5$; (*b*) 5.5 Hz, 11.0 Hz, 16.4 Hz

85. (*a*) 720 N; (*b*) 2880 N, 6480 N, 11,520 N

87. 338 m/s. This method is not very accurate because the antinode generally does not occur exactly at the end of an open pipe.

89. 9.1 g

91. (a) $I_1 = 1.99 \times 10^{-5}$ W/m^2, $I_2 = 8.84 \times 10^{-6}$ W/m^2; (b) 5.53×10^{-5} W/m^2; (c) 2.21×10^{-6} W/m^2; (d) 2.87×10^{-5} W/m^2

93. (a) Answer given in the problem. (b) 203.4 Hz

95. (a) $K = \frac{1}{4}\mu L\omega_n^2 A_n^2 \sin^2 \omega_n t$; (b) $K_{max} = \frac{1}{4}\mu L\omega_n^2 A_n^2$; (c) $y = 0$; (d) Since $\omega_n = n\omega_1$, $K_{max} \propto n^2 A_n^2$.

97. $y_1 = A_0 \cos(kx - \omega t)$, $y_2 = A_0 \cos(kx - \omega t + k\,\Delta x + \delta_0)$; (b) $y = 2A_0 \cos\frac{1}{2}(k\,\Delta x + \delta_0) \cos\frac{1}{2}[kx - \omega t + \frac{1}{2}(k\,\Delta x + \delta_0)]$; $A = 2A_0 \cos\frac{1}{2}(\delta + \delta_0)$, where $\delta = 2\pi\,\Delta x/\lambda$.

(c)

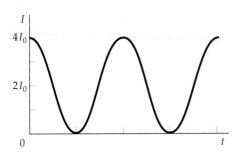

The time-average intensity $= 2I_0$.

(d)

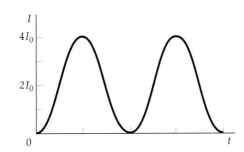

99. (a) 0.02 J; (b) 0; (c) dK_{max} at midpoint: $x = 1$ m; (d) dU_{max} at midpoint: $x = 1$ m.

Chapter 17

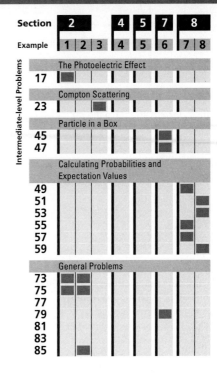

1. (c)

3. (a) 6.63×10^{-26} J, 4.14×10^{-7} eV; (b) 5.96×10^{-28} J, 3.72×10^{-9} eV

5. (a) 2.42×10^{14} Hz; (b) 2.42×10^{17} Hz; (c) 2.42×10^{20} Hz

7. (a) 12 keV; (b) 1.2 GeV

9. (a) True; (b) False; (c) True; (d) True

11. (a)

13. (a) 1.11×10^{15} Hz, 270 nm; (b) 1.62 eV; (c) 0.38 eV

15. (a) 4.73 eV; (b) 2.36 eV

17. 1.52 eV

19. 30°

21. (a) 17.4 keV; (b) 0.0760 nm; (c) 16.3 keV

23. (a) 2.43 pm; (b) 59.6 keV

25. (a) True; (b) True; (c) True; (d) False

27. (c)

29. 2.9 nm

31. (a) 0.061 eV; (b) 15 keV

33. 2.02×10^{-14} m

35. (a) 8.2×10^{-4} eV; (b) 8.2×10^8 eV

37. 0.167 nm

39. 4.6 pm

41. Aperture $\approx 1.7 \times 10^{-33}$ m. The size of an atomic nucleus is on the order of 10^{-15}, which is much larger than the size of the aperture.

43. 0.087 nm, atoms in crystals

45. (a) $E_1 = 205$ MeV, $E_2 = 821$ MeV, $E_3 = 1846$ MeV

(b) 2.01 fm; (c) 1.21 fm; (d) 0.758 fm

47. (a) 5.6×10^{-55} J, 2.2×10^{-54} J, 5.0×10^{-54} J; (b) 5×10^{-16} J, 3×10^{19}

49. (a) 0; (b) 0.003; (c) 0

51. $L/2$, $L^2/3$ for box between 0 and L

53. (a) $L/2$; (b) $0.328L^2$

55. (a) $A = \sqrt{1/a}$; (b) 0.865

57. (a) 0.5; (b) 0.402; (c) 0.75

59. $\langle x \rangle = 0$, $\langle x^2 \rangle = 0.0327L^2$

61. Yes

63. (a) 0; (b) 1.5

65. Quantum mechanics predicts only probabilities. Change "results" to "probabilities of various results."

67. 3×10^{19}

69. 1.0×10^{22} photons

71. 4.2×10^{-20} nm

73. 6800 km

75. 1.7×10^{-14} W/m^2

77. 1.9 eV

79. 5

81. 1.04 eV, 554 nm

83. (a) $\dfrac{E_{n+1} - E_n}{E_n} = \dfrac{(n+1)^2 - n^2}{n^2} = \dfrac{2}{n} + \dfrac{1}{n^2} \approx \dfrac{2}{n}$ for large n.

(b) 0.2%; (c) For large quantum numbers n, the fractional difference between adjacent energy levels here is proportional to $1/n$, so as n approaches infinity, the quantized energy levels approach a continuum of levels as in classical physics.

85. (a) 6.25×10^{-4} eV/s; (b) 3200 s

Chapter 18

1. (a) False; (b) False; (c) True; (d) False

3. 1 C° > 1 F°

5. 10°F to 19°F

7. 57°C, −62°C

9. (a) 8.4 cm; (b) 107°C

11. −320.4°F

13. (a) 54.9 torr; (b) 3700 K

15. −40°

17. −183°C, −297°F

19. (a) $R_0 = 3.89$ mΩ, $B = 3.94 \times 10^3$ K; (b) 1.32 kΩ; (c) −389 Ω/K at ice point, −4.37 Ω/K at steam point; (d) more sensitive at ice point

21. Pressure increases

23. 1.15

25. 3.2×10^8 molecules

27. (a) n = 3.66×10^3 mol; (b) 60 mol

29. 0.86 L; (b) 60 L

31. (a) 230 kPa; (b) 200 kPa

33. (a) 776 mol; (b) 4.86 km; (c) yes; (d) 6.0 km

35. 4

37. helium molecules

39. (a) 276 m/s; (b) 872 m/s

41. 5×10^5 m/s, 1.29 keV

43. $\lambda = 1/\sqrt{2}n_v \pi d^2$; since $n_v = N/V = P/KT$, $\lambda = KT/P\sqrt{2}\pi d^2$

45. (a) 1.24 km/s; (b) 0.31 km/s; (c) 0.26 km/s; (d) All three gases are likely to be present.

47. $K/mgh = 8.0 \times 10^4$

49. Answer given in the problem.

51. $v_{\text{av}} = \sqrt{8kT/\pi m}$

53. False

55. The Fahrenheit and Celsius scales emphasize biologically significant temperatures; 0° is "cold" and 100° is "hot" in everyday experience.

57. (*d*)

59. (*d*)

61. $v_2/v_1 = \sqrt{M_1/M_2}$, $K_{2,av}/K_{1,av} = 1$

63. The rate of molecule–wall collisions increases with increased density.

65. 8.79 K

67. (*a*) 122 K; (*b*) 244 K; (*c*) 1.43 atm

69. 110 mol of H_2, 55 mol of O_2

71. $m_N = 7m_H$

73. $(18/11)P_0$

75. 400.5 K

Chapter 19

1. $\Delta T_A/\Delta T_B = 1/4$

3. (*c*)

5. 5×10^5 kJ

7. 311 kJ

9. 100 g

11. 6.25 kg

13. 0.092 cal/g·K

15. (*a*) 0°C; (*b*) 125 g

17. (*a*) 4.9°C; (*b*) no

19. (*a*) 3.01°C; (*b*) 200 g; (*c*) no

21. 18 ice cubes

23. (*a*) 28.5°C; (*b*) 15.5°C

25. Yes

27. 2.2 kJ

29. 176°C

31. 54 J

33. (*a*) 34 km; (*b*) yes; (*c*) The snowflakes reach terminal velocity and hit without melting.

35. For an ideal gas, $\Delta U = 0$ implies $\Delta T = 0$ because U is a function of T alone. A real gas is likely to have small, long-range, attractive interactions, which may introduce a dependence on volume (so that molecular kinetic energies decrease slightly as volume increases).

37. Since $Q = 0$ and $W = 0$, $\Delta U = 0$. Thus the temperature must increase to offset the decrease of potential energy from the increase in average distance between the ions.

39. (*a*) 608 J; (*b*) 1060 J

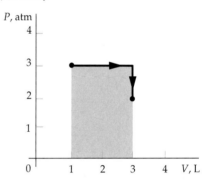

41. (*a*) 334 J; (*b*) 790 J

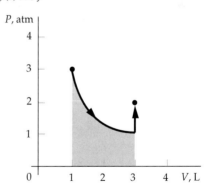

43. 100 L·atm

45. (*a*) −1.57 kJ; (*b*) −1.57 kJ

47. (*a*) 4.00 mol; (*b*) 14.9 kJ; (*c*) 83.0 J/K

49. (*a*) 0.713 J/g·K; (*b*) 252 J/L

51. $5P_0V$

53. (*a*) 3.50 mol; (*b*) $C_v = 43.7$ J/K, $C_p = 72.7$ J/K; (*c*) $C_v = 72.7$ J/K, $C_p = 102$ J/K

55. 1740 K

57. (*a*) $V_i = 2.2$ L, $V_f = 5.9$ L; (*b*) 143 K; (*c*) 1.62 kJ

59. 739 K, 10.1 atm

61. (a) 300 K, 7.79×10^{-3} m^3, $W = 1.14$ kJ, $Q = 1.14$ J; (b) 231 K, 6.00×10^{-3} m^3, $W = 287$ J, $Q = 0$

63. 575 J

65. (a)

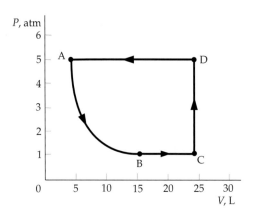

(b) $W \approx -64$ L·atm; (c) -65.1 L·atm; (d) $W = -65.1$ L·atm

67. D to A: $W = 0$, $Q = 89$ L·atm; A to B: $W = 130$ L·atm, $Q = 130$ L·atm; B to C: $W = 0$, $Q = -89$ L·atm; C to D: $W = -65$ L·atm, $Q = -65$ L·atm; Total $W = 65$ L·atm, total $Q = 65$ L·atm

69. D to A: $W = 0$, $Q = 148$ L·atm; A to B: $W = 105$ L·atm, $Q = 0$; B to C: $W = 0$, $Q = -95$ L·atm; C to D: $W = -52$ L·atm, $Q = 0$; Total $W = 53$ L·atm, Total $Q = 53$ L·atm

71. (a)

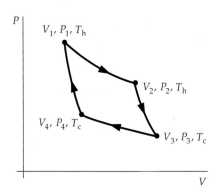

(b)–(f) Answer given in the problem.

73. (a) False; (b) False; (c) False; (d) True; (e) True; (f) False; (g) True

75. (d)

77. The temperature decreases.

79. 43 kcal

81. (a) $T_A = 65.2$ K, $T_C = 81.3$ K; (b) 16.0 L·atm; (c) 21.9 L·atm

83. (a) $T_A = 65.2$ K, $T_C = 81.3$ K; (b) 26.2 L·atm; (c) 32.1 L·atm

85. $W = 21.0$ L·atm, $Q = 26.9$ L·atm

87. $W = -170$ cal, $\Delta U = 0$, $T_f = T_i = 53$ K

89. $W = -170$ cal, $\Delta U = 0$, $T_f = T_i = 53$ K

91. (a) 3.91 kJ; (b) 5.49 kJ

93. (a) 2.74 kJ; (b) 4.91 kJ

95. (a) For an ideal gas, ΔU depends only on the states of the gas (n, T) and not on the path taken to go between the states. (b) Answer given in the problem.

97. (a) 8.6 K; (b) 143 J; (c) 1.03

99. 0.20 g

101. $4RT$

103. 4650 J/mol

105. For adiabatic expansion, $PV^\gamma = $ constant. Taking the derivative of both sides, $V^\gamma dP + \gamma PV^{\gamma-1} dV = 0$. Thus $dP/dV = -\gamma PV^{\gamma-1}/V^\gamma = -\gamma P/V$.

For isothermal expansion, $PV = nRT = $ constant. Taking the derivative, $V dP + P dV = 0$. Thus $dP/dV = -P/V$. $(-P/V)_{\text{isothermal}} = \gamma(-P/V)_{\text{adiabatic}}$.

107. (a) $T = 7418$ K, $V = 1832$ L; (b) $P = 0.0403$ atm

109. (a) $P = 218.2$ kPa; (b) $T = 3426$ K, $P = 2136$ kPa; (c) $P = 170.2$ kPa. Since N_2 is a diatomic gas, the contribution to specific heat from vibrations is R only, not $3R$ as for the triatomic gases.

111. (a) Answer given in the problem. (b) 4650 J

Chapter 20

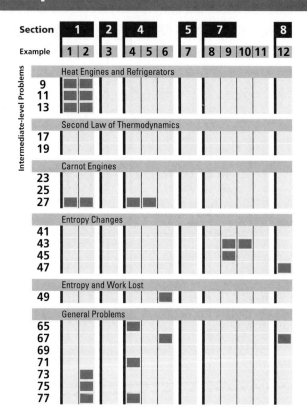

1. In an internal combustion engine, fuel is burned internally to produce hot gases which press a piston. In a steam engine, an external heat source converts water to hot steam, which then presses against a piston.

3. A refrigerator exhausts more heat into the kitchen than it absorbs from its interior.

5. (a) 500 J; (b) 400 J

7. (a) 40%; (b) 80 W

9.

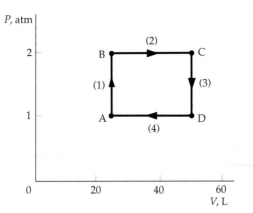

(a)	Step	W, L·atm	Q, L·atm	ΔU, L·atm
	1	0	36.9	36.9
	2	49.2	123.6	74.4
	3	0	−74.4	−74.4
	4	−24.6	−61.5	−36.9

(b) 15.3%

11.

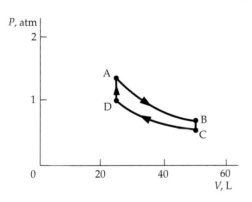

$\varepsilon = 13\%$

13. (a) 600 K, 1800 K, 600 K; (b) 15.4%

15. $\varepsilon = \varepsilon_C/\{1 + C_v\varepsilon_C/[R \ln(V_a/V_b)]\}$, where ε_C = Carnot efficiency = $(T_h - T_c)/T_h$.

17. This engine takes 200 J from a hot reservoir, does 60 J of work, and rejects the remaining 140 J to a cold reservoir. If the refrigerator statement of the second law of thermodynamics is false, then it would be possible to build a perfect refrigerator that would transfer the 140 J of heat from the cold to the hot reservoir with no other effects. The net result is that 60 J of heat is taken from the hot reservoir, 60 J of work is done, and no heat is rejected to the cold reservoir, a violation of the heat-engine statement of the second law.

19. If the proposed cycle is performed in the clockwise sense, then positive net work is done during the cycle. On the other hand, heat is exchanged only during the isothermal expansion. In this process, heat is drawn in from a high-temperature source. Note, however, that no heat is ever rejected to a low-temperature reservoir in the cycle, so the cycle would violate the heat-engine statement of the second law, namely, that it is impossible to have a cycle that uses heat to do work without exhausting waste heat in the process.

21. (a) 13.7; (b) 8.77

23. Answer given in the problem.

25. (a) 33.3%; (b) Answer given in the problem.

27. (a) 373 K; (b) 3.12 kJ, 0, −2.91 kJ; (c) 7%; (d) 35%

29. (a) 5.26; (b) 3.2 kW; (c) 4.8 kW

31. (a) 303 kJ/min; (b) 212 kJ

33. (c)

35. (a) 11.5 J/K; (b) 0

37. 6.05 kJ/K

39. 1.22 kJ/K

41. (a) 0; (b) 267 K

43. (a) 244 kJ/K; (b) −244 kJ/K; (c) 0

45. (a) −24 J/K; (b) 138 J/K; (c) 114 J/K

47. 1.98 kJ/K

49. (a) 0.42 J/K; (b) 125 J

51. (c)

53. (d)

55. The diagram is an Otto cycle, which represents an internal combustion engine.

57.

59.

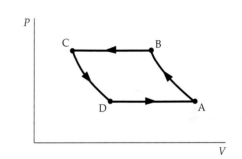

AB, CD are adiabatic; BC, DA are isobaric.

61. The 5-K decrease in the temperature of the cold reservoir

63. (a) 51%; (b) 102 kJ; (c) 98 kJ

65. 60%

67. (a) (1); (b) 7.66 J/K; 0.83 J/K

69. 313 K

71. 10 W

73. (a) 2.5 atm; (b) 462 K; (c) 68.7 L·atm, 26%

75. (a) 2.5 atm; (b) 415 K; (c) 65.3 L·atm, 35%

77. $\varepsilon = \varepsilon_C/\{1 + C_v\varepsilon_C/[R \ln(V_a/V_b)]\}$, which is less than the Carnot efficiency ε_C.

79. (a) Perfect refrigerator = $\Delta S_u = Q(T_h - T_c)/(T_hT_c) < 0$
(b) Perfect heat engine: $\Delta S_u = -Q/T_h < 0$; (c) $\Delta S \geq 0$ implies both statements, but the converse has not been proven here.

81. $\varepsilon = \varepsilon_1 + \varepsilon_2 (1 - \varepsilon_1)$. Substitute $W/Q_h = (1 - T_m/T_h) + (1 - T_c/T_m) (T_m/T_h) = 1 - T_c/T_h$.

83. 2.30×10^{-22} J/K

Chapter 21

1. The glass of the thermometer expands first, causing an increased volume of space and a corresponding dip in the level of mercury.

3. 30.026 cm

5. (a) $(1/A)(dA/dT)$; (b) 2α in each case

7. 217°C

9. $15 \times 10^{-6}\,\text{K}^{-1}$

11. (a) 1.99935 m; (b) 2.00065 m

13. 0.78 L

15. 6.54 cm^3

17. 395°C

19. (c)

21. (a) For boiling, the temperature and pressure values must lie on the OF curve. As the altitude increases, the pressure decreases. The OF curve shows that at lower pressures, lower temperatures are required for boiling to occur. The OH curve shows the temperature and pressure values required for melting ice to water. As the pressure decreases (with increased altitude), higher temperatures are required for melting. (b) Because at higher altitudes water boils at lower temperatures, foods boiled in water would take a longer time to heat thoroughly. Also, more heat would have to be applied to heat foods to a certain temperature.

23. (a) 30.6 L; (b) 374 K

25. $3.94 \times 10^{-23}\,\text{cm}^3$, $2.1 \times 10^{-8}\,\text{cm}$

27. (a) 16 K/W; (b) 6.3 W; (c) 50 K/m; (d) 87.5°C

29. (a) Cu: 0.083 K/W, Al: 0.14 K/W; (b) 0.22 K/W; (c) 360 W; (d) 70°C

31. (a) Because of conservation of energy, the thermal current into an element must equal the thermal current out of the element. (b) $I = 4\pi r^2 k\, dT/dr$; (c) $dT = (I/4\pi k)(dr/r^2)$; integrating from r_1 to r_2 gives $I = 4\pi k r_1 r_2\, (T_2 - T_1)/(r_2 - r_1)$; (d) Answer given in the problem.

33. 665 m

35. 4.4×10^{-4}

37. 9470 nm

39. 0.022 K/s

41. 97 g/h

43. (a) True; (b) True; (c) False; (d) False; (e) True

45. (d) assuming that the atmosphere is part of the earth.

47. radiation

49. 2.1 km

51. Rearranging $\beta = (1/V)\,(\Delta V/\Delta T)$ gives $\Delta V/V = \beta\,\Delta T$; $\rho = m/V$. Since m = constant, $\Delta\rho/\rho = -\Delta V/V = -\beta\,\Delta T$; hence $\Delta\rho = -\rho\beta\,\Delta T$

53. 360 s

55. 1.2 cm

57. (a) $\beta = (1/V)\,(dV/dT)$, where $V = nRT/P$ and $dV/dT = nR/P$. Thus $\beta = (P/nRT)/(nR/P) = 1/T$; (b) $\beta_t = 3.663 \times 10^{-3}\,\text{K}^{-1}$

59. 1.26×10^{13} W; $P_{lost}/P_{absorbed} = 7.3 \times 10^{-5}$ (Note that the effective area for absorption of energy from the sun is πR^2 whereas the loss is through area $4\pi R^2$.)

61. 142 W

63. $\omega_2 = \omega_1/(1 + \alpha\,\Delta T)^2$, $K_2 = MR_1^2\,\omega_1^2/4\,(1 + \alpha\,\Delta T)^2$, $L_2 = MR_1^2\,\omega_1/2$

65. Answer given in the problem.

67. 3.1×10^{-6} W/m·K

INDEX

Numbers in **bold** indicate additional display material, such as diagrams; *n* indicates a footnote; AP indicates material in the Appendixes.

Pages 1–655 are found in Volume 1; pages 656–1141 are found in Volume 2; pages 1142–1335 are found in Volume 3.

Aberrations in optical images, 1073, 1090
Absolute temperature scale, 544–546, 551, 613–614
Absorption spectra of diatomic molecules, 1212, 1217–1219
Absorption spectrum, 1031
ac circuits [*see* Alternating current (ac)]
ac Josephson effect, 845
Accelerated reference frame, 357–358, 418, 1243
Acceleration (*see also* Velocity)
  angular, 257–260
  average and instantaneous, 27, 62
  and center of mass, 218–221
  centripetal, 125–126
  constant, 29–38, 149–150
  definition, 27–28
  electric force, 674
  and gravity, 30, 87, 89
  and harmonic motion, 404, 405
  and Lorentz transformation, 1247
  Newton's laws and, 83–84, 85, 88–89
  and rotation, 275
  tangential, 258
  vectors, 59–62
Accelerators of particles, 1294–1295, 1313, **1316**
Acceptor levels in semiconductors, 1226
Accommodation, eye, 1091
Action at a distance, 92, 667
Action-reaction pair, 84, 89–90, 100
Adiabatic process, 276, 588–590
Allowed energy, 524
Alpha decay, 1293–1294
Alternating current (ac) [*see also* Direct current (dc); *RLC* circuit]
  in capacitors, conductors and inductors, 964–968
  vs. direct current, 959
  and electric motors, 985–988
  in generators, 960–961, 972, 973–981
  LC circuits, 969–971
  phasors, 968–969
  in resistors, 961–964
  root-mean-square (rms) values, 962–964

transformer, 982–984
Altitude and pressure, 380
Ammeter, 809–810, 896, 962
Ammonia (NH_3) molecule, 1211
Amorphous solid, 1219–1220
Ampère, André-Marie, 883, 895, 1017
Ampere (A)
  and Coulomb, 659
  definition, 895–897
  unit of current, 4, 787, AP1
Ampère's law, 898–901, 1000–1001, 1003
Amperian current, 904
Amplifier, *pnp* transistor as, **1230,** 1231
Amplitude, 404, 427, 448, 482
Analyzer, polarization, 1054
Anderson, Carl, 1317
Angle of incidence, refraction, 1041, 1042
Angle of minimum deviation, rainbows, 1052
Angles, conversion factors for, AP2
Angular acceleration, 257–259
Angular displacement, 258–259
Angular frequency, 405–407, 449
Angular magnification, 1094
Angular momentum (*see also* Conservation of momentum; Momentum)
  atomic spin, 1183–1184, 1316–1319
  conservation of, 304–309, 1179
  definition, 297–300
  of doublet, 1193–1194
  gyroscope, 303
  vs. magnetic moment, 906
  particle, 297
  quantization, 309–311, 1213
  quantum numbers, 1178
  and rotation, 210, 295–297, 312
  spin, 300, 310, 312
  and torque, 300–302
  unit of, 310, 312
  z component of, 1177
Angular speed, 258, AP2
Angular velocity, 258, 297
Anisotropic material, 1057
Anode in battery, 798
Antenna, electric dipole, 1005–1007
Antiderivative, 39
Antinode, waves, **488,** 489, 492
Antiparticles (*see also* Particles)
  antiproton/proton collision, **239**
  creation, 1317, 1318, 1330
  electric charge, 1328
  leptons, 1314
  mass of, 1314–1315, 1328
  neutrino, 1291, 1314–1315, 1320
  quarks, 1323, **1324**
  spin, 1316–1319, 1328

Antiquarks, **1324**
Aphelion, 322
Apparent depth, lenses, 1080
Apparent weight, 88
Arc discharge, 740
Archimedes, 381, **382**
Archimedes' principle, 380–382
Area, 7, AP2, AP14–15
Aristotle, 2
Armature, electric motor, 985
Astigmatism, 1090, 1091
Aston, Francis William, 865
Astronomical numerical data, AP3
Astronomical telescope, 1094, 1096–1099, **1098,** 1128
Astronomical unit (AU), 322
Asymmetric wave function, 1206–1208
Atmosphere (*see also* Pressure)
  escape speed, 330, 331, 558
  law of, 380
  units of, 376
Atomic magnetic moments, 906–908
Atomic mass, **1287**
Atomic number, 1169
Atomic orbitals, 1211
Atomic spectra, 1170–1171
Atomic theory of matter, 1313
Atoms (*see also* Electrons; Elementary particles; Molecular bonding; Neutrons; Nuclear physics; Protons)
  Bohr model of hydrogen, 1169–1176
  as elementary particles, 1313
  fine structure, 1183–1185
  nuclear, 1170–1171
  nuclei, properties of, 1284–1288
  optical atomic spectra, 1192–1194
  periodic table, 1185–1192
  plum pudding model, **1171**
  polyatomic molecules, 1210–1212
  quantization, 515
  quantum theory of atoms, 1176–1178
  quantum theory of hydrogen atom, 1178–1183
  rest energies of, **1266**
  selection rules, 1179
  spin, 1316–1319
  spin-orbit effect, 1183–1185
  X-ray spectra, 1194–1195
Atwood's machine, 111
AU (astronomical unit), 322
Avalanche breakdown current, 1228
Average acceleration, 27
Average force, 226–227
Average power, 962–963, 974–975
Average speed, 21
Average velocity, 19–20, 29

Average-acceleration vector, 62
Average-velocity vector, 60
Avogadro's number, 546–547, AP4
Axis of rotation, 257, 260, 271

Back emf, 935
Background radiation, 1329–1330
Ballistic pendulum, 230, 250–251
Balmer, Johann, 1170
Balmer series, 1175
Band, 841
Band energy, 841
Band theory of solids, 841–843
Banked curves, 131, 134–135, 145
Bar, unit of pressure, 379
Bardeen, John, 843
Bardeen, Walter H., 1229
Barn, unit of nuclear cross section, 1295
Barometer, **379**
Barrier penetration, electron waves, 461,
    1153–1155, 1160
Baryon number, 1320, 1323
Baryons
    and quarks, 1323, 1325
    spin 1/2 fermion, 1314, 1327
    strange, 1321
Base, transistor semiconductor region, 1229
Base-collector junction, 1230
Batteries [see also Direct current (dc)]
    and capacitors, 757
    emf and, 794–797
    ideal, 794–795
    internal resistance, 796
    Kirchhoff's rules, 804–806
    real, 795
    schematics, **798**
    terminal voltage, 795–796
BCS theory of superconductivity, 843–845
Beat frequency, 183
Beats, sound waves, 483–484
Becquerel, Antoine Henri, 2
Becquerel (Bq), unit of radioactive decay,
    1291
Bednorz, Johannes Georg, 843
Bernoulli's equation, 385–389
Beryllium (Z=4) electron configuration,
    1189
Beta decay, 1291–1292, 1320
Big Bang model, 1330–1331
Binding energy, 197, 332, 1268, 1286–1288
Binomial expansion, review, AP21
Biot, Jean Baptiste, 883
Biot-Savart law, 885–897, 901, 1000
Bipolar junction transistor, 1229
Birefringence, polarization by, 1057–1058
Black holes, 1272–1273
Black-body radiation, 647, 1329–1330
Body-centered-cubic (bcc) crystal structure,
    1223
Bohr, Niels, 515, 1169, 1175, 1299
Bohr magneton, 907
Bohr model of hydrogen atom
    energy in circular orbit, 1171–1172
    energy levels, 1174–1176
    of nuclear atom, 1313
    postulates for, 1172–1174

and quantum-mechanical theory,
    1169–1170, 1176
wavelengths emitted by, 1174–1175
Bohr orbit, 1172
Bohr radius, 1173–1174
Bohr's correspondence principle, 526
Boiling point, normal, 368–639, 542
Boltzmann, Ludwig, 646, 1016, 1018
Boltzmann factor, 559, 1219
Boltzmann's constant, 546, AP4
Bonding mechanism, molecular (see
    Molecular bonds)
Boron to neon (Z=4 to Z=10) electron
    configuration, 1189
Bosons, 834, 1164, 1317, 1326, 1327 (see also
    Elementary particles)
Bottomonium mesons, 1324
Bound charge, 772, 774
Boundary condition, standing waves, 524
Boyle, Robert, 546
Boyle's law, 546
Brackett, F., 1175
Brahe, Tycho, **1**, 321–322
Brattain, Walter H., 1229
Breeder reactor, fission, 1303
Bremsstrahlung, 1005
Brewster, Sir David, 1055
Brewster's law, 1055
Brush assembly electric motor, 985
Btu (British thermal unit), unit of heat, 567
Bubble as thin film, 1112–1115
Bubble-chamber tracks
    creation of proton-antiproton pair, **1318**
    kaon, **1317**
    lambda particle, **1321**
    proton collision, **238, 239, 1313**
Buckminsterfullerenes, **1224**
Bulk modulus (B), 376–377, 590
Buoyant force, 380
Burntime, rocket, 242

Calculus (see also Derivatives)
    fundamental theorem of, 39
    integration, 38–42, 217, 247
    review, AP22–27
Calorie, unit of heat energy, 566–567
Calorimetry, 568–569
Candela (cd), unit of luminosity, 4, AP1
Capacitance (C)
    of conductors, 752
    definition, 755
    dielectrics and, 767
    and electrostatic energy, 755–759
    equivalent, 756–759, 763–766
    unit of, 755, AP1
Capacitive reactance, 967
Capacitors
    alternating current (ac) in, 966–968
    charging, 812–814
    combinations of, 763–766
    cylindrical, 757–759
    discharging, 810–812
    integrated circuits (ICs), 1232–1233
    LC circuit, 969–971
    Leyden jar, 752–753
    parallel, 763

parallel-plate, 756–757, 767
phase relations, 968–969
RC circuit, 810–815
RLC circuit, 972
series, 763–766
time constant, 811
Carbon atoms, 1211–1212, **1224**
Carbon dating, 1292
Carnot, Nicolas L., 2
Carnot, Sadi, 607
Carnot cycle, 607, 609
Carnot efficiency, 608, 611, 612
Carnot engine, 607–614
Carnot theorem, 607
Cathode in battery, 798
Cathode-ray tube, 516, **516, 675**
Cavendish, Henry, 325
Cavendish apparatus, **326**
Cavendish experiment, 325, 663n
Celsius temperature scale, 542–545
Center of gravity, 352–353
Center of mass (see also Mass)
    calculation of, 217
    conservation of momentum, 213–221,
        240–241
    definition, 213
    description of, 212–215
    gravitational potential of, 216
    kinetic energy of, 225–226
    motion of, 218–221
    of objects, **216**, 277
    and systems of particles, 213–216
Center-of-mass reference frame, 240–241
Central diffraction maximum, 1118
Central force, 327
Central ray, lenses, 1085, 1086
Centrifugal force, 128–129
Centripetal acceleration, 125–126
Centripetal force, 126–127, 130–131
Cerenkov radiation, 468, **1098**
CERN (European Laboratory for Particle
    Physics), **239, 1318–1319**, 1326
Cgs (centimeter, gram, second) system of
    units, 5
Chamberlain, O., 1317
Characteristic rotational energy, 1213
Charge, electric (see also Electrostatics;
    Motion of point charges)
    antiparticles, 1328
    conservation, 659–660
    electric fields, 658–660
    per unit volume, 688–689
    point charges, 723–728, 753
    quantization, 658–659
    sharing and separation, 738
    unit of, 659, AP1
Charge-coupled devices (CCDs), 1234–1235
Charge-to-mass ratio, 674, 864–865
Charging by induction, 661–662
Charm, 1324
Charmed quark, 1324
Chemical energy, 152, 193
Chips, 1231, 1232–1233
Chromatic aberration, 1090
Circle of least confusion, optical images,
    1090
Circuit, electric (see also RLC circuit)
    and batteries, 794–798

Kirchhoff's rules, 803–808
LC circuit, 969–970
RC circuit, 810–815
resistor combinations, 799–802
RL circuit, 944–947
series, 969
simple alternating current (ac), 961
source of emfs, 794
unit of, 658–659
Circuits, integrated (ICs), 1232–1233
Circular motion
banked curves, 131, 134–135
centripetal force, 126–127, 130–131
Coriolis effect, 128, 129
drag forces, 135–136
Euler's method, 134–135
and harmonic motion, 409
and Newton's laws, 125–135
speed and period, 125–126
Circularly polarized electromagnetic waves, 1053
Classical electromagnetism, 999
Classical mechanics, 83, 199, 1263
Classical physics, 1–3, 19, 199
Classically forbidden region in Schrödinger equation, 1148
Classification of orbits, 331–332
Clausius statement, 601
Clock synchronization, 1253–1254, 1256–1257
Cloud chamber tracks, **91d**
Cockcroft, J. D., 1294
Coefficient of
friction, 115, 117, 123
kinetic friction, 115
performance (COP), refrigerator, 605
restitution, 236, 251
thermal expansion, 634
viscosity, 390
Coherence in harmonic waves, 1111–1112
Coherent sources, wave interference, 487
Cold reservoir, heat engine, 603
Collector, transistor semiconductor region, 1229–1231
Collisions
center-of-mass reference frame, 240–241
elastic, 226, 233–237, 1263–1264
extreme scale, 239
inelastic, 226, 615, 619–620, 1268
off-center, **237,** 238
in one dimension, 229–236
rocket propulsion, 241–243
in three dimensions, 236–238
time in conduction, 831
in two dimensions, 236–237
Color charge, field particles, 1326
Coma aberration, 1090
Compass, magnetic field, 856
Complex impedances in *RLC* circuits, 980–981
Complex numbers, review, AP21–22
Complex particles, 1323 (*see also* Elementary particles)
Compound microscope, 1094, 1095–1099
Compressive strength, 360
Compressive stress, 360
Compton, Arthur H., 514
Compton scattering, 514, **1031,** 1032

Compton wavelength, 514, AP4
Concave lens, 1083
Concave mirror, 1073, 1076
Conduction, microscopic theory of electrical (*see also* Semiconductors)
band theory of solids, 841–843
Fermi electron gas, 832–839
Fermi-Dirac distribution, 846
mean free path, 831–832
mean speed, 831–832
model of, 830–832
quantum theory of conduction, 839–840
resistivity, 791
Conduction band, 841
Conduction of thermal energy, 620, 640–646
Conductors (*see also* Dielectrics; Superconductivity)
alternating current (ac), 964–968
band theory of solids, 842
capacitance of, 752
charge and field at, 707–710
charge on nonspherical object, 741
charging by inductance, 660–662
dielectrics, 767–775, 768
electrostatic potential energy, 754
and equipotential surfaces, 736–742
free electrons in, 660–661, 707, 787–790
integrated circuits (ICs), 1232–1233
intrinsic semiconductor, 842
isolated, 755
polarization of, 661
and potential differences, 738
power dissipated in, 794
RL circuit, 944–947
RLC circuit, 972
surface charge and field, 707–710
Cones and rods, eye, 1091
Confinement, inertial and magnetic, 1304
Conservation laws and elementary particles, 1319–1322
Conservation of baryon number, 1320
Conservation of charge, 659–660
Conservation of energy (*see also* Energy)
chemical energy systems, 193–194
description of, 178–179, 185–186
and elementary particles, 1319
kinetic friction and, 188–192
law of, 186
mass and energy, 196–199
mechanical, 179–185
quantization of energy, 199–200
and thermodynamics, 573
work-energy theorem, 186–187
Conservation of lepton number, 1320
Conservation of momentum (*see also* Angular momentum; Momentum)
center of mass, 213–221, 240–241
collisions, 226–239
and elementary particles, 1319
kinetic energy of system, 225–226
law of, 221–225
magnetic force, 902–903
relativistic, 1264
and rocket propulsion, 241–243
Conservative force, 163, 166, 178–179, 185
Constant acceleration (*see also* Acceleration)
motion and, 29–38
one object problems, 30–34

two object problems, 34–38
and work-kinetic energy theorem, 149–150
Constant force, work as, 148–152
Constant velocity and special relativity theory, 1243
Constants
amplitude, position, and phase, 427
Boltzmann's, 546
Coulomb's, 663, 698, 1000
decay constant, 1288
dielectric, 767
effective force, 1215
Gauss's, 1000
Hubble, 1329
initial condition, 38
Madelung, 1220, 1223
phase, 427
physical, AP4
Planck's, 200, 310, 511–512, 1028
reproductive constant in nuclear reactor, 1300
Stefan's, 646
time, 422, 811, 945
universal gas, 547
universal gravitational, 324, 325–326
Von Klitzing, 874
Constant-volume gas thermometer, 544
Constraints, free-body diagrams, 94
Constructive interference, wave motion, 482
Contact forces, 92–94 (*see also* Friction)
Contact potential in Fermi electron gas, 838
Continuity equation, fluids, 384
Continuous object, 213, 261, 263–267
Continuous spectrum, 1029, 1030
Convection, thermal energy, 640, 646
Converging lens, 1082, 1093–1095
Conversion factors, units of, 6, AP2
Convex lens, 1082
Convex mirror, 1076–1077
Cooper, Leon, 843
Cooper pair, 844
Coriolis effect, 128, 129
Cosmic radiation, 1330
Coulomb, Charles, 663
Coulomb attractive force, Bohr model of hydrogen, 1171
Coulomb barrier, 1294, 1303
Coulomb (C), unit of electric charge, 659, AP1
Coulomb potential, 723
Coulomb repulsive force, 1286, 1303
Coulomb's constant, 663, 698, 1000, 1172
Coulomb's law
derivation of, 710–711
electric field, 663–666, 668, 689–696
vs. Gauss's law, 698–699
Couples, 356–357
Covalent bonds, 1206–1209
Critical angle for total internal reflection, 1045
Critical point, phase diagram, 639
Critical temperature and superconductivity, 843
Critically damped oscillations, 422
Cross product, 296–297
Cross section, unit of nucleus effective size, 1295
Crossed fields, 863

Crystal structure
  body-centered-cubic (bcc), 1223
  of carbon, **1224**
  crystalline, 1219–1220
  dendrites, **1203**
  diamond, **1223**
  dissociation energy of, 122
  face-centered-cubic (fcc), 1220
  hexagonal, 1223
  hexagonal close-packed (hcp), 1223
  photo essay, **1221**
  polycrystalline, 1220
  unit cell, 1220
Curie, Pierre, 909
Curie, unit of radioactivity, 1291
Curie temperature, 910
Curie's laws, **908,** 909
Current, electric [*see also* Alternating current
    (ac); Direct current (dc)]
  avalanche breakdown, 1228
  definition, 787
  vs. drift velocity, 788
  eddy, 938–939
  energy in electric circuits, 793–798
  induced, 927
  Kirchhoff's rules, 803–810
  light switch description, 789
  measuring devices, 809
  motion of charges, 787–790
  RC circuit, 810–815
  resistance and Ohm's law, 790–793
  resistor combinations, 799–802
  root-mean-square, 962–964
  sinusoidal, 959, 960, 962
  tunneling, 1228
  unit of, 4, 659, 787, 895–897, AP1
Current, magnetic field (*see also* Magnetic
    field)
  cyclotron frequency and period, 861
  loop, 886–889
  solenoid, 889–891, 940
  straight line, 892–895
  toroid, 899, 1304, **1305**
Current balance, magnetic field, 896
Current element, magnetic field, 858
Current gain, transistor, 1230
Current loops
  electric field at center, 886–889
  magnetic dipole moment, 868
  potential energy, 870–871
  torque, 868
Cyclotron, 1294
Cyclotron frequency, 861
Cyclotron period, 861
Cylinder, uniform, 265, 278

Dalton, John, 1313
Dalton's atomic theory of matter, 1313
Damped oscillations, **403,** 421–424, 425
Damped oscillator, 428
Daughter nucleus, beta decay, 1291
Davisson, C. J., 480, 518
Davy, Humphrey, 798
dc circuit [*see* Direct current (dc)]
dc Josephson effect, 845
De Broglie, Louis, 516

De Broglie hypothesis, 516–518
De Broglie wavelength, 516–517
De Maricourt, Pierre, 855
Decay, radioactive, 1288–1294
Decay constant, 1288
Decay rate, 1289
Decay time, 422
Deceleration, 32 (*see also* Acceleration)
Decibels (db), unit of sound intensity,
    457–458
Decimal system, 4–5
Deep inelastic scattering, 1323
Dees, particles in, 866–867
Deformation forces, 185
Degenerate energy level, 1161, 1180
Degree of freedom in equipartition theorem,
    553
Delayed neutrons, nuclear fission reactor,
    1301
Dendrites, **1203**
Density, 375–376, 549, AP2
Density of states, 559
Depletion region, semiconductors, 1227
Depth inversion, 1071, 1072
Derivatives (*see also* Calculus)
  conversion factors for, AP2
  definition, 24, 25
  integration of, 38–41
  partial, 446–447
  properties of, **AP23**
Descartes, René, 1042, 1048, **1049**
Destructive interference, wave motion,
    482
Deuterium, 197, 1285, 1303
Deuteron, **196,** 197
Devices, semiconductors, 1227–1231
Diamagnetic material, 904
Diamagnetism, 913–914
Diamond crystal structure, **1223**
Diamond crystalline form, **1224**
Diatomic molecules
  absorption spectra of, 1217–1219
  effective force constant of, 1215
  emission spectra of, 1216–1217
  energy levels of, 1212–1219
  energy quantization of, 199–200
  moment of inertia, 1213–1214
  reduced mass, 1214
Dielectric breakdown, 740
Dielectric constant, 767
Dielectric strength, 740
Dielectrics (*see also* Conductors)
  macroscopic behavior, 767–771
  molecular view of, 771–775
  piezoelectric effect, 774–775
  uses of, 768
Differential calculus review, AP22–26
Diffraction (*see also* Interference; Light)
  definition, 1110
  of electron waves, 518–519
  Fraunhofer patterns, 1126–1127
  Fresnel patterns, 1126–1127
  gratings, 1129–1133
  phasors, 1121–1126
  Rayleigh's criterion, 1128
  and resolution, 1128–1129
  single-slit pattern, 1118–1120, 1121,
    1124–1126

  two-slit pattern, 1115–1117, 1120,
    1124–1126
  wave motion, 462–463
Diffuse reflection, 1043
Dimensions of physical quantities, **7**
Diodes (*see also* Junctions)
  forward biased junction, 1227–1228, 1230
  integrated circuits (ICs), 1232–1233
  light-emitting diodes (LEDs), 1229
  reversed biased junction, 1228, 1230
  in semiconductors, 1125, 1227–1229
  tunnel, 1228–1229
  Zener, 1228
Diopters (D), 1084
Dipole moment (*see* Electric dipole moment;
    Magnetic dipole moment)
Dirac, Paul A., 906*n,* 1317
Dirac equation, 1317
Direct current (dc) [*see also* Alternating
    current (ac); Batteries]
  vs. alternating current (ac), 959, 964
  charge current and motion, 787–790
  in electric circuits, 793–798
  HVDC (high-voltage direct current), **959**
  Kirchhoff's rules, 803–810
  measuring devices, 809
  resistance and Ohm's law, 790–793
  resistor combinations, 799–802
  shunt motor, 987
Direction of acceleration, 85 (*see also* Vectors)
Dispersion, 499–500, 1047–1052
Displacement
  angular, 258
  definition, 19
  integration of, 42
  and rotation, 275
  vectors of, 54–55, 59–60
  velocity and speed, 19–26
Dissociation energy, 1205, 1222
Distortion of lens, 1090
Distribution of molecular speeds, 554–559
Diverging lens, 1083, 1086
Donor levels and semiconductors, 1225
Doping, semiconductors, 1225
Doppler effect
  redshift, 1272, 1329
  relativistic, 1252–1253
  wave motion, 463–468
Dot product, 155–156, 172
Double slit experiment, light waves,
    487–488, 510, 522–523
Doublet, spin angular momentum,
    1193–1194
Down-quark, 1323, **1324**
Drag forces, 135–136
Drift chamber, **1316**
Drift velocity, 787
Driven oscillations, 425, 427, 428–430
Driven oscillator, 429
Dude, Paul K., 829, 831*n*
Dulong-Petit law, 583

Eddy currents, 938–939
Efficiency
  Carnot, 608, 611, 612
  heat engine, 603

Einstein, Albert, **1243**
  Bohr model, 1171
  Einstein equation, 512
  particle nature of light, **200**
  photoelectric effect, 511–513
  photon energy equation, 1028
  postulates of, 1245–1250, 1251
  relativity, theory of, 2, 196, 1270–1273
  rest energy, 1265–1266, 1267
Einstein equation for photon energy, 1028
Elastic collision, 226, 233–237, 1263–1264
Elastic limit, 360
Elastic scattering, **1031**
Elasticity, stress and strain, 360–362
Electric capacitance [see Capacitance (C); Capacitors]
Electric charge (see Charge, electric)
Electric circuit (see Circuit, electric)
Electric conduction (see Conduction, microscopic theory of electrical; Conductors)
Electric current (see Current, electric)
Electric dipole moment
  antenna for, 1005–1007
  electric field, 671, 676–678
  of the molecule, 1208
Electric energy storage, 759–762
Electric field ($\vec{E}$)
  avalanche breakdown, 1228
  on axis of a disk charge, 694
  on axis of a ring charge, 693–694
  on axis of finite line charge, 689–690
  and conductors, 660–662, 706–710
  continuous charge distribution, 688–711
  Coulomb's law, 663–666, 689–696, 699
  definition, 667
  discrete charge distribution, 657–678
  from electric potential, 728–729
  energy storage, 759–762
  equipotential surfaces, 737
  flux and Maxwell's displacement current, 1001
  from Gauss's law, 698–706
  of infinite plane of charge, 695–696, 700
  insulators, 660–662
  lines, 672–674, 722–723
  off axis of finite line charge, 690–691
  of point charges, 668, 674–676
  radial, 728
  of a solid sphere of charge, 704–705, 734
  television cathode-ray tube schematic, **675**
  unit of, 667
  wave equations for, 1011–1012
Electric flux, 697–698
Electric force, 664, 667, 668, 720
Electric ground, 662
Electric inductance [see Inductance (L); Inductors]
Electric motor, 985–988
Electric potential (see also Electric dipole moment)
  on axis of charged disk, 731–732
  on axis of charged ring, 730–731
  on the axis of uniformly charged disk, 731–732
  charge on nonspherical object, 741
  continuity of voltage, 730–736
  continuous charge distribution, 730–736

Coulomb potential, 723
  electric field calculation, 728–729
  equipotential surfaces, 736–742
  due to an infinite line charge, 736
  due to an infinite plane of charge, 732–736
  of an infinite plane of charge, 695–696, 700
  potential difference, 720–723, 728–729
  potential function, 721, 734
  due to a system of point charges, 723–728
  unit of, 722
Electric power, transformers, 982–984
Electric resistance (see Resistance; Resistors)
Electrical wire, 792
Electrodynamics of moving bodies, 1245
Electrolyte in battery, 798
Electromagnetic force/interaction, 91–94, 200, 1314, **1326**, 1327–1328
Electromagnetic spectrum, 1004–1005, 1017 (see also Light)
Electromagnetic theory, 1172 (see also Electromagnetism)
Electromagnetic waves
  circularly polarized, 1053
  electric-dipole radiation, 1005–1007
  electromagnetic spectrum, 1004–1005, 1017
  energy and momentum in, 1008–1011
  intensity of, 1008
  light, theory of, 1017
  linearly polarized, 1052–1053
  and Maxwell's displacement current, 1000–1002
  and Maxwell's equations, 1000, 1003
  Poynting vector, 1008
  production of, 1005
  radiation, 1212
  radiation pressure, 1008–1011
  wave equation for, 1011–1015
  wave motion, 454
  wave speed, 1000
Electromagnetism
  electromagnetic spectrum, 1004–1005, 1017
  laws of, 2
  molecular radiation, 1212
  theory of, 1172
  and virtual photons, 1325
Electromotive force (emf) [see emf (electromotive force)]
Electron gas (see Fermi electron gas)
Electron microscope, 519, 1129
Electron neutrino, 1314–1315
Electron probability distribution, 1206–1207
Electron volt (eV), unit of energy, 149, 196, 722
Electron waves (see also Schrödinger equation)
  barrier penetration, 1153–1155, 1160
  de Broglie hypothesis, 516–518
  diffraction, 518–519
  functions, 1204, 1211
  reflection and transmission of, 1151–1155, 1160
  scattering, 840
Electronic molecular energy levels, 1213, 1215, 1216, **1216**
Electron-Positron collider (LEP) tunnel, **1318**
Electrons (see also Atoms; Conduction, microscopic theory of electrical;

Diffraction; Motion of point charges; Spin; Wave function)
  affinity of, 1204
  antineutrino, 1291, 1320
  in atom, 1169
  atomic orbitals charge distribution, 1211
  bubble chamber tracks, **91d, 1313**
  charge-to-mass ratio, 674, 864–865
  configurations of, 1185–1190, **1190–1192**
  covalent bonds, 1206–1209
  electric charge quantization, 658–659
  electric field deflection, 674
  electromagnetic waves, 1005
  as elementary particle, 1313
  emitted, **1031**
  Fermi electron gas, 832–839
  free in conductor, 660–661, 707, 787–790
  ion, 661
  ionic bonds, 1224–1225
  ionization energy, 1175
  line spectra, 1029–1030
  magnetic moment of, 906
  mass of, 1314–1315
  matter waves, 516–520
  orbits and electromagnetic theory, 1172
  particle-antiparticle pairs, 1317
  radioactive decay, 1288
  rest energies of, **196**
  and scanning tunneling microscope (STC), 1155
  semiconductors, 1225–1226
  tunneling, 844
  Z particle decay, **239**
Electroscope, 661
Electrostatics (see also Charge, electric)
  attraction and repulsion, 1204–1205
  definition, 657
  equilibrium, 707
  field energy, 761–762
  potential energy, 753–755, 758, 1207–1208
Electrotonic function, 1016
Electroweak theory, 1326–1328, 1330
Elementary particles (see also Antiparticles; Atoms; Baryons; Hadrons; Leptons; Mesons; Muons; Quarks)
  bosons, 834, 1164, 1317, 1326, 1327
  cloud chamber photograph, **196**
  and conservation laws, 1319–1322
  fermions, 834, 1164, 1314–1315, 1317, 1327
  field particles, 1325–1326
  gluons, 1326
  graviton, 1326
  kaon, **1317**
  lambda particle, **1321**
  neutrino, 1291, 1314-1315, 1320
  nucleon, 1285, 1321, 1323
  nuclide, 1285
  photons, 1172–1173, 1288
  pion, 1313, 1317, 1321, **1322**
  positron, 1288, 1291, 1313
  rest energies of, **196**
  in Standard Model, 1314, 1327–1328
  strangeness, 1321–1322
  tau particle, 1291, 1314
  W particle, 1326, 1327
  weak nuclear force, **91d**
  Z particle, **239**, 1326, 1327

Elements, periodic table of, 7, 1185–1187, AP6–7
Ellipse, planetary orbits, 322–323
$E = mc^2$, 196
emf (electromotive force) [see also Alternating current (ac); Forces]
    back, 935
    and batteries, 794–797
    definition, 929
    Faraday's law, 929–930
    induced, 927
    Lenz's law, 933–936
    magnetic induction, 929–933, 936–938
    self-induced, 941
Emission of light (see Light, emission of)
Emission spectra of diatomic molecules, 1212, 1217–1219
Emissivity, radiation, 646
Emitter, transistor semiconductor region, 1229–1230
Emitter-base junction, 1230
Endothermic reaction, nuclear, 1295
Energy (see also Conservation of energy; Heat; Kinetic energy; Potential energy)
    bands of, 841
    batteries, 796
    binding, 197, 332, 1268, 1286–1288
    in circular orbit, 1171–1172
    conversion factors for, AP2
    dissociation energy of crystal, 1222
    distribution function, 558–559
    in electric circuits, 793–798, 971
    electric field storage, 759–862
    in electromagnetic waves, 1008–1011
    and Fermi, 834–836
    and harmonic motion, 410–412
    ionization of, 1175
    magnetic, 942–944
    mass and, 196–201
    mechanical, 179–185
    and power, 159–162
    relativistic, 1264–1269, 1274–1275
    rest, 1265–1266, 1286
    rest mass, 1267–1269, 1274–1275
    of sound waves, 453
    thermal, 178, 185, 188
    transducers, 195
    units of, 149, 159, 196, 566–567, AP1
    of waves, 451–452
    and work, 155–159
    zero-point, 525
Energy levels
    Bohr model of hydrogen atom, 1174–1176
    degenerative, 1161, 1180
    of diatomic molecules, 1212–1219
    hydrogen atom quantum theory, 1179
    molecular, 1213–1216
    and three dimensional Schrödinger equations, 1160–1162
    and wave functions, 1149–1150
Energy quantization
    atoms, 515
    conservation of energy, 199–200
    Fermi electron gas, 833
    hydrogen atom, 531–532
    in microscopic systems, 199–200
    and standing waves, 519–520

Energy-level diagrams
    diatomic molecule, **1216**
    fine-structure, **1184**
    hydrogen atom, **532, 1179**
    optical transitions in sodium, 1193
    oscillator, 200, **531**
    particle in a box, **524**
    pn semiconductor junction, **1227**
    tunnel diode, **1228**
Engines
    electric motors, 960, 985–988
    heat, 601, 603
    internal combustion, **602**
    steam, **601**
    and thermodynamics, 606–614
Entropy
    changes in, 616, 617–622
    and energy availability, 622–623
    and probability, 623–625
    second law of thermodynamics, 616–622
Equation of state for ideal gas, 547
Equilibrium (see also Static equilibrium)
    center of gravity, 352–353
    conditions for, 351–352
    couples, 356–357
    and harmonic motion, 411
    indeterminate problems and, 359
    neutral, 167
    stability of, 167, 358–359
    static, 92, 353–358
Equipartition theorem, 552–553, 581–587, 1018
Equipotential surfaces, 736–742
Equipotential volume, 736
Equivalence, principle of, 329
Equivalent capacitance, 756–759, 763–766
Equivalent molecular orbitals, 1212
Equivalent resistance, 642, 799–802
Escape speed, 330, 331
Ether, 1244–1245
Euler's method, 134–135
European Laboratory for Particle Physics (CERN), **239, 1318–1319,** 1326
Exchange interaction, 913
Excited state, quantum theory, 1182–1183, 1192
Exclusion principle, 834, 1029, 1204, 1286
Exothermic reaction, nuclear, 1295
Expectation values, 528–530
Exponential time dependence, radioactivity, 1288
Exponents, **5,** 8–9, 11, AP12–14
External forces, 83–84, 212, 218–220
Eye as optical instrument, 1090, 1091–1093
Eyepiece, microscope, 1095

Face-centered-cubic (fcc) structure, 1220
Factoring, equations, AP12
Fahrenheit, Daniel, 543*n*
Fahrenheit temperature scale, 542–544
Farad (F), unit of capacitance, 755, AP1
Faraday, Michael, 755, 927, 1016
Faraday's law, 929–933, 1001, 1003
Farsightedness, 1091
Fermat, Pierre de, 1040

Fermat's principle, 1041, 1059–1061
Fermi, Enrico, 13
Fermi electron gas
    and conduction, 832–839
    contact potential, 838
    energy quantization in a box, 833
    Fermi factors, 836–837
    heat capacity in metal, 839
    Pauli exclusion principle, 833–834
Fermi energy, 834–836
Fermi factors, 836–837, 847
Fermi temperature, 837
Fermi-Dirac distribution, 832–833
Fermions, 834, 1164, 1314–1315, 1317, 1327
Ferromagnetic material, 904
Ferromagnetism, 909–913
Fiber optics, 1046
Field particles, 1325–1326
Field point, 338, 668
Field quanta, 1325–1326
Field-effect transistor, 1229*n*
Fields
    electric [see Electric field ($\vec{E}$)]
    gravitational, 87, 92, 334–341
    magnetic [see Magnetic field ($\vec{B}$)]
Fine structure of atoms, 1183–1185
Fine-structure splitting, 1184
Finite potential difference, 721
Finite square-well potential, 1146
Finnegans Wake (Joyce), 1323*n*
First excited state, quantum theory, 1182–1183
First focal point, 1084
First harmonics, standing wave, **488,** 492, 497
First law of thermodynamics (see Thermodynamics, first law of)
First-order spectrum, 1131
Fission, 197, 1297–1303
FitzGerald, George Francis, 1251
Fixed amount of gas, 548
Fizeau, Armand H. L., 1038
Flavors of quarks, 1323, **1324**
Flip coil, 933
Fluids
    Archimedes' principle, 380–382
    Bernoulli's equation, 385–389
    bulk modulus, 376–377, 590
    continuity equation, 384
    density, 375–376
    in motion, 384–392
    pressure in, 376–380
    Reynolds' number, 391–392
    Torricelli's law, 387
    turbulence, 391–392
    Venturi effect, 387–389
    viscous flow, 389–391
    volume flow rate, 384
Fluorescence, 1031
Flux
    electric, 697
    electric field, 1001
    magnetic, 928–929, 934
    quantization of, 949
Fluxon, 949
Focal length
    lens, 1083
    mirror, 1071, 1074

Focal plane, 1084
Focal point, 1074, 1075, 1084
Focal ray
  lens, 1085, 1086
  mirror, 1075
Foot-pond, unit of energy, 159
Forbidden energy band, 841
Forces [*see also* emf (electromotive force);
    Gravity; Newton's laws; Strong nuclear
    force/interaction; Weak nuclear
    force/interaction]
  average, 226–227
  and Big Bang, 1329
  buoyant, 380
  central, 327
  centrifugal, 128–129
  centripetal, 126–127, 130–131
  conservative, 163, 166, 178–179, 184
  constant, 148–152, 153
  contact, 92–94
  conversion factors for, AP2
  Coulomb, 1171, 1286, 1303
  couples, 356–357
  definition, 85
  of deformation, 185
  of drag, 134–136, 135–136
  effective in diatomic molecules, 1215
  electric, 664, 667, 720
  electric field, 667, 668, 672–674
  electromagnetic force/interaction, 91–94,
    200, 1314, **1326**, 1327–1328
  electroweak force/interaction, 1326–1328,
    1330
  external, 83–84, 212, 218–220
  free-body diagrams, 94–102, 106–111
  of friction, 92, 135, 185
  fundamental, 4, 91–94
  gravitational force/interaction, 1314, **1326**,
    1327–1328
  and gravity, 87–89
  hadronic, 1285, 1314
  internal, 218–221
  lines of, 672–674, 722–723, 859, 897
  magnetic field, 856–860, 897, 902–903
  magnitude of, 85
  nonconservative, 166, 185–186
  normal, 92, 115
  pseudoforces, 128–129
  shear, 362
  tensile, 360
  tidal, 340–341
  units of, 4, 5, 85, 88–89, AP1
  van der Waals, 1219
  variable, 153–154
  and vectors, 226–227
  viscous, 389
  and work, 148–154, 171–172
Forward, Robert, 1273
Forward-biased junction, 1227–1228, 1230
Foucault, Jean, 1038–1039
Fourier analysis, 498*n*
Franklin, Benjamin, 658, 752
Fraunhofer diffraction patterns, 1126–1127
Free electrons, 660–661, 707, 787–790
Free expansion of gases, 575
Free fall, 87
Free space, permeability of, 884, 1000

Free-body diagrams, 94–99, 106–111
Freezing point, normal, 542
Frequency
  angular, 405
  beat, 183
  electromagnetic spectrum, 1004–1005
  electron wave, 516
  harmonic wave, 482, 483
  mass on a spring, 405–406, 407
  natural, 425, 490, 492
  oscillation, 199–200, 404
  photon threshold, 512
  resonance of, 425, 488, 489, 492
  unit of, 404, AP1
Fresnel, Augustin, 511, 1040–1041
Fresnel diffraction patterns, 1126–1127
Fresnel lens, **1085**
Friction
  coefficients of, 115, 117, 123
  as contact force, 92–94
  and inertia, 84
  kinetic, 115–124, 188–192
  and mechanical energy, 178–179
  as nonconservative force, 185
  ordinary vs. drag forces, 135
  oscillations and, 421
  static, 114–115, 130
Fringes in thin film, 1112
Fullerenes crystalline form, **1224**
Fundamental forces, 4, 91–94 (*see also* Forces)
Fundamental frequency, 488–498
Fundamental mode of vibration, 49, 488, 497
Fundamental node, 488–498
Fusion, 1297–1298, 1303–1306

Galilean transformation, 1246
Galileo, 2, 84, **1098**, 1244
Gallium atom in semiconductors, 1226
Galvanometer, 809–810
Gamma rays, **1004**
Gamow, George, 1155, 1294
Gas
  diatomic ideal, 582
  and entropy, 616
  gas constant, AP4
  gas plasma, 1304, **1305**
  heat capacities of, 578–583
  ideal-gas law, 546–549
  internal energy of, 574–575
  kinetic theory of, 550–559
  monatomic ideal, 580
  speed of sound waves in, 443–446, 590
  sublimation of, 639
  temperature scales and thermometers,
    541–546
  work and *PV* diagram for, 575–578
Gas phase of matter, 1219
Gauge pressure, 379
Gauss (G), unit of magnetic field, 857
Gaussian surface, 700–706
Gauss's constant, 1000
Gauss's law
  vs. Coulomb's law, 698–699
  cylindrical geometry, 705–706
  definition, 698

  derivation of, 710–711
  electric field flux, 1001
  electric flux, 697
  energy field calculation, 700–706
  for magnetism, 897
  Maxwell's equations, 1003
  plane geometry, 700
  quantitative statement of, 698–699
  solid sphere of charge, 704–705
  spherical shell of charge, 701–704
Geiger, H. W., 1171
Gell-Mann, M., 1321
General relativity, theory of, 1243, 1270–1273
Generator
  alternating current (ac), 960–961, 972,
    973–981
  average power delivered by, 962–963
  resonance of, 974
  Van de Graaff, 739, 1294
Geometry and Gaussian surfaces, 700–707
Geometry review, AP14–15
Germer, L. H., 480, 518
Gilbert, William, 855
Glashow, S., 1326
Gluons, 1326
Gradient, potential vector, 728
Gram (g), unit of mass, 4
Grand unification theories (GUTs), 1328
Graphite crystalline form, **1224**
Gratings, diffraction, 1129–1133
Gravitational constant, universal (*G*), 324,
    325–326, AP4
Gravitational field, 87, 92, 334–341
Gravitational force/interaction, 87–89,
    91–92, 321, 1314, **1326**, 1327–1328 (*see
    also* Forces)
Gravitational lensing, **1244**
Gravitational mass vs. inertial mass, 329
Gravitational potential, 1271
Gravitational redshift, 1272
Graviton, 1326
Gravity
  and acceleration, 30
  center of, 352–353
  and general relativity theory, 1243
  and Kepler's laws, 321–323, 327–328
  Newton's laws of, 324–326
  potential energy of, 164, 216, 330, 331–332
Greenler, Robert, 1050–1052
Ground, electrical, 662
Ground state for electron configurations,
    1190–1192
Ground-state energy, 200, 524
Ground-state energy level, 1160–1161
Ground-state wave function, 1149–1150,
    1180–1182
Group velocity, wave packet, 500
(GUTs) grand unification theories, 1328
Gyroscope, 303

Hadronic force, 91, 1285
Hadrons
  antiparticles of, 1328
  in Standard Model, 1327
  strangeness of, 1321, **1322**

strong force/interaction, 1285, 1314–1315
weak nuclear force, **91d**
Hahn, Otto, 1299
Hale reflecting telescope, 1098
Half-life, radioactive decay, 1289–1290
Half-wave plate, 1057
Hall effect, 872–874, 1226
Hall voltage, 872
Harmonic motion, simple, 403–412
Harmonic oscillator, 531, 1148–1150, 1215
Harmonic series, 490, 496
Harmonic wave function, 449
Harmonics (*see also* Waves)
　analysis and synthesis of, 499
　coherence in, 1111–1112
　interference, 480, 481–488
　phasors adding to, 1121–1126
　simple motion, 403–412
　sound waves, 453
　standing waves, **488**, 488–498, 492
　superposition of, 481–488, 497
Haskel, Richard E., 1126*n*
Heat (*see also* Temperature; Thermal
　　Properties and Processes)
　adiabatic expansion, 587–590
　caloric theory of, 566–567
　definition, 566
　energy (*Q*), 567
　and equipartition theorem, 584–587
　internal energy of, 574–575
　phase change and latent heat, 569–572
　thermal transfer of, 640–648
　thermodynamics, 572–574
　units of, 542–545, 567, AP1
　work and the *PV* diagram, 575–578
Heat capacity
　and equipartition theorem, 581–587
　Fermi electron gas, 839
　of gases, 578–583
　of solids, 583–584
　and specific heat, 567–569
Heat engine, 601, 603
Heat pumps, 614–615
Heat reservoir, 603
Heat-engine statement, second law of
　　thermodynamics, 603, 606–607
Heisenberg, Werner, 523
Helium (He) atoms, 1208, 1329–1330
Helium (Z=2) electron configuration,
　　1186–1187
Henry, Joseph, 927
Henry (H), unit of inductance, 939–940,
　　AP1
Hertz, Heinrich, 1000
Hertz (Hz), unit of frequency, 404, AP1
Hexagonal close-packed (hcp) crystal
　　structure, 1223
Higgs boson, 1327
Higgs field, 1327
High-voltage direct current (HVDC), **959**
Holograms, 1132–1133
Holographic interferograms, **496**
Hooke, Robert, 510
Hooke's law, 92, 403
Hoover Dam, **961**
Horsepower (hp), unit of power, 159
Hot reservoir, heat engine, 603
Hubble, Edwin P., 1098, **1098**, 1329

Hubble age, 1329
Hubble Space Telescope, **307, 1099**
Hubble's law, 1329
Huygens, Christian, 510, 1040–1041
Huygens' construction of light propagation,
　　1040–1041
Huygens' principle of light propagation,
　　1040–1041
HVDC (high-voltage direct current), **959**
Hybrid atomic orbitals, 1212
Hybridization of atomic orbitals, 1212
Hydrogen
　atomic energy quantization of, 531–532
　Bohr model of, 1169–1170, 1171–1176
　energy levels, 1174–1176, 1179
　energy-level diagram for, **1175, 1179**
　isotopes of, 1285
　line spectra of, **1170**
　probability densities, 1180–1183
　quantum numbers for, 1177–1178
　quantum theory of, 1178–1183
　and Schrödinger equation, 1176–1177
　wave functions, 1180
Hydrogen bond, 1209–1210
Hydrostatic paradox, 379
Hysteresis, 911
Hysteresis curve, 911

Ice-point temperature, 542
Ideal batteries, 794–795
Ideal gas
　definition, 547
　entropy changes in, 616–622
　internal energy in, 574–575
　isotherms for, 548
Ideal-gas law, 546–549
Ideal-gas temperature scale, 545
Images
　equation for locating, 1071
　of object in plane mirror, 1070
　optical, 1070–1077, 1078–1089, 1090
　real image, 1073, 1076, 1078
　virtual image, 1070, 1073, 1076, 1078
Impact parameter, 237
Impedance, 973
Impulse, 226–227
Impurity semiconductors, 1225–1226
Incident side, sign convention for refraction,
　　1078
Incoherent sources, wave interference, 487
Independence of motion, 64
Index of refraction, 1041, 1080, 1081, 1090
Induced current, 927 (*see also* Magnetic
　　induction)
Induced emfs, 927 (*see also* Magnetic
　　induction)
Inductance (*L*)
　LC circuit, 969–971
　mutual, 941–942
　RLC circuit, 972
　self, 935, 939–941
　unit of, 939–940, AP1
Induction, electrostatic, 661–662
Induction, magnetic (*see* Magnetic induction)
Induction motor, 988
Inductive reactance, 965

Inductors (*see also RLC* circuit)
　alternating current (ac) in, 964–968
　definition, 941
　energy stored in, 943
　phase relations, 968–969
　RL circuit, 944–947
Inelastic collisions, 226, 615, 619–620, 1268
Inelastic scattering, 1031
Inertia, 84–85, 261–266
Inertial confinement, 1304
Inertial mass vs. gravitational mass, 329
Inertial reference frame, 84–85, 1243, 1244
Infinite square-well potential, 530, 1145
Infrared absorption technique, 1217
Infrared waves, 1004
Initial conditions, 38
Initial-value problem, 38
Instantaneous acceleration, 27
Instantaneous speed, 24
Instantaneous velocity, 23–25, 27
Instantaneous-acceleration vector, 62
Instantaneous-velocity vector, 60
Insulators, 660–662, 842
Integral calculus review, AP26–27 (*see also*
　　Calculus)
Integrated circuits (ICs), 1232–1233
Integration, 38–41, 217, 247
Intensity
　diffraction pattern, 1119, 1126
　of electromagnetic waves, 1008
　in terms of phase difference, 1116–1117
　of waves, 455–458
Intercept, linear equation, AP10
Interference (*see also* Diffraction; Light)
　beats, sound waves, 483–484
　coherence, 1110–1112
　definition, 1110
　electrons, 518–519
　harmonic waves, 480, 481–488,
　　1121–1126
　light waves, 510–511
　pattern of three or more sources,
　　1122–1124
　phase difference, 1110–1112, 1116
　and phasors, 1121–1126
　single-slit diffraction pattern, 1124–1126
　in thin films, 1112–1115
　two-slit diffraction pattern, 1115–1117,
　　1120, 1124–1126
Interference maxima, 1115, 1130
Interference minima, 1115
Internal combustion engine, **602**
Internal energy of gases, 574–575
Internal force, 218–221
Internal reflection, 1044–1046
Internal resistance in battery, 796
International System of measurement (*see* SI
　　units of measure)
Intrinsic semiconductors, 842, 1225–1226
Inverse-square laws, 663
Ionic bonds, 1204, 1220, 1224–1225
Ionization energy, 1175, 1186
Ions, 661, 672–674, 1169, 1204, 1222 (*see also*
　　Electrons)
Irreversible process, 607–609, 617, 622
Isobaric expansion, 576, 617
Isothermal expansion, 576
Isotherms, 548

Isotopes, 1285, **1287**
Isotropic material, 1057

Jet propulsion, 241–243
Josephson, Brian, 845
Josephson effect, 845
Josephson junction, 845
Joule, James P., 2, 566, 572
Joule heat, 793
Joule (J), unit of work and energy, 149, 567, AP1
Joule's experiment, 572–573
Joyce, James, 1323*n*
Junction rule, Kirchhoff's rules, 803
Junctions in semiconductors, 1227–1231

K shell, electron configuration, 1185
Kaon, **1317**
Keck Observatory, **1099**
Kelvin, Lord, 1018 (*see also* Thomson, William)
Kelvin (K), unit of temperature, 4, 545, AP1
Kelvin statement, 600
Kepler, Johannes, **321**
Kepler's laws, 321–323, 327–328
Kilogram (kg), unit of mass, 4, 85, 88, AP1
Kinematics, 19
Kinetic energy (*see also* Energy; Potential energy)
    absolute temperature and, 544–546
    and collisions, 226
    definition, 150
    and electric field lines, 722
    and electrostatic potential energy, 724
    and fusion, 1303–1304
    and harmonic motion, 410
    and mechanical energy, 178–179
    of molecular rotation, 1213
    negative, 1148
    in one dimension, 148–149
    of particle system, 225–226, 231
    particles and magnetic fields, 861, 866–867
    phases of matter, 1219
    proton-antiproton creation, 1318
    relativistic, 1264–1268
    of rotation, 271–276, 304, 312
    in three dimensions, 155–159
    of translation, 551–552
    and work, 149–154
Kinetic friction, 115–124, 188–192
Kinetic theory of gases, 550–559
Kirchhoff, Gustav Robert, 1040–1041
Kirchhoff's rules
    ammeters, voltmeters, ohmmeters, 809–810
    junction rule, 803
    multiloop circuit, 806–808
    single-loop circuit, 803–806
Klitzing, Klaus von, 873–874
Kohlrausch, G., 1017

L shell, electron configuration, 1185
Lambda particle, **1321**
Land, E. H., 1053

Laser (light amplification by stimulated emission of radiation), 1033–1036, 1111
Latent heat, 570
Lateral magnification, 1071, 1076
Lawrence, E. O., 866, 1294
Laws (*see also* Coulomb's law; Gauss's law; Newton's laws; Thermodynamics)
    Ampère's, 898–901, 1000–1001, 1003
    of atmospheres, 380
    Biot-Savart, 885–897, 901, 1000
    Brewster's, 1055
    conservation and elementary particles, 1319–1322
    conservation of charge, 659
    conservation of energy, 186
    conservation of momentum, 222, 304
    Curie's, **908**, 909
    of electromagnetism, 2
    of equal areas, 322, 327
    Faraday's, 929–933, 1001, 1003
    Hubble's, 1329
    of inertia, 84
    inverse-square, 663
    Kepler's, 321–323, 327–328
    Lenz's, 933–936
    Malus's, 1054
    Newton's, 2, 83–84, 1244–1245
    Ohm's, 790–793, 1231
    of reflection/refraction, 1042, 1058–1061
    Snell's, 1042, 1060
    Stefan-Boltzmann, 1030*n*
    for velocity, 1246–1247
    Wien's displacement, 1030
Lawson, J. D., 1034
Lawson's criteria, 1034
LC circuit, 969–971
LCR circuit (*see RLC* circuit)
LEDs (light-emitting diodes), 1229
Length, 4, AP1, AP2
Length contraction, 1250–1252
Lenses (*see also* Images; Optical instruments; Refraction)
    combinations of, 1087–1089
    concave, 1083
    converging, 1082, 1093–1095
    convex, 1082
    diopter (D), 1084
    diverging, 1083, 1086
    ray diagrams for, 1085–1087
    thin, 1081–1085
Lens-maker's equation, 1082
Lenz's law, 933–936
LEP (Electron-Positron collider) tunnel, **1318**
Lepton era, 1330
Lepton number, 1320
Leptons (*see also* Elementary particles)
    antiparticles of, 1328
    and the Big Bang, 1330
    conservation of, 1320
    mass of, **1325**
    Standard Model, 1327–1328
    as truly elementary particles, 1323
    weak force/interaction, **91**, 1314–1315
Lever arm, 260
Leyden jar, 752 (*see also* Capacitors)
Lick Observatory, 1098, **1098**

Light (*see also* Diffraction; Interference; Optical instruments)
    calculation of intensity, 1116
    double slit experiment, 487–488, 510, 522–523
    electromagnetic theory of, 1017
    emission of, 1029–1036
    energy as quantized, 2, 510
    hologram, 1132–1133
    laser, 1033–1036, 1111
    metastable state, 1031
    photons, 1172–1173, 1288
    as photons, 511–515
    photons as particle nature of, 511–515
    polarization, 1052–1058
    propagation, 1028, 1040–1041, 1244–1245
    rainbows, 1050–1052
    reflection and refraction, 1041–1052, 1058–1061
    relativistic Doppler effect, 1252–1253
    scattering, 1031–1032, 1057
    sources, 1029–1036
    spectrum, 1028–1029, **1048**
    speed, 1036–1040, 1244–1246
    theories of, 510–511
    visible, 1004
    wave-particle duality, 1027–1028
Light-emitting diodes (LEDs), 1229
Light-in-flight recording, **1082**
Light-sensitive semiconductors, 1234
Light-year, unit of distance, 1040
Line spectra, 1029–1030, 1170
Linear charge density, 689
Linear equation review, AP10–11
Linear momentum, 221*n*
Linear velocity, 258
Linear vs. rotational motion, **274**
Linearly polarized electromagnetic waves, 1052–1053
Lines of force
    electric field, 672–674, 722–723
    magnetic field, 859, 897
Liquid phase of matter, 1219
Liquid-drop model, 1285, 1299
Liquids (*see* Fluids)
Liquid-vapor isotherms, 638–639
Liter (L), unit of volume, 375, AP1
Lithium (Z=3) electron configuration, 1187–1188
Livingston, M. S., 866, 1294
Lloyd's mirror, 1117
Logarithm review, AP13, **AP14**
Longitudinal waves, 443
Long-range order, phases of matter, 1219
Loop rule, 803
Loops
    current, 886–889
    in magnetic field, 868–871
    multiloop circuit, 806–808
    single-loop circuit, 803–806
Lorentz, Hendrik A., 829, 1251
Lorentz transformation
    and Galilean transformation, 1246–1248
    length contraction, 1250–1252
    relativistic Doppler effect, 1252–1253
    relativistic velocity transformation, 1260–1262
    time dilation, 1248–1250, 1251

Lorentz-FitzGerald contraction, 1251
Loschmidt, Joseph, 1018
Loudness, 457–458
Luminous intensity, unit of, AP1
Lyman, T., 1175
Lyman series, **1175**

Mach number, 468
Macroscopic state variables, 547
Macroscopic systems, 185–194, 624
Madelung constant, 1220, 1223
Magnetic bottle, 862, **863**
Magnetic braking system, 939
Magnetic bubble memory chips, 1233
Magnetic confinement, 1304
Magnetic dipole moment, 868, 887 (*see also*
    Magnetic moment)
Magnetic domain, 910
Magnetic energy
    density of, 943, 1008
    through magnetic induction, 942–944
Magnetic field ($\vec{B}$)
    Ampere definition, 895–897
    changing of, 927
    current, 886–895, 899
    force exerted by, 856–860
    Hall effect, 872–874
    laws pertaining to, 885–892, 898–901,
        933–936
    lines of, 859, 897
    and magnetic confinement in fusion,
        1304
    in matter, 901, 904–914
    nonuniform, 862
    point charge motion, 861–867
    and torque on current loops and magnets,
        868–871
    uniform, 861, 868
    unit of, 857, AP1–2
    velocity sector, 863
    wave equation for, 1011–1012
Magnetic field sources
    Ampère's law, 898–901
    Biot-Savart law, 885–897
    Faraday's law and, 929–933
    Gauss's law, 897
    Lenz's law, 933–936
    magnetism in matter, 901, 904–914
    moving point charges, 884–885
Magnetic flux
    due to current in circuit, 934, 939, 941
    definition, 928
    quantization of, 949
    unit of, 929, AP1
Magnetic force, 856–860, 902–903
Magnetic inductance, units of, 939–940
Magnetic induction
    eddy current, 938–939
    Faraday's law, 929–933
    induced emf, 929–933
    Lenz's law, 933–936
    and magnetic energy, 942–944
    and magnetic flux, 928–929, 934
    and motional emf, 936–938
    mutual inductance, 941–942
    as process, 927

RL circuit, 944–947
    self-inductance, 939–941
    superconduction, 948–949
Magnetic moment
    vs. angular momentum, 906
    atomic, 906–908
    of atomic spin, 1184
    current loops and magnets, 868–871
    induced, 934
    unit of, 868
Magnetic poles, 897
Magnetic quantum number, 1177
Magnetic susceptibility, 904–905
Magnetically hard/soft, 912
Magnetization ($\vec{M}$), 904–905
Magnification (*see also* Optical instruments)
    angular, 1094
    lateral, 1071, 1076
    simple magnifier, 1093–1094
    spherical surface, 1079
Magnifier, 1093–1094
Magnifying power (M), 1094
    definition, 1094
    of lens, 1079
    of microscope, 1095
    of telescope, 1097
Magnitude, order of, 11, 85
Magnitude of uncertainty, 10
Maiman, Theodore, 1033
Malus, E. L., 1054
Malus's law, 1054
Manometer, **379**
Maricourt, Pierre de, 855
Mark, Robert, 1056
Marsden, E., 1171
Mass (*see also* Center of mass)
    of antiparticles, 1314–1315
    atomic, **1287**
    conversion factors for, AP2
    definition, 85
    density of, 443
    and energy, 196–201, 1286–1288
    gravitational and inertial, 329
    leptons, **1325**
    mesons, 1317
    molar, 548
    and Newton's laws, 83–87, 104–105
    and period, 405–406, 407
    quarks, **1325**
    reduced, 1214
    rest, 1267–1269, 1274–1275
    units of, 4, 85, 88–89, 1214, AP1
    W and *Z* particles, 1326
Mass spectrometer, 865–866
Mathematical symbols, **AP8**
Mathematics, review of, AP8–27
Matter
    atomic magnetic moment, 906–908
    Bohr magneton, 907
    composed of quarks and leptons, **1324**,
        1324–1325
    diamagnetism, 913–914
    electric charge quantization, 658–659
    ferromagnetism, 909–913
    and magnetism, 906–914
    magnetization and magnetic susceptibility,
        904–905
    paramagnetism, 908–909

phases of, 1219
    and wave-particle duality, 516–520
Maxwell, James Clerk, 2, 511, 1016–1018
Maxwell-Boltzmann distribution, 557–559,
    831–832, 840
Maxwell's displacement current, 1000–1002
Maxwell's equations
    electromagnetic waves, 1003–1011
    Maxwell's displacement current,
        1000–1002
    wave equation for electromagnetic waves,
        1011–1015
Mean free path, 553–554, 831–832, 840
Mean lifetime, 1289
Mean speed, 831–832
Measurement (*see* Units of measurement)
Mechanical energy, conservation of, 179–
    185
Mechanics, classical, 83, 199 (*see also*
    Newton's laws)
Mechanics, quantum (*see* Quantum
    mechanics)
Meissner, W., 948
Meissner effect, 948–949
Mesons (*see also* Elementary particles)
    antiparticles of, 1328
    bottomonium, 1324
    integral spin, 1314–1315, 1317
    mass of, 1317
    and quarks, 1321, 1323
    strangeness of, **1322**
Metallic bond, 1210
Metal-oxide-semiconductor (MOS)
    technology, *1232*
Metastable state
    and gamma decay, 1293
    of light, 1031
Meter (m), unit of length, 4, AP1
Methane (CH_4) molecule, 1212
Metric system of units, 4–5
Michelson, Albert A., 1038, 1245
Michelson-Morley experiment, 1245*n*,
    1251
Microscope
    compound, 1094, 1095–1099, 1128
    electron, **519**, 1129
Microscopic state of gas, 547
Microscopic systems and quantization of
    energy, 199–200
Microscopic theory of electrical conduction
    (*see* Conduction, microscopic theory of
    electrical)
Microwaves, 1004–1005
Millibar, unit of pressure, 379
Millikan, Robert Andrews, 512, 1018
Mirages, 1047
Mirror equation, 1074
Mirrors (*see also* Optical Instruments;
    Reflection)
    concave, 1073, 1076
    convex, 1076–1077
    plane, 1070–1072
    ray diagrams for, 1075–1077
    spherical, 1073–1075
Mode of vibration, standing wave, 488
Moderator, nuclear fission reactor, 1300
Modern physics, 1–3, 19
Modern telescope, 1097, **1098**

Modulus
    bulk, 376–377, 590
    shear, 362
    torsion, 362
    Young's (Y), 360–361
Molar mass, 548
Molar specific heat, 567
Mole (mol), unit of substance amount, 4, 546
Molecular bonding, 1203–1210
Molecular bonds
    covalent, 1206–1209
    hydrogen, 1209–1210
    ionic, 1224–1225
    metallic, 1210
    in polyatomic molecules, 1210–1212
    tetravalent, 1212
    van der Waals, 1209
Molecular interpretation of temperature,
        551–552
Molecular mass, 548n
Molecular orbitals, 1204
Molecular spectroscopy, 1217
Molecular speed, distribution of, 554–559
Molecular wave functions, 1204
Molecular weight, 548n
Molecules (see also Crystal structure)
    bonding of, 1203–1210
    charge-coupled devices (CCDs), 1234–1235
    diatomic, 1212–1219
    electric dipole moment, 1208
    integrated circuits (ICs), 1232–1233
    phases of matter, 1219
    polyatomic, 1210–1212
    radiation, 1212
    semiconductors, 1225–1231
    solids, structure of, 1219–1225
Moment of inertia, 261–266, **264**, 1213–1214
Momentum (see also Angular momentum;
        Conservation of momentum)
    defined, 212
    in electromagnetic waves, 1008–1011
    and kinetic energy of particle, 231
    and Newton's laws, 221–222
    of photon, 514
    relativistic, 1263–1264
    zero-momentum reference frame, 240
Monkey and ranger problem, 70–71
Morley, Edward, 1245
MOS (metal-oxide-semiconductor)
        technology, 1232, *1233*
Moseley, H., 1195
Motion (See also Newton's laws; Oscillation;
        Rotation; Torque; Wave motion)
    center of mass system, 212, 218–221
    circular, 125–136, 409
    and constant acceleration, 29–38
    of fluids, 384–392
    of gyroscope, 303
    kinematics, 19
    motional emf, 936–937
    in one dimension, 148–149
    rotational vs. linear, **274**
    study of, 2, 19
Motion in two and three dimensions
    displacement, 54–55
    position, velocity and acceleration, 59–64
    projectile motion, 64–72
    and vectors, 55–59

Motion of point charges (see Point charges,
        motion of)
Motional emf, 936–937
Motors, 960, 985–988 (see also Engines)
Müller, Karl Alexander, 843
Multiflash photographs
    acceleration, **88, 136**
    angular momentum, **304**
    center of mass, **218**
    elastic collision, **238**
    energy, **148**
    inelastic collision, **233**
    kinetic and potential energy, **218**
Multiloop circuits, 806–808
Multiple images, mirror, 1072
Muons (see also Atoms)
    detection of, **1316**
    discovery of, 1313
    mass of, 1314
    and radiation, 1291
    and time-dilation, 1251–1252, 1291
    weak nuclear force, **91d**
Mutual inductance, 941–942

Natural frequency, 425, 490, 492, 974
Natural logarithms, AP13
Near point, retinal, 1091
Nearsightedness, 1091
Negative lens, 1083, 1086
Neutral equilibrium for displacement, 167
Neutral rotational equilibrium, 358
Neutrino, **239**, 1291, 1314–1315, 1320
Neutron star, **271**
Neutrons
    electric charge quantization, 658–659
Neutrons (see also Atoms)
    in atom, 1169
    atomic mass of, **1287**
    as elementary particle, 1313
    N and Z numbers, 1285–1286
    in nuclear fission reactors, 1296–1297,
        1300–1303
    within nuclei, 1284–1285
    rest energy of, **196**
Newton, Sir Isaac, **83**
    and acceleration, 125
    and gravitational theory, 92, 322
    laws of motion, 2, 83–84
    light spectrum, 1028
    particle theory of light, 510
    Principia, 1018
Newton (N), unit of force, 4, 85, 88, AP1
Newton per coulomb, unit of electric field,
        667
Newtonian mechanics, 199
Newtonian reality and relativity, 1244–1245
Newton's first law of motion, 83, 84–85,
        1244–1245
Newton's second law of motion
    and center of mass systemic motion, 218
    description of, 83–84
    and forces in nature, 91
    gravity and weight, 87–89
    mass and force, 85–87
    and mechanical energy, 185
    and momentum of particle, 221–222

and rotation, 260–262, 267–270, 277, 301
    torque and angular momentum, 300–302
    and work-kinetic energy theorem,
        149–150, 155–159
Newton's third law of motion, 84, 89–90, 100,
        218
Newton's law of cooling, 640
Newton's law of gravity, 324–328
Newton's rings in thin films, 1112
Nishijima, K., 1321
Nodes, wave, 486, 489
Nonconservative force, 166, 185–186 (see also
        Conservative force)
Nondispersion medium, wave, 499–500
Noninertial reference frame, 128–129
Nonohmic materials, 791
Nonparaxial rays, 1073
Nonpolar molecules, 677
Nonradiating orbits, 1172
Normal boiling point, 368–639, 542
Normal force, 92, 115
Normal freezing point, 542
Normalization condition, 520–521, 555, 1146
Nova target chamber, **1306**
Npn transistor, 1230
N-type semiconductor, 1225, 1227
Nuclear atoms, 1170–1171
Nuclear energy, 197
Nuclear force, 91
Nuclear physics
    fission, 1297–1303
    fusion, 1297–1298, 1303–1306
    nuclear reactions, 1294–1297
    properties of nuclei, 1284–1288
    radioactivity, 1288–1294
Nuclear radioactivity, 2
Nuclear radius, 1285
Nuclei, properties of, 197, 1284–1288 (see also
        Atoms)
Nucleon, 1285, 1321, 1323
Nucleosynthesis period, 1331
Nuclide, 1285
Number density, 788
Numerical data, terrestrial and astronomical,
        AP3

Objective, microscope, 1095
Ochenfeld, R., 948
Ocular for microscope, 1095
Oculars, 1094
Oersted, Hans Christian, 883, **885**, 895
Ohm (Ω)
    unit of inductive reactance, 965
    unit of resistance, 790, AP
Ohmic materials, 790
Ohmmeter, 809–810
Ohm's law, 790–793, 1231 (see also
        Conduction, microscopic theory of
        electrical)
Onnes, H. Kamerlingh, 843
Oppenheimer, J. Robert, 1272
Optic axis of birefringence, 1057
Optical images
    aberrations, 1090
    lens, 1078–1089
    mirror, 1070–1077

Optical instruments (*see also* Lenses; Light; Mirrors; Telescopes)
  compound microscope, 1084, 1095–1096
  the eye, 1091–1093
  resolving power of, 1128, 1132
  simple magnifier, 1093–1094
Optical spectra of atoms, 1192–1194
Optically flat thin films, 1114
Optics, coherence of, 1111
Orbital angular momentum, 1177
Orbital quantum number, 1177
Orbits
  angular momentum of, 300
  atomic magnetic moments, 906
  classification of, 331–332
  and gravitational force, 91
  of planets, 322–323, 327–328
Order number of interference maxima, 1130
Order of magnitude, 11
Organ pipe and standing sound waves, 494
Orrery, **321**
Oscillation (*see also* Motion; Pendulum)
  damped, **403,** 421–425
  driven, 425, 427, 428–430
  energy of, 200
  in *LC* circuit, 970, 971
  in *RLC* circuit, 972, 973
  and simple harmonic motion, 403–412
  systems of, 413–421
Oscillator, 1148–1150, 1215
Otto cycle, 602
Overdamped oscillation, 422
Overtone in music terminology, 488*n*

Parabola in quadratic equation, AP12
Parabolic surface, 1090
Parallel capacitors, 763
Parallel circuits, 969
Parallel connection, electric motor, 985
Parallel force, 92
Parallel light, 1084
Parallel ray, 1075, 1085, 1086
Parallel resistors, 799–801
Parallel *RLC* circuit, 979
Parallel-axis theorem, 265–266
Parallelogram method of adding vectors, 55
Parallel-plate capacitors, 756–757
Paramagnetic material, 904
Paramagnetism, 908–909
Paraxial rays, 1073, 1078
Particle nature of light, 511–515, 1028
Particles (*see also* Antiparticles; Elementary particles)
  accelerators of, 1294–1295, 1313, **1316**
  angular momentum of, 297
  in a box, 524–527, 1145–1148
  charge-to-mass ratio, 674, 864–865
  classical behavior, 522
  in dees, 866–867
  definition, 19
  elementary, **196,** 221, **239**
  finite/infinite square-well potential, 1146–1148
  and harmonic oscillator, 1148–1150

interference and diffraction, 1110
  Schrödinger equation applications, 1146–1148
Particles, systems of
  and center of mass, 213–221, 240–241
  collisions, 226–239
  and gravitational potential energy, 216
  kinetic energy of, 225–226
  law of, 221–225
  and moment of inertia, 261, 262–263
  and momentum, 221–222
  and rocket propulsion, 241–243
  and rotation, 262
Pascal, Blaise, 378
Pascal, unit of pressure, 376
Pascal's principle, 378
Path difference, wave, 484–487
Path of projectile, 66
Pauli, Wolfgang, 1029, 1164, 1291
Pauli exclusion principle, 833–834, 1164, 1185–1186, 1317, 1327
Payload, rocket, 242
Pendulum (*see also* Oscillation)
  in accelerated reference frame, 418
  ballistic, 230, 250–251
  energy of, **180**
  physical, 419–421
  simple, 416–419
Penzias, Arno, 1330
Perfectly inelastic collisions, 226, 229–233
Performance characteristic, electric motor, 985
Perihelion, 322
Period
  and centripetal acceleration, 125
  circular motion, 906
  cyclotron, 861
  and harmonic motion, 404
  mass on a spring, 405–406, 407
  and oscillation, 199–200
  pendulum, 417, 418, 419
Periodic table of elements, 1185–1192, AP6–7
Perl, Martin Lewis, 1314
Permeability
  of free space, 884, 1000
  and magnetic susceptibility, 911
  relative, 905
Permittivity
  of a dielectric, 767
  of free space, 698, 1000
Perpendicular force, 92
Perturbation theory, 1185*n*
Pfund, H. A., 1175
Phase change, heat, 569
Phase constant, 404, 427
Phase diagrams, thermal properties and processes, 639–640
Phase difference, 484–487, 1111–1112
Phase in harmonic motion, 404
Phase velocity, 500
Phasors, 968–969, 1121–1126
Phosphorescent state, 1031
Photoelectric effect, 511–513, **1031**
Photon energy, Einstein equation for, 1028
Photons (*see also* Elementary particles; Light)
  antiparticle creation, 1317
  as bosons, **1326**

as elementary particle, 1313
  as force carrier in Standard Model, 1327
  frequency from energy conservation, 1172–1173
  as particle nature of light, 511–515
  quantum of radiation energy, 200
  radioactive decay, 1288
  virtual, 1325
Physical constants, AP4
Physical pendulum, 419–421
Physics, classical vs. modern, 1–3, 19
Piezoelectric effect, 774–775
Pion, 1313, 1317, 1321, **1322**
Pitch in harmonics, 498
Planck, Max, 200, 512*n*, 647, 1171
Planck's constant, 200, 310, 511–512, 1028, AP4
Planck's quantum hypothesis, 1018
Plane mirror, 1070–1072, 1080
Plane of incidence, reflection, 1041
Plane wave, 455, **462,** 1011
Planetary motion, 321–323 (*see also* Orbits)
Plasmas, 862–863, 1304, **1305**
Platinum-iridium cylinder, 4, 85, 88
Plum pudding model of atom, **1171**
Plutonium, 1298
Pn semiconductor junction, 1227–1229
Pnp transistor, 1230
Point charge, 723–728, 753 (*see also* Point charges, motion of)
Point charges, motion of
  cyclotron, 866–867
  in electric field, 676–677
  electron charge-to-mass ratio, 864–865
  in magnetic field, 861–867
  mass spectrometer, 865–866
  perpendicular particle velocity, 861–863
  velocity selector, 863
Poise, unit of viscosity, 390
Poiseuille, Jean Marie, 391
Poiseuille's law for viscous flow, 391
Polarization of conductor, 661
Polarization of light
  by absorption, 1053–1054
  by birefringence, 1057–1058
  circular, 1053
  linear, 1052–1053
  Malus's law, 1054
  of nonpolar molecules, 677
  by reflection, 1055
  by scattering, 1057
Polarizer, 1054
Polaroid film, 1053
Poloidal coils, **1305**
Polyatomic molecules, 1210–1212
Polycrystalline solids, 1220
Position function, 404, 427
Position vectors, 59–62, **125**
Positive lens, 1082, 1085
Positrons, **196,** 1288, 1291, 1313
Postulates of Einstein, 1245–1250, 1251
Potential, electric (*see* Electric potential)
Potential energy (*U*), 677, 870–871 (*see also* Energy; Kinetic energy)
  alpha decay, **1294**
  bound-state problems and Schrödinger application, 1151–1155, 1160

conservative force, 178–179
definition, 162
electric dipole in electric field, 677
electrostatic, 753–755, 758, 1207–1208
and equilibrium, 166–168
gravitational, 164, 216
and harmonic motion, 410, **531**
and harmonic oscillator, 1148–1150
of ion in crystal, 1220, 1222
magnetic dipole in magnetic field, 870–871
vs. separation in ionic bonding, 1205
of a spring, 165–166, 416
and three dimensional Schrödinger equations, 1160–1162
Potential-energy curve, 167
Potential-energy function, 163
Pound (lb), unit of force, 5, 89
Power
    conversion factors for, AP2
    and energy, 159–162
    and kinetic energy of rotation, 274–275
    and torque, 274
    unit of, 4, 159, AP1
Power, electric
    average, 962–963, 974–975
    dissipated in conductors, 794
    RLC circuit, 974–975
    transformers, 982–984
Power, optical instruments
    lens, 1084
    magnifying power, 1094, 1095, 1097
    resolving power, 1128, 1132
Power factor, RLC circuit, 975
Powers of x and 10 (exponents), **5**, 8–9, 11, AP12–14
Poynting, Sir John, 1008
Poynting vector, 1008
Prefixes for SI units, 4–5
Pressure
    altitude vs., 380
    conversion factors for, AP2
    definition, 376
    fluid, 376–380
    gas, 548, 550–551
    gauge, 379
    ideal gas and, 617–618
    PV diagrams, 576–578
    radiation, 1008–1011
    standard conditions, 548
    unit of, 376, 379
Principal quantum number, 1177
Principal rays
    for mirror, 1075
    for negative lens, 1086
    for positive lens, 1085
Principia (Newton), 1018
Principle of equivalence, 329, 1270–1273
Principle of Newtonian reality, 1244
Prism, light spectra, 1028, **1048**
Probability, 520–521, 623–625
Probability densities, 1180–1183
Projectile motion, 64–72
Propagation of light, 1028, 1040–1041, 1244–1245
Proper length, Lorentz transformation, 1250

Proportion review, direct and inverse, AP9–10
Propulsion, 241–243
Protons (*see also* Atoms)
    accelerated, 1294–1295, 1313, **1316**
    antiproton, 1317
    in atom, 1169
    bubble chamber tracks, **238, 239, 1313**
    electric charge quantization, 658–659
    as elementary particle, 1313, 1320, 1321
    N and Z numbers, 1285–1286
    nuclei, 1284–1285
    rest energies of, **196**
    sharing in hydrogen bond, 1209–1210
Pseudoforces, 128–129
P-type semiconductor, 1226, 1227
PV (pressure/volume) diagrams, gas, 576–578
Pythagorean theorem, 57, 238

Q factor (quality factor), 424, 975
Q value, nuclear reaction, 1295
QCD (quantum chromodynamics), 1326, 1327–1328
Quadratic equation review, AP9–10, AP12
Quality factor (Q factor), 424, 975
Quantization
    of angular momentum, 309–311
    of electric charge, 658–659
    of magnetic flux, 949
Quantization of energy
    in atoms, 515
    in hydrogen atom, 531–532
    in microscopic systems, 199–200
    particle in a box, 1145–1146
    and standing waves, 519–520
Quantum chromodynamics (QCD), 1326, 1327–1328
Quantum electrodynamics, 1325
Quantum gravity, theory of, 1330
Quantum Hall effect, 873–874
Quantum mechanics (*see also* Elementary particles)
    and classical physics, 2–3
    Schrödinger and, 520
    bound-state problem, 1151
    and covalent bonds, 1206
    polyatomic molecules, 1210–1212
    and spin-orbit effect, 1184
    and wave packet representation, 1152–1153
Quantum number
    angular momentum, 1178, 1183–1185, 1316
    covalent bonds, 1206
    definition, 526
    and energy quantization, 200
    hydrogen atom, 1177–1178
    magnetic, 1177
    orbital, 1177
    principal, 1177
    rotational, 1213
    in spherical coordinates, 1177–1178
    vibrational, 1215
Quantum states, 1161, 1204–1205

Quantum theory
    of atoms, 1176–1178
    electrical conduction, 839–840
    for hydrogen atom, 1178–1183
    and Schrödinger, 520–521, 525
    superconductivity, 843–844
Quantum-mechanical system and molecular bonding, 1203–1210
Quark confinement, 1325
Quarks (*see also* Elementary particles)
    and the Big Bang, 1330
    as elementary particles, 1323–1325, 1327
    and field quanta, 1326
    hadrons composed of, 1314
    in Standard Model, 659n, 1323, 1327–1328
Quarter-wave plate, 1057
Quasar, **196**
Quasi-static adiabatic process, 576, 588

R factor, 644
Radial electric field, 728
Radial equation, 1177
Radial probability density, 1181
Radial ray, 1075
Radiation (*see also* Radioactivity)
    background and black-body, 1329–1330
    Cerenkov, 468, **1098**
    electric-dipole, 1005–1007
    electromagnetic, 200
    and light sources, 1031–1033
    molecular absorption and emittance, 1212
    muons, 1251–1252, 1291
    nuclear, 2
    from photons, 511–515
    synchrotron, 1005
    thermal energy, 640, 646–648
Radiation era, 1331
Radiation frequency, 1173
Radiation pressure, 1008–1011
Radio waves, 1005
Radioactive carbon dating, 1292
Radioactivity
    alpha decay, 1293–1294
    beta decay, 1291–1292
    gamma decay, 1293
    rate of, 1288–1291
Radius of allowed orbit, 1173
Radius of curvature, plane mirror, 1076, 1080
Rainbows, 1048–1052
Raman, C. V., 1031
Raman scattering, 1031
Range of projectile, 64, 66
Ranger and monkey problem, 70–71
Rate of change, acceleration, 27
Rayleigh, Lord, 1031 (*see also* Strutt, John William)
Rayleigh scattering, 1031
Rayleigh's criterion for resolution, 1128
Rays
    approximation in diffraction, 463
    diagrams for lenses and mirrors, 1075–1077, 1085–1087
    principal types, 1075, 1085, 1086
    wavefronts of, 454

RC circuit
  capacitor charging, 812–815
  capacitor discharge, 810–812
  exponential decrease, 811
  time constant, 811
Reactance
  capacitive, 967
  inductive, 965
  total, 973
  unit of, 965
Reaction, action pair, 84, 89–90, 100
Reactors, nuclear fission, 1300–1303
Real image, 1073, 1076, 1078
Real object, mirror, 1076
Redshift, 1253, 1272, 1329
Reduced mass, 1214
Reference frame
  accelerated, 357–358, 418, 1243, 1270
  center-of-mass, 240–241
  clock synchronization, 1253–1254,
    1256–1257
  Galilean transformation, 1246–1247
  inertial, 84–85
  noninertial, 128–129
  relativity theory, 1243, 1244
  zero-momentum, 240
Reflecting telescope, 1097, **1098**
Reflection (*see also* Mirrors)
  derivation of laws for, 1058–1061
  diffuse, 1043
  of electron waves, 1151–1155, 1160
  Fermat's principle, 1059
  fiber optics, 1046
  Huygens' principle, 1058–1059
  law of, 1042
  mirror sign conventions, 1076
  physical mechanism for, 1043
  polarization by, 1055
  and refraction of waves, 459–461
  relative intensity of, 1044
  specular, 1043
  total internal, 1044–1046
Reflection coefficient, 1151
Refraction (*see also* Lenses)
  definition, 1041
  derivation of law for, 1058–1061
  dispersion, 1047–1052
  Fermat's principle, 1060–1061
  Huygens' principle, 1059
  index of, 1041
  lenses, 1078–1081
  magnification at spherical surface, 1079
  mirages, 1047
  physical mechanism for, 1043
  rainbows, 1048–1052
  and reflection of waves, 459–461
  at a single surface, 1078
  Snell's law of, 1042, 1060
Refrigerator, 605
Refrigerator statement, thermodynamics,
  605, 606–607
Relative permeability, magnetic material,
  905
Relative velocity, 26, 59–62, 233
Relativistic Doppler effect, 1252–1253
Relativistic energy, 1264–1269, 1274–1275
Relativistic momentum, 1263–1264
Relativistic transformation, 1247–1248

Relativistic velocity transformation,
  1260–1262
Relativity, theory of
  clock synchronization and simultaneity,
    1253–1257
  description of, 2, 26
  and Doppler effect, 466–467
  Einstein's postulates, 1245–1246
  general, 1243, 1270–1273
  Lorentz transformation, 1246–1253
  mass and energy, 199
  Newtonian reality, 1244–1245
  principle of equivalence, 329
  relativistic energy, 1264–1269, 1274–1275
  relativistic momentum, 1263–1264
  special theory of, 196, 1243
  twin paradox, 1257–1259
  velocity transformation, 1260–1262
Remnant field, 911
Reproductive constant, nuclear fission
  reactor, 1300
Residual strong nuclear force/interaction,
  1327–1328
Resistance (*R*)
  within battery, 796
  definition, 790
  equivalent, 799–802
  and Ohm's law, 790–793
  resistivity, 791
  RLC circuit and, 972
  temperature coefficient of, 791–792
  thermal, 641, 642, 644
  unit of, 790, AP1
Resistivity in electrical conduction, 791
Resistors (*see also RLC* circuit)
  alternating current (ac) in, 961–964
  combinations of, 799–802
  in integrated circuits (ICs), 1232–1233
  parallel, 799–802
  power dissipated in, 794
  RC circuit, 810–815
  RL circuit, 944–947
  root-mean-square (rms) values, 962–964
  series, 799
  shunt, 809–810
Resolution, Rayleigh's criterion for, 1128
Resolving power, optical, 1128, 1132
Resonance
  absorption of light, 1031
  alternating current (ac) circuit, 974–978
  mathematical treatment of, 426–428
  neutron reactions, 1296
Resonance curves, 425, 975
Resonance frequency, 425, 488, 489, 492, 974
Resonance width, 425, 975
Rest energy, 196, **196**, 1265–1266, 1286, 1326
Rest mass, 1267–1269, 1274–1275
Retina of the eye, 1091–1092
Reversed biased junction, 1228, 1230
Reversibility of waves, 1074
Reversible engine, 607–609
Reversible process and entropy, 617
Reynolds number, 391–392
Right-hand rule, 296, **856, 868**
Rigid body system, 258
Ritz, Walter, 1170
RL circuit, 944–947
RLC circuit (*see also* Circuit, electric)

alternating current (ac) and generators,
  972, 973–981
average power, 974–975
complex impedances, 980–981
current, 973
impedance, 973
parallel, 979
phase angle, 973
power factor, 975
Q factor, 975
resonance, 974–978
series, 973–974
solving using complex numbers, 980–981
rms (root-mean-square) current, 962
rms (root-mean-square) values, 962–964
Roche limit, 340–341
Rocket equation, 242
Rocket propulsion, 241–243
Rods and cones, eye, 1091
Roentgen, Wilhelm K., 2
Rolling friction, coefficient of, 123
Rolling objects, 275–279, 280–281
Römer, Ole, 1036
Root-mean-square (rms), 551, 555, 962–964
Rotation (*see also* Motion)
  and angular momentum, 295–297, 310, 312
  angular velocity and acceleration, 257–260
  axis of, 257, 260, 271
  centripetal acceleration, 125–126
  characteristic energy of, 1213
  and equilibrium, 358
  gyroscope, 303
  kinetic energy, 271–276, 304, 312
  vs. linear motion, **274**
  and Newton's laws, 267–270, 277, 301
  rolling objects, 275–281
  and torque, 260–262
  vector nature of, 295–297
Rotational molecular energy levels,
  1213–1215, **1216**
Rotational quantum number, 1213
Rotational spectrum, 1213
Rutherford, E., 1171
Rydberg, Johannes R., 1170
Rydberg-Ritz formula, 1170

Salam, A., 1326
Saturated bond, 1208
Saturation magnetization, 907
Savart, Felix, 883
Scalars (*see also* Vectors)
  definition, 55
  dot products, 155–156, 172
  kinetic energy, 150
  multiplying by vector, 56
Scanning tunneling microscope (STC), 1155,
  1156–1159, **1169**
Scattering
  Compton, 514
  deep inelastic, 1323
  elastic, **1031**
  of photons, 1031–1032
  polarization, 1057
  Raman, 1031
Schrieffer, Robert, 843
Schrödinger, Erwin, 519–520

Schrödinger equation
  applications of, 1143–1164
  barrier penetration, 1153–1155, 1160
  and Dirac equation, 1317
  electron wave reflection and transmission, 1151–1155, 1160
  energy quantization, 530
  and hydrogen atom, 1176–1177
  interpretation of, 520, 521
  particle in a box, 1143–1148
  for rotational energy level, 1213
  and simple harmonic oscillator, 1148–1150
  in spherical coordinates, 1177–1178
  step potential of electron wave, 1151–1153
  in three dimensions, 1160–1162
  time-dependent/independent, 1144
  for two identical particles, 1162–1164
Schwarzschild radius, 1272
Scientific notation, 8–9
Second focal point, 1084
Second law of thermodynamics (see Thermodynamics, second law of)
Second (s), unit of time, 4, AP1
Second-order spectrum, 1131
Segré, E., 1317
Selection rules, atoms, 1179
Self-inductance, 935, 939–941
Semiconductor devices
  diodes, 1225, 1227–1229
  junctions, 1227–1231
  transistors, 1225, 1229–1231
Semiconductors
  and band theory of solids, 842
  doping of, 1225
  impurity, 1225–1226
  integrated circuits (ICs), 1232–1233
  intrinsic, 842, 1225–1226
  n-type, 1225, 1227
  p-type, 1226, 1227
  transistor regions, 1229
Series capacitors, 763–766
Series circuit, 969
Series connection, electric motor, 985
Series resistors, 799
Shaded pole, 988
Shear force, 362
Shear modulus, 362
Shear strain and stress, 362
Shock waves, 467–468
Shockley, William, 1229
Short-range order, phases of matter, 1219
Shunt connection, electric motor, 985
Shunt resistor, Kirchhoff's rules, 809–810
SI units of measure, 3–5, 20, 88, AP1 (see also Units of measurement)
Sign conventions for reflection, 1076, 1078
Significant figures, 10–13
Simple harmonic motion, 403–412 (see also Harmonics)
Simple magnifier, 1093–1094
Simple pendulum, 416–419
Simple wave motion, 442–448
Simultaneity, 1254–1255
Single-loop circuits, 803–806
Single-slit interference-diffraction pattern, 1118–1120, 1121, 1124–1126
Sinusoidal current, 959, 960, 962

SLAC (Stanford Linear Accelerator Center), **1316**
Slope, 23, AP10
Slug, unit of mass, 89
Snell, Willebrod, 1042
Snell's law of refraction, 1042, 1060
Sodium chloride (NaCl) crystal, 1220
Sodium to argon (Z=11 to Z=18) electron configuration, 1189
Solar cell, pn semiconductor junction, 1229
Solenoid, 889–891, 940
Solid angle, 710–711
Solids (see also Crystal structure)
  charge-coupled devices (CCDs), 1234–1235
  and contact forces, 92
  integrated circuits (ICs), 1232–1233
  model of, **93**
  phase diagram, 639–640
  phases of matter, 1219
  semiconductors, 1225–1231
  structure of, 1219–1225
Solid-state devices, 1225
Sound waves (see also Waves)
  beats, 183, 483–484
  coherent and incoherent sources, 487
  diffraction, 462–463
  Doppler effect, 463–468
  harmonic, 453
  reflection and refraction sources, 459–461
  speed of, 443–446, 590
  standing waves, 494–496
  unit of, 457–458
  wave function, 520–521
Sources of light (see Light)
Special vs. general relativity theory, 1243 (see also Relativity, theory of)
Specific gravity, 375, 381
Specific heat, 567–569
Spectral line, 1131
Spectrometer, mass, 865–866
Spectroscopy, molecular, 1217
Spectrum (see also Light)
  absorption, 1031, 1217–1219
  continuous, 1029, 1030
  of diatomic molecules, 1212–1219
  electromagnetic, 1004–1005, 1017
  emission, 1216–1217
  first order, 1131
  line, 1029–1030, 1170
  optical, 1192–1194
  redshift, 1329
  rotational, molecular, 1213
  second order, 1131
  x-ray, 1194–1195
Specular reflection, 1043
Speed (see also Velocity)
  angular, 258
  of approach and recession, 234
  average, 21
  conversion factors for, AP2
  escape, 330, 331
  of gas molecules, 551–552
  instantaneous, 24
  of light, 1036–1040, 1244–1245, 1246
  molecular distribution of, 554–559
  rocket, 242
  root-mean-square (rms), 551
  of sound waves, 443–446, 590

  terminal, 135–136
  unit of, 20
  velocity and displacement, 19–26
Speed of light (c), 1036–1040, 1244–1245, 1246
Spherical aberration, 1073, 1090
Spherical coordinates, Schrödinger equation, 1177–1178
Spherical mirrors, 1073–1075
Spherical shell, 336, 338–339
Spin
  and angular momentum, 300, 310, 312
  and antiparticles, 1316–1319
  atomic magnetic moments, 906
  doublet angular momentum, 1193–1194
  fermions, 1314, 1327
  hadrons, 1314
  and wave function, 1164, 1206–1208
Spin-1/2 particles, 1316
Spin state, 1206
Spin-orbit effect, 1183–1185
Spontaneous emission, 1030
Springs
  and contact forces, 92–93
  and oscillating systems, 413–421
  potential energy of, 165–166, 167, 416
  and simple harmonic motion, 405–406, 407
Stable equilibrium, 167, 358
Standard conditions, 375, 548
Standard deviation, 556
Standard Model of elementary particles, 1314, 1327–1328
Standing waves
  and energy quantization, 519–520
  sound waves, 494–496
  string, 488–493
  superposition of, 497–498
  wave functions for, 493, 525–527
Standing-wave condition, 489, 524
Stanford Linear Accelerator Center (SLAC), **1316**
Static electricity (see Electrostatics)
Static equilibrium, 92, 353–358
Static friction, 114–115, 117, 130
Stator field, electric motor, 985
STC (scanning tunneling microscope), 1155, **1169**
Steady-state solution, 426
Steam engine, **601**
Steam-point temperature, 542
Stefan, Josef, 646
Stefan-Boltzmann law, 646, 1030n
Stefan's constant, 646
Step potential of electron waves, 1151–1153
Step-down transformer, 982, 984
Step-up transformer, 982
Steradian (sr), unit of solid angle, 710–711
Stimulated emissions of light, 1031–1033
Stopping distance, 31–33
Strange particles, 1321–1322
Strangeness, 1321–1322
Strange-quark, 1323
Strassmann, Fritz, 1299
Stress and strain, 360–362
Strings
  and contact forces, 94
  energy of waves on, 451–452
  harmonic waves on, 448–450

speed of waves on, 443–446
standing waves, 488–493
wave equation for, 447, **481**
Strong nuclear force/interaction (*see also* Forces)
as fundamental force, 91
and hadrons, 1314, **1315**
as mediated by bosons, **1326**
within nucleus, 1285
quantum chromodynamics (QCD), 1326, 1327–1328
between quarks, 1326
residual, 1327–1328
and strangeness, 1321
Structure of solids (*see* Solids)
Strutt, John William, 1031 (*see also* Rayleigh, Lord)
Sublimation, 639
Sunspots, **541**
Superconductivity (*see also* Conductors)
BCS theory, 843–845
and diamagnetism, 914
energy gap, 844
Josephson effect, 845
magnetic properties of, 948–949
Meissner effect, 948–949
microscopic theory of electrical conduction, 843–845
tunneling, 844
type I and II superconductors, 948
Superposition (*see also* Interference)
electric field, 665, 725
principle of, 481
of waves, 481–488, 497
Surface charge density, 688
Surface-barrier detectors, 1229
Symbols, mathematical, **AP8**
Symmetric wave function, 1164, 1207, 1208, 1209
Symmetry axis, 298
Synchrotron radiation, 1005
Synder, Hartland S., 1272
Système International (SI) (*see* SI units of measure)
Systems of particles (*see* Particles, systems of)

Tables, list of, AP4–5
Tangential acceleration and velocity, 258
Tau particle, 1291, 1314
Telescopes (*see also* Optical instruments)
astronomical, 1094, 1096–1099, **1098,** 1128
Hale reflecting, 1098
Hubble Space, **307, 1099**
magnifying power (*M*) of, 1097
modern, 1097, **1098**
reflecting, 1097, **1098**
Television, cathode-ray tube schematic, **675**
Temperature
absolute, 544–546, 613–614
during Big Bang, 1329–1331
of gases, 541–549
gradient, 640–641
molecular interpretation, 551–552
scales of, 542–544
standard conditions, 548
units of, 542–545, AP1

Temperature coefficient of resistivity, 791–792
Tensile forces, 360
Terminal speed, 135–136
Terminal voltage, 795–796
Terrestrial numerical data, AP3
Tesla (T), unit of magnetic field, 857, AP1
Test charge, electric field, 667
Tetravalent molecular bonds, 1212
Theory of relativity (*see* Relativity, theory of)
Thermal contact, 542
Thermal current, 641
Thermal equilibrium, 541–542
Thermal expansion, 633–637
Thermal neutron, 1296
Thermal properties and processes (*see also* Heat)
conductivity, 620, 645–646, AP2
energy of, 152, 178, 185, 188
energy transfer, 640–648
liquid-vapor isotherms, 637–639
phase diagrams, 639–640
van der Waals equation, 637–639
Thermal resistance (*R*), 641, 642
Thermodynamics, laws of, 2
Thermodynamics, zeroth law of, 542
Thermodynamics, first law of
definition, 573
equipartition theorem, 584–587
heat capacities, 567–569, 578–584
internal energy of ideal gas, 574–575
and Joule's experiment, 572–574
phase and latent heat, 569–572
quasi-static adiabatic expansion, 587–590
work and *PV* diagrams, 575–578
Thermodynamics, second law of
Carnot engine, 607–614
Clausius statement, 601
entropy, 616–625
heat engines and, 601–607
heat pumps, 614–615
irreversibility and disorder, 615
Kelvin statement, 600
refrigerators, 605–606
Thermometer, 541–546
Thermometric property, 542
Thin films, interference in, 1112–1115
Thin lenses, 1081–1085
Thin-lens equation, 1082
Thomson, G. P., 519
Thomson, J. J., 516, 522, 674, 864, 1171, 1313
Thomson, William, 1016 (*see also* Kelvin, Lord)
Thorium series, 1294
Threshold frequency/wavelength, photons, 512
Thrust, rocket, 242
Tidal forces, 340–341
Time
clock synchronization, 1253–1254, 1256–1257
in conduction, 831
constants of, 422, 811, 945
conversion factors for, AP2
dilation and Lorentz transformation, 1248–1250, 1251
unit of, 4, AP1

Time-dependent/independent Schrödinger equation, 1144, 1176
Tokamak, 1304, **1305**
Tone quality, harmonics, 498
Toroid, 899, 1304, **1305**
Torque (*see also* Motion)
and angular momentum, 300–302
cancellation of internal, 304
and center of mass, 277
couples, 356–357
cross or vector product, 296–297
electric dipoles, 676
internal, 304
magnetic dipoles, 868–871
and power, 274
and rotation, 260–262
Torr, unit of pressure, 379
Torricelli, Evangelista, 379
Torricelli's law, 387
Torsion modulus, 362
Total internal reflection, 1044–1046
Total reactance, 973
Transducers, 195
Transformer, 982–984
Transient solution, 426
Transistors
integrated circuits (ICs), 1232–1233
npn transistor, 1230
pnp transistor, 1230
semiconductors, 1125, 1229–1231
Transition elements, 1190
Translational kinetic energy of molecules, 551–552
Transmission axis, 1053
Transmission coefficient, 1151
Transmission side, sign convention for refraction, 1078
Transmission through a barrier, 1153
Transmitted light, 1044
Transverse waves, 443, 1003
Trigonometric formulas and review, AP15–20, **AP17**
Triple point, **639**
Tritium, 1285, 1303
Triton, rest energies of, **196**
Tube length, microscope, 1095
Tuned-mass damper, **403**
Tunnel diode, 1228–1229
Tunneling, 461, 844
Tunneling current, 1228
Turbulence in fluids, 391–392
Turning points in harmonic motion, 411
Twin paradox, 1257–1259
Two finite square wells, covalent bonds, 1206
Two-slit experiment, light waves, 487–488, 510, 522–523
Two-slit interference-diffraction pattern, 1115–1117, 1120, 1124–1126
Type I and II superconductors, 948

Ultrasonic waves, 463
Ultraviolet rays, 1004
Unbanked curves, 144–145
Uncertainty principle, 523, 524
Unified mass unit, 1214, 1286
Unit cell, crystal, 1220

Unit vectors, 58
Units of measurement, AP1
  angular momentum, 310, 312
  astronomical unit (AU), 322
  atomic mass, 1286
  capacitance, 755
  cgs (centimeter/gram/second) system, 5
  charge, 658–659
  conversion factors, 6, AP2
  current, 659, 787, 895–897
  distance, 1040
  electric charge, 659
  electric field, 667
  electric potential, 722
  energy, 149, 159, 196, 566–567
  force, 4, 5, 85, 88–89
  frequency, 404
  heat, 542–545, 567
  inductance, 939–940
  inductive reactance, 965
  luminosity, 4
  magnetic field, 857
  magnetic flux, 929
  magnetic inductance, 939–940
  magnetic moment, 868, 869
  mass, 4, 85, 88–89, 1214
  metric system of units, 4–5
  nuclear cross section, 1295
  nucleus effective size, 1295
  power, 4, 159
  pressure, 376, 379
  radioactivity, 1291
  reactance, 965
  resistance, 790
  SI system, 3–5, 20, 88, AP1
  solid angle, 710–711
  sound intensity, 457–458
  sound waves, 457–458
  speed, 20
  substance amount, 4, 546
  temperature, 4, 542–545
  time, 4
  U.S. customary system, 5, 20, 89, 159
  vectors, 58
  velocity, 20
  viscosity, 390
  volume, 375
  work, 149, 567
Universal evolution, 1328–1331
Universal gas constant, 547
Universal gravitational constant (G), 324,
    325–326, AP4
Universal motor, 988
Unstable equilibrium, 167, 358
Up-quark, 1323, **1324**
Uranium, 1298, 1303
U.S. customary system of units, 5, 20, 89, 159

Valence band, 841
Van Allen belts, 863
Van de Graaff, R., 1294
Van de Graaff generator, 739, 1294
Van der Waals bond, 1209
Van der Waals equation of state, 637
Van der Waals forces, 1219
Vapor pressure, 638, 639n

Variable force, work, 153–154
Vector bosons, 1326
Vector product, 296–297
Vectors (*see also* Scalars)
  acceleration, 62–64, **126**
  and center of mass, 213
  components of, 56–58
  definition, 55
  displacement of, 54–55, 59
  dot product of, 155–156, **156**, 172
  impulse and average force, 226–227
  momentum, 221
  and Newton's laws, 86
  phasors, 968, 1121
  position and velocity, 59–61, **125**
  potential gradient, 728
  Poynting vector, 1008
  properties of, 55–58, **59**
  and rotation, 295–297
  spin angular momentum diagram, **1184**
  unit of, 58
  and velocity, 59–62
Velocity (*see also* Acceleration; Speed)
  angular, 257–260, 296
  average, 19–20, 29
  definition, 20
  displacement and speed, 19–26
  drift, 787–790
  and inertia, 84
  instantaneous, 23–24
  and integration, 38–41
  law for, 1246–1247
  motion of point charges, 863
  and Newtonian relativity, 1244–1245
  and Newton's first law, 83, 84–85
  and nonslip rotation, 275
  perpendicular particle, 861–863
  relative, 26, 59–62, 233
  relativistic transformation, 1260–1262
  in simple harmonic motion, 405
  and special relativity theory, 1243
  tangential, 258
  unit of, 20
  and vectors, 59–62, **66**, 125
  wave packet, 500
Velocity selector, 863
Velocity transformation, 1260–1262
Venturi effect, 387–389
Venturi meter, **387**
Vertex of lens, 1085
Vibration, fundamental mode of, 49, 488, 497
Vibrational molecular energy levels,
    1215–1216, **1216**
Vibrational quantum number, 1215
Virtual image, 1070, 1073, 1076, 1078
Virtual object, mirrors, 1076, 1081n
Virtual photons, 1325
Viscosity, coefficient of, 390
Viscous forces, fluids, 389
Visible light, 1004
Volt (V)
  unit of charge, AP1
  unit of electric potential, 722
Voltage (*see* Electric potential)
Voltage drop and alternating current (ac),
    965, 967, 968
Voltage gain and transistors, 1321
Voltmeter, 809–810, 962

Volume
  charge density, 688
  conversion factors for, AP2
  flow rate, 384
  geometric, AP14–15
  PV diagrams, 576–578
Von Klitzing, Klaus, 873–874
Von Klitzing constant, 874
Vortex shedding, turbulence, **392**

W particle, 1326, 1327
Walton, E. T. S., 1294
Water (H$_2$O) molecule, 1210–1211
Watt (W), unit of power, 4, AP1
Wave equations
  derivation of, 1012–1014
  for electric and magnetic field vectors,
    1000
  for electromagnetic waves, 1011–1015
  and simple harmonic motion, 446–448, 481
Wave functions (*see also* Schrödinger
    equation)
  asymmetric and symmetric, 1164,
    1206–1209
  description of, 443
  for electrons, 1204, 1211
  first excited state, 1182–1183
  ground state, 1149–1150, 1180–1182
  interpretation of, 520–521
  molecular orbitals, 1204
  particle in finite square well, 1146–1148
  and periodic table, 1185
  and quantum states, 1161
  quantum theory of hydrogen atom,
    1180–1183
  standing waves, 493, 525–527
  and three dimensional Schrödinger
    equations, 1160–1162
  for two identical particles, 1162–1164
Wave intensity, 455–458
Wave mechanics, 520
Wave motion
  and barriers, 459–463
  diffraction, 462–463
  and Doppler effect, 463–468
  harmonic, 448–458
  simple, 442–448
  simple harmonic, 403–412
Wave nature of light, 1027
Wave number, 448
Wave packet, 499, 500, 1152–1153
Wave pulse, 443, 499
Waveforms, 498
Wavefronts, 454, 1082
Wavelengths
  electromagnetic spectrum, 1004–1005
  electron and matter waves, 516–520
  emitted by hydrogen atom, 1174–1175
  harmonic waves, 448
Wave-particle duality, 509–510, 522–523,
    528–530, 1027–1028
Waves (*see also* Frequency; Interference;
    Reflection; Refraction; Sound waves;
    Standing waves)
  classical behavior of, 522
  coherence in, 1111–1112

de Broglie, 516–517
diffraction, 462–463, 518–519
dispersion of, 499–500
Einstein's postulates, 1245
electromagnetic, 454, 1011–1015
harmonic, 448–450, 499
phasors adding to, 1121–1126
plane, 455, **462**, 1011
pulses of, 443
reflection and refraction, 459–461
reversibility, 1074
speed of, 443–446, 448–450
superposition of, 481–488, 497
in three dimensions, 454–458
transverse and longitudinal, 443
velocity and Newtonian relativity,
    1244–1245
Weak nuclear force/interaction
cloud chamber tracks, **91d**
and electroweak theory, 1326
hadrons and leptons, 1314–1316
Standard Model, 1327–1328
strangeness, 1321, 1322
Webber, Joseph, 1273
Weber, Wilhelm, 1017

Weber (Wb), unit of magnetic flux, 929,
    AP1
Weight, 5, 87–89
Weightlessness, 88
Weinberg, S., 1326
Wheeler, John A., 1299
Wien's displacement law, 647, 1030
Williams, Ellen, 1156–1159
Wilson, Robert, 1330
Wire, electrical, 792
Wobble motor, **258**
Work
adiabatic, 588, 589
by a constant force, 148
definition of, 157
and electrostatic energy, 752
in one dimension, 148–152, 153
and photoelectric effect, 512
and potential energy, 148, 162
and power, 159–162
PV (pressure/volume) diagrams, 576–578
relativistic energy, 1264
rotation and power, 274–275
thermodynamics and, 575–578
in three dimensions, 155–159, 172

unit of, 149, AP1
by a variable force, 153–154, 171–172
Work-energy theorem, 186–187
Working substance, heat engine, 601
Work-kinetic energy theorem, 149–152, 155

X-rays, 1005, 1194–1195

Young, Thomas, 480, 488, 510, 522, 1027
Young's modulus (Y), 360–361

z component of angular momentum, 1177
Z particle, 1326, 1327
Zener diode, 1228
Zero-momentum reference frame, 240
Zero-point energy, 525
Zeroth law of thermodynamics, 542
Zippy, David, 1273

Prefixes for Powers of 10	Multiple	Prefix	Abbreviation
	10^{18}	exa	E
	10^{15}	peta	P
	10^{12}	tera	T
	10^{9}	giga	G
	10^{6}	mega	M
	10^{3}	kilo	k
	10^{2}	hecto	h
	10^{1}	deka	da
	10^{-1}	deci	d
	10^{-2}	centi	c
	10^{-3}	milli	m
	10^{-6}	micro	μ
	10^{-9}	nano	n
	10^{-12}	pico	p
	10^{-15}	femto	f
	10^{-18}	atto	a

Some Physical Data

Acceleration of gravity at earth's surface	g	$9.81 \text{ m/s}^2 = 32.2 \text{ ft/s}^2$	
Radius of earth	R_E	6370 km = 3960 mi	
Mass of earth	M_E	5.98×10^{24} kg	
Mass of sun		1.99×10^{30} kg	
Mass of moon		7.36×10^{22} kg	
Escape speed at earth's surface		11.2 km/s = 6.95 mi/s	
Standard temperature and pressure (STP)		0°C = 273.15 K 1 atm = 101.3 kPa	
Earth–moon distance		$3.84 \times 10^8 \text{ m} = 2.39 \times 10^5 \text{ mi}$	
Earth–sun distance (mean)		$1.50 \times 10^{11} \text{ m} = 9.30 \times 10^7 \text{ mi}$	
Speed of sound in dry air (at STP)		331 m/s	
Density of air		1.29 kg/m^3	
Density of water		1000 kg/m^3	
Heat of fusion of water	L_f	333.5 kJ/kg	
Heat of vaporization of water	L_v	2.257 MJ/kg	

The Greek Alphabet

Alpha	A	α	Iota	I	ι	Rho	P	ρ
Beta	B	β	Kappa	K	κ	Sigma	Σ	σ
Gamma	Γ	γ	Lambda	Λ	λ	Tau	T	τ
Delta	Δ	δ	Mu	M	μ	Upsilon	Y	υ
Epsilon	E	ϵ	Nu	N	ν	Phi	Φ	ϕ
Zeta	Z	ζ	Xi	Ξ	ξ	Chi	X	χ
Eta	H	η	Omicron	O	o	Psi	Ψ	ψ
Theta	Θ	θ	Pi	Π	π	Omega	Ω	ω

Abbreviations for Units

A	ampere	lb	pound
Å	angstrom (10^{-10} m)	L	liter
atm	atmosphere	m	meter
Btu	British thermal unit	MeV	mega-electron volt
Bq	becquerel	Mm	megameter (10^6 m)
C	coulomb	mi	mile
°C	degree Celsius	min	minute
cal	calorie	mm	millimeter
Ci	curie	ms	millisecond
cm	centimeter	N	newton
dyn	dyne	nm	nanometer (10^{-9} m)
eV	electron volt	pt	pint
°F	degree Fahrenheit	qt	quart
fm	femtometer, fermi (10^{-15} m)	rev	revolution
ft	foot	R	roentgen
Gm	gigameter (10^9 m)	Sv	seivert
G	gauss	s	second
Gy	gray	T	tesla
g	gram	u	unified mass unit
H	henry	V	volt
h	hour	W	watt
Hz	hertz	Wb	weber
in	inch	y	year
J	joule	yd	yard
K	kelvin	μm	micrometer (10^{-6} m)
kg	kilogram	μs	microsecond
km	kilometer	μC	microcoulomb
keV	kilo-electron volt	Ω	ohm